To our spouses, children, parents, and friends, who much of the time have had to manage without us while we work as well as cope with our struggles and frustrations.

The Doenges families: Dean, Jim, Barbara, and Bob Lanza; David, Monita, Matthew, and Tyler; John, Holly, Nicole, and Kelsey; and the Daigle family, Nancy, Jim, Jennifer, and Jonathan.

The Moorhouse family: Jan, Paul, Jason, Ellaina, and Alexa.

To Mary and Marilynn, couldn't have done it without you— Alice.

In loving memory of my mother, Norma Loughmiller, who was my biggest promoter in my early days of writing.

To our FAD family, especially Bob Martone, Ruth De George, Herb Powell, and Bob Butler, whose support is so vital to the completion of a project of this magnitude.

To the nurses we are writing for, who daily face the challenge of caring for the acutely ill patient and are looking for a practical way to organize and document this care. We believe that nursing diagnosis and these guides will help.

To NANDA and to the International nurses who are developing and using nursing diagnoses—here we come!

Finally, to the late Mary Lisk Jeffries, who initiated the original project. The memory of our early friendship and struggles remains with us. We miss her and wish she were here to see the growth of the profession and how nursing diagnosis has contributed to the process.

KEY TO ESSENTIAL TERMINOLOGY

PATIENT ASSESSMENT DATA BASE

Provides an overview of the more commonly occurring etiology and coexisting factors associated with a specific medical/surgical diagnosis as well as the signs/symptoms and corresponding diagnostic findings.

NURSING PRIORITIES

Establishes a general ranking of needs/concerns on which the Nursing Diagnoses are ordered in constructing the plan of care. This ranking would be altered according to the individual patient situation.

DISCHARGE GOALS

Identifies generalized statements that could be developed into short-term and intermediate goals to be achieved by the patient before being "discharged" from nursing care. They may also provide guidance for creating long-term goals for the patient to work on after discharge.

NURSING DIAGNOSES

The general problem/concern (diagnosis) is stated without the distinct cause and signs/symptoms, which would be added to create a patient diagnostic statement when specific patient information is available. For example, when a patient displays increased tension, apprehension, quivering voice, and focus on self, the nursing diagnosis of Anxiety could be stated: Anxiety, severe, related to unconscious conflict, threat to self-concept as evidenced by statements of increased tension, apprehension; observations of quivering voice, focus on self.

In addition, diagnoses identified within these guides for planning care as actual or risk can be changed or deleted and new diagnoses added, depending entirely on the specific patient information.

MAY BE RELATED TO/POSSIBLY EVIDENCED BY

These lists provide the usual/common reasons (etiology) why a particular problem may occur with probable signs/symptoms, which would be used to create the "related to" and "evidenced by" portions of the *patient diagnostic statement* when the specific patient situation is known.

When a risk diagnosis has been identified, signs/symptoms have not yet developed and therefore are not included in the nursing diagnosis statement. However, interventions are provided to prevent progression to an *actual* problem. The exception to this occurs in the nursing diagnosis *Violence, risk for*, which has possible indicators that reflect the patient's risk status.

DESIRED OUTCOMES/EVALUATION CRITERIA—PATIENT WILL

These give direction to patient care as they identify what the patient or nurse hopes to achieve. They are stated in general terms to permit the practitioner to modify/individualize them by adding time lines and individual patient criteria so they become "measurable." For example, "Patient will appear relaxed and report anxiety is reduced to a manageable level within 24 hours."

ACTIONS/INTERVENTIONS

Activities are divided into independent and collaborative and are ranked in this book from most to least common. When creating the individual plan of care, interventions would normally be ranked to reflect the patient's specific needs/situation. In addition, the division of independent/collaborative is arbitrary and is actually dependent on the individual nurse's capabilities and hospital/community standards.

RATIONALE

Although not commonly appearing in patient plans of care, rationale has been included here to provide a pathophysiologic basis to assist the nurse in deciding about the relevance of a specific intervention for an individual patient situation.

CLINICAL PATHWAY

This abbreviated plan of care or care map is event- (task-)oriented and provides outcome-based guidelines for goal achievement within a designated length of stay. Several samples have been included to demonstrate alternative planning formats.

NURSING DIAGNOSES
(THROUGH 12TH NANDA CONFERENCE)†

Activity Intolerance
Activity Intolerance, risk for
Adaptive Capacity: Intracranial, decreased
Adjustment, impaired
Airway Clearance, ineffective
Anxiety [specify level]*
Aspiration, risk for
Body Image disturbance
Body Temperature, altered, risk for
Bowel Incontinence
Breastfeeding, effective
Breastfeeding, ineffective
Breastfeeding, interrupted
Breathing Pattern, ineffective
Cardiac Output, decreased
Caregiver Role Strain
Caregiver Role Strain, risk for
Communication, impaired verbal
Community Coping, potential for enhanced
Community Coping, ineffective
Confusion, acute
Confusion, chronic
Constipation
Constipation, colonic
Constipation, perceived
Coping, defensive
Coping, Individual, ineffective
Decisional Conflict (specify)
Denial, ineffective
Diarrhea
Disuse Syndrome, risk for
Diversional Activity deficit
Dysreflexia
Energy Field disturbance
Environmental Interpretation Syndrome, impaired
Family Coping: ineffective, compromised
Family Coping: ineffective, disabling
Family Coping: potential for growth
Family Process, altered: alcoholism
Family Processes, altered
Fatigue
Fear
Fluid Volume deficit [active loss]*
Fluid Volume deficit [regulatory failure]*
Fluid Volume deficit, risk for
Fluid Volume excess
Gas Exchange, impaired
Grieving, anticipatory
Grieving, dysfunctional
Growth and Development, altered
Health Maintenance, altered
Health-Seeking Behaviors (specify)
Home Maintenance Management, impaired
Hopelessness
Hyperthermia
Hypothermia
Incontinence, functional
Incontinence, reflex
Incontinence, stress
Incontinence, total
Incontinence, urge
Infant Behavior, disorganized
Infant Behavior, disorganized, risk for
Infant Behavior, organized, potential for enhanced
Infant Feeding Pattern, ineffective
Infection, risk for

Injury, risk for
Knowledge deficit [learning need]* (specify)
Loneliness, risk for
Memory, impaired
Noncompliance [Compliance, altered]* (specify)
Nutrition: altered, less than body requirements
Nutrition: altered, more than body requirements
Nutrition: altered, risk for more than body requirements
Oral Mucous Membrane, altered
Pain [acute]
Pain, chronic
Parental Role Conflict
Parent/Infant/Child Attachment, altered, risk for
Parenting, altered
Parenting, altered, risk for
Perioperative Positioning Injury, risk for
Peripheral Neurovascular dysfunction, risk for
Personal Identity disturbance
Physical Mobility, impaired
Poisoning, risk for
Post-Trauma Response
Powerlessness
Protection, altered
Rape-Trauma Syndrome
Rape-Trauma Syndrome: compound reaction
Rape-Trauma Syndrome: silent reaction
Relocation Stress Syndrome
Role Performance, altered
Self Care Deficit, feeding, bathing/hygiene, dressing/
    grooming, toileting
Self Esteem, chronic low
Self Esteem disturbance
Self Esteem, situational low
Self-Mutilation, risk for
Sensory/Perceptual alterations (specify): visual, auditory,
    kinesthetic, gustatory, tactile, olfactory
Sexual dysfunction
Sexuality Patterns, altered
Skin Integrity, impaired
Skin Integrity, impaired: risk for
Sleep Pattern disturbance
Social Interaction, impaired
Social Isolation
Spiritual Distress (distress of the human spirit)
Spiritual Well-Being, potential for enhanced
Spontaneous Ventilation, inability to sustain
Suffocation, risk for
Swallowing, impaired
Therapeutic Regimen: Community, ineffective management
Therapeutic Regimen: Families, ineffective management
Therapeutic Regimen: Individuals, effective management
Therapeutic Regimen (Individuals), ineffective
    management
Thermoregulation, ineffective
Thought Processes, altered
Tissue Integrity, impaired
Tissue Perfusion, altered (specify): cerebral,
    cardiopulmonary, renal, gastrointestinal, peripheral
Trauma, risk for
Unilateral Neglect
Urinary Elimination, altered
Urinary Retention [acute/chronic]*
Ventilatory Weaning Response, dysfunctional (DVWR)
Violence, risk for, directed at self/others

---

* [Author recommendations]

†Permission from North American Nursing Diagnosis Association (1994). NANDA Nursing Diagnoses: Definitions and Classifications 1995–1996. Philadelphia: NANDA. Copyright 1994 by the North American Nursing Diagnosis Association.

NURSING CARE PLANS

GUIDELINES FOR INDIVIDUALIZING PATIENT CARE
Edition 4

MARILYNN E. DOENGES, RN, BSN, MA, CS
Clinical Specialist
Adult Psychiatric/Mental Health Nursing
Former Instructor
Beth-El College of Nursing
Colorado Springs, Colorado

MARY FRANCES MOORHOUSE, RN, CRRN, CLNC
Nurse Consultant
TNT-RN Enterprises
Colorado Springs, Colorado

ALICE C. GEISSLER, RN, BSN
Contract Practitioner
Nurse Consultant
Colorado Springs, Colorado

 F. A. DAVIS COMPANY • Philadelphia

F. A. Davis Company
1915 Arch Street
Philadelphia, PA 19103

Printed in the United States of America

Last digit indicates print number: 10 9 8 7 6 5 4 3 2 1

Publisher, Nursing: Robert G. Martone
Production Editor: Jessica Howie Martin
Cover Designer: Louis J. Forgione

As new scientific information becomes available through basic and clinical research, recommended treatments and drug therapies undergo changes. The authors and publisher have done everything possible to make this book accurate, up to date, and in accord with accepted standards at the time of publication. The authors, editors, and publisher are not responsible for errors or omissions or for consequences from application of the book, and make no warranty, expressed or implied, in regard to the contents of the book. Any practice described in this book should be applied by the reader in accordance with professional standards of care used in regard to the unique circumstances that may apply in each situation. The reader is advised always to check product information (package inserts) for changes and new information regarding dose and contraindications before administering any drug. Caution is especially urged when using new or infrequently ordered drugs.

Library of Congress Cataloging-in-Publication Data

Doenges, Marilynn E., 1922–
    Nursing care plans : guidelines for individualizing patient care /
Marilynn E. Doenges, Mary Frances Moorhouse, Alice C. Geissler. —
Ed. 4.
        p.   cm.
    Includes bibliographical references and index.
    ISBN 0-8036-0158-1 (pbk.)
    1. Nursing care plans. I. Moorhouse, Mary Frances, 1947– .
II. Geissler, Alice C., 1946– . III. Title.
    [DNLM: 1. Patient Care Planning—handbooks.   2. Nursing Process-
-handbooks.
WY 49 D651na 1997]
RT49.D64   1997
610.73—dc21
DNLM/DLC
for Library of Congress   96-46196
                                                              CIP

PREFACE

One of the most significant achievements in the healthcare field during the past 20 years has been the emergence of the professional nurse as an active coordinator and initiator of patient care. While the transition from helpmate to healthcare professional has been painfully slow and is not yet complete, the importance of the nurse within the system can no longer be denied or ignored. Today's nurse designs nursing care interventions that will move the total patient toward the goal of improved health.

The current state of the theory of Nursing Process, Diagnosis, and Intervention has been brought to the clinical setting to be implemented by the nurse. This book gives definition and direction to the development and use of individualized nursing care. The book is therefore not an end in itself but a beginning for the future growth and development of the profession.

Professional care standards, other healthcare professionals, and patients will continue to increase expectations for nurses' performance as each day brings advances in the struggle to understand the mysteries of normal body function and human response to actual and potential health problems. With this increased knowledge comes greater responsibility for the nurse. To meet these challenges competently, the nurse must have up-to-date physical assessment skills and a working knowledge of pathophysiologic concepts concerning the more common diseases/conditions encountered in general healthcare. This book is a tool, a means of attaining that competency.

In the past, plans of care were viewed principally as learning tools for students and seemed to have little relevance after graduation. However, the need for a written format to communicate and document individualized patient care has been recognized in all care settings. In addition, governmental regulations and third-party payor requirements have created the need to validate the appropriateness of the care provided, as well as the need to justify patient care charges and staffing patterns. Thus, although the student's "case studies" were too cumbersome to be practical in the clinical setting, the patient plan of care meets the aforementioned identified needs. The practicing nurse, as well as the nursing student, will welcome this text as a ready reference in clinical practice. The book is designed for use in the acute medical/surgical setting, as well as the community setting, and is organized by systems for easy reference. Rationales (which state not only why an intervention is important but also provide a brief related pathophysiology, when applicable) enhance the reader's understanding of the intervention. This information also serves as a catalyst for thought in planning and evaluating the care being rendered.

Chapter 1 discusses some current issues and trends affecting the nursing profession. An overview of cultural, community, sociologic, and ethical concepts affecting the nurse is included. The important concept of cooperation and coordination with other healthcare professionals is integrated throughout the plans of care.

Chapter 2 reviews the historic use of the nursing process in formulating plans of care and the nurse's role in the delivery of that care. Nursing diagnosis is discussed to assist the nurse in understanding its role in the nursing process.

Chapter 3 demonstrates construction of the plan of care and the use and adaptation of the guides for care planning presented in this book. A nursing-based assessment tool is presented with a sample patient situation, data base, and corresponding plan of care to aid the nurse to make the transition from theory to practice. Additionally, a clinical pathway reflecting the sample situation is included to demonstrate another method of evaluating and documenting the patient's response to care.

Chapters 4 through 15 present guides for planning care that include information from multiple disciplines to help the nurse provide holistic care. Each plan of care is developed by identifying nursing diagnoses with "related to" and "evidenced by" factors that provide an explanation of patient problems/needs. Each plan includes a patient assessment data base (presented in a nursing format) and associated diagnostic studies. After the data base is collected, nursing priorities are sifted from the information to help focus and structure the patient care provided. Discharge goals are also listed to identify the general goals that should be accomplished by the time of discharge from care. In addition, mean length of stay has been identified to provide a general idea of time constraints for achieving discharge goals in the inpatient setting. Desired patient outcomes are stated in behavioral terms that can be measured to evaluate the patient's progress and the effectiveness of care provided. (Time lines have been omitted here because they are individually determined by specific patient data.) The interventions are designed to assist with problem resolution. Rationales for these actions are provided to enable the nurse to decide whether the intervention applies to a particular patient situation. Additional information is provided to assist the nurse in identifying and planning for rehabilitation/care in the community setting as the patient progresses toward discharge. As in Chapter 3, samples of clinical pathways have been included to demonstrate alternative plan-of-care formats and enhance the learning experience.

As a final note, this book is not intended to be a procedure manual, and efforts have been made to avoid detailed descriptions of techniques/protocols that might be viewed as individual/regional in nature. Instead, the reader is referred to procedure manual/standards of care resources for in-depth direction for these concerns.

CONTRIBUTORS

Nancy Lea Carter, RN, MA, ONC
Clinical Nurse, Orthopedics
Presbyterian Medical Center
Albuquerque, New Mexico

Rebecca D. Ellis, RN, MS, NP
Multiple Sclerosis Nurse Practitioner/
    Coordinator
Department of Veterans Affairs
Medical Center, Denver, Colorado

Christie A. Hinds, RN, NP
Director: HIV Patient Care
FHL Health Care, Inc.
Colorado Springs, Colorado

Laura Ruth Johnson, RN, BSN, MNED
Clinical Educator, Surgery
Penrose Community Hospital
Colorado Springs, Colorado

Ginger Pittman, RN, CNN
Education Coordinator
Pikes Peak Dialysis Center, Inc.
Colorado Springs, Colorado

Tracy Steinberg, RN, MSN, CNS
Transplant Coordinator
Division of Transplant Surgery
University of Colorado Health Sciences
    Center
Denver, Colorado

Geri L. Tierney, RN, ONC
Coordinator, Total Joint Program
The Penrose-St. Francis Healthcare
    System
Colorado Springs, Colorado

Anne Zobec, RN, MS, CS, OCN
Clinical Nurse Specialist
Medical/Surgical/Oncology
Penrose-St. Francis Health Care System
Colorado Springs, Colorado

CONTENTS IN BRIEF

A table of contents including nursing diagnoses follows.

DETAILED CONTENTS

INDEX OF NURSING DIAGNOSES appears on pages 941–945

INDEX OF NURSING DIAGNOSES appears on pages 941–945

Issues and Trends in Medical/Surgical Nursing

Healthcare reform has become the focus of much writing and debate in the 1990s, but few decisions have been reached about what constitutes healthcare reform. Whether brought about by federal or state law, or by third-party payors and healthcare providers, the changes in healthcare delivery (or healthcare system reform) are continuing and will be far-reaching. To achieve cost containment, many innovations such as downsizing, unlicensed assistive personnel, healthcare networks, managed care and capitation, advanced practice nurses, and alternative therapies are fast moving from concept to reality.

DOWNSIZING

Today, hospitals are expected to deliver the same quality and quantity of services as they did in yesteryear, for less money, to a patient population that is, on the average, older with greater care needs (higher acuity). To achieve this goal, hospitals are changing the way they do business and evaluating the cost-effectiveness of every service they provide. Unprofitable or marginal services are discontinued or merged with those of other providers. Studies (Prescott, 1993) show that having a higher ratio of professional nurses on staff improves patient outcomes and lowers mortality rates; however, hospitals are downsizing professional staff through attrition, early retirement, and layoffs. RNs are being replaced by LPNs or unlicensed assistive personnel (UAP).

This cutting of staff requires that registered nurses be more flexible and able to work in more than one area as needed. Nurses must be technically competent, skilled at critical thinking and problem solving, able to work with a variety of people, and cross-trained to be competent in more than one setting. Additionally, nurses must be fiscally responsible, aware of the cost of services, and able to find cost-effective ways of providing required care.

NETWORKS

The need to lower costs has forced hospitals to seek alternatives to inpatient care. Currently the emphasis is on outpatient services and affiliations with other provider groups. Healthcare networks are being created, some of which encompass a major hub or tertiary hospital, smaller affiliating hospitals, freestanding emergency and surgical centers, subacute units, rehabilitation centers, long-term care facilities, and home care agencies. The networks are designed to meet all the patient's healthcare needs while keeping all the revenue within the network. These networks have the potential of limiting competition, thereby causing the decline of independent healthcare agencies and practitioners as doctors, insurance companies, pharmacies, and equipment supply houses join the network. Current predictions are that 1 in 10 acute-care hospitals will close by the year 2000.

MANAGED CARE

Healthcare delivery systems use managed care to keep patients out of acute-care hospitals by using other, less costly services within the network. Whether the ''case manager'' is a physician, nurse, or insurance adjustor, all individuals involved in care are responsible for evaluating both the therapeutic benefit and cost-effectiveness of the services provided. This is especially critical for end-of-life care, in which a high percentage of healthcare dollars are spent. In response, medicine is developing criteria such as computer program APACHE (Acute Physiology and Chronic Health Evaluation) to help allocate resources and choose appropriate treatment options. This computer program provides data on the likely outcomes of various treatments in specific patient populations. Thus, reimbursement could be tied to a scoring system reflecting the likelihood of survival. Another cost-control measure is capitation, in which providers contract to provide services to a specific population (e.g., insured group) for a preset fee, regardless of actual cost.

In the acute care setting, the coordination and evaluation of interdisciplinary care may be reflected in clinical or critical pathways. Clinical pathways are currently being developed for specific conditions/procedures based on the DRG or the agency expected length of stay (ELOS). They comprise a flow sheet of common activities/tasks and general goals that must be achieved so that patient discharge occurs within the agency's predetermined time frame. Variance from the standardized pathway indicates a need for further evaluation and additional intervention. The lack of flexibility to accommodate preexisting multiple diagnoses (e.g., coronary bypass surgery in a patient with COPD and chronic renal insufficiency) or the development of complications generally precludes the use of clinical pathways when greater individualization of care is required. Additionally, since pathways address a specific episode of care, they presently cannot focus on care over a continuum.

NURSING CARE COSTS

The profession's attention is focused on the cost of providing nursing care to patients within the setting of prospective reimbursement/capitation, fewer dollars, limited time, and reduced beds and staff. Quantification of nursing's contribution to patient care can be used to determine the cost of providing care to specific patients and patient populations. Quantifying nursing time requires the identification of the level of nursing care necessary for each patient, which can be used for direct "billing" of services rendered. In those hospitals already billing for nursing services, the patient plan of care is an integral part of the justification of nursing care costs.

Describing the work of nursing has been an ongoing challenge since the beginning of our profession. The *what* and *how* of the work of nursing have been explained in part in a number of existing publications that help to operationalize the work of nursing. The 1980 ANA *Nursing's Social Policy Statement* described nursing as the diagnosis and treatment of human responses to actual or potential health problems. The North American Nursing Diagnosis Association's

TABLE 1–1. **Standards of Clinical Nursing Practice***

Standards of Care

1. Assessment: The nurse collects client health data.
2. Diagnosis: The nurse analyzes the assessment data in determining diagnoses.
3. Outcome identification: The nurse identifies expected outcomes individualized to the client.
4. Planning: The nurse develops a plan of care that prescribes interventions to attain expected outcomes.
5. Implementation: The nurse implements the interventions identified in the plan of care.
6. Evaluation: The nurse evaluates the client's progress toward attainment of outcome.

Standards of Professional Performance

1. Quality of Care: The nurse systematically evaluates the quality and effectiveness of nursing practice.
2. Performance Appraisal: The nurse evaluates his or her own nursing practice in relation to professional practice standards and relevant statutes and regulations.
3. Education: The nurse acquires and maintains current knowledge in nursing practice.
4. Collegiality: The nurse contributes to the professional development of peers, colleagues, and others.
5. Ethics: The nurse's decisions and actions on behalf of clients are determined in an ethical manner.
6. Collaboration: The nurse collaborates with the client, significant others, and healthcare providers in providing client care.
7. Research: The nurse uses research findings in practice.
8. Resource utilization: The nurse considers factors related to safety, effectiveness, and cost in planning and delivering client care.

---

*Measurement criteria have also been developed for each standard and are included in the document *Standards of Clinical Nursing Practice*, 1991, available from the American Nurses Association.

(NANDA) development of a taxonomy (1989) began a classification schema to categorize and classify nursing diagnostic labels. NANDA's definition of nursing diagnosis (1990) further clarified the second step of the nursing process (i.e., problem identification/diagnosis). The *ANA Standards of Clinical Nursing Practice* (1991) describes the patient care process and identifies standards for professional performance (Table 1–1).

The advancement of knowledge continues with the work of the US Department of Health and Human Services' Agency for Health Care Policy and Research (AHCPR), whose purpose is to enhance the quality, appropriateness, and effectiveness of healthcare services and access to these services. To this end, multidisciplinary panels of clinicians (including nurses) have begun the arduous process of creating clinical practice guidelines addressing specific patient care situations. These guidelines are intended to assist healthcare providers in the prevention, diagnosis, treatment, and management of clinical conditions. They provide a resource by which patient care can be evaluated, the provider held accountable, and reimbursement justified. There are more than 16 clinical practice guidelines published and available free of charge to help nurses structure the care they provide.

In 1992, the *Iowa Intervention Project: Nursing Interventions Classification* (NIC) directed our focus to the content and process of nursing care by identifying and standardizing some of the direct care activities nurses perform. Now this group is extending its scope by focusing on the classification of nursing outcomes (NOC).

EARLY DISCHARGE

Patients are being discharged from acute care as soon as they are out of danger or their condition is stabilized. Many still require specialized care, however. Subacute or transitional units can provide routine monitoring; ongoing therapies; and complex care such as IV therapy, pain and wound management, airway care, ventilator weaning, neurologic rehabilitation, or additional postsurgical recovery. As the need for complex care decreases, the patient may be discharged home with support services or transferred to a rehabilitation or long-term care facility as appropriate.

Shorter hospital stays have shifted the burden of recovery to the home setting. Families are expected to be more involved in postdischarge care, and patients could be "abandoned" or recovery delayed or prolonged if the family's personal resources cannot meet these new challenges.

AGING POPULATION

The increase in the mean age of patients requiring hospitalization also necessitates some changes in the way health care is provided. A general lack of knowledge among healthcare providers regarding special needs of the elderly, limited resources to meet these needs, and the high incidence of adverse events (such as confusion, falls, and incontinence) have contributed to suboptimal patient care. At the least, this has resulted in prolonged facility stays and increases in the number and complexity of procedures and therapies, readmissions, and adverse outcomes. To this end, the nursing profession is working to develop models that will improve the care provided to this population (Nurses Improving Care to the Hospitalized Elderly [NICHE] Project).

Another area of concern for nurses in elder care is the use of advance directives, which may create ethical concerns regarding the withdrawal or withholding of treatment or care. Living wills and advance directives cannot be expected to anticipate all situations patients may encounter; however, they can provide information to a proxy (named in a medical durable power of attorney) to help in the decision-making process.

TECHNOLOGIC ADVANCES

In the near future, expanded use of monoclonal antibodies to carry chemotherapy agents or radionuclides to cancer cells will reduce adverse reactions and the need for acute care. Endotoxin antibodies (immune system molecules that can mediate sepsis) and gene therapy to manage or even eliminate hereditary diseases will reduce other high-cost therapy needs. Equipment developments are creating user-friendly ventilators, smaller implantable ventricular-assist devices, and artificial hearts that allow patients to leave acute care settings. The cost of care and the likelihood of complications or adverse outcomes are lowered by the use of such procedures as noninvasive monitoring of pulmonary pressures and cardiac output by Doppler, near-infrared spectroscopy for noninvasive intracranial pressure monitoring, tube locators to verify placement of catheters or enteral tubes, and bedside monitoring of many laboratory studies (such as electrolytes, BUN, hematocrit, glucose, and coagulation times). Additionally, point-of-care computer systems are being refined in an effort to cut documentation time and track nursing time for costing of care. Computers can also provide real-time updating of the patient plan of care and by enabling the nurse to process large amounts of data from monitoring activities, facilitate evaluation of the effectiveness of nursing actions and other therapies.

As technology changes and more people become knowledgeable partners in health care, many are choosing alternative therapies and modalities. Billions of dollars are spent yearly for multiple types of therapies, ranging from guided imagery and meditation to homeopathy and acupuncture. Nurses have long placed emphasis on the psychosocial, spiritual, and physical needs of their patients within the medical regimen. Now nurses need to be knowledgeable and open-minded regarding alternative therapies, supporting patient choices and learning new techniques as appropriate.

FUTURE OF NURSING

In general, the public's image of nursing remains positive; however, expectations may be limited because people are not usually aware of nursing's varied capabilities and advanced practice potential. While the public expects nurses to demonstrate technical competence and academic knowledge, it is also demanding "consumer service," that is, friendliness, attention to the patient's personal or special needs, concern for privacy, information about tests and therapies, and inclusion of the family in the information loop.

As the number of RNs in acute care facilities declines and as they are replaced with less experienced and knowledgeable LPNs and UAPs, nurses need to learn to delegate, using the team members effectively and *safely*. Nurses, who now have less time for nonclinical activities, are spending more time collaborating with a variety of healthcare professionals in order to coordinate care, clarify patient needs, and communicate data regarding effectiveness of therapies. To ensure that patients are getting what they need without wasting healthcare dollars RNs must be more knowledgeable about costs and reimbursement plans, as well as the relative benefits of treatment options. Nurses need to interact more with families, providing them with the information they need to make decisions reflecting the patient's goals and values, and to incorporate families into the caregiving process in preparation for the patient's discharge.

Downsizing has become an additional stimulus to nurses to broaden their skill base through cross-training and to acquire certification documenting their expertise in a given area. Certification in itself is not enough, however, rather the outcomes of nursing care are the true measurement of the ability to provide appropriate care. Healthcare systems can no longer employ individuals (e.g., RNs) in roles that do not directly, critically, and clearly contribute to the outcomes of the organization. Nursing's contribution must be defined in the language of outcomes, for that is how services will be evaluated and reimbursed. If nursing cannot define its contribution, then, as far as the reimburser is concerned, the contribution does not exist.

As nurses adapt to the changes in healthcare delivery, they are identifying new practice environments in which to use their skills and working to further define nursing practice and the special contribution nursing will continue to offer.

In the midst of this whirlwind of change, as we experiment with new ways to provide cost-effective care within a specified time frame, it is imperative for nurses to build on the foundation of the profession. Nursing is a science as well as an art, and nursing practice is rooted in the scientific process. Whether or not we choose to rename the steps we engage in (assessing patients' needs, choosing actions to meet those needs, and evaluating the effectiveness of those actions), our purpose remains the same—the diagnosis and treatment of human responses to health and illness. If we allow our nursing focus to be replaced by the medical model, our practice will be subsumed and more will be lost than the essence of our profession. Our patients will lose the holistic coordination of individualized care and professional nurses will no longer be required for the provision of *mere* task-oriented care.

Therefore, as we work collaboratively with other disciplines to provide holistic patient care, we need to continue to identify and document the nursing-care needs of our patients through the use of the nursing process and nursing diagnosis. This journey into change is not optional, but nursing does have the opportunity and responsibility to take an active role in shaping that change.

CONCLUSION

Rapid changes in the healthcare environment, with continuous technologic advances, increasing severity of illness, budget constraints, and expanding nursing knowledge, have greatly increased the responsibilities facing today's nurse. To fulfill these responsibilities, planning and documentation of care are essential to satisfy patient needs and meet legal obligations. Documentation of the impact of nursing on patient care also provides a basis for evaluating continuing care needs, dealing with legal concerns, and determining payment.

What lies ahead for nursing and care planning? Definitely, a tremendously exciting and exacting challenge!

The Nursing Process

Nursing care is a key factor in patient survival and in the maintenance, rehabilitative, and preventive aspects of health care. To this end, the nursing profession has identified a problem-solving process that "combines the most desirable elements of the art of nursing with the most relevant elements of systems theory, using the scientific method" (Shore, 1988).

This nursing process was introduced in the 1950s as a three-step process of *assessment, planning,* and *evaluation* based on the scientific method of observing, measuring, gathering data, and analyzing the findings. Years of study, use, and refinement have led nurses to the expansion of the nursing process to five concrete steps (assessment, problem/need identification, planning, implementation, and evaluation), which provide an efficient method of organizing thought processes for clinical decision making. These five steps are central to nursing actions and the delivery of higher quality, individualized patient care in any setting. The nursing process is included in the conceptual framework of all nursing curricula and is accepted as part of the legal definition of nursing in the Nurse Practice Acts of most states.

When a patient enters the healthcare system, the nurse, using the steps of the nursing process, collects data, identifies problems/needs (nursing diagnoses), establishes goals, identifies outcomes, and chooses nursing interventions to achieve these outcomes and goals. After interventions have been carried out, the nurse evaluates the effectiveness of the plan of care in reaching the desired outcomes and goals by determining whether or not the problems have been resolved. If some of the identified problems remain unresolved at the time of discharge, plans must be made for further assessment, additional problem/need identification, alteration of outcomes and goals, and/or changes of interventions in the home-care settings.

Although we use the terms assessment, problem/ need identification, planning, implementation, and evaluation as separate, progressive steps, they are, in reality, interrelated elements. Together, they form a continuous circle of thought and action throughout the patient's contact with the healthcare system. Figure 2–1 gives some idea of how this cycling process works. The nursing process, combining all of the skills of critical thinking, creates a method of active problem solving that is both dynamic and cyclic.

The critical element for providing effective planned nursing care is its relevance as identified in patient assessments. According to the American Nurses Association *Standards of Clinical Nursing Practice* (ANA, 1991), patient assessment is required in the following areas: physical, psychologic, sociocultural, spiritual, cognitive, functional abilities, developmental, economic, and lifestyle. These assessments, combined with the results of medical findings and diagnostic studies, are documented in the patient data base and form a strong basis for developing the patient's plan of care.

PATIENT DATA BASE

Assessment includes data collected through the history-taking interview, physical assessment, diagnostic studies, and review of prior records.

In this book each selected medical condition has an accompanying patient data base that includes subjective ("may report") and objective ("may exhibit") data. The patient data base is organized within the 13 categories of the Diagnostic Divisions. A sample medical/surgical assessment tool, definitions of the divisions, and a patient situation are included in Chapter 3.

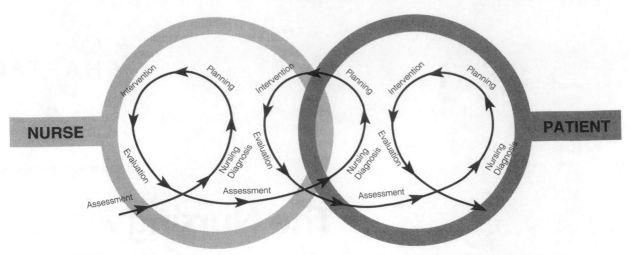

FIGURE 2–1. Diagram of the nursing process. The steps of the nursing process are interrelated, forming a continuous circle of though and action that is both dynamic and cyclic.

Interviewing

Interviewing provides data the nurse obtains from the patient and significant others through conversation and observation. The data may be collected during one or more contact periods and should include all relevant information. Organizing and updating this data assists in the ongoing identification of patient care needs and nursing diagnoses. All participants in the interview process need to know that collected data are used in planning the patient's care.

Physical Assessment

During this aspect of information gathering, the nurse exercises perceptual and observational skills, using the senses of sight, hearing, touch, and smell. The duration and depth of any physical assessment depends on the current condition of the patient and the urgency of the situation but usually includes *inspection, palpation, percussion,* and *auscultation.* In this book the physical assessment data are presented within the patient data base as *objective* data.

Diagnostic Studies

Laboratory and other diagnostic studies are included as part of the data-gathering process. The nurse needs to be aware of significant test results that require reporting to the physician and/or initiation of specific nursing interventions. Some tests are used to diagnose disease, whereas others are useful in following the course of a disease or in adjusting therapies. In many cases, the relationship of the test to the pathologic physiology is clear, but in other cases it is not. This is the result of the interrelationship between various organs and body systems. Interpretation of diagnostic test results should be integrated with the history and physical findings.

NURSING PRIORITIES

In this book, nursing priorities are listed in a certain order to facilitate the ranking of selected associated nursing diagnoses that appear in the plan-of-care guidelines. In any given patient situation, nursing priorities differ on the basis of specific patient need and can vary from minute to minute. A nursing diagnosis that is a priority today may be less of a priority tomorrow, depending on the fluctuating physical and psychosocial condition of the patient or the patient's changing responses to the existing condition.

An example of nursing priorities for a patient diagnosed with severe hypertension would include:

1. Maintain/enhance cardiovascular functioning.
2. Prevent complications.
3. Provide information about disease process, prognosis, and treatment regimen.
4. Support active patient control of condition.

DISCHARGE GOALS

Once the nursing priorities are determined, the next step is to establish goals of treatment. In this book, each medical condition has established *discharge goals,* which are broadly stated and reflect the desired general status of the patient on discharge or transfer to another care setting.

An example of discharge goals for a patient with severe hypertension would include:

1. Blood pressure within acceptable limits for individual
2. Cardiovascular and systemic complications prevented/minimized
3. Disease process/prognosis and therapeutic regimen understood
4. Necessary lifestyle/behavioral changes initiated

NURSING DIAGNOSIS (PROBLEM/NEED IDENTIFICATION)

Nursing diagnoses are a uniform way of identifying, focusing on, and dealing with specific patient needs and responses to actual and high-risk problems. Nursing diagnosis labels provide a format for expressing the problem identification portion of the nursing process. The current working definition of nursing diagnosis developed by the North American Nursing Diagnosis Association (NANDA) is presented in Box 2–1.

BOX 2–1. NANDA Working Definition of Nursing Diagnosis

Nursing diagnosis is a clinical judgment about individual, family, or community responses to actual and potential health problems/life processes. Nursing diagnoses provide the basis for selection of nursing interventions to achieve outcomes for which the nurse is accountable.

There are several steps involved in the process of problem/need identification. Integrating these steps provides a systematic approach to accurately identifying nursing diagnoses.

1. Collecting a patient data base (nursing interview, physical assessment, and diagnostic studies) combined with information collected by other healthcare providers.
2. Reviewing and analyzing the patient data.
3. Synthesizing the gathered patient data as a whole and then labeling your clinical judgment about the patient's response to these actual or high-risk problems.
4. Comparing and contrasting the relationships among your clinical judgments against related factors and defining characteristics for the selected nursing diagnosis. This step is crucial to choosing the appropriate nursing diagnosis label to be used in creating a specific patient diagnostic statement.

5. Combining the nursing diagnosis with the related factors and defining characteristics to create the patient diagnostic statement. For example, the diagnostic statement for a paraplegic patient with a decubitus ulcer could read: Skin Integrity, impaired, related to pressure, circulatory impairment, and decreased sensation evidenced by draining wound, sacral area.

The nursing diagnosis is as correct as the present information will allow because it is supported by the immediate data collected. It documents what the patient's situation is at the present time and should reflect changes as they occur in the patient's condition. Accurate need identification and diagnostic labeling provide the basis for selecting nursing interventions.

The nursing diagnosis may be a physical or a psychosocial response. Physical nursing diagnoses can include those that pertain to physical processes, such as circulation (Altered Tissue Perfusion); ventilation (Impaired Gas Exchange); and elimination (Constipation). Psychosocial nursing diagnoses can include those that pertain to the mind (Acute Confusion); emotion (Fear); or lifestyle/relationship (Altered Role Performance). Unlike medical diagnoses, nursing diagnoses change as the patient progresses through various stages of illness/maladaptation to resolution of the problem or to the conclusion of the condition. Each decision the nurse makes is time-dependent and, with additional information gathered at a later point in time, decisions may change. For example, the initial problems/needs for a patient undergoing cardiac surgery may be Pain, Cardiac Output, Airway Clearance, and Risk for Infection. As the patient progresses, problems/needs will likely shift to Activity Intolerance, Knowledge Deficit, and Role Performance.

Diagnostic reasoning is used to ensure the accuracy of the patient diagnostic statement. The defining characteristics and related factors associated with the chosen nursing diagnosis are reviewed and compared with the patient data. If the diagnosis is not consistent with a majority of the cues, or is not supported by relevant cues, additional data may be required or another nursing diagnosis needs to be investigated.

DESIRED PATIENT OUTCOMES

A desired patient outcome is defined as the result of nursing interventions and patient responses that is achievable, desired by the patient and/or caregiver, and attainable within a defined time period, given the present situation and resources. These desired outcomes are the measurable steps toward achieving the previously established discharge goals and are used to evaluate the patient's response to nursing interventions. (The fifth step of the nursing process, *evaluation*, is addressed in the sample patient situation provided in Chapter 3.)

Useful desired patient outcomes must:

1. Be specific.
2. Be realistic.
3. Be measurable.
4. Indicate a definite time frame for achievement.
5. Consider patient's desires and resources.

Desired patient outcomes are written by listing items and/or behaviors that can be observed and monitored to determine whether or not an acceptable outcome has been achieved within a specified time frame. Action verbs and time frames are used, for example, "patient will ambulate, using cane, within 48 hours of surgery." The action verbs describe the patient's behavior to be evaluated. Time frames are dependent on the patient's projected or anticipated length of stay, often determined by diagnosis-related group (DRG) classification and considering the presence of complications or extenuating circumstances (e.g., age, debilitating disease process).

When outcomes are properly written, they provide direction for planning and validating the selected nursing interventions. Consider the two following patient outcomes: "Identifies individual nutritional needs within 36 hours" and "Formulates a dietary plan based on identified nutritional needs within 72 hours." Based on the clarity of these outcomes, the nurse can select nursing interventions to ensure that the patient's dietary knowledge is assessed, individual needs identified, and nutritional education presented.

NURSING ACTIONS/ INTERVENTIONS

Nursing interventions are prescriptions for specific behaviors expected from the patient and/or actions to be carried out by nurses. Nursing actions/interventions are selected to assist the patient in achieving the stated desired patient outcomes and discharge goals. The expectation is that the prescribed behavior will benefit the patient and family in a predictable way, related to the identified problem and chosen outcomes. These interventions have the intent of individualizing care by meeting a specific patient need and should incorporate identified patient strengths when possible.

Nursing interventions should be specific and clearly stated, beginning with an action verb. Qualifiers of *how, when, where, time/frequency,* and *amount* provide the content of the planned activity. For example, "Assist as needed with self-care activities each morning." "Record respiratory and pulse rates before, during, and after activity." "Measure intake/output hourly." "Active-listen patient's concerns regarding diagnosis." "Instruct family in postdischarge care."

This book divides the nursing interventions/actions into *independent* (nurse-initiated) and *collaborative* (initiated by other care providers). Examples of these two different professionally initiated actions are:

Independent: Provide calm, restful surroundings, minimize environmental activity/noise, and limit numbers of visitors and length of stay.

Collaborative: Administer antianxiety medication as indicated.

RATIONALE

Although rationales do not appear on agency plans of care, they are included to assist the student and practicing nurse in associating the pathophysiologic and/ or psychologic principles with the selected nursing intervention.

Applying Theory to Practice

In the previous chapter, we discussed the theory of nursing process, incorporating nursing diagnosis. In this chapter, given the formative stage of nursing diagnosis, the nurse is encouraged to learn to tailor the plan of care to the individual patient. The plans of care presented here are guides for the nurse in the use of this process. They are designed to give the nurse a sampling of information about general patient situations, and to identify many factors that may or may not need to be given consideration in caring for any particular patient.

Patient assessment is the foundation on which identification of individual needs, responses, and problems is based. To facilitate the steps of assessment and problem identification in the nursing process, we have constructed an assessment tool (Fig. 3–1) using a nursing focus instead of the more familiar medical approach ("review of systems"). This has the advantage of identifying and validating nursing diagnoses as opposed to medical diagnoses.

To achieve this nursing focus, we grouped the North American Nursing Diagnosis Association (NANDA) nursing diagnoses into related categories entitled "Diagnostic Divisions" (Table 3–1), which reflect a blending of theories, primarily Maslow's Hierarchy of Needs and a self-care philosophy. These divisions serve as the framework or outline for data collection and clustering that focuses attention on the nurse's phenomena of concern—the human responses to actual and potential health problems—and direct the nurse to the corresponding nursing diagnosis labels. Because these divisions are based on human responses/needs and are not specific "systems," information may be recorded in more than one area. For this reason, the nurse is encouraged to keep an open mind and to collect as much data as possible

before choosing the nursing diagnosis label. The results (synthesis) of the collected data are written concisely (patient diagnostic statements) to best reflect the patient's situation.

Desired patient outcomes are then identified to facilitate choosing appropriate interventions and to serve as evaluators of both nursing care and patient response. These outcomes also form the framework for documentation.

Interventions are designed to specify the action of the nurse, the patient, and/or significant other(s). They are not all-inclusive, because such basic nursing actions as "bathe the patient" or "notify the physician of changes" have been left out. It is expected that these are included in routine patient care. Sometimes controversial issues or treatments are presented for the sake of information and/or because alternate therapies may be used in different care settings or geographic locations.

In addition to achieving physiologic stability, interventions need to promote the patient's movement toward health and independence. This requires that the patient be involved in his or her own care, including participation in decisions about care activities and projected outcomes. This promotes patient responsibility, negating the idea that healthcare providers control patients' lives.

To assist you in visualizing the tailoring of a plan of care, a prototype Patient Situation (pp 19–23) is provided as an example of data collection and care plan construction. As you review the patient assessment database, you can identify the etiologic/risk factors and defining characteristics that were used to formulate the patient diagnostic statements. Time lines were added to specific patient outcomes to reflect anticipated length of stay and individual patient/nurse expectations. The choice of interventions is based on the concerns and needs identified by the patient and nurse during data collection, in addition to physician orders. Although not normally included in a plan of care, rationales are included in this sample for the purpose of explaining or clarifying the choice of interventions.

Finally, to complete the learning experience, we present samples of the evaluation step based on the patient situation.

ADULT MEDICAL/SURGICAL ASSESSMENT TOOL

General Information

Name: _____

Age: _____ DOB: _____ Sex: _____ Race: _____

Admission Date: _____ Time: _____ From: _____

Source of Information: _____

Reliability (1–4 with 4 = very reliable): _____

Activity/Rest

Subjective (Reports)

Occupation: _____ Usual activities: _____

  Leisure time activities/hobbies: _____

Limitations imposed by condition: _____

Sleep: Hours: _____ Naps: _____ Aids: _____

  Insomnia: _____ Related to: _____

  Rested on awakening: _____

  Excessive grogginess: _____

Feelings of boredom/dissatisfaction: _____

Objective (Exhibits)

Observed response to activity:

  Cardiovascular: _____

  Respiratory: _____

Mental status (i.e., withdrawn/lethargic): _____

Neuromuscular assessment: Muscle mass/tone: _____

  Posture: _____ Tremors: _____ ROM: _____

  Strength: _____ Deformity: _____

Circulation

Subjective (Reports)

History of: Hypertension: _____

  Heart trouble: _____ Rheumatic fever: _____

  Ankle/leg edema: _____ Phlebitis: _____

  Slow healing: _____ Claudication: _____

  Dysreflexia: _____ Bleeding tendencies/

  episodes: _____ Palpitations: _____

  Syncope: _____

Extremities: Numbness: _____ Tingling: _____

Cough/hemoptysis: _____

Change in frequency/amount of urine: _____

Objective (Exhibits)

BP: R and L: Lying/sit/stand: _____

  Pulse pressure: _____ Auscultatory gap: _____

Pulses (palpation): Carotid: _____ Temporal: _____

  Jugular: _____ Radial: _____ Femoral: _____

  Popliteal: _____ Post-tibial: _____

  Dorsalis pedis: _____

Cardiac (palpation): Thrill: _____ Heaves: _____

Heart sounds: Rate: _____ Rhythm: _____

  Quality: _____ Friction rub: _____

  Murmur: _____

Vascular bruit: _____

  Jugular vein distention: _____

Breath sounds: _____

Extremities: Temperature: _____ Color: _____

  Capillary refill: _____ Homan's sign: _____

  Varicosities: _____ Nail abnormalities: _____

FIGURE 3–1. Adult medical-surgical assessment tool. This is a suggested guide and tool for creating a data base reflecting a nursing focus. Although the diagnostic divisions are alphabetized here for ease of presentation, they can be prioritized or rearranged in any manner to meet individual needs. In addition, this assessment tool can be adapted to meet the needs of specific patient populations.

Edema: _____

Distribution/quality of hair: _____

Trophic skin changes: _____

Color: General: _____ Mucous membranes: _____

 Lips: _____ Nail beds: _____ Conjunctiva: _____

 Sclera: _____

Diaphoresis: _____

Ego Integrity

Subjective (Reports)

Stress factors: _____

Ways of handling stress: _____

Financial concerns: _____

Relationship status: _____

Cultural factors: _____

Religion: _____ Practicing: _____

Lifestyle: _____ Recent changes: _____

Sense of connectedness/harmony with self: _____

Feelings of: Helplessness: _____

 Hopelessness: _____

 Powerlessness: _____

Objective (Exhibits)

Emotional status (check those that apply):

 Calm: _____ Anxious: _____ Angry: _____

 Withdrawn _____ Fearful: _____

 Irritable: _____ Restive: _____

 Euphoric: _____

Observed physiologic response(s): _____

Changes in energy field: Temperature: _____

 Color: _____ Distribution: _____

 Movement: _____ Sounds: _____

Elimination

Subjective (Reports)

Usual bowel pattern: _____

Laxative use: _____

Character of stool: _____ Last BM: _____

History of bleeding: _____ Hemorrhoids: _____

Constipation: _____ Diarrhea: _____

Usual voiding pattern: _____

 Incontinence/when: _____ Urgency: _____

 Frequency: _____ Retention: _____

Character of urine: _____

Pain/burning/difficulty voiding: _____

History of kidney/bladder disease: _____

 Diuretic use: _____

Objective (Exhibits)

Abdomen: Tender: _____ Soft/firm: _____

 Palpable mass: _____ Size/girth: _____ Bowel

 sounds: _____ location: _____ type: _____

Hemorrhoids: _____ Stool guaiac: _____

Bladder palpable: _____ Overflow voiding: _____

CVA tenderness: _____

Food/Fluid

Subjective (Reports)

Usual diet (type): _____

Number of meals daily: _____

Last meal/intake: _____

Dietary pattern/content: B: _____ L: _____ D: _____

Fat intake: _____ g/d

Objective (Exhibits)

Current weight: _____ Height: _____

 Body build: _____

Skin turgor: _____

 Mucous membranes moist/dry: _____

Breath sounds: Crackles: _____ Wheezes: _____

FIGURE 3–1. (continued)

Vitamin/food supplement use: _____

Loss of appetite: _____ Nausea/vomiting: _____

Heartburn/indigestion: _____ Related to: _____

    Relieved by: _____

Allergy/food intolerance: _____

Mastication/swallowing problems: _____

    Dentures: _____

Usual weight: _____ Changes in weight: _____

Diuretic use: _____

Edema: General _____ Dependent: _____

    Periorbital: _____ Ascites: _____

Jugular vein distention: _____

Thyroid enlarged: _____

Condition of teeth/gums: _____

Appearance of tongue: _____

    Mucous membranes: _____ Halitosis: _____

Bowel sounds: _____

Hernia/masses: _____

Urine S/A or Chemstix: _____

Serum glucose (Glucometer): _____

Hygiene

Subjective (Reports)

Activities of daily living: Independent/dependent

    (level): Mobility: _____ Feeding: _____

    Hygiene: _____ Dressing/Grooming: _____

    Toileting: _____

Preferred time of personal care/bath: _____

Equipment/prosthetic devices required: _____

Assistance provided by: _____

Objective (Exhibits)

General appearance: _____

Manner of dress: _____ Personal habits: _____

    Body odor: _____ Condition of scalp: _____

    Presence of vermin: _____

Neurosensory

Subjective (Reports)

Fainting spells/dizziness: _____

Headaches: Location: _____ Frequency: _____

Tingling/numbness/weakness (location): _____

Stroke/Brain injury (residual effects): _____

Seizures: Type: _____ Aura: _____

    Frequency: _____ Postictal state: _____

    How controlled: _____

Eyes: Vision loss: _____ Last exam: _____

    Glaucoma: _____ Cataract: _____

Ears: Hearing loss: _____ Last exam: _____

Sense of smell: _____

Epistaxis: _____

Objective (Exhibits)

Mental status (Note duration of change):

    Oriented/disoriented: Person: _____

    Place: _____ Time: _____ Situation: _____

    Alert: _____ Drowsy: _____ Lethargic: _____

    Stuporous: _____ Comatose: _____

    Cooperative: _____ Combative: _____

    Delusions: _____ Hallucinations: _____

    Affect (describe): _____

    Memory: Recent: _____ Remote: _____

Glasses: _____ Contacts: _____

    Hearing aids: _____

Pupil: Shape: _____ Size/reaction: R/L: _____

Facial droop: _____ Swallowing: _____

Handgrasp/release, R/L: _____

Posturing: _____

Deep tendon reflexes: _____

Paralysis: _____

Pain/Discomfort

Subjective (Reports)

Location: _____

    Intensity (0–10 with 10 most severe): _____

    Frequency: _____

Objective (Exhibits)

Facial grimacing: _____

    Guarding affected area: _____

    Emotional response: _____

FIGURE 3–1. (continued)

Quality: _____

Duration: _____

Radiation: _____

Precipitating/aggravating factors: _____

How relieved: _____

Associated symptoms: _____

Effect on activities: _____ Relationships: _____

Narrowed focus: _____

Change in blood pressure: _____ Pulse: _____

Respiration

Subjective (Reports)

Dyspnea/related to: _____

Cough/sputum: _____

History of bronchitis: _____ Asthma: _____

    Emphysema: _____ Tuberculosis: _____

    Recurrent pneumonia: _____

    Exposure to noxious fumes: _____

Smoker: pack/day: _____ # of pack-years: _____

Use of respiratory aids: _____ Oxygen: _____

Objective (Exhibits)

Respiratory: Rate: _____ Depth: _____

    Symmetry: _____

Use of accessory muscles: _____ Nasal flaring: _____

Fremitus: _____

Breath sounds: _____ Egophony: _____

Cyanosis: _____ Clubbing of fingers: _____

Sputum characteristics: _____

Mentation/restlessness: _____

Safety

Subjective (Reports)

Allergics/sensitivity: _____ Reaction: _____

Exposure to infectious diseases: _____

Previous alteration of immune system: _____

    Cause: _____

History of sexually transmitted disease

    (date/type): _____ Testing: _____

    High-risk behaviors: _____

Blood transfusion/number: _____ When: _____

    Reaction: _____ Describe: _____

Geographic areas lived in/visited: _____

Seat belt/helmet use: _____

History of accidental injuries: _____

    Fractures/dislocations: _____

Arthritis/unstable joints: _____

    Back problems: _____

Changes in moles: _____ Enlarged nodes: _____

Delayed healing: _____

Cognitive limitations: _____

    Impaired vision/hearing: _____

Prosthesis: _____ Ambulatory devices: _____

Objective (Exhibits)

Temperature: _____ Diaphoresis: _____

Skin integrity: Scars: _____ Rashes: _____

    Lacerations: _____ Ulcerations: _____

    Ecchymosis: _____ Blisters: _____ Burns

    (degree/percent): _____ Drainage: _____

Mark location of above on diagram:

General strength: _____ Muscle tone: _____

    Gait: _____ ROM: _____

    Paresthesia/paralysis: _____

Results of cultures: _____

    Immune system testing: _____

    Tuberculosis testing: _____

FIGURE 3–1. (continued)

Sexuality (component of Ego Integrity and Social Interaction)

Subjective (Reports)

Sexually active: _____ Use of condoms: _____

Birth control method: _____

Sexual concerns/difficulties: _____

Recent change in frequency/interest: _____

Objective (Exhibits)

Comfort level with subject matter: _____

Female:

Subjective (Reports)

Age at menarche: _____ Length of cycle: _____

    Duration: _____ Number of pads uses/d: _____

    Last menstrual period: _____ Pregnant now: _____

Bleeding between periods: _____

Menopause: _____ Vaginal lubrication: _____

Vaginal discharge: _____

Surgeries: _____

Hormonal therapy/calcium use: _____

Practices breast self-exam: _____

    Mammogram: _____

Last PAP smear: _____

Objective (Exhibits)

Breast exam: _____

Genital warts/lesions: _____

Discharge: _____

Male:

Subjective (Reports)

Penile discharge: _____

Prostate disorder: _____

Circumcised: _____ Vasectomy: _____

Practice self-exam: Breast: _____ Testicles: _____

Last proctoscopic/prostate exam: _____

Objective (Exhibits)

Breast: _____ Penis: _____

Testicles: _____

Genital warts/lesions: _____

Discharge: _____

Social Interactions

Subjective (Reports)

Marital status: _____ Years in relationship: _____

    Living with: _____ Concerns/stresses: _____

Extended family: _____

    Other support person(s): _____

Role within family structure: _____

Perception of relationships with family

    members: _____

Feelings of: Mistrust: _____ Rejection: _____

    Unhappiness: _____ Loneliness/isolation: _____

Problems related to illness/condition: _____

Problems with communication: _____

    Use of communication aids: _____

Objective (Exhibits)

Speech: Clear: _____ Slurred: _____

    Unintelligible: _____ Aphasic: _____

    Usual speech pattern/impairment: _____

    Use of speech aids: _____

    Laryngectomy present: _____

Verbal/nonverbal communication with

    family/SO(s): _____

    Family interaction (behavioral) pattern: _____

FIGURE 3–1. (continued)

Teaching/Learning

Subjective (Reports)

Dominant language (specify): _____ Literate: _____

    Education level: _____ Learning disabilities:

    (specify): _____ Cognitive limitations: _____

Health beliefs/practices: _____

Special healthcare concerns (e.g., impact of

    religious/cultural practices): _____

    Health goals: _____

Familial risk factors (indicate relationship):

    Diabetes: _____ Thyroid (specify): _____

    Tuberculosis: _____ Heart disease: _____

    Strokes: _____ High BP: _____

    Epilepsy: _____

Kidney disease: _____ Cancer: _____

    Mental illness: _____ Other: _____

Prescribed medications: Drug: _____ Dose: _____

    Times (circle last dose): _____

    Take regularly: _____ Purpose: _____

    Side effects/ problems: _____

Nonprescription drugs: OTC drugs: _____

    Street drugs: _____ Tobacco: _____

    Smokeless tobacco: _____

Alcohol (amount/frequency): _____

Admitting diagnosis per provider: _____

Reason for hospitalization per patient: _____

History of current complaint: _____

Patient expectations of this hospitalization: _____

Previous illnesses and/or hospitalizations/

    surgeries: _____

Evidence of failure to improve: _____

Last complete physical exam: _____

Discharge Plan Considerations

DRG projected mean length of stay: _____

Date information obtained: _____

Anticipated date of discharge: _____

Resources available: Persons: _____ Financial: _____

    Community: _____ Support groups: _____

    Socialization: _____

Areas that may require alteration/assistance: Food

    preparation: _____ Shopping: _____

    Transportation: _____ Ambulation:

    Medication/IV therapy: _____

    Treatments: _____ Wound care: _____

    Supplies: _____ Self-care (specify): _____

    Homemaker/maintenance (specify): _____

    Physical layout of home (specify): _____

Anticipated changes in living situation after

    discharge: _____

Living facility other than home (specify): _____

Referrals (date, source, services): Social

    services: _____ Rehab services: _____

    Dietary: _____ Home care: _____

    Resp/O_2: _____ Equipment: _____

    Supplies: _____ Other: _____

FIGURE 3–1. (continued)

TABLE 3–1. **Nursing Diagnoses Organized According to Diagnostic Divisions***

After data are collected and areas of concern/need identified, the nurse is directed to the Diagnostic Divisions to review the list of nursing diagnoses that fall within the individual categories. This will assist the nurse in choosing the specific diagnostic label to describe the data accurately. Then, with the addition of etiology (when known) and signs and symptoms/cues (defining characteristics), the patient diagnostic statement emerges.

Activity/rest—Ability to engage in necessary/desired activities of life (work and leisure) and to obtain adequate sleep/rest

    Activity intolerance

    Activity intolerance, risk for

    Disuse Syndrome, risk for

    Diversional Activity deficit

Activity/rest—Ability to engage in necessary/desired activities of life (work and leisure) and to obtain adequate sleep/rest (*Continued*)

Fatigue
Sleep Pattern disturbance

Circulation–Ability to transport oxygen and nutrients necessary to meet cellular needs

Adaptive Capacity: Intracranial, decreased
Cardiac Output, decreased
Dysreflexia
Tissue Perfusion, altered (specify): renal, cerebral, cardiopulmonary, gastrointestinal, peripheral

Ego Integrity—Ability to develop and use skills and behaviors to integrate and manage life experiences

Adjustment, impaired
Anxiety [specify level]
Body Image disturbance
Coping, defensive
Coping, Individual, ineffective
Decisional Conflict (specify)
Denial, ineffective
Fear
Grieving, anticipatory
Grieving, dysfunctional
Hopelessness
Personal Identity disturbance
Post-trauma Response
Powerlessness
Rape-Trauma Syndrome
Rape-Trauma Syndrome: compound reaction
Rape-Trauma Syndrome: silent reaction
Relocation Stress Syndrome
Self Esteem, chronic low
Self Esteem, disturbance
Self Esteem, situational low
Spiritual Distress (distress of the human spirit)
Spiritual Well-Being, potential for enhanced

Elimination—Ability to excrete waste products

Bowel Incontinence
Constipation
Constipation, colonic
Constipation, perceived
Diarrhea
Incontinence, functional
Incontinence, reflex
Incontinence, stress
Incontinence, total
Incontinence, urge
Urinary Elimination, altered
Urinary Retention [acute/chronic]

Food/Fluid—Ability to maintain intake of and utilize nutrients and liquids to meet physiologic needs

Breastfeeding, effective
Breastfeeding, ineffective
Breastfeeding, interrupted
Fluid Volume deficit [active loss]
Fluid Volume deficit [regulatory failure]
Fluid Volume deficit, risk for
Fluid Volume excess

Food/Fluid—Ability to maintain intake of and utilize nutrients and liquids to meet physiologic needs (*Continued*)

Infant Feeding Pattern, ineffective
Nutrition: altered, less than body requirements
Nutrition: altered, more than body requirements
Nutrition: altered, risk for more than body requirements
Oral Mucous Membrane, altered
Swallowing, impaired

Hygiene—Ability to perform activities of daily living

Self Care deficit: feeding, bathing/hygiene, dressing/grooming, toileting

Neurosensory—Ability to perceive, integrate, and respond to internal and external cues

Confusion, acute
Confusion, chronic
Infant Behavior, disorganized
Infant Behavior, disorganized, risk for
Infant Behavior, organized, potential for enhanced
Memory, impaired
Peripheral Neurovascular dysfunction, risk for
Sensory/Perceptual alterations (specify): visual, auditory, kinesthetic, gustatory, tactile, olfactory
Thought Processes, altered
Unilateral Neglect

Pain/Discomfort—Ability to control internal/external environment to maintain comfort

Pain [acute]
Pain, chronic

Respiration—Ability to provide and use oxygen to meet physiologic needs

Airway Clearance, ineffective
Aspiration, risk for
Breathing Pattern, ineffective
Gas Exchange, impaired
Spontaneous Ventilation, inability to sustain
Ventilatory Weaning Response, dysfunctional (DVWR)

Safety—Ability to provide safe, growth-promoting environment

Body Temperature, altered, risk for
Environmental Interpretation Syndrome, impaired
Health Maintenance, altered
Home Maintenance Management, impaired
Hyperthermia
Hypothermia
Infection, risk for
Injury, risk for
Perioperative Positioning Injury, risk for
Physical Mobility, impaired
Poisoning, risk for
Protection, altered
Self-mutilation, risk for
Skin Integrity, impaired
Skin Integrity, impaired, risk for
Suffocation, risk for
Thermoregulation, ineffective
Tissue Integrity, impaired
Trauma, risk for
Violence, risk for, directed at self/others

Sexuality [Component of Ego Integrity and Social Interaction]—Ability to meet requirements/characteristics of male/female role

Sexual dysfunction
Sexuality Patterns, altered

Social Interaction—Ability to establish and maintain relationships

Caregiver Role Strain
Caregiver Role Strain, risk for
Communication, impaired verbal
Community Coping, ineffective

Social Interaction—Ability to establish and maintain relationships (*Continued*)

Community Coping, potential for enhanced
Family Coping: ineffective, compromised
Family Coping: ineffective, disabling
Family Coping: potential for growth
Family Process, altered: alcoholism
Family Processes, altered
Loneliness, risk for
Parent/Infant/Child Attachment, altered, risk for
Parental Role conflict
Parenting, altered
Parenting, altered, risk for
Role Performance, altered
Social Interaction, impaired
Social Isolation

Teaching/Learning—Ability to incorporate and use information to achieve healthy lifestyle/optimal wellness

Growth and Development, altered
Health-Seeking Behaviors (specify)
Knowledge deficit [learning need] (specify)
Noncompliance [Compliance, altered] (specify)
Therapeutic Regimen: Community, ineffective management
Therapeutic Regimen: Families, ineffective management
Therapeutic Regimen: Individual, effective management
Therapeutic Regimen: Individual, ineffective management

*Permission from North American Nursing Diagnosis Association (1994). NANDA Nursing Diagnoses: Definitions and Classifications 1995–1996. Philadelphia: NANDA. Copyright 1994 by the North American Nursing Diagnosis Association.

PATIENT SITUATION: Diabetes Mellitus

Mr. R.S., a non–insulin-dependent diabetic (NIDDM, Type II) for 5 years, presented to his physician's office with a nonhealing ulcer of 3 weeks' duration on his left foot. Laboratory studies at the doctor's office revealed blood glucose of 256/fingerstick and urine Chemstix of 1% and small.

Admitting Physician's Orders

Culture/sensitivity and Gram's stain of foot ulcer.
Random blood glucose on admission and fingerstick BG every AM.
CBC, electrolytes, glycosylated Hb in AM.
Chest x-ray and ECG in AM.
Humulin N 15 U q AM, SC. Begin insulin instruction for postdischarge self-care.
Dicloxacillin 500 mg po, q6h, start after culture obtained.
Darvocet-N 100 mg q4h prn, pain.
Diet—2400 calories ADA/3 meals with 2 snacks.
Up in chair ad lib with feet elevated.
Foot cradle for bed.
Betadine soak L foot tid × 15 minutes, then cover with dry sterile dressing.
Vital signs qid.

Patient Assessment Data Base

Name: R.S. Informant: Patient. Reliability (Scale 1–4): 3.
Age 67. DOB: 5/3/27. Race: Caucasian. Sex: M.
Admission date: 6/28/94 Time: 7 PM From: Home.

ACTIVITY/REST

Reports (Subjective):	Occupation: Farmer. Usual activities/hobbies: Reading, playing cards. "Don't have time to do much. Anyway I'm too tired most of the time to do anything after the chores." Limitations imposed by illness: "Have to watch what I order if I eat out." Sleep: Hours: 6–8 h/night. Naps: No. Aids: No. Insomnia: "Not unless I drink coffee after supper." Usually feels rested when awakens at 4:30 AM.
Exhibits (Objective):	Observed response to activity: Limps, favors L foot when walking. Mental status: Alert/active. Neuromuscular assessment: Muscle mass/tone: bilaterally equal/firm. Posture: Erect. ROM: Full. Strength: Equal 3 extremities/favors L leg currently.

CIRCULATION

Reports (Subjective):	Slow healing: lesion L foot, 3 weeks' duration. Extremities: Numbness/tingling: "My feet feel cold and tingly when I walk a lot." Cough/character of sputum: Occasional/white. Change in frequency/amount of urine: Yes, voiding more lately.
Exhibits (Objective):	Peripheral pulses: Radials 3+, popliteal, dorsalis, posttibial/pedal, all 1+. BP: R: Lying: 146/90. Sit: 140/86. Stand: 138/90 L: Lying: 142/88. Sit: 138/88. Stand: 138/84.

Pulse: Apical: 86. Radial: 86. Quality: Strong. Rhythm: Regular.
Chest auscultation: Few wheezes clear with cough, no murmurs/rubs.
JVD: -0-.
Extremities: Temperature: Feet cool bilat/legs warm.
  Color—skin: Legs pale. Capillary refill: Slow both feet.
  Homan's sign: -0-. Varicosities: Few enlarged superficial veins both calves.
    Nails: Toenails thickened, yellow, brittle. Distribution and quality of hair:
    Coarse hair to midcalf, none on ankles/toes.
  Color—general: Ruddy face/arms. Mucous membranes/lips: Pink.
  Nail beds: Blanch well. Conjunctiva and sclera: White.

EGO INTEGRITY

Reports (Subjective):

Report of stress factors: "Normal farmer's problems: weather, pests, bankers, and so on."
Ways of handling stress: "I get busy with the chores and talk things over with my livestock; they listen real good."
Financial concerns: No insurance; needs to hire someone to do chores while in hospital.
Relationship status: Married.
Cultural factors: Rural/agrarian, Eastern European descent.
Religion: Protestant/practicing.
Lifestyle: Middle class/self-sufficient farmer.
Recent changes: -0-.
Feelings: "I'm in control of most things, except the weather and this diabetes."
Concerned regarding possible therapy change "from pills to shots."

Exhibits (Objective):

Emotional status: Generally calm.
Observed physiologic response(s): Occasionally sighs deeply/frowns, shrugs shoulders/throws up hands, appears frustrated.

ELIMINATION

Reports (Subjective):

Usual bowel pattern: Most every PM.
Last bowel movement: Last night. Character of stool: Firm/brown.
Bleeding: -0-. Hemorrhoids: -0-. Constipation: Occasional.
Laxative used: Hot prune juice.
Urinary: No problems. Character of urine: Pale yellow.

Exhibits (Objective):

Abdomen tender: No. Soft/Firm: Soft. Palpable mass: None.
Bowel sounds: Active all 4 quads.

FOOD/FLUID

Reports (Subjective):

Usual diet (type): 2400 ADA (occasionally "cheats" with dessert, "My wife watches it pretty closely"). Number of meals daily: 3.
Dietary Pattern: Breakfast: Fruit juice, toast, ham, coffee. Lunch: Meat, potatoes, vegetables, fruit, milk. Dinner: Meat sandwich, soup, fruit, coffee. Snack: milk/crackers at HS. Usual beverage: Skim milk, 2–3 cups decaf coffee. Drinks a lot of water.
Last meal/intake: Dinner: roast beef sandwich, vegetable soup, pear with cheese, decaf coffee.
Loss of appetite: "Never, but lately I don't feel as hungry as usual."
Nausea/Vomiting: -0-. Food Allergies: None.
Heartburn/food intolerance: Cabbage causes gas, coffee after supper causes heartburn.
Mastication/swallowing problems: No. Dentures: Partial upper plate.
Usual weight: 175 lb.
Recent changes: Has lost about 3 lb this month.
Diuretic therapy: No.

Exhibits (Objective):

Wt: 171 lb. Ht: 5'10". Build: Stocky. Skin turgor: Good/leathery.
Appearance of tongue: Midline, pink. Mucous membranes: Pink, intact.

Condition of teeth/gums: Good; no irritation/bleeding noted.
Breath sounds: Few wheezes cleared with cough.
Bowel sounds: Active all 4 quads.
Urine Chemstix: 1%/small. Fingerstick: 256 (Dr. office).

HYGIENE

Reports (Subjective): Activities of daily living: Independent in all areas.
Preferred time of bath: PM.

Exhibits (Objective): General appearance: Clean, shaven, short-cut hair, hands rough and dry.
Scalp and eyebrows: Scaly white patches.

NEUROSENSORY

Reports (Subjective): Headaches: "Occasionally behind my eyes when I worry too much."
Tingling/Numbness: Feet, once or twice a week.
Eyes: Vision loss, far-sighted. Examination: 2 years ago.
Ears—Hearing loss: R: "Some" L: No (Has not been tested).
Nose: Epistaxis: -0-. Sense of smell: "No problems."

Exhibits (Objective): Mental status: Alert, oriented to time, place, person, situation. Affect: Concerned.
Memory: Remote and recent: clear and intact
Speech: Clear, coherent, appropriate
Pupil reaction: PERLA/small. Glasses: Reading. Hearing aid: No.
Handgrip/release: Strong/equal.

PAIN/DISCOMFORT

Reports (Subjective): Location: Lateral aspect, heel of L foot.
Intensity (0–10): 4–5. Quality: Dull ache with occasional sharp stabbing sensation.
Frequency/Duration: "Seems like all the time." Radiation: No.
Precipitating factors: Shoes, walking. How relieved: ASA, not helping.
Other complaints: Sometimes has back pain following chores/heavy lifting relieved by ASA/liniment rubdown.

Exhibits (Objective): Facial grimacing: When lesion border palpated.
Guarding affected area: Pulls foot away. Narrowed focus: No.
Emotional response: Tense, irritated.

RESPIRATORY

Reports (Subjective): Dyspnea: -0-. Cough: Occasional morning cough, white sputum.
Emphysema: -0-. Bronchitis: -0-. Asthma: -0-. Tuberculosis: -0-.
Smoker: Filters. Packs/day: 1/2. Number of years: 25+.
Use of respiratory aids: -0-.

Exhibits (Objective): Respiratory rate: 22. Depth: Good. Symmetry: Equal, bilateral.
Auscultation: Few wheezes, clear with cough.
Cyanosis: -0-. Clubbing of fingers: -0-.
Sputum characteristics: None to observe.
Mentation/restlessness: Alert/oriented/relaxed.

SAFETY

Reports (Subjective): Allergies: -0-. Blood transfusions: -0-.
Sexually transmitted disease: None.
Fractures/dislocations: L clavicle, 1962, fell getting off tractor.
Arthritis/unstable joints: "Think I've got some arthritis in my knees."

Back problems: Occasional lower back pain.
Vision impaired: Requires glasses for reading.
Hearing impaired: Slightly (R), compensates by turning "good ear" toward speaker.

Exhibits (Objective): Temperature: 99.4°F, tympanic.
Skin integrity: Impaired L foot. Scars: R Ing, surgical.
Rashes: -0-. Bruises: -0-. Lacerations: -0-. Blisters: -0-.
Ulcerations: Medial aspect L foot, 2.5 cm diameter, approximately 3 mm deep, draining small amount cream color/pink tinged matter, no odor noted.
Strength (general): Equal all extremities. Muscle tone: Firm.
ROM: Good. Gait: Favors L foot. Paresthesia/Paralysis: -0-.

SEXUALITY: MALE

Reports (Subjective): Sexually active: Yes. Use of condoms: No (monogamous).
Recent changes in frequency/interest: "I've been too tired lately."
Penile discharge: -0-. Prostate disorder: -0-. Vasectomy: -0-.
Last proctoscopic examination: 2 years ago. Prostate examination: 1 year ago.
Practice self-examination: Breast/testicles: No.
Problems/complaints: "I don't have any problems, but you'd have to ask my wife if there are any complaints."

Exhibits (Objective): Examination—Breast: No masses. Testicles: Deferred. Prostate: Deferred.

SOCIAL INTERACTIONS

Reports (Subjective): Marital status: Married, 43 years. Living with: Wife.
Report of problems: None.
Extended family: 1 daughter lives in town (30 miles away); 1 daughter married/grandson, living out of state.
Other: Several couples; he and wife play cards/socialize 2 or 3 times a month.
Role: Works farm alone; husband/father/grandfather.
Report of problems related to illness/condition: None until now.
Coping behaviors: "My wife and I have always talked things out. You know the 11th commandment is 'Thou shalt not go to bed angry.'"

Exhibits (Objective): Speech: Clear, intelligible.
Verbal/Nonverbal communication with family/SO(s): Speaks quietly with wife, looking her in the eye; relaxed posture.
Family interaction patterns: Wife sitting at bedside, relaxed, both reading paper, making occasional comments to each other.

TEACHING/LEARNING

Reports (Subjective): Dominant language: English. Literate: Yes.
Education level: 2 years of college.
Health beliefs/practices: "I take care of the minor problems and only see the doctor when something's broken."
Familial risk factors/relationship:
 Diabetes: Maternal uncle. Tuberculosis: Brother died age 27.
 Heart Disease: Father died age 78, heart attack.
 Strokes: Mother died age 81. High BP: Mother.
Prescribed medications:

Drug	Dose	Schedule	Time/last dose	Purpose
Orinase	250 mg	8 AM/6 PM	Last dose 6 PM today	Diabetes

Home urine glucose monitoring: "Stopped several months ago when I ran out of TesTape. It was always negative anyway."

Take medications regularly: Yes.

Nonprescription (OTC) drugs: Occasionally ASA.

Use of alcohol (amount/frequency): Socially, occasionally beer.

Tobacco: ½ pack/d

Admitting Diagnosis (physician): Hyperglycemia with nonhealing lesion L foot.

Reason for hospitalization (patient): Sore on foot and "My sugar is up."

History of current complaint: "Three weeks ago, I got a blister on my foot from breaking in my new boots. It got sore so I lanced it, but it isn't getting any better."

Patient's expectations of this hospitalization: "Clear up this infection and control my diabetes."

Other relevant illness and/or previous hospitalizations/surgeries: 1965 R Ing. hernia repair.

Evidence of failure to improve: Lesion L foot, 3 weeks.

Last physical examination: Complete 1 year ago, office follow-up 3 months ago.

Discharge Considerations (as of 6/28):

Anticipated discharge: 7/1/94 (3 days).

Resources: Person: Self, wife. Financial: "If this doesn't take too long to heal, we got some savings to cover things." Community supports: Diabetic support group (has not participated).

Anticipated lifestyle changes: None.

Assistance needed: May require farm help for several days.

Teaching: Learn new medication regimen and wound care, review diet.

Referrals: Supplies: Downtown Pharmacy or AARP. Equipment: Glucometer—AARP.

Follow-up: Primary care provider 1 wk after discharge to evaluate wound healing and additional changes in diabetic regimen.

PLAN OF CARE: Mr. R.S.

ACTIONS/INTERVENTIONS	RATIONALE
Obtain sterile specimen of wound drainage on admission.	Identifies pathogens and therapy of choice.
Administer dicloxacillin 500 mg po q6h, starting 10 PM. Observe for signs of hypersensitivity, i.e., pruritus, urticaria, rash.	Treatment of infection/prevention of complications. Food interferes with drug absorption requiring scheduling around meals. Although no prior history of penicillin reaction, it may occur at any time.
Soak foot in room-temperature sterile water with betadine solution tid × 15 minutes.	Local germicidal effective for surface wounds.
Assess wound with each dressing change.	Provides information about effectiveness of therapy and identifies additional needs.
Massage area around wound site gently.	Stimulates circulation and delivery of white blood cells, fibroblasts, and nutrients required for healing and removal of phagocytized debris.
Dress wound with dry sterile dressing. Use paper tape.	Keeps wound clean/minimizes cross-contamination. Adhesive tape may be abrasive to fragile tissues.
Administer 15 U Humulin N insulin SC q AM after daily fingerstick BG.	Treats underlying metabolic dysfunction, reducing hyperglycemia and promoting healing.

ACTIONS/INTERVENTIONS

Determine pain characteristics through patient's description.

Place foot cradle on bed/encourage use of loose-fitting slipper, when up.

Administer Darvocet-N 100 mg po q4h as needed. Document effectiveness.

RATIONALE

Establishes baseline for assessing improvement/changes.

Avoids direct pressure to area of injury, which could result in vasoconstriction/increased pain.

Provides relief of discomfort when unrelieved by other measures.

PATIENT DIAGNOSTIC STATEMENT:

Altered peripheral tissue perfusion, related to decreased arterial flow, evidenced by decreased pulses, pale/cool feet, thick brittle nails, numbness/tingling of feet "when walks a lot."

DESIRED OUTCOMES—PATIENT WILL:

Verbalize understanding of relationship between chronic disease (diabetes mellitus) and circulatory changes within 48 hours (6/30 1900).

Demonstrate awareness of safety factors/proper foot care within 48 hours (6/30 1900).

Maintain adequate level of hydration to maximize perfusion (ongoing), as evidenced by balanced intake/output, moist skin/mucous membranes, adequate capillary refill.

ACTIONS/INTERVENTIONS

Elevate feet when up in chair. Avoid long periods with feet dependent.

Assess for signs of dehydration. Monitor intake/output. Encourage oral fluids.

Instruct patient to avoid constricting clothing/socks and ill-fitting shoes.

Reinforce safety precautions regarding use of heating pads, hot water bottles/soaks.

Discuss complications of disease that result from vascular changes, i.e., ulceration, gangrene, muscle or bony structure changes.

Review proper foot care as outlined in teaching plan.

RATIONALE

Minimizes interruption of blood flow, reduces venous pooling.

Glycosuria may result in dehydration with consequent reduction of circulating volume and further impairment of peripheral circulation.

Compromised circulation and decreased pain sensation may precipitate or aggravate tissue breakdown.

Heat increases metabolic demands on compromised tissues. Vascular insufficiency alters pain sensation increasing risk of injury.

Proper control of diabetes mellitus may not prevent complications but may minimize severity of effect.

Altered perfusion of lower extremities may lead to serious/persistent complications at the cellular level.

ACTIONS/INTERVENTIONS	RATIONALE
Determine patient's level of knowledge, priorities of learning needs, desire/need for including wife in instruction.	Establishes baseline and direction for teaching/planning. Involvement of wife, if desired, will provide additional resource for recall/understanding and may enhance patient's follow-through.
Provide teaching guide, "Understanding Your Diabetes" 6/28 AM. Show film "Living with Diabetes" 6/29 4 PM when wife is visiting. Include in group teaching session 6/30 AM. Review information and obtain feedback from patient and wife.	Provides different methods for accessing/reinforcing information and enhances opportunity for learning/understanding.
Discuss factors related to/altering diabetic control, e.g., stress, illness, exercise.	Drug therapy/diet may need to be altered in response to both short- and long-term stressors.
Review signs/symptoms of hyperglycemia, (e.g., fatigue, nausea/vomiting, polyuria/dypsia). Discuss how to prevent and evaluate this situation, and when to seek medical care. Have patient identify appropriate interventions.	Recognition/understanding of these signs/symptoms and timely intervention will aid patient in avoiding recurrences and preventing complications.
Review and provide information about necessity for routine examination of feet, and proper foot care, e.g., daily inspection for injuries, pressure areas, corns, calluses; proper nail cutting; daily washing. Recommend wearing loose-fitting socks and properly fitting shoes (break new shoes in gradually) and avoiding going barefoot. If foot injury/skin break occurs, wash with soap and water, cover with sterile dressing, inspect wound and change dressing daily; report redness, swelling, or presence of drainage.	Reduces risk of tissue injury, promotes understanding and prevention of stasis ulcer formation and wound healing difficulties.
Instruct regarding prescribed insulin therapy:	May be a temporary treatment of hyperglycemia with infection, or may be permanent replacement of oral hypoglycemic agent.
Humulin N insulin, sc;	Intermediate-acting insulin generally lasts 18–28 hours, with peak effect 6–12 hours.
Keep vial in current use at room temperature, store extra vials in refrigerator.	Refrigeration prevents wide fluctuations in temperature prolonging the drug shelf-life; cold can impede absorption.

Roll bottle and invert to mix. Do not shake vigorously;

Vigorous shaking may create foam, which can interfere with accurate dose withdrawal and may damage the insulin molecule.

Choice of injection sites (e.g., across abdomen in "Z" pattern).

Provides for steady absorption of medication; site is easily visualized and accessible by patient; "Z" pattern minimizes tissue damage.

Demonstrate, then observe patient in drawing insulin into syringe, reading syringe markings, and administering dose. Assess for accuracy.

May require several instruction sessions and practice before patient and wife feel comfortable drawing up and injecting medication.

Instruct in signs/symptoms of insulin reaction/hypoglycemia, i.e., fatigue, nausea, headache, hunger, sweating, irritability, shakiness, anxiety, difficulty concentrating.

Knowing what to watch for and appropriate treatment (such as grape juice for immediate response and cheese for sustained effect) may prevent or minimize complications.

ACTIONS/INTERVENTIONS

RATIONALE

Review "Sick Day Rules," e.g., call doctor if too sick to eat normally/stay active; take insulin as ordered. Keep record as noted on Sick Day Guide.

Understanding of necessary actions in the event of mild/severe illness promotes competent self-care and reduces risk of hyper/hypoglycemia.

Instruct patient and wife in fingerstick glucose monitoring and observe return demonstrations of the procedure.

Fingerstick monitoring provides accurate and timely information regarding diabetic status. Return demonstration verifies correct learning.

Recommend patient maintain record of fingerstick testing, insulin dosage/site, unusual physiologic response, dietary intake.

Provides accurate record for review by caregivers for assessment of therapy effectiveness/needs.

Refer to dietician for consultation regarding diet.

Calories are unchanged on new orders but have been redistributed to 3 meals and 2 snacks. Dietary choices (e.g., increased vitamin C) may enhance healing.

Discuss other healthcare issues, e.g., smoking habits, self-monitoring for cancer (breasts/testicles), and reporting changes in general well-being.

Encourages patient involvement, awareness, and responsibility for own health; promotes wellness.

EVALUATION

As nursing care is provided, ongoing assessment evaluates the patient's response to therapy and progress toward accomplishing the desired outcomes. This activity serves as the feedback and control part of the nursing process, through which the status of the individual patient diagnostic statement is judged to be resolved, continuing, or requiring revision.

This process is visualized in Figure 3–2. Observation of Mr. R.S.'s wound reveals that edges are clean and pink and drainage is scant. Therefore, he is progressing *toward* achieving wound healing, and this problem will continue to be addressed although no revision in the treatment plan is required at this time.

DOCUMENTATION

A way to evaluate and document the patient's progress (response to care) is through the use of clinical pathways. These were originally developed as a tool for providing care in case management systems and are now used in many settings. A clinical pathway is a type of abbreviated plan of care that is event-oriented (task-oriented) and provides outcome-based guidelines for goal achievement within a designated length of stay. The pathway incorporates agency and professional standards of care and may be interdisciplinary, depending on the care setting. As a rule, however, the standarized clinical pathways address a specific diagnosis/condition or procedure (e.g., myocardial infarc-

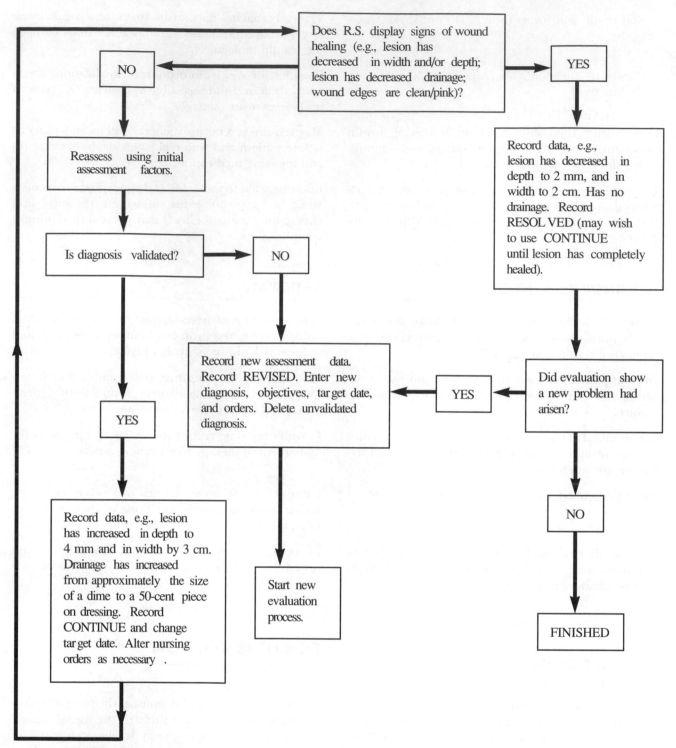

FIGURE 3–2. Outcome-based evaluation of the patient's response to therapy. (Adapted from Cox, HC, et al: Clinical Applications of Nursing Diagnosis, ed 3. F. A. Davis Co., Philadelphia, 1996.)

CP: Non-healing Lesion—Diabetic. ELOS: 3 Days—Variations from Designated Pathway Should Be Documented in Progress Notes

ND and categories of care	Adm Day	Day 1	Day 2	Day 3
Impaired skin/ tissue integrity R/T	Actions: Goals:	Actions: Goals: Verbalize understanding of condition; Display blood glucose WNL (ongoing)	Actions: Goals: Be free of signs of dehydration; Wound free of purulent drainage; Verbalize understanding of treatment need; Perform self-care tasks #1 & 3 correctly; Explain reasons for actions	Actions: Goals: Wound edges show signs of healing process; Perform self-care tasks: #2 correctly; Explain reason for actions; Plan in place to meet discharge needs
Referrals		Dietician: Determine need for: Home care; Physical therapy; Visiting nurse		
Diagnostic studies	Wound culture; Gram's stain; Random blood glucose; Fingerstick BG Ø	→ CBC, electrolytes; Glycosylated Hb; → Fingerstick BG qAM; → Chest X ray (if indi); → ECG (if indi)	Fingerstick BG qAM	Fingerstick BG qAM
Additional assessments	VS qid; I & O/level of hydration qd; Character of wound tid; Level of knowledge and priorities of learning needs; Observe for signs of antibiotic hypersensitivity reaction	→ ; → ; →	→ VS Qshift; → ; →	→ ; → D/C; →
Medications	Antibiotic: Dicloxacillin 500 mg po q6h; Antidiabetic: none; Other: Betadine soaks tid	Anticipated discharge needs; Antibiotic: same; Antidiabetic: Humulin Ni insulin 15 u SC q AM; Other: same	Antibiotic: same; Antidiabetic: same; Other: same	Antibiotic: same; Antidiabetic: same; Other: same

FIGURE 3–3. Sample clinical pathway.

CP: Non-healing Lesion—Diabetic. ELOS: 3 Days—Variations from Designated Pathway Should Be Documented in Progress Notes (*Continued*)

ND and categories of care	Adm Day	Day 1	Day 2	Day 3
Patient education	Provide "Understanding Your Diabetes"	Film "Living with Diabetes" Demonstrate and practice self-care activities: 1. Fingerstick BG 2. Insulin admin 3. Wound care 4. Routine foot care	Actions: Group sessions: *Diabetic management*	Actions: Practice self-care activities *2-insulin admin* Review discharge instructions
Goals: Perform self-care tasks: #2 correctly Explain reason for actions Plan in place to meet discharge needs
Additional nursing actions Pain	Up ad lib Dressing change TID State pain relieved or minimized with *1hr* of analgesic administration (ongoing) Verbalize understanding of when to report pain and rating scale used Verbalize understanding of S/C measures: *#1–2* Explain reason for actions	→ → Verbalize understanding of S/C measures: *#3* Explain reason for actions	→ → Goals: Able to participate at usual level: *ambulate full wt. bearing*	→ → State pain-free/controlled w/ medication Verbalize understanding of correct medication use
Additional assessments	Characteristics of pain Level of participation in activities Individual analgesic needs	→ → →	→ → →	→ → →
Medications Allergies: _____	Analgesic: Darvocet-N 100 mg po q4h prn	Analgesic: same	Analgesic: same	Analgesic: same
Patient education	Orient to unit/room Guidelines for self-report of pain and rating scale 0–10 Safety/comfort measures: *1 elevation of feet 2 proper footwear*	Safety/comfort measures: *3 prevention of injury*		Review discharge medication instructions: dosage, route, frequency, side effects
Additional nursing actions	Bed cradle as indicated	→	→	→

FIGURE 3–3. (continued)

tion, total hip replacement, chemotherapy) and do not provide for inclusion of secondary diagnoses or complications (e.g., asthmatic patient in alcohol withdrawal). In short, if the patient does not achieve the daily outcomes or goals of care, the variance is identified and a separate plan of care must be developed to meet the patient's individual needs. Therefore, while clinical pathways are becoming common in the clinical setting, they have limited value (in place of more in-depth plans of care) as learning tools for students who are working to practice the nursing process, critical thinking, and a holistic approach to meeting patient needs.

A sample clinical pathway (Fig. 3–3) has been created reflecting Mr. R.S.'s primary diagnostic problem—nonhealing lesion, diabetic.

Cardiovascular

HYPERTENSION: SEVERE

Hypertension is defined by the Joint National Committee on Detection, Evaluation and Treatment of High Blood Pressure as pressure greater than 140/90 mm Hg and is classified according to the degree of severity, ranging from high normal BP (130–139/85–89) to very severe hypertension ($\geq$210/$\geq$120). Hypertension is categorized as primary/essential (constituting approximately 90% of all cases) or secondary, which occurs as a result of an identifiable, often correctable pathologic condition. The goal of treatment is to prevent the long-term sequelae of this disease (i.e., target organ disease [TOD]).

CARE SETTING

Although hypertension is usually treated in a community setting, symptoms of complications/compromise may require inpatient care. The majority of interventions included here can be used in either setting.

RELATED CONCERNS

Cerebrovascular Accident/Stroke, p 242
Myocardial Infarction, p 71
Psychosocial Aspects of Care, p 783
Renal Failure: Acute, p 555
Renal Failure: Chronic, p 568

Patient Assessment Data Base

ACTIVITY/REST

May report: Weakness, fatigue, shortness of breath, sedentary lifestyle

May exhibit: Elevated heart rate
Change in heart rhythm
Tachypnea

CIRCULATION

May report: History of hypertension, atherosclerosis, valvular/coronary artery heart disease and cerebrovascular disease
Episodes of palpitations, diaphoresis

May exhibit: Elevated BP (serial elevated measurements are necessary to confirm diagnosis)
Postural hypotension (may be related to drug regimen)

Pulse: Bounding carotid, jugular, radial pulsations; pulse disparities, e.g., femoral delay as compared with radial or brachial pulsation; absence of/diminished popliteal, posterior tibial, pedal pulses

Apical pulse: PMI possibly displaced and/or forceful

Rate/rhythm: Tachycardia, various dysrhythmias

Heart sounds: Accentuated S_2 at base; S_3 (early HF); S_4 (rigid left ventricle/left ventricular hypertrophy)

Murmurs of valvular stenosis

Vascular bruits audible over carotid, femoral, or epigastrium (artery stenosis) JVD (venous congestion)

Extremities: Discoloration of skin, cool temperature (peripheral vasoconstriction); capillary refill possibly slow/delayed (vasoconstriction)

Skin: Pallor, cyanosis, and diaphoresis (congestion, hypoxemia); flushing (pheochromocytoma)

EGO INTEGRITY

May report: History of personality changes, anxiety, depression, euphoria, or chronic anger (may indicate cerebral impairment)

Multiple stress factors (relationship, financial, job-related)

May exhibit: Mood swings, restlessness, irritability, narrowed attention span, outbursts of crying

Emphatic hand gestures, tense facial muscles (particularly around the eyes), quick physical movement, expiratory sighs, accelerated speech pattern

ELIMINATION

May report: Past or present renal insult (e.g., infection/obstruction or past history of kidney disease)

FOOD/FLUID

May report: Food preferences, which may include high-salt, high-fat, high-cholesterol foods (e.g., fried foods, cheese, eggs); licorice; high caloric content; or low dietary intake of potassium, calcium, and magnesium

Nausea, vomiting

Recent weight changes (gain/loss)

History of diuretic use

May exhibit: Normal weight or obesity

Presence of edema (may be generalized or dependent); venous congestion, JVD

Glycosuria (almost 10% of hypertensive patients are diabetic)

NEUROSENSORY

May report: Fainting spells/dizziness

Throbbing, suboccipital headaches (present on awakening and disappearing spontaneously after several hours)

Episodes of numbness and/or weakness on one side of the body, brief periods of confusion or difficulty with speech (TIA); or history of CVA

Visual disturbances (diplopia, blurred vision)

Episodes of epistaxis

May exhibit: Mental status: Changes in alertness, orientation, speech pattern/content, affect, thought process, or memory

Motor responses: Decreased strength, hand grip and/or deep tendon reflexes

Optic retinal changes: From mild sclerosis/arterial narrowing to marked retinal and sclerotic changes with edema or papilledema, exudates, hemorrhages, and arterial nicking dependent on severity/duration of hypertension

33

PAIN/DISCOMFORT

May report: Angina (coronary artery disease/cardiac involvement)

Intermittent pain in legs/claudication (indicative of arteriosclerosis of lower extremity arteries)

Severe occipital headaches as previously noted

Abdominal pain/masses (pheochromocytoma)

RESPIRATION (Generally associated with advanced cardiopulmonary effects of sustained/severe hypertension.)

May report: Dyspnea associated with activity/exertion

Tachypnea, orthopnea, paroxysmal nocturnal dyspnea

Cough with/without sputum production

Smoking history

May exhibit: Respiratory distress/use of accessory muscles

Adventitious breath sounds (crackles/wheezes)

Cyanosis

SAFETY

May report/ exhibit: Impaired coordination/gait

Transient episodes of unilateral paresthesia

Postural hypotension

TEACHING/LEARNING

May report: Familial risk factors: Hypertension, atherosclerosis, heart disease, diabetes mellitus, cerebrovascular/kidney disease

Ethnic/racial risk factors, e.g., African-American, Southeast Asian

Use of birth control pills or other hormones; drug/alcohol use

Discharge plan considerations: **DRG projected mean length of inpatient stay: 4.2 days**

Assistance with self-monitoring of BP

Alterations in medication therapy

Refer to section at end of plan for postdischarge considerations.

DIAGNOSTIC STUDIES

Hemoglobin/hematocrit: Not diagnostic but assesses relationship of cells to fluid volume (viscosity) and may indicate risk factors such as hypercoagulability, anemia.

BUN/creatinine: Provides information about renal perfusion/function.

Glucose: Hyperglycemia (diabetes mellitus is a precipitator of hypertension) may result from elevated catecholamine levels (increases hypertension).

Serum potassium: Hypokalemia may indicate the presence of primary aldosteronism (cause) or be a side effect of diuretic therapy.

Serum calcium: Imbalance may contribute to hypertension.

Lipid panel (total lipids, HDL, LDH, cholesterol, triglycerides, phospholipids): Elevated level may indicate predisposition for/presence of atheromatous plaquing (cardiovascular effect).

Thyroid studies: Hyperthyroidism may lead or contribute to vasoconstriction and hypertension.

Serum/urine aldosterone level: To assess for primary aldosteronism (cause).

Urinalysis: Blood, protein, glucose suggest renal dysfunction and/or presence of diabetes.

Creatinine clearance: May be reduced, reflecting renal damage.

Urine VMA (catecholamine metabolite): Elevation may indicate presence of pheochromocytoma (cause); 24-hour urine VMA may be done for assessment of pheochromocytoma if hypertension is intermittent.

Uric acid: Hyperuricemia has been implicated as a risk factor for the development of hypertension.

Renin: Elevated in renovascular and malignant hypertension, salt-wasting disorders.

Urine steroids: Elevation may indicate hyperadrenalism, pheochromocytoma or pituitary dysfunction, Cushing's syndrome; renin levels may also be elevated.

IVP: May identify cause of hypertension, e.g., renal parenchymal disease, renal/ureteral calculi.

Kidney and renography nuclear scan: Evaluates renal status (TOD).

Chest x-ray: May demonstrate obstructing calcification in valve areas; deposits in and/or notching of aorta; cardiac enlargement.

CT scan: Assesses for cerebral tumor, CVA, encephalopathy, or to rule out pheochromocytoma.

ECG: May demonstrate enlarged heart, strain patterns, conduction disturbances. *Note:* Broad, notched P wave is one of the earliest signs of hypertensive heart disease.

NURSING PRIORITIES

1. Maintain/enhance cardiovascular functioning.
2. Prevent complications.
3. Provide information about disease process/prognosis and treatment regimen.
4. Support active patient control of condition.

DISCHARGE GOALS

1. BP within acceptable limits for individual.
2. Cardiovascular and systemic complications prevented/minimized.
3. Disease process/prognosis and therapeutic regimen understood.
4. Necessary lifestyle/behavioral changes initiated
5. Plan in place to meet needs after discharge.

NURSING DIAGNOSIS: Cardiac Output, decreased, risk for

Risk factors may include
Increased vascular resistance, vasoconstriction
Myocardial ischemia
Ventricular hypertrophy/rigidity

Possibly evidenced by
[Not applicable; presence of signs and symptoms establishes an *actual* diagnosis]

DESIRED OUTCOMES/EVALUATION CRITERIA—PATIENT WILL:
Participate in activities that reduce BP/cardiac workload.
Maintain BP within individually acceptable range.
Demonstrate stable cardiac rhythm and rate within patient's normal range.

ACTIONS/INTERVENTIONS

Independent

Monitor BP. Measure in both arms/thighs for initial evaluation. Use correct cuff size and accurate technique.

RATIONALE

Comparison of pressures provides a more complete picture of vascular involvement/scope of problem. Severe hypertension is classified in the adult as a diastolic pressure elevation to 110 mm Hg; progressive diastolic readings above 120 mm Hg are considered first accelerated, then malignant (very severe). Systolic hypertension also is an established risk factor for cerebrovascular disease and ischemic heart disease, when diastolic pressure is elevated.

ACTIONS/INTERVENTIONS	RATIONALE
Independent	
Note presence, quality of central and peripheral pulses.	Bounding carotid, jugular, radial and femoral pulses may be observed/palpated. Pulses in the legs may be diminished, reflecting effects of vasoconstriction (increased SVR) and venous congestion.
Auscultate heart tones and breath sounds.	S_4 is common in severely hypertensive patients due to the presence of atrial hypertrophy (increased atrial volume/pressure). Development of S_3 indicates ventricular hypertrophy and impaired functioning. Presence of crackles, wheezes may indicate pulmonary congestion secondary to developing or chronic heart failure.
Observe skin color, moisture, temperature, and capillary refill time.	Presence of pallor, cool, moist skin and delayed capillary refill time may be due to peripheral vasoconstriction or reflect cardiac decompensation/decreased output.
Note dependent/general edema.	May indicate heart failure, renal or vascular impairment.
Provide calm, restful surroundings, minimize environmental activity/noise. Limit the number of visitors and length of stay.	Helps to reduce sympathetic stimulation; promotes relaxation.
Maintain activity restrictions, e.g., bed/chair rest; schedule periods of uninterrupted rest; assist patient with self-care activities as needed.	Reduces stress and tension that affect blood pressure and the course of hypertension.
Provide comfort measures, e.g., back and neck massage, elevation of head.	Decreases discomfort and may reduce sympathetic stimulation.
Instruct in relaxation techniques, guided imagery, distractions.	Can reduce stressful stimuli, produce calming effect, thereby reducing BP.
Monitor response to medications to control blood pressure.	Response to "stepped" drug therapy (consisting of diuretics, angiotensin inhibitors, vascular smooth muscle relaxants and adrenergic blockers) is dependent on both the individual and synergistic effects of the drugs. Because of side effects, it is important to use the smallest number and lowest dosage of medications.
Collaborative	
Administer medications as indicated, e.g.:	
Thiazide diuretics, e.g., chlorothiazide (Diuril); hydrochlorothiazide (Esidrix/HydroDIURIL); bendroflumethiazide (Naturetin);	Thiazides may be used alone or in association with other drugs to reduce BP in patients with relatively normal renal function. These diuretics potentiate other antihypertensive agents by limiting fluid retention and reduce the incidence of strokes and heart failure.
Loop diuretics, e.g., furosemide (Lasix); ethacrynic acid (Edecrin); bumetanide (Bumex);	These drugs produce marked diuresis by inhibiting resorption of sodium and chloride and are effective antihypertensives, especially in patients who are resistant to thiazides or have renal impairment.

ACTIONS/INTERVENTIONS	RATIONALE
Independent	
Potassium-sparing diuretics, e.g., spironolactone (Aldactone); triamterene (Dyrenium); amilioride (Midamor);	May be given in combination with a thiazide diuretic to minimize potassium loss.
α and β or centrally acting adrenergic antagonists, e.g., propranolol (Inderal); metoprolol (Lopressor); atenolol (Tenormin); nadolol (Corgard); methyldopa (Aldomet); clonidine (Catapres); methyldopa (Aldomet); prazosin (Minipress); tetazosin (Hytrin);	Specific actions of these drugs vary, but they generally reduce BP through the combined effect of decreased total peripheral resistance, reduced cardiac output, inhibited sympathetic activity, and suppression of renin release.
Calcium channel blockers, e.g., nifedipine (Procardia); verapamil (Calan); diltiazem (Cardizem);	May be necessary to treat severe hypertension when a combination of a diuretic and a sympathetic inhibitor has not sufficiently controlled BP. Vasodilation of healthy cardiac vasculature and increased coronary blood flow are secondary benefits of vasodilator therapy.
Adrenergic neuron blockers: guanadrel (Hylorel); quanethidine (Ismelin); reserpine (Serpasil);	Reduce arterial and venous constriction activity at the sympathetic nerve endings.
Direct-acting oral vasodilators: hydralazine (Apresoline); minoxidil (Loniten);	Relax vascular smooth muscle.
Direct-acting parenteral vasodilators: diazoxide (Hyperstat); nitroprusside (Nipride, Nitropress);	These are given intravenously for management of hypertensive emergencies.
Ganglion blockers, e.g., guanethidine (Ismelin); trimethaphan (Arfonad), or ACE inhibitors, e.g., captopril (Capoten).	The use of an additional sympathetic inhibitor may be required (for its cumulative effect) when other measures have failed to control BP and patient cooperation with the therapeutic regimen has been verified.
Implement fluid and dietary sodium restrictions as indicated.	These restrictions can help manage fluid retention with associated hypertensive response, thereby decreasing myocardial workload.
Prepare for surgery when indicated.	When hypertension is due to the presence of pheochromocytoma, removal of the tumor will correct condition.

NURSING DIAGNOSIS: Activity intolerance

May be related to
Generalized weakness
Imbalance between oxygen supply and demand

Possibly evidenced by
Verbal report of fatigue or weakness
Abnormal heart rate or BP response to activity
Exertional discomfort or dyspnea
ECG changes reflecting ischemia; dysrhythmias

DESIRED OUTCOMES/EVALUATION CRITERIA—PATIENT WILL:
Participate in necessary/desired activities.
Report a measurable increase in activity tolerance.
Demonstrate a decrease in physiologic signs of intolerance.

ACTIONS/INTERVENTIONS

Independent

Assess the patient's response to activity, noting pulse rate over 20 bpm above resting rate; marked increase in BP during/after activity (systolic pressure increase of 40 mm Hg or diastolic pressure increase of 20 mm Hg); dyspnea or chest pain; excessive fatigue and weakness; diaphoresis; dizziness or syncope.

Instruct patient in energy-saving techniques, e.g., using chair when showering, sitting to brush teeth or comb hair, carrying out activities at a slower pace.

Encourage progressive activity/self-care when tolerated. Provide assistance as needed.

RATIONALE

The stated parameters are helpful in assessing physiologic responses to the stress of activity and, if present, are indicators of overexertion associated with the activity level.

Energy-saving techniques reduce the energy expenditure, thereby assisting in equalization of oxygen supply and demand.

Gradual activity progression prevents a sudden increase in cardiac workload. Providing assistance only as needed encourages independence in performing activities.

NURSING DIAGNOSIS: Pain [acute], headache

May be related to
Increased cerebral vascular pressure

Possibly evidenced by
Reports of throbbing pain located in suboccipital region, present on awakening, and disappearing spontaneously after being up and about
Reluctance to move head, rubbing head, avoidance of bright lights and noise, wrinkled brow, clenched fists
Reports of stiffness of neck, dizziness, blurred vision, nausea, and vomiting

DESIRED OUTCOMES/EVALUATION CRITERIA—PATIENT WILL:
Report pain/discomfort is relieved/controlled.
Verbalize methods that provide relief.
Follow prescribed pharmacologic regimen.

ACTIONS/INTERVENTIONS

Independent

Encourage/maintain bed rest during acute phase.

Provide/recommend nonpharmacologic measures for relief of headache, e.g., cool cloth to forehead; back and neck rubs; quiet, dimly lit room; relaxation techniques (guided imagery, distraction); and diversional activities.

Eliminate/minimize vasoconstricting activities that may aggravate headache, e.g., straining at stool, prolonged coughing, bending over.

Assist patient with ambulation as needed.

RATIONALE

Minimizes stimulation/promotes relaxation.

Measures that reduce cerebral vascular pressure and that slow/block sympathetic response are effective in relieving headache and associated complications.

Activities that increase vasoconstriction accentuate the headache in the presence of increased cerebral vascular pressure.

Dizziness and blurred vision frequently are associated with headache. The patient may also experience episodes of postural hypotension.

ACTIONS/INTERVENTIONS

Independent

Provide liquids, soft foods, frequent mouth care if nosebleeds occur or nasal packing has been done to stop bleeding.

Collaborative

Administer medications as indicated:

Analgesics;

Antianxiety agents, e.g., lorazepam (Ativan), diazepam (Valium).

RATIONALE

Promotes general comfort. Nasal packing may interfere with swallowing or require mouth breathing, leading to stagnation of oral secretions and drying of mucous membranes.

Reduces/controls pain and decreases stimulation of the sympathetic nervous system.
May aid in the reduction of tension and discomfort that is intensified by stress.

NURSING DIAGNOSIS: Nutrition: altered, more than body requirements

May be related to
Excessive intake in relation to metabolic need
Sedentary lifestyle
Cultural preferences

Possibly evidenced by
Weight 10%–20% over ideal for height and frame
Triceps skin fold greater than 15 mm in men and 25 mm in women (maximum for age and sex)
Reported or observed dysfunctional eating patterns

DESIRED OUTCOMES/EVALUATION CRITERIA—PATIENT WILL:
Identify correlation between hypertension and obesity.
Demonstrate change in eating patterns (e.g., food choices, quantity, and so on), to attain desirable body weight with optimal maintenance of health.
Initiate/maintain individually appropriate exercise program.

ACTIONS/INTERVENTIONS

Independent

Assess patient understanding of direct relationship between hypertension and obesity.

Discuss necessity for decreased caloric intake and limiting intake of fats, salt, and sugar as indicated.

RATIONALE

Obesity is an added risk with high blood pressure because of the disproportion between fixed aortic capacity and increased cardiac output associated with increased body mass. Reduction in weight may obviate the need for drug therapy or decrease the amount of medication needed for control of BP.

Faulty eating habits contribute to atherosclerosis and obesity, which predispose to hypertension and subsequent complications, e.g., stroke, kidney disease, heart failure. Excessive salt intake expands the intravascular fluid volume and may damage kidneys, which can further aggravate hypertension.

ACTIONS/INTERVENTIONS	RATIONALE

Independent

Determine patient's desire to lose weight.	Motivation for weight reduction is internal. The individual must want to lose weight, or program most likely will not succeed.
Review usual daily caloric intake and dietary choices.	Identifies current strengths/weaknesses in dietary program. Aids in determining individual need for adjustment/teaching.
Establish a realistic weight reduction plan with the patient, e.g., 1 lb weight loss/wk.	Reducing one's caloric intake by 500 calories daily theoretically yields a weight loss of 1 lb/wk. Slow reduction in weight is therefore indicative of fat loss with muscle sparing and generally reflects a change in eating habits.
Encourage patient to maintain a diary of food intake including when and where eating takes place and the circumstances and feelings around which the food was eaten.	Provides a data base for both the adequacy of nutrients eaten, as well as the emotional conditions of eating. Helps to focus attention on factors that patient has control over/can change.
Instruct and assist in appropriate food selection, avoiding foods high in saturated fat (butter, cheese, eggs, ice cream, meat), and cholesterol (fatty meats, egg yolks, whole dairy products, shrimp, organ meats).	Avoiding foods high in saturated fat and cholesterol is important in preventing progressing atherogenesis. Moderation and use of low-fat products in place of total abstinence from certain food items may prevent sense of deprivation and enhance cooperation with dietary regimen.

Collaborative

Refer to dietitian as indicated.	Can provide additional counseling and assistance with meeting individual dietary needs.

NURSING DIAGNOSIS: Coping, Individual, ineffective

May be related to

Situational/maturational crisis; multiple life changes
Inadequate relaxation; little or no exercise
Inadequate support systems
Poor nutrition
Unmet expectations; unrealistic perceptions
Work overload
Inadequate coping methods

Possibly evidenced by

Verbalization of inability to cope or ask for help
Inability to meet role expectations/basic needs or problem-solve
Destructive behavior toward self; overeating, lack of appetite; excessive smoking/drinking, proneness to alcohol abuse
Chronic fatigue/insomnia; muscular tension; frequent head/neck aches; chronic worry/irritability/anxiety/emotional tension, depression

DESIRED OUTCOMES/EVALUATION CRITERIA—PATIENT WILL:

Identify ineffective coping behaviors and consequences.
Verbalize awareness of own coping abilities/strengths.
Identify potential stressful situations and steps to avoid/modify them.
Demonstrate the use of effective coping skills/methods.

ACTIONS/INTERVENTIONS	RATIONALE
Independent	
Assess effectiveness of coping strategies by observing behaviors, e.g., ability to verbalize feelings and concerns, willingness to participate in the treatment plan.	Adaptive mechanisms are necessary to appropriately alter one's lifestyle, deal with the chronicity of hypertension, and integrate prescribed therapies into daily living.
Note reports of sleep disturbances, increasing fatigue, impaired concentration, irritability, decreased tolerance of headache, inability to cope/problem-solve.	Manifestations of maladaptive coping mechanisms may be indicators of repressed anger and have been found to be major determinants of diastolic BP.
Assist patient to identify specific stressors and possible strategies for coping with them.	Recognition of stressors is the first step in altering one's response to the stressor.
Include patient in planning of care and encourage maximum participation in treatment plan.	Involvement provides the patient with an ongoing sense of control, improves coping skills, and can enhance cooperation with therapeutic regimen.
Encourage patient to evaluate life priorities/goals. Ask questions such as, "Is what you are doing getting you what you want?"	Focuses patient's attention on reality of present situation relative to patient's view of what is wanted. Strong work ethic, need for "control," and outward focus may have led to lack of attention to personal needs.
Assist patient to identify and begin planning for necessary lifestyle changes. Assist to adjust, rather than abandon, personal/family goals.	Necessary changes should be realistically prioritized to avoid being overwhelmed and feeling powerless.

NURSING DIAGNOSIS: Knowledge deficit [learning need] regarding condition, treatment plan, self care and discharge needs

May be related to
Lack of knowledge/recall
Information misinterpretation
Cognitive limitation
Denial of diagnosis

Possibly evidenced by
Verbalization of the problem
Request for information
Statement of misconception
Inaccurate follow-through of instructions; inadequate performance of procedures
Inappropriate or exaggerated behaviors, e.g., hostile, agitated, apathetic

DESIRED OUTCOMES/EVALUATION CRITERIA—PATIENT WILL:
Verbalize understanding of disease process and treatment regimen.
Identify drug side effects and possible complications that necessitate medical attention.
Maintain BP within individually acceptable parameters.

Independent

Assess readiness and blocks to learning. Include SO.

Misconceptions and denial of the diagnosis because of longstanding feelings of well-being may interfere with patient/SO willingness to learn about disease, progression, and prognosis. If the patient does not accept the reality of a life condition requiring continuing treatment, lifestyle/behavioral changes will not be initiated/sustained.

Define and state the limits of normal BP. Explain hypertension and its effects on the heart, blood vessels, kidneys, and brain.

Provides basis for understanding elevations of BP and clarifies frequently used medical terminology. Understanding that high BP can exist without symptoms is central to enabling patient to continue treatment even when feeling well.

Avoid saying "normal" BP, and use the term "well-controlled" when describing patient's BP within desired limits.

Because treatment for hypertension is lifelong, conveying the idea of "control" helps the patient to understand the need for continued treatment/medication.

Assist the patient in identifying modifiable risk factors, e.g., obesity, diet high in saturated fats and cholesterol, sedentary lifestyle, smoking, alcohol intake (more than 2 oz/d on a regular basis), stressful lifestyle.

These risk factors have been shown to contribute to hypertension and cardiovascular and renal disease.

Problem-solve with patient to identify ways in which appropriate lifestyle changes can be made to reduce the above factors.

Changing "comfortable/usual" behavior patterns can be very stressful. Support, guidance, and empathy can enhance the patient's success in accomplishing these tasks.

Discuss importance of eliminating smoking and assist patient in formulating a plan to quit smoking.

Nicotine increases catecholamine discharge, resulting in increased heart rate, BP, vasoconstriction, and myocardial workload, and reduces tissue oxygenation.

Reinforce the importance of cooperation with treatment regimen and keeping follow-up appointments.

Lack of cooperation is a common reason for failure of antihypertensive therapy. Therefore, ongoing evaluation for patient cooperation is critical to successful treatment. Compliance usually improves when the patient understands causative factors as well as consequences of inadequate intervention and health maintenance.

Instruct and demonstrate technique of BP self-monitoring. Evaluate patient's hearing, visual acuity, manual dexterity, and coordination.

Monitoring BP at home is reassuring to the patient, as it provides visual/positive reinforcement for patient efforts in following the medical regimen and promotes early detection of deleterious changes.

Help patient to develop a simple, convenient schedule for taking medications.

Individualizing medication schedule to fit the patient's personal habits/needs may facilitate cooperation with long-term regimen.

Explain prescribed medications along with their ractionale, dosage, expected and adverse side effects, and idiosyncrasies, e.g.:

Adequate information and understanding that side effects (e.g., mood changes, initial weight gain, dry mouth) are common and often subside with time enhances cooperation with treatment plan.

Diuretics: Take daily doses (or larger dose) in the early morning;

Scheduling minimizes nighttime urination.

ACTIONS/INTERVENTIONS	RATIONALE
Independent	
Weigh self on a regular schedule and record;	Primary indicator of effectiveness of diuretic therapy.
Avoid/limit alcohol intake;	The combined vasodilating effect of alcohol and the volume-depleting effect of a diuretic greatly increases the risk of orthostatic hypotension.
Notify physician if unable to tolerate food or fluid;	Dehydration can develop rapidly if intake is poor and patient continues to take a diuretic.
Antihypertensives: Take prescribed dose on a regular schedule, avoid skipping, altering, or making up doses, and do not discontinue without notifying the healthcare provider; rise slowly from a lying to standing position, sitting for a few minutes before standing. Sleep with the head slightly elevated.	Abruptly discontinuing drug causes rebound hypertension that may lead to severe complications. Measures reduce severity of orthostatic hypotension associated with the use of vasodilators and diuretics.
Suggest frequent position changes, leg exercises when lying down.	Decreases peripheral venous pooling that may be potentiated by vasodilators and prolonged sitting/stand0ing.
Recommend avoiding hot baths, steam rooms and saunas, and concomitant use of alcoholic beverages.	Prevents unnecessary vasodilation with dangerous side effect of syncope and hypotension.
Instruct the patient to consult healthcare provider before taking other prescription or nonprescription medication.	Precaution is important in preventing potentially dangerous drug interactions. Any drug that contains a sympathetic nervous stimulant may increase BP or counteract antihypertensive effects.
Instruct patient about increasing intake of foods/fluids high in potassium, e.g., oranges, bananas, figs, dates, tomatoes, potatoes, raisins, apricots, Gatorade, fruit juices; and foods/fluids high in calcium, e.g., low-fat milk, yogurt or calcium supplements, as indicated.	Diuretics can deplete potassium levels. Dietary replacement is more palatable than drug supplements and may be all that is needed to correct deficit. Some studies show that 400–2000 mg of calcium/d can lower systolic and diastolic BP. Correcting mineral deficiencies can also affect BP.
Review signs/symptoms requiring notification of healthcare provider, e.g., headache present on awakening; sudden and continued increase of BP; chest pain/shortness of breath; irregular/increased pulse rate; significant weight gain (2 lb/d or 5 lb/wk) or peripheral/abdominal swelling; visual disturbances; frequent, uncontrollable nose bleeds; depression/emotional lability; severe dizziness or episodes of fainting, muscle weakness/cramping, nausea/vomiting; excessive thirst, decreased libido/impotence.	Early detection of developing complications of, decreased effectiveness of, or adverse reactions to drug regimen allows for timely intervention.
Explain rationale for prescribed dietary regimen (usually a diet low in sodium, saturated fat, and cholesterol).	Excess saturated fats, cholesterol, sodium, alcohol, and calories have been defined as nutritional risks in hypertension. A low-fat and high polyunsaturated-fat diet reduces BP, possibly through prostaglandin balance, in both normotensive and hypertensive people.
Help patient to identify sources of sodium intake, (e.g., table salt, salty snacks, processed meats and cheeses, sauerkraut, sauces, canned soups and vegetables, baking soda, baking powder, monosodium glutamate). Stress importance of reading ingredient labels of foods and OTC drugs.	Two years on a moderately low-salt diet may be sufficient to control mild hypertension or reduce the amount of medication required.

43

ACTIONS/INTERVENTIONS	RATIONALE

Independent

Encourage patient to decrease or eliminate caffeine, e.g., coffee, tea, cola, chocolate.	Caffeine is a cardiac stimulant and may adversely affect cardiac function/reserves.
Stress importance of planning/accomplishing daily rest periods.	Alternating rest and activity increases tolerance to activity progression.
Recommend that patient monitor own physiological response to activity (e.g., pulse rate, shortness of breath); report a decreased tolerance to activity; and stop activity that causes chest pain, shortness of breath, dizziness, extreme fatigue, or weakness.	The patient's involvement in monitoring his or her own activity tolerance is vital to safely resuming and/or modifying activities of daily living.
Encourage patient to establish an individual exercise program incorporating aerobic exercise (walking, swimming) within the patient's capabilities. Stress the importance of avoiding isometric activity.	Besides helping to lower BP, aerobic activity aids in toning the cardiovascular system. Isometric exercise can increase serum catecholamine levels, further elevating BP.
Demonstrate application of ice pack to the back of the neck and pressure over the distal third of nose, and recommend that patient lean the head forward, if nose bleed occurs.	Nasal capillaries may rupture as a result of excessive vascular pressure. Cold and pressure constrict capillaries, which slows or halts bleeding. Leaning forward reduces the amount of blood that is swallowed.
Provide information regarding community resources and support the patient in making lifestyle changes. Initiate referrals as indicated.	Community resources such as the American Heart Association, "coronary clubs," stop smoking clinics, alcohol rehabilitation, weight loss programs, stress management classes, and counseling services may be helpful to the patient's efforts to initiate and maintain lifestyle changes.

POTENTIAL CONSIDERATIONS following acute hospitalization (dependent on patient's age, physical condition/presence of complications, personal resources and life responsibilities)

Activity intolerance—frequently occurs as a result of alterations in cardiac output and side effects of medication.
Nutrition: altered, more than body requirements—obesity is often present and a factor in blood pressure control.
Therapeutic Regimen: Individual, ineffective management—result of the complexity of the therapeutic regimen, required lifestyle changes, side effects of medication, and frequent feelings of general well-being ("I'm not really sick").
Sexuality Patterns, altered—interference in sexual functioning may occur due to activity intolerance and side effects of medication.
Family Coping: potential for growth—opportunity exists for family members to support patient while reducing risk factors for themselves and improving quality of life for family as a whole.

HEART FAILURE: CHRONIC

Failure of the left and/or right chambers of the heart results in inability to provide sufficient output to meet tissue needs and causes the development of pulmonary and systemic congestion. Despite diagnostic and therapeutic advances, HF continues to be associated with high morbidity and mortality. (AHCPR Guidelines [6/94] promote the term heart failure [HF] in place of congestive heart failure [CHF] as many patients with heart failure do not manifest pulmonary or systemic congestion.)

CARE SETTING

Although generally managed at the community level, inpatient stay may be required for periodic exacerbation of failure/development of complications.

RELATED CONCERNS

Cardiac Surgery, p 95
Dysrhythmias, p 85
Psychosocial Aspects of Care, p 783

Patient Assessment Data Base

ACTIVITY/REST

May report: Fatigue/exhaustion progressing throughout the day; exercise intolerance
Insomnia
Chest pain with activity
Dyspnea at rest or with exertion

May exhibit: Restlessness, mental status changes, e.g., lethargy
Vital sign changes with activity

CIRCULATION

May report: History of hypertension, recent/acute multiple MIs, previous episodes of HF, valvular heart disease, cardiac surgery, endocarditis, SLE, anemia, septic shock
Swelling of feet, legs, abdomen, "belt too tight" (right-sided failure)

May exhibit: BP: May be low (pump failure); normal (mild or chronic HF); or high (fluid overload/increased SVR)
Pulse pressure: May be narrow, reflecting reduced stroke volume
Heart rate: Tachycardia (left-sided failure)
Heart rhythm: Dysrhythmias, e.g., atrial fibrillation, premature ventricular contractions/tachycardia, heart blocks
Apical pulse: PMI may be diffuse and displaced inferiorly to the left
Heart sounds: S_3 (gallop) is diagnostic; S_4 may occur; S_1 and S_2 may be softened
Systolic and diastolic murmurs may indicate the presence of valvular stenosis or insufficiency
Pulses: Peripheral pulses diminished; alteration in strength of beat may be noted; central pulses may be bounding, e.g., visible jugular, carotid, abdominal pulsations
Color: Ashen, pale, dusky, cyanotic
Nailbeds: Pale or cyanotic with slow capillary refill
Liver: Enlarged/palpable, positive hepatojugular reflex
Breath sounds: Crackles, rhonchi
Edema: May be dependent, generalized, or pitting, especially in extremities; JVD may be present

EGO INTEGRITY

May report: Anxiety, apprehension, fear
Stress related to illness/financial concerns (job/cost of medical care)

May exhibit: Various behavioral manifestations, e.g., anxiety, anger, fearful, irritable

ELIMINATION

May report: Decreased voiding, dark urine
Night voiding (nocturia)
Diarrhea/constipation

FOOD/FLUID

May report: Loss of appetite/anorexia
Nausea/vomiting
Significant weight gain (may not respond to diuretic use)
Lower extremity swelling
Tight clothing/shoes
Diet high in salt/processed foods, fat, sugar, and caffeine
Use of diuretics

May exhibit: Rapid weight gain
Abdominal distention (ascites); edema (general, dependent, pitting, brawn)
Abdominal tenderness (ascites, hepatic engorgement)

HYGIENE

May report: Fatigue/weakness, exhaustion during self-care activities

May exhibit: Appearance indicative of neglect of personal care

NEUROSENSORY

May report: Weakness, dizziness, fainting episodes

May exhibit: Lethargy, confusion, disorientation
Behavior changes, irritability

PAIN/DISCOMFORT

May report: Chest pain, chronic or acute angina
Right upper abdominal pain (RVF)
Generalized muscle aches/pains

May exhibit: Nervousness, restlessness
Narrowed focus (withdrawal)
Guarding behavior

RESPIRATION

May report: Dyspnea on exertion, sleeping sitting up or with several pillows.
Cough with/without sputum production, dry/hacking—especially when recumbent.
History of chronic lung disease.
Use of respiratory aids, e.g., oxygen and/or medications.

May exhibit: Respirations: Tachypnea; shallow, labored breathing; use of accessory muscles, nasal flaring.

Cough: Dry/hacking/nonproductive or may be gurgling with/without sputum production.
Sputum: May be blood-tinged, pink/frothy (pulmonary edema).
Breath sounds: May be diminished, with bibasilar crackles and wheezes.
Mentation: May be diminished; lethargy; restlessness.
Color: Pallor or cyanosis.

SAFETY

May exhibit: Changes in mentation/confusion
Loss of strength/muscle tone
Skin excoriations, rashes

SOCIAL INTERACTION

May report: Decreased participation in usual social activities

TEACHING/LEARNING

May report: Use/misuse of cardiac medications, e.g., β-blockers, calcium channel blockers
Recent/recurrent hospitalizations

May exhibit: Evidence of failure to improve

Discharge plan considerations: **DRG projected mean length of inpatient stay: 8.2 days.**
Assistance with shopping, transportation, self-care needs, homemaker/maintenance tasks
Alteration in medication use/therapy
Changes in physical layout of home

Refer to section at end of plan for postdischarge considerations.

DIAGNOSTIC STUDIES

ECG: Ventricular or atrial hypertrophy, axis deviation, ischemia, and damage patterns may be present. Dysrhythmias, e.g., tachycardia, atrial fibrillation, frequent PVCs may be present. Persistent ST/T segment elevation 6 weeks or more after myocardial infarction suggests presence of ventricular aneurysm (may cause cardiac dysfunction/failure).

Sonograms (echocardiogram, Doppler and transesophageal echocardiogram): May reveal enlarged chamber dimensions, alterations in valvular function/structure, or areas of decreased ventricular contractility.

Heart scan (Multigated acquisition [MUGA]): Measures ejection fraction and estimates wall motion.

Exercise or pharmacologic stress myocardial perfusion scintigraphy (e.g., thallium scan): Determines presence of myocardial ischemia.

PET scan: More sensitive test than scintigraphy for evaluation of myocardial ischemia/detecting viable myocardium.

Cardiac catheterization: Abnormal pressures are indicative and help differentiate right-versus left-sided heart failure, and valve stenosis or insufficiency. Also assess patency of coronary arteries. Contrast injected into the ventricles reveals abnormal size and ejection fraction/altered contractility.

Chest x-ray: May show enlarged cardiac shadow reflecting chamber dilatation/hypertrophy, or changes in blood vessels reflecting increased pulmonary pressure. Abnormal contour, e.g., bulging of left cardiac border, may suggest ventricular aneurysm.

Liver enzymes: Elevated in liver congestion/failure.

Digoxin and other cardiac drug levels: Determine therapeutic range and correlate with patient response.

Bleeding and clotting times: Determine therapeutic range, identify those at risk for excessive clot formation.

Electrolytes: May be altered due to fluid shifts/decreased renal function, diuretic therapy.

Pulse oximetry: Oxygen saturation may be low, especially when acute HF is imposed on COPD or chronic HF.

ABGs: Left ventricular failure is characterized by mild respiratory alkalosis (early) or hypoxemia with an increased Pco_2 (late).

BUN, creatinine: Elevated BUN suggests decreased renal perfusion. Elevation of both BUN and creatinine is indicative of renal failure.

Serum albumin/transferrin: May be decreased as a result of reduced protein intake or reduced protein synthesis in congested liver.

CBC: May reveal anemia, polycythemia, or dilutional changes indicating water retention. WBCs may be elevated, reflecting recent/acute MI, pericarditis, or other inflammatory or infectious states.

Sedimentation rate (ESR): May be elevated, indicating acute inflammatory reaction.

Thyroid studies: Increased thyroid activity suggests thyroid hyperactivity as precipitator of HF.

NURSING PRIORITIES

1. Improve myocardial contractility/systemic perfusion.
2. Reduce fluid volume overload.
3. Prevent complications.
4. Provide information about disease/prognosis, therapy needs and prevention of recurrences.

DISCHARGE GOALS

1. Cardiac output adequate for individual needs.
2. Complications prevented/resolved.
3. Optimum level of activity/functioning attained.
4. Disease process/prognosis and therapeutic regimen understood.
5. Plan in place to meet needs after discharge.

NURSING DIAGNOSIS: Cardiac Output, decreased

May be related to

Altered myocardial contractility/inotropic changes

Alterations in rate, rhythm, electrical conduction

Structural changes (e.g., valvular defects, ventricular aneurysm)

Possibly evidenced by

Increased heart rate (tachycardia); dysrhythmias; ECG changes

Changes in BP (hypotension/hypertension)

Extra heart sounds (S_3, S_4)

Decreased urine output

Diminished peripheral pulses

Cool, ashen skin; diaphoresis

Orthopnea, crackles, JVD, liver engorgement, edema

Chest pain

DESIRED OUTCOMES/EVALUATION CRITERIA—PATIENT WILL:

Display vital signs within acceptable limits, dysrhythmias absent/controlled, and no symptoms of failure (e.g., hemodynamic parameters within acceptable limits, urinary output adequate).

Report decreased episodes of dyspnea, angina.

Participate in activities that reduce cardiac workload.

ACTIONS/INTERVENTIONS	RATIONALE
Independent	
Auscultate apical pulse; assess heart rate, rhythm; (Document dysrhythmia if telemetry available).	Tachycardia is usually present (even at rest) to compensate for decreased ventricular contractility. PACs, PAT, MAT, PVCs, and AF are common dysrhythmias associated with HF, although others may also occur. *Note:* Intractable ventricular dysrhythmias unresponsive to medication suggest ventricular aneurysm.

ACTIONS/INTERVENTIONS	RATIONALE
Independent	
Note heart sounds.	S_1 and S_2 may be weak because of diminished pumping action. Gallop rhythms are common (S_3 and S_4), produced as blood flows into noncompliant/distended chambers. Murmurs may reflect valvular incompetence/stenosis.
Palpate peripheral pulses.	Decreased cardiac output may be reflected in diminished radial, popliteal, dorsalis pedis, and posttibial pulses. Pulses may be fleeting or irregular to palpation, and pulsus alternans (strong beat alternating with weak beat) may be present.
Monitor BP.	In early, moderate, or chronic HF, BP may be elevated due to increased SVR. In advanced HF, the body may no longer be able to compensate, and profound/irreversible hypotension may occur.
Inspect skin for pallor, cyanosis.	Pallor is indicative of diminished peripheral perfusion secondary to inadequate cardiac output, vasoconstriction, and anemia. Cyanosis may develop in refractory HF. Dependent areas are often blue or mottled as venous congestion increases.
Monitor urine output, noting decreasing output and dark/concentrated urine.	Kidneys respond to reduced cardiac output by retaining water and sodium. Urine output is usually decreased during the day because of fluid shifts into tissues but may be increased at night as fluid returns to circulation when patient is recumbent.
Note changes in sensorium, e.g., lethargy, confusion, disorientation, anxiety, and depression.	May indicate inadequate cerebral perfusion secondary to decreased cardiac output.
Provide rest semirecumbent in bed or chair. Assist with physical care as indicated.	Physical rest should be maintained during acute or refractory HF to improve efficiency of cardiac contraction and to decrease myocardial oxygen demand/consumption and workload.
Provide for psychological rest by quiet environment; explaining medical/nursing management; helping patient avoid stressful situations, listening/responding to expressions of feelings/fears.	Emotional stress produces vasoconstriction, which elevates BP and increases heart rate/work.
Provide bedside commode. Have patient avoid activities eliciting a vasovagal response, e.g., straining during defecation, holding breath during position changes.	Commode use decreases work of getting to bathroom or struggling to use bedpan. Vasovagal maneuver causes vagal stimulation followed by rebound tachycardia, which further compromises cardiac function/output.
Elevate legs, avoiding pressure under knee. Encourage active/passive exercises. Increase ambulation/activity as tolerated.	Decreases venous stasis and may reduce incidence of thrombus/embolus formation.
Check for calf tenderness, diminished pedal pulse, swelling, local redness, or pallor of extremity.	Reduced cardiac output, venous pooling/stasis, and enforced bed rest increases risk of thrombophlebitis.
Withhold digitalis preparation as indicated and notify physician if marked changes occur in cardiac rate or rhythm or signs of digitalis toxicity occur.	Incidence of toxicity is high (20%) because of narrow margin between therapeutic and toxic ranges. Digoxin may have to be discontinued in the presence of toxic drug levels, a slow heart rate, or low potassium level. (Refer to CP: Dysrhythmias, ND: Poisoning, risk for digitalis toxicity, p 91.)

ACTIONS/INTERVENTIONS	RATIONALE
Collaborative	
Administer supplemental oxygen as indicated.	Increases available oxygen for myocardial uptake to combat effects of hypoxia/ischemia.
Administer medications as indicated:	A variety of medications may be used to increase stroke volume, improve contractility, and reduce congestion.
Diuretics, e.g., furosemide (Lasix); ethacrynic acid (Edecrin); bumetanide (Bumex); spironolactone (Aldactone);	Type and dosage of diuretic depends on cause and degree of heart failure and state of renal funtion. Preload reduction is most useful in treating patients with a relatively normal cardiac output accompanied by congestive symptoms. Loop diuretics block chloride reabsorption, thus interfering with the reabsorption of sodium and water. *Note:* Recent research suggests that diuretic therapy may not be as beneficial as previously believed and, depending on practitioner/patient situation, may not be a first-line therapy choice.
Vasodilators, e.g., nitrates (Nitro-Dur, Isordil); arteriodilators, e.g., hydralazine (Apresoline); combination drugs, e.g., prazosin (Minipress);	Vasodilators are used to increase cardiac output, reducing circulating volume (venodilators) and decreasing systemic vascular resistance (arteriodilators), thereby reducing ventricular workload.
Digoxin (Lanoxin);	Increases force of myocardial contraction and slows heart rate by decreasing conduction velocity and prolonging refractory period of the AV junction to increase cardiac efficiency/output.
Captopril (Capoten); lisinopril (Prinivil); enalapril (Vasotec), quinapril (Accupril);	ACE inhibitors may be used to control heart failure by inhibiting angiotensin conversion in the lungs and reduce vasoconstriction, SVR, and BP.
Inotropic agents, e.g., amrinone (Inocor); milrinone (Primacor); vesnarinone (Arkin-Z);	Short-term treatment of heart failure unresponsive to therapy with cardiac glycoside (e.g., digitalis), vasodilators, and diuretics. Quinoline derivative currently being tested (in combination with digoxin and ACE inhibitors) for long-term oral use. Positive inotropic properties have reduced mortality rates 50% and improved quality of life.
Morphine sulfate;	Decreases vascular resistance and venous return reducing myocardial workload. Allays anxiety and breaks the feedback cycle of anxiety/catecholamine release/anxiety.
Antianxiety agents/sedatives;	Promotes rest/relaxation reducing oxygen demand and myocardial workload.
Anticoagulants, e.g., low-dose heparin; warfarin (Coumadin).	May be used prophylactically to prevent thrombus/emboli formation in presence of risk factors such as venous stasis, enforced bed rest, cardiac dysrhythmias, and history of previous thrombolic episodes.
Administer IV solutions, restricting total amount as indicated. Avoid saline solutions.	Because of existing elevated left ventricular pressure, patient may not tolerate increased fluid volume (preload). HF patients also excrete less sodium, which causes fluid retention and increases myocardial workload.
Monitor/replace electrolytes.	Fluid shifts and use of diuretics can alter electrolytes (especially potassium and chloride), which affect cardiac rhythm and contractility.

ACTIONS/INTERVENTIONS	RATIONALE
Collaborative	
Monitor serial ECG and chest x-ray changes.	ST segment depression and T wave flattening can develop because of increased myocardial oxygen demand, even if no coronary artery disease is present. Chest x-ray may show enlarged heart and changes of pulmonary congestion.
Measure cardiac output and other functional parameters as indicated.	Cardiac index, preload/afterload, contractility, and cardiac work can be measured noninvasively using thoracic electrical bioimpedance (TEB) technique. Useful in determining effectiveness of therapeutic interventions, response to activity, and so on.
Monitor laboratory studies, e.g., BUN, creatinine;	Elevation of BUN/creatinine reflects kidney hypoperfusion/failure.
Liver function studies (AST, LDH);	AST/LDH may be elevated due to liver congestion and indicate need for smaller dosages of medications that are detoxified by the liver.
PT/APTT/coagulation studies.	Measures changes in coagulation processes or effectiveness of anticoagulant therapy.
Prepare for insertion/maintain pacemaker, if indicated.	May be necessary to correct bradydysrhythmias unresponsive to drug intervention, which can aggravate congestive failure/produce pulmonary edema.
Prepare for surgery as indicated.	Heart failure due to ventricular aneurysm or valvular dysfunction may require aneurysectomy or valve replacement to improve myocardial contractility/function. With end-stage heart failure, cardiac transplantation may be indicated. Cardiomyoplasty, an experimental procedure in which the latissimus dorsi muscle is wrapped around the heart and electrically stimulated to contract with each heartbeat, may be done to augment ventricular function while the patient is awaiting cardiac transplantation or when transplantation is not an option. Other new surgical techniques include transmyocardial revascularization using CO_2 laser technology, in which a laser is used to create multiple 1-mm diameter channels in viable but underperfused cardiac muscle; and implantation of a battery-powered LV assist system, which is positioned between the cardiac apex and the descending thoracic or abdominal aorta. This device receives blood from the LV and ejects it into the systemic circulation, often allowing the patient to resume a nearly normal lifestyle while awaiting heart transplantation.

NURSING DIAGNOSIS: Activity intolerance

May be related to
Imbalance between oxygen supply/demand
Generalized weakness
Prolonged bed rest/immobility

Possibly evidenced by
Weakness, fatigue
Changes in vital signs, presence of dysrhythmias
Dyspnea
Pallor, diaphoresis

DESIRED OUTCOMES/EVALUATION CRITERIA—PATIENT WILL:
Participate in desired activities; meet own self-care needs
Achieve measurable increase in activity tolerance, evidenced by reduced fatigue and weakness and vital signs within acceptable limits during activity.

ACTIONS/INTERVENTIONS

Independent

Check vital signs before and immediately after activity, especially if patient is on vasodilators, diuretics, or β-blockers.

Document cardiopulmonary response to activity. Note tachycardia, dysrhythmias, dyspnea, diaphoresis, pallor.

Assess for other precipitators/causes of fatigue, e.g., treatments, pain, medications.

Evaluate accelerating activity intolerance.

Provide assistance with self-care activities as indicated. Intersperse activity periods with rest periods.

Collaborative

Implement graded cardiac rehabilitation/activity program.

RATIONALE

Orthostatic hypotension can occur with activity because of medication effect (vasodilation); fluid shifts (diuresis); or compromised cardiac function.

Compromised myocardium/inability to increase stroke volume during activity may cause an immediate increase in heart rate and oxygen demands, thereby aggravating weakness and fatigue.

Fatigue is a side effect of some medications (β-blockers, tranquilizers, and sedatives). Pain and stressful regimens also extract energy and produce fatigue.

May denote increasing cardiac decompensation rather than overactivity.

Meets patient's personal care needs without undue myocardial stress/excessive oxygen demand.

Gradual increase in activity avoids excessive myocardial workload and oxygen consumption. Strengthens and improves cardiac function under stress, if cardiac dysfunction is not irreversible.

NURSING DIAGNOSIS: Fluid Volume excess

May be related to
Reduced glomerular filtration rate (decreased cardiac output)/increased ADH production, and sodium/water retention

Possibly evidenced by
Orthopnea, S_3 heart sound
Oliguria, edema, JVD, positive hepatojugular reflex
Weight gain
Hypertension
Respiratory distress, abnormal breath sounds

> **DESIRED OUTCOMES/EVALUATION CRITERIA—PATIENT WILL:**
> Demonstrate stabilized fluid volume with balanced intake and output, breath sounds clear/clearing, vital signs within acceptable range, stable weight, and absence of edema.
> Verbalize understanding of individual dietary/fluid restrictions.

ACTIONS/INTERVENTIONS	RATIONALE
Independent	
Monitor urine output, noting amount and color, as well as time of day when diuresis occurs.	Urine output may be scanty and concentrated (especially during the day) because of reduced renal perfusion. Recumbency favors diuresis; therefore urine output may be increased at night/during bed rest.
Monitor/calculate 24-hour intake and output balance.	Diuretic therapy may result in sudden/excessive fluid loss (circulating/hypovolemia) even though edema/ascites remains.
Maintain chair or bed rest in semi-Fowler's position during acute phase.	Recumbency increases glomerular filtration and decreases production of ADH, thereby enhancing diuresis.
Establish fluid intake schedule, incorporating beverage preferences when possible. Give frequent mouth care/ice chips as part of fluid allotment.	Involving patient in therapy regimen may enhance sense of control and cooperation with restrictions.
Weigh daily.	Documents changes in/resolution of edema in response to therapy. A gain of 5 lb represents approximately 2 L of fluid. Conversely, diuretics can result in rapid/excessive fluid shifts and weight loss.
Assess for distended neck and peripheral vessels. Inspect dependent body areas for edema with/without pitting; note presence of generalized body edema (anasarca).	Excessive fluid retention may be manifested by venous engorgement and edema formation. Peripheral edema begins in feet/ankles (or dependent areas) and ascends as failure worsens. Pitting edema is generally obvious only after retention of at least 10 lb of fluid. Increased vascular congestion (associated with right-sided heart failure) eventually results in systemic tissue edema.
Change position frequently. Elevate feet when sitting. Inspect skin surface, keep dry and provide padding as indicated. (Refer to ND: Skin Integrity, impaired, risk for, p 55.)	Edema formation, slowed circulation, altered nutritional intake and prolonged immobility/bed rest are cumulative stressors that affect skin integrity and require close supervision/preventive interventions.
Auscultate breath sounds, noting decreased and/or adventitious sounds, e.g., crackles, wheezes. Note presence of increased dyspnea, tachypnea, orthopnea, paroxysmal nocturnal dyspnea, persistent cough.	Excess fluid volume often leads to pulmonary congestion. Symptoms of pulmonary edema may reflect acute left-sided heart failure. Right-sided heart failure's respiratory symptoms (dyspnea, cough, orthopnea) may have slower onset but are more difficult to reverse.

ACTIONS/INTERVENTIONS	RATIONALE
Independent	
Investigate reports of sudden extreme dyspnea/air hunger, need to sit straight up, sensation of suffocation, feelings of panic or impending doom.	May indicate development of complications (pulmonary edema/embolus) and differs from orthopnea and paroxysmal nocturnal dyspnea in that it develops much more rapidly and requires immediate intervention.
Monitor BP and CVP (if available).	Hypertension and elevated CVP suggests fluid volume excess and may reflect developing/increasing pulmonary congestion, heart failure.
Assess bowel sounds. Note complaints of anorexia, nausea, abdominal distention, constipation.	Visceral congestion (occurring in progressive HF), can alter gastric/intestinal function.
Provide small, frequent easily digestible meals.	Reduced gastric motility can adversely affect digestion and absorption. Small, frequent meals may enhance digestion/prevent abdominal discomfort.
Measure abdominal girth, as indicated.	In progressive right-sided heart failure, fluid may shift into the peritoneal space, causing increasing abdominal girth (ascites).
Encourage verbalization of feelings regarding limitations.	Expression of feelings/concerns may decrease stress/anxiety, which is an energy drain and can contribute to feelings of fatigue.
Palpate for hepatomegaly. Note reports of right upper quadrant pain/tenderness.	Advancing heart failure leads to venous congestion, resulting in abdominal distention, liver engorgement, and pain. This can alter liver function and impair/prolong drug metabolism.
Note increased lethargy, hypotension, muscle cramping.	Signs of potassium and sodium deficits that may occur due to fluid shifts and diuretic therapy.
Collaborative	
Administer medications as indicated:	
Diuretics, e.g., furosemide (Lasix); bumetanide (Bumex);	Increases rate of urine flow and may inhibit reabsorption of sodium/chloride in the renal tubules.
Thiazides with potassium-sparing agents, e.g., spironolactone (Aldactone);	Promotes diuresis without excessive potassium losses.
Potassium supplements, e.g., K Dur.	Replaces potassium that is lost as a common side effect of diuretic therapy, which can adversely affect cardiac function.
Maintain fluid/sodium restrictions as indicated.	Reduces total body water/prevents fluid reaccumulation.
Consult with dietitian.	May be necessary to provide diet acceptable to patient that meets caloric needs within sodium restriction.
Monitor chest x-ray.	Reveals changes indicative of increase/resolution of pulmonary congestion.
Assist with rotating tourniquets/phlebotomy, dialysis, or ultrafiltration as indicated.	Although not frequently used, mechanical fluid removal may be carried out to rapidly reduce circulating volume, especially in pulmonary edema refractory to other therapies.

NURSING DIAGNOSIS: Gas Exchange, impaired, risk for

Risk factors may include
Alveolar-capillary membrane changes, e.g., fluid collection/shifts into interstitial space/
     alveoli

Possibly evidenced by
[Not applicable; presence of signs and symptoms establishes an *actual* diagnosis]

DESIRED OUTCOMES/EVALUATION CRITERIA—PATIENT WILL:
Demonstrate adequate ventilation and oxygenation of tissues by ABGS/oximetry
     within patient's normal ranges and free of symptoms of respiratory distress.
Participate in treatment regimen within level of ability/situation.

ACTIONS/INTERVENTIONS	RATIONALE
Independent	
Auscultate breath sounds noting crackles, wheezes.	Reveals presence of pulmonary congestion/collection of secretions indicating need for further intervention.
Instruct patient in effective coughing, deep breathing.	Clears airways and facilitates oxygen delivery.
Encourage frequent position changes.	Helps prevent atelectasis and pneumonia.
Maintain chair/bed rest with head of bed elevated 20 to 30 degrees, semi-Fowler's position. Support arms with pillows.	Reduces oxygen consumption/demands and promotes maximal lung inflation.
Collaborative	
Monitor/graph serial ABGs, pulse oximetry.	Hypoxemia can be severe during pulmonary edema. Compensatory changes are usually present in chronic HF.
Administer supplemental oxygen as indicated.	Increases alveolar oxygen concentration, which may correct/reduce tissue hypoxemia.
Administer medications as indicated.	
Diuretics, e.g., furosemide (Lasix);	Reduces alveolar congestion, enhancing gas exchange.
Bronchodilators, e.g., aminophylline.	Increases oxygen delivery by dilating small airways and exerts mild diuretic effect to aid in reducing pulmonary congestion.

NURSING DIAGNOSIS: Skin Integrity, impaired, risk for

Risk factors may include
Prolonged bed rest
Edema, decreased tissue perfusion

Possibly evidenced by
[Not applicable; presence of signs and symptoms establishes an *actual* diagnosis]

DESIRED OUTCOMES/EVALUATION CRITERIA—PATIENT WILL:
Maintain skin integrity.
Demonstrate behaviors/techniques to prevent skin breakdown.

ACTIONS/INTERVENTIONS	RATIONALE

Independent

Inspect skin, noting skeletal prominences, presence of edema, areas of altered circulation/pigmentation, or obesity/emaciation.

Skin is at risk because of impaired peripheral circulation, physical immobility, and alterations in nutritional status.

Provide gentle massage around reddened or blanched areas.

Improves blood flow, minimizing tissue hypoxia. *Note:* Direct massage of compromised area may cause tissue injury.

Reposition frequently in bed/chair, assist with active/passive ROM exercises.

Reduces pressure on tissues, improving circulation and reducing time any one area is deprived of full blood flow.

Provide frequent skin care, minimize contact with moisture/excretions.

Excessive dryness or moisture damages skin and hastens breakdown.

Check fit of shoes/slippers and change as needed.

Dependent edema may cause shoes to fit poorly, increasing risk of pressure and skin breakdown on feet.

Avoid intramuscular route for medication.

Interstitial edema and impaired circulation impede drug absorption and predispose to tissue breakdown/development of infection.

Collaborative

Provide alternating pressure/egg-crate mattress, sheepskin elbow/heel protectors.

Reduces pressure to skin, may improve circulation.

NURSING DIAGNOSIS: Knowledge deficit [learning need] regarding condition, treatment regimen, self care and discharge needs

May be related to
Lack of understanding/misconceptions about interrelatedness of cardiac function/disease/failure

Possibly evidenced by
Questions
Statements of concern/misconceptions
Recurrent, preventable episodes of HF

DESIRED OUTCOMES/EVALUATION CRITERIA—PATIENT WILL:
Identify relationship of ongoing therapies (treatment program) to reduction of recurrent episodes and prevention of complications.
List signs/symptoms that require immediate intervention.
Identify own stress/risk factors and some techniques for handling.
Initiate necessary lifestyle/behavioral changes.

ACTIONS/INTERVENTIONS	RATIONALE

Independent

Discuss normal heart function. Include information regarding patient's variance from normal function. Explain difference between heart attack and HF.

Knowledge of disease process and expectations can facilitate adherence to prescribed treatment regimen.

ACTIONS/INTERVENTIONS

Independent

ACTIONS/INTERVENTIONS	RATIONALE
Reinforce treatment rationale.	Patient may believe it is acceptable to alter postdischarge regimen when feeling well and symptom-free or when feeling below par, which can increase the risk of exacerbation of symptoms. Understanding of regimen, medications, and restrictions may augment cooperation with control of symptoms.
Encourage developing a regular home exercise program, and provide guidelines for sexual activity.	Promotes maintenance of muscle tone and organ function for overall sense of well-being. Changing sexual habits may be difficult (e.g., sex in morning when well rested, patient on top, inclusion of other physical expressions of affection) but provides opportunity for continuing satisfying sexual relationship.
Discuss importance of being as active as possible without becoming exhausted and of rest between activities.	Excessive physical activity or overexertion can further weaken the heart, exacerbating failure, and necessitates adjustment of exercise program.
Discuss importance of sodium limitation. Provide list of sodium content of common foods that are to be avoided/limited. Encourage reading of labels on food and drug packages.	Dietary intake of sodium above 3 g/d can offset effect of diuretic. Most common source of sodium is table salt and obviously salty foods, although canned soups/vegetables, luncheon meats, and dairy products also may contain high levels of sodium.
Refer to dietician for counseling specific to individual needs/dietary customs.	Identifies dietary needs, especially in presence of nausea/vomiting and resulting wasting syndrome (cardiac cachexia). Eating 6 small meals, use of liquid dietary supplements and vitamin supplements can limit inappropriate weight loss.
Review medications, purpose and side effects. Provide both oral and written instructions.	Understanding therapeutic needs and importance of prompt reporting of side effects can prevent occurrence of drug-related complications. Anxiety may block comprehension of input or details and patient/SO may refer to written material at later date to refresh memory.
Recommend taking diuretic early in morning.	Provides adequate time for drug effect before bedtime to prevent/limit interruption of sleep.
Instruct and receive return demonstration of ability to take and record daily pulse and when to notify healthcare provider, e.g., pulse above/below preset rate, changes in rhythm/regularity.	Promotes self-monitoring of condition/drug effect. Early detection of changes allows for timely intervention and may prevent complications, such as digitalis toxicity.
Explain and discuss patient's role in control of risk factors (e.g., smoking) and precipitating or aggravating factors, (e.g., high-salt diet, inactivity/over-exertion, exposure to extremes in temperature).	Adds to body of knowledge and permits patient to make informed decisions regarding control of condition and prevention of recurrence/complications. Smoking potentiates vasoconstriction; sodium intake promotes water retention/edema formation; improper balance between activity/rest and exposure to extremes in temperature may result in exhaustion/increased myocardial workload and increased risk of respiratory infections. Alcohol can depress cardiac contractility. Limitation of alcohol use to social occasions or maximum of 1 drink/d may be tolerated unless cardiomyopathy is alcohol-induced (requiring complete abstinence).

ACTIONS/INTERVENTIONS

Independent

ACTIONS/INTERVENTIONS	RATIONALE
Review signs/symptoms that require immediate medical attention, e.g., rapid/significant weight gain, edema, shortness of breath, increased fatigue, cough, hemoptysis, fever.	Self-monitoring increases patient responsibility in health maintenance and aids in prevention of complications, e.g., pulmonary edema, pneumonia. Weight gain of more than 3 lb since last clinical evaluation requires medical evaluation/adjustment of diuretic therapy. *Note:* Patient should weigh self daily in AM without clothing, after voiding and before eating.
Provide opportunities for patient/SO to ask questions, discuss concerns, and make necessary lifestyle changes.	Chronicity and recurrent/debilitating nature of HF often exhausts coping abilities and supportive capacity of both patient and SO, leading to depression.
Discuss general health risks (such as infection), recommending avoidance of crowds and individuals with respiratory infections, obtaining yearly influenza immunization and 1-time pneumonia immunization.	This population is at increased risk for infection due to circulatory compromise.
Stress importance of reporting signs/symptoms of digitalis toxicity, e.g., development of GI and visual disturbances, changes in pulse rate/rhythm, worsening of heart failure.	Early recognition of developing complications and involvement of healthcare provider may prevent toxicity/hospitalization.
Identify community resources/support groups and visiting home health nurse as indicated.	May need additional assistance with self-monitoring/home management.
Discuss importance of advance directives and of communicating plan/wishes to family and primary care providers.	Up to 50% of all deaths from heart failure are sudden, with many occurring at home, possibly without significant worsening of symptoms. If patient chooses to refuse life-support measures, an alternative contact person (rather than 911) needs to be designated should cardiac arrest occur.

POTENTIAL CONSIDERATIONS following discharge from care setting (dependent on patient's age, physical condition/presence of complications, personal resources and life responsibilities)

Activity intolerance—poor cardiac reserve, side effects of medication, generalized weakness.
Fluid Volume excess or deficit—changes in glomerular filtration rate, diuretic use, individual fluid/salt intake.
Skin Integrity, impaired—decreased activity level, prolonged sitting, presence of edema, altered circulation.
Therapeutic Regimen: Individual, ineffective management—complexity of regimen, economic limitations.
Home Maintenance Management, impaired—chronic/debilitating condition, insufficient finances, inadequate support systems.
Self Care deficit—decreased strength/endurance, depression.

Sample CP: Heart Failure, Hospital. ELOS 4 days Cardiology or Medical Unit

ND and Categories of Care	Day 1 _____	Day 2 _____	Day 3 _____	Day 4 _____
Decreased cardiac output R/T decreased myocardial contractility, altered electrical conduction, structural changes	Goals Participate in actions to reduce cardiac workload	Display VS within acceptable limits; dysrhythmias controlled; pulse oximetry within acceptable range Meet own self-care needs with assist as necessary Verbalize understanding of general condition and healthcare needs	→ Dysrhythmias controlled or absent → Free of signs of respiratory distress → Demonstrate measurable increase in activity tolerance Plan for lifestyle/ behavior changes	→ Plan in place to meet postdischarge needs.
Fluid Volume Excess R/T compromised regulatory mechanism	Verbalize understanding of fluid/food restrictions	Breath sounds clearing Urinary output adequate Wt loss (reflecting fluid loss)	Breath sounds clear Balanced I & O Edema resolving	Wt stable (continued loss if edema present)
Referrals	Cardiology Dietitian	Cardiac Rehab Occupational therapist (for ADLs) Social Services Home care	Community Resources	
Diagnostic studies	ECG Echo-Doppler CXR ABGs/Pulse oximetry Cardiac enzymes BUN/Cr CBC, lytes, Mg++ PT/aPTT Liver function studies Serum glucose Albumin Uric Acid Digoxin level (as indi) UA	Echo-Doppler (if not done day 1) or MUGA Cardiac enzymes (if ↑) BUN/Cr Electrolytes PT/aPTT (if on anticoagulents)	CXR BUN/Cr Electrolytes PT/aPTT (as indi) Repeat digoxin level (if indi)	
Additional assessments	Apical pulse, heart/ breath sounds q8h → Cardiac rhythm (Telemetry) q4h → B/P, P, R q2h til stable, q4h → q8h Temp q8h → I & O q8h → Weight qAM → Peripheral edema q8h → Peripheral pulses q8h → Sensorium q8h → DVT check qd → Response to activity → Response to therapeutic interventions →		→ bid → D/C → → → → → bid → bid → bid → → →	→ → → → → D/C → → qd → D/C → D/C → → →

ND and Categories of Care	Day 1 _____	Day 2 _____	Day 3 _____	Day 4 _____

Medications
  Allergies:
  _____
  _____
	IV diuretic
	ACE inhibitor
	Digoxin
	PO/Cutaneous nitrates
	Morphine sulfate
	Daytime/HS sedation
	PO/low dose
	  anticoagulant
	IV/PO potassium
	Stool softener/laxative
		→ po
		→
		→
		→
		→
		→
		→
		
		→
		→
			→
			→
			→
			→
			→ D/C
			→
			→ po or D/C
			
			→ D/C
			→
				→
				→
				→
				→
				
				→ D/C
				→
				
				→

Patient education	Orient to unit/room
	Review advanced
	  directives
	Discuss expected
	  outcomes, diagnostic
	  tests/results
	Fluid/nutritional
	  restrictions/needs
		Cardiac education per
		  protocol
		Review medications:
		  Dose, time, route,
		  purpose, side effects
		Progressive activity
		  program
		Skin care
			Signs/symptoms to
			  report to heathcare
			  provider
			Plan for homecare
			  needs
				Provide written
				  instructions for
				  homecare
				Schedule for follow-
				  up appointments

Additional nursing actions	Bed/chair rest
	
	Assist with physical
	  care
	Egg-crate mattress
	Dysrhythmia/angina
	  care per protocol
	Supplemental O$_2$
	Cardiac diet
		→ BPR/Ambulate as tol,
		  cardiac program
		→
		
		→
		
		→
		→
		→
			→ Up ad lib/graded
			  program
			→
			
			→
			
			→
			→ D/C
			→
				→
				
				→
				
				→ (send home)
				
				→
				
				→

ANGINA PECTORIS

The classic symptom of coronary artery disease is angina—pain caused by inadequate flow of oxygen to the myocardium. Angina has three major forms, (1) stable (percipitated by effort of short duration and relieved easily); (2) unstable (longer lasting, more severe, may not be relieved by rest/nitroglycerin or, new onset of pain with exertion, or recent acceleration/increase in severity of pain); and (3) variant (chest pain at rest with ECG changes).

CARE SETTING

Patients judged to be at intermediate or high likelihood of significant CAD are often hospitalized for further evaluation and therapeutic intervention. Classification of angina (as provided by Canadian Cardiovascular Society) aids in determining the risk of adverse outcomes for patients with unstable angina and, thereby, level of treatment needs. Class III angina occurs when patient can walk less than 2 blocks and normal activity is markedly limited, and Class IV angina occurs at rest or with minimal activity and level of activity is severely limited. These 2 classes generally require inpatient evaluation/therapeutic adjustments.

RELATED CONCERNS

Cardiac Surgery, p 95
Heart Failure: Chronic, p 45
Dysrhythmias, p 85
Myocardial Infarction, p 71
Psychosocial Aspects of Care, p 783

Patient Assessment Data Base

ACTIVITY/REST

May report:	Sedentary lifestyle, weakness
	Fatigue, feeling incapacitated after exercise
	Chest pain with exertion
	Being awakened with chest pain
May exhibit:	Exertional dyspnea

CIRCULATION

May report:	History of heart disease, hypertension, obesity
May exhibit:	Tachycardia, dysrhythmias
	Blood pressure normal, elevated, or decreased
	Heart sounds: May be normal; late S_4 or transient late systolic murmur (papillary muscle dysfunction) may be evident during pain
	Moist, cool, pale skin/mucous membranes in presence of vasoconstriction

FOOD/FLUID

May report:	Nausea, "heartburn"/epigastric distress with eating
	Diet high in cholesterol/fats, salt, caffeine, liquor
May exhibit:	Belching, gastric distention

EGO INTEGRITY

May report: Stressors of work, family, others

May exhibit: Apprehension, uneasiness

PAIN/DISCOMFORT

May report: Substernal, anterior chest pain that may radiate to jaw, neck, shoulders, and upper extremities (to left side more than right)

Quality: Varies; mild to moderate, heavy pressure, tightness, squeezing, burning

Duration: Usually less than 15 minutes, rarely more than 30 minutes (average 3 minutes)

Precipitating factors: Pain may be related to physical exertion or great emotion, such as anger or sexual arousal; exercise in weather extremes; or may be unpredictable and/or occur during rest

Relieving factors: Pain may be responsive to particular relief mechanisms (e.g., rest, antianginal medications)

New or ongoing chest pain that has changed in frequency, duration, character or predictability (i.e., unstable, variant, Prinzmetal's)

May exhibit: Facial grimacing, placing fist over midsternum, rubbing left arm, muscle tension, restlessness

Autonomic responses, e.g., tachycardia, blood pressure changes

RESPIRATION

May report: Dyspnea with exertion

History of smoking

May exhibit: Respirations: Increased rate/rhythm and alteration in depth

TEACHING/LEARNING

May report: Family history of heart disease, hypertension, stroke, diabetes

Use/misuse of cardiac, hypertensive, or OTC drugs

Regular alcohol use, illicit drug use, e.g., cocaine, amphetamines

Discharge Plan Considerations: **DRG projected mean length of inpatient stay: 3.8 days**

Alteration in medication use/therapy

Assistance with homemaker/maintenance tasks

Changes in physical layout of home

Refer to section at end of plan for postdischarge considerations.

DIAGNOSTIC STUDIES

Cardiac enzymes (AST, CPK, CK and CK-MB; LDH and isoenzymes LD$_1$, LD$_2$): usually WNL, elevation indicates myocardial damage.

ECG: Usually normal when patient at rest but flattening or depression of the ST segment of T wave signifies ischemia. Transient ST elevation, or decrease greater than 1 mm during pain with no abnormalities when pain-free, demonstrates transient myocardial ischemia. Dysrhythmias and heart block may also be present.

24-hour ECG monitoring (Holter): Done to see whether pain episodes correlate with ST segment changes. ST depression without pain is highly indicative of ischemia.

Exercise or pharmacological stress electrocardiography: Provides more diagnostic information, such as duration and level of activity before onset of angina, degree of ST depression, duration of abnormal ST response.

Chest x-ray: Usually normal; however, infiltrates may be present, reflecting cardiac decompensation or pulmonary complications.

PCO_2, potassium and myocardial lactate: May be elevated during anginal attack (all play a role in myocardial ischemia and may perpetuate it).

Serum lipids (total lipids, lipoprotein electrophoresis [HDL, LDL, VLDL]; cholesterol, triglycerides; phospholipids): May be elevated (CAD risk factor).

Echocardiogram: May reveal abnormal valvular action as cause of chest pain.

Nuclear imaging studies (rest or stress scan)
> ***Thallium 201:*** Ischemic regions appear as areas of decreased thallium uptake.
> ***Multigated imaging (MUGA):*** Evaluates specific and general ventricle performance, regional wall motion, and ejection fraction.

Cardiac catheterization with angiography: Definitive test in patients with known ischemic disease with angina, or incapacitating chest pain, in patients with cholesteremia and familial heart disease who are experiencing chest pain, and in patients with abnormal resting ECGs. Abnormal results are present in valvular disease, altered contractility, ventricular failure, and circulatory abnormalities. *Note:* 10% of patients with unstable angina have normal-appearing coronary arteries.

Ergonovine (Ergotrate) injection: Patients who have angina at rest may demonstrate hyperspastic coronary vessels. (Patients with resting angina usually experience chest pain, ST elevation, or depression and/or pronounced rise in LVEDP, fall in systemic systolic pressure, and/or high-grade coronary artery narrowing. Some patients may also have severe ventricular dysrhythmias.)

NURSING PRIORITIES

1. Relieve/control pain.
2. Prevent/minimize development of myocardial complications.
3. Provide information about disease process/prognosis and treatment.
4. Support patient/SO in initiating necessary lifestyle/behavioral changes.

DISCHARGE GOALS

1. Achieves desired activity level; meets self-care needs with minimal or no pain.
2. Free of complications.
3. Disease process/prognosis and therapeutic regimen understood.
4. Participating in treatment program, behavioral changes.
5. Plan in place to meet needs after discharge.

NURSING DIAGNOSIS: Pain [acute]

May be related to
Decreased myocardial blood flow
Increased cardiac workload/oxygen consumption

Possibly evidenced by
Reports of pain varying in frequency, duration, and intensity (especially as condition worsens)
Narrowed focus
Distraction behaviors (moaning, crying, pacing, restlessness)
Autonomic responses, e.g., diaphoresis, blood pressure and pulse rate changes, pupillary dilation, increased/decreased respiratory rate

DESIRED OUTCOMES/EVALUATION CRITERIA—PATIENT WILL:
Verbalize/demonstrate relief of pain
Report anginal episodes decreased in frequency, duration, and severity.

ACTIONS/INTERVENTIONS	RATIONALE
Independent	
Instruct patient to notify nurse immediately when chest pain occurs.	Pain and decreased cardiac output may stimulate the sympathetic nervous system to release excessive amounts of norepinephrine, which increases platelet aggregation and release of thromboxane A_2. This potent vasoconstrictor causes coronary artery spasm, which can precipitate, complicate, and/or prolong an anginal attack. Unbearable pain may cause vasovagal response, decreasing BP and heart rate.
Assess and document patient response/effects of medication.	Provides information about disease progression. Aids in evaluating effectiveness of interventions and may indicate need for change in therapeutic regimen.
Identify precipitating event, if any; frequency, duration, intensity, and location of pain.	Helps differentiate this chest pain and aids in evaluating possible progression to unstable angina. (Stable angina usually lasts 3–5 minutes while unstable angina is more intense and may last up to 45 minutes.)
Observe for associated symptoms, e.g., dyspnea, nausea/vomiting, dizziness, palpitations, desire to micturate.	Decreased cardiac output (which may occur during ischemic myocardial episode) stimulates sympathetic/parasympathetic nervous system, causing a variety of vague aches/sensations that patient may not identify as related to anginal episode.
Evaluate reports of pain in jaw, neck, shoulder, arm, or hand (typically on left side).	Cardiac pain may radiate, e.g., pain is often referred to more superficial sites served by the same spinal cord nerve level.
Place patient at complete rest during anginal episodes.	Reduces myocardial oxygen demand to minimize risk of tissue injury/necrosis.
Elevate head of bed if patient is short of breath.	Facilitates gas exchange to decrease hypoxia and resultant shortness of breath.
Monitor heart rate/rhythm.	Patients with unstable angina have an increased risk of acute life-threatening dysrhythmias, which occur in response to ischemic changes and/or stress.
Monitor vital signs every 5 minutes during anginal attack.	Blood pressure may rise initially due to sympathetic stimulation, then fall if cardiac output is compromised. Tachycardia also develops in response to sympathetic stimulation and may be sustained as a compensatory response if cardiac output falls.
Stay with patient who is experiencing pain or appears anxious.	Anxiety releases catecholamines, which increase myocardial workload and can escalate/prolong ischemic pain. Presence of nurse can reduce feelings of fear and helplessness.
Maintain quiet, comfortable environment; restrict visitors as necessary.	Mental/emotional stress increases myocardial workload.
Provide light meals. Have patient rest for 1 hour after meals.	Decreases myocardial workload associated with work of digestion, reducing risk of anginal attack.
Collaborative	
Provide supplemental oxygen as indicated.	Increases oxygen available for myocardial uptake/reversal of ischemia.

64

ACTIONS/INTERVENTIONS	RATIONALE

Collaborative

Administer antianginal medication(s) promptly as indicated:

Nitroglycerin: Sublingual (Nitrostat), buccal or oral tablets, sublingual spray;

Nitroglycerin has set the standard for treating and preventing anginal pain for more than 100 years. Today it is still the cornerstone of antianginal therapy. Rapid vasodilator effect lasts 10–30 minutes and can be used prophylactically to prevent, as well as abort, anginal attacks. *Note:* May enhance vasospastic angina.

Sustained release tablets, caplets, patches, transmucosal ointment, chewable tablets (long-acting), e.g., Nitro-Dur, Transderm-Nitro, isosorbide (Isordil, Sorbitrate);

Reduces frequency and severity of attack by producing prolonged/continuous vasodilation. May cause headache, dizziness, lightheadedness—symptoms that usually pass quickly. If headache is intolerable, alteration of dose or discontinuation of drug may be necessary.

β-blockers, e.g., atenolol (Tenormin), nadolol (Corgard), metroprolol (Lopressor), propranolol (Inderal);

Reduces angina by reducing the heart's workload. (Refer to following ND: Cardiac Output, decreased.)

Analgesics, i.e., acetaminophen (Tylenol);

Usually sufficient analgesia for relief of headache caused by dilatation of cerebral vessels in response to nitrates.

Morphine sulphate.

Potent narcotic analgesic that has several beneficial effects, e.g., causes peripheral vasodilation and reduces myocardial workload; has a sedative effect to produce relaxation; interrupts the flow of vasoconstricting catecholamines and thereby effectively relieves severe chest pain. MS is given IV for rapid action, and because decreased cardiac output compromises peripheral tissue absorption.

Monitor serial ECG changes.

Ischemia during anginal attack may cause transient ST segment depression or elevation and T wave inversion. Serial tracings verify ischemic changes, which may disappear when patient is pain-free. They also provide a baseline with which to compare later pattern changes.

NURSING DIAGNOSIS: Cardiac Output, decreased

May be related to
Inotropic changes (transient/prolonged myocardial ischemia, effects of medications)
Alterations in rate/rhythm and electrical conduction

Possibly evidenced by
Changes in hemodynamic readings; diminished peripheral pulses
Dyspnea
Restlessness; change in mental status
Decreased tolerance for activity; fatigue
Cool/pale skin
Continued chest pain

DESIRED OUTCOMES/EVALUATION CRITERIA—PATIENT WILL:
Report/display decreased episodes of dyspnea, angina, and dysrhythmias.
Demonstrate increased activity tolerance.
Participate in behaviors/activities that reduce the workload of the heart.

ACTIONS/INTERVENTIONS	RATIONALE

Independent

Monitor vital signs (e.g., heart rate, BP) and cardiac rhythm.

Tachycardia may be present because of pain, anxiety, hypoxemia, and reduced cardiac output. Changes may also occur in BP (hypertension or hypotension) because of cardiac response. ECG changes reflecting ischemia/dysrhythmias indicate need for additional evaluation and therapeutic intervention.

Evaluate mental status, noting development of confusion, disorientation.

Reduced perfusion of the brain can produce observable changes in sensorium.

Note skin color and presence/quality of pulses.

Peripheral circulation is reduced when cardiac output falls, giving the skin a pale or gray color (depending on level of hypoxia) and diminishing the strength of peripheral pulses.

Auscultate breath sounds and heart sounds. Listen for murmurs.

S_3, S_4, or crackles can occur with cardiac decompensation or some medications (especially β-blockers). Development of murmurs may reveal a valvular cause for chest pain (e.g., aortic stenosis, mitral stenosis), or papillary muscle rupture.

Maintain bed rest in position of comfort during acute episodes.

Decreases oxygen consumption/demand reducing myocardial workload and risk of decompensation.

Provide for adequate rest periods. Assist with/perform self-care activities, as indicated.

Conserves energy, reduces cardiac workload.

Stress importance of avoiding straining/bearing down, especially during defecation.

Valsalva maneuver causes vagal stimulation, reducing heart rate (bradycardia), which may be followed by rebound tachycardia, both of which may impair cardiac output.

Encourage immediate reporting of pain for prompt administration of medications as indicated.

Timely interventions can reduce oxygen consumption and myocardial workload and may prevent/minimize cardiac complications.

Monitor for and document effects of/adverse response to medications, noting BP, heart rate and rhythm (especially when giving combination of calcium antagonists, β-blockers, and nitrates).

Desired effect is to decrease myocardial oxygen demand by decreasing ventricular stress. Drugs with negative inotropic properties can decrease perfusion to an already ischemic myocardium. Combination of nitrates and β-blockers may have cumulative effect on cardiac output.

Assess for signs and symptoms of HF.

Angina is only a symptom of underlying pathology causing myocardial ischemia. Disease may compromise cardiac function to point of decompensation.

Collaborative

Administer supplemental oxygen as needed.

Increases oxygen available for myocardial uptake to improve contractility, reduce ischemia, and reduce lactic acid levels.

Monitor pulse oximetry or ABGs as indicated.

Determines adequacy of O_2 therapy.

Measure cardiac output and other functional parameters as indicated.

Cardiac index, preload/afterload, contractility, and cardiac work can be measured noninvasively using thoracic electrical bioimpedance (TEB) technique. Useful in evaluating response to therapeutic interventions and identifying need for more aggressive/emergency care.

ACTIONS/INTERVENTIONS	RATIONALE
Collaborative	
Administer medications as indicated:	
Calcium channel blockers, e.g., diltiazem (Cardizem), nifedipine (Procardia), verapamil (Calan);	Although differing in mode of action, calcium channel blockers play a major role in preventing and terminating ischemia induced by coronary artery spasm and in reducing vascular resistance, thereby decreasing BP and cardiac workload. *Note:* Procardia should be used in conjunction with β-blockers.
β-blockers, e.g., atenolol (Tenormin), nadolol (Corgard), propranolol (Inderal), esmolol (Brevibloc);	These medications decrease cardiac workload by reducing heart rate and systolic BP. *Note:* Overdosage produces cardiac decompensation.
ASA, other antiplatelet agents, e.g., ticlopidine (Ticlid);	Useful in unstable angina, ASA diminishes platelet aggregation/clot formation. For patients with major GI intolerance, alternate drugs may be indicated.
IV heparin.	Bolus, followed by continuous infusion, is recommended to help reduce risk of subsequent MI and recurrent unstable angina for patients diagnosed with intermediate or high-risk unstable angina.
Monitor lab studies e.g., aPTT.	Evaluates therapy needs/effectiveness.
Discuss purpose and prepare for stress testing and cardiac catheterization, when indicated.	Stress testing provides information about the health/strength of the ventricles, which is useful in determining appropriate levels of activity. Angiography may be indicated to identify areas of coronary artery obstruction/damage that may require surgical intervention.
Prepare for surgical intervention (PTCA, intracoronary stent placement, valve replacement, CABG), if indicated.	PTCA has become a fairly common procedure in the last 15 years. PTCA increases coronary blood flow by compression of atheromatous lesions and dilatation of the vessel lumen in an occluded coronary artery. This procedure is preferred over the more invasive cardiac surgery (CABG). CABG is recommended when testing confirms myocardial ischemia as a result of left main coronary artery disease or symptomatic two-vessel disease. Intracoronary stents may be placed at the time of PTCA to provide structural support within the coronary artery and improve the odds of long-term patency.
Prepare for transfer to critical care unit if condition warrants.	Profound/prolonged chest pain with decreased cardiac output reflects development of complications requiring more intense/emergency interventions.

NURSING DIAGNOSIS: Anxiety [specify level]

May be related to

Situational crises

Threat to self-concept (altered image/abilities)

Underlying pathophysiologic response

Threat to or change in health status (disease course which can lead to further compromise, debility, even death)

Negative self-talk

67

ACTIONS/INTERVENTIONS	RATIONALE
Independent	
Explain purpose of tests and procedures, e.g., stress testing.	Reduces anxiety attributable to fear of unknown diagnosis and prognosis.
Promote expression of feelings and fears, e.g., denial, depression, and anger. Let patient/SO know these are normal reactions. Note statements of concern, e.g., ''Heart attack is inevitable.''	Unexpressed feelings may create internal turmoil and affect self-image. Verbalization of concerns reduces tension, verifies level of coping, and facilitates dealing with feelings. Presence of negative self-talk can increase level of anxiety and may contribute to exacerbation of angina attacks.
Encourage family and friends to treat patient as before.	Reassures patient that role in the family and business has not been altered.
Tell patient the medical regimen has been designed to reduce/limit future attacks and increase cardiac stability.	Encourages patient to test symptom control (e.g., no angina with certain levels of activity), to increase confidence in medical program, and integrate abilities into perceptions of self. (Refer to CP: Psychosocial Aspects of Care, ND: Anxiety [specify level]/Fear for additional considerations, p 785).
Collaborative	
Administer sedatives, tranquilizers, as indicated.	May be desired to help patient to relax until physically able to reestablish adequate coping strategies.

> **DESIRED OUTCOMES/EVALUATION CRITERIA—PATIENT WILL:**
> Participate in learning process.
> Assume responsibility for own learning, looking for information and asking questions.
> Verbalize understanding of condition/disease process and treatment.
> Participate in treatment regimen.
> Initiate necessary lifestyle changes.

ACTIONS/INTERVENTIONS

Independent

Review pathophysiology of condition. Stress need for preventing anginal attacks.

Encourage avoidance of factors/situations that may precipitate anginal episode, e.g., emotional stress, physical exertion, ingestion of large/heavy meal, exposure to extremes in environmental temperature.

Assist patient/SO to identify sources of physical and emotional stress and discuss ways that they can be avoided.

Review importance of weight control, cessation of smoking, dietary changes, and exercise.

Encourage patient to follow prescribed reconditioning program; caution to avoid exhaustion.

Discuss impact of illness on desired lifestyle and activities, including work, driving, sexual activity, and hobbies. Provide information, privacy, or consultation, as indicated.

Demonstrate/encourage patient to monitor own pulse during activities, schedule/simplify activities, avoid strain.

Discuss steps to take when anginal attacks occur, e.g., cessation of activity, administration of prn medication, use of relaxation techniques.

Review prescribed medications for control/prevention of anginal attacks.

Stress importance of checking with physician prior to taking OTC drugs.

Discuss ASA and other antiplatelet agents as indicated.

RATIONALE

Patients with angina need to learn why it occurs and what they can do to control it. This is the focus of therapeutic management in order to reduce likelihood of myocardial infarction.

May reduce incidence/severity of ischemic episodes.

This is a crucial step in limiting/preventing anginal attacks.

Knowledge of the significance of risk factors provides patient with opportunity to make needed changes.

Fear of triggering attacks may cause patient to avoid participation in activity that has been prescribed to enhance recovery (increase myocardial strength and form collateral circulation).

Patient may be reluctant to resume/continue usual activities because of fear of anginal attack or death. Patient should take nitroglycerin prophylactically before any activity that is known to precipitate angina.

Allows patient to identify those activities that can be modified to avoid cardiac stress and stay below the anginal threshold.

Being prepared for an event takes away the fear that patient will not know what to do if attack occurs.

Angina is a complicated condition that often requires the use of many drugs given to decrease myocardial workload, improve coronary circulation, and control the occurrence of attacks.

OTC drugs may potentiate or negate prescribed medications.

May be given prophylactically on a daily basis to decrease platelet aggregation and improve coronary circulation.

ACTIONS/INTERVENTIONS	RATIONALE
Independent	
Review symptoms to be reported to physician, e.g., increase in frequency/duration of attacks, changes in response to medications.	Knowledge of expectations can avoid undue concern for insignificant reasons or delay in treatment of important symptoms.
Discuss importance of follow-up appointments.	Angina is a symptom of progressive coronary artery disease that should be monitored and may require occasional adjustment of treatment regimen.

POTENTIAL CONSIDERATIONS following discharge from care setting (dependent on patient's age, physical condition/presence of complications, personal resources and life responsibilities)

Pain [acute]—episodes of decreased myocardial blood flow/ischemia.

Activity intolerance—imbalance between oxygen supply/demand, sedentary/stressful lifestyle.

Denial, ineffective—learned response patterns (e.g., avoidance), cultural factors, personal and family value systems.

Family Process, altered—situational transition and crisis.

Home Maintenance Management, impaired—altered ability to perform tasks, inadequate support systems, reluctance to request assistance.

MYOCARDIAL INFARCTION

Myocardial infarction (MI) is caused by reduced blood flow through one or more of the coronary arteries, resulting in myocardial ischemia and necrosis.

CARE SETTING

Inpatient acute hospital, step-down or medical unit.

RELATED CONCERNS

Angina Pectoris, p 61
Heart Failure: Chronic, p 45
Dysrhythmias, p 85
Psychosocial Aspects of Care, p 783
Thrombophlebitis: Deep Vein Thrombosis, p 107

Patient Assessment Data Base

ACTIVITY/REST

May report: Weakness, fatigue, loss of sleep
Sedentary lifestyle, sporadic exercise schedule

May exhibit: Tachycardia, dyspnea with rest/activity

CIRCULATION

May report: History of previous MI, coronary artery disease, HF, BP problems, diabetes mellitus.

May exhibit: BP: May be normal or increased/decreased; postural changes may be noted from lying to sitting/standing.
Pulse: May be normal; full/bounding, or weak/thready quality with delayed capillary refill; irregularities (dysrhythmias) may be present.
Heart sounds: Extra heart sounds: S_3/S_4 may reflect cardiac failure/decreased ventricular contractility, or compliance.
Murmurs: If present, may reflect valvular insufficiency or papillary muscle dysfunction.
Friction rub: Suggests pericarditis.
Heart rate: May be abnormal (tachycardia, bradycardia).
Heart rhythm: Can be regular or irregular.
Edema: Jugular vein distention, peripheral/dependent edema, generalized edema, crackles may be present with cardiac/ventricular failure.
Color: Pallor or cyanosis/mottling of skin, nailbeds, mucous membranes, and lips may be noted.

EGO INTEGRITY

May report: Denial of significance of symptoms/presence of condition
Fear of dying, feelings of impending doom
Anger at inconvenience of illness/"unnecessary" hospitalization
Worry about family, job, finances

May exhibit: Denial, withdrawal, anxiety, lack of eye contact
Irritability, anger, combative behavior
Focus on self/pain

ELIMINATION

May exhibit: Normal or decreased bowel sounds

FOOD/FLUID

May report: Nausea, loss of appetite, belching, indigestion/heartburn

May exhibit: Decreased skin turgor; dry/diaphoretic skin
Vomiting
Weight change

HYGIENE

May report/exhibit: Difficulty performing care tasks

NEUROSENSORY

May report: Dizziness, fainting spells in or out of bed (upright or at rest)

May exhibit: Changes in mentation
Weakness

PAIN/DISCOMFORT

May report: Sudden onset of chest pain (may/may not be associated with activity), unrelieved by rest or nitroglycerin. (Although most pain is deep and visceral, 20% of the MIs are painless.)
Location: Typically anterior chest, substernal, precordium; may radiate to arms, jaws, face. May have atypical location such as epigastrium, elbow, jaw, abdomen, back, neck.
Quality: Crushing, constricting, viselike, squeezing, heavy, steady.
Intensity: Usually 10 on a scale of 1–10; may be "worst pain ever experienced." *Note:* Pain may be absent in postoperative patients, those with diabetes mellitus or hypertension, or the elderly.

May exhibit: Facial grimacing, changes in body posture, may place clenched fist on midsternum when describing pain
Crying, groaning, squirming, stretching
Withdrawal, loss of eye contact
Autonomic responses: Changes in heart rate/rhythm, BP, respirations, skin color/moisture, level of consciousness

RESPIRATION

May report: Dyspnea with/without exertion, nocturnal dyspnea
Cough with/without sputum production
History of smoking, chronic respiratory disease

May exhibit: Increased respiratory rate, shallow/labored breathing
Pallor or cyanosis
Breath sounds: Clear or crackles/wheezes
Sputum: Clear, pink-tinged

SOCIAL INTERACTION

May report: Recent stress, e.g., work, family
Difficulty coping with current stressors, e.g., illness, hospitalization

May exhibit:	Difficulty resting quietly, overemotional responses (intense anger, fear)
	Withdrawal from family

TEACHING/LEARNING

May report:	Family history of heart disease/MI, diabetes, stroke, hypertension, peripheral vascular disease
	Use of tobacco
Discharge plan considerations:	**DRG projected length of inpatient stay: 7.3 days; (2–4 days/CCU)** Assistance with food preparation, shopping, transportation, homemaking/maintenance tasks; physical layout of home

DIAGNOSTIC STUDIES

ECG: Shows S-T elevation, signifying ischemia; depressed or inverted T wave, indicating injury; and presence of Q waves, signifying necrosis.

Cardiac enzymes and isoenzymes

CPK-MB (isoenzyme found in heart muscle): Elevates within 4–8 hours, peaks in 12–20 hours, returns to normal in 48–72 hours.

LDH_1: Elevates within 8–24 hours, peaks within 72–144 hours, and may take as long as 14 days to return to normal. An LDH_1 greater than LDH_2 (flipped ratio) helps confirm/diagnose MI if not detected in acute phase.

Electrolytes: Imbalances of sodium and potassium can alter conduction and can compromise contractility.

WBC: Leukocytosis (10,000–20,000) usually appears on the 2nd day after MI due to inflammatory process.

Sedimentation rate (ESR): Rises on 2nd–3rd day after MI, indicating inflammation.

Chemistry profiles: May be abnormal depending on acute/chronic abnormal organ function/perfusion.

ABGs/pulse oximetry: May indicate hypoxia or acute/chronic lung disease processes.

Lipids (total lipids, HDL, LDL, cholesterol, triglycerides, phospholipids): Elevations may reflect arteriosclerosis as a cause for MI.

Chest x-ray: May be normal or show an enlarged cardiac shadow suggestive of HF or ventricular aneurysm.

Echocardiogram: May be done to determine dimensions of chambers, septal/ventricular wall motion, and valve configuration/function.

Nuclear imaging studies

Thallium: Evaluates myocardial blood flow and status of myocardial cells, e.g., location/extent of acute/previous MI.

Technetium: Accumulates in ischemic cells outlining necrotic area(s).

Cardiac blood imaging/MUGA: Evaluates specific and general ventricular performance, regional wall motion, and ejection fraction (blood flow).

Coronary angiography: Visualizes narrowing/occlusion of coronary arteries and is usually done in conjunction with measurements of chamber pressures and assessment of left ventricular function (ejection fraction). Procedure is not usually done in acute phase of MI unless angioplasty/emergency heart surgery is imminent.

Digital subtraction angiography (DSA): Technique used to visualize status of arterial bypass grafts and to detect peripheral artery disease.

MRI: Allows visualization of blood flow, cardiac chambers/intraventricular septum, valves, vascular lesions, plaque formations, areas of necrosis/infarction, and blood clots.

Exercise stress test: Determines cardiovascular response to activity (often done in conjunction with thallium imaging in the recovery phase).

NURSING PRIORITIES

1. Relieve pain, anxiety.
2. Reduce myocardial workload.
3. Prevent/detect and assist in treatment of life-threatening dysrhythmias or complications.
4. Promote cardiac health, self-care.

DISCHARGE GOALS

1. Chest pain absent/controlled.
2. Heart rate/rhythm sufficient to sustain adequate cardiac output/tissue perfusion.
3. Achievement of activity level sufficient for basic self-care.
4. Anxiety reduced/managed.
5. Disease process treatment plan, and prognosis understood.
6. Plan in place to meet needs after discharge.

NURSING DIAGNOSIS: Pain [acute]

May be related to
Tissue ischemia secondary to coronary artery occlusion

Possibly evidenced by
Reports of chest pain with/without radiation
Facial grimacing
Restlessness, changes in level of consciousness
Changes in pulse, BP

DESIRED OUTCOMES/EVALUATION CRITERIA—PATIENT WILL:
Verbalize relief/control of chest pain.
Demonstrate use of relaxation techniques.
Display reduced tension, relaxed manner, ease of movement.

ACTIONS/INTERVENTIONS	RATIONALE
Independent	
Monitor/document characteristics of pain, noting verbal reports, nonverbal cues, (e.g., moaning, crying, restlessness, diaphoresis, clutching chest, rapid breathing) and hemodynamic response (BP/heart rate changes).	Variation of appearance and behavior of patients in pain may present a challenge in assessment. Most patients with an acute MI appear ill, distracted, and focused on pain. Verbal history and deeper investigation of precipitating factors should be postponed until pain is relieved. Respirations may be increased as a result of pain and associated anxiety, while release of stress induced catecholamines will increase heart rate and BP.
Obtain full description of pain from patient including location; intensity (0–10); duration; quality (dull/crushing); and radiation.	Pain is a subjective experience and must be described by the patient. Assist patient to quantify pain by comparing it to other experiences.
Review history of previous angina, anginal equivalent, or MI pain. Discuss family history if pertinent.	May differentiate current pain from preexisting patterns, as well as identify complications such as extension of infarction, pulmonary embolus, or pericarditis.
Instruct patient to report pain immediately.	Delay in reporting pain hinders pain relief/may require increased dosage of medication to achieve relief. In addition, severe pain may induce shock by stimulating the sympathetic nervous system, thereby creating further damage and interfering with diagnostics and relief of pain.

ACTIONS/INTERVENTIONS	RATIONALE
Independent	
Provide quiet environment, calm activities, and comfort measures (e.g., dry/winkle-free linens, backrub). Approach the patient calmly and confidently.	Decreases external stimuli, which may aggravate anxiety and cardiac strain and limit coping abilities and adjustment to current situation.
Assist/instruct in relaxation techniques, e.g., deep/slow breathing, distraction behaviors, visualization, guided imagery.	Helpful in decreasing perception of/response to pain. Provides a sense of having some control over the situation, increase in positive attitude.
Check vital signs before and after narcotic medication.	Hypotension/respiratory depression can occur as a result of narcotic administration. These problems may increase myocardial damage in presence of ventricular insufficiency.
Collaborative	
Administer supplemental oxygen by means of nasal cannula or face mask, as indicated.	Increases amount of oxygen available for myocardial uptake and thereby may relieve discomfort associated with tissue ischemia.
Administer medications as indicated, e.g.:	
Antianginals, e.g., nitroglycerin (Nitro-Bid, Nitrostat, Nitro-Dur);	Nitrates are useful for pain control by coronary vasodilating effects, which increase coronary blood flow and myocardial perfusion. Peripheral vasodilation effects reduce the volume of blood returning to the heart (preload), thereby decreasing myocardial work and oxygen demand.
β-blockers, e.g., atenolol (Tenormin), pindolol (Visken), propranolol (Inderal);	Important second-line agents for pain control through effect of blocking sympathetic stimulation, thereby reducing heart rate, systolic BP, and myocardial oxygen demand. May be given alone or with nitrates. *Note:* β-blockers may be contraindicated if myocardial contractility is severely impaired, because negative inotropic properties can further reduce contractility.
Analgesics, e.g., morphine, meperidine (Demerol);	Although IV morphine is the usual drug of choice, other injectable narcotics may be used in acute phase/recurrent chest pain unrelieved by nitroglycerin to reduce severe pain, provide sedation, and decrease myocardial workload. IM injections should be avoided, if possible, because they can alter the CPK diagnostic indicator and are not well absorbed in underperfused tissue.
Calcium channel blockers, e.g., verapamil (Calan), diltiazem (Cardizem), nifedipine (Procardia);	Vasodilation effects can increase coronary blood flow, encourage collateral circulation, and reduce preload and myocardial oxygen demands. Some of these agents also have antidysrhythmic properties.
Prepare for PTCA angioplasty, also called balloon angioplasty, possibly with intracoronary stints.	This procedure is employed to open partially blocked coronary arteries before they become totally blocked. The mechanism seems to include a combination of vessel stretching and plaque compression. Intracoronary stents may be placed at the time of PTCA to provide structural support within the coronary artery, to improve the odds of long-term patency.

ACTIONS/INTERVENTIONS	RATIONALE
Independent	
Record/document heart rate, rhythm, and BP changes before, during, after activity, as indicated. Correlate with reports of chest pain/shortness of breath. (Refer to ND: Cardiac Output, decreased risk for, p 78.)	Trends determine patient's response to activity and may indicate myocardial oxygen deprivation that may require decrease in activity level/return to bed rest, changes in medication regimen, use of supplemental oxygen.
Promote rest (bed/chair) initially. Limit activity on basis of pain/hemodynamic response. Provide nonstress diversional activities.	Reduces myocardial workload/oxygen consumption, reducing risk of complications (e.g., extension of MI).
Limit visitors and/or visiting by patient, initially.	Lengthy/involved conversations can be very taxing for the patient; however, periods of quiet visitation can be therapeutic.
Instruct patient to avoid increasing abdominal pressure, e.g., straining during defecation.	Activities that require holding the breath and bearing down (Valsalva maneuver) can result in bradycardia, temporarily reduced cardiac output, and rebound tachycardia with elevated BP.
Explain pattern of graded increase of activity level, e.g., getting up in chair when there is no pain, progressive ambulation, and resting for 1 hour after meals.	Progressive activity provides a controlled demand on the heart, increasing strength and preventing overexertion.
Review signs/symptoms reflecting intolerance of present activity level or requiring notification of nurse/physician.	Palpitations, pulse irregularities, development of chest pain, or dyspnea may indicate need for changes in exercise regimen or medication.
Collaborative	
Refer to cardiac rehabilitation program.	Provides continued support/additional supervision and participation in recovery and wellness process.

NURSING DIAGNOSIS: Anxiety [specify level]/Fear

May be related to
Threat to or change in health and socioeconomic status
Threat of loss/death
Unconscious conflict about essential values, beliefs, and goals of life
Interpersonal transmission/contagion

Possibly evidenced by
Fearful attitude
Apprehension, increased tension, restlessness, facial tension
Uncertainty, feelings of inadequacy
Somatic complaints/sympathetic stimulation
Focus on self, expressions of concern about current and future events
Fight (e.g., belligerent attitude) or flight behavior

DESIRED OUTCOMES/EVALUATION CRITERIA—PATIENT WILL:
Recognize feelings.
Identify causes, contributing factors.
Verbalize reduction of anxiety/fear.
Demonstrate positive problem-solving skills.
Identify/use resources appropriately.

ACTIONS/INTERVENTIONS

Independent

Identify and acknowledge patient's perception of threat/situation. Encourage expressions of and do not deny feelings of anger, grief, sadness, fear, etc.

Note presence of hostility, withdrawal, and/or denial (inappropriate affect or refusal to comply with medical regimen).

Maintain confident manner (without false reassurance).

Observe for verbal/nonverbal signs of anxiety and stay with patient. Intervene if patient displays destructive behavior.

RATIONALE

Coping with pain and emotional trauma of an MI is difficult. Patient may fear death and/or be anxious about immediate environment. Ongoing anxiety (related to concerns about impact of heart attack on future lifestyle, matters left unattended/unresolved, and effects of illness on family) may be present in varying degrees for some time and may be manifested by symptoms of depression.

Research into survival rates between type A/type B individuals and the impact of denial has been ambiguous; however, studies show some correlation between degree/expression of anger or hostility and an increased risk for MI.

Patient and SO can be affected by the anxiety/uneasiness displayed by health team members. Honest explanations can alleviate anxiety.

Patient may not express concern directly, but words/actions may convey sense of agitation, aggression, and hostility. Intervention can help patient to regain control of own behavior.

ACTIONS/INTERVENTIONS	RATIONALE
Independent	
Accept but do not reinforce use of denial. Avoid confrontations.	Denial can be beneficial in decreasing anxiety but can postpone dealing with the reality of the current situation. Confrontation can promote anger and increase use of denial, reducing cooperation and possibly impeding recovery.
Orient patient/SO to routine procedures and expected activities. Promote participation when possible.	Predictability and information can decrease anxiety for patient.
Answer all questions factually. Provide consistent information; repeat as indicated.	Accurate information about the situation reduces fear, strengthens nurse-patient relationship, and assists patient/SO to deal realistically with situation. Attention span may be short, and repetition of information helps with retention.
Encourage patient/SO to communicate with one another, sharing questions and concerns.	Sharing information elicits support/comfort and can relieve tension of unexpressed worries.
Provide rest periods/uninterrupted sleep time, quiet surroundings, with patient controlling type, amount of external stimuli.	Conserves energy and enhances coping abilities.
Support normality of grieving process, including time necessary for resolution.	Can provide reassurance that feelings are normal response to situation/perceived changes.
Provide privacy for patient and SO.	Allows needed time for expression of feelings, relief of anxiety, and the establishing of more adaptive behaviors.
Encourage independence, self-care, and decision making within accepted treatment plan.	Increased independence from staff promotes self-confidence and reduces feelings of abandonment that can accompany transfer from coronary unit/discharge from hospital.
Encourage discussion about postdischarge expectations.	Helps patient/SO identify realistic goals, thereby reducing risk of discouragement in face of the reality of limitations of condition/pace of recuperation.
Collaborative	
Administer antianxiety/hypnotics as indicated, e.g., diazepam (Valium), lorazepam (Ativan), flurazepam (Dalmane).	Promotes relaxation/rest and reduces feelings of anxiety.

NURSING DIAGNOSIS: Cardiac Output, decreased, risk for

Risk factors may include
Changes in rate, rhythm, electrical conduction
Reduced preload/increased SVR
Infarcted/dyskinetic muscle, structural defects, e.g., ventricular aneurysm, septal defects

Possibly evidenced by
[Not applicable; presence of signs and symptoms establishes *actual* diagnosis]

DESIRED OUTCOMES/EVALUATION CRITERIA—PATIENT WILL:
Maintain hemodynamic stability, e.g., BP, cardiac output within normal range, adequate urinary output, decreased/absent dysrhythmias.
Report decreased episodes of dyspnea, angina.
Demonstrate an increase in activity tolerance.

ACTIONS/INTERVENTIONS	RATIONALE
Independent	
Auscultate BP. Compare both arms and obtain lying, sitting, and standing pressures when able.	Hypotension may occur related to ventricular dysfunction, hypoperfusion of the myocardium, and vagal stimulation. However, hypertension is also a common phenomenon, possibly related to pain, anxiety, catecholamine release, and/or preexisting vascular problems. Orthostatic (postural) hypotension may be associated with complications of infarct, e.g., HF.
Evaluate quality and equality of pulses, as indicated.	Decreased cardiac output results in diminished weak/thready pulses. Irregularities suggest dysrhythmias, which may require further evaluation/monitoring.
Auscultate heart sound: Note development of S$_3$, S$_4$;	S$_3$ is usually associated with HF, but it may also be noted with mitral insufficiency (regurgitation) and left ventricular overload that can accompany severe infarction. S$_4$ may be associated with myocardial ischemia, ventricular stiffening, and pulmonary or systemic hypertension.
Presence of murmurs/rubs.	Indicates disturbances of normal blood flow within the heart, e.g., incompetent valve, septal defect, or vibration of papillary muscle/chordae tendonae (complication of MI). Presence of rub with an infarction is also associated with inflammation, e.g., pericardial effusion and pericarditis.
Auscultate breath sounds.	Crackles reflecting pulmonary congestion may develop because of depressed myocardial function.
Monitor heart rate and rhythm. Document dysrhythmias via telemetry.	Heart rate and rhythm respond to medication and activity, as well as developing complications/dysrhythmias (especially premature ventricular contractions or progressive heart blocks), which could compromise cardiac function or increase ischemic damage. Acute or chronic atrial flutter/fibrillation may be seen with coronary artery or valvular involvement and may or may not be pathologic.
Note response to activity and promote rest appropriately. (Refer to ND: Activity intolerance, p 76.)	Overexertion increases oxygen consumption/demand and can compromise myocardial function.
Provide bedside commode if unable to use bathroom facilities.	Attempts at using bedpan can be exhausting and psychologically stressful, thereby increasing oxygen demand and cardiac workload.
Provide small/easily digested meals. Restrict caffeine intake, e.g., coffee, chocolate, cola.	Large meals may increase myocardial workload and cause vagal stimulation resulting in bradycardia/ectopic beats. Caffeine is a direct cardiac stimulant that can increase heart rate.
Have emergency equipment/medications available.	Sudden coronary occlusion, lethal dysrhythmias, extension of infarct, or unrelenting pain are situations that may precipitate cardiac arrest, requiring immediate life-saving therapies/transfer to critical care unit.

Collaborative

Administer supplemental oxygen, as indicated.	Increases amount of oxygen available for myocardial uptake, reducing ischemia and resultant dysrhythmias.
Measure cardiac output and other functional parameters as appropriate.	Cardiac index, preload/afterload, contractility, and cardiac work can be measured noninvasively using thoracic electrical bioimpedance (TEB) technique. Useful in evaluating response to therapeutic interventions, and identifying need for more aggressive/emergency care.
Maintain IV/hep-lock access as indicated.	Patent line is important for administration of emergency drugs in presence of persistent dysrhythmias or chest pain.
Review serial ECGs.	Provides information regarding progression/resolution of infarction, status of ventricular function, electrolyte balance, and effects of drug therapies.
Review chest x-ray.	May reflect pulmonary edema related to ventricular dysfunction.
Monitor laboratory data: e.g., cardiac enzymes, ABGs, electrolytes.	Enzymes monitor resolution/extension of infarction. Presence of hypoxia indicates need for supplemental oxygen. Electrolyte imbalance, e.g., hypokalemia/hyperkalemia adversely affects cardiac rhythm/contractility.
Prepare patient for additional diagnostic testing, e.g., Cine scan.	A CT scan of the heart provides images of muscle contraction/ventricular function aiding in diagnosis of heart failure.
Administer antidysrhythmic drugs and ACE inhibitors as indicated.	Dysrhythmias are usually treated symptomatically, except for PVCs, which are often treated prophylactically. Early inclusion of ACE inhibitor therapy (especially in presence of large anterior MI, ventricular aneurysm or heart failure) enhances ventricular output, increases survival and may slow progression of heart failure.
Assist with insertion/maintain pacemaker, when used.	Pacing may be a temporary support measure during acute/healing phase or may be needed permanently if infarction severely damages conduction system, impairing systolic function. Evaluation is based on echocardiography or radionuclide ventriculography.

NURSING DIAGNOSIS: Tissue Perfusion, altered, risk for

Risk factors may include
Reduction/interruption of blood flow, e.g., vasoconstriction, hypovolemia/shunting, and thromboembolic formation

Possibly evidenced by
[Not applicable; presence of signs and symptoms establishes an *actual* diagnosis]

DESIRED OUTCOMES/EVALUATION CRITERIA—PATIENT WILL:
Demonstrate adequate perfusion as individually appropriate, e.g., skin warm and dry, peripheral pulses present/strong, vital signs within patient's normal range, patient alert/oriented, balanced intake/output, absence of edema, free of pain/discomfort.

ACTIONS/INTERVENTIONS	RATIONALE
Independent	
Investigate sudden changes or continued alterations in mentation, e.g., anxiety, confusion, lethargy, stupor.	Cerebral perfusion is directly related to cardiac output and is also influenced by electrolyte/acid-base variations, hypoxia, or systemic emboli.
Inspect for pallor, cyanosis, mottling, cool/clammy skin. Note strength of peripheral pulse.	Systemic vasoconstriction resulting from diminished cardiac output may be evidenced by decreased skin perfusion and diminished pulses. (Refer to ND: Cardiac Output, decreased, risk for, p 78.)
Assess for Homans' sign (pain in calf on dorsiflexion), erythema, edema.	Indicators of deep vein thrombosis.
Encourage active/passive leg exercises, avoidance of isometric exercises.	Enhances venous return, reduces venous stasis, and decreases risk of thrombophlebitis; however, isometric exercises can adversely affect cardiac output by increasing myocardial work and oxygen consumption.
Instruct patient in application/periodic removal of antiembolic hose, when used.	Limits venous stasis, improves venous return and reduces risk of thrombophlebitis in patient who is limited in activity.
Monitor respirations, note work of breathing.	Cardiac pump failure may precipitate respiratory distress; however, sudden/continued dyspnea may indicate thromboembolic pulmonary complications.
Assess gastrointestinal function, noting anorexia, decreased/absent bowel sounds, nausea/vomiting, abdominal distention, constipation.	Reduced blood flow to mesentery can produce gastrointestinal dysfunction, e.g., loss of peristalsis. Problems may be potentiated/aggravated by use of analgesics, decreased activity, and dietary changes.
Monitor intake, note changes in urine output. Record urine specific gravity as indicated.	Decreased intake/persistent nausea may result in reduced circulating volume, which negatively affects perfusion and organ function. Specific gravity measurements reflect hydration status and renal function.
Collaborative	
Monitor laboratory data, e.g., ABGs, BUN, creatinine, electrolytes, coagulation studies (PT, aPTT, clotting times).	Indicators of organ perfusion/function. Abnormalities in coagulation may occur as a result of therapeutic measures (e.g., heparin/Coumadin use and some cardiac drugs such as quinidine).
Administer medications as indicated, e.g.:	
Heparin/warfarin sodium (Coumadin);	Low-dose heparin may be given prophylactically in high-risk patients (e.g., atrial fibrillation, obesity, ventricular aneurysm, or history of thrombophlebitis) to reduce risk of thrombophlebitis or mural thrombus formation. Coumadin is the drug of choice for long-term/postdischarge anticoagulant therapy.
Cimetidine (Tagamet), ranitidine (Zantac), antacids.	Reduces or neutralizes gastric acid, preventing discomfort and gastric irritation, especially in presence of reduced mucosal circulation.

ACTIONS/INTERVENTIONS

Collaborative

Prepare for/assist with administration of thrombolytic agents, e.g., alteplase (t-PA), streptokinase (Streptase). Transfer to critical care, and other measures as indicated.

RATIONALE

In the event of infarct extension, or new MI, thrombolytic therapy is the treatment of choice (when initiated within 6 hours) to dissolve the clot (if that is the cause of the MI) and restore perfusion of the myocardium. *Note:* t-PA has a better outcome (compared with streptokinase) if begun within 3 hours of vascular occlusion/onset of chest pain.

NURSING DIAGNOSIS: Fluid Volume excess, risk for

Risk factors may include
Decreased organ perfusion (renal)
Increased sodium/water retention
Increased hydrostatic pressure or decreased plasma proteins (sequestering of fluid in interstitial space/tissues)

Possibly evidenced by
[Not applicable; presence of signs and symptoms establishes an *actual* diagnosis]

DESIRED OUTCOMES/EVALUATION CRITERIA—PATIENT WILL:
Maintain fluid balance as evidenced by BP within patient's normal limits.
Be free of peripheral/venous distention and dependent edema, with lungs clear and weight stable.

ACTIONS/INTERVENTIONS

Independent

Auscultate breath sounds for presence of crackles.

Note JVD, development of dependent edema.

Measure intake/output, noting decrease in output, concentrated appearance. Calculate fluid balance.

Weigh daily.

Maintain total fluid intake at 2000 ml/24 h within cardiovascular tolerance.

Collaborative

Provide low-sodium diet/beverages.

Administer diuretics, e.g., furosemide (Lasix), spirolactone with hydrochlorothiazide (Aldactazide), hydralazine (Apresoline).

RATIONALE

May indicate pulmonary edema secondary to cardiac decompensation.

Suggests developing congestive failure/fluid volume excess.

Decreased cardiac output results in impaired kidney perfusion, sodium/water retention, and reduced urine output. Recurrent positive fluid balance in presence of other symptoms suggests volume excess/cardiac failure.

Sudden changes in weight reflect alterations in fluid balance.

Meets normal adult body fluid requirements but may require alteration/restriction in presence of cardiac decompensation.

Sodium enhances fluid retention and should therefore be restricted.

May be necessary to correct fluid overload. Drug choice is usually dependent on acute/chronic nature of symptoms.

ACTIONS/INTERVENTIONS	RATIONALE
Collaborative	
Monitor potassium as indicated.	Hypokalemia can limit effectiveness of therapy and can occur with use of potassium-depleting diuretics.

> **NURSING DIAGNOSIS: Knowledge deficit [learning need] regarding condition, treatment needs, self care and discharge needs**
>
> **May be related to**
> Lack of factual information regarding cardiac functioning/implications of heart disease and future health status
> Need for lifestyle changes
> Unfamiliarity with postdischarge therapy/self-care needs
>
> **Possibly evidenced by**
> Statements of concern/misconceptions, questions
> Development of preventable complications
>
> **DESIRED OUTCOMES/EVALUATION CRITERIA—PATIENT WILL:**
> Verbalize understanding of own heart disease, treatment plan, purpose of medications, and side effects/adverse reactions.
> Relate symptoms that require immediate attention.
> Identify/plan for necessary lifestyle changes.

ACTIONS/INTERVENTIONS	RATIONALE
Independent	
Assess patient/SO level of knowledge and ability/desire to learn.	Necessary for creation of individual instruction plan. Reinforces expectation that this will be a "learning experience." Verbalization identifies misunderstandings and allows for clarification.
Be alert to signs of avoidance, e.g., changing subject away from information being presented or extremes of behavior (withdrawal/euphoria).	Natural defense mechanisms, such as anger, denial of significance of situation, can block learning, affecting patient's response and ability to assimilate information. Changing to a less formal/structured style may be more effective until patient/SO is ready to accept/deal with current situation.
Present information in varied learning formats, e.g., programmed books, audio/visual tapes, question/answer sessions, group activities.	Using multiple learning methods enhances retention of material.
Reinforce explanations of risk factors, dietary/activity restrictions, medications, and symptoms requiring immediate medical attention.	Provides opportunity for patient to retain information and to assume control/participate in rehabilitation program.
Encourage identification/reduction of individual risk factors, e.g., smoking/alcohol consumption, obesity.	These behaviors/chemicals have direct adverse effect on cardiovascular function and may impede recovery, increase risk for complications.
Warn against isometric activity, Valsalva maneuver, and activities requiring arms positioned above head.	These activities greatly increase cardiac work/myocardial oxygen consumption and may adversely affect myocardial contractility/output.

Independent

ACTIONS/INTERVENTIONS	RATIONALE
Review programmed increases in levels of activity. Educate patient regarding gradual resumption of activities, e.g., walking, work, recreational and sexual activity. Provide guidelines for gradually increasing activity and instruction regarding target heart rate and pulse taking, as appropriate.	Gradual increase in activity increases strength and prevents overexertion, may enhance collateral circulation, and allows return to normal lifestyle.
Identify alternate activities for "bad weather" days, such as measured walking in house or shopping mall.	Provides for continuing daily activity program.
Review signs/symptoms requiring reduction in activity and notification of healthcare provider.	Pulse elevations beyond established limits, development of chest pain, or dyspnea may require changes in exercise and medication regimen.
Stress importance of follow-up care and identify community resources/support groups, e.g., cardiac rehabilitation programs, "Coronary Clubs," smoking cessation clinics.	Emphasizes that this is an ongoing/continuing health problem for which support/assistance is available postdischarge.
Emphasize importance of contacting physician if chest pain, change in anginal pattern, or other symptoms recur.	Timely evaluation/intervention may prevent complications.
Stress importance of reporting development of fever in association with diffuse/atypical chest pain (pleural, pericardial) and joint pain.	Post-MI complication of pericardial inflammation (Dressler's syndrome) requires further medical evaluation/intervention.

POTENTIAL CONSIDERATIONS following discharge from care setting (dependent on patient's age, physical condition/presence of complications, personal resources, and life responsibilities)

Activity intolerance—imbalance between myocardial oxygen supply/demand.

Grieving, anticipatory—perceived loss of general well-being, required changes in lifestyle, confronting mortality.

Decisional Conflict (treatment)—multiple/divergent sources of information, perceived threat to value system, support system deficit.

Family Processes, altered—situational transition and crisis.

Home Maintenance Management, impaired—altered ability to perform tasks, inadequate support systems, reluctance to request assistance.

DYSRHYTHMIAS

Cardiac dysrhythmias are changes in heart rate and rhythm caused by abnormal electrical conduction or auto-maticity. Dysrhythmias vary in severity and in their effects on cardiac function, which is partially influenced by the site of origin (ventricular or supraventricular).

CARE SETTING

Generally, minor dysrhythmias are monitored and treated in the physician's office/clinic setting; however, potential life-threatening situations usually require a short inpatient stay.

RELATED CONCERNS

Heart Failure: Chronic, p 45
Myocardial Infarction, p 71
Psychosocial Aspects of Care, p 783

Patient Assessment Data Base

ACTIVITY/REST

May report:	Weakness, generalized and exertional fatigue
May exhibit:	Changes in heart rate/BP with activity/exercise

CIRCULATION

May report:	History of previous/acute MI (90%–95% experience dysrhythmias), cardiomyopathy, HF, valvular heart disease, hypertension History of pacemaker insertion Pulse: Fast, slow, or irregular; palpitations, skipped beats
May exhibit:	BP changes, e.g., hypertension or hypotension during episodes of dysrhythmia Pulses: May be irregular, e.g., skipped beats; pulsus alternans (regular strong beat/weak beat); bigeminal pulse (irregular strong beat/weak beat) Pulse deficit (difference between apical pulse and radial pulse) Heart sounds: Irregular rhythm, extra sounds, dropped beats Skin: Color and moisture changes, e.g., pallor, cyanosis, diaphoresis (heart failure, shock) Edema: Dependent, generalized, JVD (in presence of heart failure) Urine output: Decreased if cardiac output is severely diminished

EGO INTEGRITY

May report:	Feeling nervous (certain tachydysrhythmias), sense of impending doom Stressors related to current medical problems
May exhibit:	Anxiety, fear, withdrawal, anger, irritability, crying

FOOD/FLUID

May report:	Loss of appetite, anorexia Food intolerance (with certain medications) Nausea/vomiting Changes in weight

May exhibit: Weight gain or loss
                     Edema
                     Changes in skin moisture/turgor
                     Respiratory crackles

NEUROSENSORY

May report: Dizzy spells, fainting, headaches

May exhibit: Mental status/sensorium changes, e.g., disorientation, confusion, loss of memory;
                    changes in usual speech pattern/consciousness, stupor, coma
                    Behavioral changes, e.g., combativeness, lethargy, hallucinations
                    Pupil changes (equality and reaction to light)
                    Loss of deep tendon reflexes with life-threatening dysrhythmias (ventricular tachycardia,
                    severe bradycardia)

PAIN/DISCOMFORT

May report: Chest pain, mild to severe, which may or may not be relieved by antianginal medication
May exhibit: Distraction behaviors, e.g., restlessness

RESPIRATION

May report: Chronic lung disease
                    History of or current tobacco use
                    Shortness of breath
                    Coughing (with/without sputum production)

May exhibit: Changes in respiratory rate/depth during dysrhythmia episode
                    Breath sounds: Adventitious sounds (crackles, rhonchi, wheezing) may be present indi-
                    cating respiratory complications, such as left heart failure (pulmonary edema) or
                    pulmonary thromboembolic phenomena
                    Hemoptysis

SAFETY

May exhibit: Fever
                    Skin: Rashes (medication reaction)
                    Loss of muscle tone/strength

TEACHING/LEARNING

May report: Familial risk factors, e.g., heart disease, stroke
                    Use/misuse of prescribed medications, e.g., heart medications (digitalis); anticoagulants
                    (Coumadin); or OTC medications, e.g., cough syrup and analgesics containing ASA
                    Lack of understanding about disease process/therapeutic regimen
                    Evidence of failure to improve, e.g., recurrent/intractable dysrhythmias that are life-
                    threatening

Discharge plan   DRG projected mean length of inpatient stay: 3.2 days
considerations: Alteration of medication use/therapy

                    Refer to section at end of plan for postdischarge considerations.

DIAGNOSTIC STUDIES

ECG: Demonstrates patterns of ischemic injury and conduction aberrance. Reveals type/source of dysrhythmia and effects of electrolyte imbalances and cardiac medications. *Note:* Exercise ECG can reveal dysrhythmias occurring only when patient is not at rest (can be diagnostic for cardiac cause of syncope).

Holter monitor: Extended ECG tracing (24 hours) may be desired to determine which dysrhythmias may be causing specific symptoms when patient is active (home/work). May also be used to evaluate pacemaker function, antidysrhythmia drug effect, or effectiveness of cardiac rehabilitation.

Signal-averaged ECG (SAE): May be used to screen high-risk patients (especially post-MI or with unexplained syncope) for ventricular dysrhythmias. Diagnoses presence of delayed conduction and late potentials (as occurs with sustained ventricular tachycardia).

Chest x-ray: May show enlarged cardiac shadow due to ventricular or valve dysfunction.

Myocardial imaging scans: May demonstrate ischemic/damaged myocardial areas that could impede normal conduction or impair wall motion and pumping capabilities.

HIS bundle study: Provides a cardiac mapping of entire conduction system to evaluate normal and abnormal pathways of electrical conduction. Used to diagnose dysrhythmias and evaluate effectiveness of medication or pacemaker therapies.

Electrolytes: Elevated or decreased levels of potassium, calcium, and magnesium can cause dysrhythmias.

Drug screen: May reveal toxicity of cardiac drugs, presence of street drugs, or suggest interaction of drugs, e.g., digitalis, quinidine, and so on.

Thyroid studies: Elevated or depressed serum thyroid levels can cause/aggravate dysrhythmias.

Sedimentation rate: Elevation may indicate acute/active inflammatory process, e.g., endocarditis, as a precipitating factor for dysrhythmias.

ABGs/pulse oximetry: Hypoxemia can cause/exacerbate dysrhythmias.

NURSING PRIORITIES

1. Prevent/treat life-threatening dysrhythmias.
2. Support patient/SO in dealing with anxiety/fear of potentially life-threatening situation.
3. Assist in identification of cause/precipitating factors.
4. Review information regarding condition/prognosis/treatment regimen.

DISCHARGE GOALS

1. Free of life-threatening dysrhythmias and complications of impaired cardiac output/tissue perfusion.
2. Anxiety reduced/managed.
3. Disease process, therapy needs, and prevention of complications understood.
4. Plan in place to meet needs after discharge.

NURSING DIAGNOSIS: Cardiac Output, decreased, risk for

Risk factors may include
Altered electrical conduction
Reduced myocardial contractility

Possibly evidenced by:
[Not applicable; presence of signs and symptoms establishes an *actual* diagnosis.]

DESIRED OUTCOMES/EVALUATION CRITERIA—PATIENT WILL:
Maintain/achieve adequate cardiac output as evidenced by BP/pulse within normal range, adequate urinary output, palpable pulses of equal quality, usual level of mentation.
Display reduced frequency/absence of dysrhythmia(s).
Participate in activities that reduce myocardial workload.

ACTIONS/INTERVENTIONS	RATIONALE

Independent

Palpate pulses (radial, carotid, femoral, dorsalis pedis) noting rate, regularity, amplitude (full/thready), and symmetry. Document presence of pulsus alternans, bigeminal pulse, or pulse deficit.

Differences in equality, rate, and regularity of pulses are indicative of the effect of altered cardiac output on systemic/peripheral circulation.

Auscultate heart sounds noting rate, rhythm. Note presence of extra heart beats, dropped beats.

Specific dysrhythmias are more clearly detected audibly than by palpation. Hearing extra heart beats or dropped beats helps identify dysrhythmias in the unmonitored patient.

Monitor vital signs and assess adequacy of cardiac output/tissue perfusion. Report significant variations in BP/pulse rate equality, respirations, changes in skin color/temperature, level of consciousness/sensorium, and urine output during episodes of dysrhythmias.

Although not all dysrhythmias are considered life-threatening, immediate treatment to terminate dysrhythmia may be required in the presence of alterations in cardiac output and tissue perfusion.

Determine type of dysrhythmia and document with rhythm strip (if cardiac/telemetry monitoring is available):

Useful in determining need for/type of intervention required.

Tachycardia;

Tachycardia can occur in response to stress, pain, fever, infection, coronary artery blockage, valvular dysfunction, hypovolemia, hypoxia, or as a result of decreased vagal tone or increased sympathetic nervous system activity with the release of catecholamines. Persistent tachycardia may worsen underlying pathology in patients with ischemic heart disease because of shortened diastolic filling time and increased oxygen demands.

Bradycardia;

Bradycardia is common in patients with acute MI (especially inferior) and is the result of excessive parasympathetic activity, blocks in conduction to the SA or AV nodes, or loss of automaticity of the heart muscle. Patients with severe heart disease may not be able to compensate for a slow rate by increasing stroke volume. Therefore, decreased cardiac output, HF, and potentially lethal ventricular dysrhythmias may occur.

Atrial dysrhythmias;

PACs can occur as a response to ischemia and are normally harmless but can precede or precipitate AF. Acute and chronic atrial flutter and/or fibrillation can occur with coronary artery or valvular disease and may or may not be pathologic. Rapid atrial flutter/fibrillation reduces cardiac output as a result of incomplete ventricular filling (shortened cardiac cycle) and increased oxygen demand.

Ventricular dysrhythmias;

PVCs or VPBs reflect cardiac irritability and are commonly associated with MI, digitalis toxicity, coronary vasospasm, and misplaced temporary pacemaker leads. Frequent, multiple, or multifocal PVCs result in diminished cardiac output and may lead to potentially lethal dysrhythmias, e.g., VT or sudden death/cardiac arrest from ventricular flutter/fibrillation. *Note:* Intractable ventricular dysrhythmias unresponsive to medication may reflect ventricular aneurysm.

ACTIONS/INTERVENTIONS	RATIONALE

Independent

Heart blocks.

Reflect altered transmission of impulses through normal conduction channels (slowed, altered), and may be the result of MI, coronary artery disease with reduced blood supply to SA or AV nodes, drug toxicity, and sometimes cardiac surgery. Progressing heart block is associated with slowed ventricular rates, decreased cardiac output, and potentially lethal ventricular dysrrhythmias or cardiac standstill.

Provide calm/quiet environment. Review reasons for limitation of activities during acute phase.

Reduces stimulation and release of stress-related catecholamines, which cause/aggravate dysrhythmias and vasoconstriction and increase myocardial workload.

Demonstrate/encourage use of stress management behaviors, e.g., relaxation techniques, guided imagery, slow/deep breathing.

Promotes patient participation in exerting some sense of control in a stressful situation.

Investigate reports of chest pain, documenting location, duration, intensity, and relieving/aggravating factors. Note nonverbal pain cues, e.g., facial grimacing, crying, changes in BP/heart rate.

Reasons for chest pain are variable and depend on underlying cause of dysrhythmias. However, chest pain may indicate ischemia due to decreased myocardial perfusion or increased oxygen need (impending/evolving MI).

Be prepared for/initiate CPR as indicated.

Development of life-threatening dysrythmias requires prompt intervention to prevent ischemic damage/death.

Collaborative

Monitor laboratory studies, e.g.

Electrolytes;

Imbalance of electrolytes such as potassium, magnesium, and calcium, adversely affects cardiac rhythm and contractility.

Drug levels.

Reveals therapeutic/toxic level of prescription medications or street drugs that may affect/contribute to presence of dysrhythmias.

Administer supplemental oxygen as indicated.

Increases amount of oxygen available for myocardial uptake, which decreases irritability caused by hypoxia.

Administer medications as indicated:

Dysrhythmias are generally treated symptomatically, except for ventricular prematures, which may be treated prophylactically in acute MI.

Potassium;

Correction of hypokalemia may be sufficient to terminate some ventricular dysrhythmias.

Antidysrhythmics, such as:

Group Ia, e.g., disopyramide (Norpace), procainamide (Pronestyl, Procan SR), quinidine (Quinaglute);

These drugs *increase* action potential, duration, and effective refractory period, and *decrease* membrane responsiveness prolonging both QRS complex and QT interval. Useful for treatment of atrial and ventricular premature beats, repetitive dysrhythmias (e.g., atrial tachycardias and atrial flutter/fibrillation). *Note:* Myocardial depressant effects may be potentiated when Group Ia drugs are used in conjunction with any drugs possessing similar properties.

Collaborative

Group Ib, e.g., lidocaine (Xylocaine), phenytoin (Dilantin), tocainide (Tonocard), mexiletine (Mexitil);

These drugs shorten duration of refractory period (QT interval), and their action depends on the tissue affected and the level of extracellular potassium. Drugs of choice for ventricular dysrhythmias, they are also effective for automatic and reentrant dysrhythmias and digitalis-induced dysrhythmias. *Note:* These drugs may aggravate myocardial depression.

Group Ic, e.g., flecainide (Tambocor), propafenone (Rhythmol), encainide (Enkaid);

These drugs slow conduction by depressing SA node automaticity and decreasing conduction velocity through the atria, ventricles, and Purkinje fibers. The result is prolongation of the P-R interval and lengthening of the QRS complex. They suppress and prevent all types of ventricular dysrhythmias. *Note:* Flecainide increases risk of drug-induced dysrhythmias post MI. Propafenone can worsen or cause new dysrhythmias, a tendency called the "proarrhythmic effect." Encainde is available only for patients who demonstrated a good result prior to drug being removed from the market.

Group II, e.g., propranolol (Inderal), nadolol (Corgard), acebutolol (Monitan), esmolol (Brevibloc), sotalol (Betapace);

β-adrenergic blockers have antiadrenergic properties and decrease automaticity. Therefore, they are useful in the treatment of dysrhythmias occurring because of SA and AV node dysfunction (e.g., supraventricular tachycardias, atrial flutter or fibrillation). *Note:* These drugs may exacerbate bradycardia and cause myocardial depression, especially when combined with drugs with similar properties.

Group III e.g.; bretylium tosylate (Bretylol), amiodarone (Cordarone), sotalol (Betapace);

These drugs prolong refractory period and action potential duration, consequently prolonging Q-T interval. They are used to terminate ventricular fibrillation as well as other life-threatening ventricular dysrhythmias/sustained ventricular tachyarrhythmias, especially when lidocaine/pronestyl is not effective. *Note:* Sotalol is a nonselective β-blocker with characteristics of both Class II and III.

Group IV e.g., verapamil (Calan), nifedipine (Procardia), diltiazem (Cardizem);

Calcium antagonists slow conduction time through the AV node (prolonging P-R interval) to decrease ventricular response in supraventricular tachycardias, atrial flutter/fibrillation.

Miscellaneous e.g., atropine sulfate, isoproterenol (Isuprel), cardiac glycosides: digitalis (Lanoxin);

Useful in treating bradycardia by increasing SA and AV conduction and enhancing automaticity. Cardiac glycosides may be used alone or in combination with other antidysrhythmic drugs to reduce ventricular rate in presence of uncontrolled/poorly tolerated atrial tachycardias or flutter/fibrillation.

Adenosine (Adenocard).

Unclassified first-line treatment for paroxysmal supraventricular tachycardia. Slows conduction and interrupts reentry pathways in AV node. *Note:* Contraindicated in patients with 2° or 3° heart block or those with sick sinus syndrome who do not have a functioning pacemaker.

ACTIONS/INTERVENTIONS	RATIONALE
Collaborative	
Prepare for/assist with elective cardioversion.	May be used in atrial fibrillation or certain unstable dysrhythmias to restore normal heart rate/relieve symptoms of heart failure.
Assist with insertion/maintain pacemaker function.	Temporary pacing may be necessary to accelerate impulse formation or override tachydysrhythmias and ectopic activity, in order to maintain cardiovascular function until spontaneous pacing is restored, or permanent pacing is initiated.
Insert/maintain IV access.	Patent access line may be required for administration of emergency drugs.
Prepare for invasive diagnostic procedures/surgery as indicated.	Differential diagnosis of underlying cause may be required to formulate appropriate treatment plan. Resection of ventricular aneurysm may be required to correct intractable ventricular dysrhythmias unresponsive to medical therapy. CABG may be indicated to enhance circulation to myocardium and conduction system.
Prepare for implantation of cardioverter/defibrillator (ICD) when indicated.	This device may be surgically implanted in those patients with recurrent, life-threatening ventricular dysrhythmias despite carefully tailored drug therapy. Third-generation devices can provide multilevel ("tiered") therapy, i.e., pacing, cardioversion, and/or defibrillation, depending on how each device is programmed.

NURSING DIAGNOSIS: Poisoning, risk for digitalis toxicity

Risk factors may include:
Limited range of therapeutic effectiveness, lack of education/proper precautions, reduced vision/cognitive limitations

Possibly evidenced by:
[Not applicable; presence of signs and symptoms establishes an *actual* diagnosis]

DESIRED OUTCOMES/EVALUATION CRITERIA—PATIENT WILL:
Verbalize understanding of individual prescription, how it interacts with other drugs/substances, and importance of maintaining prescribed regimen.
Be free of signs of toxicity, display serum drug level within individually acceptable range.
Recognize signs of digitalis overdose and developing heart failure, and what to report to physician.

ACTIONS/INTERVENTIONS	RATIONALE
Independent	
Explain patient's specific type of digitalis preparation.	Reduces confusion due to digitalis preparations varying in name (although they may be similar), dosage strength, and onset and duration of action. Up to 15% of all patients receiving digitalis develop toxicity some time during the course of therapy.

ACTIONS/INTERVENTIONS	RATIONALE
Independent	
Instruct patient not to change dose for any reason, not to omit dose (unless instructed to depend on pulse rate), not to increase dose or take extra doses, and to contact doctor if more than one dose is omitted.	Alterations in drug regimen can reduce therapeutic effects/result in toxicity and cause complications.
Advise patient that digitalis may react with many other drugs (e.g., barbiturates, neomycin, quinidine) and that physician should be informed that digitalis is taken whenever new medications are prescribed. Advise patient not to use OTC drugs (e.g., laxatives, antidiarrheals, antacids, cold remedies, diuretics) without first checking with the pharmacist or healthcare provider.	Knowledge may help prevent dangerous drug interactions.
Review importance of dietary and supplemental intake of potassium, calcium, and magnesium.	Maintaining electrolytes at normal ranges may prevent or limit development of toxicity/correct many associated dysrhythmias.
Provide information and have the patient/SO verbalize understanding of toxic signs/symptoms to report to the healthcare provider.	Nausea, vomiting, diarrhea, unusual drowsiness, confusion, very slow or very fast irregular pulse, thumping in chest, double/blurred vision, yellow/green tint or halos around objects, flickering color forms or dots, altered color perception and worsening heart failure (e.g., dependent/generalized edema, dyspnea, decreased amount/frequency of voiding), indicate need for prompt evaluation/intervention. Mild symptoms of toxicity may be managed with a brief drug holiday. *Note:* In severe/refractory heart failure, altered cardiac binding of digitalis may result in toxicity even with previously appropriate drug doses.
Discuss necessity of periodic laboratory evaluation:	
Serum digoxin (Lanoxin) or digitoxin (Crystodigin) level;	Digitalis has a narrow therapeutic serum range, with toxicity occurring at levels that are dependent on individual response. Laboratory levels are evaluated in conjunction with clinical manifestations and ECG to determine individual therapeutic levels/resolution of toxicity.
Electrolytes, BUN, creatinine, liver function studies.	Abnormal levels of potassium, calcium, or magnesium increase the heart's sensitivity to digitalis. Impaired kidney function can cause Lanoxin (mainly excreted by the kidney) to accumulate to toxic levels. Crystodigin levels (mainly excreted by the bowel) are affected by impaired liver function.
Collaborative	
Administer other appropriate antidysrhythmia medications, e.g., Lidocaine, propanalol, and procanamide.	May be necessary to maintain/improve cardiac output in presence of excess effect of digitalis.
Prepare patient for transfer to critical care unit as indicated (e.g., dangerous dysrhythmias/exacerbation of heart failure).	In the presence of digitalis toxicity, patients frequently require intensive monitoring until therapeutic levels have been restored. Because all digitalis preparations have long serum half-lives, stabilization can take several days.

NURSING DIAGNOSIS: Knowledge deficit [learning need] regarding cause/treatment of condition, self care and discharge needs

May be related to

Lack of information/misunderstanding of medical condition/therapy needs

Unfamiliarity with information resources

Lack of recall

Possibly evidenced by

Questions; statement of misconception

Failure to improve on previous regimen

Development of preventable complications

DESIRED OUTCOMES/EVALUATION CRITERIA—PATIENT WILL:

Verbalize understanding of condition, treatment regimen, and function of pacemaker (if used).

List desired action and possible adverse side effects of medications.

Correctly perform necessary procedures and explain reasons for actions.

Relate signs of pacemaker failure.

ACTIONS/INTERVENTIONS	RATIONALE
Independent	
Review normal cardiac function/electrical conduction.	Provides a knowledge base to understand individual variations and to understand reasons for therapeutic interventions.
Explain/reinforce specific dysrhythmia problem and therapeutic measures to patient/SO.	Ongoing/updated information (e.g., whether or not the problem is resolving or may require long-term control measures) can decrease anxiety associated with the unknown and prepare patient/SO to make necessary lifestyle adaptations. Educating the SO may be especially important if the patient is elderly, visually or hearing impaired, or unable or even unwilling to learn/follow instructions. Repeated explanations may be needed, because anxiety and/or bulk of new information can block/limit learning.
Identify adverse effects/complications of specific dysrhythmias, e.g., fatigue, dependent edema, progressing changes in mentation, vertigo.	Dysrhythmias may decrease cardiac output manifested by symptoms of developing cardiac failure/altered cerebral perfusion. Tachydysrhythmias may also be accompanied by debilitating anxiety/feelings of impending doom.
Instruct/document teaching regarding medications. Include why the drug is needed (desired action); how and when to take the drug; what to do if a dose is forgotten (dosage and usage information); expected side effects or possible adverse reactions/interactions with other prescribed/OTC drugs or substances (alcohol, tobacco); as well as what and when to report to the physician.	Information necessary for patient to make informed choices and to manage medication regimen.
Encourage development of regular exercise routine, avoiding overexertion. Identify signs/symptoms requiring immediate cessation of activities, e.g., dizziness, lightheadedness, dyspnea, chest pain.	When dysrhythmias are properly managed, normal activity should not be affected. Exercise program is useful in improving overall cardiovascular well-being.

Review individual dietary needs/restrictions, e.g., potassium, caffeine.

Depending on specific problem, patient may need to increase dietary potassium, such as when potassium-depleting diuretics are used. Caffeine may be limited to prevent cardiac excitation.

Provide information in written form for patient/SO to take home.

Follow-up reminders may enhance patient's understanding and cooperation with the desired regimen. Written instructions are a helpful resource when patient is not in direct contact with healthcare team.

Instruct patient in proper pulse-taking technique. Encourage daily recording of pulse before medication and during exercise. Identify situations requiring immediate medical intervention.

Continued self-observation/monitoring provides for timely intervention to avoid complications. Medication regimen may be altered or further evaluation may be required when heart rate varies from desired rate or pacemaker's preset rate.

Review safety precautions, techniques to evaluate/maintain pacemaker or ICD function, and symptoms requiring medical intervention.

Promotes self-care, provides for timely interventions to prevent serious complications. Instructions/concerns will be dependent on function and type of device, as well as the patient's condition and presence/absence of family or caregivers.

Review procedures to terminate PAT e.g., carotid/sinus massage, Valsalva maneuver, if appropriate.

On occasion, these procedures may be deemed necessary in some patients to restore regular rhythm/cardiac output in emergency situations.

POTENTIAL CONSIDERATIONS following discharge from care setting (dependent on patient's age, physical condition/presence of complications, personal resources and life responsibilities)

Activity intolerance—imbalance between oxygen supply/demand.

Therapeutic Regimen: Individual, ineffective management—complexity of therapeutic regimen, decisional conflicts, economic difficulties, inadequate number/types of cues to action.

CARDIAC SURGERY: CORONARY ARTERY BYPASS GRAFT; CARDIOMYOPLASTY; VALVE REPLACEMENT (POSTOPERATIVE CARE)

The goal of treatment for heart disease is to maximize cardic output. Surgically, this may be done by improving myocardial muscle function and blood flow through procedures such as coronary artery bypass grafting, wrapping the latissimus dorsi muscle around the heart, and/or repair or replacement of defective valves. Of the three types of cardiac surgery: (1) reparative (e.g., closure of atrial or ventricular septal defect, repair of mitral stenosis); (2) reconstructive (e.g., CABG, reconstruction of an incompetent valve) and; (3) substitutional (e.g., valve replacement, cardiac transplant), reparative surgeries are more likely to produce cure or prolonged improvement.

CARE SETTING

Inpatient acute hospital on a surgical or post-ICU stepdown unit.

RELATED CONCERNS

Angina Pectoris, p 61
Heart Failure: Chronic, p 45
Dysrhythmias, p 85
Hemothorax/Pneumothorax, p 154
Myocardial Infarction, 71
Psychosocial Aspects of Care, p 783
Surgical Intervention, p 802

Patient Assessment Data Base

The preoperative data presented here are dependent on the specific disease process and underlying cardiac condition/reserve.

ACTIVITY/REST

May report: History of exercise intolerance
Generalized weakness, fatigue
Inability to perform expected/usual life activities

May exhibit: Abnormal heart rate, BP changes with activity
Exertional discomfort or dyspnea
ECG changes/dysrhythmias

CIRCULATION

May report: History of recent/acute MI, three (or more) vessel coronary artery disease, valvular heart disease, hypertension

May exhibit: Variations in BP, heart rate/rhythm
Abnormal heart sounds: S_3/S_4 murmurs
Pallor/cyanosis of skin or mucous membranes
Cool/cold, clammy skin
Edema, JVD
Diminished peripheral pulses
Crackles
Restlessness/other changes in mentation or sensorium (severe cardiac decompensation)

95

EGO INTEGRITY

May report: Feeling frightened/apprehensive, helpless
Distress over current events (anger/fear)
Fear of death/eventual outcome of surgery, possible complications
Fear about changes in lifestyle/role functioning

May exhibit: Apprehension
Restlessness
Insomnia/sleep disturbance
Facial/general tension
Withdrawal/lack of eye contact
Crying
Focus on self, hostility, anger
Changes in heart rate, BP, breathing patterns

FOOD/FLUID

May report: Change in weight
Loss of appetite
Abdominal pain, nausea/vomiting
Change in urine frequency/amount

May exhibit: Weight gain/loss
Dry skin, poor skin turgor
Postural hypotension
Diminished/absent bowel sounds
Edema (generalized, dependent, pitting)

NEUROSENSORY

May report: Fainting spells, vertigo

May exhibit: Changes in orientation or usual response to stimuli
Restlessness; irritability
Apathy; exaggerated emotional responses

PAIN/DISCOMFORT

May report: Chest pain, angina
Postoperative
    Incisional discomfort
    Pain/paresthesia of shoulders, arms, hands, legs

May exhibit: **Postoperative**
    Guarding
    Facial mask of pain; grimacing
    Distraction behaviors; moaning; restlessness
    Changes in BP/pulse/respiratory rate

RESPIRATION

May report: Shortness of breath
Postoperative
    Inability to cough or take a deep breath

May exhibit: **Postoperative**
    Decreased chest expansion
    Splinting/muscle guarding
    Dyspnea (normal response to thoractomy)

Areas of diminished or absent breath sounds (atelectasis)
Anxiety
Changes in ABGs/pulse oximetry

SAFETY

May report: Infectious episode with valvular involvement

May exhibit: **Postoperative**
Oozing/bleeding from chest or donor site incisions

TEACHING/LEARNING

May report: Familial risk factors of diabetes, heart disease, hypertension, strokes
Use of various cardiovascular drugs
Failure to improve

Discharge plan considerations: **DRG projected mean length of inpatient stay: 11.2 days. (may be divided among multiple levels of care)**
Assistance with food preparation, shopping, transportation, self-care needs and home-maker/home maintenance tasks

Refer to section at end of plan for postdischarge considerations.

DIAGNOSTIC STUDIES (POSTOPERATIVE)

Hemoglobin/hematocrit: Decreased Hb reduces oxygen-carrying capacity and indicates need for red blood cell replacement. Elevation of Hct suggests dehydration/need for fluid replacement.

Coagulation studies: Various studies may be done (e.g., platelet count, bleeding and clotting time) to determine possible problems before surgery.

Electrolytes: Imbalances (hyperkalemia/hypokalemia, hypernatremia/hyponatremia, and hypocalcemia) can affect cardiac function and fluid balance.

ABGs: Identifies oxygenation status/effectiveness of respiratory function and acid/base balance.

Pulse oximetry: Noninvasive measure of oxygenation at tissue level.

BUN/creatinine: Reflects adequacy of renal and liver perfusion/function.

Amylase: Elevation is occasionally seen in high-risk patients, e.g., those with heart failure undergoing valve replacement.

Glucose: Fluctuations may occur due to preoperative nutritional status, presence of diabetes/organ dysfunction, rate of dextrose infusions.

Cardiac enzymes/isoenzymes: Elevated in the presence of acute, recent, or perioperative MI.

Chest x-ray: Reveals heart size and position, pulmonary vasculature, and changes indicative of pulmonary complications (e.g., atelectasis). Verifies condition of valve prosthesis and sternal wires, position of pacing leads, intravascular/cardiac lines.

ECG: Identifies changes in electrical/mechanical function such as might occur in immediate postoperative phase, acute/perioperative MI, valve dysfunction, and/or pericarditis.

Cardiac echocardiogram/catheterization: Abnormal chamber pressures and pressure gradients across valves are present with valve disease. Findings in coronary artery disease include occlusions of arteries, impaired coronary perfusion, and possible wall-motion abnormalities.

Nuclear studies (e.g., thallium 201, DPY-thallium/Persantine): Heart scans demonstrate coronary artery disease, heart chamber dimensions, and presurgical/postsurgical functional capabilities.

NURSING PRIORITIES

1. Support hemodynamic stability/ventilatory function.
2. Promote relief of pain/discomfort.
3. Promote healing.
4. Provide information about postoperative expectations and treatment regimen.

DISCHARGE GOALS

1. Activity tolerance adequate to meet self-care needs.
2. Pain alleviated/managed.
3. Complications prevented/minimized.
4. Incisions healing.
5. Postdischarge medications, exercise, diet, therapy understood.
6. Plan in place to meet needs after discharge.

NURSING DIAGNOSIS: Cardiac Output, decreased, risk for

Risk factors may include

Decreased myocardial contractility secondary to temporary factors (e.g., ventricular wall surgery, recent MI, response to certain medications/drug interactions)
Decreased preload (hypovolemia)
Alterations in electrical conduction (dysrhythmias)

Possibly evidenced by

[Not applicable; presence of signs and symptoms establishes an *actual* diagnosis]

DESIRED OUTCOMES/EVALUATION CRITERIA—PATIENT WILL:

Report/display decreased episodes of angina and dysrhythmias.
Demonstrate an increase in activity tolerance.
Participate in activities that maximize/enhance cardiac function.

ACTIONS/INTERVENTIONS	RATIONALE
Independent	
Monitor/document trends in heart rate and BP, especially noting hypertension. Be aware of specific systolic/diastolic limits defined for patient.	Tachycardia is a common response to discomfort and anxiety, inadequate blood/fluid replacement, and the stress of surgery; however, sustained tachycardia increases cardiac workload and can decrease effective cardiac output. Hypertension can occur (fluid excess or preexisting condition) placing stress on suture lines of new grafts and changing blood flow/pressure within heart chambers and across valves, with increased risk for various complications. Hypotension may result from fluid deficit, dysrhythmias, heart failmture/shock.
Monitor/document cardiac dysrhythmias. Observe patient response to dysrhythmias, e.g., drop in BP.	Life-threatening dysrhythmias can occur due to electrolyte imbalance, myocardial ischemia, or alterations in the heart's electrical conduction. Decreased cardiac output and hemodynamic compromise occurring with dysrhythmias require prompt intervention.
Observe for changes in usual mental status/orientation/body movement or reflexes, e.g., onset of confusion, disorientation, restlessness, reduced response to stimuli, stupor.	May indicate decreased cerebral blood flow or oxygenation as a result of diminished cardiac output (sustained or severe dysrhythmias, low BP, heart failure, or thromboembolic phenomena).
Record skin temperature/color, and quality/equality of peripheral pulses.	Warm, pink skin and strong, equal pulses are general indicators of adequate cardiac output.
Measure/document intake, output, and fluid balance.	Useful in determining fluid needs or identifying fluid excesses, which can compromise cardiac output/oxygen consumption.

ACTIONS/INTERVENTIONS

Independent

Schedule uninterrupted rest/sleep periods. Assist with self-care activities.

Monitor graded activity program. Note patient response, vital signs before/during/after activity, development of dysrhythmias.

Evaluate presence/degree of anxiety/emotional duress. Encourage the use of relaxation techniques, e.g., deep breathing, diversional activities.

Inspect for JVD, peripheral or dependent edema, congestion in lungs, shortness of breath, change in mental status.

Investigate reports of angina/severe chest pain, accompanied by restlessness, diaphoresis, ECG changes.

Investigate/report profound hypotension (unresponsive to fluid challenge), tachycardia, distant heart sounds, stupor/coma.

Collaborative

Review serial ECGs.

Measure cardiac output and other functional parameters as indicated.

Administer IV fluids/blood transfusions as indicated.

Administer supplemental oxygen as indicated.

Administer electrolytes and medications as indicated, e.g., electrolyte solutions/potassium, antidysrhythmics, β-blockers, digitalis, diuretics, anticoagulants.

RATIONALE

Prevents fatigue/overexhaustion and excessive cardiovascular stress.

Regular exercise stimulates circulation/cardiovascular tone and promotes feeling of well-being. Progression of activity is dependent on cardiac tolerance.

Excessive/escalating emotional reactions can affect vital signs and systemic vascular resistance, eventually affecting cardiac function.

May be indicative of heart failure (acute or chronic).

Although not a common complication of CABG, perioperative or postoperative MI can occur.

Development of cardiac tamponade can rapidly progress to cardiac arrest due to inability of the heart to fill adequately for effective cardiac output. *Note:* This is a relatively rare life-threatening complication that usually occurs in the immediate postoperative period but can occur later in the recovery phase.

Most frequently done to follow the progress in normalization of electrical conduction patterns/ventricular function after surgery or to identify complications, e.g., perioperative MI.

Cardiac index, preload/afterload, contractility, and cardiac work can be measured noninvasively using thoracic electrical bioimpedance (TEB) technique. Useful in evaluating response to therapeutic interventions and identifying need for more aggressive/emergency care.

IV fluids may be discontinued prior to discharge from the intensive care unit, or 1 line (central/peripheral) may remain in place for fluid replacement and/or emergency cardiac medications. Red blood cell replacement may be indicated on occasion to restore/maintain adequate circulating volume and enhance oxygen-carrying capacity.

Promotes maximal oxygenation, which can reduce cardiac workload, aid in resolving myocardial ischemia and dysrhythmias.

Patient needs are variable, depending on type of surgery (CABG or valve replacement), response to surgical intervention, and preexisting conditions (e.g., general health, age, type of heart disease). Electrolytes, antidysrhythmics, and other heart medications may be required on a short-term or long-term basis to maximize cardiac contractility/output.

99

ACTIONS/INTERVENTIONS

Collaborative

Maintain surgically placed pacing wires (atrial/ventricular), and initiate pacing if indicated.

RATIONALE

May be required to support cardiac output in presence of conduction disturbances (severe dysrhythmias) which compromise cardiac function.

NURSING DIAGNOSIS: Pain [acute]/[Discomfort]

May be related to
Sternotomy (mediastinal incision) and/or donor site (leg/arm incision)
Myocardial ischemia (acute MI, angina)
Tissue inflammation/edema formation
Intraoperative nerve trauma

Possibly evidenced by
Reports of incisional discomfort/pain, paresthesia, pain in hand, arm, shoulder
Anxiety, restlessness, irritability
Distraction behaviors
Increased heart rate

DESIRED OUTCOMES/EVALUATION CRITERIA—PATIENT WILL:
Verbalize relief/absence of pain.
Demonstrate relaxed body posture, ability to rest/sleep appropriately.
Differentiate surgical discomfort from angina/preoperative heart pain.

ACTIONS/INTERVENTIONS

Independent

Note type/location of incision(s).

Encourage patient to report type, location, and intensity of pain, rating on a scale of 0–10. Ask the patient how this compares with preoperative chest pain.

Observe for anxiety, irritability, crying, restlessness, sleep disturbances.

Monitor vital signs.

Identify/promote position of comfort using adjuncts as necessary.

RATIONALE

Newer procedures may require only a "mini" chest incision, with minimal pain.

Pain is perceived, manifested, and tolerated individually. It is important for the patient to differentiate incisional pain from other types of chest pain, e.g., angina. Many CABG patients do not experience severe discomfort in chest incision and may complain more often of donor site incision discomfort. Severe pain in either area should be investigated further for possible complications.

These nonverbal cues may indicate the presence/degree of pain being experienced.

Heart rate usually increases with pain, although a bradycardiac response can occur in a severely diseased heart. BP may be elevated slightly with incisional discomfort but may be decreased or unstable if chest pain is severe and/or myocardial damage is occurring.

Pillows/blanket rolls are useful in supporting extremities, maintaining body alignment, and splinting incisions to reduce muscle tension/promote comfort.

ACTIONS/INTERVENTIONS	RATIONALE
Independent	
Provide comfort measures (e.g., back rubs, position changes), assist with self-care activities and encourage diversional activities as indicated.	May promote relaxation/redirect attention and reduce analgesic dosage needs/frequency.
Schedule care activities to balance with adequate periods of sleep/rest.	Rest and sleep are vital for cardiac healing (balance between oxygen demand and consumption), and can enhance coping with stress and discomfort.
Identify/encourage use of behaviors such as guided imagery, distractions, visualizations, deep breathing.	Relaxation techniques aid in management of stress, promote sense of well-being, may reduce analgesic needs, and promote healing.
Tell patient that it is acceptable, even preferable, to request analgesics as soon as discomfort becomes noticeable.	Presence of pain causes muscle tension, which can impair circulation, slow healing process, and intensify pain.
Medicate prior to procedures/activities as indicated.	Patient comfort and cooperation in respiratory treatments, ambulation, and procedures (e.g., removal of chest tubes, pacemaker wires and suture removal) are facilitated by prior analgesic administration.
Investigate reports of pain in unusual areas (e.g., calves of legs, abdomen) or vague complaints of discomfort, especially when accompanied by changes in mentation, vital signs, respiratory rate.	May be an early manifestation of developing complication, e.g., thrombophlebitis, infection, gastrointestinal dysfunction.
Note reports of pain and/or numbness in ulnar area (fourth and fifth digits) of the hand often accompanied by pain/discomfort of the arms and shoulders. Tell the patient that the problem usually resolves with time.	Indicative of a stretch injury of the brachial plexus as a result of the position of the arms during surgery. No specific treatment is currently useful.
Collaborative	
Administer medications as indicated, e.g., propoxyphene and acetaminophen (Darvocet-N), acetaminophen and oxycodone (Tylox).	Usually provides for adequate control of pain and reduces muscle tension, which improves patient comfort and promotes healing.

NURSING DIAGNOSIS: Role Performance, altered

May be related to
Situational crisis (dependent role)/recuperative process
Uncertainty about future

Possibly evidenced by
Delay/alteration in physical capacity to resume role
Change in usual role or responsibility
Change in self/others' perception of role

DESIRED OUTCOMES/EVALUATION CRITERIA—PATIENT WILL:
Verbalize realistic perception and acceptance of self in changed role.
Talk with SO about situation and changes that have occurred.
Develop realistic plans for adapting to perceived role changes.

ACTIONS/INTERVENTIONS

Independent

Assess patient role in family constellation. Identify concerns about role dysfunction/interruption, e.g., recuperation, health-illness transitions.

Assess level of anxiety, patient's perception of degree of threat to self/life.

Note cultural factors affecting role changes.

Maintain positive attitude toward the patient, providing opportunities for the patient to exercise control as much as possible.

Assist patient/SO to develop strategies for dealing with changes, e.g., shift responsibilities to other family members/friends or neighbors; acquire temporary assistance (homemaker/yardwork); investigate avenues for financial assistance.

Acknowledge reality of grieving process related to change in usual role (even if only temporary) and help patient to deal realistically with feelings of anger and sadness.

RATIONALE

Helps to know patient responsibilities and how illness affects this role. Dependent role of the patient provokes anxiety and concern about how the patient will be able to manage usual role responsibilities.

Information provides baseline for identifying/individualizing plan of care.

Cultural expectations regarding male/female illness role can determine how patient/SO react to and deal with current situation and may affect future adaptation to perceived changes.

Helps patient to accept changes that are occurring and to begin to realize that control over self is possible.

Planning for changes that may occur/be required promotes sense of control and accomplishment without loss of self-esteem.

Cardiac surgery constitutes a dramatic point in the patient's life, which will never be the same again. Patient needs to recognize these feelings in order to deal with them and move forward.

NURSING DIAGNOSIS: Breathing Pattern, ineffective, risk for

Risk factors may include
Inadequate ventilation (pain/muscular weakness)
Diminished oxygen-carrying capacity (blood loss)
Decreased lung expansion (atelectasis or pneumothorax/hemothorax)

Possibly evidenced by
[Not applicable; presence of signs and symptoms establishes an *actual* diagnosis]

DESIRED OUTCOMES/EVALUATION CRITERIA—PATIENT WILL:
Maintain a normal/effective respiratory pattern free of cyanosis and other signs/symptoms of hypoxia with breath sounds equal bilaterally, lung fields clearing.
Display complete reexpansion of lungs with absence of pneumothorax/hemothorax.

ACTIONS/INTERVENTIONS

Independent

Evaluate respiratory rate and depth. Note respiratory effort, e.g., presence of dyspnea, use of accessory muscles, nasal flaring.

RATIONALE

Patient responses are variable. Rate and effort may be increased by pain, fear, fever, diminished circulating volume (blood or fluid loss), accumulation of secretions, hypoxia, or gastric distention. Respiratory suppression (decreased rate) can occur from excessive use of narcotic analgesics. Early recognition and treatment of abnormal ventilation may prevent complications.

ACTIONS/INTERVENTIONS	RATIONALE
Independent	
Auscultate breath sounds. Note areas of diminished/absent breath sounds and presence of adventitious sounds, e.g., crackles or rhonchi.	Breath sounds are often diminished in lung bases for a period of time following surgery due to normally occurring atelectasis. Loss of active breath sounds in an area of previous ventilation may reflect collapse of the lung segment, especially if chest tubes have recently been removed. Crackles or rhonchi may be indicative of fluid accumulation (interstitial edema, pulmonary edema, or infection) or partial airway obstruction (pooling of secretions).
Observe chest excursion. Investigate decreased expansion or lack of symmetry in chest movement.	Air or fluid in the pleural space prevents complete expansion (usually on one side) and requires further assessment of ventilation status.
Observe character of cough and sputum production.	Frequent coughing may simply be throat irritation from operative ET tube placement or can reflect pulmonary congestion. Purulent sputum suggests onset of pulmonary infection.
Inspect skin and mucous membranes for cyanosis.	Cyanosis of lips, nailbeds, or earlobes or general duskiness may indicate a hypoxic condition due to heart failure or pulmonary complications. General pallor (commonly present in immediate postoperative period) may indicate anemia from blood loss/insufficient blood replacement or red blood cell destruction from cardiopulmonary bypass pump.
Elevate head of bed, place in upright or semi-Fowler's position. Assist with early ambulation/increased time out of bed.	Stimulates respiratory function/lung expansion. Effective in preventing and resolving pulmonary congestion.
Encourage patient participation/responsibility for deep-breathing exercises, use of adjuncts (blow bottles), and coughing, as indicated.	Aids in reexpansion/maintaining patency of small airways especially after removal of chest tubes. Coughing is not necessary unless wheezes/rhonchi are present, indicating retention of secretions.
Reinforce splinting of chest with pillows during deep breathing/coughing.	Reduces incisional tension, promotes maximal lung expansion, and may enhance effectiveness of cough effort.
Explain that coughing/respiratory treatments will not loosen/damage grafts or reopen chest incision.	Provides reassurance that injury will not occur and may enhance cooperation with therapeutic regimen.
Encourage maximal fluid intake within cardiac reserves.	Adequate hydration helps liquefy secretions, facilitating expectoration.
Medicate with analgesic before respiratory treatments, as indicated.	Allows for easier chest movement and reduces discomfort related to incisional pain, facilitating patient cooperation with/effectiveness of respiratory treatments.
Record response to deep-breathing exercises or other respiratory treatment noting breath sounds (before/after treatment), cough/sputum production.	Documents effectiveness of therapy or need for more aggressive interventions.
Investigate/report respiratory distress, diminished or absent breath sounds, tachycardia, severe agitation, drop in BP.	Although not a common complication, hemothorax/pneumothorax may occur following removal of the chest tubes and requires prompt intervention to maintain respiratory function.

103

Collaborative

ACTIONS/INTERVENTIONS	RATIONALE
Review chest x-ray reports and laboratory studies (ABGs, hemoglobin) as indicated.	Monitors effectiveness of respiratory therapy and/or documents developing complications. A blood transfusion may be needed if blood loss is the reason for respiratory hypoxemia.
Assist with use of incentive spirometer/blow bottles.	Used to maximize lung inflation, reduce atelectasis, and prevent pulmonary complications.
Administer supplemental oxygen by cannula or mask, as indicated.	Enhances oxygen delivery to the lungs for circulatory uptake, especially in presence of reduced/altered ventilation.
Assist with reinsertion of chest tubes or thoracentesis if indicated.	Reexpands lung by removal of accumulated blood/air and restoration of negative pleural pressure.

NURSING DIAGNOSIS: Skin Integrity, impaired

May be related to
Surgical incisions, puncture wounds

Possibly evidenced by
Disruption of skin surface

DESIRED OUTCOMES/EVALUATION CRITERIA—PATIENT WILL:
Demonstrate behaviors/techniques to promote healing, prevent complications.
Display timely wound healing.

ACTIONS/INTERVENTIONS

RATIONALE

Independent

Inspect all incisions. Evaluate healing progress. Review expectations for healing with patient.	Healing begins immediately, but complete healing will take time. Chest incision heals first (minimal muscle tissue), but donor site incision (when saphenous vein used) will require more time (more muscle tissue, longer incision, slower circulation). As healing progresses, the incision lines may appear dry with crusty scabs. Underlying tissue may look bruised and feel tense, warm, and lumpy (resolving hematoma).
Suggest wearing soft cotton shirts and loose-fitting clothing, cover/pad incisions as indicated, leave incisions open to air as much as possible.	Reduces suture line irritation and pressure from clothing. Leaving incisions open to air promotes healing process and may reduce risk of infection.
Have patient shower in warm water, washing incisions gently. Tell patient to avoid tub baths until approved by physician.	Keeps incision clean, promotes circulation/healing. *Note:* "Climbing" out of tub requires use of arms and pectoral muscles, which can put undue stress on sternotomy.
Support incisions with Steri-strips (as needed) when sutures are removed.	Aids in maintaining approximation of wound edges to promote healing when saphenous vein is used.
Encourage elevation of legs when sitting up in chair.	Promotes circulation, reduces edema to improve tissue healing.

ACTIONS/INTERVENTIONS

Independent

Watch for/report to physician: places in incision that do not heal; reopening of healed incision; any drainage (bloody or purulent); localized area that is swollen with redness, feels increasingly painful, and is hot to touch.

Promote adequate nutritional and fluid intake.

Collaborative

Obtain specimen of wound drainage as indicated.

RATIONALE

Signs/symptoms indicating failure to heal; development of complications requiring further evaluation/intervention.

Helps to maintain good circulating volume for tissue perfusion and meets cellular energy requirements to facilitate tissue regeneration/healing process.

If infection occurs, local and systemic treatments may be required, e.g., peroxide/saline/Betadine soaks, antibiotic therapy.

NURSING DIAGNOSIS: Knowledge deficit [learning need] regarding condition, postoperative care, self care and discharge needs

May be related to
Lack of exposure
Information misinterpretation
Lack of recall

Possibly evidenced by
Questions/requests for information
Verbalization of problem
Statement of misconception
Inaccurate follow-through of instructions

DESIRED OUTCOMES/EVALUATION CRITERIA—PATIENT WILL:
Participate in learning process.
Assume responsibility for own learning.
Begin to look for information/ask questions.
Verbalize understanding of condition, prognosis, and therapeutic needs.

ACTIONS/INTERVENTIONS

Independent

Reinforce surgeon's explanation of particular surgical procedure, providing diagram as appropriate.

Incorporate this information into discussion about short-/long-term recovery expectations.

Review prescribed exercise program and progress to date. Assist patient/SO to set realistic goals.

RATIONALE

Provides individually specific information creating knowledge base for subsequent learning regarding home management.

Length of rehabilitation and prognosis is dependent on type of surgical procedure, preoperative physical condition, and duration/severity of complications.

Individual capabilities and expectations are dependent on type of surgery, underlying cardiac function, and prior physical conditioning.

105

ACTIONS/INTERVENTIONS	RATIONALE

Independent

Encourage alternating rest periods with activity and light tasks with heavy tasks. Avoid heavy lifting, isometric/strenuous upper-body exercise.	Prevents excessive fatigue/overexhaustion. *Note:* Strenuous use of arms can place undue stress on sternotomy.
Problem-solve with patient/SO ways to continue progressive activity program during temperature exntremes and high wind/pollution days, e.g., walking predetermined distance within own house or local indoor shopping mall/exercise tract.	Having a plan will forestall giving up exercise because of interferences such as weather.
Schedule rest periods and short naps several times a day.	Rest and sleep enhance coping abilities, reduce nervousness (common in this phase), and promote healing.
Reinforce physician's time limitations about lifting, driving, returning to work, and resumption of sexual activity.	These restrictions are present until after the first postoperative office visit for assessment of sterum healing.
Discuss issues concerning resumption of sexual activity, e.g., comparison of stress of sexual intercourse with other activities;	Concerns about sexual activity often go unexpressed, but patients usually desire information about what to expect. In general, patient can safely engage in sexual act when activity level has advanced to point where patient can climb two flights of stairs (which is about the same amount of energy expenditure).
Position recommendations;	Patient should avoid positions that restrict breathing (sexual activity increases oxygen demand and consumption). Patient should not support self or partner with arms (breast bone healing, support muscles stretched).
Expectations of sexual performance;	Impotence appears to occur with some regularity in postoperative cardiac surgery patients. Although etiology is unknown, condition usually resolves in time without specific intervention. If situation persists, may require further evaluation.
Appropriate timing, e.g., avoid sexual intercourse following heavy meal; during periods of emotional distress; when patient is fatigued/exhausted;	Timing of activity may reduce occurrence of complications/angina.
Pharmacologic considerations.	Some patients may require antianginal medications (prophylactically) before sexual activity.

POTENTIAL CONSIDERATIONS following discharge from care setting (dependent on patient's age, physical condition/presence of complications, personal resources and life responsibilities)

Activity intolerance—generalized weakness, sedentary lifestyle.
Skin/Tissue Integrity, impaired—surgical incisions, puncture wounds.
Home Maintenance Management, impaired—altered ability to perform tasks, inadequate support systems, reluctance to request assistance.
Infection, risk for—broken skin, traumatized tissue, invasive procedures, decreased hemoglobin.
Self Care deficit—decreased strength and endurance, discomfort.
Role Performance, altered—situational crisis/recuperative process, uncertainty about future.

THROMBOPHLEBITIS: DEEP VEIN THROMBOSIS

Thrombophlebitis is a condition in which a clot forms in a vein secondary to inflammation/trauma of the vein wall or because of a partial obstruction of the vein. Clot formation is related to (1) stasis of blood flow, (2) abnormalities in the vessel walls, and (3) alterations in the clotting mechanism (Virchow's triad). *Note:* Approximately 50% of patients with DVT are asymptomatic.

Thrombophlebitis can affect superficial or deep veins, and while both conditions can cause symptoms, DVT is more serious in terms of potential complications, including pulmonary embolism, postphlebotic syndrome, chronic venous insufficiency, and vein valve destruction.

CARE SETTING

Primarily treated at the community level with short inpatient stay generally indicated in the presence of embolization.

RELATED CONCERNS:

Psychosocial Aspects of Care, p 783

Patient Assessment Data Base

ACTIVITY/REST

May report: Occupation that requires sitting or standing for long periods of time
Lengthy immobility, (e.g., orthopedic trauma, long hospitalization/bedrest, complicated pregnancy); paralysis/progressive debilitating condition
Pain with activity/prolonged standing
Fatigue/weakness of affected extremity, general malaise

May exhibit: Generalized or extremity weakness

CIRCULATION

May report: History of previous vascular disease, venous thrombosis, preexisting varices
Presence of other predisposing factors, e.g., hypertension (pregnancy-induced); diabetes mellitus, MI/valvular heart disease; thrombotic cerebrovascular accident

May exhibit: Tachycardia
Peripheral pulse may be diminished in the affected extremity (DVT)
Varicosities and/or hardened, bumpy/knotty vein (thrombus)
Skin color/temperature in affected extremity (calf/thigh): pale, cool, edematous (DVT); pinkish red, warm along the course of the vein (superficial)
Positive Homans' sign (absence does not rule out DVT as only about 20% of patients have a positive sign)

FOOD/FLUID

May exhibit: Poor skin turgor, dry mucous membranes (dehydration predisposes to hypercoagulability)
Obesity (predisposes to stasis and pelvic vein pressure)
Edema of affected extremity (dependent on location of thrombus)

PAIN/DISCOMFORT

May report: Throbbing, tenderness, aching pain aggravated by standing or movement (affected extremity)

May exhibit: Guarding of affected extremity

SAFETY

May report: History of direct or indirect injury to extremity or vein (e.g., major trauma/fractures, orthopedic/pelvic surgery, prolonged labor with fetal head pressure on pelvic veins, intravenous therapy)

Presence of malignancy (particularly of the pancreas, lung, GI system)

May exhibit: Fever, chills

TEACHING/LEARNING

May report: Use of oral contraceptives/estrogens; recent anticoagulant therapy (predisposes to hypercoagulability)

Recurrence/lack of resolution of previous thrombophlebotic episode

Discharge plan considerations: **DRG projected mean length of inpatient stay: 7.7 days**

Assistance with shopping, transportation, and homemaker/maintenance tasks

Properly fitted antiembolic hose

DIAGNOSTIC STUDIES

Hematocrit: Hemoconcentration (elevated Hct) potentiates risk of thrombus formation.

Coagulation studies: May reveal hypercoagulability.

Noninvasive vascular studies (Doppler oscillometry, exercise tolerance, impedance plethysmography, and real-time (duplex) ultrasonography): Changes in blood flow and volume identify venous occlusion, vascular damage, and vascular insufficiency. Ultrasonography appears to be most accurate noninvasive method for diagnosing multiple proximal DVT (iliac, femoral, popliteal), but is less reliable in detecting isolated calf vein thrombi.

Trendelenburg test: May demonstrate vessel valve incompetence.

Venography: Radiographically confirms diagnosis through changes in blood flow and/or size of channels.

MRI: May be useful in assessing blood flow turbulence and movement, venous valvular competence.

NURSING PRIORITIES

1. Maintain/enhance tissue perfusion, facilitate resolution of thrombus.
2. Promote optimal comfort.
3. Prevent complications.
4. Provide information about disease process/prognosis and treatment regimen.

DISCHARGE GOALS

1. Tissue perfusion improved in affected limb.
2. Pain/discomfort relieved.
3. Complications prevented/resolved.
4. Disease process/prognosis and therapeutic needs understood.
5. Plan in place to meet needs after discharge.

NURSING DIAGNOSIS: Tissue Perfusion, altered, peripheral

May be related to

Decreased blood flow/venous stasis (partial or complete venous obstruction)

Possibly evidenced by
Tissue edema, pain
Diminished peripheral pulses, slow/diminished capillary refill
Skin color changes (pallor, erythema)

DESIRED OUTCOMES/EVALUATION CRITERIA—PATIENT WILL:
Demonstrate improved perfusion as evidenced by peripheral pulses present/equal, skin color and temperature normal, absence of edema.
Engage in behaviors/actions to enhance tissue perfusion.
Display increasing tolerance to activity.

ACTIONS/INTERVENTIONS

Independent

Evaluate neurological function of extremity—both sensory and motor. Inspect for skin color and temperature changes, as well as edema (from groin to foot). Note symmetry of calves; measure and record calf circumference. Report proximal progression of inflammatory process, traveling pain.

Examine extremity for obviously prominent veins. Palpate (gently) for local tissue tension, stretched skin, knots/bumps along course of vein.

Assess capillary refill and check for Homans' sign.

Promote bed rest with legs elevated 6″ above heart level during acute phase.

Elevate legs when in bed or chair, as indicated. Periodically elevate feet and legs above heart level.

Initiate active or passive exercises while in bed (e.g., flex/extend/rotate foot periodically). Assist with gradual resumption of ambulation (e.g., walking 10 min/h) as soon as patient is permitted out of bed.

RATIONALE

Symptoms help distinguish between superficial thrombophlebitis and DVT. Redness, heat, tenderness, and localized edema are characteristic of superficial involvement. Pallor and coolness of extremity are characteristic of DVT. Calf-vein involvement of DVT is associated with absence of edema; femoral-vein involvement is associated with mild to moderate edema; iliofemoral-vein thrombosis is characterized by severe edema.

Distention of superficial veins can occur in DVT because of backflow through communicating veins. Evidence of thrombophlebitis in superficial veins may be visible or palpable.

Diminished capillary refill usually present in DVT. Positive Homans' sign (deep calf pain in affected leg upon dorsiflexion of foot) is not as consistent a clinical manifestation as once thought and may or may not be present.

Until treatment is instituted, limitation of activity reduces oxygen and nutrient demands on affected extremity and minimizes the possibility of dislodging thrombus/creating emboli, elevation of legs 6″ (6 degrees) can increase peak blood velocity by 33%. *Note:* Caution is required in presence of leg ischemia.

Reduces tissue swelling and rapidly empties superficial and tibial veins, preventing overdistention and thereby increasing venous return. *Note:* Some physicians believe that elevation may potentiate release of thrombus, thus increasing risk of embolization and decreasing circulation to the most distal portion of the extremity.

These measures are designed to increase venous return from lower extremities and reduce venous stasis, as well as improve general muscle tone/strength. They also promote normal organ function, and enhance general well-being.

ACTIONS/INTERVENTIONS	RATIONALE
Independent	
Caution patient to avoid crossing legs or hyperflexion at knee (seated position with legs dangling, or lying in jackknife position).	Physical restriction of circulation impairs blood flow and increases venous stasis in pelvic, popliteal, and leg vessels, thus increasing swelling and discomfort.
Instruct patient to avoid rubbing/massaging the affected extremity.	This activity potentiates risk of fragmenting/dislodging thrombus, causing embolization and increasing risk of complications.
Encourage deep-breathing exercises.	Increases negative pressure in thorax, which assists in emptying large veins.
Increase fluid intake to at least 2000 ml/d, within cardiac tolerance.	Dehydration increases blood viscosity and venous stasis, predisposing to thrombus formation.
Collaborative	
Apply warm, moist compresses, or heat cradle to affected extremity if indicated.	May be prescribed to promote vasodilation and venous return and resolution of local edema. *Note:* May be contraindicated in presence of arterial insufficiency, in which heat can increase cellular oxygen consumption/nutritional needs, furthering imbalance between supply and demand.
Administer anticoagulants, e.g.:	
Heparin via continuous or intermittent IV, intermittent subcutaneous (SC) injections; and/or coumarin derivatives (Coumadin);	Heparin is preferred initially because of its prompt, predictable antagonistic action on thrombin as it is formed and also because it removes activated coagulation factors XII, XI, IX, X (intrinsic pathway), preventing further clot formation. Coumadin has a potent depressant effect on liver formation of prothrombin from vitamin K and impairs formation of factors VII, IX, X (extrinsic pathway). Coumadin may be used for long-term/postdischarge therapy. *Note:* A new low-molecular-weight heparin derivative, Enoxaparin (Lovenex) is a fast-acting substance (given SQ for 7–10 days), which prevents the conversion of factor Xa to thrombin. Currently used to prevent DVT after hip replacement surgery, it is also under investigation for treating proximal DVT.
Thrombolytic agents, e.g., streptokinase, urokinase.	May be used for treatment of acute (less than 5 days old) or massive DVT to prevent valvular damage and development of chronic venous insufficiency. Heparin is usually begun several hours after the completion of thrombolytic therapy.
Monitor laboratory studies as indicated: prothrombin time (PT), partial thromboplastin time (PTT), activated partial thromboplastin time (aPTT), CBC.	Monitors anticoagulant therapy and presence of risk factors, e.g., hemoconcentration and dehydration, which potentiate clot formation. *Note:* Enoxaparin does not require serial monitoring as PT or aPTT are not affected.
Apply/regulate graduated compression stockings, intermittent pneumatic compression, if indicated.	Sequential compression devices may be used to improve blood flow velocity and emptying of vessels by providing artificial muscle-pumping action.

ACTIONS/INTERVENTIONS

Collaborative

Apply elastic support hose following acute phase. Take care to avoid tourniquet effect.

Prepare for surgical intervention when indicated.

RATIONALE

Properly fitted support hose are useful (once ambulation has begun) to minimize or delay development of postphlebotic syndrome. They must exert a sustained, evenly distributed pressure over entire surface of calves and thighs to reduce the caliber of superficial veins and increase blood flow to deep veins.

Thrombectomy (excision of thrombus) is occasionally necessary if inflammation extends proximally or circulation is severely restricted. Multiple/recurrent thrombotic episodes unresponsive to medical treatment (or when anticoagulant therapy is contraindicated) may require insertion of a vena caval screen/umbrella.

NURSING DIAGNOSIS: Pain [acute]/[Discomfort]

May be related to
Diminished arterial circulation and oxygenation of tissues with production/accumulation of lactic acid in tissues
Inflammatory process

Possibly evidenced by
Reports of pain, tenderness, aching/burning
Guarding of affected limb
Restlessness, distraction behaviors

DESIRED OUTCOMES/EVALUATION CRITERIA—PATIENT WILL:
Report pain/discomfort is alleviated or controlled.
Verbalize methods that provide relief.
Display relaxed manner; be able to sleep/rest and engage in desired activity.

ACTIONS/INTERVENTIONS

Independent

Assess degree and characteristics of discomfort/pain. Note guarding of extremity. Palpate leg with caution.

Maintain bed rest during acute phase.

Elevate affected extremity.

Provide foot cradle.

RATIONALE

Degree of pain is directly related to extent of circulatory deficit, inflammatory process, degree of tissue ischemia, and extent of edema associated with thrombus development. Changes in characteristics of pain may indicate progression of problem/development of complications.

Reduces discomfort associated with muscle contraction and movement.

Encourages venous return to facilitate circulation, reducing stasis/edema formation.

Cradle keeps pressure of bedclothes off the affected leg, thereby reducing pressure discomfort.

ACTIONS/INTERVENTIONS	RATIONALE

Independent

Encourage patient to change position frequently.	Decreases/prevents muscle fatigue, helps minimize muscle spasm, maximizes circulation to tissues.
Monitor vital signs, noting elevated temperature.	Elevations in heart rate may indicate increased pain/discomfort or occur in response to fever and inflammatory process. Fever can also increase patient's discomfort.
Investigate reports of sudden and/or sharp chest pain, accompanied by dyspnea, tachycardia, and apprehension.	These signs/symptoms suggest presence of pulmonary emboli as a complication of DVT.

Collaborative

Administer medications, as indicated:	
Analgesics (narcotic/non-narcotic);	Relieves pain and decreases muscle tension.
Antipyretics, e.g., acetaminophen.	Reduces fever and inflammation. *Note:* Risk of bleeding may be increased by concurrent use of drugs that affect platelet function, e.g., ASA and NSAIDs.
Apply moist heat to extremity, if indicated.	Causes vasodilation, which increases circulation; relaxes muscles; and may stimulate release of natural endorphins.

NURSING DIAGNOSIS: Gas Exchange, impaired (in presence of pulmonary embolus)

May be related to:
Altered blood flow to alveoli or to major portions of the lung
Alveolar-capillary membrane changes (atelectasis, airway/alveolar collapse, pulmonary edema/effusion, excessive secretions/active bleeding)

Possibly evidenced by:
Profound dyspnea, restlessness, apprehension, somnolence, cyanosis
Changes in ABGs/pulse oximetry, e.g., hypoxemia and hypercapnia

DESIRED OUTCOMES/EVALUATION CRITERIA—PATIENT WILL:
Demonstrate adequate ventilation/oxygenation by ABGs within patient's normal range.
Report/display resolution/absence of symptoms of respiratory distress.

ACTIONS/INTERVENTIONS	RATIONALE

Independent

Note respiratory rate and depth, work of breathing (use of accessory muscles/nasal flaring, pursed-lip breathing).	Tachypnea and dyspnea accompany pulmonary obstruction. Dyspnea ("air hunger") and increased work of breathing may be first or only sign of subacute PE. More severe respiratory failure accompanies moderate to severe loss of functional lung units.

ACTIONS/INTERVENTIONS

Independent

Auscultate lungs for areas of decreased/absent breath sounds and the presence of adventitious sounds, e.g., crackles.

Observe for generalized duskiness and cyanosis in "warm tissues" such as earlobes, lips, tongue, and buccal membranes.

Institute measures to restore/maintain patent airways, e.g., coughing, suctioning.

Elevate head of bed as patient requires/tolerates.

Assist with frequent changes of position, and get patient out of bed/ambulate as tolerated.

Assist patient to deal with fear/anxiety that may be present:

Encourage expression of feelings, inform patient/SOs of normalcy of anxious feelings, sense of impending doom;

Provide brief explanations of what is happening and expected effects of interventions;

Monitor frequently, arrange for individual (volunteer, family, etc) to stay with patient as indicated.

Monitor vital signs. Note changes in cardiac rhythm.

Assess level of consciousness/mentation changes.

Assess activity tolerance, e.g., reports of weakness/fatigue, or vital sign changes, increased dyspnea during exertion. Encourage rest periods and limit activities to patient tolerance.

Collaborative

Prepare for lung scan.

Administer supplemental oxygen by appropriate method.

RATIONALE

Nonventilated areas may be identified by absence of breath sounds. Crackles occur in fluid-filled tissues/airways or may reflect cardiac decompensation.

Indicative of systemic hypoxemia.

Plugged/collapsed airways reduce number of functional alveoli, negatively affecting gas exchange.

Promotes maximal chest expansion, making it easier to breathe and enhancing physiological/psychological comfort.

Turning and ambulation enhance aeration of different lung segments, thereby improving gas diffusion.

Feelings of fear and severe anxiety are associated with inability to breathe and may actually increase oxygen consumption/demand.

Understanding basis of feelings may help patient regain some sense of control over emotions.

Allays anxiety related to unknown and may help reduce fears concerning personal safety.

Provides assurance that changes in condition will be noted, and that assistance is readily available.

Tachycardia, tachypnea, and changes in BP are associated with advancing hypoxemia and acidosis. Rhythm alterations and extra heart sounds may reflect increased cardiac work-load related to worsening ventilation imbalance.

Systemic hypoxemia may be demonstrated initially by restlessness and irritability, then by progressively decreased mentation.

These parameters assist in determining patient response to resumed activities and ability to participate in self-care.

May reveal pattern of abnormal perfusion in areas of ventilation (ventilation/perfusion mismatch) confirming diagnosis of PE and degree of obstruction. Absence of both ventilation and perfusion reflects alveolar congestion/airway obstruction.

Maximizes available oxygen for gas exchange, reducing work of breathing. *Note:* If obstruction is large, or hypoxemia does not respond to supplemental oxygenation, it may be necessary to move patient to critical care area for intubation and mechanical ventilation.

Collaborative

ACTIONS/INTERVENTIONS	RATIONALE
Monitor serial ABGs/pulse oximetry.	Hypoxemia is present in varying degrees, depending on the amount of airway obstruction, usual cardiopulmonary function, and presence/degree of shock. Respiratory alkalosis and metabolic acidosis may also be present.
Administer fluids (IV/PO) as indicated.	Increased fluids may be given to reduce hyperviscosity of blood (potentiates thrombus formation) or to support circulating volume/tissue perfusion.
Administer medications as indicated:	
Thrombolytic agents, e.g., streptokinase (Kabikinase, Streptase), urokinase (Abbokinase, Breakinase), alteplase (t-PA, Activase);	Indicated in massive pulmonary obstruction when the patient is seriously hemodynamically threatened. *Note:* These patients will probably be initially cared for in/transferred to the critical care setting.
Morphine sulfate, antianxiety agents.	May be necessary initially to control pain/anxiety and improve work of breathing, maximizing gas exchange.
Provide supplemental humidification, e.g., ultrasonic nebulizers.	Delivers moisture to mucous membranes and helps liquefy secretions to facilitate airway clearance.
Assist with chest physiotherapy (e.g., postural drainage and percussion of nonaffected area, blow bottles/incentive spirometer).	Facilitates deeper respiratory effort and promotes drainage of secretions from lung segments into bronchi, where they may more readily be removed by coughing/suctioning.
Prepare for/assist with bronchoscopy.	May be done to remove blood clots and clear airways.
Prepare for surgical intervention if indicated.	Vena caval ligation or insertion of an intracaval umbrella may be useful for patients who experience recurrent emboli despite adequate anticoagulation, when anticoagulation is contraindicated, or when septic emboli arising from below the renal veins do not respond to treatment. Additionally, pulmonary embolectomy may be considered in life-threatening situations.

NURSING DIAGNOSIS: Knowledge deficit [learning need] regarding condition, treatment program, self care and discharge needs

May be related to
Lack of exposure or recall
Misinterpretation of information
Unfamiliarity with information resources

Possibly evidenced by
Request for information
Statement of misconception
Inaccurate follow-through of instructions
Development of preventable complications

DESIRED OUTCOMES/EVALUATION CRITERIA—PATIENT WILL:
Verbalize understanding of disease process, treatment regimen, and limitations.
Participate in learning process.
Identify signs/symptoms requiring medical evaluation.
Correctly perform therapeutic procedure(s) and explain reasons for actions.

ACTIONS/INTERVENTIONS	RATIONALE
Independent	
Review pathophysiology of condition and signs/symptoms of possible complications, e.g., pulmonary emboli, chronic venous insufficiency, venous stasis ulcers (postphlebotic syndrome).	Provides a knowledge base from which patient can make informed choices and understand/identify healthcare needs. Up to 33% will experience a recurrence of DVT.
Explain purpose of activity restrictions and need for balance between activity/rest.	Rest reduces oxygen and nutrient needs of compromised tissues and decreases risk of fragmentation of thrombosis. Balancing rest with activity prevents exhaustion and further impairment of cellular perfusion.
Establish appropriate exercise/activity program.	Aids in developing collateral circulation, enhances venous return, and prevents recurrence.
Problem-solve solutions to predisposing factors that may be present, e.g., employment that requires prolonged standing/sitting; wearing of restrictive clothing (girdles/garters); use of oral contraceptives; obesity, prolonged bed rest/immobility; dehydration.	Actively involves patient in identifying and initiating lifestyle/behavior changes to promote health and prevent recurrence of condition/development of complications.
Recommend sitting with feet touching the floor, avoiding crossing of legs.	Prevents excess pressure on the popliteal space.
Discuss purpose, dosage of anticoagulant. Emphasize importance of taking drug as prescribed.	Promotes patient safety by reducing risk of inadequate therapeutic response/deleterious side effects.
Identify safety precautions, e.g., use of soft toothbrush, electric razor for shaving, gloves for gardening, avoiding sharp objects (including toothpicks), walking barefoot, engaging in rough sports/activities, or forceful blowing of nose.	Reduces the risk of traumatic injury, which potentiates bleeding/clot formation.
Review possible drug interactions and stress need to read ingredient labels of OTC drugs.	Salicylates and excess alcohol decrease prothrombin activity, whereas vitamin K (multivitamins, bananas, green leafy vegetables) increases prothrombin activity. Barbiturates increase metabolism of coumarin drugs; antibiotics alter intestinal flora and may interfere with vitamin K synthesis.
Identify untoward anticoagulant effects requiring medical attention, e.g., bleeding from mucous membranes (nose, gums), continued oozing from cuts/punctures, severe bruising after minimal trauma, development of petechiae.	Early detection of deleterious effects of therapy (prolongation of clotting time) allows for timely intervention and may prevent serious complications.
Stress importance of medical follow-up/laboratory testing.	Understanding that close supervision of anticoagulant therapy is necessary (therapeutic dosage range is narrow and complications may be deadly) promotes patient participation.
Encourage wearing of medical-alert identification bracelet/tag, as indicated.	Alerts emergency healthcare providers to use of anticoagulants.
Review purpose and demonstrate correct application/removal of antiembolic hose.	Understanding may enhance cooperation with prescribed therapy and prevent improper/ineffective use.

ACTIONS/INTERVENTIONS	RATIONALE

Independent

Instruct in meticulous skin care of lower extremities, e.g., prevent/promptly treat breaks in skin and report development of lesions/ulcers or changes in skin color.

Chronic venous congestion/postphlebotic syndrome may develop (especially in presence of severe vascular involvement and/or recurrent episodes) potentiating risk of stasis ulcers/infection.

POTENTIAL CONSIDERATIONS following discharge from care setting (dependent on patient's age, physical condition/presence of complications, personal resources and life responsibilities)

Therapeutic Regimen: Individual, ineffective management—perceived seriousness of condition susceptibility to recurrence, benefit of therapy.

CHAPTER 5

Respiratory

CHRONIC OBSTRUCTIVE PULMONARY DISEASE (COPD)

All respiratory diseases characterized by chronic obstruction to airflow fall under the broad classification of COPD, also known as chronic airflow limitations (CAL). Within that broad category the primary cause of the obstruction may vary, e.g., airway inflammation, mucus plugging, narrowed airway lumina, or airway destruction.

Asthma: Characterized by reversible constriction of bronchial smooth muscle, hypersecretion of mucus, and mucosal inflammation and edema. Precipitating factors include allergens, emotional upheaval, cold weather, exercise, chemicals, medications, and infections.

Chronic bronchitis: Widespread inflammation of airways with narrowing or blocking of airways, increased production of mucoid sputum, and marked cyanosis.

Emphysema: Most severe form of COPD, characterized by recurrent inflammation that damages and eventually destroys alveolar walls to create large blebs or bullae (air spaces) and collapsed bronchioles on expiration (air-trapping).

Note: Chronic bronchitis and emphysema coexist in many patients and are the two diseases most commonly seen in hospitalized COPD patients. Both diseases are characterized by chronic airflow limitation. Chronic bronchitis and emphysema are usually irreversible, although some effects can be mediated.

CARE SETTING

Primarily community level; however, severe exacerbations may necessitate emergency and/or inpatient stay.

RELATED CONCERNS

Heart Failure: Chronic, p 45
Pneumonia: Microbial, p 130
Psychosocial Aspects of Care, p 783
Ventilatory Assistance (Mechanical), p 176
Surgical Intervention, p 802

Patient Assessment Data Base

ACTIVITY/REST

May report:	Fatigue, exhaustion, malaise
	Inability to perform basic ADLs because of breathlessness
	Inability to sleep, need to sleep sitting up
	Dyspnea at rest or in response to activity or exercise

May exhibit: Fatigue
Restlessness, insomnia
General debilitation/loss of muscle mass

CIRCULATION

May report: Swelling of lower extremities

May exhibit: Elevated BP
Elevated heart rate/severe tachycardia, dysrhythmias
Distended neck veins (advanced disease)
Dependent edema, may not be related to heart disease
Faint heart sounds (due to increased AP chest diameter)
Skin color/mucous membranes: Normal or bluish/cyanotic; clubbing of nails and peripheral cyanosis
Pallor can indicate anemia

EGO INTEGRITY

May report: Increased stress factors
Changes in lifestyle
Feelings of hopelessness, loss of interest in life

May exhibit: Anxious, fearful, irritable behavior, emotional distress
Apathy, dull affect, withdrawal

FOOD/FLUID

May report: Nausea (side effect of medication/mucus production)
Poor appetite/anorexia (emphysema)
Inability to eat because of respiratory distress
Persistent weight loss (emphysema) or weight gain may reflect edema (bronchitis, prednisone use)

May exhibit: Poor skin turgor
Dependent edema
Diaphoresis
Weight loss (or gain), decreased muscle mass/subcutaneous fat (emphysema)
Abdominal palpation may reveal hepatomegaly (bronchitis)

HYGIENE

May report: Decreased ability/increased need for assistance with ADLs

May exhibit: Poor hygiene, body odor

RESPIRATION

May report: Variable levels of dyspnea:
Insidious and progressive onset (predominant symptom in emphysema) especially on exertion; seasonal or episodic occurrence of breathlessness (asthma); sensation of chest tightness, inability to breathe (asthma)
Chronic ''air hunger''
Persistent cough with sputum production (gray, white, or yellow), which may be copious (chronic bronchitis)
Intermittent cough episodes, usually nonproductive in early stages, although they may become productive (emphysema)
History of recurrent pneumonia, long-term exposure to chemical pollution/respiratory

irritants (e.g., cigarette smoke), or occupation dust/fumes (e.g., cotton, hemp, as-bestos, coal dust, sawdust)
Familial and hereditary factors, i.e., deficiency of α_1-antitrypsin (emphysema)
Use of oxygen at night or continuously

May exhibit: Respirations: Usually rapid, may be shallow; prolonged expiratory phase with grunting, pursed-lip breathing (emphysema)
Assumption of 3-point ("tripod") position for breathing (especially with acute exacerbation of chronic bronchitis)
Use of accessory muscles for respiration, e.g., elevated shoulder girdle, retraction of supraclavicular fossae, flaring of nares
Chest: May appear hyperinflated with increased AP diameter (barrel-shaped); minimal diaphragmatic movement
Breath sounds: May be faint with expiratory wheezes (emphysema); scattered, fine, or coarse moist crackles (bronchitis); rhonchi, wheezing throughout lung fields on expiration, and possibly during inspiration, progressing to diminished or absent breath sounds (asthma)
Percussion: Hyperresonant over lung fields (e.g., air-trapping with emphysema); dull over lung fields (e.g., consolidation, fluid, mucus)
Difficulty speaking sentences or more than 4 or 5 words at one time
Color: Pallor with cyanosis of lips, nail beds; overall duskiness; ruddy color (chronic bronchitis, "blue bloaters"). Patients with moderate emphysema are often called "pink puffers" because of normal skin color despite abnormal gas exchange and rapid respiratory rate
Clubbing of the fingers (emphysema)

SAFETY:

May report: History of allergic reactions or sensitivity to substances/environmental factors
Recent/recurrent infections
Flushing/perspiration (asthma)

SEXUALITY

May report: Decreased libido

SOCIAL INTERACTION

May report: Dependent relationship(s)
Lack of support systems
Insufficient support from/to partner/SO
Prolonged disease or disability progression

May exhibit: Inability to converse/maintain voice because of respiratory distress
Limited physical mobility
Neglectful relationships with other family members

TEACHING/LEARNING

May report: Use/misuse of respiratory drugs
Difficulty stopping smoking
Regular use of alcohol
Failure to improve

Discharge plan considerations: **DRG projected mean length of inpatient stay: 5.9 days**
Assistance with shopping, transportation, self-care needs, homemaker/home maintenance tasks
Changes in medication/therapeutic treatments, use of supplemental oxygen, ventilator support

Refer to section at end of plan for postdischarge considerations.

DIAGNOSTIC STUDIES

Chest x-ray: May reveal hyperinflation of lungs; flattened diaphragm; increased retrosternal air space; decreased vascular markings/bullae (emphysema); increased bronchovascular markings (bronchitis); normal findings during periods of remission (asthma).

Pulmonary function tests: Done to determine cause of dyspnea, to determine whether functional abnormality is obstructive or restrictive, to estimate degree of dysfunction and to evaluate effects of therapy, e.g., bronchodilators. Exercise pulmonary function studies may also be done to evaluate activity tolerance in those with known pulmonary impairment/progression of disease.

TLC: Increased in advanced bronchitis and occasionally in asthma; decreased in emphysema.

Inspiratory capacity: Reduced in emphysema.

Residual volume: Increased in emphysema, chronic bronchitis, and asthma.

FEV_1/FVC: Ratio of forced expiratory volume to forced vital capacity is decreased in bronchitis and asthma.

ABGs: Estimates progression of chronic disease process, e.g., most often PaO_2 is decreased, and $PaCO_2$ is normal or increased (chronic bronchitis and emphysema) but is often decreased in asthma; pH normal or acidotic, mild respiratory alkalosis secondary to hyperventilation (moderate emphysema or asthma).

Bronchogram: Can show cylindrical dilation of bronchi on inspiration; bronchial collapse on forced expiration (emphysema); enlarged mucous ducts seen in bronchitis.

Lung scan: Perfusion/ventilation studies may be done to differentiate between the various pulmonary diseases. COPD is characterized by a mismatch of perfusion and ventilation (i.e., areas of abnormal ventilation in area of perfusion defect).

CBC and differential: Increased hemoglobin (advanced emphysema), increased eosinophils (asthma).

Blood chemistry: α_1-antitrypsin done to verify deficiency and a diagnosis of primary emphysema.

Sputum: Culture to determine presence of infection, identify pathogen; cytologic examination to rule out underlying malignancy or allergic disorder.

ECG: Right axis deviation, peaked P waves (severe asthma); atrial dysrhythmias (bronchitis), tall, peaked P waves in leads II, III, AVF (bronchitis, emphysema); vertical QRS axis (emphysema).

Exercise ECG, stress test: Helps in assessing degree of pulmonary dysfunction, evaluating effectiveness of bronchodilator therapy, planning/evaluating exercise program.

NURSING PRIORITIES

1. Maintain airway patency.
2. Assist with measures to facilitate gas exchange.
3. Enhance nutritional intake.
4. Prevent complications, slow progression of condition.
5. Provide information about disease process/prognosis and treatment regimen.

DISCHARGE GOALS

1. Ventilation/oxygenation adequate to meet self-care needs.
2. Nutritional intake meeting caloric needs.
3. Infection treated/prevented.
4. Disease process/prognosis and therapeutic regimen understood.
5. Plan in place to meet needs after discharge.

NURSING DIAGNOSIS: Airway Clearance, ineffective

May be related to
Bronchospasm
Increased production of secretions, retained secretions, thick, viscous secretions.
Decreased energy/fatigue

Possibly evidenced by
Statement of difficulty breathing
Changes in depth/rate of respirations, use of accessory muscles

Abnormal breath sounds, e.g., wheezes, rhonchi, crackles
Cough (persistent), with/without sputum production

DESIRED OUTCOMES/EVALUATION CRITERIA—PATIENT WILL:
Maintain patent airway with breath sounds clear/clearing.
Demonstrate behaviors to improve airway clearance, e.g., cough effectively and expectorate secretions.

ACTIONS/INTERVENTIONS	RATIONALE
Independent	
Auscultate breath sounds. Note adventitious breath sounds, e.g., wheezes, crackles, rhonchi.	Some degree of bronchospasm is present with obstructions in airway and may/may not be manifested in adventitious breath sounds, e.g., scattered, moist crackles (bronchitis); faint sounds, with expiratory wheezes (emphysema); or absent breath sounds (severe asthma).
Assess/monitor respiratory rate. Note inspiratory/expiratory ratio.	Tachypnea is usually present in some degree and may be pronounced on admission or during stress/concurrent acute infectious process. Respirations may be shallow and rapid with prolonged expiration in comparison to inspiration.
Note presence/degree of dyspnea, e.g., reports of "air hunger," restlessness, anxiety, respiratory distress, use of accessory muscles.	Respiratory dysfunction is variable dependent on stage of chronic process in addition to acute process that precipitated hospitalization, e.g., infection, allergic reaction.
Assist the patient to assume position of comfort, e.g., elevate head of bed, sitting on edge of bed.	Elevation of the head of the bed facilitates respiratory function by use of gravity; however, the patient in severe distress will seek the position that most eases breathing. Supporting arms/legs with table, pillows, and so on helps reduce muscle fatigue and can aid chest expansion.
Keep environmental pollution to a minimum, e.g., dust, smoke, and feather pillows according to individual situation.	Precipitators of allergic type of respiratory reactions that can trigger onset of acute episode.
Encourage/assist with abdominal or pursed-lip breathing exercises.	Provides the patient with some means to cope with and control dyspnea and reduce air-trapping.
Observe characteristics of cough, e.g., persistent, hacking, moist. Assist with measures to improve effectiveness of cough effort.	Cough can be persistent but ineffective, especially if the patient is elderly, acutely ill, or debilitated. Coughing is most effective in an upright or in a head-down position after chest percussion.
Increase fluid intake to 3000 ml/d *within cardiac tolerance.* Provide warm/tepid liquids. Recommend intake of fluids between, instead of during, meals.	Hydration helps decrease the viscosity of secretions, facilitating expectoration. Using warm liquids may decrease bronchospasm. Fluids during meals can increase gastric distention and pressure on the diaphragm.

121

ACTIONS/INTERVENTIONS	RATIONALE
Collaborative	
Administer medications as indicated:	
Bronchodilators: e.g., anticholinergic agents: ipratropium (Atrovent); β-agonists: epinephrine (Adrenalin, Vaponefrin), albuterol (Proventil, Ventolin), terbutaline (Brethine, Brethaire), isoetharine (Bronkosol, Bronkometer);	Relaxes smooth muscles and reduces local congestion, reducing airway spasm, wheezing, and mucous production. Medications may be oral, injected, or inhaled. *Note:* Inhaled anticholinergic agents are now considered the first-line drugs for patients with stable COPD since studies indicate they have a longer duration of action with less toxicity while still providing the effective relief of the β-agonists.
Xanthines, e.g., aminophylline, oxtriphylline (Choledyl), theophylline (Bronkodyl, Theo-Dur);	Decreases mucosal edema and smooth muscle spasm (bronchospasm) by indirectly increasing cyclic AMP. May also reduce muscle fatigue/respiratory failure by increasing diaphragmatic contractility. Although theophylline has been the cornerstone of therapy, use of theophylline may be of little or no benefit in presence of adequate β-agonist regimen; however, it may sustain bronchodilation as effect of β-agonist diminishes between doses. Recent research suggests theophylline use may correlate with reduced frequency of hospitalization.
Cromolyn (Intal), flunisolide (Aerobid);	Decreases local airway inflammation and edema by inhibiting effects of histamine and other mediators.
Oral, IV, and inhaled steroids: methylprednisolone (Medrol), dexamethasone (Decadral); antihistamines, e.g., beclomethasone (Vanceril, Beclonent), triamcinolone (Azmacort);	May be used to prevent allergic reactions/inhibit release of histamine, reducing severity and frequency of airway spasm, respiratory inflammation, and dyspnea.
Antimicrobials;	Various antimicrobials may be indicated for control of respiratory infection/pneumonia. *Note:* Even in the absence of pneumonia, therapy may enhance airflow and improve outcome.
Analgesics, cough suppressants/antitussives, e.g., codeine, dextromethorphan products (Benylin DM, Comtrex, Novahistine).	Persistent, exhausting cough may need to be suppressed to conserve energy and permit the patient to rest.
Provide supplemental humidification, e.g., ultrasonic nebulizer, aerosol room humidifier.	Humidity helps reduce viscosity of secretions facilitating expectoration and may reduce/prevent formation of thick mucous plug in bronchioles.
Assist with respiratory treatments, e.g., IPPB, spirometry, chest physiotherapy.	Breathing exercises help enhance diffusion; aerosol/nebulizer medications can reduce bronchospasm and stimulate expectoration. Postural drainage and percussion enhance removal of excessive/sticky secretions and improve ventilation of bottom lung segments. *Note:* Chest physiotherapy may aggravate bronchospasms in asthmatics.
Monitor/graph serial ABGs, pulse oximetry, chest x-ray.	Establishes baseline for monitoring progression/regression of disease process and complications.

NURSING DIAGNOSIS: Gas Exchange, impaired

May be related to

Altered oxygen supply (obstruction of airways by secretions, bronchospasm; air-trapping)

Alveoli destruction

Possibly evidenced by

Dyspnea

Confusion, restlessness

Inability to move secretions

Abnormal ABG values (hypoxia and hypercapnia)

Changes in vital signs

Reduced tolerance for activity

DESIRED OUTCOMES/EVALUATION CRITERIA—PATIENT WILL:

Demonstrate improved ventilation and adequate oxygenation of tissues by ABGs within patient's normal range and be free of symptoms of respiratory distress.

Participate in treatment regimen within level of ability/situation.

ACTIONS/INTERVENTIONS	RATIONALE
Independent	
Assess respiratory rate, depth. Note use of accessory muscles, pursed-lip breathing, inability to speak/converse.	Useful in evaluating the degree of respiratory distress, and/or chronicity of the disease process.
Elevate head of bed, assist patient to assume position to ease work of breathing. Include periods of time in prone position as tolerated. Encourage deep-slow or pursed-lip breathing as individually needed/tolerated.	Oxygen delivery may be improved by upright position and breathing exercises to decrease airway collapse, dyspnea, and work of breathing. Note: Recent research supports use of prone position to increase PaO_2.
Assess/routinely monitor skin and mucous membrane color.	Cyanosis may be peripheral (noted in nail beds) or central (noted around lips/or earlobes). Duskiness and central cyanosis would indicate advanced hypoxemia.
Encourage expectoration of sputum; suction when indicated.	Thick, tenacious, copious secretions are a major source of impaired gas exchange in small airways. Deep suctioning may be required when cough is ineffective for expectoration of secretions.
Auscultate breath sounds, noting areas of decreased airflow and/or adventitious sounds.	Breath sounds may be faint because of decreased airflow or areas of consolidation. Presence of wheezes may indicate bronchospasm/retained secretions. Scattered moist crackles may indicate interstitial fluid/cardiac decompensation.
Palpate for fremitus.	Decrease of vibratory tremors suggests fluid collection or air-trapping.

123

ACTIONS/INTERVENTIONS	RATIONALE

Independent

Monitor level of consciousness/mental status. Investigate changes.	Restlessness and anxiety are common manifestations of hypoxia. Worsening ABGs accompanied by confusion/somnolence are indicative of cerebral dysfunction due to hypoxemia.
Evaluate level of activity tolerance. Provide calm, quiet environment. Limit patient's activity or encourage bed/chair rest during acute phase. Have patient resume activity gradually and increase as individually tolerated.	During severe/acute/refractory respiratory distress the patient may be totally unable to perform basic self-care activities because of hypoxemia and dyspnea. Rest interspersed with care activities remains an important part of treatment regimen. An exercise program is aimed at increasing endurance and strength without causing severe dyspnea, and can enhance sense of well-being.
Evaluate sleep patterns, note reports of difficulties and whether patient feels well rested. Provide quiet environment, group care/monitoring activities to allow periods of uninterrupted sleep; limit stimulants, e.g., caffeine; encourage position of comfort.	Multiple external stimuli and presence of dyspnea may prevent relaxation and inhibit sleep.
Monitor vital signs and cardiac rhythm.	Tachycardia, dysrhythmias, and changes in BP can reflect effect of systemic hypoxemia on cardiac function.

Collaborative

Monitor/graph serial ABGs and pulse oximetry.	$PaCO_2$ usually elevated (bronchitis, emphysema) and PaO_2 is generally decreased, so that hypoxia is present in a lesser or greater degree. *Note:* A "normal" or increased $PaCO_2$ signals impending respiratory failure for asthmatics.
Administer supplemental oxygen judiciously as indicated by ABG results and patient tolerance.	May correct/prevent worsening of hypoxia. *Note:* In chronic emphysema, patient's respiratory drive is determined by the CO_2 level and may be eliminated by excess elevation of PaO_2.
Administer drugs causing depression (e.g., antianxiety, sedative, or narcotic) with caution.	May be used to control anxiety/restlessness which increases oxygen consumption/demand, exacerbating dyspnea. Must be monitored closely as respiratory failure can occur.
Assist with noninvasive positive pressure ventilation (NIPPV), or intubation, institution/maintenance of mechanical ventilation; transfer to critical care area dependent on patient directives.	Development of/impending respiratory failure requires prompt life-saving measures. *Note:* NIPPV provides periodic ventilatory support without intubation, and may be useful in the home setting as well, to treat chronic failure or limit acute exacerbations in patients who are able to maintain spontaneous respiratory effort.
Prepare for surgical intervention as appropriate.	Screened candidates may benefit from lung volume reduction surgery (LVRS) in which hyperinflated giant bullae/cysts occupying at least 1/3 of the involved lobe, or areas of lung tissue with small cystic disease are removed. In the absence of fibrosis, this procedure removes ineffective lung tissue, allowing for better expansion and maximal blood flow to healthy tissues, thus increasing alveolar gas exchange.

> **NURSING DIAGNOSIS: Nutrition: altered, less than body requirements**
>
> **May be related to**
> Dyspnea
> Fatigue
> Medication side effects
> Sputum production
> Anorexia, nausea/vomiting
>
> **Possibly evidenced by**
> Weight loss
> Loss of muscle mass, poor muscle tone
> Fatigue
> Reported altered taste sensation
> Aversion to eating, lack of interest in food
>
> **DESIRED OUTCOMES/EVALUATION CRITERIA—PATIENT WILL:**
> Display progressive weight gain toward goal as appropriate.
> Demonstrate behaviors/lifestyle changes to regain and/or maintain appropriate weight.

ACTIONS/INTERVENTIONS	RATIONALE
Independent	
Assess dietary habits, recent food intake. Note degree of difficulty with eating. Evaluate weight and body size (mass).	The patient in acute respiratory distress is often anorectic because of dyspnea, sputum production, medications. In addition, many COPD patients habitually eat poorly, even though respiratory insufficiency creates a hypermetabolic state with increased caloric needs. As a result, patient often is admitted with some degree of malnutrition. People who have emphysema are often thin with wasted musculature.
Auscultate bowel sounds.	Diminished/hypoactive bowel sounds may reflect decreased gastric motility and constipation (common complication) related to limited fluid intake, poor food choices, decreased activity, and hypoxemia.
Give frequent oral care, remove expectorated secretions promptly, provide specific container for disposal of secretions and tissues.	Noxious tastes, smells, and sights are prime deterrents to appetite and can produce nausea and vomiting with increased respiratory difficulty.
Encourage a rest period of 1 hour before and after meals. Provide frequent small feedings.	Helps to reduce fatigue during mealtime and provides opportunity to increase total caloric intake.
Avoid gas-producing foods and carbonated beverages.	Can produce abdominal distention, which hampers abdominal breathing and diaphragmatic movement, and can increase dyspnea.
Avoid very hot or very cold foods.	Extremes in temperature can precipitate/aggravate coughing spasms.
Weigh as indicated.	Useful in determining caloric needs, setting weight goal, and evaluating adequacy of nutritional plan. *Note:* Weight loss may continue initially, despite adequate intake, as edema is resolving.

125

Collaborative

Consult dietician/nutritional support team to provide easily digested, nutritionally balanced meals by appropriate means, e.g., oral, supplemental/tube feedings, parenteral nutrition. (Refer to CP: Total Nutritional Support: Parenteral/Enteral Feeding, p 491.)	Method of feeding and caloric requirements is based on individual situation/needs to provide maximal nutrients with minimal patient effort/energy expenditure.
Review laboratory studies, e.g., serum albumin/prealbumin, transferrin, amino acid profile, iron, nitrogen balance studies, glucose, liver function studies, electrolytes. Administer vitamins/minerals/electrolytes as indicated.	Evaluates/treats deficits and monitors effectiveness of nutritional therapy.
Administer supplemental oxygen during meals, as indicated.	Decreases dyspnea and increases energy for eating, enhancing intake.

NURSING DIAGNOSIS: Infection, risk for

Risk factors may include
Inadequate primary defenses (decreased ciliary action, stasis of secretions)
Inadequate acquired immunity (tissue destruction, increased environmental exposure)
Chronic disease process
Malnutrition

Possibly evidenced by
[Not applicable; presence of signs and symptoms establishes an *actual* diagnosis]

DESIRED OUTCOMES/EVALUATION CRITERIA—PATIENT WILL:
Verbalize understanding of individual causative/risk factors.
Identify interventions to prevent/reduce risk of infection.
Demonstrate techniques, lifestyle changes to promote safe environment.

ACTIONS/INTERVENTIONS	RATIONALE
Independent	
Monitor temperature.	Fever may be present because of infection and/or dehydration.
Review importance of breathing exercises, effective cough, frequent position changes, and adequate fluid intake.	These activities promote mobilization and expectoration of secretions to reduce risk of developing pulmonary infection.
Observe color, character, odor of sputum.	Odorous, yellow, or greenish secretions suggest the presence of pulmonary infection.
Demonstrate and assist the patient in disposal of tissues and sputum. Stress proper hand-washing (nurse and patient), and use gloves when handling/disposing of tissues, sputum containers.	Prevents spread of fluid-borne pathogens.
Monitor visitors; provide masks as indicated.	Reduces potential for exposure to infectious illnesses (e.g., URI).
Encourage balance between activity and rest.	Reduces oxygen consumption/demand imbalance and improves patient's resistance to infection, promoting healing.

ACTIONS/INTERVENTIONS

Independent

Discuss need for adequate nutritional intake.

Collaborative

Obtain sputum specimen by deep coughing or suctioning for Gram's stain, culture/sensitivity.

Administer antimicrobials as indicated.

RATIONALE

Malnutrition can affect general well-being and lower resistance to infection.

Done to identify causative organism and susceptibility to various antimicrobials.

May be given for specific organisms identified by culture and sensitivity, or be given prophylactically because of high risk.

NURSING DIAGNOSIS: Knowledge deficit [learning need] regarding condition, treatment, self care and discharge needs

May be related to
Lack of information/unfamiliarity with information resources
Information misinterpretation
Lack of recall/cognitive limitation

Possibly evidenced by
Request for information
Statement of concerns/misconception
Inaccurate follow-through of instructions
Development of preventable complications

DESIRED OUTCOMES/EVALUATION CRITERIA—PATIENT WILL:
Verbalize understanding of condition/disease process and treatment.
Identify relationship of current signs/symptoms to the disease process and correlate these with causative factors.
Initiate necessary lifestyle changes and participate in treatment regimen.

ACTIONS/INTERVENTIONS

Independent

Explain/reinforce explanations of individual disease process. Encourage patient/SO to ask questions.

Instruct/reinforce rationale for breathing exercises, coughing effectively, and general conditioning exercises.

Discuss respiratory medications, side effects, adverse reactions.

RATIONALE

Decreases anxiety and can lead to improved participation in treatment plan.

Pursed-lip and abdominal/diaphragmatic breathing exercises strengthen muscles of respiration, help minimize collapse of small airways, and provide the individual with means to control dyspnea. General conditioning exercises increase activity tolerance, muscle strength, and sense of well-being.

Frequently these patients are simultaneously on several respiratory drugs that have similar side effects and potential drug interactions. It is important that the patient understand the difference between nuisance side effects (medication continued), and untoward or adverse side effects (medication possibly discontinued/changed).

127

ACTIONS/INTERVENTIONS	RATIONALE
Independent	
Demonstrate technique for using a metered-dose inhaler (MDI), such as how to hold it, taking 2–5 minutes between puffs, cleaning the inhaler.	Proper administration of drug enhances delivery and effectiveness.
Devise system for recording prescribed intermittent drug/inhaler usage.	Reduces risk of improper use/overdosage of prn medications, especially during acute exacerbations, when cognition may be impaired.
Recommend avoidance of sedative antianxiety agents unless specifically prescribed/approved by physician treating respiratory condition.	Although the patient may be nervous and feel the need for sedatives, these can depress respiratory drive and protective cough mechanisms.
Stress importance of oral care/dental hygiene.	Decreases bacterial growth in the mouth, which can lead to pulmonary infections.
Discuss importance of avoiding people with active respiratory infections. Stress need for routine influenza/pneumococcal vaccinations.	Decreases exposure to and incidence of acquired acute upper respiratory infections.
Discuss individual factors that may aggravate condition, e.g., excessively dry air, wind, environmental temperature extremes, pollen, tobacco smoke, aerosol sprays, air pollution. Encourage patient/SO to explore ways to control these factors in and around the home.	These environmental factors can induce/aggravate bronchial irritation leading to increased secretion production and airway blockage.
Review the harmful effects of smoking and advise cessation of smoking by patient and/or SO.	Cessation of smoking may slow/halt progression of COPD. Even when patient wants to stop smoking, support groups and medical monitoring may be needed. *Note:* Research studies indicate that "side-stream" or "second-hand" smoke can be as detrimental as actually smoking.
Provide information about activity limitations and alternating activities with rest periods to prevent fatigue; ways to conserve energy during activities (e.g., pulling instead of pushing, sitting instead of standing while performing tasks); use of pursed-lip breathing, side-lying position, and possible need for supplemental oxygen during sexual activity.	Having this knowledge can enable patient to make informed choices/decisions to reduce dyspnea, maximize activity level, perform most desired activities, and prevent complications.
Discuss importance of medical follow-up care, periodic chest x-rays, sputum cultures.	Monitoring disease process allows for alterations in therapeutic regimen to meet changing needs and may help prevent complications.
Review oxygen requirements/dosage for patient who is discharged on supplemental oxygen. Discuss safe use of oxygen and refer to supplier as indicated.	Reduces risk of misuse (too little/too much) and resultant complications. Promotes environmental/physical safety.
Instruct patient/SO in use of NIPPV as appropriate. Problem-solve possible side effects and identify adverse signs/symptoms, e.g., increased dyspnea, fatigue, daytime drowsiness, or headaches on awakening.	NIPPV may be used at night/periodically during day to decrease CO_2 levels, improve quality of sleep, and enhance functional level during the day. Preventing/reducing risk of skin breakdown (pressure from headgear), gastric distention, and nasal congestion/irritation, increases likelihood of positive outcome. Signs of increasing CO_2 levels indicate need for more aggressive therapy.

ACTIONS/INTERVENTIONS	RATIONALE
Independent	
Provide information/encourage participation in support groups, e.g., American Lung Association, public health department.	These patients and their SOs may experience anxiety, depression, and other reactions as they deal with a chronic disease that has an impact on their desired lifestyle. Support groups and/or home visits may be desired or needed to provide assistance, emotional support, and respite care.
Refer for evaluation of home care if indicated. Provide a detailed plan of care and baseline physical assessment to home care nurse as needed on discharge from acute care.	Provides for continuity of care. May help reduce frequency of rehospitalization.

POTENTIAL CONSIDERATIONS following acute hospitalization (dependent on patient's age, physical condition/presence of complications, personal resources, and life responsibilities)

Self Care deficit, specify—intolerance to activity, decreased strength/endurance, depression, severe anxiety.

Home Maintenance Management, impaired—intolerance to activity, inadequate support system, insufficient finances, unfamiliarity with neighborhood resources.

Infection, risk for—decreased ciliary action, stasis of secretions, tissue destruction, increased environmental exposure, chronic disease process, malnutrition.

PNEUMONIA: MICROBIAL

Pneumonia is an inflammation of the lung parenchyma, usually associated with the filling of the alveoli with fluid. Likely causes include various infectious agents, chemical irritants, and radiation therapy. This plan of care deals with bacterial and viral pneumonias, e.g., pneumococcal pneumonia, pneumocystis carinni, haemophilus influenza, mycoplasma, Gram-negative.

CARE SETTING

Hospitalization is not always necessary for people with pneumonia; however, persons at higher risk, (e.g., with ongoing/chronic health problems) are treated in hospital, as are those already hospitalized for other reasons.

RELATED CONCERNS

AIDS, p 739
Chronic Obstructive Pulmonary Disease (COPD), p 117
Psychosocial Aspects of Care, p 783
Sepsis/Septicemia, p 719
Surgical Intervention, p 802

Patient Assessment Data Base

ACTIVITY/REST

May report:	Fatigue, weakness Insomnia
May exhibit:	Lethargy Decreased tolerance to activity

CIRCULATION

May report:	History of recent/chronic HF
May exhibit:	Tachycardia Flushed appearance or pallor

EGO INTEGRITY

May report:	Multiple stressors, financial concerns

FOOD/FLUID

May report:	Loss of appetite, nausea/vomiting
May exhibit:	Distended abdomen Hyperactive bowel sounds Dry skin with poor turgor Cachectic appearance (malnutrition)

NEUROSENSORY

May report:	Frontal headache (influenza)
May exhibit:	Changes in mentation (confusion, somnolence)

PAIN/DISCOMFORT

May report:
Headache
Chest pain (pleuritic), aggravated by cough; substernal chest pain (influenza)
Myalgia, arthralgia

May exhibit:
Splinting/guarding over affected area. (Patient commonly lies on affected side to restrict movement.)

RESPIRATION

May report:
History of recurrent/chronic URI, COPD, cigarette smoking
Tachypnea, progressive dyspnea; shallow grunting respirations, use of accessory muscles, nasal flaring
Cough: Dry hacking (initially) progressing to productive cough

May exhibit:
Sputum: Pink, rusty, or purulent
Percussion: Dull over consolidated areas
Fremitus: Tactile and vocal, gradually increases with consolidation
Pleural friction rub
Breath sounds: Diminished or absent over involved area, or bronchial breath sounds over area(s) of consolidation; coarse inspiratory crackles
Color: Pallor or cyanosis of lips/nail beds

SAFETY

May report:
History of altered immune system: i.e., SLE, AIDS, steroid or chemotherapy use, institutionalization, general debilitation
Fever (e.g., 102°F–104°F)

May exhibit:
Diaphoresis
Shaking/recurrent chills
Rash may be noted in cases of rubeola or varicella

TEACHING/LEARNING

May report:
History of recent surgery; chronic alcohol use

Discharge plan considerations:
DRG projected mean length of inpatient stay: 6.8 days
Assistance with self-care, homemaker tasks.
Oxygen may be needed if predisposing condition exists.

Refer to section at end of plan for postdischarge considerations.

DIAGNOSTIC STUDIES

Chest x-ray: Identifies structural distribution (e.g., lobar, bronchial); may also reveal multiple abscesses/infiltrates, empyema (staphylococcus); scattered or localized infiltration (bacterial); or diffuse/extensive nodular infiltrates (more often viral). In mycoplasmal pneumonia, chest x-ray may be clear.

ABGs/pulse oximetry: Abnormalities may be present, depending on extent of lung involvement and underlying lung disease.

Gram's stain/cultures: Sputum collection; needle aspiration of empyema, pleural, and transtracheal or transthoracic fluids; lung biopsies; and blood cultures may be done to recover causative organism. More than 1 type of organism may be present; common bacteria include *Diplococcus pneumoniae, Staphylococcus aureus,* α-hemolytic *streptococcus, Haemophilus influenzae; CMV. Note:* Sputum cultures may not identify all offending organisms. Blood cultures may show transient bacteremia.

CBC: Leukocytosis usually present, although a low WBC may be present in viral infection, immunosuppressed conditions such as AIDS, overwhelming bacterial pneumonia. ESR is elevated.

Serologic studies, e.g., viral or Legionella titers, cold agglutinins: Assist in differential diagnosis of specific organism.

131

Lung function studies: Volumes may be decreased (congestion and alveolar collapse); airway pressure may be increased and compliance decreased. Shunting will be present (hypoxemia).

Electrolytes: Sodium and chloride may be low.

Bilirubin: May be increased.

Percutaneous aspiration/open biopsy of lung tissues: May reveal typical intranuclear and cytoplasmic inclusions (CMV); characteristic giant cells (rubeola).

NURSING PRIORITIES

1. Maintain/improve respiratory function.
2. Prevent complications.
3. Support recuperative process.
4. Provide information about disease process/prognosis and treatment.

DISCHARGE GOALS

1. Ventilation and oxygenation adequate for individual needs.
2. Complications prevented/minimized.
3. Disease process/prognosis and therapeutic regimen understood.
4. Lifestyle changes identified/initiated to prevent recurrence.
5. Plan in place to meet needs after discharge.

NURSING DIAGNOSIS: Airway Clearance, ineffective

May be related to
Tracheal bronchial inflammation, edema formation, increased sputum production
Pleuritic pain
Decreased energy, fatigue

Possibly evidenced by
Changes in rate, depth of respirations
Abnormal breath sounds, use of accessory muscles
Dyspnea, cyanosis
Cough, effective or ineffective; with/without sputum production

DESIRED OUTCOMES/EVALUATION CRITERIA—PATIENT WILL:
Identify/demonstrate behaviors to achieve airway clearance.
Display patent airway with breath sounds clearing, absence of dyspnea, cyanosis.

ACTIONS/INTERVENTIONS	RATIONALE
Independent	
Assess rate/depth of respirations and chest movement.	Tachypnea, shallow respirations, and asymmetric chest movement are frequently present because of discomfort of moving chest wall and/or fluid in lung.
Auscultate lung fields, noting areas of decreased/absent airflow and adventitious breath sounds, e.g., crackles, wheezes.	Decreased airflow occurs in areas consolidated with fluid. Bronchial breath sounds (normal over bronchus) can also occur in consolidated areas. Crackles, rhonchi, and wheezes are heard on inspiration and/or expiration in response to fluid accumulation, thick secretions, and airway spasm/obstruction.
Elevate head of bed, change position frequently.	Lowers diaphragm, promoting chest expansion, aeration of lung segments, mobilization and expectoration of secretions.

ACTIONS/INTERVENTIONS	RATIONALE
Independent	
Assist patient with frequent deep-breathing exercises. Demonstrate/help patient learn to perform activity, e.g., splinting chest and effective coughing while in upright position.	Deep breathing facilitates maximum expansion of the lungs/smaller airways. Coughing is a natural self-cleaning mechanism, assisting the cilia to maintain patent airways. Splinting reduces chest discomfort, and an upright position favors deeper, more forceful cough effort.
Suction as indicated.	Stimulates cough or mechanically clears airway in patient who is unable to do so because of ineffective cough or decreased level of consciousness.
Force fluids to at least 2500 ml/d (unless contraindicated). Offer warm, rather than cold, fluids.	Fluids (especially warm liquids) aid in mobilization and expectoration of secretions.
Collaborative	
Assist with/monitor effects of nebulizer treatments and other respiratory physiotherapy, e.g., incentive spirometer, IPPB, blow bottles, percussion, postural drainage. Perform treatments between meals and limit fluids when appropriate.	Facilitates liquefication and removal of secretions. Postural drainage may not be effective in interstitial pneumonias or those causing alveolar exudate/destruction. Coordination of treatments/schedules and oral intake reduces likelihood of vomiting with coughing, expectorations.
Administer medications as indicated: mucolytics, expectorants, bronchodilators, analgesics.	Aids in reduction of bronchospasm as well as mobilization of secretions. Analgesics are given to improve cough effort by reducing discomfort, but should be used cautiously, as they can decrease cough effort/depress respirations.
Provide supplemental fluids, e.g., IV, humidified oxygen, and room humidification.	Fluids are required to replace losses (including insensible) and aid in mobilization of secretions.
Monitor serial chest x-rays, ABGs, pulse oximetry readings. (Refer to ND: Gas Exchange, impaired, below.)	Follows progress and effects of disease process and facilitates necessary alterations in therapy.
Assist with bronchoscopy/thoracentesis, if indicated.	Occasionally needed to remove mucus plugs, drain purulent secretions, and/or prevent atelectasis.

NURSING DIAGNOSIS: Gas Exchange, impaired

May be related to
Alveolar-capillary membrane changes (inflammatory effects)
Altered oxygen-carrying capacity of blood/release at cellular level (fever, shifting oxy-hemoglobin curve)
Altered delivery of oxygen (hypoventilation)

Possibly evidenced by
Dyspnea, cyanosis
Tachycardia
Restlessness/changes in mentation
Hypoxia

DESIRED OUTCOMES/EVALUATION CRITERIA—PATIENT WILL:
Demonstrate improved ventilation and oxygenation of tissues by ABGs within patient's acceptable range and absence of symptoms of respiratory distress.
Participate in actions to maximize oxygenation.

ACTIONS/INTERVENTIONS	RATIONALE
Independent	
Assess respiratory rate, depth, and ease.	Manifestations of respiratory distress are dependent on/and indicative of the degree of lung involvement and underlying general health status.
Observe color of skin, mucous membranes, and nail beds, noting presence of peripheral cyanosis (nail beds), or central cyanosis (circumoral).	Cyanosis of nail beds may represent vasoconstriction or the body response to fever/chills; however, cyanosis of earlobes, mucous membranes, and skin around the mouth ("warm membranes") is indicative of systemic hypoxemia.
Assess mental status.	Restlessness, irritation, confusion, and somnolence may reflect hypoxemia/decreased cerebral oxygenation.
Monitor heart rate/rhythm.	Tachycardia usually present as a result of fever/dehydration but may represent a response to hypoxemia.
Monitor body temperature, as indicated. Assist with comfort measures to reduce fever and chills, e.g., addition/removal of bedcovers, comfortable room temperature, tepid or cool water sponge bath.	High fever (common in bacterial pneumonia and influenza) greatly increases metabolic demands and oxygen consumption and alters cellular oxygenation.
Maintain bed rest. Encourage use of relaxation techniques and diversional activities.	Prevents overexhaustion and reduces oxygen consumption/demands to facilitate resolution of infection.
Elevate head and encourage frequent position changes, deep breathing, and effective coughing.	These measures promote maximal inspiration, enhance expectoration of secretions to improve ventilation. (Refer to ND: Airway Clearance, ineffective, p 132.)
Assess level of anxiety. Encourage verbalization of concerns/feelings. Answer questions honestly. Visit frequently, arrange for SO/visitors to stay with patient as indicated.	Anxiety is a manifestation of psychologic concerns as well as physiologic responses to hypoxia. Providing reassurance and enhancing sense of security can reduce the psychologic component, thereby decreasing oxygen demand and adverse physiologic response.
Observe for deterioration in condition, noting hypotension, copious amounts of pink/bloody sputum, pallor, cyanosis, change in level of consciousness, severe dyspnea, restlessness.	Shock and pulmonary edema are the most common causes of death in pneumonia and require immediate medical intervention.
Collaborative	
Administer oxygen therapy by appropriate means, e.g., nasal prongs, mask, Venturi mask.	The purpose of oxygen therapy is to maintain PaO_2 above 60 mm Hg. Oxygen is administered by the method that provides appropriate delivery within the patient's tolerance.
Monitor ABGs, pulse oximetry.	Follows progress of disease process and facilitates alterations in pulmonary therapy.
Prepare for/transfer to critical care setting if indicated.	Intubation and mechanical ventilation may be required in the event of severe respiratory insufficiency.

> **NURSING DIAGNOSIS: Infection, risk for [spread]**
>
> **Risk factors may include:**
> Inadequate primary defenses (decreased ciliary action, stasis of respiratory secretions)
> Inadequate secondary defenses (presence of existing infection, immunosuppression), chronic disease, malnutrition
>
> **Possibly evidenced by:**
> [Not applicable; presence of signs and symptoms establishes an *actual* diagnosis]
>
> **DESIRED OUTCOMES/EVALUATION CRITERIA—PATIENT WILL:**
> Achieve timely resolution of current infection without complications.
> Identify interventions to prevent/reduce risk of infection.

ACTIONS/INTERVENTIONS	RATIONALE
Independent	
Monitor vital signs closely, especially during initiation of therapy.	During this period of time, potentially fatal complications (hypotension/shock) may develop.
Instruct patient concerning the disposition of secretions (e.g., raising and expectoration versus swallowing) and reporting changes in color, amount, odor of secretions.	Although patient may find expectoration offensive and attempt to limit or avoid it, it is essential that sputum be disposed of in a safe manner. Changes in characteristics of sputum reflect resolution of pneumonia or development of secondary infection.
Demonstrate/encourage good hand-washing technique.	Effective means of reducing spread/acquisition of infection.
Change position frequently and provide good pulmonary toilet.	Promotes expectoration, clearing of infection.
Limit visitors as indicated.	Reduces likelihood of exposure to other infectious pathogens.
Institute isolation precautions as individually appropriate.	Dependent on type of infection, response to antibiotics, patient's general health, and development of complications, isolation techniques may be desired to prevent spread/protect patient from other infectious processes.
Encourage adequate rest balanced with moderate activity. Promote adequate nutritional intake.	Facilitates healing process and enhances natural resistance.
Monitor effectiveness of antimicrobial therapy.	Signs of improvement in condition should occur within 24–48 hours.
Investigate sudden changes/deterioration in condition, such as increasing chest pain; extra heart sounds, altered sensorium, recurring fever, changes in sputum characteristics.	Delayed recovery or increase in severity of symptoms suggest resistance to antibiotics or secondary infection. Complications affecting any/all organ systems include lung abscess/empyema, bacteremia, pericarditis/endocarditis, meningitis/encephalitis, and superinfections.

Collaborative

Administer antimicrobials as indicated by results of sputum/blood cultures: e.g., penicillins, erythromycin, tetracycline, amikacin (Amikin); cephalosporins: amantadine (Symmetrel).

These drugs are used to combat most of the microbial pneumonias. Combinations of antiviral and antifungal agents may be used when the pneumonia is a result of mixed organisms. *Note:* Vancomycin and third-generation cephalosporins are the treatment of choice for penicillin-resistant streptococcal pneumonia.

Prepare for/assist with diagnostic studies as indicated.

Fiberoptic bronchoscopy (FOB) may be done in patients who do not respond rapidly (within 1–3 days) to antimicrobial therapy to clarify diagnosis and therapy needs.

NURSING DIAGNOSIS: Activity intolerance

May be related to
Imbalance between oxygen supply and demand
General weakness
Exhaustion associated with interruption in usual sleep pattern due to discomfort, excessive coughing, and dyspnea

Possibly evidenced by
Verbal reports of weakness, fatigue, exhaustion
Exertional dyspnea, tachypnea
Tachycardia in response to activity
Development/worsening of pallor/cyanosis

DESIRED OUTCOMES/EVALUATION CRITERIA—PATIENT WILL:
Report/demonstrate a measurable increase in tolerance to activity with absence of dyspnea and excessive fatigue, and vital signs within patient's acceptable range.

ACTIONS/INTERVENTIONS	RATIONALE
Independent	
Evaluate patient's response to activity. Note reports of dyspnea, increased weakness/fatigue, and changes in vital signs during and after activities.	Establishes patient's capabilities/needs and facilitates choice of interventions.
Provide a quiet environment and limit visitors during acute phase as indicated. Encourage use of stress management and diversional activities as appropriate.	Reduces stress and excess stimulation, promoting rest.
Explain importance of rest in treatment plan and necessity for balancing activities with rest.	Bed rest is maintained during acute phase to decrease metabolic demands, thus conserving energy for healing. Activity restrictions thereafter are determined by individual patient response to activity and resolution of respiratory insufficiency.
Assist the patient to assume comfortable position for rest/sleep.	Patient may be comfortable with head of bed elevated, sleeping in a chair, or leaning forward on overbed table with pillow support.
Assist with self-care activities as necessary. Provide for progressive increase in activities during recovery phase.	Minimizes exhaustion and helps to balance oxygen supply and demand.

NURSING DIAGNOSIS: Pain [acute]

May be related to
Inflammation of lung parenchyma
Cellular reactions to circulating toxins
Persistent coughing

Possibly evidenced by
Pleuritic chest pain
Headache, muscle/joint pain
Guarding of affected area
Distraction behaviors, restlessness

DESIRED OUTCOMES/EVALUATION CRITERIA—PATIENT WILL:
Verbalize relief/control of pain.
Demonstrate relaxed manner, resting/sleeping and engaging in activity appropriately.

ACTIONS/INTERVENTIONS	RATIONALE
Independent	
Determine pain characteristics, e.g., sharp, constant, stabbing. Investigate changes in character/location/intensity of pain.	Chest pain, usually present to some degree with pneumonia, may also herald the onset of complications of pneumonia, such as pericarditis and endocarditis.
Monitor vital signs.	Changes in heart rate or BP may indicate that the patient is experiencing pain, especially when other reasons for changes in vital signs have been ruled out.
Provide comfort measures, e.g., back rubs, change of position, quiet music/conversation, relaxation/breathing exercises.	Nonanalgesic measures administered with a gentle touch can lessen discomfort and augment therapeutic effects of analgesics.
Offer frequent oral hygiene.	Mouth breathing and oxygen therapy can irritate and dry out mucous membranes, potentiating general discomfort.
Instruct and assist patient in chest splinting techniques during coughing episodes. (Refer to ND: Airway Clearance, ineffective, p 132.)	Aids in control of chest discomfort while enhancing effectiveness of cough effort.
Collaborative	
Administer analgesics and antitussives as indicated.	These medications may be used to suppress nonproductive/paroxysmal cough or reduce excess mucus, thereby enhancing general comfort/rest.

NURSING DIAGNOSIS: Nutrition: altered, risk for less than body requirements

Risk factors may include
Increased metabolic needs secondary to fever and infectious process
Anorexia associated with bacterial toxins, the odor and taste of sputum, and certain aerosol treatments
Abdominal distention/gas associated with swallowing air during dyspneic episodes

ACTIONS/INTERVENTIONS	RATIONALE
Independent	
Identify factors that are contributing to nausea/vomiting, e.g., copious sputum, aerosol treatments, severe dyspnea, pain.	Choice of interventions is dependent on the underlying cause of the problem.
Provide covered container for sputum and remove at frequent intervals. Assist with/encourage oral hygiene after emesis, after aerosol and postural drainage treatments, and before meals.	Eliminates noxious sights, tastes, smells from the patient environment and can reduce nausea.
Schedule respiratory treatments at least 1 hour before meals.	Reduces effects of nausea associated with these treatments.
Auscultate for bowel sounds. Observe/palpate for abdominal distention.	Bowel sounds may be diminished/absent if the infectious process is severe/prolonged. Abdominal distention may occur as a result of air swallowing or reflect the influence of bacterial toxins on the GI tract.
Provide small, frequent meals, including dry foods (toast, crackers) and/or foods that are appealing to patient.	These measures may enhance intake even though appetite may be slow to return.
Evaluate general nutritional state, obtain baseline weight.	Presence of chronic conditions (such as COPD or alcoholism) or financial limitations can contribute to malnutrition, lowered resistance to infection, and/or delayed response to therapy.

ACTIONS/INTERVENTIONS

Independent

Assess vital sign changes, e.g., increased temperature/prolonged fever, tachycardia, orthostatic hypotension.

Assess skin turgor, moisture of mucous membranes (lips, tongue).

Note reports of nausea/vomiting.

Monitor intake and output, noting color, character of urine. Calculate fluid balance. Be aware of insensible losses. Weigh as indicated.

Force fluids to at least 2500 ml/d or as individually appropriate.

Collaborative

Administer medications as indicated, e.g., antipyretics, antiemetics.

Provide supplemental IV fluids as necessary.

RATIONALE

Elevated temperature/prolonged fever increases metabolic rate and fluid loss through evaporation. Orthostatic BP changes and increasing tachycardia may indicate systemic fluid deficit.

Indirect indicators of adequacy of fluid volume, although oral mucous membranes may be dry because of mouth-breathing and supplemental oxygen.

Presence of these symptoms reduces oral intake.

Provides information about adequacy of fluid volume and replacement needs.

Meets basic fluid needs, reducing risk of dehydration.

Useful in reducing fluid losses.

In presence of reduced intake/excessive loss, use of parenteral route may correct/prevent deficiency.

NURSING DIAGNOSIS: Knowledge deficit [learning need] regarding condition and treatment needs, self care and discharge needs

May be related to
Lack of exposure
Misinterpretation of information
Altered recall

Possibly evidenced by
Requests for information
Statement of misconception
Failure to improve/recurrence

DESIRED OUTCOMES/EVALUATION CRITERIA—PATIENT WILL:
Verbalize understanding of condition, disease process, and treatment.
Initiate necessary lifestyle changes and participate in treatment program.

ACTIONS/INTERVENTIONS

Independent

Review normal lung function, pathology of condition.

Discuss debilitating aspects of disease, length of convalescence, and recovery expectations. Identify self-care and homemaker needs/resources.

RATIONALE

Promotes understanding of current situation and importance of cooperating with treatment regimen.

Information can enhance coping and help reduce anxiety and excessive concern. Respiratory symptoms may be slow to resolve, and fatigue and weakness can persist for an extended period. These factors may be associated with depression and the need for various forms of support and assistance.

139

ACTIONS/INTERVENTIONS	RATIONALE
Independent	
Provide information in written as well as verbal form.	Fatigue and depression can affect ability to assimilate information/follow medical regimen.
Stress importance of continuing effective coughing/deep-breathing exercises.	During initial 6–8 weeks after discharge, patient is at greatest risk for recurrence of pneumonia.
Emphasize necessity for continuing antibiotic therapy for prescribed period.	Early discontinuation of antibiotics may result in failure to completely resolve infectious process.
Review importance of cessation of smoking.	Smoking destroys tracheobronchial ciliary action, irritates bronchial mucosa, and inhibits alveolar macrophages, compromising body's natural defense against infection.
Outline steps to enhance general health and well-being, e.g., balanced rest and activity, well-rounded diet, avoidance of crowds during cold/flu season and persons with upper respiratory infections.	Increase natural defenses/immunity, limits exposure to pathogens.
Stress importance of continuing medical follow-up and obtaining vaccinations/immunizations as appropriate.	May prevent recurrence of pneumonia and/or related complications.
Identify signs/symptoms requiring notification of healthcare provider, e.g., increasing dyspnea, chest pain, prolonged fatigue, weight loss, fever/chills, persistence of productive cough, changes in mentation.	Prompt evaluation and timely intervention may prevent/minimize complications.

POTENTIAL CONSIDERATIONS following acute hospitalization (dependent on patient's age, physical condition/presence of complications, personal resources, and life responsibilities)

Fatigue—increased energy requirements to perform ADLs, discomfort, effects of antimicrobial therapy.

Infection, risk for—inadequate secondary response (e.g., leukopenia, suppressed inflammatory response), chronic disease, malnutrition, current use of antibiotics.

Therapeutic Regimen: Individual, ineffective management—complexity of therapeutic regimen, economic difficulties, perceived seriousness/susceptibility.

Sample CP: Bacterial Pneumonia, Hospital. ELOS: 5 days Medical Unit

ND and categories of care	Day 1	Day 2	Day 3	Day 4	Day 5
Impaired gas exchange R/T alveolar congestion, inflammation, hypoventilation	**Goals** Participate in activities to maximize oxygenation and airway clearance	Demonstrate improving ventilation and oxygenation by lessening symptoms of respiratory distress, ABGs approaching acceptable levels	Verbalize understanding of general healthcare needs	Initiate activities accepting responsibility for therapeutic regimen within level of ability Plan in place to meet postdischarge needs	Demonstrate ABGs within pt's acceptable range and absence of respiratory distress
Referrals	Pulmonary specialist		Home care Home O$_2$/Resp. Therapist		
Diagnostic studies	CXR				
	ABGs	→ Repeat if pulse ox <87%			
	CBC, lytes		Repeat if WBC elevated, febrile, or ABGs not WNL Hb/Hct		
	Sputum C & S/gram stain				
	Blood culture				
	Pulse oximetry q4h	→ DC if >92%			
Additional assessments	Respiratory rate, rhythm, depth, use of accessory muscles, color of skin/mucous membranes q4h	→	→ q8h	↑	↑
	Breath sounds q4h	→	→ q8h	↑	↑
	Cough/sputum characteristics	→ q4h as indicated	→ q8h	↑	↑
	Vital signs	→	→	↑	↑
	I & O q8h	→	→	↑	↑
	Weight qd	→	→ PO	↑	↑
Medications Allergies: _____ _____	IV antibiotics	→	→	↑	↑
	Bronchodilator via MDI or nebulizer	→ MDI			
	Mucolytic	→	→	↑	↑
	Antitussives-prn	→	→ D/C		
	Acetaminophen if temp above 101°	→ D/C		Medications post-discharge: dose, time, route, purpose, side effects	
	Analgesics-prn	→ D/C			

Sample CP: Bacterial Pneumonia, Hospital. ELOS: 5 days Medical Unit (Continued)

ND and categories of care	Day 1	Day 2	Day 3	Day 4	Day 5
Patient education	Orient to unit/room; Review advance directives; Diagnostic tests/results; Pulmonary hygiene: T,C,DB, splinting techniques; Use of incentive spirometer, MDI; Proper handling of secretions, handwashing techniques; Relaxation techniques	Adaptive breathing techniques as indicated; Pacing of activities; Smoking cessation; Fluid/nutritional needs, balancing activity/rest	Individual risk factors, prevention of recurrence, vaccinations/immunizations; Signs/symptoms to report to healthcare provider	Proper use and care of home care equipment (eg, O_2 concentrator, nebulizer)	Provide written instructions; Schedule for follow-up appointments
Additional nursing actions	Position for maximal respiratory effort	→ per self			
	Assist with physical care	→	→ as necessary	→ per self	
	Incentive spirometry q4h	→	→ per self WA	→ D/C	
	Supplemental O_2	→ per self			
	Oral care—prn	→	→	→ D/C	
	Suction as indicated	→		→ D/C	
	Screen visitors/staff for URI	→		→	
	Encourage fluid to 2500 ml/d as tol	→		→ per self	

LUNG CANCER: SURGICAL INTERVENTION (POSTOPERATIVE CARE)

Lung cancer usually develops within the wall or epithelium of the bronchial tree. The two major categories are small cell lung cancers (SCLC), e.g., oat cell; and non–small cell cancers (NSCLC), such as squamous cell, adenocarcinoma, and large cell. Prognosis is generally poor, varying with the type of cancer and extent of involvement at time of diagnosis. Survival rates are better with NSCLC, especially with treatment in early stages. Although NSCLC tumors are frequently associated with metastases, they are generally slow-growing.

Treatment options can include combinations of surgery, radiation, and chemotherapy. Surgery is the primary treatment for stage I, stage II, or selected stage III carcinomas, if the tumor is resectable. Surgical procedures for operable tumors of the lung include:

1. Pneumonectomy (removal of an entire lung), performed for lesions originating in the mainstem bronchus or lobar bronchus
2. Lobectomy (removal of one lobe), preferred for peripheral carcinoma localized in a lobe
3. Wedge or segmental resection, performed for lesions that are small and well-contained within one segment

CARE SETTING

Inpatient surgical and possibly subacute units.

RELATED CONCERNS

Cancer, p 875
Hemothorax/Pneumothorax, p 154
Psychosocial Aspects of Care, p 783
Radical Neck Surgery: Laryngectomy (Postoperative Care), p 162
Surgical Intervention, p 802

Patient Assessment Data Base (Preoperative)

Findings are dependent on type, duration of cancer, and extent of metastasis.

ACTIVITY/REST

May report:	Fatigue, inability to maintain usual routine, dyspnea with activity
May exhibit:	Lassitude (usually in advanced stage)

CIRCULATION

May exhibit:	JVD (vena caval obstruction) Heart sounds: Pericardial rub (indicating effusion) Tachycardia/dysrhythmias Clubbing of fingers

EGO INTEGRITY

May report:	Frightened feelings, fear of outcome of surgery Denial of severity of condition/potential for malignancy
May exhibit:	Restlessness, insomnia, repetitive questioning

ELIMINATION

May report:	Intermittent diarrhea (hormonal imbalance, small cell carcinoma) Increased frequency/amount of urine (hormonal imbalance, epidermoid tumor)

FOOD/FLUID

May report: Weight loss, poor appetite, decreased food intake
Difficulty swallowing
Thirst/increased fluid intake

May exhibit: Thin, emaciated or wasted appearance (late stages)
Edema of face/neck, chest, back (vena caval obstruction); facial/periorbital edema (hormonal imbalance, small-cell carcinoma)
Glucose in urine (hormonal imbalance, epidermoid tumor)

PAIN/DISCOMFORT

May report: Chest pain (not usually present in early stages and not always in advanced stages), which may/may not be affected by position change
Shoulder/arm pain (particularly with large cell or adenocarcinoma)
Bone/joint pain: Cartilage erosion secondary to increased growth hormones (large cell or adenocarcinoma)
Intermittent abdominal pain

May exhibit: Distraction behaviors (restlessness, withdrawal)
Guarding/protective actions

RESPIRATION

May report: Mild cough or change in usual cough pattern and/or sputum production
Shortness of breath
Occupational exposure to pollutants, industrial dusts (e.g., asbestos, iron oxides, coal dust), radioactive material
Hoarseness/change in voice (vocal cord paralysis)
History of smoking

May exhibit: Dyspnea, aggravated by exertion
Increased tactile fremitus (indicating consolidation)
Brief crackles/wheezes on inspiration or expiration (impaired airflow)
Persistent crackles/wheezes; tracheal shift (space-occupying lesion)
Hemoptysis

SAFETY

May exhibit: Fever may be present (large cell or adenocarcinoma)
Bruising, discoloration of skin (hormonal imbalance, small cell carcinoma)

SEXUALITY

May exhibit: Gynecomastia (neoplastic hormonal changes, large cell carcinoma)
Amenorrhea/impotence (hormonal imbalance, small cell carcinoma)

TEACHING/LEARNING

May report: Familial risk factors: Cancer (especially lung), tuberculosis
Failure to improve

Discharge plan considerations: DRG projected mean length of inpatient stay: 11.7 days
Assistance with transportation, medications, treatments, self-care, homemaker/maintenance tasks

Refer to section at end of plan for postdischarge considerations.

DIAGNOSTIC STUDIES

Chest x-ray (PA and lateral), chest tomography: Outlines shape, size and location of lesion. May reveal mass of air in hilar region, pleural effusion, atelectasis, erosion of ribs or vertebrae.

Cytologic examinations (sputum, pleural, or lymph node): Performed to assess presence/stage of carcinoma.

Fiberoptic bronchoscopy: Allows for visualization, regional washings, and cytologic brushing of lesions (large percent of bronchogenic carcinomas may be visualized).

Biopsy: May be performed on scalene nodes, hilar lymph nodes, or pleura to establish diagnosis.

Mediastinoscopy: Used for staging of carcinoma.

Lung scan: Helpful in determining tumor size/location and for staging.

Pulmonary function studies and ABGs: Assess lung capacity to meet postoperative ventilatory needs.

Skin tests, absolute lymphocyte counts: May be done to evaluate for immunocompetence (common in lung cancers).

Bone scan; CT scan of brain, liver; gallium scan of liver, spleen, bone: To detect metastasis.

NURSING PRIORITIES

1. Maintain/improve respiratory function.
2. Control/alleviate pain.
3. Support efforts to cope with diagnosis/situation.
4. Provide information about disease process/prognosis and therapeutic regimen.

DISCHARGE GOALS

1. Oxygenation/ventilation adequate to meet individual activity needs.
2. Pain controlled.
3. Anxiety/fear decreased to manageable level.
4. Free of preventable complications.
5. Disease process/prognosis and planned therapies understood.
6. Plan in place to meet needs after discharge.

NURSING DIAGNOSIS: Gas Exchange, impaired

May be related to
Removal of lung tissue
Altered oxygen supply (hypoventilation)
Decreased oxygen-carrying capacity of blood (blood loss)

Possibly evidenced by
Dyspnea
Restlessness/changes in mentation
Hypoxemia and hypercapnea
Cyanosis

DESIRED OUTCOMES/EVALUATION CRITERIA—PATIENT WILL:
Demonstrate improved ventilation and adequate oxygenation of tissues by ABGs within patient's normal range.
Be free of symptoms of respiratory distress.

ACTIONS/INTERVENTIONS	RATIONALE

Independent

Note respiratory rate, depth, and ease of respirations. Observe for use of accessory muscles, pursed-lip breathing, changes in skin/mucous membrane color, e.g., pallor, cyanosis.	Respirations may be increased as a result of pain or as an initial compensatory mechanism to accommodate for loss of lung tissue; however, increased work of breathing and cyanosis may indicate increasing oxygen consumption and energy expenditures and/or reduced respiratory reserve, e.g., elderly patient or extensive chronic obstructive lung disease.
Auscultate lungs for air movement and abnormal breath sounds.	Consolidation and lack of air movement on operative side is normal in the pneumonectomy patient; however, the lobectomy patient should demonstrate normal airflow in remaining lobes.
Investigate restlessness and changes in mentation/level of consciousness.	May indicate increased hypoxia or complications such as mediastinal shift in pneumonectomy patient when accompanied by tachypnea, tachycardia, and tracheal deviation.
Maintain patent airway by positioning, suctioning, use of airway adjuncts.	Airway obstruction impedes ventilation, impairing gas exchange. (Refer to ND: Airway Clearance, ineffective, p 147.)
Reposition frequently, placing patient in sitting positions as well as supine to side positions.	Maximizes lung expansion and drainage of secretions.
Avoid positioning the patient with a pneumonectomy on the nonoperative side with the remaining lung dependent.	This position reduces lung expansion and decreases perfusion to the "good" lung and could foster the development of a tension pneumothorax secondary to a mediastinal shift and accumulation of fluid in the remaining lung.
Encourage/assist with deep-breathing exercises and pursed-lip breathing as appropriate.	Promotes maximal ventilation and oxygenation and reduces/prevents atelectasis.
Maintain patency of chest drainage system for lobectomy, segmental/wedge resection patient.	Drains fluid from pleural cavity to promote reexpansion of remaining lung segments.
Note changes in amount/type of chest tube drainage.	Bloody drainage should decrease in amount and change to a more serous composition as recovery progresses. A sudden increase in amount of bloody drainage or return to frank bleeding suggests thoracic bleeding/hemothorax; sudden cessation suggests blockage of tube, requiring further evaluation and intervention.
Observe presence/degree of bubbling in water-seal chamber.	Air leaks immediately postoperative are not uncommon, especially following lobectomy or segmental resection; however, this should diminish as healing progresses. Prolonged or new leaks require evaluation to identify problems in the patient versus the drainage system.
Assess patient response to activity. Encourage rest periods/limit activities to patient tolerance.	Increased oxygen consumption/demand and stress of surgery can result in increased dyspnea and changes in vital signs with activity; however, early mobilization is desired to help prevent pulmonary complications and to obtain and maintain respiratory and circulatory efficiency. Adequate rest balanced with activity can prevent respiratory compromise.

ACTIONS/INTERVENTIONS

Independent

Note development of fever.

Collaborative

Administer supplemental oxygen via nasal cannula, partial rebreathing mask, or high-humidity face mask, as indicated.

Assist with/encourage use of incentive spirometer or blow bottles.

Monitor/graph ABGs, pulse oximetry readings. Note Hb levels.

RATIONALE

Fever within the first 24 hours after surgery is frequently due to atelectasis. Temperature elevation within the 5th–10th postoperative day usually indicates an infection, e.g., wound or systemic.

Maximizes available oxygen, especially while ventilation is reduced from anesthetic depression or pain, as well as during period of compensatory physiologic shift of circulation to remaining functional alveolar units.

Prevents/reduces atelectasis and promotes reexpansion of small airways.

Decreasing PaO_2 or increasing $PaCO_2$ may indicate need for ventilatory support. Significant blood loss can result in decreased oxygen-carrying capacity, reducing PaO_2.

NURSING DIAGNOSIS: Airway Clearance, ineffective

May be related to
Increased amount/viscosity of secretions
Restricted chest movement/pain
Fatigue/weakness

Possibly evidenced by
Changes in rate/depth of respiration
Abnormal breath sounds
Ineffective cough
Dyspnea

DESIRED OUTCOMES/EVALUATION CRITERIA—PATIENT WILL:
Demonstrate patent airway, with fluid secretions easily expectorated, clear breath sounds, and noiseless respirations.

ACTIONS/INTERVENTIONS

Independent

Auscultate chest for character of breath sounds and presence of secretions.

Assist patient with/instruct in effective deep breathing and coughing with upright position (sitting) and splinting of incision.

RATIONALE

Noisy respirations, rhonchi, and wheezes are indicative of retained secretions and/or airway obstruction.

Upright position favors maximal lung expansion, and splinting improves force of cough effort to mobilize and remove secretions. Splinting may be done by nurse (placing hands anteriorly and posteriorly over chest wall) and by patient (with pillows) as strength improves.

147

ACTIONS/INTERVENTIONS	RATIONALE
Independent	
Observe amount and character of sputum/aspirated secretions. Investigate changes as indicated.	Increased amounts of colorless (or blood-streaked)/watery secretions are normal initially and should decrease as recovery progresses. Presence of thick/tenacious, bloody, or purulent sputum suggests development of secondary problems (e.g., dehydration, pulmonary edema, local hemorrhage, or infection) requiring correction/treatment.
Suction if cough is weak or rhonchi not cleared by cough effort. Avoid deep endotracheal/nasotracheal suctioning in pneumonectomy patient if possible.	"Routine" suctioning increases risk of hypoxemia and mucosal damage. Deep tracheal suctioning is generally contraindicated following pneumonectomy to reduce the risk of rupture of the bronchial stump suture line. If suctioning is unavoidable, it should be done gently only to induce effective coughing.
Encourage oral fluid intake (at least 2500 ml/d) within cardiac tolerance.	Adequate hydration aids in keeping secretions loose/enhances expectoration.
Assess for pain/discomfort and medicate on a routine basis and prior to breathing exercises.	Encourages the patient to move, cough more effectively, and breathe more deeply to prevent respiratory insufficiency.
Collaborative	
Provide/assist with IPPB, incentive spirometer, blow bottles, postural drainage/percussion as indicated.	Improves lung expansion/ventilation and facilitates removal of secretions. *Note:* Postural drainage may be contraindicated in some patients and in any event must be performed cautiously to prevent respiratory embarrassment and incisional discomfort.
Use humidified oxygen/ultrasonic nebulizer. Provide additional fluids via IV as indicated.	Providing maximal hydration helps loosen/liquefy secretions to promote expectoration. Impaired oral intake necessitates IV supplementation to maintain hydration.
Administer bronchodilators, expectorants, and/or analgesics as indicated.	Relieves bronchospasm to improve airflow. Expectorants increase mucous production to liquefy and reduce viscosity of secretions, facilitating removal. Alleviation of chest discomfort promotes cooperation with breathing exercises and enhances effectiveness of respiratory therapies.

NURSING DIAGNOSIS: Pain [acute]

May be related to
Surgical incision, tissue trauma, and disruption of intercostal nerves
Presence of chest tube(s)
Cancer invasion of pleura, chest wall

Possibly evidenced by
Verbal reports of discomfort
Guarding of affected area
Distraction behaviors, e.g., restlessness
Narrowed focus (withdrawal)
Changes in BP, heart/respiratory rate

ACTIONS/INTERVENTIONS	RATIONALE
Independent	
Ask patient about pain. Determine pain characteristics, e.g., continuous, aching, stabbing, burning. Have patient rate intensity on a 0–10 scale.	Helpful in evaluating cancer-related pain symptoms, which may involve viscera, nerve, or bone tissue. Use of rating scale aids patient in assessing level of pain and provides tool for evaluating effectiveness of analgesics, enhancing patient control of pain.
Assess patient's verbal and nonverbal pain cues.	Discrepancy between verbal/nonverbal cues may provide clues to degree of pain, need for/effectiveness of interventions.
Note possible pathophysiologic and psychologic causes of pain.	A posterolateral incision is more uncomfortable for the patient than an anterolateral incision. The presence of chest tubes can greatly increase discomfort. In addition, fear, distress, anxiety, and grief over confirmed diagnosis of cancer can impair ability to cope.
Evaluate effectiveness of drug regimen. Encourage sufficient medication to control pain; change medication or time span as appropriate.	Pain perception and pain relief are subjective and thus pain management is best left to the patient's discretion. If the patient is unable to provide input, the nurse should observe physiologic and nonverbal signs of pain and administer medications on a regular basis.
Encourage verbalization of feelings about the pain.	Fears/concerns can increase muscle tension and lower threshold of pain perception. (Refer to ND: Fear/Anxiety [specify level], p 150.)
Provide comfort measures, e.g., frequent changes of position, back rubs, support with pillows. Encourage use of relaxation techniques, e.g., visualization, guided imagery, and appropriate diversional activities.	Promotes relaxation and redirects attention. Relieves discomfort and augments therapeutic effects of analgesia.
Schedule rest periods, provide quiet environment.	Decreases fatigue and conserves energy, enhancing coping abilities.
Assist with self-care activities, breathing/arm exercises, and ambulation.	Prevents undue fatigue and incisional strain. Encouragement and physical assistance/support may be needed for some time before the patient is able or confident enough to perform these activities because of pain or fear of pain.
Collaborative	
Administer analgesics routinely as indicated, especially 45–60 minutes before respiratory treatments, deep-breathing/coughing exercises. Assist with PCA or analgesia through epidural catheter.	Maintaining a more constant drug level avoids cyclic periods of pain, aids in muscle healing, and improves respiratory function and emotional comfort/coping.

ACTIONS/INTERVENTIONS	RATIONALE
Independent	
Evaluate patient/SO level of understanding of diagnosis.	Patient and SO are hearing and assimilating new information that includes changes in self-image and lifestyle. Understanding perceptions of those involved sets the tone for individualizing care and provides information necessary for choosing appropriate interventions.
Acknowledge reality of patient's fears/concerns and encourage expression of feelings.	Support may enable the patient to begin exploring/dealing with the reality of cancer and its treatment. Patient may need time to identify feelings and even more time to begin to express them.
Provide opportunity for questions and answer them honestly. Be sure that patient and care providers have the same understanding of terms used.	Establishes trust and reduces misperceptions/misinterpretation of information.
Accept, but do not reinforce, patient's denial of the situation.	When extreme denial or anxiety is interfering with progress of recovery, the issues facing the patient need to be explained and resolutions explored.
Note comments/behaviors indicative of beginning acceptance and/or use of effective strategies to deal with situation.	Fear/anxiety will diminish as patient begins to accept/deal positively with reality. Indicator of patient's readiness to accept responsibility for participation in recovery and to "resume life."
Involve patient/SO in care planning. Provide time to prepare for events/treatments.	May help restore some feeling of control/independence to patient who feels powerless in dealing with diagnosis and treatment.
Provide for patient's physical comfort.	It is difficult to deal with emotional issues when experiencing extreme/persistent physical discomfort.

> **NURSING DIAGNOSIS: Knowledge deficit [learning need] regarding condition, treatment, prognosis, self care and discharge needs**
>
> **May be related to**
> Lack of exposure, unfamiliarity with information/resources
> Information misinterpretation
> Lack of recall
>
> **Possibly evidenced by**
> Statements of concern
> Request for information
> Inadequate follow-through of instruction
> Inappropriate or exaggerated behaviors, e.g., hysterical, hostile, agitated, apathetic
>
> **DESIRED OUTCOMES/EVALUATION CRITERIA—PATIENT WILL:**
> Verbalize understanding of ramifications of diagnosis, treatment regimen.
> Correctly perform necessary procedures and explain reasons for the actions.
> Participate in learning process.
> Initiate necessary lifestyle changes.

ACTIONS/INTERVENTIONS	RATIONALE
Independent	
Discuss diagnosis, current/planned therapies and expected outcomes.	Provides individually specific information, creating knowledge base for subsequent learning regarding home management. Radiation or chemotherapy may follow surgical intervention and information is essential to enable the patient/SO to make informed decisions.
Reinforce surgeon's explanation of particular surgical procedure providing diagram as appropriate. Incorporate this information into discussion about short-/long-term recovery expectations.	Length of rehabilitation and prognosis is dependent on type of surgical procedure, preoperative physical condition, and duration/degree of complications.
Discuss necessity of planning for follow-up care prior to discharge.	Follow-up assessment of respiratory status and general health is imperative to assure optimal recovery. Also provides opportunity to readdress concerns/questions at a less stressful time.
Identify signs/symptoms requiring medical evaluations, e.g., changes in appearance of incision, development of respiratory difficulty, fever, increased chest pain, changes in appearance of sputum.	Early detection and timely intervention may prevent/minimize complications.
Help patient determine activity tolerance and set goals.	Weakness and fatigue should lessen as lung(s) heal and respiratory function improves during recovery period, especially if cancer was completely removed. If cancer is advanced, it is emotionally helpful for the patient to be able to set realistic activity goals to achieve optimal independence.
Evaluate availability/adequacy of support system(s) and necessity for assistance in self-care/home management.	General weakness and activity limitations may reduce individual's ability to meet own needs.

151

ACTIONS/INTERVENTIONS	RATIONALE
Independent	
Recommend alternating rest periods with activity and light tasks with heavy tasks. Stress avoidance of heavy lifting, isometric/strenuous upper-body exercise. Reinforce physician's time limitations about lifting.	Generalized weakness and fatigue are usual in the early recovery period but should diminish as respiratory function improves and healing progresses. Rest and sleep enhance coping abilities, reduce nervousness (common in this phase), and promote healing. *Note:* Strenuous use of arms can place undue stress on incision because chest muscles may be weaker than normal for 3–6 months following surgery.
Recommend stopping any activity that causes undue fatigue or increased shortness of breath.	Exhaustion aggravates respiratory insufficiency.
Encourage inspection of incisions. Review expectations for healing with patient.	Healing begins immediately, but complete healing will take time. As healing progresses, incision lines may appear dry, with crusty scabs. Underlying tissue may look bruised and feel tense, warm, and lumpy (resolving hematoma).
Instruct patient/SO to watch for/report places in incision that do not heal or reopening of healed incision, any drainage (bloody or purulent), localized area of swelling with redness, increased pain, hot to touch.	Signs/symptoms indicating failure to heal, development of complications requiring further medical evaluation/intervention.
Suggest wearing soft cotton shirts and loose-fitting clothing, cover/pad portion of incision as indicated, leave incision open to air as much as possible.	Reduces suture line irritation and pressure from clothing. Leaving incisions open to air promotes healing process and may reduce risk of infection.
Shower in warm water, washing incision gently. Avoid tub baths until approved by physician.	Keeps incision clean, promotes circulation/healing. *Note:* "Climbing" out of tub requires use of arms and pectoral muscles, which can put undue stress on incision.
Support incision with Steri-strips as needed when sutures/staples are removed.	Aids in maintaining approximation of wound edges to promote healing.
Instruct in/provide rationale for arm/shoulder exercises. Have patient/SO demonstrate exercises. Encourage following graded increase in number/intensity of routine repetitions.	Simple arm circles and lifting arms over the head or out to the affected side are initiated on the 1st or 2nd postoperative day to restore normal range of motion of shoulder and to prevent ankylosis of the affected shoulder.
Stress importance of avoiding exposure to smoke, air pollution, and contact with individuals with upper respiratory infections.	Protects lung(s) from irritation and reduces risk of infection.
Review nutritional/fluid needs. Suggest increasing protein and use of high-calorie snacks as appropriate.	Meeting cellular energy requirements and maintaining good circulating volume for tissue perfusion facilitates tissue regeneration/healing process.
Identify individually appropriate community resources, e.g., American Cancer Society, visiting nurse, social services, home care.	Agencies such as these offer a broad range of services that can be tailored to provide support and meet individual needs.

POTENTIAL CONSIDERATIONS following hospitalization (dependent on patient's age, physical condition/presence of complications, personal resources, and life responsibilities)

Airway Clearance, ineffective—increased amount/viscosity of secretions, restricted chest movement/pain, fatigue/weakness.

Pain [acute]—surgical incision, tissue trauma, disruption of intercostal nerves, presence of distress/anxiety.

Self Care deficit—decreased strength/endurance, presence of pain, intolerance to activity, depression, presence of therapeutic devices, e.g., IV lines.

Refer to CP, Cancer for other considerations, p 875

153

HEMOTHORAX/PNEUMOTHORAX

The lung may collapse partially/completely due to collection of air (pneumothorax), blood (hemothorax), or other fluid (pleural effusion) in the pleural/potential space. The intrathoracic pressure changes induced by increased pleural space volumes reduce lung capacity, causing respiratory distress and gas exchange problems, and producing tension on mediastinal structures that can impede cardiac and systemic circulation. Pneumothorax may be traumatic (open or closed) or spontaneous.

CARE SETTING:

Inpatient medical or surgical unit.

RELATED CONCERNS

Cardiac Surgery: Coronary Artery Bypass Graft; Cardiomyoplasty; Valve Replacement (Postoperative Care), p 95
Chronic Obstructive Pulmonary Disease (COPD), p 117
Psychosocial Aspects of Care, p 783
Pulmonary Tuberculosis (TB), p 190
Ventilatory Assistance (Mechanical), p 176

Patient Assessment Data Base

Findings vary, depending on the amount of air and/or fluid accumulation, rate of accumulation, and underlying lung function.

ACTIVITY/REST

May report:	Dyspnea with activity or even at rest

CIRCULATION

May exhibit:	Tachycardia; irregular rate/dysrhythmias
	S_3 or S_4/gallop heart rhythm (heart failure secondary to effusion)
	Apical pulse (PMI) displaced in presence of mediastinal shift (with tension pneumothorax)
	Hamman's sign (crunching sound correlating with heart beat, reflecting air in mediastinum)
	BP: hypertension/hypotension
	JVD

EGO INTEGRITY

May exhibit:	Apprehension, irritability

FOOD/FLUID

May exhibit:	Recent placement of central venous IV/pressure line (causative factor)

PAIN/DISCOMFORT

May report (dependent on the size/area involved):	Unilateral chest pain, aggravated by breathing, coughing
	Sudden onset of symptoms while coughing or straining (spontaneous pneumothorax)
	Sharp, stabbing pain aggravated by deep breathing, possibly radiating to neck, shoulders, abdomen (pleural effusion)

May exhibit:	Guarding affected area
	Distraction behaviors
	Facial grimacing

RESPIRATION

May report:	Difficulty breathing, "air hunger"
	Coughing (may be presenting symptom)
	History of recent chest surgery/trauma; chronic lung disease, lung inflammation/infection (empyema/effusion); diffuse interstitial disease (sarcoidosis); malignancies, (e.g., obstructive tumor)
	Previous spontaneous pneumothorax; spontaneous rupture of emphysematous bulla, subpleural bleb (COPD)
May exhibit:	Respirations: Increased rate/tachypnea
	Increased work of breathing, use of accessory muscles in chest, neck; intercostal retractions, forced abdominal expiration
	Breath sounds decreased or absent (involved site)
	Fremitus decreased (involved site)
	Chest percussion: Hyperresonance over air-filled area (pneumothorax); dullness over fluid-filled area (hemothorax)
	Chest observation and palpation: Unequal (paradoxic) chest movement (if trauma, flail); reduced thoracic excursion (affected side)
	Skin: Pallor, cyanosis, diaphoresis, subcutaneous crepitation (air in tissues on palpation)
	Mentation: Anxiety, restlessness, confusion, stupor
	Use of positive pressure mechanical ventilation/PEEP therapy

SAFETY

| **May report:** | Recent chest trauma |
| | Radiation/chemotherapy for malignancy |

TEACHING/LEARNING

May report:	History of familial risk factors: Tuberculosis, cancer
	Recent intrathoracic surgery/lung biopsy
	Evidence of failure to improve
Discharge plan considerations:	**DRG projected length of inpatient stay: 7.2 days**
	Assistance with self-care, homemaker/maintenance tasks
	Refer to section at end of plan for postdischarge considerations.

DIAGNOSTIC STUDIES

Chest x-ray: Reveals air and/or fluid accumulation in the pleural space; may show shift of mediastinal structures (heart).

ABGs: Variable dependent on degree of compromised lung function, altered breathing mechanics, and ability to compensate. $PaCO_2$ occasionally elevated. PaO_2 may be normal or decreased; oxygen saturation usually decreased.

Thoracentesis: Reveals blood/serosanguinous fluid (hemothorax).

Hb: May be decreased, indicating blood loss.

NURSING PRIORITIES

1. Promote/maintain lung reexpansion for adequate oxygenation/ventilation.
2. Minimize/prevent complications.
3. Reduce discomfort/pain.
4. Provide information about disease process, treatment regimen, and prognosis.

DISCHARGE GOALS

1. Adequate ventilation/oxygenation maintained.
2. Complications prevented/resolved.
3. Pain absent/controlled.
4. Disease process/prognosis and therapy needs understood.
5. Plan in place to meet needs after discharge.

NURSING DIAGNOSIS: Breathing Pattern, ineffective

May be related to
Decreased lung expansion (air/fluid accumulation)
Musculoskeletal impairment
Pain/anxiety
Inflammatory process

Possibly evidenced by
Dyspnea, tachypnea
Changes in depth/equality of respirations; altered chest excursion
Use of accessory muscles, nasal flaring
Cyanosis, abnormal ABGs

DESIRED OUTCOMES/EVALUATION CRITERIA—PATIENT WILL:
Establish a normal/effective respiratory pattern with ABGs within patient's normal range.
Be free of cyanosis and other signs/symptoms of hypoxia.

ACTIONS/INTERVENTIONS	RATIONALE
Independent	
Identify etiology/precipitating factors, e.g., spontaneous collapse, trauma, malignancy, infection, complication of mechanical ventilation.	Understanding the cause of lung collapse is necessary for proper chest tube placement and choice of other therapeutic measures.
Evaluate respiratory function, noting rapid/shallow respirations, dyspnea, reports of ''air hunger,'' development of cyanosis, changes in vital signs.	Respiratory distress and changes in vital signs may occur as a result of physiologic stress and pain or may indicate development of shock due to hypoxia/hemorrhage.
Monitor for synchronous respiratory pattern when using mechanical ventilator. Note changes in airway pressures.	Difficulty breathing ''with'' ventilator and/or increasing airway pressures suggests worsening of condition/development of complications (e.g., spontaneous rupture of a bleb creating a new pneumothorax).
Auscultate breath sounds.	Breath sounds may be diminished or absent in a lobe, lung segment, or entire lung field (unilateral). Atelectatic area will have no breath sounds, and partially collapsed areas have decreased sounds. Evaluation also establishes areas of good air exchange and provides a baseline to evaluate resolution of pneumothorax.
Note chest excursion and position of trachea.	Chest excursion is unequal until lung reexpands. Trachea deviates away from affected side with tension pneumothorax.

ACTIONS/INTERVENTIONS	RATIONALE
Independent	
Assess fremitus.	Voice and tactile fremitus (vibration) is reduced in fluid-filled/consolidated tissue.
Assist patient with splinting painful area when coughing, deep breathing.	Supporting chest and abdominal muscles makes coughing more effective/less traumatic.
Maintain position of comfort, usually with head of bed elevated. Turn to affected side. Encourage patient to sit up as much as possible.	Promotes maximal inspiration; enhances lung expansion and ventilation in unaffected side.
Maintain a calm attitude, assisting patient to "take control" by the use of slower/deeper respirations.	Assists the patient to deal with the physiologic effects of hypoxia, which may be manifested as anxiety and/or fear.
Once chest tube is inserted:	
Check suction control chamber for correct amount of suction (determined by water level, wall/table regulator at correct setting);	Maintains prescribed intrapleural negativity, which promotes optimum lung expansion and/or fluid drainage. Note: Dry suction setups with *automatic control valve (AVC)* provide flow rate similar to that achieved with water seal system. However, the presence of a graduated inline connector (Christmas tree) in a dry system without AVC can reduce suction pressure to less than 5 LPM flow at -20 cm H_2O, necessitating replacement of connector.
Check fluid level in water-seal chamber; maintain at prescribed level;	Water in a sealed chamber serves as a barrier that prevents atmospheric air from entering the pleural space should the suction source be disconnected and aids in evaluating whether the chest drainage system is functioning appropriately. *Note:* Underfilling the water-seal chamber leaves it exposed to air, putting the patient at risk for pneumothorax or tension pneumothorax. Overfilling (a more common mistake) prevents air from exiting the pleural space and prevents correction of pneumothorax or tension pneumothorax.
Observe water-seal chamber bubbling;	Bubbling during expiration reflects venting of pneumothorax (desired action). Bubbling usually decreases as the lung expands or may occur only during expiration or coughing as the pleural space diminishes. Absence of bubbling may indicate complete lung reexpansion (normal) or represent complications, e.g., obstruction in the tube.
Evaluate for abnormal/continuous water-seal chamber bubbling;	With suction applied, this indicates a persistent air leak that may be from a large pneumothorax at the chest insertion site (patient-centered), or chest drainage unit (system-centered).
Determine location of air leak (patient- or system-centered) by clamping thoracic catheter just distal to exit from chest;	If bubbling stops when catheter is clamped at insertion site, leak is patient-centered (at insertion site or within the patient).
Place petrolatum gauze and/or other appropriate material around the insertion as indicated;	Usually corrects insertion site air leak.
Clamp tubing in stepwise fashion downward toward drainage unit if air leak continues;	Isolates location of a system-centered air leak.

157

ACTIONS/INTERVENTIONS	RATIONALE

Independent

Seal drainage tubing connection sites securely with lengthwise tape or bands according to established policy.	Prevents/corrects air leaks at connector sites.
Monitor water-seal chamber "tidaling." Note whether change is transient or permanent.	The water-seal chamber serves as an intrapleural manometer (gauges intrapleural pressure); therefore, fluctuation (tidaling) reflects pressure differences between inspiration and expiration. Tidaling of 2–6 cm during inspiration is normal, and may increase briefly during coughing episodes. Continuation of excessive tidal fluctuations may indicate airway obstruction exists or presence of a large pneumothorax.
Position drainage system tubing for optimal function, e.g., shorten tubing/coil extra tubing on bed, making sure tubing is not kinked or hanging below entrance to drainage container. Drain accumulated fluid as necessary.	Improper position, kinking, or accumulation of clots/fluid in the tubing changes the desired negative pressure and impedes air/fluid evacuation.
Note character/amount of chest tube drainage.	Useful in evaluating resolution of condition/development of complication or hemorrhage requiring prompt intervention. *Note:* Some drainage systems are equipped with an auto-transfusion device, which allows for salvage of shed blood.
Evaluate need for tube stripping ("milking").	Although it is unlikely that serous or serosanguinous drainage will obstruct tubes, stripping may be necessary occasionally to maintain drainage in the presence of fresh bleeding/large blood clots or purulent exudate (empyema).
Strip tubes carefully per protocol, in a manner that minimizes excess negative pressure.	Stripping is usually uncomfortable for the patient because of the change in intrathoracic pressure, which may induce coughing or chest discomfort. Vigorous stripping can create very high intrathoracic suction pressure, which can be injurious (e.g., invagination of tissue into catheter eyelets, collapse of tissues around the catheter, and/or bleeding from rupture of small blood vessels).

If thoracic catheter is disconnected/dislodged:

Observe for signs of respiratory distress. If possible, reconnect thoracic catheter to tubing/suction, using clean technique. If the catheter is dislodged from the chest, cover insertion site immediately with petrolatum dressing and apply firm pressure. Notify physician at once.	Pneumothorax may recur requiring prompt intervention to prevent fatal pulmonary and circulatory impairment.

After thoracic catheter is removed:

Cover insertion site with sterile occlusive dressing. Observe for signs/symptoms that may indicate recurrence of pneumothorax, e.g., shortness of breath, reports of pain. Inspect insertion site, note character of drainage.	Early detection of developing complication is essential, e.g., recurrence of pneumothorax, presence of infection.

Collaborative

Review serial chest x-rays.

Monitors progress of resolving hemothorax/pneumothorax and reexpansion of lung. Can identify malposition of endotracheal tube affecting lung reexpansion.

Monitor/graph serial ABGs and pulse oximetry. Review vital capacity/tidal volume measurements.

Assesses status of gas exchange and ventilation, need for continuation or alterations in therapy.

Administer supplemental oxygen via cannula/mask as indicated.

Aids in reducing work of breathing; promotes relief of respiratory distress and cyanosis associated with hypoxemia.

NURSING DIAGNOSIS: Trauma/Suffocation, risk for

Risk factors may include
Concurrent disease/injury process
Dependence on external device (chest drainage system)
Lack of safety education/precautions

Possibly evidenced by
[Not applicable; presence of signs and symptoms establishes an *actual* diagnosis]

DESIRED OUTCOMES/EVALUATION CRITERIA—PATIENT WILL:
Recognize need for/seek assistance to prevent complications.

CAREGIVER WILL:
Correct/avoid environmental and physical hazards.

ACTIONS/INTERVENTIONS

RATIONALE

Independent

Review with patient purpose/function of chest drainage unit, taking note of safety features.

Information on how system works provides reassurance, reducing patient anxiety.

Anchor thoracic catheter to chest wall and provide extra length of tubing before turning or moving patient:

Prevents thoracic catheter dislodgment or tubing disconnection and reduces pain/discomfort associated with pulling or jarring of tubing.

Secure tubing connection sites;

Prevents tubing disconnection.

Pad banding sites with gauze/tape.

Protects skin from irritation/pressure.

Secure drainage unit to patient's bed or on stand/cart placed in low-traffic area.

Maintains upright position and reduces risk of accidental tipping/breaking of unit.

Provide safe transportation if patient is sent off unit for diagnostic purposes. Before transporting: check water-seal chamber for correct fluid level, presence/absence of bubbling; presence/degree/timing of tidaling. Ascertain whether or not chest tube can be clamped or disconnected from suction source.

Promotes continuation of optimal evacuation of fluid/air during transport. If patient is draining large amounts of chest fluid or air, tube should not be clamped or suction interrupted because of risk of reaccumulation of fluid/air, compromising respiratory status.

159

ACTIONS/INTERVENTIONS	RATIONALE

Independent

Monitor thoracic insertion site, noting condition of skin, presence/characteristics of drainage from around the catheter. Change/reapply sterile occlusive dressing as needed.	Provides for early recognition and treatment of developing skin/tissue erosion or infection.
Instruct patient to refrain from lying/pulling on tubing.	Reduces risk of obstructing drainage/inadvertently disconnecting tubing.
Identify changes/situations that should be reported to caregivers, e.g., change in sound of bubbling, sudden "air hunger" and chest pain, disconnection of equipment.	Timely intervention may prevent serious complications.
Observe for signs of respiratory distress if thoracic catheter is disconnected/dislodged. (Refer to ND: Breathing Pattern, ineffective, p 156.)	Pneumothorax may recur/worsen, compromising respiratory function and requiring emergency intervention.

NURSING DIAGNOSIS: Knowledge deficit [learning need] regarding condition, treatment regimen, self care and discharge needs

May be related to
Lack of exposure to information

Possibly evidenced by
Expressions of concern, request for information
Recurrence of problem

DESIRED OUTCOMES/EVALUATION CRITERIA—PATIENT WILL:
Verbalize understanding of cause of problem (when known).
Identify signs/symptoms requiring medical follow-up.
Follow treatment regimen and demonstrate lifestyle changes if necessary to prevent recurrence.

ACTIONS/INTERVENTIONS	RATIONALE

Independent

Review pathology of individual problem.	Information reduces fear of unknown. Provides knowledge base for understanding underlying dynamics of condition and significance of therapeutic interventions.
Identify likelihood for recurrence/long-term complications.	Certain underlying lung diseases such as severe COPD and malignancies may increase incidence of recurrence. In otherwise healthy patients who suffered a spontaneous pneumothorax, incidence of recurrence is 10%–50%. Those who have a second spontaneous episode are at high risk for a third incident (60%).
Review signs/symptoms requiring immediate medical evaluation, e.g., sudden chest pain, dyspnea/air hunger, progressive respiratory distress.	Recurrence of pneumothorax/hemothorax requires medical intervention to prevent/reduce potential complications.

ACTIONS/INTERVENTIONS

Independent

Review significance of good health practices, e.g., adequate nutrition, rest, exercise.

RATIONALE

Maintenance of general well-being promotes healing and may prevent/limit recurrences.

POTENTIAL CONSIDERATIONS following acute hospitalization (dependent on patient's age, physical condition/presence of complications, personal resources, and life responsibilities)

Infection, risk for—invasive procedure, traumatized tissue/broken skin, decreased ciliary action.
Breathing Pattern, ineffective—recurrence of condition, inflammatory process.

RADICAL NECK SURGERY: LARYNGECTOMY (POSTOPERATIVE CARE)

Head and neck cancer refers to a malignancy that lies above the clavicle but excludes the brain, spinal cord, axial skeleton, and vertebrae. Head and neck cancer accounts for 5.5% of all malignant disease. The majority of the laryngeal neoplasms (95%) are squamous cell carcinomas that arise from the oral cavity. When cancer is limited to the vocal cords (intrinsic), spread may be slow. When the cancer involves the epiglottis (extrinsic), metastasis is more common. Current treatment choices include surgery, radiation, and chemotherapy. Carbon dioxide laser may be used for early stage disease. This plan of care focuses on nursing care of the patient undergoing radical surgery of the neck including laryngectomy.

Partial laryngectomy: Tumors that are limited to only 1 vocal cord are removed and a temporary tracheotomy is performed to maintain the airway. After recovery from surgery, the patient's voice will be hoarse.

Hemilaryngectomy: When there is a possibility the cancer includes 1 true and 1 false vocal cord, they are removed along with an arytenoid cartilage and half of the thyroid cartilage. Temporary tracheotomy is performed, and the patient's voice will be hoarse after surgery.

Supraglottic laryngectomy: When the tumor is located in the epiglottis or false vocal cords, radical neck dissection is done and tracheotomy performed. The patient's voice remains intact; however, swallowing is more difficult because the epiglottis has been removed.

Total laryngectomy: Advanced cancers that involve a large portion of the larynx require removal of the entire larynx, the hyoid bone, the cricoid cartilage, 2 or 3 tracheal rings, and the strap muscles connected to the larynx. A permanent opening is created in the neck for the trachea, and a laryngectomy tube inserted to keep the stoma open. The lower portion of the posterior pharynx is removed when the tumor extends beyond the epiglottis, with the remaining portion sutured to the esophagus after a nasogastric tube is inserted. The patient must breathe through a permanent tracheostomy, with normal speech no longer possible. Swallowing is not a long-term problem because there is no connection between the esophagus and trachea.

CARE SETTING

Inpatient surgical and possibly subacute units.

RELATED CONCERNS

Cancer, p 875
Psychosocial Aspects of Care, p 783
Surgical Intervention, p 802
Total Nutritional Support: Parenteral/Enteral Feeding, p 491

Patient Assessment Data Base

Preoperative data presented here is dependent on specific type/location of cancer process and underlying complications.

EGO INTEGRITY

May report:	Feelings of fear about loss of voice, dying, occurrence/recurrence of cancer
	Concern about how surgery will affect family relationships, ability to work, and finances
May exhibit:	Anxiety, depression, anger, and withdrawal
	Denial

FOOD/FLUID

May report: Difficulty swallowing

May exhibit: Difficulty handling oral secretions, chokes easily
Swelling, ulcerations, masses may be noted dependent on location of cancer
Oral inflammation/drainage, poor dental hygiene
Leukoplakia, erythroplasia of oral cavity
Halitosis
Swelling of tongue
Altered gag reflex and facial paralysis

HYGIENE

May exhibit: Neglect of dental hygiene
Need for assistance in basic care

NEUROSENSORY

May report: Diplopia (double vision)
Deafness
Tingling, paresthesia of facial muscles

May exhibit: Hemiparalysis of face (parotid and submandibular involvement); persistent hoarseness
or loss of voice (dominant and earliest symptom of intrinsic laryngeal cancer)
Difficulty swallowing
Conduction deafness
Disruption of mucous membranes

PAIN/DISCOMFORT

May report: Chronic sore throat, "lump in throat"
Referred pain to ear, facial pain (late stage, probably metastatic)
Pain/burning sensation with swallowing (especially with hot liquids or citrus juices), local
pain in oropharynx
Postoperative
Sore throat or mouth (pain is not usually reported as severe following head and neck
surgery, as compared with pain noted prior to surgery)

May exhibit: Guarding behaviors
Restlessness
Facial mask of pain
Alteration in muscle tone

RESPIRATION

May report: History of smoking/chewing tobacco
Occupation working with hardwood sawdust, toxic chemicals/fumes, heavy metals
History of voice overuse, e.g., professional singer or auctioneer
History of chronic lung disease
Cough with/without sputum
Bloody nasal drainage

May exhibit: Blood-tinged sputum, hemoptysis
Dyspnea (late)

SAFETY

May report: Excessive sun exposure over a period of years or radiation therapy
Visual/hearing changes

May exhibit: Masses/enlarged nodes

SOCIAL INTERACTION

May report: Lack of family/support system (may be result of age group or behaviors, e.g., alcoholism)
Concerns about ability to communicate, engage in social interactions

May exhibit: Persistent hoarseness, change in voice pitch
Muffled/garbled speech, reluctance to speak
Hesitancy/reluctance of significant others to provide care/be involved in rehabilitation

TEACHING/LEARNING

May report: Nonhealing of oral lesions
Concurrent use of alcohol/history of alcohol abuse

Discharge plan considerations: **DRG projected mean length of inpatient stay: 7.4 days**
Assistance with wound care, treatments, supplies; transportation, shopping; food preparation; self-care, homemaker/maintenance tasks

Refer to section at end of plan for postdischarge considerations.

DIAGNOSTIC STUDIES

Direct/indirect laryngoscopy; laryngeal tomography and biopsy: Are the most reliable diagnostic indicators.
Laryngography: May be performed with contrast to study blood vessels and lymph nodes.
Pulmonary function studies, bone scans, or other organ scans: May be indicated if distant metastasis is suspected.
Chest x-ray: Done to establish baseline lung status and/or identify metastases.
CBC: May reveal anemia, which is a common problem.
Immunologic surveys: May be done for patients receiving chemotherapy/immunotherapy.
Biochemical profile: Changes may occur in organ function as a result of cancer, metastasis, and therapies.
ABGs/pulse oximetry: May be done to establish baseline/monitor status of lungs (ventilation).

NURSING PRIORITIES

1. Maintain patent airway, adequate ventilation.
2. Assist patient in developing alternate communication methods.
3. Restore/maintain skin integrity.
4. Reestablish/maintain adequate nutrition.
5. Provide emotional support for acceptance of altered body image.
6. Provide information about disease process/prognosis and treatment.

DISCHARGE GOALS

1. Ventilation/oxygenation adequate for individual needs.
2. Communicating effectively.
3. Complications prevented/minimized.
4. Beginning to cope with change in body image.
5. Disease process/prognosis and therapeutic regimen understood.
6. Plan in place to meet needs after discharge.

NURSING DIAGNOSIS: Airway Clearance, ineffective/Aspiration, risk for

May be related to

Partial/total removal of the glottis, altering ability to breathe, cough, and swallow

Temporary or permanent change to neck breathing (dependent on patent stoma)

Edema formation (surgical manipulation and lymphatic accumulation)

Copious and thick secretions

Possibly evidenced by (Airway Clearance)

Dyspnea/difficulty breathing

Changes in rate/depth of respiration

Use of accessory respiratory muscles

Abnormal breath sounds

Cyanosis

DESIRED OUTCOMES/EVALUATION CRITERIA—PATIENT WILL:

Maintain patent airway with breath sounds clear/clearing.

Expectorate/clear secretion and be free of aspiration.

Demonstrate behaviors to improve/maintain airway clearance within level of ability/ situation.

ACTIONS/INTERVENTIONS	RATIONALE
Independent	
Monitor respiratory rate/depth; note ease of breathing. Auscultate breath sounds. Investigate restlessness, dyspnea, development of cyanosis.	Changes in respirations, use of accessory muscles, and/or presence of rhonchi/wheezes suggests retention of secretions. Airway obstruction (even partial) can lead to ineffective breathing patterns and impaired gas exchange resulting in complications, e.g., pneumonia, respiratory arrest.
Elevate head of bed 30–45 degrees.	Facilitates drainage of secretions, work of breathing, and lung expansion.
Encourage swallowing, if patient is able.	Prevents pooling of oral secretions reducing risk of aspiration. *Note:* Swallowing is impaired when the epiglottis is removed and/or significant postoperative edema and pain are present.
Encourage effective coughing and deep breathing.	Mobilizes secretions to clear airway and helps prevent respiratory complications.
Suction laryngectomy/tracheostomy tube, oral and nasal cavities. Note amount, color, and consistency of secretions.	Prevents secretions from obstructing airway, especially when swallowing ability is impaired and patient cannot blow nose. Changes in character of secretions may indicate developing problems (e.g., dehydration, infection) and need for further evaluation/treatment.
Demonstrate and encourage patient to begin self-suction procedures as soon as possible. Educate patient in "clean" techniques.	Assists patient to exercise some control in postoperative care and prevention of complications. Reduces anxiety associated with difficulty in breathing or inability to handle secretions when alone.

165

ACTIONS/INTERVENTIONS

Independent

Maintain proper position of laryngectomy/tracheostomy tube. Check/adjust ties as indicated.

Observe tissue surrounding tube for bleeding. Change patient's position to check for pooling of blood behind neck or on posterior dressings.

Change tube/inner cannula as indicated. Instruct patient in cleaning procedures.

Collaborative

Provide supplemental humidification, e.g., compressed air/oxygen mist collar, room humidifier, increased fluid intake.

Resume oral intake with caution. (Refer to ND: Nutrition: altered, less than body requirements, p 171.)

Monitor serial ABGs/pulse oximetry; chest x-ray.

RATIONALE

As edema develops/subsides, tube can be displaced, compromising airway. Ties should be snug but not constrictive to surrounding tissue or major blood vessels.

Small amount of oozing may be present; however, continued bleeding or sudden eruption of uncontrolled hemorrhage presents a sudden and very real possibility of airway obstruction/suffocation.

Prevents accumulation of secretions and thick mucus plugs from obstructing airway. *Note:* This is a common cause of respiratory distress/arrest in later postoperative period.

Normal physiologic (nose/nasal passages) means of filtering/humidifying air are bypassed. Supplemental humidity decreases mucous crusting and facilitates coughing/suctioning of secretions through stoma.

Changes in muscle mass/strength and nerve inervation increase likelihood of aspiration.

Pooling of secretions/presence of atelectasis may lead to pneumonia requiring more aggressive therapeutic measures.

NURSING DIAGNOSIS: Communication, impaired verbal

May be related to
Anatomic deficit (removal of vocal cords)
Physical barrier (tracheostomy tube)
Required voice rest

Possibly evidenced by
Inability to speak
Change in vocal characteristics

DESIRED OUTCOMES/EVALUATION CRITERIA—PATIENT WILL:
Communicate needs in an effective manner.
Identify/plan for appropriate alternate speech methods after healing.

ACTIONS/INTERVENTIONS

Independent

Review preoperative instructions/discussion of why speech and breathing are altered, using anatomic drawings or models to assist in explanations.

Determine whether patient has other communication impairment, e.g., hearing, vision, literacy.

RATIONALE

Reinforces teaching at a time when fear of surviving surgery is past.

Presence of other problems will influence plan for alternate communication.

ACTIONS/INTERVENTIONS	RATIONALE
Independent	
Provide immediate and continual means to summon nurse, e.g., call light/bell. Let the patient know the summons will be answered immediately. Stop by to check on patient periodically without being summoned. Post notice at central answering system/nursing station that patient is unable to speak.	Patient needs assurance that nurse is vigilant and will respond to summons. Trust and self-esteem are fostered when the nurse cares enough to come at times other than when called by the patient.
Prearrange signals for obtaining immediate help.	May decease patient's anxiety about inability to speak.
Provide alternate means of communication appropriate to patient need, e.g., pad and pencil, magic slate, alphabet/picture board, sign language. Consider placement of IV.	Permits patient to "express" needs/concerns. *Note:* IV positioned in hand/wrist may limit ability to write or sign.
Allow sufficient time for communication.	Loss of speech and stress of alternate communication can cause frustration and block expression, especially when caregivers seem "too busy" or preoccupied.
Provide nonverbal communication, e.g., touching and physical presence. Anticipate needs.	Communicates concern and meets need for contact with others. Touch is believed to generate complex biochemical events, with possible release of endorphins contributing to reduction of anxiety.
Encourage ongoing communication with "outside world," e.g., newspapers, television, radio, calendar, clock.	Maintains contact with "normal lifestyle" and continued communication through other avenues.
Refer to loss of speech as temporary after a partial laryngectomy and/or depending on availability of voice prosthetics.	Provides encouragement and hope for future with the thought that alternate means of communication and speech are available and possible.
Caution patient not to use voice until physician gives permission.	Promotes healing of vocal cord and limits potential for permanent cord dysfunction.
Arrange for meeting with other persons who have experienced this procedure, as appropriate.	Provides role model, enhancing motivation for problem solving and learning new ways to communicate.
Collaborative	
Consult with appropriate health team members/therapists/rehabilitation agency (e.g., speech pathologist, social services, laryngectomee clubs) for hospital-based rehabilitation as well as community resources, such as Lost Chord/NewVoice Club, International Association of Laryngectomees, American Cancer Society.	Ability to use alternate voice and speech methods (e.g., electrolarynx, 1-way valved voice prosthesis, esophageal speech) varies greatly, dependent on extent of surgical procedures, patient's age, emotional state, and motivation to return to an active life. Rehabilitation time may be lengthy and require a number of agencies/resources to facilitate/support learning process.

NURSING DIAGNOSIS: Skin/Tissue Integrity, impaired

May be related to

Surgical removal of tissues/grafting

Radiation or chemotherapeutic agents

Altered circulation/reduced blood supply

Compromised nutritional status

Edema formation

Pooling/continuous drainage of secretions (oral, lymph, or chyle)

ACTIONS/INTERVENTIONS	RATIONALE
Independent	
Assess skin color/temperature and capillary refill in operative and skin graft areas.	Skin should be pink or similar to color of surrounding skin. Skin graft flaps should be pink and warm and should blanch (when gentle finger pressure is applied), with return to color within seconds. Cyanosis and slow refill may indicate venous congestion, which can lead to tissue ischemia/necrosis.
Keep head of bed elevated 30–45 degrees. Monitor facial edema (usually peaks by 3rd–5th postoperative day).	Minimizes postoperative tissue congestion and edema related to excision of lymph channels.
Protect skin flaps and suture lines from tension or pressure. Provide pillows/rolls and instruct patient to support head/neck during activity.	Pressure from tubings and tracheostomy tapes or tension on suture lines can alter circulation/cause tissue injury.
Monitor bloody drainage from surgical sites, suture lines, drains. Measure drainage from hemovac device (if used).	Bloody drainage usually declines steadily after first 24 hours. Steady oozing or frank bleeding indicates problem requiring medical attention.
Note/report any milky-appearing drainage.	Milky drainage may indicate thoracic lymph duct leakage (can result in depletion of body fluids and electrolytes). Such a leak may heal spontaneously or require surgical closure.
Change dressings as indicated.	Damp dressings increase risk of tissue damage/infection. *Note:* Pressure dressings are not used over skin flaps, because blood supply is easily compromised.
Cleanse incisions with sterile saline and peroxide (mixed 1:1) after dressings have been removed.	Prevents crust formation, which can trap purulent drainage, destroy skin edges, and increase size of wound. Peroxide is not used full strength because it may cauterize wound edges and impair healing.
Monitor donor site if graft performed; check dressings as indicated.	Donor site may be adjacent to operative site or a distant site (e.g., thigh). Pressure dressings are usually removed within 24–48 hours and wound is left open to air to promote healing.
Cleanse thoroughly around stoma and neck tubes (if in place) avoiding soap or alcohol. Show patient how to do self-stoma/tube care with clean water and peroxide, using cloth, not tissue or cotton.	Keeping area cleansed promotes healing and comfort. Soap and other drying agents can lead to stomal irritation and possible inflammation. Materials other than cloth may leave fibers in stoma that can irritate or be inhaled into lungs.
Monitor all sites for signs of wound infection, e.g., unusual redness, increasing edema, pain, exudates, and temperature elevation.	Impedes healing, which may already be slow because of changes induced by cancer, cancer therapies, and/or malnutrition.

Collaborative

Administer oral, IV, and topical antibiotics as indicated.

Prevents/controls infection.

Cover donor sites with petroleum gauze or moisture-impermeable dressing.

Nonadherent dressing covers exposed sensory nerve endings and protects site from contamination.

NURSING DIAGNOSIS: Oral Mucous Membranes, altered

May be related to
Dehydration/absence of oral intake
Poor/inadequate oral hygiene
Pathologic condition (oral cancer)
Mechanical trauma (oral surgery)
Decreased saliva production secondary to radiation (common) or surgical procedure (rare)
Difficulty swallowing and pooling of secretions/drooling
Nutritional deficits

Possibly evidenced by
Xerostomia (dry mouth), oral discomfort
Thick/mucoid saliva, decreased saliva production
Dry, crusted, coated tongue; inflamed lips
Absent teeth/gums, poor dental health, halitosis

DESIRED OUTCOMES/EVALUATION CRITERIA—PATIENT WILL:
Report/demonstrate a decrease in symptoms.
Identify specific interventions to promote healthy oral mucosa.
Demonstrate techniques to restore/maintain mucosal integrity.

ACTIONS/INTERVENTIONS	RATIONALE
Independent	
Inspect oral cavity and note changes in:	
Saliva;	Damage to salivary glands may decrease production of saliva, resulting in dry mouth. Pooling and drooling of saliva may occur because of compromised swallowing capability or pain in throat and mouth.
Tongue;	Surgery may have included partial resection of tongue, soft palate, and pharynx. This patient will have decreased sensation and movement of tongue, with difficulty swallowing and increased risk of aspiration of secretions, as well as potential for hemorrhage.
Lips;	Surgical removal of part of lip may result in uncontrollable drooling.
Teeth and gums;	Teeth may not be intact (surgical) or may be in poor condition because of malnutrition, chemical therapies, and neglect. Gums may also be surgically altered or inflamed because of poor hygiene, long history of smoking/chewing tobacco, or chemical therapies.
Mucous membranes.	May be excessively dry, ulcerated, erythematous, edematous.

169

ACTIONS/INTERVENTIONS	RATIONALE

Independent

Suction oral cavity gently/frequently. Have patient perform self-suctioning when possible or use gauze wick to drain secretions.	Saliva contains digestive enzymes that may be erosive to exposed tissues. Since drooling may be constant, patient can promote own comfort and enhance oral hygiene.
Show patient how to brush inside of mouth, palate, tongue, and teeth frequently.	Reduces bacteria and risk of infection, promotes tissue healing and comfort.
Apply lubrication to lips; provide oral irrigations as indicated.	Counteracts drying effects of therapeutic measures; negates erosive nature of secretions.

NURSING DIAGNOSIS: Pain [acute]

May be related to
Surgical incisions
Tissue swelling
Presence of nasogastric/orogastric feeding tube

Possibly evidenced by
Discomfort in surgical areas/pain with swallowing
Facial mask of pain
Distraction behaviors, restlessness
Guarding behavior

DESIRED OUTCOMES/EVALUATION CRITERIA—PATIENT WILL:
Report/indicate pain is relieved/controlled.
Demonstrate relief of pain/discomfort by reduced tension and relaxed manner, sleeping/resting appropriately.

ACTIONS/INTERVENTIONS	RATIONALE

Independent

Support head and neck with pillows. Show patient how to support neck during activity.	Muscle weakness results from muscle and nerve resection in the structures of the neck and/or shoulders. Lack of support aggravates discomfort and may result in injury to suture areas.
Provide comfort measures (e.g., back rub, position change) and diversional activities (e.g., television, visiting, reading).	Promotes relaxation and helps the patient refocus attention on something besides self/discomfort. May reduce analgesic dosage needs/frequency.
Encourage patient to expectorate saliva or to suction mouth gently if unable to swallow.	Swallowing causes muscle activity that may be painful because of edema/strain on suture lines.
Investigate changes in characteristics of pain. Check mouth, throat suture lines for fresh trauma.	May reflect developing complications requiring further evaluation/intervention. Tissues are inflamed and congested and may be easily traumatized by suction catheter, feeding tube, and so on.
Note nonverbal indicators and autonomic responses to pain. Evaluate effects of analgesics.	Aids in determining presence of pain, need for/effectiveness of medication.

ACTIONS/INTERVENTIONS

Independent

Medicate before activity/treatments as indicated.

Schedule care activities to balance with adequate periods of sleep/rest.

Recommend use of stress management behaviors, e.g., relaxation techniques, guided imagery.

Collaborative

Provide oral irrigations, anesthetic sprays, and gargles. Instruct patient in self-irrigations.

Administer analgesics, e.g., codeine, ASA, and Darvon, as indicated.

RATIONALE

May enhance cooperation and participation in therapeutic regimen.

Prevents fatigue/exhaustion and may enhance coping with stress/discomfort.

Promotes sense of well-being, may reduce analgesic needs and enhance healing.

Improves comfort, promotes healing, and reduces halitosis. *Note:* Commercial mouthwashes containing alcohol or phenol are to be avoided because of their drying effect.

Degree of pain is related to extent and psychologic impact of surgery as well as general body condition. Studies appear to support the idea that many patients experience more pain before than after head and neck surgery.

NURSING DIAGNOSIS: Nutrition: altered, less than body requirements

May be related to
Temporary or permanent alteration in mode of food intake
Altered feedback mechanisms of desire to eat, taste, and smell because of surgical/ structural changes, radiation, or chemotherapy

Possibly evidenced by
Inadequate food intake, perceived inability to ingest food
Aversion to eating, lack of interest in food
Reported altered taste sensation
Weight loss
Weakness of muscles required for swallowing or mastication

DESIRED OUTCOMES/EVALUATION CRITERIA—PATIENT WILL:
Indicate understanding of importance of nutrition to healing process and general well-being.
Make dietary choices to meet nutrient needs within individual situation.
Demonstrate progressive weight gain toward goal, with normalization of laboratory values and timely healing of tissues/incisions.

ACTIONS/INTERVENTIONS

Independent

Auscultate bowel sounds.

RATIONALE

Feedings are usually begun after bowel sounds are restored postoperatively. Note: In more aggressive therapy, tube feeding may be started earlier if gastric residuals are closely monitored.

171

ACTIONS/INTERVENTIONS	RATIONALE
Independent	
Maintain feeding tube, e.g., check for tube placement, flush with warm water as indicated.	Tube is inserted during surgery and usually sutured in place. Initially the tube may be attached to suction to reduce nausea and/or vomiting. Flushing aids in maintaining patency of tube.
Monitor intake and weigh as indicated. Show patient how to monitor and record weight on a scheduled basis.	Provides information regarding nutritional needs and effectiveness of therapy.
Instruct patient/SO in self-feeding techniques, e.g., bulb syringe, bag and funnel method, and blending soft foods if the patient is to go home with a feeding tube. Make sure patient and SO are able to perform this procedure prior to discharge and that appropriate food and equipment are available at home.	Helps promote nutritional success and preserves dignity in the adult who is now forced to be dependent on others for very basic needs in the social setting of meals.
Begin with small feedings and advance as tolerated. Note signs of gastric fullness, regurgitation, diarrhea.	Content of feeding may result in GI intolerance, requiring change in rate or type of formula.
Provide supplemental water by feeding tube or orally if patient can swallow.	Keeps patient hydrated to offset insensible losses and drainage from surgical areas. Meets free water needs associated with enteral feeding.
Encourage patient when relearning swallowing; e.g., maintain quiet environment, have suction equipment on standby, and demonstrate appropriate breathing techniques.	Helps patient to deal with the frustration and safety concerns involved with swallowing. Provides reassurance that measures are available to prevent/limit aspiration.
Resume oral feedings when feasible. Stay with patient during meals the first few days.	Oral feedings can usually resume after suture lines are healed (8–10 days) unless further reconstruction is required or patient will be going home with feeding tube. The patient may experience pain or difficulty with chewing and swallowing initially and may require suctioning during meals, in addition to support and encouragement.
Develop and encourage a pleasant environment for meals.	Promotes socialization and maximizes patient comfort when eating difficulties cause embarrassment.
Help patient/SO develop nutritionally balanced home meal plans.	Promotes understanding of individual needs and significance of nutrition in healing and recovery process.
Collaborative	
Consult with dietitian/nutritional support team as indicated. Incorporate and reinforce dietitian's teaching.	Useful in identifying individual nutritional needs to promote healing and tissue regeneration. Discharge teaching and follow-up by the dietitian may be needed to evaluate patient needs for diet/equipment modifications and meal planning in the home setting.
Provide nutritionally balanced diet (e.g., semisolid/soft foods) or tube feedings (e.g., blended soft food or commercial preparations) as indicated.	Variations can be made to add or limit certain factors, such as fat and sugar, or to provide a food that the patient prefers.
Monitor laboratory studies, e.g., BUN, glucose, liver function, prealbumin/protein, electrolytes.	Indicators of utilization of nutrients as well as organ function.

172

NURSING DIAGNOSIS: Body Image disturbance/Role Performance, altered

May be related to

Loss of voice

Changes in anatomic contour of face and neck (disfigurement and/or severe functional impairment)

Presence of chronic illness

Possibly evidenced by

Report of fear of rejection by/reaction of others

Negative feelings about body change

Refusal to verify actual change or preoccupation with change/loss, not looking at self in mirror

Change in social involvement; discomfort in social situations

Change in self/others' perception of role

Anxiety, depression, lack of eye contact

Failure of family members to adapt to change or deal with experience constructively

DESIRED OUTCOMES/EVALUATION CRITERIA—PATIENT WILL:

Identify feelings and methods for coping with negative perception of self.

Demonstrate initial adaptation to body changes as evidenced by participating in self-care activities and positive interactions with others.

Communicate with SO about changes in role that have occurred.

Begin to develop plans for altered lifestyle.

Participate in team efforts toward rehabilitation.

ACTIONS/INTERVENTIONS	RATIONALE
Independent	
Discuss meaning of loss/change with patient, identifying perceptions of current situation/future expectations.	Aids in identifying/defining the problem(s) to focus attention and interventions constructively.
Note nonverbal body language, negative attitudes/self-talk. Assess for self-destructive/suicidal behavior.	May indicate depression/despair, need for further assessment/more intense intervention.
Note emotional reactions, e.g., grieving, depression, anger. Allow patient to progress at own rate.	The patient may experience immediate depression after surgery, or react with shock and denial. Acceptance of changes cannot be forced, and the grieving process needs time for resolution.
Maintain calm, reassuring manner. Acknowledge and accept expression of feelings of grief, hostility.	May help allay patient's fears of dying, suffocation, inability to communicate, or mutilation. Patient and SO need to feel supported and know that all feelings are appropriate for the type of experience they are going through.
Allow but do not participate in patient's use of denial, e.g., when patient is reluctant to participate in self-care (e.g., suctioning stoma). Provide care in a nonjudgmental manner.	Denial may be the most helpful defense for the patient in the beginning, permitting the individual to begin to deal slowly with difficult adjustment.
Set limits on maladaptive behaviors, assisting patient to identify positive behaviors that will aid recovery.	Acting out can result in lowered self-esteem and impede adjustment to new self-image.

ACTIONS/INTERVENTIONS	RATIONALE
Independent	
Encourage SO to treat patient normally and not as an invalid.	Distortions of body image may be unconsciously reinforced.
Alert staff that facial expressions and other nonverbal behaviors need to convey acceptance and not revulsion.	The patient is very sensitive to nonverbal communication and may make negative assumptions about others' body language.
Encourage identification of anticipated personal/work conflicts that may arise.	Expressions of concern bring problems into the open where they can be examined/dealt with.
Recognize behavior indicative of overconcern with future lifestyle/relationship functioning.	Ruminating about anticipated losses/reactions of others is nonproductive and is a block to problem solving.
Encourage patient to deal with situation in small steps.	May feel overwhelmed/have difficulty coping with larger picture but can manage 1 piece at a time.
Provide positive reinforcement for efforts/progress made.	Encourages patient to feel a sense of movement toward recovery.
Encourage patient/SO to communicate feelings to each other.	All those involved may have difficulty in this area (because of the loss of voice function and/or disfigurement) but need to understand that they may gain courage and help from one another.
Collaborative	
Refer patient/SO to supportive resources, e.g., psychotherapy, social worker, family counseling, pastoral care.	A multifaceted approach is required to assist patient toward rehabilitation and wellness. Families need assistance in understanding the processes that the patient is going through and to help them with their own emotions. The goal is to enable them to guard against the tendency to withdraw from/isolate the patient from social contact.

NURSING DIAGNOSIS: Knowledge deficit [learning needs] regarding condition and treatment, self care and discharge needs

May be related to
Lack of information/recall
Misinterpretation of information
Poor assimilation of material presented
Lack of interest in learning

Possibly evidenced by
Indications of concern/request for information
Inaccurate follow-through of instructions
Inappropriate or exaggerated behaviors, e.g., hostile, agitated, apathetic

DESIRED OUTCOMES/EVALUATION CRITERIA—PATIENT WILL:
Indicate basic understanding of disease process, surgical intervention, prognosis, treatment needs.
Demonstrate ability to provide safe care.
Use resources (rehabilitation team members) appropriately.
Identify symptoms requiring medical evaluation/intervention.
Develop plan for/schedule follow-up appointments.

ACTIONS/INTERVENTIONS	RATIONALE

Independent

Ascertain amount of preoperative preparation and retention of information. Assess level of anxiety related to diagnosis and surgery.

Information can provide clues to patient's postoperative reactions. Anxiety may have interfered with understanding of information given before surgery.

Provide/repeat explanations at patient's level of acceptance. Discuss inaccuracies in perception of disease process and therapies with patient and SO.

Overwhelming stressors are present and may be coupled with limited knowledge. Misconceptions are inevitable, but failure to explore and correct them can result in the patient's failing to progress toward health.

Provide written directions for the patient/SO to read and have available for future reference.

Reinforces proper information and may be used as a home reference.

Educate the patient and SO about basic information regarding stoma, e.g.:

Tub baths instead of showers (initially), shampoo by leaning forward, no swimming or water sports;

Prevents water from entering airway/stoma.

Cover stoma with bib/natural fiber scarf (e.g., cotton or silk);

Prevents dust and particles from being inhaled.

Cover stoma when coughing or sneezing;

Normal airways are bypassed, and mucus will exit from stoma.

Reinforce necessity of not smoking.

Necessary to preserve lung function. *Note:* Patient may need extra support and encouragement to understand that quality of life can be improved by cessation of smoking.

Discuss importance of reporting to caregiver/physician immediately such symptoms as stoma narrowing, presence of "lump" in throat, dysphagia, or bleeding.

May be signs of tracheal stenosis, recurrent cancer, or carotid erosion.

Develop a means of emergency communication at home.

Permits patient to summon assistance when needed.

Recommend wearing medical-alert identification tag/bracelet. Encourage family members to become CPR-certified if they are interested/able to do so.

Provides for appropriate care if the patient becomes unconscious or suffers a pulmonary arrest.

Give careful attention to the provision of needed rehabilitative measures, e.g., temporary/permanent prosthesis, dental care, speech therapy, surgical reconstruction; vocational, sexual/marital counseling; financial assistance.

These services can contribute to patient's well-being and have a positive effect on patient's quality of life.

Identify homecare needs and available resources.

Provides support for transition from hospital setting.

POTENTIAL CONSIDERATIONS following acute hospitalization (dependent on patient's age, physical condition/presence of complications, personal resources and life responsibilities)

Aspiration, risk for—presence of tracheostomy, tube feedings, impaired swallowing, decreased muscle mass/strength (status after neck surgery).

Communication, impaired verbal—anatomic presence of tracheostomy.

Infection, risk for—broken skin/traumatized tissue, stasis of secretions, suppressed inflammatory response, chronic disease, malnutrition.

Nutrition: altered, less than body requirements—temporary alteration in mode of food intake, altered feedback mechanisms relative to senses of taste and smell.

Self Care deficit—decreased strength/endurance, presence of pain, depression.

VENTILATORY ASSISTANCE (MECHANICAL)

More and more patients on ventilators are being transferred from the ICU to medical-surgical units with problems such as (1) neuromuscular deficits, e.g., quadriplegia with phrenic nerve injury or high C-spine injuries, Guillain-Barré, and ALS; (2) COPD with respiratory muscle atrophy and malnutrition (inability to wean); and (3) restrictive conditions of chest or lungs, e.g., kyphoscoliosis, interstitial fibrosis.

The expectation is that the majority of patients will be weaned prior to discharge. That is the focus of this plan of care. However, it is known that some patients are unsuccessful at weaning, or are not candidates for weaning. For those patients, portions of this plan of care would need to be modified.

Volume-cycled ventilators are the primary choice for long-term ventilation of patients whose permanent changes in lung compliance and resistance require increased pressure to provide adequate ventilation (e.g., COPD).

Pressure-cycled ventilators are desirable for patients with relatively normal lung compliance who cannot initiate or sustain respiration because of muscular/phrenic nerve involvement (e.g., quadriplegics).

CARE SETTING

Patients on ventilators may be cared for in any setting; however, weaning is usually attempted/accomplished in the acute, subacute, or rehabilitation setting.

RELATED CONCERNS

Cardiac Surgery: Coronary Artery Bypass Graft; Cardiomyoplasty; Valve Replacement (Postoperative Care), p 95
Chronic Obstructive Pulmonary Disease (COPD), p 117
Hemothorax/Pneumothorax, p 154
Psychosocial Aspects of Care, p 783
Spinal Cord Injury (Acute Rehabilitative Phase), p 278
Total Nutritional Support: Parenteral/Enteral Feeding, p 491

Patient Assessment Data Base

Data gathered are dependent on the underlying pathophysiology and/or reason for ventilatory support. Refer to the appropriate plan of care.

Discharge plan considerations:
DRG projected mean length of inpatient stay: 13.1 days
If ventilator-dependent, may require changes in physical layout of home, acquisition of equipment/supplies, provision of a backup power source, instruction of SO/caregivers, provision for continuation of plan of care, assistance with transportation, and coordination of resources/support systems

Refer to section at end of plan for postdischarge considerations.

DIAGNOSTIC STUDIES

Pulmonary function studies: Determine the ability of the lungs to exchange oxygen and carbon dioxide and include but are not limited to the following:

Vital capacity (VC): Is reduced in restrictive chest or lung conditions; is normal or increased in COPD; normal to decreased in neuromuscular diseases (Guillain-Barré); decreased in conditions limiting thoracic movement (kyphoscoliosis).

Forced vital capacity (FVC): measured by spirometry, is reduced in restrictive conditions and in asthma, normal to reduced in COPD.

Tidal volume (V_T): May be decreased in both restrictive and obstructive processes.

Negative inspiratory force (NIF): Can be substituted for vital capacity to help determine whether the patient can initiate a breath.

Minute ventilation (V_E): Measures volume of air inhaled and exhaled in 1 minute of normal breathing. This reflects muscle endurance and is a major determinant of work of breathing.

Inspiratory pressure (Pi_{max}): Measures respiratory muscle strength (less than -20 cm H_2O is considered insufficient for weaning).

Forced expiratory volume (FEV): Usually decreased in chronic obstructive lung diseases.

Flow-volume (F-V) loops: Abnormal loops are indicative of large and small airway obstructive disease and restrictive diseases, when far advanced.

ABGs: Assesses status of oxygenation and ventilation and of acid-base balance.

Chest x-ray: Monitors resolution/progression of underlying condition (e.g., ARDS) or complications (e.g., atelectasis, pneumonia).

Nutritional assessment: Done to identify nutritional and electrolyte imbalances which might interfere with successful weaning.

NURSING PRIORITIES

1. Promote adequate ventilation and oxygenation.
2. Prevent complications.
3. Provide emotional support for patient/SO.
4. Provide information about disease process/prognosis and treatment needs.

DISCHARGE GOALS

1. Respiratory function adequate to meet individual needs.
2. Complications prevented/minimized.
3. Effective means of communication established.
4. Disease process/prognosis and therapeutic regimen understood (including home ventilatory support if indicated).
5. Plan in place to meet needs after discharge.

NURSING DIAGNOSIS: Breathing Pattern, ineffective/Spontaneous Ventilation, inability to sustain

May be related to

Respiratory center depression

Respiratory muscle weakness/paralysis

Noncompliant lung tissue (decreased lung expansion)

Alteration of patient's usual O_2/CO_2 ratio

Possibly evidenced by

Changes in rate and depth of respirations

Dyspnea/increased work of breathing, use of accessory muscles

Reduced vital capacity/total lung volume

Tachypnea/bradypnea or cessation of respirations when off the ventilator

Cyanosis

Decreased Po_2 and Sao_2; increased Pco_2

Increased restlessness, apprehension, and metabolic rate

DESIRED OUTCOMES/EVALUATION CRITERIA—PATIENT WILL:

Reestablish/maintain effective respiratory pattern via ventilator with absence of retractions/use of accessory muscles, cyanosis, or other signs of hypoxia; ABGs/oxygen saturation within acceptable range.

Participate in efforts to wean (as appropriate) within individual ability.

CAREGIVER WILL:

Demonstrate behaviors necessary to maintain patient's respiratory function.

ACTIONS/INTERVENTIONS	RATIONALE

Independent

Investigate etiology of respiratory failure.

Understanding the underlying cause of the patient's particular ventilatory problem is essential to the care of the patient, e.g., decisions about future patient capabilities/ventilation needs and most appropriate type of ventilatory support.

Observe overall breathing pattern. Note respiratory rate, distinguishing between spontaneous respirations and ventilator breaths.

Patients on ventilator can experience hyperventilation/hypoventilation, dyspnea/"air hunger," and attempt to correct deficiency by overbreathing.

Auscultate chest periodically, noting presence/absence and equality of breath sounds, adventitious breath sounds, as well as symmetry of chest movement.

Provides information regarding airflow through the tracheobronchial tree and the presence/absence of fluid, mucus obstruction. *Note:* Frequent crackles or rhonchi that do not clear with coughing/suctioning may indicate developing complications (atelectasis, pneumonia, acute bronchospasm, pulmonary edema). Changes in chest symmetry may indicate improper placement of endotracheal tube, development of barotrauma.

Count patient's respirations for 1 full minute and compare to desired/ventilator set rate.

Respirations vary, depending on problem requiring ventilatory assistance, e.g., patient may be totally ventilator-dependent, or be able to take breath(s) on own between ventilator-delivered breaths. Rapid patient respirations can produce respiratory alkalosis and/or prevent desired volume from being delivered by ventilator. Slow patient respirations/hypoventilation increases $PaCO_2$ levels and may cause acidosis.

Verify that patient's respirations are in phase with the ventilator.

Adjustments may be required in tidal volume, respiratory rate, and/or dead space of the ventilator, or the patient may need sedation to synchronize respirations and reduce work of breathing/energy expenditure.

Elevate head of bed or place in orthopedic chair if possible.

Elevation of the patient's head or getting out of bed while still on the ventilator is both physically and psychologically beneficial.

Inflate tracheal/endotracheal tube cuff properly using minimal leak/occlusive technique. Check cuff inflation every 4–8 hours and whenever cuff is deflated/reinflated.

The cuff must be properly inflated to ensure adequate ventilation/delivery of desired tidal volume. *Note:* In long-term patients, the cuff may be deflated most of the time or a noncuffed tracheostomy tube used.

Check tubing for obstruction, e.g., kinking or accumulation of water. Drain tubing as indicated, avoiding draining toward the patient or back into the reservoir.

Kinks in tubing prevent adequate volume delivery and increase airway pressure. Water prevents proper gas distribution and predisposes to bacterial growth.

Check ventilator alarms for proper functioning. Do not turn off alarms, even for suctioning. Remove from ventilator and ventilate manually if source of ventilator alarm cannot be quickly identified and rectified. Ascertain that alarms can be heard in the nurses' station.

Ventilators have a series of visual and audible alarms, e.g., oxygen, low/high pressure, I:E ratio. Turning off/failure to reset alarms places patient at risk for unobserved ventilator failure or respiratory distress/arrest.

Keep resuscitation bag at bedside and ventilate manually whenever indicated.

Provides/restores adequate ventilation when patient or equipment problems require that the patient be temporarily removed from the ventilator.

ACTIONS/INTERVENTIONS

Independent

Assist patient in "taking control" of breathing if weaning is attempted/ventilatory support is interrupted during procedure/activity.

Collaborative

Assess ventilator settings routinely and readjust as indicated:

Note operating mode of ventilation, i.e., assist control (ACV), intermittent mandatory (IMV), pressure support (PSU), inverse ratio (IRV);

Observe oxygen concentration percentage (FIO_2); verify that oxygen line is in proper outlet/tank; monitor in-line oxygen analyzer or perform periodic oxygen analysis;

Assess minute ventilation (respiratory rate and tidal volume);

Assess tidal volume (10–15 ml/kg). Verify proper function of spirometer, bellows or computer readout of delivered volume. Note alterations from desired volume delivery;

Note airway pressure;

RATIONALE

Coaching the patient to take slower, deeper breaths, practice abdominal/pursed-lip breathing, assume position of comfort, and use relaxation techniques, can be helpful in maximizing respiratory function.

Controls/settings are adjusted according to patient's primary disease and results of diagnostic testing in order to maintain parameters within appropriate limits.

The patient's respiratory requirements, presence or absence of an underlying disease process, and the extent to which the patient can participate in ventilatory effort determines parameters of each setting. PSV, a relatively new mode, has shown advantages for patients who are ventilated long-term, as it allows the patient to strengthen pulmonary musculature without compromising oxygenation and ventilation during the weaning process. One recent study suggests that intermittent trials of unassisted breathing work faster (for weaning) than methods involving partial ventilatory support.

FIO_2 is adjusted to maintain an acceptable oxygen percentage and saturation for patient's condition (may be 21%–100%). Because machine dials are not always accurate, an oxygen analyzer may be used to ascertain that patient is receiving the desired concentration of oxygen.

Respiratory rate of 10–15/m may be appropriate except for patient with COPD and CO_2 retention. In these patients, minute ventilation should be adjusted to achieve patient's baseline $PaCO_2$, not necessarily a "normal" $PaCO_2$.

Monitors amount of air inspired and expired. Changes may indicate alteration in lung compliance or leakage through machine/around tube cuff (if used). *Note:* Smaller tidal volume may be required in patients with decreased lung compliance (e.g., ARDS).

Airway pressure should remain relatively constant. Increased pressure alarm reading reflects (1) increased airway resistance as may occur with bronchospasm; (2) retained secretions; and/or (3) decreased lung compliance as may occur with obstruction of the ET tube, development of atelectasis, ARDS, pulmonary edema, worsening COPD, or pneumothorax. Low airway pressure alarms may be triggered by pathophysiologic conditions causing hypoventilation, e.g., disconnection from ventilator, low ET cuff pressure, ET displaced above the vocal cords, patient "overbreathing" or out of phase with the ventilator.

ACTIONS/INTERVENTIONS	RATIONALE
Collaborative	
Monitor inspiratory and expiratory (I:E) ratio;	Expiratory phase is usually twice the length of the inspiratory rate, but may be longer to compensate for air-trapping to improve gas exchange in the COPD patient.
Check sigh rate intervals (usually 1½–2 times tidal volume);	Sighing promotes maximal ventilation of alveoli to prevent/reduce atelectasis, and enhances movement of secretions.
Note inspired humidity and temperature.	Usual warming and humidifying function of nasopharynx is bypassed with intubation. Dehydration can dry up normal pulmonary fluids, cause secretions to thicken, and increase risk of infection. Temperature should be maintained at about body temperature to reduce risk of damage to cilia and hyperthermia reactions.

NURSING DIAGNOSIS: Airway Clearance, ineffective

May be related to
Foreign body (artificial airway) in the trachea
Inability to cough/ineffective cough

Possibly evidenced by
Changes in rate or depth of respiration
Cyanosis
Abnormal breath sounds
Anxiety/restlessness

DESIRED OUTCOMES/EVALUATION CRITERIA—PATIENT WILL:
Maintain patent airway with breath sounds clear.
Be free of aspiration.

CAREGIVER WILL:
Identify potential complications and initiate appropriate actions.

ACTIONS/INTERVENTIONS	RATIONALE
Independent	
Assess airway patency.	Obstruction may be caused by accumulation of secretions, mucus plugs, hemorrhage, bronchospasm, and/or problems with the position of tracheostomy/endotracheal tube.
Evaluate chest movement and auscultate for bilateral breath sounds.	Symmetrical chest movement with breath sounds throughout lung fields indicates proper tube placement/unobstructed airflow. Lower airway obstruction (e.g., pneumonia/atelectasis) produces changes in breath sounds such as rhonchi, wheezing.

ACTIONS/INTERVENTIONS

Independent

Monitor endotracheal tube placement. Note lip line marking and compare with desired placement. Secure tube carefully with tape or tube holder. Obtain assistance when retaping or repositioning tube.

Note excessive coughing, increased dyspnea, high-pressure alarm sounding on ventilator, visible secretions in endotracheal/tracheostomy tube, increased rhonchi.

Suction as needed when patient is coughing or experiencing respiratory distress, limiting duration of suction to 15 seconds or less. Choose appropriate suction catheter. Hyperventilate before and after each catheter pass, using 100% oxygen if appropriate.

Instruct patient in coughing techniques during suctioning, e.g., splinting, timing of breathing, and "quad cough" as indicated.

Reposition/turn periodically.

Encourage/provide fluids within individual capability.

Collaborative

Provide chest physiotherapy as indicated, e.g., postural drainage, percussion.

Administer IV and aerosol bronchodilators as indicated, e.g., aminophylline, metaproterenol sulfate (Alupent); isoetharine hydrochloride (Bronkosol).

Assist with fiberoptic bronchoscopy, if indicated.

RATIONALE

The endotracheal tube may slip into the right mainstem bronchus, thereby obstructing airflow to the left lung and putting patient at risk for a tension pneumothorax.

The intubated patient often has an ineffective cough reflex, or the patient may have neuromuscular or neurosensory impairment, altering ability to cough. These patients are dependent on alternate means such as suctioning to remove secretions.

Suctioning should not be *routine*, and duration should be limited to reduce hazard of hypoxia. Suction catheter diameter should be less than 50% of the internal diameter of the endotracheal/tracheostomy tube for prevention of hypoxia. Hyperoxygenation with bag or ventilator sigh on 100% oxygen may be desired to reduce atelectasis and to reduce accidental hypoxia. *Note:* Instilling NS is no longer recommended for "routine use," as research reveals that the fluid pools at the distal end of the ET/tracheal tube; this impairs oxygenation and increases the risk of infection.

Enhances effectiveness of cough effort and secretion clearing.

Promotes drainage of secretions and ventilation to all lung segments, reducing risk of atelectasis.

Helps liquefy secretions, enhancing expectoration.

Promotes ventilation of all lung segments and aids drainage of secretions.

Promotes ventilation and removal of secretions by relaxation of smooth muscle/bronchospasm.

May be performed to remove secretions/mucus plugs.

NURSING DIAGNOSIS: Communication, impaired verbal

May be related to
Physical barrier, e.g., endotracheal/tracheostomy tube
Neuromuscular weakness/paralysis

Possibly evidenced by
Inability to speak

DESIRED OUTCOMES/EVALUATION CRITERIA—PATIENT WILL:
Establish method of communication in which needs can be understood.

ACTIONS/INTERVENTIONS	RATIONALE
Independent	
Assess patient's ability to communicate by alternate means.	Reasons for long-term ventilatory support are various; patient may be alert and be adept at writing (e.g., chronic COPD with inability to be weaned) or may be lethargic, comatose, or paralyzed. Method of communicating with patient is therefore highly individualized.
Establish means of communication, e.g., maintain eye contact; ask yes/no questions; provide magic slate, paper/pencil, picture/alphabet board; use sign language as appropriate; validate meaning of attempted communications.	Eye contact assures patient of interest in communicating; if patient is able to move head, blink eyes, or is comfortable with simple gestures, a great deal can be done with yes/no questions. Pointing to letter boards or writing is often tiring to patients, who can then become frustrated with the effort needed to attempt conversations. Use of picture boards that express a concept or routine needs may simplify communication. Family members/other caregivers may be able to assist/interpret needs.
Consider form of communication when placing IV.	IV positioned in hand/wrist may limit ability to write or sign.
Place call light/bell within reach, making certain patient is alert and physically capable of using it. Answer call light/bell immediately. Anticipate needs. Tell patient that nurse is immediately available should assistance be required.	Ventilator-dependent patient may be better able to relax, feel safe (not abandoned), and breathe with the ventilator knowing that nurse is vigilant and needs will be met.
Place note at central call station informing staff that patient is unable to speak.	Alerts all staff members to respond to the patient at the bedside instead of over the intercom.
Encourage family/SO to talk with patient, providing information about family and daily happenings.	SO may feel self-conscious in one-sided conversation, but knowledge that he or she is assisting patient to regain/maintain contact with reality as well as enabling patient to feel part of family unit can reduce feelings of awkwardness.
Collaborative	
Evaluate need for/appropriateness of talking tracheostomy tube.	Patients with adequate cognitive/muscular skills may have the ability to manipulate talking tracheostomy tube.

NURSING DIAGNOSIS: Anxiety [specify level]/Fear

May be related to
Situational crises; threat to self-concept
Threat of death/dependency on mechanical support
Change in health/socioeconomic/role functioning
Interpersonal transmission/contagion

Possibly evidenced by
Increased muscle/facial tension
Insomnia; restlessness
Hypervigilance

Feelings of inadequacy
Fearfulness, uncertainty, apprehension
Focus on self/negative self-talk
Expressed concern regarding changes in life events

DESIRED OUTCOMES/EVALUATION CRITERIA—PATIENT WILL:
Verbalize/communicate awareness of feelings and healthy ways to deal with them.
Demonstrate problem-solving skills/behaviors to cope with current situation.
Report anxiety/fear is reduced to manageable level.
Appear relaxed and sleeping/resting appropriately.

ACTIONS/INTERVENTIONS	RATIONALE
Independent	
Identify patient's perception of threat represented by situation.	Defines scope of individual problem and influences choice of interventions.
Observe/monitor physical responses, e.g., restlessness, changes in vital signs, repetitive movements. Note congruency of verbal/nonverbal communication.	Useful in evaluating extent/degree of concerns, especially when compared with "verbal" comments.
Encourage patient/SO to acknowledge and express fears.	Provides opportunity for dealing with concerns, clarifies reality of fears, and reduces anxiety to a more manageable level.
Acknowledge the anxiety and fear of the situation. Avoid meaningless reassurance that everything will be all right.	Validates the reality of the situation without minimizing the emotional impact. Provides opportunity for the patient/SO to accept and begin to deal with what has happened, reducing anxiety.
Identify/review with patient/SO the safety precautions being taken, e.g., backup power and oxygen supplies, emergency equipment at hand for suction. Discuss/review the meanings of alarm system.	Provides reassurance to help allay unnecessary anxiety, reduce concerns of the unknown and preplan for response in emergency situation.
Note reactions of SO. Provide opportunity for discussion of personal feelings/concerns and future expectations.	Family members have individual responses to what is happening, and their anxiety may be communicated to the patient, intensifying these emotions.
Identify previous coping strengths of patient/SO and current areas of control/ability.	Focuses attention on own capabilities, increasing sense of control.
Demonstrate/encourage use of relaxation techniques, e.g., focused breathing, guided imagery, progressive relaxation.	Provides active management of situation to reduce feelings of helplessness.
Provide/encourage sedentary diversional activities within individual capabilities, e.g., handicrafts, writing, television.	Although handicapped by dependence on ventilator, activities that are normal/desired by the individual should be encouraged to enhance quality of life.
Collaborative	
Refer to support groups and therapy as needed.	May be necessary to provide additional assistance if patient/SO is not managing anxiety or when patient is "identified with the machine."

ACTIONS/INTERVENTIONS	RATIONALE
Independent	
Routinely inspect oral cavity, teeth, gums for sores, lesions, bleeding.	Early identification of problems provides opportunity for appropriate intervention/preventive measures.
Administer mouth care routinely and as needed, especially in the patient with an oral intubation tube, e.g., cleanse mouth with water, saline, or preferred mouthwash. Brush teeth with soft toothbrush, Waterpik, or moistened swab.	Prevents drying/ulceration of mucous membrane and reduces medium for bacterial growth. Promotes comfort.
Change position of endotracheal tube/airway on a regular/prn schedule as appropriate.	Reduces risk of lip and oral mucous membrane ulceration.
Apply lip balm; administer oral lubricant solution.	Maintains moisture, prevents drying.

ACTIONS/INTERVENTIONS	RATIONALE
Independent	
Evaluate ability to eat.	Patient with a tracheostomy tube may be able to eat, but patients with endotracheal tubes must be tube fed or parenterally nourished.
Observe/monitor for generalized muscle wasting, loss of subcutaneous fat.	These symptoms are indicative of depletion of muscle energy and can reduce respiratory muscle function.
Weigh as indicated.	Significant and recent weight loss (7%–10% body weight) and poor nutritional intake provide clues regarding catabolism, muscle glycogen stores, and ventilatory drive sensitivity.
Document oral intake if/when resumed. Offer foods that patient enjoys.	Appetite is usually poor and intake of essential nutrients may be reduced. Offering favorite foods can enhance oral intake.
Provide small frequent feedings of soft/easily digested foods if able to swallow.	Prevents excessive fatigue, enhances intake, and reduces risk of gastric distress.
Encourage/administer fluid intake of at least 2500 ml/d within cardiac tolerance.	Prevents dehydration that can be exacerbated by increased insensible losses (e.g., ventilator/intubation) and reduces risk of constipation.
Assess GI function: Presence/quality of bowel sounds; note changes in abdominal girth, nausea/vomiting. Observe/document changes in bowel movements, e.g., diarrhea/constipation. Test all stools for occult blood.	A functioning GI system is essential for the proper utilization of enteral feedings. Mechanically ventilated patients are at risk of developing abdominal distention (trapped air or ileus) and gastric bleeding (stress ulcers).
Collaborative	
Adjust diet to meet respiratory needs as indicated.	High carbohydrates, protein, and calories may be desired/needed during ventilation to improve respiratory muscle function. Carbohydrates may be reduced and fat somewhat increased just prior to weaning attempts to prevent excessive CO_2 production and reduced respiratory drive.
Monitor laboratory studies as indicated, e.g., prealbumin, serum, transferrin, BUN/Cr, glucose.	Provides information about adequacy of nutritional support/need for change.

NURSING DIAGNOSIS: Infection, risk for

Risk factors may include
Inadequate primary defenses (traumatized lung tissue, decreased ciliary action, stasis of body fluids)
Inadequate secondary defenses (immunosuppression)
Chronic disease, malnutrition
Invasive procedure (intubation)

Possibly evidenced by
[Not applicable; presence of signs and symptoms establishes an *actual* diagnosis.]

DESIRED OUTCOMES/EVALUATION CRITERIA—PATIENT/CAREGIVER WILL:
Indicate understanding of individual risk factors.
Identify interventions to prevent/reduce risk of infection.
Demonstrate techniques to promote safe environment.

ACTIONS/INTERVENTIONS	RATIONALE

Independent

Note risk factors for occurrence of infection.	Intubation, prolonged mechanical ventilation, general debilitation, malnutrition, age, and invasive procedures are factors that potentiate patient's risk of acquiring infection and prolonging recovery. Awareness of individual risk factors provides opportunity to limit effects.
Observe color/odor/characteristics of sputum. Note drainage around tracheostomy tube.	Yellow/green, purulent odorous sputum is indicative of infection; thick, tenacious sputum suggests dehydration.
Reduce nosocomial risk factors via proper handwashing by all caregivers, maintaining sterile suction techniques.	These factors may be the simplest but are the most important keys to prevention of hospital-acquired infection.
Encourage deep breathing, coughing, and frequent position changes.	Maximizes lung expansion and mobilization of secretions to prevent/reduce atelectasis and accumulation of sticky, thick secretions.
Auscultate breath sounds.	Presence of rhonchi/wheezes suggests retained secretions requiring expectoration/suctioning.
Monitor/screen visitors. Avoid contact with persons with upper respiratory infection.	Individual is already compromised and is at increased risk for development of infections.
Instruct patient in proper secretion disposal, e.g., tissues, soiled tracheostomy dressings.	Reduces transmission of fluid-borne organisms.
Provide respiratory isolation when indicated.	Depending on specific diagnosis the patient may require protection from others or must prevent transmission of infection to others (e.g., tuberculosis).
Maintain adequate hydration and nutrition. Encourage fluids to 2500 ml/d within cardiac tolerance.	Helps improve general resistance to disease and reduces risk of infection from static secretions.
Encourage self-care/activities to limit of tolerance. Assist with graded exercise program.	Improves general well-being and muscle strength and may stimulate immune system recovery.

Collaborative

Obtain sputum cultures as indicated.	May be needed to identify pathogens and appropriate antimicrobials.
Administer antimicrobials as indicated.	If infection does occur, 1 or more agents may be used, depending on identified pathogen(s).

NURSING DIAGNOSIS: Ventilatory Weaning Response, dysfunctional (DVWR), risk for

Risk factors may include
Sleep disturbance
Limited/insufficient energy stores
Pain or discomfort
Adverse environment (e.g., inadequate monitoring/support)
Patient-perceived inability to wean; decreased motivation
History of extended weaning

Possibly evidenced by
[Not applicable; presence of signs and symptoms establishes an *actual* diagnosis]

> **DESIRED OUTCOMES/EVALUATION CRITERIA—PATIENT WILL:**
> Actively participate in the weaning process.
> Reestablish independent respiration with ABGs within acceptable range and free of signs of respiratory failure.
> Demonstrate increased tolerance for activity/participate in self-care within level of ability.

ACTIONS/INTERVENTIONS	RATIONALE
Independent	
Assess physical factors involved in weaning, e.g.:	
Stable heart rate/rhythm, BP, and clear breath sounds;	The heart will have to work harder to meet increased energy needs associated with weaning. Physician may defer weaning if tachycardia, pulmonary crackles, and hypertension are present.
Fever;	Increase of 1°F in body temperature raises metabolic rate and oxygen demands by 7%.
Nutritional status and muscle strength.	Weaning is hard work. Patient not only must be able to withstand the stress of weaning but also must have the stamina to breathe spontaneously for extended periods.
Determine psychologic readiness.	Weaning provokes anxiety for the patient regarding concerns about ability to breathe on own and long-term need of ventilator.
Explain weaning techniques, e.g., T-piece, SIMV, CPAP, or NIPPV. Discuss individual plan and expectations.	Assists patient to prepare for weaning process, helps limit fear of unknown, promotes cooperation, and enhances likelihood of a successful outcome.
Provide undisturbed rest/sleep periods. Avoid stressful procedures/situations or nonessential activities.	Maximizes energy for weaning process; limits fatigue and oxygen consumption.
Evaluate/document patient's progress. Note restlessness; changes in BP, heart rate, respiratory rate; use of accessory muscles; discoordinated breathing with ventilator; increased concentration on breathing (mild dysfunction); patient's concerns about possible machine malfunction; inability to cooperate/respond to coaching; color changes.	Indicators that patient may require slower weaning/opportunity to stabilize or may need to stop program.
Recognize/provide encouragement for patient's efforts.	Positive feedback provides reassurance and support for continuation of weaning process.
Monitor response to activity.	Excessive oxygen consumption/demand increases the possibility of failure.
Collaborative	
Consult with dietitian, nutritional support team for adjustments of composition of diet.	Reduction of carbohydrates/fats may be required to prevent excessive production of CO_2, which could alter respiratory drive.
Monitor CBC, serum albumin and prealbumin, transferrin, total iron-binding capacity, and electrolytes (especially potassium, calcium, and phosphorus).	Verifies that nutrition is adequate to meet energy requirements for weaning.

ACTIONS/INTERVENTIONS

Collaborative

Review chest x-ray and ABGs.

RATIONALE

Chest x-rays should show clear lungs or marked improvement in pulmonary congestion or infiltrates. ABGs should document satisfactory oxygenation on an FIO_2 of 40% or less.

NURSING DIAGNOSIS: Knowledge deficit [learning need] regarding condition, prognosis and therapy, self care and discharge needs

May be related to
Lack of exposure/recall
Misinterpretation of information
Unfamiliarity with information resources
Stress of situational crisis

Possibly evidenced by
Questions about care, request for information
Reluctance to learn new skills
Inaccurate follow-through of instructions
Development of preventable complications

DESIRED OUTCOMES/EVALUATION CRITERIA—PATIENT/SO/CAREGIVER WILL:
Participate in learning process.
Exhibit increased interest, shown by verbal/nonverbal cues.
Assume responsibility for own learning and begin to look for information and to ask questions.
Indicate understanding of mechanical ventilation therapy.
Demonstrate behaviors/new skills to meet individual needs/prevent complications.

ACTIONS/INTERVENTIONS

Independent

Determine ability and willingness to learn.

Discuss specific condition requiring ventilatory support, what measures are being tried for weaning, short- and long-term goals of treatment.

Encourage patient/SO to evaluate impact of ventilatory dependence on their lifestyle and what changes they are willing or unwilling to make. Problem-solve solutions to issues raised.

RATIONALE

Physical condition may preclude patient involvement in care before and after discharge. SO/caregiver may feel inadequate and afraid of machinery and have reservations about ability to learn or deal with overall situation.

Provides knowledge base to aid patient/SO in making informed decisions. Weaning efforts may continue for several weeks (extended period of time). Dependence is evidenced by repeatedly increased PCO_2, and/or decline in PaO_2 during weaning attempts, presence of dypsnea, anxiety, tachycardia, perspiration, cyanosis.

Quality of life must be resolved by the ventilator-dependent patient and caregivers who need to understand that home ventilatory support is a 24-hour job that will affect everyone.

ACTIONS/INTERVENTIONS	RATIONALE
Independent	
Promote participation in self-care/diversional activities and socialization as appropriate.	Refocuses attention back toward more normal life activities, increases endurance, and helps to prevent depersonalization.
Review issues of general well-being: role of nutrition; assistance with feeding/meal preparation; graded exercise/specific restrictions; rest periods alternated with activity.	Enhances recuperation and ensures that individual needs will be met.
Recommend that SO/caregivers learn CPR.	Provides sense of security about ability to handle emergency situations that might arise until help can be obtained.
Schedule team conference. Establish in-hospital training for caregivers if patient is to be discharged home on ventilator.	Team approach is needed to coordinate patient's care and teaching program to meet individual needs.
Instruct caregiver and patient in hand-washing techniques, use of sterile technique for suctioning, tracheostomy/stoma care, and chest physiotherapy.	Reduces risk of infection and promotes optimal respiratory function.
Provide both demonstration and ''hands-on'' sessions as well as written material about specific type of ventilator to be used, function, and care of equipment.	Enhances familiarity, reducing anxiety and promoting confidence in implementation of new tasks/skills.
Discuss what/when to report to the healthcare provider, e.g., signs of respiratory distress, infection.	Helps to reduce general anxiety while promoting timely/appropriate evaluation and intervention to prevent complications.
Ascertain that all needed equipment is in place and that safety concerns have been addressed, e.g., alternate power source (generator, batteries); backup equipment; patient call/alarm system.	Predischarge preparations can ease the transfer process. Planning for potential problems increases sense of security for patient/SO.
Contact community/hospital-based services.	Suppliers of home equipment, physical therapy, care providers, emergency power provider, social services; financial assistance, aid in procuring equipment/personnel, and facilitating transition to home.
Refer to vocational/occupational therapist.	Some ventilator-dependent patients are able to resume vocations, either while on the ventilator or during the day (while ventilator-dependent at night).

POTENTIAL CONSIDERATIONS following acute hospitalization (dependent on patient's age, physical condition/presence of complications, personal resources, and life responsibilities).

If patient is discharged on ventilator, the patient's needs/concerns remain the same as noted in this plan of care, in addition to:

Self Care deficit—decreased strength/endurance, inability to perform ADLs, depression, restrictions imposed by therapeutic intervention.

Family Processes, altered—situational crisis.

Caregiver Role Strain, risk for—severity of illness of care receiver, discharge of family member with significant home care needs, presence of situational stressors (economic vulnerability, changes in roles/responsibilities), duration of caregiving required, inexperience in caregiving.

PULMONARY TUBERCULOSIS (TB)

TB is on the rise today, although many still believe it to be a problem of the past. Although most frequently seen as a pulmonary disease, TB may be extrapulmonary and affect organs and tissues other than the lungs. In the United States, incidence is higher among the homeless, drug-addicted, and impoverished populations, as well as among immigrants from or visitors to countries where TB is endemic. In addition, persons at highest risk include those who may have been exposed to the bacillus in the past and those who are debilitated or have lowered immunity because of chronic conditions, such as AIDS, cancer, advanced age, malnutrition, and so on. When the immune system weakens, dormant TB organisms can reactivate and multiply. When this latent infection develops into active disease, it is known as reactivation TB, which is often drug-resistant.

CARE SETTING

Most patients are treated as outpatients, but may be hospitalized for diagnostic evaluation/initiation of therapy, adverse drug reactions, or severe illness/debilitation.

RELATED CONCERNS

Long-Term Care, p 824
Pneumonia: Microbial, p 130
Psychosocial Aspects of Care, p 783

Patient Assessment Data Base

Data are dependent on stage of disease and degree of involvement.

ACTIVITY/REST

May report: Generalized weakness and fatigue
Shortness of breath with exertion
Difficulty sleeping with evening or night fever, chills, and/or sweats
Nightmares

May exhibit: Tachycardia, tachypnea/dyspnea on exertion
Muscle wasting, pain, and stiffness (advanced stages)

EGO INTEGRITY

May report: Recent/long-standing stress factors
Financial concerns, poverty
Feelings of helplessness/hopelessness
Cultural/ethnic populations: Native American or recent immigrants from Central America, Southeast Asia, Indian subcontinent

May exhibit: Denial (especially during early stages)
Anxiety, apprehension, irritability

FOOD/FLUID

May report: Loss of appetite
Indigestion
Weight loss

May exhibit: Poor skin turgor, dry/flaky skin
Muscle wasting/loss of subcutaneous fat

PAIN/DISCOMFORT

May report: Chest pain aggravated by recurrent cough

May exhibit: Guarding of affected area
Distraction behaviors, restlessness

RESPIRATION

May report: Cough, productive or nonproductive
Shortness of breath
History of tuberculosis/exposure to infected individual

May exhibit: Increased respiratory rate (extensive disease or fibrosis of the lung parenchyma and pleura)
Asymmetry in respiratory excursion (pleural effusion)
Dullness to percussion and decreased fremitus (pleural fluid or pleural thickening)
Breath sounds: Diminished/absent bilaterally or unilaterally (pleural effusion/pneumothorax). Tubular breath sounds and/or whispered pectoriloquies over large lesions. Crackles may be noted over apex of lungs during quick inspiration after a short cough (post-tussive crackles)
Sputum characteristics: Green/purulent, yellowish mucoid, or blood-tinged
Tracheal deviation (bronchogenic spread)
Inattention, marked irritability, change in mentation (advanced stages)

SAFETY

May report: Presence of immunosuppressed conditions, e.g., AIDS, cancer
HIV infection
Visit to/immigration from or close contact with persons in countries with high prevalence of TB

May exhibit: Low-grade fever or acute febrile illness
Positive HIV test

SOCIAL INTERACTION

May report: Feelings of isolation/rejection because of communicable disease
Change in usual patterns of responsibility/change in physical capacity to resume role

TEACHING/LEARNING

May report: Familial history of TB
General debilitation/poor health status
Use/abuse of substances such as IV drugs, alcohol, cocaine, and crack
Failure to improve/reactivation of TB
Nonparticipation in therapy

Discharge plan considerations: **DRG projected mean length of inpatient stay: 6.8 days.**
May require assistance with/alteration in drug therapy and also assistance in self-care and homemaker/maintenance tasks

Refer to section at end of plan for postdischarge considerations.

DIAGNOSTIC STUDIES

Sputum culture: Positive for *Mycobacterium tuberculosis* in the active stage of the disease.
Ziehl-Neelsen (acid-fast stain applied to a smear of body fluid): Positive for acid-fast bacilli.

191

Skin tests (purified protein derivative [PPD] or old tuberculin [OT] administered by intradermal injection [Mantoux] or multipuncture technique [Tine]): A positive reaction (area of induration 10 mm or greater, occurring 48–72 hours after interdermal injection of the antigen) indicates past infection and the presence of antibodies but is not necessarily indicative of active disease. A significant reaction in a patient who is clinically ill means that active TB cannot be dismissed as a diagnostic possibility. A significant reaction in healthy persons usually signifies dormant TB or an infection caused by a different mycobacterium.

ELISA/Western blot: May reveal presence of HIV.

Chest x-ray: May show small infiltrations of early lesions in the upper-lung field, calcium deposits of healed primary lesions, or fluid of an effusion. Changes indicating more advanced TB may include cavitation, fibrous areas.

Histologic or tissue cultures (including gastric washings; urine and CSF, skin biopsy): Positive for *Mycobacterium tuberculosis* and may indicate extrapulmonary involvement.

Needle biopsy of lung tissue: Positive for granulomas of TB; presence of giant cells indicating necrosis.

Electrolytes: May be abnormal depending on the location and severity of infection; e.g., hyponatremia caused by abnormal water retention may be found in extensive chronic pulmonary TB.

ABGs: May be abnormal depending on location, severity and residual damage to the lungs.

Pulmonary function studies: Decreased vital capacity, increased dead space, increased ratio of residual air to total lung capacity, and decreased oxygen saturation are secondary to parenchymal infiltration/fibrosis, loss of lung tissue, and pleural disease (extensive chronic pulmonary TB).

NURSING PRIORITIES

1. Achieve/maintain adequate ventilation/oxygenation.
2. Prevent spread of infection.
3. Support behaviors/tasks to maintain health.
4. Promote effective coping strategies.
5. Provide information about disease process/prognosis and treatment needs.

DISCHARGE GOALS

1. Respiratory function adequate to meet individual need.
2. Complications prevented.
3. Lifestyle/behavior changes adopted to prevent spread of infection.
4. Disease process/prognosis and therapeutic regimen understood.
5. Plan in place to meet needs after discharge.

NURSING DIAGNOSIS: Infection, risk for [spread/reactivation]

Risk factors may include
Inadequate primary defenses, decreased ciliary action/stasis of secretions
Tissue destruction/extension of infection
Lowered resistance/suppressed inflammatory process
Malnutrition
Environmental exposure
Insufficient knowledge to avoid exposure to pathogens

Possibly evidenced by
[Not applicable; presence of signs and symptoms establishes an *actual* diagnosis]

DESIRED OUTCOMES/EVALUATION CRITERIA—PATIENT WILL:
Identify interventions to prevent/reduce risk of spread of infection.
Demonstrate techniques/initiate lifestyle changes to promote safe environment.

ACTIONS/INTERVENTIONS	RATIONALE

Independent

Review pathology of disease (active/inactive phases; dissemination of infection through bronchi to adjacent tissues or via bloodstream/lymphatic system) and potential spread of infection via air-borne droplet during coughing, sneezing, spitting, talking, laughing, singing.

Helps patient realize/accept necessity of adhering to medication regimen to prevent reactivation/complication. Understanding of how the disease is passed and awareness of transmission possibilities help patient/SO to take steps to prevent infection of others.

Identify others at risk, e.g., household members, close associates/friends.

Those exposed may require a course of drug therapy to prevent spread/development of infection.

Instruct patient to cough/sneeze and expectorate into tissue and to refrain from spitting. Review proper disposal of tissue and good hand-washing techniques. Encourage return demonstration.

Behaviors necessary to prevent spread of infection.

Review necessity of infection control measures, e.g., temporary respiratory isolation.

May help patient to understand need for protecting others while acknowledging patient's sense of isolation and social stigma associated with communicable diseases. *Note:* AFB particles can pass through standard masks; therefore particulate respirators are required.

Monitor temperature as indicated.

Febrile reactions are indicators of continuing presence of infection.

Identify individual risk factors for reactivation of tuberculosis, e.g., lowered resistance (alcoholism, malnutrition/intestinal bypass surgery); use of immunosuppression drugs/corticosteroids; presence of diabetes mellitus, cancer; postpartum.

Knowledge about these factors helps patient to alter lifestyle and avoid/reduce incidence of exacerbation.

Stress importance of uninterrupted drug therapy. Evaluate patient's potential for cooperation.

Contagious period may last only 2–3 days after initiation of chemotherapy, but in presence of cavitation or moderately advanced disease, risk of spread of infection may continue up to 3 months. Compliance with multidrug regimens for prolonged periods is difficult, so directly observed therapy (DOT) should be considered.

Review importance of follow-up and periodic reculturing of sputum for the duration of therapy.

Aids in monitoring the effects and effectiveness of medications and the patient's response to therapy.

Encourage selection/ingestion of well-balanced meals. Provide frequent small "snacks" in place of large meals as appropriate.

Presence of anorexia and/or preexisting malnutrition lowers resistance to infectious process and impairs healing. Small snacks may enhance overall intake.

Collaborative

Administer anti-infective agents as indicated, e.g.:

Primary drugs: Isoniazid (INH), ethambutal (Myambutol), rifampin (RMP/Rifadin), rifampin with isoniazid (Rifamate), pyrazinamide (PZA/Aldinamide), streptomycin (Strycin);

Initial therapy of uncomplicated pulmonary disease usually includes 4 drugs e.g., 4 primary drugs or primary plus secondary drugs. INH is usually drug of choice for infected patient and those at risk for developing TB. Short-course chemotherapy including INH, rifampin, PZA and ethambutal for at least 2 months (or until serial sputums are clear) followed by 3 more

ACTIONS/INTERVENTIONS

Collaborative

	months of therapy with INH may be sufficient. Ethambutol should be given if CNS or disseminated disease is present, or if INH resistance is suspected. Extended therapy (up to 24 months) is indicated for reactivation cases, extrapulmonary reactivated TB, or in the presence of other medical problems, e.g., diabetes mellitus or silicosis. Prophylaxis with INH for 12 months should be considered in HIV-positive patients with positive PPD test.
Ethionamide (Trecator-SC), para-amino salicylic (PAS), cycloserine (Seromycin).	These second-line drugs may be required when infection is resistant to or intolerant of primary drugs.
Monitor laboratory studies, e.g., sputum smear results;	Patient who has three consecutive negative sputum smears (takes 3–5 months), is adhering to drug regimen, and is asymptomatic will be classified a nontransmitter.
AST/ALT.	Adverse effects of drug therapy include hepatitis.
Notify local health department.	Helpful in identifying contacts reducing spread of infection, and required by law in many states. Treatment course is long and usually handled in the community with public health nurse monitoring.

NURSING DIAGNOSIS: Airway Clearance, ineffective

May be related to
Thick, viscous, or bloody secretions
Fatigue, poor cough effort
Tracheal/pharyngeal edema

Possibly evidenced by
Abnormal respiratory rate, rhythm, depth
Abnormal breath sounds (rhonchi, wheezes), stridor
Dyspnea

DESIRED OUTCOMES/EVALUATION CRITERIA—PATIENT WILL:
Maintain patent airway.
Expectorate secretions without assistance.
Demonstrate behaviors to improve/maintain airway clearance.
Participate in treatment regimen, within the level of ability/situation.
Identify potential complications and initiate appropriate actions.

ACTIONS/INTERVENTIONS

Independent

Assess respiratory function, e.g., breath sounds, rate, rhythm and depth, and use of accessory muscles.	Diminished breath sounds may reflect atelectasis. Rhonchi, wheezes indicate accumulation of secretions/inability to clear airways that may lead to use of accessory muscles and increased work of breathing.

ACTIONS/INTERVENTIONS	RATIONALE
Independent	
Note ability to expectorate mucous/cough effectively; document character, amount of sputum, presence of hemoptysis.	Expectoration may be difficult when secretions are very thick (i.e., effect of the infection and/or inadequate hydration). Blood-tinged or frankly bloody sputum results from tissue breakdown (cavitation) in the lungs or from bronchial ulceration and may require further evaluation/intervention.
Place patient in semi- or high-Fowler's position. Assist patient with coughing and deep-breathing exercises.	Positioning helps maximize lung expansion and decreases respiratory effort. Maximal ventilation may open atelectic areas and promote movement of secretions into larger airways for expectoration.
Clear secretions from mouth and trachea; suction as necessary.	Prevents obstruction/aspiration. Suctioning may be necessary if patient is unable to expectorate secretions.
Maintain fluid intake of at least 2500 ml/d unless contraindicated.	High fluid intake helps to thin secretions, making them easier to expectorate.
Collaborative	
Humidify inspired air/oxygen.	Prevents drying of mucous membranes; helps to thin secretions.
Administer medications as indicated:	
Mucolytic agents, e.g., acetylcysteine (Mucomyst);	Reduces the thickness and stickiness of pulmonary secretions to facilitate clearance.
Bronchodilators, e.g., oxtriphylline (Choledyl), theophylline (Theo-Dur);	Increases lumen size of the tracheobronchial tree, thus decreasing resistance to airflow and improving oxygen delivery.
Corticosteroids (Prednisone).	May be useful in presence of extensive involvement with profound hypoxemia and when inflammatory response is life-threatening.
Be prepared for/assist with emergency intubation.	Intubation may be necessary in rare cases of bronchogenic TB accompanied by laryngeal edema or acute pulmonary bleeding.

NURSING DIAGNOSIS: Gas Exchange, impaired, risk for

Risk factors may include
Decrease in effective lung surface, atelectasis
Destruction of alveolar-capillary membrane
Thick, viscous secretions
Bronchial edema

Possibly evidenced by
[Not applicable; presence of signs and symptoms establishes an *actual* diagnosis]

DESIRED OUTCOMES/EVALUATION CRITERIA—PATIENT WILL:
Report absence of/decreased dyspnea.
Demonstrate improved ventilation and adequate oxygenation of tissues by ABGs within acceptable ranges.
Be free of symptoms of respiratory distress.

ACTIONS/INTERVENTIONS	RATIONALE
Independent	
Assess for dyspnea, tachypnea, abnormal/diminished breath sounds, increased respiratory effort, limited chest wall expansion, and fatigue.	Pulmonary TB can cause a wide range of effects in the lungs ranging from a small patch of bronchopneumonia to diffuse intense inflammation, caseous necrosis, pleural effusion, and extensive fibrosis. Respiratory effects can range from mild dyspnea to profound respiratory distress.
Evaluate change in level of mentation. Note cyanosis and/or change in skin color, including mucous membranes and nail beds.	Accumulation of secretions/airway compromise can impair oxygenation of vital organs and tissues. (Refer to ND: Airway Clearance, ineffective, p 194.)
Demonstrate/encourage pursed-lip breathing during exhalation, especially for patients with fibrosis or parenchymal destruction.	Creates resistance against outflowing air, to prevent collapse/narrowing of the airways, thereby helping to distribute air throughout the lungs and relieve/reduce shortness of breath.
Promote bed rest/limit activity and assist with self-care activities as necessary.	Reducing oxygen consumption/demand during periods of respiratory compromise may reduce severity of symptoms.
Collaborative	
Monitor serial ABGs/pulse oximetry.	Decreased oxygen content (PaO_2), and/or saturation or increased $PaCO_2$ indicates need for intervention/change in therapeutic regimen.
Provide supplemental oxygen as appropriate.	Aids in correcting the hypoxemia that may occur secondary to decreased ventilation/diminished alveolar lung surface.

NURSING DIAGNOSIS: Nutrition: altered, less than body requirements

May be related to
Fatigue
Frequent cough/sputum production; dyspnea
Anorexia
Insufficient financial resources

Possibly evidenced by
Weight 10%–20% below ideal for frame and height
Reported lack of interest in food, altered taste sensation
Poor muscle tone

DESIRED OUTCOMES/EVALUATION CRITERIA—PATIENT WILL:
Demonstrate progressive weight gain toward goal with normalization of laboratory values and free of signs of malnutrition.
Initiate behaviors/lifestyle changes to regain and/or to maintain appropriate weight.

ACTIONS/INTERVENTIONS	RATIONALE
Independent	
Document patient's nutritional status on admission, noting skin turgor, current weight and degree of weight loss, integrity of oral mucosa, ability/inability to swallow, presence of bowel tones, history of nausea/vomiting or diarrhea.	Useful in defining degree/extent of problem and appropriate choice of interventions.
Ascertain patient's usual dietary pattern, likes/dislikes.	Helpful in identifying specific needs/strengths. Consideration of individual preferences may improve dietary intake.
Monitor intake/output and weight periodically.	Useful in measuring effectiveness of nutritional and fluid support.
Investigate anorexia, nausea, and vomiting and note possible correlation to medications. Monitor frequency, volume, consistency of stools.	May affect dietary choices and identify areas for problem solving to enhance intake/utilization of nutrients.
Encourage and provide for frequent rest periods.	Helps to conserve energy especially when metabolic requirements are increased with fever.
Provide oral care before and after respiratory treatments.	Reduces bad taste left from sputum or medications used for respiratory treatments that can stimulate the vomiting center.
Encourage small, frequent meals with foods high in protein and carbohydrates.	Maximizes nutrient intake without undue fatigue/energy expenditure from eating large meals and reduces gastric irritation.
Encourage SO to bring foods from home and to share meals with patient unless contraindicated.	Creates a more normal social environment during mealtime and helps meet personal, cultural preferences.
Collaborative	
Refer to dietitian for adjustments in dietary composition.	Provides assistance in planning a diet with nutrients adequate to meet patient's metabolic requirements and dietary preferences.
Consult with respiratory therapy to schedule treatments 1–2 hours before/after meals.	May help to reduce the incidence of nausea and vomiting associated with medications or the effects of respiratory treatments on a full stomach.
Monitor laboratory studies, e.g., BUN, serum protein, and prealbumin/albumin.	Low values reflect malnutrition and indicate need for intervention/change in therapeutic regimen.
Administer antipyretics as appropriate.	Fever increases metabolic needs and therefore calorie consumption.

NURSING DIAGNOSIS: Knowledge deficit [learning need] regarding condition, treatment, prevention, self care and discharge needs

May be related to
Lack of exposure to/misinterpretation of information
Cognitive limitations
Inaccurate/incomplete information presented

ACTIONS/INTERVENTIONS	RATIONALE
Independent	
Assess patient's ability to learn, e.g., level of fear, concern, fatigue, participation level, best environment in which patient can learn, how much content, best media and language, who should be included.	Learning is dependent on emotional and physical readiness and is achieved at an individual pace.
Identify symptoms that should be reported to healthcare provider, e.g., hemoptysis, chest pain, fever, difficulty breathing, hearing loss, vertigo.	May indicate progression or reactivation of disease or side effects of medications requiring further evaluation.
Emphasize the importance of maintaining high-protein and carbohydrate diet and adequate fluid intake. (Refer to ND: Nutrition: altered, less than body requirements, p 196.)	Meeting metabolic needs helps to minimize fatigue and promote recovery. Fluids aid in liquefying/expectorating of secretions.
Provide instruction and specific written information for the patient to refer to, e.g., schedule for medications and follow-up sputum testing for documenting response to therapy.	Written information relieves the patient of the burden of having to remember large amounts of information. Repetition strengthens learning.
Explain medication dosage, frequency of administration, expected action, and the reason for prolonged treatment. Review potential interactions with other drugs/substances.	Enhances cooperation with therapeutic regimen and may prevent discontinuation of medication as patient's condition improves.
Review potential side effects of treatment (e.g., dryness of mouth, constipation, visual disturbances, headache, orthostatic hypertension) and problem-solve solutions.	May prevent/reduce discomfort associated with therapy and enhance cooperation with regimen.
Stress need to abstain from alcohol while on INH.	Combination of INH and alcohol has been linked with increased incidence of hepatitis.
Refer for eye examination after starting and then monthly while taking ethambutal.	Major side effect is reduced visual acuity; initial sign may be decreased ability to perceive green.
Encourage patient/SO to verbalize fears/concerns. Answer questions factually. Note prolonged use of denial.	Provides opportunity to correct misconceptions/alleviate anxiety. Inadequate finances/prolonged denial may affect coping with/managing the tasks necessary to regain/maintain health.

ACTIONS/INTERVENTIONS	RATIONALE

Independent

Evaluate job-related risk factors, e.g., working in foundry/rock quarry, sandblasting.

Excessive exposure to silicone dust enhances risk of silicosis, which may negatively affect respiratory function/bronchitis.

Encourage abstaining from smoking.

Although smoking does not stimulate recurrence of TB, it does increase the likelihood of respiratory dysfunction/bronchitis.

Review how TB is transmitted (e.g., primarily by inhalation of airborne organisms but may also spread through stools or urine if infection is present in these systems) and hazards of reactivation.

Knowledge may reduce risk of transmission/reactivation. Complications associated with reactivation include cavitation, abscess formation, destructive emphysema, spontaneous pneumothorax, diffuse interstitial fibrosis, serous effusion, empyema, bronchiectasis, hemoptysis, GI ulceration, bronchopleural fistula, tuberculous laryngitis, and miliary spread.

Refer to public health agency.

Directly observed therapy by community nurses is often the most effective way to ensure patient adherence to therapy. Monitoring can include pill counts and urine dipstick testing for presence of antitubercular drug.

POTENTIAL CONSIDERATIONS following acute hospitalization (dependent on patient's age, physical condition/presence of complications, personal resources, and life responsibilities)

Therapeutic Regimen: Individual, ineffective management—complexity of therapeutic regimen, economic difficulties, family patterns of health care, perceived seriousness/benefits.

Infection, risk for (secondary)—decrease in ciliary action, stasis of body fluids, suppressed inflammatory response, tissue destruction, chronic disease, malnutrition, increased environmental exposure.

Fatigue—increased energy requirements to perform ADLs, discomfort.

Therapeutic Regimen: Families, ineffective management—complexity of therapeutic regimen, decisional conflicts, economic difficulties, family conflict.

RESPIRATORY ACID-BASE IMBALANCES

The body has the remarkable ability to maintain plasma pH within a narrow range of 7.35–7.45. It does so by means of chemical buffering mechanisms by the lungs and kidneys. Although single acid/base imbalances (e.g., respiratory acidosis) do occur, mixed acid/base imbalances are more common (e.g., respiratory acidosis/metabolic acidosis as occurs with cardiac arrest).

RESPIRATORY ACIDOSIS (PRIMARY CARBONIC ACID EXCESS)

Respiratory acidosis represents an elevated $PaCO_2$ caused by hypoventilation with resultant excess of carbonic acid (H_2CO_3). It can be due to primary defects in lung function or changes in normal respiratory pattern. Compensatory mechanisms include (1) an increased respiratory rate; (2) Hb buffering, forming bicarbonate ions and deoxygenated Hb; and (3) increased renal ammonia acid excretions with reabsorption of bicarbonate. The disorder may be acute or chronic.

Acute respiratory acidosis: Associated with acute pulmonary edema, aspiration of foreign body, overdose of sedatives/barbiturate poisoning, smoke inhalation, acute laryngospasm, hemothorax/pneumothorax, atelectasis, ARDS, anesthesia, mechanical ventilators, excessive CO_2 intake (e.g., use of rebreathing mask), CVA therapy; Pickwickian syndrome.

Chronic respiratory acidosis: Associated with emphysema, asthma, bronchiectasis; neuromuscular disorders (such as Guillain-Barré syndrome and myasthenia gravis), botulism, spinal cord injuries.

CARE SETTING:

This condition does not occur in isolation but rather is a complication of a broader problem and usually requires inpatient care in a medical/surgical or subacute unit.

RELATED CONCERNS

Plans of care specific to predisposing factors.
Fluid and Electrolyte Imbalances, p 899
Metabolic Acidosis, p 506
Metabolic Alkalosis, p 510

Patient Assessment Data Base

(Dependent on underlying cause)

ACTIVITY/REST

May report:	Fatigue
May exhibit:	Generalized weakness, ataxia, loss of coordination (chronic)

CIRCULATION

May exhibit:	Hypotension with bounding pulses, pinkish color, warm skin (reflects vasodilation of severe acidosis)
	Tachycardia, dysrhythmias
	Diaphoresis, pallor, and cyanosis (late stage)

FOOD/FLUID

May report:	Nausea/vomiting

NEUROSENSORY

May report: Feeling of fullness in head (acute—associated with vasodilation)
Headache, dizziness, visual disturbances

May exhibit: Confusion, apprehension, agitation, restlessness, somnolence; coma (acute)
Tremors: Decreased reflexes (severe acidosis)

RESPIRATION

May report: Dyspnea with exertion

May exhibit: Increased respiratory effort with nasal flaring/yawning, use of neck and upper body muscles
Decreased respiratory rate/hypoventilation (associated with decreased function of respiratory center as in head trauma, oversedation, general anesthesia, metabolic alkalosis)
Adventitious breath sounds (crackles, wheezes), stridor, crowing

TEACHING/LEARNING

Refer to predisposing/contributing factors

Discharge plan considerations: **DRG projected mean length of inpatient stay: 4.1 days**
May require assistance with changes in therapies for underlying disease process/condition

Refer to section at end of plan for postdischarge considerations.

DIAGNOSTIC STUDIES

Arterial pH: Decreased, less than 7.35.
Paco$_2$: Increased, greater than 45 mm Hg (primary acidosis).
Bicarbonate (HCO$_3$): Normal or increased, greater than 26 mEq/L (compensated/chronic stage).
Pao$_2$: Normal or decreased.
Oxygen saturation: Decreased.
Serum potassium: May be normal or increased.
Serum chloride: Decreased.
Serum calcium: Increased.
Lactic acid: May be elevated.
Urine pH: Decreased, 6.0.
Screening tests: As indicated to determine underlying cause.

NURSING PRIORITIES

1. Achieve homeostasis.
2. Prevent/minimize complications.
3. Provide information about condition/prognosis and treatment needs as appropriate.

DISCHARGE GOALS

1. Physiologic balance restored.
2. Free of complications.
3. Condition, prognosis, and treatment needs understood.
4. Plan in place to meet needs after discharge.

ACTIONS/INTERVENTIONS	RATIONALE
Independent	
Monitor respiratory rate, depth and effort. Note pulse oximetry readings.	Hypoventilation and associated hypoxemia lead to respiratory distress/failure. Use of bedside pulse oximetry monitoring can show early progression of hypoxia/response to therapy before other signs or symptoms are observed.
Auscultate breath sounds.	Identifies area(s) of decreased ventilation (e.g., atelectasis) or airway obstruction, and therapy needs/effectiveness.
Note decreased level of awareness/consciousness.	Signals severe acidotic state, which requires immediate attention. *Note:* Sensorium clears slowly because it takes longer for hydrogen ions to clear from cerebrospinal fluid.
Monitor heart rate/rhythm.	Tachycardia develops early in an attempt to increase oxygen delivery to the tissues. Dysrhythmias may occur due to hypoxia (myocardial ischemia) and electrolyte imbalances.
Note skin color, temperature, moisture.	Diaphoresis, pallor, cool/clammy skin are late changes associated with hypoxemia.
Encourage/assist with breathing exercises, turning, and coughing. Suction as necessary. Provide airway adjunct as indicated. Place in semi-Fowler's position.	These measures improve ventilation and reduce/prevent airway obstruction.
Limit use of hypnotic sedatives or tranquilizers.	In the presence of hypoventilation, respiratory depression can occur with the use of sedatives, and CO_2 narcosis may develop.
Discuss cause of condition (if known) and appropriate interventions/self-care activities.	Promotes participation in therapeutic regimen and may reduce recurrence of disorder.

Collaborative

Assist with identification/treatment of underlying cause.	Treatment of disorder is directed at improving ventilation. Addressing the primary condition (e.g., oversedation, pulmonary edema, aspiration) promotes correction of the acid/base disorder.
Monitor/graph serial ABGs; serum electrolyte levels.	Evaluates therapy needs/effectiveness.
Administer supplemental oxygen as indicated. Increase respiratory rate or tidal volume of ventilator if used.	Prevents/corrects hypoxemia and respiratory failure. *Note:* Must be used with caution in presence of emphysema/COPD because respiratory depression/failure may result.
Maintain hydration (IV/PO)/provide humidification.	Assists in thinning/mobilization of respiratory secretions.
Provide aggressive chest physiotherapy, including postural drainage, and breathing exercises.	Aids in clearing secretions which may improve ventilation, allowing excess CO_2 to be eliminated.
Assist with ventilatory aids, e.g., IPPB in conjunction with bronchodilators.	Increases lung expansion and opens airways to improve ventilation preventing respiratory failure.
Administer IV solutions of lactated Ringer's solution or 0.6 M solution of sodium lactate.	May be useful in nonemergency situations to help control acidosis, until underlying respiratory problem can be corrected.
Administer medications as indicated, e.g.: Naloxone hydrochloride (Narcan);	May be useful in arousing patient and stimulating respiratory function in presence of drug overdose/sedation, or acidosis resulting from cardiac arrest.
Sodium bicarbonate ($NaHCO_3$);	May be given in small IV doses in emergency situations to quickly correct acidosis if pH is less than 7.25 and hyperkalemia coexists. *Note:* Rebound alkalosis or tetany may occur.
Potassium chloride (KCl).	Acidosis causes potassium to shift out of cells into circulation. Correction of acidosis may then cause a relative serum hypokalemia as potassium shifts back into cells. Potassium imbalance can impair neuromuscular/respiratory function.

POTENTIAL CONSIDERATIONS following acute hospitalization (dependent on patient's age, physical condition/presence of complications, personal resources, and life responsibilities)

Refer to Potential Considerations relative to underlying cause of acid/base disorder.

RESPIRATORY ALKALOSIS
(PRIMARY CARBONIC ACID DEFICIT)

Respiratory alkalosis is represented by a decrease in P_{CO_2} with a deficit of carbonic acid (H_2CO_3) due to a marked increase in the rate of respirations. Compensatory mechanisms include decreased respiratory rate (if the body is able to respond to the drop in Pa_{CO_2}), increased renal excretion of bicarbonate, and retention of hydrogen.

CARE SETTING

This condition does not occur in isolation but rather is a complication of a broader problem and usually requires inpatient care in a medical/surgical or subacute unit.

RELATED CONCERNS

Plans of care specific to predisposing factors.
Fluid and Electrolyte Imbalances, p 899
Metabolic Acidosis, p 506
Metabolic Alkalosis, p 510

Patient Assessment Data Base
(Dependent on underlying cause)

CIRCULATION

May report: Palpitations

May exhibit: Hypotension
Tachycardia, irregular pulse/dysrhythmias

ELIMINATION

May report: Concurrent peritoneal dialysis (causing too-rapid correction of metabolic acidosis)

FOOD/FLUID

May report: Dry mouth
Nausea/vomiting

May exhibit: Abdominal distention (elevating diaphragm as with ascites, pregnancy)

NEUROSENSORY

May report: Headache, tinnitus
Numbness/tingling of face, hands, and toes; circumoral paresthesia
Lightheadedness, syncope, vertigo, blurred vision

May exhibit: Anxiety, confusion, restlessness, obtundation, coma
Hyperactive reflexes, positive Chvostek's sign, tetany, seizures (thyrotoxicosis)
Muscle weakness

PAIN/DISCOMFORT

May report: Muscle cramps, epigastric pain

RESPIRATION

May report: Dyspnea
History of asthma, pulmonary fibrosis
Recent move/visit at high altitude

May exhibit: Tachypnea; rapid, shallow breathing; intermittent periods of apnea
Hyperventilation (extreme emotions, severe pain, cerebral lesions causing overbreathing)

SAFETY

May exhibit: Fever

TEACHING/LEARNING

May report: Use of salicylates, catecholamines, theophylline

Discharge plan considerations: **DRG projected mean length of inpatient stay: 4.1 days**
May require change in treatment/therapy of underlying disease process/condition.

Refer to section at end of plan for postdischarge considerations.

DIAGNOSTIC STUDIES

Arterial pH: Greater than 7.45 (may be near normal in chronic stage).
Bicarbonate (HCO$_3$): Normal or decreased; less than 25 mEq/L (compensatory mechanism).
Paco$_2$: Decreased, less than 35 mm Hg (primary).
Serum potassium: Decreased.
Serum chloride: Increased.
Serum calcium: Decreased.
Urine pH: increased, greater than 7.0.
Screening tests as indicated to determine underlying cause, e.g.,
    CBC: May reveal severe anemia (decreasing oxygen-carrying capacity).
    Blood cultures: May identify sepsis (usually gram-negative).
    Blood alcohol: Marked elevation (acute alcoholic intoxication).
    Toxicology screen: May reveal early salicylate poisoning.
    Chest x-ray/lung scan: May reveal multiple pulmonary emboli.

NURSING PRIORITIES

1. Achieve homeostasis.
2. Prevent/minimize complications.
3. Provide information about condition/prognosis and treatment needs as appropriate.

DISCHARGE GOALS

1. Physiologic balance restored.
2. Free of complications.
3. Condition, prognosis and treatment needs understood.
4. Plan in place to meet needs after discharge.

NURSING DIAGNOSIS: Gas Exchange, impaired

May be related to

Ventilation perfusion imbalance (e.g., altered oxygen supply, altered blood flow, altered oxygen-carrying capacity of blood, alveolar-capillary membrane changes)

ACTIONS/INTERVENTIONS	RATIONALE
Independent	
Monitor respiratory rate, depth, and effort; ascertain cause for hyperventilation if possible, e.g., anxiety, pain, improper ventilator settings.	Identifies alterations from usual breathing pattern and influences choice of intervention.
Assess level of awareness/cognition and note neuromuscular status, e.g., strength, tone, reflexes and sensation.	Decreased mentation (mild to severe) and tetany or convulsions may occur when alkalosis is severe and metabolic factors are in force.
Demonstrate appropriate breathing patterns, if appropriate, and assist with respiratory aids, e.g., rebreathing mask/bag.	Decreasing the rate of respirations can elevate PCO_2 level, lowering pH.
Provide support by a calm manner and voice.	May help reassure and calm the agitated patient, thereby aiding in reduction of respiratory rate.
Provide safety/seizure precautions, e.g., bed in low position, padded side rails, frequent observation.	Changes in mentation/CNS and neuromuscular hyperirritability may result in patient harm, especially if tetany/convulsions occur.
Discuss cause of condition (if known) and appropriate interventions/self-care activities.	Promotes participation in therapeutic regimen and may reduce recurrence of disorder.
Collaborative	
Assist with identification/treatment of underlying cause.	Respiratory alkalosis is a complication, not an isolated occurrence; addressing the primary condition (e.g., hyperventilation of panic attack, organ failure, severe anemia; drug effect, such as with paraldehyde or epinephrine) promotes correction of the disorder and reduces likelihood of recurrence.
Monitor/graph serial ABGs, and pulse oximetry.	Identifies therapy needs/effectiveness.
Monitor serum potassium. Replace as indicated.	Hypokalemia may occur as potassium is lost (urine) or shifted into the cell in exchange for hydrogen in an attempt to correct alkalosis.
Provide sedation, as indicated.	May be required to reduce psychogenic cause of hyperventilation.

ACTIONS/INTERVENTIONS	RATIONALE
Collaborative	
Administer CO_2, or use rebreathing mask as indicated. Reduce respiratory rate/tidal volume, or add additional dead space (tubing) to mechanical ventilator.	Increasing CO_2 retention may correct carbonic acid deficit.

POTENTIAL CONSIDERATIONS following acute hospitalization (dependent on patient's age, physical condition/presence of complications, personal resources, and life responsibilities)

Refer to Potential Considerations relative to underlying cause of acid/base disorder.

Neurologic/Sensory Disorders

GLAUCOMA

This condition of increased intraocular pressure (IOP) is the result of inadequate drainage of aqueous humor from the anterior chamber of the eye. The increased pressure causes atrophy of the optic nerve and blindness if untreated. There are four major types of glaucoma: (1) open angle (chronic); (2) closed angle (acute); (3) congenital; and (4) secondary. Open angle (chronic) is the most common type. Chronic glaucoma has no early warning signs and the loss of peripheral vision occurs so gradually that a substantial amount of optic nerve damage can occur before glaucoma is detected.

CARE SETTING

Community, unless sudden increase in IOP requires emergency intervention and close monitoring.

RELATED CONCERNS

Psychosocial Aspects of Care, p 783

Patient Assessment Data Base

ACTIVITY/REST

May report:	Change in usual activities/hobbies due to altered vision

FOOD/FLUID

May report:	Nausea/vomiting (acute glaucoma)

NEUROSENSORY

May report:	Gradual loss of peripheral vision, difficulty adjusting to darkened room, halos around lights, mild headache (chronic glaucoma) Cloudy/blurred vision, appearance of halos/rainbows around lights, sudden loss of peripheral vision, photophobia (acute glaucoma) Glasses/treatment change does not improve vision
May exhibit:	Dilated pupils (acute glaucoma) Fixed pupil and red/hard eye with cloudy cornea (glaucoma emergency) Increased tearing Intermescent cataracts, intraocular hemorrhage (secondary glaucoma)

PAIN/DISCOMFORT

May report: Mild discomfort or aching/tired eyes (chronic glaucoma)

Sudden/persistent severe pain or pressure in and around eye(s), headache (acute glaucoma)

SAFETY

May report: History of hemorrhage, trauma, ocular disease, tumor (secondary glaucoma)

Difficulty seeing, managing activities

May exhibit: Inflammatory disease of eye (secondary glaucoma)

TEACHING/LEARNING

May report: Family history of glaucoma, diabetes, systemic vascular disorders

History of stress, allergies, vasomotor disturbances (e.g., increased venous pressure), endocrine imbalance, diabetes (glaucoma)

History of ocular surgery/cataract removal; steroid use

Discharge plan considerations: May require assistance with transportation, meal preparation, self-care, home-maker/maintenance tasks

Refer to section at end of plan for postdischarge considerations.

DIAGNOSTIC STUDIES

Ophthalmoscopy examination: Assesses internal ocular structures, noting optic disc atrophy, papilledema, retinal hemorrhage, and microaneurysms. Slit-lamp examination provides three-dimensional view of eye structures, identifies corneal abnormalities/change in shape, increased IOP, and general vision deficits associated with glaucoma.

Visual acuity tests (e.g., Snellen, Jayer): Vision may be impaired by defects in cornea, lens, aqueous or vitreous humor, refraction, or disease of the nervous or vascular system supplying the retina or optic pathway.

Visual fields (e.g., confrontation, tangent screen, perimetry): Reduction of peripheral vision may be caused by glaucoma or other conditions such as CVA, pituitary/brain tumor mass, carotid or cerebral artery pathology.

Tonography measurement: Assesses intraocular pressure (normal: 12–20 mm Hg).

Gonioscopy measurement: Helps differentiate open angle from angle-closure glaucoma.

Provocative tests: May be useful in establishing presence/type of glaucoma when IOP is normal or only mildly elevated.

CBC, sedimentation rate (ESR): Rules out systemic anemia/infection.

ECG, serum cholesterol, and lipid studies: May be done to rule out atherosclerosis, CAD.

Glucose tolerance test/FBS: Determines presence/control of diabetes.

NURSING PRIORITIES

1. Prevent further visual deterioration.
2. Promote adaptation to changes in/reduced visual acuity.
3. Prevent complications.
4. Provide information about disease process/prognosis and treatment needs.

DISCHARGE GOALS

1. Vision maintained at highest possible level.
2. Patient coping with situation in a positive manner.
3. Complications prevented/minimized.
4. Disease process/prognosis and therapeutic regimen understood.
5. Plan in place to meet needs after discharge.

ACTIONS/INTERVENTIONS	RATIONALE
Independent	
Ascertain degree/type of visual loss.	Affects patient's future expectations and choice of interventions.
Encourage expression of feelings about loss/possibility of loss of vision.	While early intervention may prevent blindness, the patient faces the possibility or may have already experienced partial or complete loss of vision. Although vision loss that has already occurred cannot be restored (even with treatment), further loss can be prevented.
Demonstrate administration of eyedrops, e.g., counting drops, adhering to schedule, not missing doses.	Controls IOP, preventing further loss of vision.
Recommend measures to assist patient to manage visual limitations, e.g., reducing clutter, arranging furniture out of travel path; turning head to view subjects; correcting for dim light and problems of night vision.	Reduces safety hazards related to changes in visual fields/loss of vision and papillary accommodation to environmental light.
Collaborative	
Assist with administration of medications as indicated:	
Chronic, simple, open-angle glaucoma:	
Pilocarpine hydrochloride (IsoptoCarpine, Ocusert [disc], Pilopine HS Gel);	These topical myotic drugs cause pupillary constriction, facilitating the outflow of aqueous humor. *Note:* Ocusert is a disc (similar to a contact) that is placed in the lower eye lid, where it can remain for up to 1 week before being replaced.
Timolol maleate (Timoptic), betaxalol (Betoptic), careteolol (Ocupress), metipranolol (Opti-Pranolol), levobunolol (Betagan);	β-blockers decrease formation of aqueous humor without changing pupil size, vision, or accommodation. *Note:* These drugs may be contraindicated, or require close monitoring for systemic effects in the presence of bradycardia or asthma.
Acetazolamide (Diamox);	Decreases the rate of production of aqueous humor.
Narrow angle (angle closure) type:	
Myotics (until pupil is constricted);	Contracts the sphincter muscles of the iris, deepens anterior chamber, and dilates vessels of outflow tract during acute attack/prior to surgery.
Carbonic anhydrase inhibitors, e.g., acetazolamide (Diamox);	Decreases secretion of aqueous humor and lowers IOP.

ACTIONS/INTERVENTIONS	RATIONALE

Independent

Dipivefrin hydrochloride (Propine);

Adrenergic drops may be of benefit when patient is unresponsive to other medications. Free of side effects such as miosis, blurred vision, and night blindness.

Hyperosmotic agents, e.g., mannitol (Osmitrol), glycerine.

Used to decrease circulating fluid volume, which will decrease production of aqueous humor if other treatments have not been successful.

Provide sedation, analgesics as necessary.

Acute glaucoma attack is associated with sudden pain, which can precipitate anxiety/agitation, further elevating IOP. *Note:* Medical management may require 4–6 hours before IOP decreases and pain subsides.

Prepare for surgical intervention as indicated, e.g.:

Laser therapy, e.g., argon laser trabeculoplasty (ALT) or trabeculectomy/trephination;

Filtering operations create an opening between the anterior chamber and the subjunctival spaces so that aqueous humor can bypass the trabecular mesh block. *Note:* Apradclonidine (Iopidine) eye drops may be used in conjunction with laser therapy to lessen/prevent postprocedure elevations of IOP.

Iridectomy;

Surgical removal of a portion of the iris facilitates drainage of aqueous humor. Upper iris usually is covered with upper eyelid, and flow of tears washes bacteria downward. *Note:* Bilateral iridectomy is performed because glaucoma usually develops in the other eye.

Malteno valve implantation;

Experimental device corrects or prevents scarring over/closure of drainage sac created by trabeculectomy.

Cyclodialysis;

Separates ciliary body from the sclera to facilitate outflow of aqueous humor.

Aqueous-venous shunt;

Used in intractable glaucoma.

Diathermy/cryosurgery.

If other treatments fail, destruction of the ciliary body will reduce formation of aqueous humor.

NURSING DIAGNOSIS: Anxiety [specify level]

May be related to
Physiologic factors, change in health status; presence of pain; possibility/reality of loss of vision
Unmet needs
Negative self-talk

Possibly evidenced by
Apprehension, uncertainty
Expressed concern regarding changes in life events

DESIRED OUTCOMES/EVALUATION CRITERIA—PATIENT WILL:
Appear relaxed and report anxiety is reduced to a manageable level.
Demonstrate problem-solving skills.
Use resources effectively.

ACTIONS/INTERVENTIONS

Independent

Assess anxiety level, degree of pain experienced/suddenness of onset of symptoms, and current knowledge of condition.

Provide accurate, honest information. Discuss probability that careful monitoring and treatment can prevent additional visual loss.

Encourage patient to acknowledge concerns and express feelings.

Identify helpful resources/people.

RATIONALE

These factors affect patient perception of threat to self, potentiate the cycle of anxiety, and may interfere with medical attempts to control IOP.

Reduces anxiety related to unknown/future expectations and provides factual basis for making informed choices about treatment.

Provides opportunity for patient to deal with reality of situation, clarify misconceptions, and problem-solve concerns.

Provides reassurance that patient is not alone in dealing with problem.

NURSING DIAGNOSIS: Knowledge deficit [learning need] regarding condition, prognosis, treatment, self care and discharge needs

May be related to
Lack of exposure/unfamiliarity with resources
Lack of recall, information misinterpretation

Possibly evidenced by
Questions; statement of misconception
Inaccurate follow-through of instruction
Development of preventable complications

DESIRED OUTCOMES/EVALUATION CRITERIA—PATIENT WILL:
Verbalize understanding of condition, prognosis, and treatment.
Identify relationship of signs/symptoms to the disease process.
Correctly perform necessary procedures and explain reasons for the actions.

ACTIONS/INTERVENTIONS

Independent

Discuss necessity of wearing identification, e.g., Medi-Alert bracelet.

Demonstrate proper technique for administration of eye drops, gels, or discs. Have patient repeat demonstration.

Review importance of maintaining drug schedule, e.g., eye drops. Discuss medications that should be avoided, e.g., mydriatic drops (atropine/propantheline bromine), overuse of topical steroids.

Identify potential side effects/adverse reactions of treatment, e.g., decreased appetite, nausea/vomiting, diarrhea, fatigue, "drugged" feeling, decreased libido, impotence, cardiac irregularities, syncope, HF.

RATIONALE

Vital to provide information for caregivers in case of emergency to reduce risk of receiving contraindicated drugs (e.g., atropine).

Enhances effectiveness of treatment. Provides opportunity for patient to show competence and ask questions.

This disease can be controlled, not cured, and maintaining consistent medication regimen is vital to control. Some drugs cause pupil dilation, increasing IOP and potentiating additional loss of vision.

Drug side/adverse effects range from uncomfortable to severe/health-threatening. Approximately 50% of patients will develop sensitivity/allergy to parasympathomimetics (e.g., pilocarpine) or anticholinesterase drugs. These problems require medical evaluation and possible change in therapeutic regimen.

ACTIONS/INTERVENTIONS	RATIONALE

Independent

Encourage patient to make necessary changes in lifestyle.

A tranquil lifestyle decreases the emotional response to stress, preventing ocular changes that push the iris forward, which may precipitate an acute attack.

Reinforce avoidance of activities, such as heavy lifting/pushing, snow shoveling, wearing tight/constricting clothing.

May increase IOP precipitating acute attack. *Note:* If patient is not experiencing pain, cooperation with drug regimen and acceptance of lifestyle changes are often difficult to sustain.

Discuss dietary considerations, e.g., adequate fluid, bulk/fiber intake.

Measures to maintain consistency of stool to avoid constipation/straining during defecation.

Stress importance of routine checkups.

Important to monitor progression/maintenance of disease to allow for early intervention and prevent further loss of vision.

Advise patient to immediately report severe eye pain, inflammation, increased photophobia, increased lacrimation, changes in visual field/veil-like curtain, blurred vision, flashes of light/particles floating in visual field.

Prompt action may be necessary to prevent further vision loss/other complications, e.g., detached retina.

Recommend family members be examined regularly for signs of glaucoma.

Hereditary tendency to shallow anterior chambers places family members at risk for developing the condition.

Identify strategies/resources for socialization, e.g., support groups, Visually Impaired Society, local library, and transportation services.

Decreased visual acuity may limit patient's ability to drive/cause patient to withdraw from usual activities.

POTENTIAL CONSIDERATIONS following acute hospitalization (dependent on patient's age, physical condition/presence of complications, personal resources, and life responsibilities)

Trauma, risk for—poor vision.
Social Interaction, impaired—limited physical mobility (poor vision), inadequate support system.
Therapeutic Regimen: Individual, ineffective management—complexity of therapeutic regimen, economic difficulties, inadequate number and types of cues to action, perceived seriousness (of condition) or benefit (versus side effects).

Seizures (convulsions) are the result of uncontrolled electrical discharges from the nerve cells of the cerebral cortex, and are characterized by sudden, brief attacks of altered consciousness, motor activity, and/or sensory phenomena. Seizures can be associated with a variety of cerebral or systemic disorders as a focal or generalized disturbance of corticol function.

The phases of seizure activity are prodromal, aura, ictal, and postictal. The prodromal phase involves mood or behavior changes that may precede seizure by hours/days. The aura is a premonition of impending seizure activity and may be visual, auditory, or gustatory. The ictal stage is seizure activity, usually musculoskeletal. The postictal stage is a period of confusion/somnolence/irritability that occurs after the seizure.

The main causes for seizures can be divided into six categories:

Toxic agents: Poisons, alcohol, overdoses of prescription/nonprescription drugs, with drugs the leading cause.

Chemical imbalances: Hyperkalemia, hypoglycemia, and acidosis.

Fever: Acute infections, heatstroke.

Cerebral pathology: Resulting from head injury, infections, hypoxia, expanding brain lesions, increased intracranial pressure.

Eclampsia: Prenatal hypertension/toxemia of pregnancy.

Idiopathic: Unknown origin.

Seizures can be divided into two major classifications (generalized and focal). Generalized seizure types include grand mal, petit mal, and minor motor seizures. Focal (partial) seizure types include (1) partial motor, (2) partial sensory, and (3) partial seizures with complex symptoms. (Partial seizures are the most common type).

CARE SETTING

Community; however, may require brief inpatient care on a medical or subacute unit for stabilization/treatment of status epilepticus.

RELATED CONCERNS

Cerebrovascular Accident/Stroke, p 242

Craniocerebral Trauma (Acute Rehabilitative Phase), p 224

Psychosocial Aspects of Care, p 783

Substance Dependence/Abuse Rehabilitation, p 862

Patient Assessment Data Base

ACTIVITY/REST

May report: Fatigue, general weakness

Limitation of activities/occupation imposed by self/SO/healthcare provider or others

May exhibit: Altered muscle tone/strength

Involuntary movement/contractions of muscles or muscle groups (generalized tonic-clonic seizures)

CIRCULATION

May exhibit: Ictal: Hypertension, increased pulse, cyanosis

Postictal: Vital signs normal; or depressed with decreased pulse and respiration

EGO INTEGRITY

May report: Internal/external stressors related to condition and/or treatment

Irritability; sense of helplessness/hopelessness

Changes in relationships

May exhibit: Wide range of emotional responses

ELIMINATION

May report: Episodic incontinence

May exhibit: Ictal: Increased bladder pressure and sphincter tone
Postictal: Muscles relaxed resulting in incontinence (urinary/fecal)

FOOD/FLUID

May report: Food sensitivity nausea/vomiting correlating with seizure activity

May exhibit: Dental/soft tissue damage (injury during seizure)
Gingival hyperplasia (side effect of long-term Dilantin use)

NEUROSENSORY

May report: History of headaches, recurring seizure activity, fainting, dizziness
History of head trauma, anoxia, cerebral infections
Presence of aura (stimulation of visual, auditory, hallucinogenic areas)
Postictal: Weakness, muscle pain, areas of paresthesia/paralysis

May exhibit: Seizure characteristics:

Prodromal phase

Vague changes in emotional reactivity or affective response preceding aura in some cases and lasting minutes to hours.

Generalized seizures

Tonic-clonic (grand mal): Rigidity and jerking posturing, vocalization, loss of consciousness, dilated pupils, stertorous respiration, excessive saliva (froth), fecal/urinary incontinence, and biting of the tongue may occur.

Postictal: Patient sleeps 30 minutes to several hours, then may be weak, confused, and amnesic concerning the episode, with nausea and stiff, sore muscles.

Absence (petit mal): Periods of altered awareness or consciousness (staring, fluttering of eyes) lasting 5–30 seconds, which may occur as much as 100 times a day. Minor motor seizures may be akinetic (loss of movement), myoclonic (repetitive motor contractions), or atonic (loss of muscle tone).

Postictal phase: Amnesia for seizure events, no confusion, able to resume activity.

Partial seizures (complex)

Psychomotor/temporal lobe: Patient generally remains conscious, with reactions such as dream state, staring, wandering, irritability, hallucinations, hostility, or fear. May display involuntary motor symptoms (lip smacking) and behaviors that appear purposeful but are inappropriate (automatism) and include impaired judgment, and on occasion, antisocial acts.

Postictal phase: Absence of memory for these events, mild to moderate confusion.

Partial seizures (simple)

Focal-motor/Jacksonian: Often preceded by aura, lasts 2–15 minutes. No loss of consciousness (unilateral) or loss of consciousness (bilateral). Convulsive movements and temporary disturbance in part controlled by the brain region involved (e.g., frontal lobe [motor dysfunction]; parietal [numbness, tingling]; occipital [bright, flashing lights]; posterotemporal [difficulty speaking]). Convulsions may march along limb or side of body in orderly progression. If restrained during seizure, patient may exhibit combative and uncooperative behavior.

Status epilepticus

Continuous seizure activity occurring spontaneously or related to abrupt withdrawal of anticonvulsants and other metabolic phenomena. *Note:* If absence seizures are the pattern, problem may go undetected for a period of time, as the patient does not lose consciousness.

215

PAIN/DISCOMFORT

May report: Headache, muscle/back soreness postictally
Paroxysmal abdominal pain during ictal phase (may occur during some partial/focal seizures without loss of consciousness)

May exhibit: Guarding behavior
Alteration in muscle tone
Distraction behavior/restlessness

RESPIRATION

May exhibit: Ictal: Clenched teeth, cyanosis, decreased or rapid respirations; increased mucous secretions
Postictal: Apnea

SAFETY

May report: History of accidental falls/injuries, fractures
Presence of allergies

May exhibit: Soft tissue injury/ecchymosis
Decreased general strength/muscle tone

SOCIAL INTERACTION

May report: Problems with interpersonal relationships within family/socially
Limitation/avoidance of social contacts

TEACHING/LEARNING

May report: Familial history of epilepsy
Drug (including alcohol) use/misuse
Increased frequency of episodes/failure to improve

Discharge plan considerations: **DRG projected mean length of inpatient stay: 3.5 days**
May require changes in medications, assistance with some homemaker/maintenance tasks relative to issues of safety and transportation

Refer to section at end of plan for postdischarge considerations.

DIAGNOSTIC STUDIES

Electrolytes: Imbalances may affect/predispose to seizure activity.
Glucose: Hypoglycemia may precipitate seizure activity.
BUN: Elevation may potentiate seizure activity or may indicate nephrotoxicity related to medication regimen.
CBC: Aplastic anemia may result from drug therapy.
Serum drug levels: To verify therapeutic range of antiepileptic drugs.
Toxicology screen: Determines potentiating factors such as alcohol or other drug use.
Skull x-rays: Identifies presence of space-occupying lesions, fractures.
Electroencephalogram (EEG): Locates area of cerebral dysfunction; measures brain activity. Brain waves take on characteristic spikes in each type of seizure activity.
Video-EEG monitoring, 24 hours (video picture obtained at same time as EEG): May identify exact focus of seizure activity (advantage of repeated viewing of event with EEG recording).
CT scan: Identifies localized cerebral lesions, infarcts, hematomas, cerebral edema, trauma, abscesses, tumor; can be done with or without contrast medium.
Positron emission tomography (PET): Demonstrates metabolic alterations, e.g., decreased metabolism of glucose at site of lesion.

MRI: Localizes focal lesions.

Single photon emission computed tomography (SPECT): May show local areas of brain dysfunction when CT and MRI are normal.

Lumbar puncture: Detects abnormal CSF pressure, signs of infections or bleeding (subarachnoid, subdural hemorrhage) as a cause of seizure activity.

Magnetoencephalogram: Maps the electrical impulses/potential of brain for abnormal discharge patterns.

Wada: Determines hemispheric dominance (done as a presurgical evaluation prior to temporal lobectomy).

NURSING PRIORITIES

1. Prevent/control seizure activity.
2. Protect patient from injury.
3. Maintain airway/respiratory function.
4. Promote positive self-esteem.
5. Provide information about disease process, prognosis, and treatment needs.

DISCHARGE GOALS

1. Seizure activity controlled.
2. Complications/injury prevented.
3. Capable/competent self-image displayed.
4. Disease process/prognosis, therapeutic regimen, and limitations understood.
5. Plan in place to meet needs after discharge.

NURSING DIAGNOSIS: Trauma/Suffocation, risk for

Risk factors may include
Weakness, balancing difficulties
Cognitive limitations/altered consciousness
Loss of large or small muscle coordination
Emotional difficulties

Possibly evidenced by
[Not applicable; presence of signs and symptoms establishes an *actual* diagnosis]

DESIRED OUTCOMES/EVALUATION CRITERIA—PATIENT WILL:
Verbalize understanding of factors that contribute to possibility of trauma, and/or suffocation and take steps to correct situation.
Demonstrate behaviors, lifestyle changes to reduce risk factors and protect self from injury.
Modify environment as indicated to enhance safety.
Maintain treatment regimen to control/eliminate seizure activity.

CAREGIVERS WILL:
Identify actions/measures to take when seizure activity occurs.

ACTIONS/INTERVENTIONS	RATIONALE
Independent	
Explore with patient the various stimuli that may precipitate seizure activity.	Alcohol, various drugs, and other stimuli (e.g., loss of sleep, flashing lights, prolonged television viewing) may increase brain activity, thereby increasing the potential for seizure activity.

217

ACTIONS/INTERVENTIONS	RATIONALE
Independent	
Keep padded side rails up with bed in lowest position or place bed up against wall and pad floor if rails not available.	Minimizes injury should seizures (frequent/generalized) occur while patient is in bed.
Encourage patient not to smoke except while supervised.	May cause burns if cigarette is accidentally dropped during aura/seizure activity.
Evaluate need for/provide protective headgear.	Use of helmet may provide added protection for individuals who suffer recurrent/severe seizures.
Use metal or tympanic thermometer when necessary to take temperature.	Reduces risk of patient biting and breaking glass thermometer or suffering injury if sudden seizure activity should occur.
Maintain strict bed rest if prodromal signs/aura experienced. Explain necessity for these actions.	Patient may feel restless/need to ambulate or even defecate during aura phase, thereby inadvertently removing self from safe environment and easy observation. Understanding importance of providing for own safety needs may enhance patient cooperation.
Stay with patient during/after seizure.	Promotes patient safety.
Insert plastic airway/bite block or soft roll between teeth (if jaw relaxed). Turn head to side/suction airway as indicated.	Helps maintain airway and reduces risk of oral trauma but should not be "forced" or inserted when teeth are clenched, because dental and soft tissue damage may result. *Note:* Wooden tongue blades should not be used, because they may splinter and break in patient's mouth. (Refer to ND: Airway Clearance/Breathing Pattern, ineffective, risk for, p 219.)
Cradle head, place on soft area, or assist to floor if out of bed. Do not attempt to restrain.	Gentle guiding of extremities reduces risk of physical injury when patient lacks voluntary muscle control. *Note:* If attempt is made to restrain patient during seizure, erratic movements may increase, and patient may injure self or others.
Document type of seizure activity (e.g., location/duration of motor activity, loss of consciousness, incontinence) and frequency/recurrence.	Helps to localize the cerebral area of involvement.
Perform neurologic/vital sign check after seizure, e.g., level of consciousness, orientation, BP, pulse/respiratory rate.	Documents postictal state and time/completeness of recovery to normal state.
Reorient patient following seizure activity.	Patient may be confused, disoriented, and possibly amnesic after the seizure and need help to regain control and alleviate anxiety.
Allow postictal "automatic" behavior without interfering while providing environmental protection.	May display behavior (of motor or psychic origin) that seems inappropriate/irrelevant for time and place. Attempts to control or prevent activity may result in patient becoming aggressive/combative.
Observe for status epilepticus, e.g., one tonic-clonic seizure after another in rapid succession.	This is a life-threatening emergency that may cause respiratory arrest, severe hypoxia, and/or brain and nerve cell damage. Immediate intervention is required to control seizure activity. *Note:* Although absence seizures may become static, they are not usually life-threatening.

ACTIONS/INTERVENTIONS	RATIONALE

Independent

Discuss seizure warning signs (if appropriate) and usual seizure pattern. Teach SO to recognize warning signs and how to care for patient during and after seizure.

Enables patient to protect self from injury and recognize changes that require notification of physician/further intervention. Knowing what to do when seizure occurs can prevent injury/complications and decrease SO's feelings of helplessness.

Collaborative

Administer medications as indicated:

Specific drug therapy is dependent on seizure type.

AEDs, e.g., phenytoin (Dilantin), primidone (Mysoline), carbamazepine (Tegretol), clonazepam (Klonopin), valproic acid (Depakote);

Antiepileptic drugs raise the seizure threshold by stabilizing nerve cell membranes, reducing the excitability of the neurons, or through direct action on the limbic system, thalamus, and hypothalamus. Goal is optimal suppression of seizure activity with lowest possible dose of drug and with fewest side effects.

Phenobarbital (Luminal);

Potentiates/enhances effects of AEDs and allows for lower dosage to reduce side effects.

Diazepam (Valium);

May be used alone (or in combination with phenobarbital) as a first-line drug to suppress status seizure activity.

Glucose, thiamine.

May be given to restore metabolic balance if seizure is induced by hypoglycemia or alcohol.

Monitor/document AED drug levels, corresponding side effects, and frequency of seizure activity.

Standard therapeutic level may not be optimal for individual patient if untoward side effects develop or seizures are not controlled.

Monitor CBC, electrolytes, glucose levels.

Identifies factors that aggravate/decrease seizure threshold.

Prepare for surgery/electrode implantation as indicated.

Vagal nerve stimulator, magnetic beam therapy, or other surgical intervention (e.g., temporal lobectomy) may be done for intractable seizures or well-localized epileptogenic lesions when patient is disabled and at high risk for serious injury.

NURSING DIAGNOSIS: Airway Clearance/Breathing Pattern, ineffective, risk for

Risk factors may include
Neuromuscular impairment
Tracheobronchial obstruction
Perceptual/cognitive impairment

Possibly evidenced by
[Not applicable; presence of signs and symptoms establishes an *actual* diagnosis]

DESIRED OUTCOMES/EVALUATION CRITERIA—PATIENT WILL:
Maintain effective respiratory pattern with airway patent/aspiration prevented.

Independent

Encourage patient to empty mouth of dentures/foreign objects if aura occurs and to avoid chewing gum/sucking lozenges if seizures occur without warning.

Reduces risk of aspiration/foreign bodies lodging in pharynx.

Place in lying position, flat surface; turn head to side during seizure activity.

Promotes drainage of secretions; prevents tongue from obstructing airway.

Loosen clothing from neck/chest and abdominal areas.

Facilitates breathing/chest expansion.

Insert bite stick/airway or soft roll as indicated.

If inserted prior to tightening of the jaw, these devices may prevent biting of tongue and facilitate suctioning/respiratory support if required. Airway adjunct may be indicated after cessation of seizure activity if patient is unconscious and unable to maintain safe position of tongue.

Suction as needed.

Reduces risk of aspiration/asphyxiation.

Collaborative

Administer supplemental oxygen/hand ventilate as needed postictally.

May reduce cerebral hypoxia resulting from decreased circulation/oxygenation secondary to vascular spasm during seizure. *Note:* Artificial ventilation during general seizure activity is of limited or no benefit as it is not possible to move air in/out of lungs during sustained contraction of respiratory musculature. As seizure abates, respiratory function will return unless a secondary problem exists (e.g., foreign body/aspiration).

Prepare for/assist with intubation, if indicated.

Presence of prolonged apnea postictally may require ventilatory support.

NURSING DIAGNOSIS: Self Esteem/Personal Identity disturbance (specify)

May be related to
Stigma associated with condition
Perception of being out of control

Possibly evidenced by
Verbalization about changed lifestyle
Fear of rejection; negative feelings about body
Change in self-perception of role
Change in usual patterns of responsibility
Lack of follow-through/nonparticipation in therapy

DESIRED OUTCOMES/EVALUATION CRITERIA—PATIENT WILL:
Identify feelings and methods for coping with negative perception of self.
Verbalize increased sense of self-esteem in relation to diagnosis.
Verbalize realistic perception and acceptance of self in changed role/lifestyle.

ACTIONS/INTERVENTIONS	RATIONALE

Independent

Discuss feelings about diagnosis, perception of threat to self. Encourage expression of feelings.

Reactions vary among individuals, and previous knowledge/experience with this condition will affect acceptance of therapeutic regimen. Verbalization of fears, anger, and concerns about future implications can help patient begin to accept/deal with situation.

Identify possible/anticipated public reaction to condition. Encourage patient to refrain from concealing problem.

Provides opportunity to problem-solve responses and provides measure of control over situation. Concealment is destructive to self-esteem (potentiates denial), blocking progress in dealing with problem and may actually increase risk of injury/negative response when seizure does occur.

Explore with patient current/past successes and strengths.

Focusing on positive aspects can help to alleviate feelings of guilt/self-consciousness and help patient begin to accept manageability of condition.

Avoid overprotecting patient; encourage activities providing supervision/monitoring when indicated.

Participation in as many experiences as possible can lessen depression about limitations. Observation/supervision needs to be provided for such activities as gymnastics, climbing, and water sports.

Determine attitudes/capabilities of SO. Help individual realize that his/her feelings are normal; however guilt and blame are not helpful.

Negative expectations from SO may affect patient's sense of competency/self-esteem and interfere with support received from SO, limiting potential for optimal management.

Stress importance of staff/SO remaining calm during seizure activity.

Anxiety of caregivers is contagious and can be conveyed to the patient, increasing/multiplying individual's own negative perceptions of situation/self.

Collaborative

Refer patient/SO to support group, e.g., Epilepsy Foundation of America and National Association of Epilepsy Centers.

Provides opportunity to gain information, support, and ideas for dealing with problems from others who share similar experiences.

Discuss referral for psychotherapy with patient/SO.

Seizures have a profound effect on personal self-esteem, and patient/SO may feel guilt over perceived limitations and public stigma. Counseling can help overcome feelings of inferiority/self-consciousness.

NURSING DIAGNOSIS: Knowledge deficit [learning need] regarding condition, treatment regimen, self care and discharge needs

May be related to
Lack of exposure
Information misinterpretation; lack of recall
Cognitive limitation
Failure to improve

Possibly evidenced by
Questions
Increased frequency/lack of control of seizure activity
Lack of follow-through of drug regimen

DESIRED OUTCOMES/EVALUATION CRITERIA—PATIENT WILL:
Verbalize understanding of disorder and various stimuli that may increase/potentiate seizure activity.
Initiate necessary lifestyle/behavior changes as indicated.
Adhere to prescribed drug regimen.

ACTIONS/INTERVENTIONS

Independent

Review pathology/prognosis of condition and life-long need for treatment as indicated.

Review medication regimen, necessity of taking drugs as ordered, and not discontinuing therapy without physician supervision. Include directions for missed dose.

Recommend taking drugs with meals if appropriate.

Discuss adverse side effects of particular drugs, e.g., drowsiness, hyperactivity, sleep disturbances, gingival hypertrophy, visual disturbances, nausea/vomiting, rashes, syncope/ataxia, birth defects, aplastic anemia.

Provide information about potential drug interactions and necessity of notifying other healthcare providers of drug regimen.

Encourage patient to wear identification tag/bracelet stating the presence of a seizure disorder.

Stress need for routine follow-up care/laboratory testing as indicated, e.g., CBC should be monitored bi-annually and in presence of sore throat/fever.

Review possible effects of hormonal changes.

Discuss significance of maintaining good general health, e.g., adequate diet, rest, moderate exercise, and avoidance of exhaustion, alcohol, caffeine, and stimulant drugs.

Review importance of good oral hygiene and regular dental care.

RATIONALE

Provides opportunity to clarify/dispel misconceptions and present condition as something that is manageable within a normal lifestyle.

Lack of cooperation with medication regimen is a leading cause of seizure breakthrough. Patient needs to know risks of status epilepticus resulting from abrupt withdrawal of anticonvulsants. Dependent on drug and frequency, patient may be instructed to take missed dose if remembered within a predetermined time frame.

May reduce incidence of gastric irritation, nausea/vomiting.

May indicate need for change in dosage/choice of drug therapy. Promotes involvement/participation in decision-making process, and awareness of potential long-term effects of drug therapy and provides opportunity to minimize/prevent complications.

Knowledge of anticonvulsant use reduces risk of prescribing drugs that may interact, thus altering seizure threshold or therapeutic effect. For example, Dilantin potentiates anticoagulant effect of Coumadin, whereas INH and chloromycetin increase the effect of Dilantin.

Expedites treatment and diagnosis in emergency situations.

Therapeutic needs may change and/or serious drug side effects (e.g., agranulocytosis or toxicity) may develop.

Alterations in hormonal levels that occur during menstruation and pregnancy may increase risk of seizures.

Regularity and moderation in activities may aid in reducing/controlling precipitating factors, enhancing sense of general well-being, and strengthening coping ability and self-esteem.

Reduces risk of oral infections and gingival hyperplasia.

ACTIONS/INTERVENTIONS	RATIONALE
Independent	
Identify necessity/promote acceptance of actual limitations; discuss safety measures concerned with driving, using mechanical equipment, climbing ladders, swimming, hobbies, and so on.	Reduces risk of injury to self or others, especially if seizures occur without warning.
Discuss local laws/restrictions pertaining to persons with epilepsy/seizure disorder. Encourage awareness but not necessarily acceptance of these policies.	Although legal/civil rights of persons with epilepsy have improved during the past decade, restrictions still exist in some states pertaining to obtaining driver's license, sterilization, worker's compensation, and required reportability to state agencies.

POTENTIAL CONSIDERATIONS following acute hospitalization (dependent on patient's age, physical condition/presence of complications, personal resources, and life responsibilities)

Injury, risk for—weakness, balancing difficulties, cognitive limitations/altered consciousness, loss of large or small muscle coordination.

Self Esteem (specify)—stigma associated with condition, perception of being out of control, personal vulnerability, negative evaluation of self/capabilities.

Therapeutic Regimen: Individual, ineffective management—social support deficits, perceived benefit (versus side effects of medication), perceived susceptibility (possible long periods of remission).

CRANIOCEREBRAL TRAUMA (ACUTE REHABILITATIVE PHASE)

Craniocerebral trauma, also called head or brain injury (open or closed) includes skull fractures, brain concussion, cerebral contusion/laceration, and hemorrhage (subarachnoid, subdural, epidural, intracerebral, brainstem). *Primary* injury may occur from direct blow to head or be indirect (acceleration/deceleration of brain). *Secondary* brain injury can result from diffuse intracerebral axonal injury, intracranial hypertension, hypoxemia, hypercapnea, or systemic hypotension.

Consequences of head injury range from no apparent neurologic disturbance to a persistent vegetative state or death. Therefore, every head injury must be considered potentially serious.

CARE SETTING

Rehabilitation following acute injury may occur in medical/surgical, subacute, and/or rehabilitation units.

RELATED CONCERNS

Cerebrovascular Accident/Stroke, p 242
Psychosocial Aspects of Care, p 783
Seizure Disorders/Epilepsy, p 214
Total Nutritional Support: Parenteral/Enteral Feeding, p 491
Upper Gastrointestinal/Esophageal Bleeding, p 315
Thrombophlebitis: Deep Vein Thrombosis, p 107

Patient Assessment Data Base

Data are dependent on type, location, and severity of injury and may be complicated by additional injury to other vital organs.

ACTIVITY/REST

May report: Weakness, fatigue, clumsiness, loss of balance

May exhibit: Altered consciousness, lethargy
Hemiparesis, quadriparesis
Unsteady gait (ataxia)
Balance problems
Orthopedic injuries (trauma)
Loss of muscle tone, muscle spasticity

CIRCULATION

May exhibit: Normal or altered BP (hypertension)
Changes in heart rate (bradycardia, tachycardia alternating with bradycardia, other dysrhythmias)

EGO INTEGRITY

May report: Behavior or personality changes (subtle or dramatic)

May exhibit: Anxiety, irritability, delirium, agitation, confusion, depression, impulsivity

ELIMINATION

May exhibit: Bowel/bladder incontinence or dysfunction

FOOD/FLUID

May report: Nausea/vomiting, changes in appetite

May exhibit: Vomiting (may be projectile)
Swallowing problems (coughing, drooling, dysphagia)

NEUROSENSORY

May report: Loss of consciousness, variable levels of awareness, amnesia surrounding trauma events
Vertigo, syncope, tinnitus, hearing loss
Tingling, numbness in extremity
Visual changes, e.g., decreased acuity, diplopia, photophobia, loss of part of visual field
Loss of/changes in senses of taste or smell

May exhibit: Alteration in consciousness, coma
Mental status changes (orientation, alertness/responsiveness, attention, concentration, problem solving, emotional affect/behavior, memory)
Pupillary changes (response to light, symmetry), deviation of eyes, inability to follow
Loss of senses, e.g., taste, smell, hearing
Facial asymmetry
Unequal, weak handgrip
Absent/weak deep tendon reflexes
Apraxia, hemiparesis, quadriparesis
Posturing (decorticate, decerebrate); seizure activity
Heightened sensitivity to touch and movement
Altered sensation to parts of body
Difficulty in understanding self/limbs in relation to environment (proprioception)

PAIN/DISCOMFORT

May report: Headache of variable intensity and location (usually long-lasting)

May exhibit: Facial grimacing, withdrawal response to painful stimuli, restlessness, moaning

RESPIRATION

May exhibit: Changes in breathing patterns (e.g., periods of apnea alternating with hyperventilation)
Noisy respirations, stridor, choking
Rhonchi, wheezes (possible aspiration)

SAFETY

May report: Recent trauma/accidental injuries

May exhibit: Fractures/dislocations
Impaired vision
Skin: Head/facial lacerations, abrasions, discoloration, e.g., raccoon eyes, Battles' sign around ears (trauma signs)
Drainage from ears/nose (CSF)
Impaired cognition
Range of motion impairment, loss of muscle tone, general strength; paralysis
Fever, altered body temperature regulation

SOCIAL INTERACTION

May exhibit: Expressive or receptive aphasia, unintelligible speech, repetitive speech, dysarthria, anomia

225

May report:	Use of alcohol/other drugs
Discharge plan considerations:	**DRG projected mean length of inpatient stay: 17.1 days (inclusive)** May require assistance with self-care, ambulation, transportation, food preparation, shopping, treatments, medications, homemaker/maintenance tasks; change in physical layout of home or placement in living facility other than home

Refer to section at end of plan for postdischarge considerations.

DIAGNOSTIC STUDIES

CT scan (with/without contrast): Identifies space-occupying lesions, hemorrhage; determines ventricular size, brain tissue shift. *Note:* Serial study may be required as ischemic injury/infarct may not be detected for 24–72 hours postinjury.

MRI: Uses similar to those of CT scan with or without use of radioactive contrast.

Cerebral angiography: Demonstrates cerebral circulatory anomalies, e.g., brain tissue shifts secondary to edema, hemorrhage, trauma.

Serial EEG: May reveal presence or development of pathologic waves.

X-rays: Detect changes in bony structure (fractures), shifts of midline structures (bleeding/edema), bone fragments.

BAER: Determines levels of cortical and brainstem function.

PET/SPECT: Detects changes in metabolic activity in the brain.

Otoneurologic tests (falling, post-pointing and Romberg): Screening for neurologic disorders affecting posture, balance, and coordination of movements.

CSF, lumbar puncture: May be diagnostic for suspected subarachnoid hemorrhage.

ABGs: Determines presence of ventilation or oxygenation problems that may exacerbate/increase intracranial pressure.

Serum chemistry/electrolytes: May reveal imbalances that contribute to increased intracranial pressure (IICP)/changes in mentation.

Toxicology screen: Detects drugs that may be responsible for/potentiate loss of consciousness.

Serum anticonvulsant levels: May be done to ensure that therapeutic level is adequate to prevent seizure activity.

NURSING PRIORITIES

1. Maximize cerebral perfusion/function.
2. Prevent/minimize complications.
3. Promote optimal functioning/return to preinjury level.
4. Support coping process and family recovery.
5. Provide information about condition/prognosis, treatment plan, and resources.

DISCHARGE GOALS

1. Cerebral function improved; neurologic deficits resolving/stabilized.
2. Complications prevented or minimized.
3. ADL needs met by self or with assistance of other(s).
4. Family acknowledging reality of situation and involved in recovery program.
5. Condition/prognosis and treatment regimen understood and available resources identified.
6. Plan in place to meet needs after discharge.

NURSING DIAGNOSIS: Tissue Perfusion, altered, cerebral

May be related to

Interruption of blood flow by space-occupying lesions (hemorrhage, hematoma); cerebral edema (localized or generalized response to injury, metabolic alterations, drug/alcohol overdose); decreased systemic BP/hypoxia (hypovolemia, cardiac dysrhythmias)

Possibly evidenced by

Altered level of consciousness; memory loss

Changes in motor/sensory responses, restlessness

Changes in vital signs

DESIRED OUTCOMES/EVALUATION CRITERIA—PATIENT WILL:

Maintain usual/improved level of consciousness, cognition, and motor/sensory function.

Demonstrate stable vital signs and absence of signs of increased ICP.

ACTIONS/INTERVENTIONS	RATIONALE
Independent	
Determine factors related to individual situation, cause for coma/decreased cerebral perfusion and potential for IICP.	Influences choice of interventions. Deterioration in neurologic signs/symptoms or failure to improve after initial insult may reflect decreased intracranial adaptive capacity requiring that the patient be transferred to critical care for monitoring of intracranial pressure and/or surgical intervention.
Monitor/document neurologic status frequently and compare with baseline, e.g., Glasgow Coma Scale during first 48 hours;	Assesses trends in LOC and potential for IICP and is useful in determining location, extent, and progression/resolution of CNS damage.
Evaluate eye opening, e.g., spontaneous (awake), opens only to painful stimuli, keeps eyes closed (coma);	Determines arousal ability/level of consciousness.
Assess verbal response; note whether patient is alert, oriented to person, place, time or is confused; uses inappropriate words/phrases that make little sense;	Measures appropriateness of speech and content of consciousness. If minimal damage has occurred in the cerebral cortex, the patient may be aroused by verbal stimuli but may appear drowsy or uncooperative. More extensive damage to the cerebral cortex may be displayed by slow response to commands, lapsing into sleep when not stimulated, disorientation, and stupor. Damage to midbrain, pons, and medulla are manifested by lack of appropriate responses to stimuli.
Assess motor response to simple commands, noting purposeful (obeys command, attempts to push stimulus away) and nonpurposeful (posturing) movement. Note limb movement and document right and left sides separately.	Measures overall awareness and ability to respond to external stimuli and best indicates state of consciousness in the patient whose eyes are closed because of trauma or who is aphasic. Consciousness and involuntary movement are integrated if the patient can both grasp and release the tester's hand, or hold up 2 fingers on command. Purposeful movement can include grimacing or withdrawing from painful stimuli or movements that the patient desires, e.g., sitting up. Other movements (posturing and abnormal flexion of extremities) usually indicate diffuse cortical damage. Absence of spontaneous movement on one side of the body indicates damage to the motor tracts in the opposite cerebral hemisphere.

227

ACTIONS/INTERVENTIONS	RATIONALE
Independent	
Monitor vital signs, e.g.: BP, noting onset of/continuing systolic hypertension and widening pulse pressure; observe for hypotension in multiple trauma patient;	Normally, autoregulation maintains constant cerebral blood flow despite fluctuations in systemic BP. Loss of autoregulation may follow local or diffuse cerebral vascular damage. Elevating systolic BP accompanied by decreasing diastolic BP (widening pulse pressure) is an ominous sign of IICP when accompanied by decreased level of consciousness. Hypovolemia/hypotension (associated with multiple trauma) may also result in cerebral ischemia/damage.
Heart rate/rhythm, noting bradycardia, alternating bradycardia/tachycardia, other dysrhythmias;	Changes in rate (most often bradycardia) and dysrhythmias may develop, reflecting brainstem pressure/injury in the absence of underlying cardiac disease.
Respirations, noting patterns and rhythm, e.g., periods of apnea after hyperventilation, Cheyne-Stokes respiration.	Irregularities can suggest location of cerebral insult/increasing ICP and need for further intervention including possible respiratory support. (Refer to ND: Breathing Pattern, ineffective, risk for, p 230.)
Evaluate pupils, noting size, shape, equality, light reactivity.	Pupil reactions are regulated by the oculomotor (III) cranial nerve and are useful in determining if the brainstem is intact. Pupil size/equality is determined by balance between parasympathetic and sympathetic enervation. Response to light reflects combined function of optic (II) and oculomotor (III) cranial nerves.
Assess for changes in vision, e.g., double vision (diplopia) blurred vision, alterations in visual field, depth perception.	Visual alterations, which can result from microscopic damage to the brain, have consequent safety concerns and influence choice of interventions.
Assess position/movement of eyes, noting whether in midposition or deviated to side or downward. Note loss of doll's eyes (oculocephalic reflex).	Position and movement of eyes help localize area of brain involvement. An early sign of increased ICP is impaired abduction of eyes, indicating pressure/injury to the fifth cranial nerve. Loss of doll's eyes indicates deterioration in brainstem function and poor prognosis.
Note presence/absence of reflexes (e.g., blink, cough, gag, Babinski).	Alterations in reflexes reflect injury at level of midbrain or brainstem and have direct implications for patient safety. Loss of blink reflex suggests damage to the pons and medulla. Absence of cough and gag reflexes reflect damage to medulla. Presence of Babinski reflex indicates injury along pyramidal pathways in the brain.
Monitor temperature and regulate environmental temperature as indicated. Limit use of blankets; administer tepid sponge bath in presence of fever. Wrap extremities in blankets when hypothermia blanket is used.	Fever may reflect damage to hypothalamus. Increased metabolic needs and oxygen consumption occur (especially with fever and shivering), which can further increase ICP.
Monitor intake and output. Weigh as indicated. Note skin turgor, status of mucous membranes.	Useful indicators of total body water, which is an integral part of tissue perfusion. Cerebral trauma/ischemia can result in diabetes insipidus (DI) or SIADH. Alterations may lead to hypovolemia or vascular engorgement, either of which can negatively affect cerebral pressure.

ACTIONS/INTERVENTIONS	RATIONALE
Independent	
Maintain head/neck in midline or neutral position, support with small towel rolls and pillows. Avoid placing head on large pillows.	Turning head to one side compresses the jugular veins and inhibits cerebral venous drainage, thereby increasing ICP.
Provide rest periods between care activities and limit duration of procedures.	Continual activity can increase ICP by producing a cumulative stimulant effect.
Decrease extraneous stimuli and provide comfort measures, e.g., back massage, quiet environment, soft voice, gentle touch.	Provides calming effect, reduces adverse physiologic response, and promotes rest to maintain/lower ICP.
Help patient avoid/limit coughing, vomiting, straining at stool/bearing down when possible.	These activities increase intrathoracic and intraabdominal pressures, which can increase ICP.
Avoid/limit use of restraints.	Mechanical restraints may enhance fight response, increasing ICP. *Note:* Cautious use may be indicated to prevent injury to patient.
Encourage SO to talk to patient.	Familiar voices of family/SO appear to have a relaxing effect on many comatose patients, which can reduce ICP.
Investigate increasing restlessness, moaning, guarding behaviors.	These nonverbal cues may indicate increasing ICP or reflect presence of pain when patient is unable to verbalize complaints. Unrelieved pain can in turn aggravate/potentiate IICP.
Palpate for bladder distention, maintain patency of urinary drainage if used. Monitor for constipation.	May trigger autonomic responses potentiating elevation of ICP.
Observe for seizure activity and protect patient from injury.	Seizures can occur as a result of cerebral irritation, hypoxia, or IICP, and seizures can further elevate ICP, compounding cerebral damage.
Assess for nuchal rigidity, twitching, increased restlessness, irritability, onset of seizure activity.	Indicative of meningeal irritation, which may occur due to interruption of dura, and/or development of infection during acute or recovery period of brain injury.
Collaborative	
Elevate head of bed 15–45 degrees as tolerated/indicated.	Promotes venous drainage from head, thereby reducing cerebral congestion and edema/risk of IICP.
Restrict fluid intake as indicated. Administer IV fluids with control device.	Fluid restriction may be needed to reduce cerebral edema; minimize fluctuations in vascular load, BP, and ICP.
Administer supplemental oxygen as indicated.	Reduces hypoxemia, which may increase cerebral vasodilation and blood volume, elevating ICP.
Monitor ABGs/pulse oximetry.	Determines respiratory sufficiency (presence of hypoxia/acidosis) and indicates therapy needs.
Administer medications as indicated:	
Diuretics, e.g., mannitol (Osmitrol), furosemide (Lasix);	Diuretics may be used in acute phase to draw water from brain cells, reducing cerebral edema and ICP.
Steroids, e.g., dexamethasone (Decadron), methylprednisolone (Medrol);	Decreases inflammation, reducing tissue edema.

229

ACTIONS/INTERVENTIONS	RATIONALE
Collaborative	
Anticonvulsant, e.g., phenytoin (Dilantin);	Dilantin is the drug of choice for treatment and prevention of seizure activity in immediate post-traumatic period. Prophylactic anticonvulsive therapy may be continued for an indeterminate period of time.
Chlorpromazine (Thorazine);	Useful in treating posturing and shivering, which can increase ICP. *Note:* This drug can lower the seizure threshold or precipitate Dilantin toxicity.
Mild analgesics, e.g., codeine;	May be indicated to relieve pain and its negative effect on ICP but should be used with caution to prevent respiratory embarrassment.
Sedatives, e.g., diphenhydramine (Benadryl);	May be used to control restlessness, agitation.
Antipyretics, e.g., acetaminophen (Tylenol).	Reduces/controls fever and its deleterious effect on cerebral metabolism/oxygen needs.
Prepare for surgical intervention, if indicated.	Craniotomy or trephination ("burr" holes) may be done to remove bone fragments, elevate depressed fractures, evacuate hematoma, control hemorrhage, and debride necrotic tissue.

NURSING DIAGNOSIS: Breathing Pattern, ineffective, risk for

Risk factors may include
Neuromuscular impairment (injury to respiratory center of brain)
Perception or cognitive impairment
Tracheobronchial obstruction

Possibly evidenced by
[Not applicable; presence of signs and symptoms establishes an *actual* diagnosis]

DESIRED OUTCOMES/EVALUATION CRITERIA—PATIENT WILL:
Maintain a normal/effective respiratory pattern, free of cyanosis, with ABGs within patient's acceptable range.

ACTIONS/INTERVENTIONS	RATIONALE
Independent	
Monitor rate, rhythm, depth of respiration. Note breathing irregularities.	Changes may indicate onset of pulmonary complications (common following brain injury) or indicate location/extent of brain involvement. Slow respiration, periods of apnea may indicate need for mechanical ventilation.
Note competence of gag/swallow reflexes and patient's ability to protect own airway. Insert airway adjunct as indicated.	Ability to mobilize or clear secretions is important to airway maintenance. Loss of swallow or cough reflex may indicate need for artificial airway/intubation. *Note:* Soft nasopharyngeal airways may be preferred to prevent stimulation of the gag reflex by hard oropharyngeal airway, which can lead to excessive coughing and increased ICP.

ACTIONS/INTERVENTIONS

Independent

Elevate head of bed as permitted, position on sides as indicated.

Encourage deep breathing if patient is conscious.

Suction with extreme caution, no longer than 10–15 seconds. Note character, color, odor of secretions.

Auscultate breath sounds, noting areas of hypoventilation and presence of adventitious sounds (crackles, rhonchi, wheezes).

Monitor use of respiratory depressant drugs, e.g., sedatives.

Collaborative

Monitor/graph serial ABGs, pulse oximetry.

Review chest x-rays.

Administer supplemental oxygen.

Assist with chest physiotherapy when indicated.

RATIONALE

Facilitates lung expansion/ventilation and reduces risk of airway obstruction by tongue.

Prevents/reduces atelectasis.

Suctioning is usually required if patient is comatose or immobile and unable to clear own airway. Deep tracheal suctioning should be done with caution, because it can cause or aggravate hypoxia, which produces vasoconstriction, adversely affecting cerebral perfusion.

Identifies pulmonary problems such as atelectasis, congestion, and airway obstruction, which may jeopardize cerebral oxygenation and/or indicate onset of pulmonary infection (common complication of head injury).

Can increase respiratory embarrassment/complications.

Determines respiratory sufficiency, acid-base balance, and therapy needs.

Reveals ventilatory state and signs of developing complications (e.g., atelectasis, pneumonia).

Maximizes arterial oxygenation and aids in prevention of hypoxia. If respiratory center is depressed, mechanical ventilation may be required.

Although contraindicated in patient with acute IICP, these measures are often necessary in acute rehabilitation phase to mobilize and clear lung fields and reduce atelectasis/pulmonary complications.

NURSING DIAGNOSIS: Sensory-Perceptual alterations (specify)

May be related to
Altered sensory reception, transmission and/or integration (neurologic trauma or deficit)

Possibly evidenced by
Disorientation to time, place, person
Change in usual response to stimuli
Motor incoordination, alterations in posture, inability to tell position of body parts (proprioception)
Altered communication patterns
Visual and auditory distortions
Poor concentration, altered thought processes/bizarre thinking
Exaggerated emotional responses, change in behavior pattern

DESIRED OUTCOMES/EVALUATION CRITERIA—PATIENT WILL:
Regain/maintain usual level of consciousness and perceptual functioning.
Acknowledge changes in ability and presence of residual involvement.
Demonstrate behaviors/lifestyle changes to compensate for/overcome deficits.

ACTIONS/INTERVENTIONS	RATIONALE

Independent

Evaluate/continually monitor changes in orientation, ability to speak, mood/affect, sensorium, thought process.

Upper cerebral functions are often the first to be affected by altered circulation, oxygenation. Damage may occur at time of initial injury or develop sometime afterward because of swelling or bleeding. Motor, perceptual, cognitive, and personality changes may develop and persist, with gradual normalization of responses or remain permanently to some degree.

Assess sensory awareness, e.g., response to touch, hot/cold, dull/sharp, and awareness of motion and location of body parts. Note problems with vision, other senses.

Information is essential to patient safety. All sensory systems may be affected with changes involving an increase or decrease in sensitivity or loss of sensation/ability to perceive and respond appropriately to stimuli.

Observe behavioral responses, e.g., hostility, crying, inappropriate affect, agitation, hallucinations. (Refer to ND: Thought Processes, altered, p 233.)

Individual responses may be variable but commonalities, such as emotional lability, lowered frustration level, apathy, and impulsiveness exist during recovery from brain injury. Documentation of behavior provides information needed for development of structured rehabilitation.

Document specific changes in abilities, e.g., focusing/tracking with both eyes, following simple verbal instructions, answering "yes" or "no" to questions, feeding self with dominant hand.

Helps localize areas of cerebral dysfunction and identifies signs of progress toward improved neurologic function.

Eliminate extraneous noise/stimuli as necessary.

Reduces anxiety, exaggerated emotional responses/confusion associated with sensory overload.

Speak in calm, quiet voice. Use short, simple sentences. Maintain eye contact.

Patient may have limited attention span/understanding during acute and recovery stages, and these measures can help patient to attend to communication.

Ascertain/validate patient's perceptions, provide feedback. Reorient patient frequently to environment, staff, and procedures, especially if vision is impaired.

Assists patient to separate reality from altered perceptions. Cognitive dysfunction and/or visual deficits can potentiate disorientation and anxiety.

Provide meaningful stimulation: verbal (talk to patient); olfactory (e.g., oil of clove, coffee); tactile (touch, hand holding); and auditory (tapes, television, radio, visitors). Avoid physical or emotional isolation of patient.

Carefully selected sensory input may be useful for coma stimulation as well as during cognitive retraining.

Provide structured environment, including therapies, activities. Write out schedule for patient (if appropriate) and refer to regularly.

Promotes consistency and reassurance, reducing anxiety associated with the unknown. Promotes sense of control/cognitive retraining.

Schedule adequate rest/uninterrupted sleep periods.

Reduces fatigue, prevents exhaustion, provides for REM sleep (absence of which can aggravate sensory-perceptual deficits).

Use day/night lighting.

Provides for normal sense of passage of time and sleep/wake pattern.

Allow adequate time for communication and performance of activities.

Reduces frustration associated with altered abilities/delayed response pattern.

Provide patient safety, e.g., padded side rails, assistance with ambulation, protection from hot/sharp objects. Note perceptual deficit on chart and at bedside.

Agitation, impaired judgment, poor balance, and sensory deficits increase risk of patient injury.

232

ACTIONS/INTERVENTIONS	RATIONALE
Independent	
Identify alternate ways of dealing with perceptual deficits, e.g., arrange bed, personal articles, food to take advantage of functional vision; describe where affected body parts are located.	Enables patient to progress toward independence, enhancing sense of control, while compensating for neurologic deficits.
Collaborative	
Refer to physical, occupational, speech, and cognitive therapists.	Interdisciplinary approach can create an integrated treatment plan based on the individual's unique combination of abilities/disabilities with focus on evaluation and functional improvement in physical, cognitive, and perceptual skills.

NURSING DIAGNOSIS: Thought Processes, altered

May be related to
Physiologic changes; psychologic conflicts

Possibly evidenced by
Memory deficit/changes in remote, recent, immediate memory
Distractibility, altered attention span/concentration
Disorientation to time, place, person, circumstances, and events
Impaired ability to make decisions, problem-solve, reason, abstract, or conceptualize
Personality changes; inappropriate social behavior

DESIRED OUTCOMES/EVALUATION CRITERIA—PATIENT WILL:
Maintain/regain usual mentation and reality orientation.
Recognize changes in thinking/behavior.
Participate in therapeutic regimen/cognitive retraining.

ACTIONS/INTERVENTIONS	RATIONALE
Independent	
Assess attention span, distractibility. Note level of anxiety.	Attention span/ability to attend/concentrate may be severely shortened, which both causes and potentiates anxiety, affecting thought processes.
Confer with SO to compare past behaviors/preinjury personality with current responses.	Recovery from head injury includes a phase of agitation, angry responses, and disordered thought sequences/conversation. Presence of hallucinations or alteration in interpretation of stimuli may have been present independent of current condition, or be part of developing sequelae of brain injury. *Note:* SOs often have difficulty accepting and dealing with patient's aberrant behavior and may require assistance in coping with situation.
Maintain consistency in staff assigned to patient as much as possible.	Provides patient with feelings of stability and control of situation.
Present reality concisely and briefly, avoid challenging illogical thinking.	Patient may be totally unaware of injury (amnesic) or of extent of injury, and therefore deny reality of injury. Structured reality orientation can reduce defensive reactions.

ACTIONS/INTERVENTIONS	RATIONALE

Independent

Explain procedures and reinforce explanations given by others. Provide information about disease process in relationship to symptoms.	Loss of internal structure (changes in memory, reasoning, and ability to conceptualize) as well as fear of the unknown affect processing and retention of information, compounding anxiety, confusion, and disorientation.
Review necessity of recurrent neurologic evaluations.	Understanding that assessments are done frequently to prevent/limit complications and do not necessarily reflect seriousness of patient's condition may help reduce anxiety.
Reduce provocative stimuli, negative criticism, arguments, and confrontations.	Reduces risk of triggering fight/flight response. Severely brain-injured patient may become violent or physically/verbally abusive.
Listen with regard to patient's verbalizations in spite of speech pattern/content.	Conveys interest and worth to individual, enhancing self-esteem and encouraging continued efforts.
Promote socialization within individual limitations.	Reinforcement of positive behaviors (e.g., appropriate interaction with others) may be helpful in relearning internal structure.
Encourage SO to provide current news/family happenings, and so on.	Promotes maintenance of contact with usual events, enhancing reality orientation and normalization of thinking.
Instruct in relaxation techniques. Provide diversional activities.	Can help refocus attention and reduce anxiety to manageable levels.
Maintain realistic expectations of patient's ability to control own behavior, comprehend, remember information.	It is important to maintain an expectation of the ability to improve and progress to a higher level of functioning to maintain hope and promote continued work of rehabilitation.
Avoid leaving patient alone when agitated, frightened.	Anxiety can lead to loss of control and escalate to panic. Support may provide calming effect, reducing anxiety and risk of injury.
Implement measures to control emotional outbursts/aggressive behavior if needed; e.g., tell patient to "stop," speak in a calm voice, remove from the situation, provide distraction. May need restraint for brief periods of time.	Patient may need help/external control to protect self or others from harm until internal control is regained. Restraints (physical holding, mechanical, pharmacologic) should be used judiciously to avoid escalating violent, irrational behavior.
Inform patient/SO that intellectual function, behavior, and emotional functioning will gradually improve but that some effects may persist for months or even be permanent.	Most brain-injured patients have problems with concentration and memory and may think more slowly; have difficulty problem solving. Recovery may be complete, or residual effects may remain.

Collaborative

Coordinate/participate in cognitive retraining or rehabilitation program as indicated.	Assists with learning methods to compensate for disruption of cognitive skills and addresses problems in concentration, memory, judgment, sequencing, and problem solving.
Refer to support groups, e.g., Brain Injury Association, social services, visiting nurse, and counseling/therapy as needed.	Additional assistance may be helpful in supporting/sustaining recovery efforts.

NURSING DIAGNOSIS: Physical Mobility, impaired

May be related to

Perceptual or cognitive impairment

Decreased strength/endurance

Restrictive therapies/safety precautions, e.g., bed rest, immobilization

Possibly evidenced by

Inability to purposefully move within the physical environment, including bed mobility, transfer, ambulation

Impaired coordination, limited range of motion, decreased muscle strength/control

DESIRED OUTCOMES/EVALUATION CRITERIA—PATIENT WILL:

Regain/maintain optimal position of function, as evidenced by absence of contractures, footdrop.

Maintain/increase strength and function of affected and/or compensatory body part(s).

Demonstrate techniques/behaviors that enable resumption of activities.

Maintain skin integrity, bladder and bowel function.

ACTIONS/INTERVENTIONS	RATIONALE
Independent	
Review functional ability and reasons for impairment.	Identifies probable functional impairments and influences choice of interventions.
Assess degree of immobility, using a scale to rate dependence (0–4).	The patient may be completely independent (0) or require minimal assistance/equipment (1); moderate assistance/supervision/teaching (2); extensive assistance/equipment, and devices (3); or be completely dependent on caregivers (4). Persons in all categories are at risk for injury, but those in categories 2–4 are at greatest risk for hazards associated with immobility.
Position patient to avoid pressure damage. Turn at regular intervals, and make small position changes between turns.	Regular turning more normally distributes body weight and promotes circulation to all areas. If paralysis or limited cognition is present, patient should be repositioned frequently and positioned on affected side for only brief periods.
Maintain functional body alignment, e.g., hips, feet, hands. Monitor for proper placement of devices and/or signs of pressure from devices.	Use of high-top tennis shoes, "space boots," and T-bar sheepskin devices can help prevent footdrop. Handsplints are variable and designed to prevent hand deformities and promote optimal function. Use of pillows, bedrolls, and sandbags can help prevent abnormal hip rotation.
Support head and trunk, arms and shoulders, feet and legs when patient is in wheelchair/recliner. Pad chair seat with foam or water-filled cushion, and assist patient to shift weight at frequent intervals.	Maintains comfortable, safe, and functional posture and prevents/reduces risk of skin breakdown.
Provide/assist with range-of-motion exercises.	Maintains mobility and function of joints/functional alignment of extremities and reduces venous stasis.

235

ACTIONS/INTERVENTIONS	RATIONALE
Independent	
Instruct/assist patient with exercise program and use of mobility aids. Increase activity and participation in self-care as tolerated.	Lengthy convalescence often follows brain injury, and physical reconditioning is an essential part of the program. Involving patient in planning and performing activities is important to promote patient cooperation/sustain program.
Provide meticulous skin care, massaging with emollients. Remove wet linen/clothing, keep bedding free of wrinkles.	Promotes circulation and skin elasticity and reduces risk of skin excoriation.
Provide eye care, artificial tears; patch eyes as indicated.	Protects delicate tissues from drying. Patient may require eye patches during sleep to protect eyes from trauma if unable to keep eyes closed.
Monitor urinary output. Note color and odor of urine. Assist with bladder retraining when appropriate.	Indwelling catheter used during the acute phase of injury may be needed for an extended period of time before bladder retraining is possible. Once the catheter is removed, several methods of continence control may be tried, e.g., intermittent catheterization (for residual and complete emptying); external catheter; planned intervals on commode; incontinence pads.
Provide fluids within individual tolerance (e.g., neurologic and cardiac), including cranberry juice, as indicated.	Once past the acute phase of head injury and if patient has no other contraindicating factors, forcing fluids will decrease risk of urinary tract infections/stone formation as well as provide other positive effects such as normal stool consistency and optimal skin turgor.
Monitor bowel elimination and provide for/assist with a regular bowel routine. Check for impacted stool; use digital stimulation as indicated. Sit patient upright on commode or stool at regular intervals. Add fiber/bulk/fruit juice to diet as appropriate.	A regular bowel routine requires simple but diligent measures to prevent complications. Stimulation of the internal rectal sphincter will stimulate bowel to empty automatically if stool is soft enough to do so. Upright position aids evacuation.
Inspect for localized tenderness, redness, skin warmth, muscle tension, and/or ropy veins in calves of legs. Observe for sudden dyspnea, tachypnea, fever, respiratory distress, chest pain.	Patient is at risk for development of DVT and PE (especially after trauma), requiring prompt medical evaluation/intervention to prevent serious complications.
Provide air/water mattress, kinetic therapy as appropriate.	Equalizes tissue pressure, enhances circulation, and helps reduce venous stasis to decrease risk of tissue injury.

NURSING DIAGNOSIS: Infection, risk for

Risk factors may include
Traumatized tissues, broken skin, invasive procedures
Decreased ciliary action, stasis of body fluids
Nutritional deficits
Suppressed inflammatory response (steroid use)
Altered integrity of closed system (CSF leak)

Possibly evidenced by
[Not applicable; presence of signs and symptoms establishes an *actual* diagnosis]

DESIRED OUTCOMES/EVALUATION CRITERIA—PATIENT WILL:
Maintain normothermia, free of signs of infection.
Achieve timely wound healing when present.

ACTIONS/INTERVENTIONS	RATIONALE
Independent	
Provide meticulous/aseptic care, maintain good hand-washing techniques.	First-line defense against nosocomial infections.
Observe areas of impaired skin integrity (e.g., wounds, suture lines, invasive line insertion sites), noting drainage characteristics and presence of inflammation.	Early identification of developing infection permits prompt intervention and prevention of further complications.
Monitor temperature routinely. Note presence of chills, diaphoresis, changes in mentation.	May indicate developing sepsis requiring further evaluation/intervention.
Encourage deep breathing, aggressive pulmonary toilet. Observe sputum characteristics.	Enhances mobilization and clearing of pulmonary secretions to reduce risk of pneumonia, atelectasis. *Note:* Postural drainage should be used with caution if risk of IICP exists.
Provide perineal care. Maintain integrity of closed urinary drainage system if used. Encourage adequate fluid intake.	Reduces potential for bacterial growth/ascending infection.
Observe color/clarity of urine. Note presence of foul odor.	Indicators of developing urinary tract infection requiring prompt intervention.
Screen/restrict access of visitors or caregivers with upper respiratory infections.	Reduces exposure of "compromised host."
Collaborative	
Administer antibiotics as indicated.	Prophylactic therapy may be used in the presence of trauma, CSF leak, or after surgical procedures to reduce risk of nosocomial infections.
Obtain specimens as indicated.	Culture/sensitivity, Gram's stain may be done to verify presence of infection and identify causative organism and appropriate treatment choices.

NURSING DIAGNOSIS: Nutrition: altered, risk for less than body requirements

Risk factors may include
Altered ability to ingest nutrients (decreased level of consciousness)
Weakness of muscles required for chewing, swallowing
Hypermetabolic state

Possibly evidenced by
[Not applicable; presence of signs and symptoms establishes an *actual* diagnosis]

DESIRED OUTCOMES/EVALUATION CRITERIA—PATIENT WILL:
Demonstrate maintenance of/progressive weight gain toward goal.
Experience no signs of malnutrition, with laboratory values within normal range.

ACTIONS/INTERVENTIONS	RATIONALE

Independent

Assess ability to chew, swallow, cough, handle secretions.

These factors determine choice of feeding as patient must be protected from aspiration.

Auscultate bowel sounds, noting decreased/absent or hyperactive sounds.

GI functioning is usually preserved in brain-injured patients, so bowel sounds help in determining response to feeding or development of complications, e.g., ileus.

Weigh as indicated.

Evaluates effectiveness or need for changes in nutritional therapy.

Provide for feeding safety, e.g., elevate head of bed while eating or during tube feeding.

Reduces risk of regurgitation and/or aspiration.

Divide feedings into small amounts and give frequently.

Enhances digestion and patient's tolerance of nutrients and can improve patient cooperation in eating.

Promote pleasant, relaxing environment, including socialization during meals. Encourage SO to bring in food that patient enjoys.

Although the recovering patient may require assistance with feeding and/or use of assistive devices, mealtime socialization with SO or friends can improve intake and normalize the life function of eating.

Check stools, gastric aspirant, vomitus for blood.

Acute/subacute bleeding may occur (Cushing's ulcer) requiring intervention and alternate method of providing nutrition.

Collaborative

Consult with dietitian/nutritional support team.

Effective resource for identifying caloric/nutrient needs dependent on age, body size, desired weight, concurrent conditions (trauma, cardiac/metabolic problems).

Monitor laboratory studies, e.g., prealbumin/albumin, transferrin, amino acid profile, iron, BUN, nitrogen balance studies, glucose, AST/ALT, electrolytes.

Identifies nutritional deficiencies, organ function, and response to nutritional therapy.

Administer feedings by appropriate means, e.g., tube feeding, oral feedings with soft foods and thick liquids.

Choice of route is dependent on patient needs/capabilities. Tube feedings (nasogastric, gastric) may be required initially. If the patient is able to swallow, soft foods or semiliquid foods may be more easily managed without aspiration.

Involve speech/occupational/physical therapists when mechanical problem exists, e.g., impaired swallow reflexes, wired jaws, contractures of hands, paralysis.

Individual strategies/devices may be needed to improve ability to eat.

NURSING DIAGNOSIS: Family Processes, altered

May be related to
Situational transition and crisis
Uncertainty about outcomes/expectations

Possibly evidenced by
Difficulty adapting to change or dealing with traumatic experience constructively
Family not meeting needs of its members
Difficulty accepting or receiving help appropriately
Inability to express or to accept feelings of members

DESIRED OUTCOMES/EVALUATION CRITERIA—FAMILY WILL:
Begin to express feelings freely and appropriately.
Identify internal and external resources to deal with the situation.
Direct energies in a purposeful manner to plan for resolution of crisis.
Encourage and allow injured member to progress toward independence.

ACTIONS/INTERVENTIONS	RATIONALE
Independent	
Note components of family unit, availability/involvement of support systems.	Defines family resources and identifies areas of need.
Encourage expression of concerns about seriousness of condition, possibility of death, or incapacitation.	Verbalization of fears gets concerns out in the open and can decrease anxiety and enhance coping with reality.
Listen for expressions of helplessness/hopelessness	Joy of survival of victim is replaced by grief/anger at "loss" and necessity of dealing with "new person that family does not know and may not even like." Prolongation of these feelings may result in depression.
Encourage expression of/acknowledge feelings. Do not deny or reassure patient/SO that everything will be all right.	Because it is not possible to predict the outcome, it is more helpful to assist the person to deal with feelings about what is happening instead of giving false reassurance.
Reinforce previous explanations about extent of injury, treatment plan, and prognosis. Provide accurate information at current level of understanding/ability to accept.	Patient/SO are unable to absorb/recall all information, and blocking can occur because of emotional trauma. As time goes by, reinforcement of information can help reduce misconceptions, fear about the unknown/future expectations.
Stress importance of continuous open dialogue between family members.	Provides opportunity to get feelings out in the open. Recognition and awareness promotes resolution of guilt, anger.
Evaluate/discuss family goals and expectations.	Family may believe that if patient is going to live, rehabilitation will bring about a cure. Despite accurate information, expectations may be unrealistic. Also, patient's early recovery may be rapid, then plateau, resulting in disappointment/frustration.
Identify individual roles and anticipated/perceived changes.	Responsibilities/roles may have to be partially or completely assumed by others, which can further complicate family coping.
Assess energy direction, e.g., whether efforts at resolution/problem solving are purposeful or scattered.	May need assistance to focus energies in an effective way/enhance coping.
Identify and encourage use of previously successful coping behaviors.	Focuses on strengths and reaffirms individual's ability to deal with current crisis.
Demonstrate and encourage use of stress management skills, e.g., relaxation techniques, breathing exercises, visualization.	Helps redirect attention toward revitalizing self to enhance coping ability.

ACTIONS/INTERVENTIONS	RATIONALE

Independent

Help family recognize needs of all members.

Attention may be so focused on injured member that other members feel isolated/abandoned, which can compromise family growth and unity.

Support family grieving for "loss" of member. Acknowledge normality of wide range of feelings and ongoing nature of process.

Although grief may never be fully resolved and family may vacillate among various stages, understanding that this is typical may help members accept/cope with the situation.

Collaborative

Include family in rehabilitation team meetings and care planning/placement decisions.

Facilitates communication, enables family to be an integral part of the rehabilitation, and provides sense of control.

Identify community resources, e.g., VNA, homemaker service, day care facility, legal/financial counselor.

Provides assistance with problems that may arise because of altered role function.

Refer to family therapy, support groups.

Cognitive/personality changes are usually very difficult for family to deal with. Decreased impulse control, emotional lability, inappropriate sexual or aggressive/violent behavior can disrupt family and result in abandonment/divorce, and so on. Trained therapists and peer role models may assist family to deal with feelings/reality of situation and provide support for decisions that are made.

NURSING DIAGNOSIS: Knowledge deficit [learning need] regarding condition, treatment, self care and discharge needs

May be related to
Lack of exposure, unfamiliarity with information/resources
Lack of recall/cognitive limitation

Possibly evidenced by
Request for information, statement of misconception
Inaccurate follow-through of instructions

DESIRED OUTCOMES/EVALUATION CRITERIA—PATIENT WILL:
Participate in learning process.
Verbalize understanding of condition, treatment regimen, potential complications.
Initiate necessary lifestyle changes and/or involvement in rehabilitation program.
Correctly perform necessary procedures.

ACTIONS/INTERVENTIONS	RATIONALE

Independent

Evaluate capabilities and readiness to learn of both patient and SO.

Permits presentation of material based on individual needs. *Note:* Patient may not be emotionally/mentally capable of assimilating information.

Review information regarding injury process and aftereffects.

Aids in establishing realistic expectations and promotes understanding of current situation and needs.

ACTIONS/INTERVENTIONS	RATIONALE

Independent

Review/reinforce current therapeutic regimen. Identify ways of continuing program after discharge.	Recommended activities, limitations, medication/therapy needs have been established on the basis of a coordinated interdisciplinary approach, and follow-through is essential to progression of recovery/prevention of complications.
Discuss plans for meeting self-care needs.	Varying levels of assistance may be required/need to be planned based on individual situation.
Provide written instructions and schedules for activity, medication, important facts.	Provides visual reinforcement and reference source after discharge.
Identify signs/symptoms of individual risks, e.g., delayed CSF leak, post-traumatic seizures, headache/chronic pain.	Recognizing developing problems provides opportunity for prompt evaluation and intervention to prevent serious complications.
Discuss with patient/SO development of symptoms, such as re-experiencing traumatic event (flashbacks, intrusive thoughts, repetitive dreams/nightmares); psychic/emotional numbness; changes in lifestyle, including adoption of self-destructive behaviors.	May indicate occurrence/exacerbation of posttrauma response, which can occur months to years after injury, requiring further evaluation and supportive interventions.
Identify community resources, e.g., head injury support groups, social services, rehabilitation facilities, outpatient programs, VNA.	May be needed to provide assistance with physical care, home management, adjustment to lifestyle changes, as well as emotional and financial concerns.
Refer/reinforce importance of follow-up care by rehabilitation team, e.g., physical/occupational/speech/vocational therapists, cognitive retrainers.	Diligent work (often for several years with these providers) may eventually overcome residual neurologic deficits and enable patient to resume desired/productive lifestyle.

POTENTIAL CONSIDERATIONS following acute hospitalization (dependent on patient's age, physical condition/presence of complications, personal resources, and life responsibilities)

Memory, impaired—neurologic disturbances, anemia, fluid/electrolyte imbalances.

Health/Home Maintenance, Management, impaired—significant alteration in communication skills, lack of ability to make deliberate/thoughtful judgments, perceptual/cognitive impairments, insufficient finances, unfamiliarity with neighborhood resources, inadequate support systems.

Pain [acute]/chronic—tissue injury/neuronal damage, stress/anxiety.

Confusion, chronic—head injury.

CEREBROVASCULAR ACCIDENT/STROKE

Cerebrovascular disease refers to any functional or structural abnormality of the brain caused by a pathologic condition of the cerebral vessels or of the entire cerebral vascular system. This pathology either causes hemorrhage from a tear in the vessel wall or impairs the cerebral circulation by a partial or complete occlusion of the vessel lumen with transient or permanent effects. Symptoms dependent on distribution of vessel(s) involved. Ischemia may be transient (TIA) and resolve within 24 hours; reversible with resolution of symptoms over a period of 1 week (RIND); or progress to cerebral infarction with variable effects and degrees of recovery.

CARE SETTING

Although the patient may be cared for in the ICU, this phase of care focuses on stepdown or medical unit; subacute/rehabilitation units to community level.

RELATED CONCERNS

Hypertension: Severe, p 32
Craniocerebral Trauma (Acute Rehabilitative Phase), p 224
Psychosocial Aspects of Care, p 783
Seizure Disorders/Epilepsy, p 214
Total Nutritional Support: Parenteral/Enteral Feeding, p 491

Patient Assessment Data Base

Data collected will be determined by location, severity, and duration of pathology.

ACTIVITY/REST

May report:	Difficulties with activity due to weakness, loss of sensation, or paralysis (hemiplegia)
	Tiring easily; difficulty resting (pain or muscle twitchings)
May exhibit:	Altered muscle tone (flaccid or spastic); paralysis (hemiplegia); generalized weakness
	Visual disturbances
	Altered level of consciousness

CIRCULATORY

May report:	History of postural hypotension, cardiac disease (e.g., MI, rheumatic/valvular heart disease, HF, bacterial endocarditis), polycythemia
May exhibit:	Arterial hypertension (frequently found unless the CVA is due to embolism or vascular malformation)
	Pulse: Rate may vary (preexisting heart conditions, medications, effect of stroke on vasomotor center)
	Dysrhythmias, ECG changes
	Bruit in carotid, femoral, and iliac arteries or abdominal aorta

EGO INTEGRITY

May report:	Feelings of helplessness, hopelessness
May exhibit:	Emotional lability and inappropriate response to anger, sadness, happiness
	Difficulty expressing self

ELIMINATION

May exhibit:	Change in voiding patterns, e.g., incontinence, anuria
	Distended abdomen (overdistended bladder); absent bowel sounds (paralytic ileus)

242

FOOD/FLUID

May report: Lack of appetite
Nausea/vomiting during acute event (increased IICP)
Loss of sensation in tongue, cheek, and throat; dysphagia
History of diabetes, elevated serum lipids

May exhibit: Mastication/swallowing problems (palatal and pharyngeal reflex involvement)
Obesity (risk factor)

NEUROSENSORY

May report: Dizziness/syncope (before CVA/transient during TIA)
Headaches: Severe with intracerebral or subarachnoid hemorrhage
Tingling/numbness/weakness (commonly reported during TIAs, found in varying degrees in other types of stroke); involved side seems "dead"
Visual deficits, e.g., blurred vision, partial loss of vision (monocular blindness), double vision (diplopia), or other disturbances in visual fields
Touch: Sensory loss on contralateral side (opposite side) in extremities and sometimes in ipsilateral side (same side) of face
Disturbance in senses of taste, smell
History of TIA, RIND (predisposing factor for subsequent infarction)

May exhibit: Mental status/LOC: Coma usually present in the initial stages of hemorrhagic disturbances; consciousness is usually preserved when the etiology is thrombotic in nature; altered behavior (e.g., lethargy, apathy, combativeness); altered cognitive function (e.g., memory, problem-solving, sequencing)
Extremities: Weakness/paralysis (contralateral with all kinds of stroke), unequal hand grasp; diminished deep tendon reflexes (contralateral)
Facial paralysis or paresis (ipsilateral)
Aphasia: Defect or loss of language function may be expressive (difficulty producing speech); receptive (difficulty comprehending speech); or global (combination of the two)
Loss of ability to recognize or appreciate import of visual, auditory, tactile stimuli (agnosia), e.g., altered body image awareness, neglect or denial of contralateral side of body, disturbances in perception
Loss of ability to execute purposeful motor acts despite physical ability and willingness to do so (apraxia)
Pupil size/reaction: Inequality; dilated and fixed pupil on the ipsilateral side (hemorrhage/herniation)
Nuchal rigidity (common in hemorrhagic etiology); seizures (common in hemorrhagic etiology)

PAIN/DISCOMFORT

May report: Headache of varying intensity (carotid artery involvement)

May exhibit: Guarding/distraction behaviors, restlessness, muscle/facial tension

RESPIRATION

May report: Smoking (risk factor)

May exhibit: Inability to swallow/cough/protect airway
Labored and/or irregular respirations
Noisy respirations/rhonchi (aspiration of secretions)

SAFETY

May exhibit: Motor/sensory: Problems with vision
Changes in perception of body spatial orientation (right CVA)
Difficulty seeing objects on left side (RCVA)
Being unaware of affected side
Inability to recognize familiar objects, colors, words, faces
Diminished response to heat and cold/altered body temperature regulation
Swallowing difficulty, inability to meet own nutritional needs
Impaired judgment, little concern for safety, impatience/lack of insight (RCVA)

SOCIAL INTERACTION

May exhibit: Speech problems, inability to communicate

TEACHING/LEARNING

May report: Family history of hypertension, strokes; African heritage (risk factor)
Use of oral contraceptives, alcohol abuse (risk factor)

Discharge plan considerations: **DRG projected mean length of inpatient stay: 7.3 days**
May require medication regimen/therapeutic treatments
Assistance with transportation, shopping, food preparation, self-care and home-maker/ maintenance tasks
Changes in physical layout of home; transition placement before return to home setting

Refer to section at end of plan for postdischarge considerations.

DIAGNOSTIC STUDIES

MRI: Shows areas of infarction, hemorrhage, arteriovenous malformations; and areas of ischemia (possibly earlier than revealed by CT scan).

CT scan: Demonstrates edema, hematomas, ischemia, and infarctions. *Note:* May not immediately reveal all changes, e.g., ischemic infarcts may not be evident on CT for 8–12 hours; however, intracerebral hemorrhage is immediately apparent.

Cerebral angiography: Helps determine specific cause of stroke, e.g., hemorrhage or obstructed artery, pinpoints site of occlusion or rupture.

Lumbar puncture: Normal pressure and usually clear in cerebral thrombosis, embolism, and TIA. Pressure elevation and grossly bloody fluid suggests subarachnoid and intracerebral hemorrhage. Total protein level may be elevated in cases of thrombosis due to inflammatory process. LP should be performed if septic embolism from bacterial endocarditis is suspected.

Doppler ultrasonography: Identifies arteriovenous disease, e.g., problems with carotid system (blood flow/presence of atherosclerotic plaques).

EEG: Identifies problems based on brain waves and may demonstrate specific areas of lesions.

X-rays (skull): May show shift of pineal gland to the opposite side from an expanding mass; calcifications of the internal carotid may be visible in cerebral thrombosis; partial calcification of walls of an aneurysm may be noted in subarachnoid hemorrhage.

Laboratory studies to rule out systemic causes: CBC, platelet and clotting studies, VDRL, ESR, chemistries (glucose, sodium).

ECG, chest x-ray and echocardiography: To rule out cardiac origin as source of embolus (20% of strokes are the result of blood or vegetative emboli associated with valvular disease, dysrhythmias, or endocarditis).

NURSING PRIORITIES

1. Promote adequate cerebral perfusion and oxygenation.
2. Prevent/minimize complications and permanent disabilities.

3. Assist patient to gain independence in ADLs.
4. Support coping process and integration of changes into self-concept.
5. Provide information about disease process/prognosis and treatment/rehabilitation needs.

DISCHARGE GOALS

1. Cerebral function improved, neurologic deficits resolving/stabilized.
2. Complications prevented or minimized.
3. ADL needs met by self or with assistance of other(s).
4. Coping with situation in positive manner, planning for the future.
5. Disease process/prognosis, and therapeutic regimen understood.
6. Plan in place to meet needs after discharge.

NURSING DIAGNOSIS: Tissue Perfusion, altered, cerebral

May be related to

Interruption of blood flow: occlusive disorder, hemorrhage; cerebral vasospasm, cerebral edema

Possibly evidenced by

Altered level of consciousness; memory loss
Changes in motor/sensory responses; restlessness
Sensory, language, intellectual, and emotional deficits
Changes in vital signs

DESIRED OUTCOMES/EVALUATION CRITERIA—PATIENT WILL:

Maintain usual/improved level of consciousness, cognition, and motor/sensory function.
Demonstrate stable vital signs and absence of signs of increased ICP
Displays no further deterioration/recurrence of deficits.

ACTIONS/INTERVENTIONS

Independent

Determine factors related to individual situation/cause for coma/decreased cerebral perfusion, and potential for increased ICP.

Monitor/document neurologic status frequently and compare with baseline. (Refer to CP: Craniocerebral Trauma (Acute Rehabilitative Phase), ND: Tissue Perfusion, altered, cerebral, p 226, for complete neurologic evaluation.)

RATIONALE

Influences choice of interventions. Deterioration in neurologic signs/symptoms or failure to improve after initial insult may reflect decreased intracranial adaptive capacity requiring the patient be transferred to critical care area for monitoring of ICP, other therapies. If the stroke is in evolution, the patient can deteriorate quickly and require repeated assessment and progressive treatment. If the stroke is "completed," the neurologic deficit is nonprogressive, and treatment is geared toward rehabilitation and preventing recurrence.

Assesses trends in LOC and potential for increased ICP, and is useful in determining location, extent, and progression/resolution of CNS damage. May also reveal presence of TIA, which may warn of impending thrombotic CVA.

ACTIONS/INTERVENTIONS	RATIONALE
Independent	
Monitor vital signs, i.e., note:	
Hypertension/hypotension, compare BP readings in both arms;	Variations may occur because of cerebral pressure/injury in vasomotor area of the brain. Hypertension or postural hypotension may have been a precipitating factor. Hypotension may occur because of shock (circulatory collapse). Increased ICP may occur (tissue edema, clot formation). Subclavian artery blockage may be revealed by difference in pressure readings between arms.
Heart rate and rhythm; auscultate for murmurs;	Changes in rate, especially bradycardia, can occur because of the brain damage. Dysrhythmias and murmurs may reflect cardiac disease, which may have precipitated CVA (e.g., stroke after MI or from valve dysfunction).
Respiration, noting patterns and rhythm, e.g., periods of apnea after hyperventilation, Cheyne-Stokes respiration.	Irregularities can suggest location of cerebral insult/increasing ICP and need for further intervention, including possible respiratory support. (Refer to CP: Craniocerebral Trauma (Acute Rehabilitative Phase), ND: Breathing Pattern, ineffective, risk for, p 230.)
Evaluate pupils, noting size, shape, equality, light reactivity.	Pupil reactions are regulated by the oculomotor (III) cranial nerve and are useful in determining whether the brainstem is intact. Pupil size/equality is determined by balance between parasympathetic and sympathetic enervation. Response to light reflects combined function of the optic (II) and oculomotor (III) cranial nerves.
Document changes in vision, e.g., reports of blurred vision, alterations in visual field/depth perception.	Specific visual alterations reflect area of brain involved, indicate safety concerns, and influence choice of interventions.
Assess higher functions, including speech, if patient is alert. (Refer to ND: Communication, impaired verbal [and/or written], p 249.)	Changes in cognition and speech content are an indicator of location/degree of cerebral involvement and may indicate deterioration/increased ICP.
Position with head slightly elevated and in neutral position.	Reduces arterial pressure by promoting venous drainage and may improve cerebral circulation/perfusion.
Maintain bed rest; provide quiet environment; restrict visitors/activities as indicated. Provide rest periods between care activities, limit duration of procedures.	Continual stimulation/activity can increase ICP. Absolute rest and quiet may be needed to prevent rebleeding in the case of hemorrhage.
Prevent straining at stool, holding breath.	Valsalva maneuver increases ICP and potentiates risk of rebleeding.
Assess for nuchal rigidity, twitching, increased restlessness, irritability, onset of seizure activity.	Indicative of meningeal irritation, especially in hemorrhagic disorders. Seizures may reflect increased ICP/cerebral injury, requiring further evaluation and intervention.
Collaborative	
Administer supplemental oxygen as indicated.	Reduces hypoxemia, which can cause cerebral vasodilation and increase pressure/edema formation.

246

ACTIONS/INTERVENTIONS	RATIONALE
Collaborative	
Administer medications as indicated:	
Anticoagulants, e.g., warfarin sodium (Coumadin), heparin; antiplatelet agents e.g., aspirin (ASA), dipyridamole (Persantine), ticlopidine (Ticlid);	May be used to improve cerebral blood flow and prevent further clotting when embolus/thrombosis is the problem. Contraindicated in hypertensive patients because of increased risk of hemorrhage.
Antifibrolytics, e.g., aminocaproic acid (Amicar);	Used with caution in hemorrhagic disorder to prevent lysis of formed clots and subsequent rebleeding.
Antihypertensives;	Preexisting/chronic hypertension requires cautious treatment, because aggressive management increases the risk of extension of tissue damage. Transient hypertension often occurs during acute stroke and resolves often without therapeutic intervention.
Peripheral vasodilators, e.g., cyclandelate (Cyclospasmol), papaverine (Pavabid/Vasospan), isoxsuprine (Vasodilan);	Used to improve collateral circulation or decrease vasospasm.
Steroids, dexamethasone (Decadron);	Use is controversial in control of cerebral edema.
Phenytoin (Dilantin), phenobarbital;	May be used to control seizures and/or for sedative action. *Note:* Phenobarbital enhances action of antiepileptics.
Stool softeners.	Prevents straining during bowel movement and corresponding increase of ICP.
Prepare for surgery: endarterectomy, microvascular bypass, cerebral angioplasty.	May be necessary to resolve situation, reduce neurologic symptoms/risk of recurrent stroke.
Monitor laboratory studies as indicated, e.g., prothrombin/aPTT time, Dilantin level.	Provides information about drug effectiveness/therapeutic level.

NURSING DIAGNOSIS: Physical Mobility, impaired

May be related to
Neuromuscular involvement: weakness, paresthesia; flaccid/hypotonic paralysis (initially); spastic paralysis
Perceptual/cognitive impairment

Possibly evidenced by
Inability to purposefully move within the physical environment; impaired coordination; limited range of motion; decreased muscle strength/control

DESIRED OUTCOMES/EVALUATION CRITERIA—PATIENT WILL:
Maintain optimal position of function as evidenced by absence of contractures, footdrop.
Maintain/increase strength and function of affected or compensatory body part.
Demonstrate techniques/behaviors that enable resumption of activities.
Maintain skin integrity.

Independent

Assess functional ability/extent of impairment initially and on a regular basis. Classify according to 0–4 scale. (Refer to CP: Craniocerebral Trauma (Acute Rehabilitative Phase), ND: Physical Mobility, impaired, p 235.)

Identifies strengths/deficiencies and may provide information regarding recovery. Assists in choice of interventions, as different techniques are used for flaccid and spastic paralysis.

Change positions at least every 2 hours (supine, side-lying) and possibly more often if placed on affected side.

Reduces risk of tissue ischemia/injury. Affected side has poorer circulation and reduced sensation and is more predisposed to skin breakdown/decubitus.

Position in prone position once or twice a day if patient can tolerate.

Helps maintain functional hip extension; however, may increase anxiety, especially about ability to breathe.

Begin active/passive range of motion to all extremities (including splinted) on admission. Encourage exercises such as quadriceps/gluteal exercise, squeezing rubber ball, extension of fingers and legs/feet.

Minimizes muscle atrophy, promotes circulation, helps prevent contractures. Reduces risk of hypercalciuria and osteoporosis if underlying problem is hemorrhage. *Note:* Excessive/imprudent stimulation can predispose to rebleeding.

Prop extremities in functional position, use footboard during the period of flaccid paralysis. Maintain neutral position of head.

Prevents contractures/footdrop and facilitates use when/if function returns. Flaccid paralysis may interfere with ability to support head, whereas spastic paralysis may lead to deviation of head to one side.

Use arm sling when patient is in upright position, as indicated.

During flaccid paralysis, use of sling may reduce risk of shoulder subluxation and shoulder-hand syndrome.

Evaluate use of/need for positional aids and/or splints during spastic paralysis:

Flexion contractures occur because flexor muscles are stronger than extensors.

Place pillow under axilla to abduct arm;

Prevents adduction of shoulder and flexion of elbow.

Elevate arm and hand;

Promotes venous return and helps prevent edema formation.

Place hard hand-rolls in the palm with fingers and thumb opposed;

Hard cones decrease the stimulation of finger flexion, maintaining finger and thumb in a functional position.

Place knee and hip in extended position;

Maintains functional position.

Maintain leg in neutral position with a trochanter roll;

Prevents external hip rotation.

Discontinue use of footboard, when appropriate.

Continued use (after change from flaccid to spastic paralysis) can cause excessive pressure on the ball of the foot, enhance spasticity, and actually increase plantar flexion.

Assist to develop sitting balance (e.g., raise head of bed; assist to sit on edge of bed, having patient use the strong arm to support body weight and strong leg to move affected leg; increase sitting time) and standing balance (e.g., put flat walking shoes on patient; support patient's lower back with hands while positioning own knees outside patient's knees; assist in using parallel bars/walkers).

Aids in retraining neuronal pathways, enhancing proprioception and motor response.

248

ACTIONS/INTERVENTIONS	RATIONALE
Independent	
Observe affected side for color, edema, or other signs of compromised circulation.	Edematous tissue is more easily traumatized and heals more slowly.
Inspect skin, particularly over bony prominences, regularly. Gently massage any reddened areas and provide aids such as sheepskin pads as necessary.	Pressure points over bony prominences are most at risk for decreased perfusion/ischemia. Circulatory stimulation and padding helps prevent skin breakdown and decubitus development.
Get up in chair as soon as vital signs are stable except following cerebral hemorrhage.	Helps stabilize BP (restores vasomotor tone), promotes maintenance of extremities in a functional position and emptying of bladder/kidneys, reducing risk of urinary stones and infections from stasis. *Note:* If stroke is not completed, activity increases risk of additional bleed/infarction.
Pad chair seat with foam or waterfilled cushion and assist patient to shift weight at frequent intervals.	Prevents/reduces coccyx pressure/skin breakdown.
Set goals with patient/SO for participation in activities/exercise and position changes.	Promotes sense of expectation of progress/improvement and provides some sense of control/independence.
Encourage patient to assist with movement and exercises using unaffected extremity to support/move weaker side.	May respond as if affected side is no longer part of body and needs encouragement and active training to "reincorporate" it as a part of own body.
Collaborative	
Provide egg-crate mattress, water bed, flotation device, or specialized beds (e.g., kinctic) as indicated.	Promotes even weight distribution decreasing pressure on bony points and helping to prevent skin breakdown/decubitus formation. Specialized beds help with positioning the extremely obese patient, enhances circulation, and reduces venous stasis to decrease risk of tissue injury and complications such as orthostatic pneumonia.
Consult with physical therapist regarding active, resistive exercises and patient ambulation.	Individualized program can be developed to meet particular needs/deal with deficits in balance, coordination, strength.
Assist with electrical stimulation, e.g., TENS unit as indicated.	May assist with muscle strengthening and increase voluntary muscle control.
Administer muscle relaxants, antispasmodics as indicated, e.g., baclofen (Lioresal), dantrolene (Dantrium).	May be required to relieve spasticity in affected extremities.

NURSING DIAGNOSIS: Communication, impaired verbal [and/or written]

May be related to

Impaired cerebral circulation; neuromuscular impairment, loss of facial/oral muscle tone/control; generalized weakness/fatigue

Possibly evidenced by

Impaired articulation; does not/cannot speak (dysarthria)

Inability to modulate speech, find and name words, identify objects; inability to comprehend written/spoken language

Inability to produce written communication

ACTIONS/INTERVENTIONS	RATIONALE
Independent	
Assess type/degree of dysfunction: e.g., patient does not seem to understand words or has trouble speaking or making self understood;	Helps determine area and degree of brain involvement and difficulty patient has with any or all steps of the communication process. Patient may have trouble understanding spoken words (receptive aphasia/damage to Wernicke's speech area); speaking words correctly (expressive aphasia/damage to Broca's speech areas); or experience damage to both areas.
Differentiate aphasia from dysarthria;	Choice of interventions is dependent on type of impairment. Aphasia is a defect in using and interpreting symbols of language and may involve sensory and/or motor components, e.g., inability to comprehend written/spoken words or write, make signs, speak. A dysarthric person can understand, read, and write language but has difficulty forming/pronouncing words due to weakness and paralysis of oral musculature.
Listen for errors in conversation and provide feedback;	Patient may lose ability to monitor verbal output and be unaware that communication is not sensible. Feedback helps patient realize why caregivers are not understanding/responding appropriately and provides opportunity to clarify content/meaning.
Ask patient to follow simple commands (e.g., "Shut your eyes," "Point to the door"), repeat simple words/sentences;	Tests for receptive aphasia.
Point to objects and ask patient to name them;	Tests for expressive aphasia; e.g., patient may recognize item but not be able to name it.
Have patient produce simple sounds, e.g., "Sh," "Cat";	Identifies dysarthria as motor components of speech (tongue, lip movement, breath control) can affect articulation and may/may not be accompanied by expressive aphasia.
Ask the patient to write name and/or a short sentence. If unable to write, have patient read a short sentence.	Tests for writing disability (agraphia) and deficits in reading comprehension (alexia), which are also part of receptive and expressive aphasia.
Post notice at nurses' station and patient's room about speech impairment. Provide special call bell if necessary.	Allays anxiety related to inability to communicate and fear that needs will not be met promptly. Call bell that is activated by minimal pressure is useful when patient is unable to use regular call system.
Provide alternative methods of communication, e.g., writing or felt board, pictures. Provide visual clues (gestures, pictures, "needs" list, demonstration).	Provides for communication of needs/desires based on individual situation/underlying deficit.

250

ACTIONS/INTERVENTIONS	RATIONALE
Independent	
Anticipate and provide for patient's needs.	Helpful in decreasing frustration when dependent on others and unable to communicate desires.
Talk directly to patient, speaking slowly and distinctly. Use yes/no questions to begin with, progressing in complexity as patient responds.	Reduces confusion/anxiety at having to process and respond to large amount of information at one time. As retraining progresses, advancing complexity of communication stimulates memory and further enhances word/idea association.
Speak in normal tones and avoid talking too fast. Give patient ample time to respond. Talk without pressing for a response.	Patient is not necessarily hearing-impaired, and raising voice may anger patient/cause irritation. Forcing responses can result in frustration and may cause patient to resort to "automatic" speech, e.g., garbled speech, obscenities.
Encourage SO/visitors to persist in efforts to communicate with patient, e.g., reading mail, discussing family happenings.	Reduces patient's social isolation and promotes establishment of effective communication.
Discuss familiar topics, e.g., job, family, hobbies.	Promotes meaningful conversation and provides opportunity to practice skills.
Respect patient's preinjury capabilities; avoid "speaking down" to patient or making patronizing remarks.	Enables patient to feel esteemed, because intellectual abilities often remain intact.
Collaborative	
Consult with/refer to speech therapist.	Assesses individual verbal capabilities and sensory, motor, and cognitive functioning to identify deficits/therapy needs.

NURSING DIAGNOSIS: Sensory-Perceptual alterations (specify)

May be related to
Altered sensory reception, transmission, integration (neurologic trauma or deficit)
Psychologic stress (narrowed perceptual fields caused by anxiety)

Possibly evidenced by
Disorientation to time, place, person
Change in behavior pattern/usual response to stimuli; exaggerated emotional responses
Poor concentration, altered thought processes/bizarre thinking
Reported/measured change in sensory acuity: hypoparesthesia; altered sense of taste/smell
Inability to tell position of body parts (proprioception)
Inability to recognize/attach meaning to objects (visual agnosia)
Altered communication patterns
Motor incoordination

DESIRED OUTCOMES/EVALUATION CRITERIA—PATIENT WILL:
Regain/maintain usual level of consciousness and perceptual functioning.
Acknowledge changes in ability and presence of residual involvement.
Demonstrate behaviors to compensate for/overcome deficits.

ACTIONS/INTERVENTIONS	RATIONALE

Independent

Review pathology of individual condition.	Awareness of type/area of involvement aids in assessing for/anticipating specific deficits and planning care.
Evaluate for visual deficits. Note loss of visual field, changes in depth perception (horizontal/vertical planes), presence of diplopia (double vision).	Presence of visual disorders can negatively affect patient's ability to perceive environment and relearn motor skills and increases risk of accident/injury.
Approach patient from visually intact side. Leave light on; position objects to take advantage of intact visual fields. Patch affected eye if indicated.	Provides for recognition of the presence of persons/objects; may help with depth perception problems; prevents patient from being startled. Patching may decrease the sensory confusion of double vision.
Simplify environment, remove excess equipment/furniture.	Decreases/limits amount of visual stimuli that may confuse interpretation of environment; reduces risk of accidental injury.
Assess sensory awareness, e.g., differentiation of hot/cold, dull/sharp; position of body parts/muscle, joint sense.	Diminished sensory awareness and impairment of kinesthetic sense negatively affects balance/positioning and appropriateness of movement, which interferes with ambulation, increasing risk of trauma.
Stimulate sense of touch; e.g., give patient objects to touch, grasp. Have patient practice touching walls/other boundaries.	Aids in retraining sensory pathways to integrate reception and interpretation of stimuli. Helps patient orient self spatially and strengthens use of affected side.
Protect from temperature extremes; assess environment for hazards. Recommend testing warm water with unaffected hand.	Promotes patient safety, reducing risk of injury.
Note inattention to body parts, segments of environment; lack of recognition of familiar objects/persons.	Presence of agnosia (loss of comprehension of auditory, visual, or other sensations, although sensory sphere is intact) may lead to/result in unilateral neglect, inability to recognize environmental cues/meaning of commonplace objects, considerable self-care deficits, and disorientation or bizarre behavior.
Encourage patient to watch feet when appropriate and consciously position body parts. Make the patient aware of all neglected body parts, e.g., sensory stimulation to affected side, exercises that bring affected side across midline, reminding person to dress/care for affected ("blind") side.	Use of visual and tactile stimuli assists in reintegration of affected side and allows patient to experience forgotten sensations of normal movement patterns.
Observe behavioral responses, e.g., hostility, crying, inappropriate affect, agitation, hallucination. (Refer to CP: Craniocerebral Trauma (Acute Rehabilitative Phase), ND: Thought Processes, altered, p 233.)	Individual responses are variable, but commonalities such as emotional lability, lowered frustration threshold, apathy, and impulsiveness may exist, complicating care.
Eliminate extraneous noise/stimuli as necessary.	Reduces anxiety and exaggerated emotional responses/confusion associated with sensory overload.
Speak in calm, quiet voice, using short sentences. Maintain eye contact.	Patient may have limited attention span or problems with comprehension. These measures can help patient to attend to communication.

ACTIONS/INTERVENTIONS

Independent

Ascertain/validate patient's perceptions. Reorient patient frequently to environment, staff, procedures.

RATIONALE

Assists patient to identify inconsistencies in reception and integration of stimuli and may reduce perceptual distortion of reality.

NURSING DIAGNOSIS: Self Care deficit (specify)

May be related to
Neuromuscular impairment, decreased strength and endurance, loss of muscle control/coordination
Perceptual/cognitive impairment
Pain/discomfort
Depression

Possibly evidenced by
Impaired ability to perform ADLs, e.g., inability to bring food from receptacle to mouth; inability to wash body part(s), regulate temperature of water; impaired ability to put on/take off clothing; difficulty completing toileting tasks

DESIRED OUTCOMES/EVALUATION CRITERIA—PATIENT WILL:
Demonstrate techniques/lifestyle changes to meet self-care needs.
Perform self-care activities within level of own ability.
Identify personal/community resources that can provide assistance as needed.

ACTIONS/INTERVENTIONS

Independent

Assess abilities and level of deficit (0–4 scale) for performing ADLs.

Avoid doing things for the patient that the patient can do for self, but provide assistance as necessary.

Be aware of impulsive behavior/actions suggestive of impaired judgment.

Maintain a supportive, firm attitude. Allow patient sufficient time to accomplish tasks.

Provide positive feedback for efforts/accomplishments.

Create plan for visual deficits that are present, e.g.:

Place food and utensils on the tray related to the patient's unaffected side;

RATIONALE

Aids in anticipating/planning for meeting individual needs.

These patients may become fearful and dependent, and although assistance is helpful in preventing frustration, it is important for the patient to do as much as possible for self to maintain self-esteem and promote recovery.

May indicate need for additional interventions and supervision to promote patient safety.

Patients will need empathy but need to know caregivers will be consistent in their assistance.

Enhances sense of self-worth, promotes independence, and encourages patient to continue endeavors.

Patient will be able to see to eat the food.

253

ACTIONS/INTERVENTIONS	RATIONALE
Independent	
Situate the bed so that the patient's unaffected side is facing the room with the affected side to the wall;	Will be able to see when getting in/out of bed, observe anyone who comes into the room.
Position furniture against wall/out of travel path.	Provides for safety when patient is able to move around the room, reducing risk of tripping/falling over furniture.
Provide self-help devices, e.g., button/zipper hook, knife-fork combinations, long-handled brushes, extensions for picking things up from floor; toilet riser, leg bag for catheter; shower chair. Assist and encourage good grooming and makeup habits.	Enables patient to manage for self, enhancing independence and self-esteem, reduces reliance on others for meeting own needs, and enables patient to be more socially active.
Encourage SO to allow patient to do as much as possible for self.	Reestablishes sense of independence and fosters self-worth and enhances rehabilitation process. *Note:* This may be very difficult and frustrating for the SO/caregiver depending on degree of disability and time required for patient to complete activity.
Assess patient's ability to communicate the need to void and/or ability to use urinal, bedpan. Take patient to the bathroom at frequent/periodic intervals for voiding if appropriate.	Patient may have neurogenic bladder, be inattentive, or be unable to communicate needs in acute recovery phase, but usually able to regain independent control of this function as recovery progresses.
Identify previous bowel habits and reestablish normal regimen. Increase bulk in diet; encourage fluid intake, increased activity.	Assists in development of retraining program (independence) and aids in preventing constipation and impaction (long-term effects).
Collaborative	
Administer suppositories and stool softeners.	May be necessary at first to aid in establishing regular bowel function.
Consult with physical/occupational therapist.	Provides expert assistance for developing a therapy plan and identifying special equipment needs.

NURSING DIAGNOSIS: Coping, Individual, ineffective

May be related to
Situational crises, vulnerability, cognitive perceptual changes

Possibly evidenced by
Inappropriate use of defense mechanisms
Inability to cope/difficulty asking for help
Change in usual communication patterns
Inability to meet basic needs/role expectations
Difficulty problem solving

DESIRED OUTCOMES/EVALUATION CRITERIA—PATIENT WILL:
Verbalize acceptance of self in situation.
Talk/communicate with SO about situation and changes that have occurred.
Verbalize awareness of own coping abilities.
Meet psychologic needs as evidenced by appropriate expression of feelings, identification of options, and use of resources.

ACTIONS/INTERVENTIONS	RATIONALE
Independent	
Assess extent of altered perception and related degree of disability.	Determination of individual factors aids in developing plan of care/choice of interventions.
Identify meaning of the loss/dysfunction/change to the patient. Note ability to understand events, provide realistic appraisal of situation.	Some patients accept and manage altered function effectively with little adjustment, while others have considerable difficulty recognizing and adjusting to deficits.
Determine outside stresses, e.g., family, work, social, future nursing/healthcare needs.	Helps identify specific needs, provides opportunity to offer information/support and begin problem-solving.
Encourage patient to express feelings including hostility or anger, denial, depression.	Demonstrates acceptance of/assists patient to recognize and begin to deal with these feelings.
Note whether patient refers to affected side as "it" or denies affected side and says it is "dead."	Suggests rejection of body part/negative feelings about body image and abilities, indicating need for intervention and emotional support.
Acknowledge statement of feelings about betrayal of body; remain matter-of-fact about reality that patient can still use unaffected side and learn to control affected side. Use words (e.g., weak, affected, right-left) that incorporate that side as part of the whole body.	Helps patient to see that the nurse accepts both sides as part of the whole individual. Allows patient to feel hopeful and begin to accept current situation.
Identify previous methods of dealing with life problems. Determine presence/quality of support systems.	Provides opportunity to use behaviors previously effective, build on past successes, and mobilize resources.
Emphasize small gains either in recovery of function or independence.	Consolidates gains, helps reduce feelings of anger and helplessness, and conveys sense of progress.
Support behaviors/efforts such as increased interest/participation in rehabilitation activities.	Suggests possible adaptation to changes and understanding about own role in future lifestyle.
Monitor for sleep disturbance, increased difficulty concentrating, statements of inability to cope, lethargy, withdrawal.	May indicate onset of depression (common after effect of stroke), which may require further evaluation and intervention.
Collaborative	
Refer for neuropsychologic evaluation and/or counseling if indicated.	May facilitate adaptation to role changes that are necessary for a sense of feeling/being a productive person.

NURSING DIAGNOSIS: Swallowing, impaired, risk for

Risk factors may include
Neuromuscular/perceptual impairment

Possibly evidenced by
[Not applicable; presence of signs and symptoms establishes an *actual* diagnosis]

DESIRED OUTCOMES/EVALUATION CRITERIA—PATIENT WILL:
Demonstrate feeding methods appropriate to individual situation with aspiration prevented.
Maintain desired body weight.

255

ACTIONS/INTERVENTIONS	RATIONALE

Independent

Review individual pathology/ability to swallow, noting extent of paralysis, clarity of speech, facial, tongue involvement, ability to protect airway/episodes of coughing or choking, presence of adventitious breath sounds, amount/character of oral secretions. Weigh periodically as indicated.

Nutritional interventions/choice of feeding route is determined by these factors.

Have suction equipment available at bedside, especially during early feeding efforts.

Timely intervention may limit amount/untoward effect of aspiration.

Promote effective swallowing, e.g.:

Schedule activities/medications to provide a minimum of 30 minutes rest before eating.

Promotes optimal muscle function, helps to limit fatigue.

Provide pleasant environment free of distractions (e.g., TV).

Promotes relaxation and allows patient to focus on task of eating/swallowing.

Assist patient with head control/support;

Counteracts hyperextension, aiding in prevention of aspiration and enhancing ability to swallow.

Place patient in upright position during and after feeding;

Uses gravity to facilitate swallowing and reduces risk of aspiration.

Stimulate lips to close or manually open mouth by light pressure on lips/under chin, if needed;

Aids in sensory retraining and promotes muscular control.

Place room-temperature food in unaffected side of mouth;

Provides sensory stimulation (including taste), which may trigger swallowing efforts and enhance intake. *Note:* Dysphagic patients may be oversensitive to heat/cold.

Touch parts of the cheek with tongue blade/apply ice to weak tongue;

Can improve tongue movement and control (necessary for swallowing) and inhibits tongue protrusion.

Feed slowly allowing 30–45 minutes, for meals;

Feeling rushed can increase stress/level of frustration, may increase risk of aspiration, and may result in patient terminating meal early.

Begin oral feedings with semiliquid, soft foods when patient can swallow water. Select/assist patient to select foods that require little or no chewing, are easy to swallow, e.g., custard, applesauce, eggs, soft finger foods, or finely chopped foods;

Soft foods/thick fluids are easier to control in mouth, reducing risk of choking/aspiration. *Note:* Pureed food is not recommended as patient may not be able to recognize what is being eaten; and most milk products, peanut butter, syrup, and bananas are avoided as they are sticky and produce mucus.

Offer solid foods and liquids at different times;

Prevents patient from swallowing food before it is thoroughly chewed.

Limit/avoid use of drinking straw for liquids;

Although use may strengthen facial and swallowing muscles, if patient lacks tight lip closure to accommodate straw or if liquid is deposited too far back in mouth, risk of aspiration may be increased.

Encourage SO to bring favorite foods.

Stimulates feeding efforts and may enhance swallowing/intake.

Maintain upright position for 45–60 minutes after eating.

Helps patient manage oral secretions and reduces risk of regurgitation.

ACTIONS/INTERVENTIONS

Independent

Maintain accurate I&O; record calorie count.

Encourage participation in exercise/activity program.

Collaborative

Review results of radiographic studies, e.g., video fluoroscopy.

Administer IV fluids and/or tube feedings.

Coordinate multidisciplinary approach to develop treatment plan that meets individual needs.

RATIONALE

If swallowing efforts are not sufficient to meet fluid/nutrition needs, alternate methods of feeding must be pursued.

May increase release of endorphins in the brain, promoting a sense of general well-being and increasing appetite.

Aids in determining phase of swallowing difficulties (i.e., oral preparatory, oral, pharyngeal or esophageal phase).

May be necessary for fluid replacement and nutrition if patient is unable to take anything orally.

Inclusion of dietician, speech and occupational therapists can increase effectiveness of plan and reduce 40% risk of silent aspiration.

NURSING DIAGNOSIS: Knowledge deficit [learning need] regarding condition, treatment, self care and discharge needs

May be related to
Lack of exposure; unfamiliarity with information resources
Cognitive limitation, information misinterpretation, lack of recall

Possibly evidenced by
Request for information
Statement of misconception
Inaccurate follow-through of instructions
Development of preventable complications

DESIRED OUTCOMES/EVALUATION CRITERIA—PATIENT WILL:
Participate in learning process.
Verbalize understanding of condition/prognosis and therapeutic regimen.
Initiate necessary lifestyle changes.

ACTIONS/INTERVENTIONS

Independent

Evaluate type/degree of sensory-perceptual involvement.

Discuss specific pathology and individual potentials.

Review current restrictions/limitations and discuss planned/potential resumption of activities (including sexual relations).

RATIONALE

Deficits affect the choice of teaching methods and content/complexity of instruction.

Aids in establishing realistic expectations and promotes understanding of current situation and needs.

Promotes understanding, provides hope for future, and creates expectation of resumption of more "normal" life.

257

ACTIONS/INTERVENTIONS	RATIONALE
Independent	
Review/reinforce current therapeutic regimen, including use of aspirin or similar-acting drugs, e.g., Ticlid, Coumadin. Identify ways of continuing program after discharge.	Recommended activities, limitations, and medication/therapy needs are established on the basis of a coordinated interdisciplinary approach. Follow-through is essential to progression of recovery/prevention of complications. *Note:* Long-term anticoagulation may be beneficial for patients over 45 years of age who are prone to clot formation; however, use of these drugs is not effective for CVA resulting from vascular aneurysm/vessel rupture.
Discuss plans for meeting self-care needs.	Varying levels of assistance may be required/need to be planned for based on individual situation.
Provide written instructions and schedules for activity, medication, important facts.	Provides visual reinforcement and reference source after discharge.
Encourage patient to refer to lists/written communications or notes instead of depending on memory.	Provides aids to support memory and promotes improvement in cognitive skills.
Suggest patient reduce/limit environmental stimuli, especially during cognitive activities.	Multiple/concomitant stimuli may aggravate confusion and impair mental abilities.
Recommend patient seek assistance in problem-solving process and validate decisions, as indicated.	Some patients (especially those with right CVA) may display impaired judgment and impulsive behavior, compromising ability to make sound decisions.
Identify individual risk factors (e.g., hypertension, obesity, smoking, atherosclerosis, use of oral contraceptives) and necessary lifestyle changes.	Promotes general well-being and may reduce risk of recurrence.
Identify signs/symptoms requiring further follow-up, e.g., changes/decline in visual, motor, sensory functions; alteration in mentation or behavioral responses; severe headache.	Prompt evaluation and intervention reduces risk of complications/further loss of function.
Refer to discharge planner/home care supervisor, visiting nurse.	Home environment may require evaluation and modifications to meet individual needs.
Identify community resources, e.g., stroke support clubs, senior services, Meals on Wheels, adult day care/respite program, and visiting nurse.	Enhances coping abilities and promotes home management and adjustment to impairments.
Refer to/reinforce importance of follow-up care by rehabilitation team, e.g., physical/occupational/speech/vocational therapists.	Diligent work may eventually overcome/minimize residual deficits.

POTENTIAL CONSIDERATIONS following acute hospitalization (dependent on patient's age, physical condition/presence of complications, personal resources, and life responsibilities)

Injury, risk for—general weakness, visual deficits, balancing difficulties, reduced large/small muscle or hand-eye coordination, cognitive impairment.

Nutrition: altered, less than body requirements—inability to ingest food, cognitive limitations, limited financial resources.

Self Care deficit—decreased strength/endurance, perceptual/cognitive impairment, neuromuscular impairment, muscular pain, depression.

Home Maintenance Management, impaired—individual physical limitations, inadequate support systems, insufficient finances, unfamiliarity with neighborhood resources.

Self-Esteem, situational low—cognitive/perceptual impairment, perceived loss of control in some aspect of life, loss of independent functioning.

HERNIATED NUCLEUS PULPOSUS (RUPTURED INTERVERTEBRAL DISC)

A herniated disc (HNP) is a major cause of severe, chronic, and recurrent back pain. Herniation, either complete or partial, of the nuclear material in the vertebral areas of L-4 to L-5, L-5 to S-1, or C-5 to C-6, C-6 to C-7 is most common and may be the result of trauma or degenerative changes associated with the aging process.

CARE SETTING

Most disc problems are treated conservatively at the community level, although diagnostics and therapy services may be provided through outpatient facilities. Brief hospitalization is restricted to episodes of severe debilitating pain/neurologic deficit.

RELATED CONCERNS

Disc Surgery, p 267
Psychosocial Aspects of Care, p 783

Patient Assessment Data Base

Data are dependent on site, severity, whether acute/chronic, effects on surrounding structures, and degree of nerve root compression.

ACTIVITY/REST

May report: History of occupation requiring heavy lifting, sitting, driving for long periods
Need to sleep on bedboard/firm mattress, difficulty falling asleep/staying asleep
Decreased range of motion of affected extremity/extremities
Inability to perform usual/desired activities

May exhibit: Atrophy of muscles on the affected side
Gait disturbances

ELIMINATION

May report: Constipation, difficulty in defecation
Urinary incontinence/retention

EGO INTEGRITY

May report: Fear of paralysis
Financial, employment concerns

May exhibit: Anxiety, depression, withdrawal from family/SO

NEUROSENSORY

May report: Tingling, numbness, weakness, of affected extremity/extremities

May exhibit: Decreased deep tendon reflexes; muscle weakness, hypotonia
Tenderness/spasm of paravertebral muscles
Decreased pain perception (sensory)

PAIN/DISCOMFORT

May report: Pain knifelike, aggravated by coughing, sneezing, bending, lifting, defecation, straight leg raising (Lasègue's sign) or neck flexion; unremitting pain or intermittent epi-

259

sodes of more severe pain; radiation to leg, buttocks area (lumbar) or shoulder; occiput with stiff neck (cervical)

Heard "snapping" sound at time of initial pain/trauma or felt "back giving way"

Limited mobility/forward bending

May exhibit: Stance: Leans away from affected area

Altered gait, walking with a limp, elevated hip on affected side

Pain on palpation

SAFETY

May report: History of previous back problems

TEACHING/LEARNING

May report: Lifestyle: Sedentary or overactive

Discharge plan   **DRG projected mean length of inpatient stay: 6.1 days**

considerations: May require assistance with transportation, self-care, and homemaker/maintenance tasks

Refer to section at end of plan for postdischarge considerations.

DIAGNOSTIC STUDIES

Spinal x-rays: May show degenerative changes in spine/intervertebral space or rule out other suspected pathology, e.g., tumors, osteomyelitis.

CT scan with/without enhancement: May reveal spinal canal narrowing, disc protrusion.

MRI: Noninvasive study can reveal changes in bone and soft tissues, and can validate disc herniation/surgical decisions.

Provocative tests (discography, nerve root blocks): Determine site of origin of pain by replicating and then relieving symptoms. Can also be used to rule out sacroiliac joint involvement.

Electrophysiologic studies—electromyoneurography (EMG and NCS): Can localize lesion to level of particular spinal nerve root involved; nerve conduction and velocity study usually done in conjunction with study of muscle response to assist in diagnosis of peripheral nerve damage and effect on skeletal muscle.

Epidural venogram: May be done for cases where myelogram accuracy is limited.

Lumbar puncture: Rules out other related conditions, infection, presence of blood.

Myelogram: May be normal or show "narrowing" of disc space, specific location and size of herniation.

NURSING PRIORITIES

1. Reduce back stress, muscle spasm, and pain.
2. Promote optimal functioning.
3. Support patient/SO in rehabilitation process.
4. Provide information concerning condition/prognosis and treatment needs.

DISCHARGE GOALS

1. Pain relieved/manageable.
2. Proper lifting, posture, exercises demonstrated.
3. Motor function/sensation restored to optimal level.
4. Disease/injury process, prognosis, and therapeutic regimen understood.
5. Plan in place to meet needs after discharge.

NURSING DIAGNOSIS: Pain [acute]/chronic

May be related to

Physical injury agents: nerve compression, muscle spasm

Possibly evidenced by
Reports of back pain, stiff neck
Walking with a limp, inability to walk
Guarding behavior, leans toward affected side when standing
Decreased tolerance for activity
Preoccupation with pain, self/narrowed focus
Altered muscle tone
Facial mask of pain; distraction
Autonomic responses (when pain is acute)
Changes in sleep patterns
Physical/social withdrawal

DESIRED OUTCOMES/EVALUATION CRITERIA—PATIENT WILL:
Report pain is relieved/controlled.
Verbalize methods that provide relief.
Demonstrate use of therapeutic interventions (e.g., relaxation skills, behavior modification) to relieve pain.

ACTIONS/INTERVENTIONS	RATIONALE
Independent	
Assess reports of pain, noting location, duration, precipitating/aggravating factors. Ask patient to rate on scale of 0–10 (or other scale as appropriate).	Helps determine choice of interventions and provides basis for comparison and evaluation of therapy.
Maintain bed rest during acute phase. Place patient in semi-Fowler's position with spine, hips, knees flexed; supine with/without head elevated 10–30 degrees; or lateral position.	Bed rest in position of comfort allows for decrease of muscle spasm, reduces stress on structures, and facilitates reduction of disc protrusion.
Logroll for position change if patient requires assistance.	Reduces flexion, twisting, and strain on back especially when nerve block impairs patient's ability to move legs.
Assist with application of brace/corset. Instruct patient in how to self-place brace with assistance, then independently.	Often used during acute phase of ruptured disc or after surgery to provide support and limit flexion/twisting. *Note:* Prolonged use can increase muscle weakness and cause further disc degeneration, nerve impairment.
Limit activity to short time periods during acute phase as indicated. Intersperse rest periods frequently; shortening rest intervals and length as patient improves.	Decreases forces of gravity and motion, which can relieve muscle spasms and reduce edema and stress on structures around affected disk.
Place needed items, call bell within easy reach.	Reduces risk of straining to reach.
Instruct in/assist with relaxation/visualization techniques.	Refocuses attention away from pain, aids in reducing muscle spasm/tension; and promotes tissue oxygenation/healing.
Instruct in/encourage correct body mechanics/body posture.	Alleviates stress on muscles and prevents further injury.
Provide opportunities to talk/listen to concerns.	Ventilation of worries can help to decrease stress factors present in illness/hospitalization. Provides opportunity to give information/correct misinformation.

Collaborative

Provide orthopedic bed or place board under mattress.	Provides support and reduces spinal flexion, decreasing spasms.
Administer medications as indicated:	
Muscle relaxants, e.g., diazepam (Valium), carisoprodol (Soma), methcarbamol (Robaxin);	Relaxes muscles, decreasing pain.
NSAIDs, e.g., ibuprofen (Motrin, Advil), diflurisal (Dolobid), Ketoproten (Orudis), meclofenamate (Meclomen);	Decreases edema and pressure on nerve root(s). *Note:* Epidural or facet joint injection of anti-inflammatory drugs may be tried if other interventions fail to alleviate pain.
Analgesics, e.g., acetaminophen (Tylenol) with codeine, meperidine (Demerol), hydrocodone (Vicodin), butorphanol (Stadol).	May be required for relief of moderate to severe pain.
Apply physical supports, e.g., lumbar brace, cervical collar.	Support of structures decreases muscle stress/spasms and reduces pain.
Maintain traction if indicated.	Removes weight bearing from affected disc area, increasing intravertebral separation and allowing disk bulge to move away from nerve root.
Consult with physical therapist.	Individual stretching/exercise program can relieve muscle spasm and strengthen back, extensor, abdominal, and quadriceps muscles to increase support to lumbar area.
Apply/monitor use of cold or moist hot packs, diathermy, ultrasound.	Increases circulation to affected muscles, promotes relief of spasms, and enhances patient's relaxation.
Instruct in postmyelogram procedures when appropriate, e.g., force fluids and lie flat or at 30-degree elevation, as indicated for specific number of hours.	Decreases risk of postprocedure headache/spinal fluid leak.
Assist with/instruct in use of TENS unit.	Decreases stimuli by blocking pain transmission.
Refer to pain clinic.	Coordinated team efforts may include physical as well as psychologic therapy to deal with all aspects of chronic pain and allow patient to increase activity and productivity.

NURSING DIAGNOSIS: Physical Mobility, impaired

May be related to
Pain and discomfort, muscle spasms
Restrictive therapies, e.g., bed rest, traction
Neuromuscular impairment

Possibly evidenced by
Reports of pain on movement
Reluctance to attempt/difficulty with purposeful movement
Impaired coordination, limited range of motion, decreased muscle strength

DESIRED OUTCOMES/EVALUATION CRITERIA—PATIENT WILL:
Verbalize understanding of situation/risk factors and individual treatment regimen.
Demonstrate techniques/behaviors that enable resumption of activities.
Maintain or increase strength and function of affected and/or compensatory body part.

ACTIONS/INTERVENTIONS	RATIONALE
Independent	
Provide for safety measures as indicated by individual situation.	Dependent on area of involvement/type of procedure, imprudent activity increases chance of spinal injury. (Refer to CP: Disc Surgery, ND: Trauma [spinal], risk for, p 268.)
Note emotional/behavioral responses to immobility. Provide diversional activities.	Forced immobility may heighten restlessness, irritability. Diversional activity aids in refocusing attention and promotes coping with limitations.
Follow activity/procedures with rest periods. Encourage participation in ADLs within individual limitations.	Enhances healing and builds muscle strength and endurance. Patient participation promotes independence and sense of control.
Provide/assist with passive and active range of motion exercises.	Strengthens abdominal muscles and flexors of spine; promotes good body mechanics.
Encourage lower leg/ankle exercises. Evaluate for edema, erythema of lower extremities, presence of Homan's sign.	Stimulates venous circulation/return decreasing venous stasis and possible thrombus formation.
Assist with activity/progressive ambulation.	Activity limitation is dependent on individual situation but usually progresses slowly according to tolerance.
Demonstrate use of adjunctive devices, e.g., walker, cane.	Provides stability and support to compensate for altered muscle tone/strength and balance.
Provide good skin care; massage pressure points after each position change. Check skin under brace periodically.	Reduces risk of skin irritation/breakdown.
Collaborative	
Administer medication for pain approximately 30 minutes prior to turning patient/ambulation, as indicated.	Anticipation of pain can increase muscle tension. Medication can relax patient, enhance comfort and cooperation during activity.
Apply antiembolism stockings as indicated.	Promotes venous return, reducing risk of DVT.

NURSING DIAGNOSIS: Anxiety [specify level]/Coping, Individual, ineffective

May be related to
Situational crisis
Threat to/change in health status, socioeconomic status, role functioning
Recurrent disorder with continuing pain
Inadequate relaxation, little or no exercise
Inadequate coping methods

Possibly evidenced by
Apprehension, uncertainty, helplessness
Expressed concerns regarding changes in life events
Verbalization of inability to cope
Muscular tension, general irritability, restlessness; insomnia/fatigue
Inability to meet role expectations

ACTIONS/INTERVENTIONS	RATIONALE
Independent	
Assess level of anxiety. Determine how patient has dealt with problems in the past as well as how he/she is coping with current situation.	Aids in identifying strengths and skills that may help patient deal with current situation and/or enable others to provide appropriate assistance.
Provide accurate information and honest answers.	Enables patient to make decisions based on knowledge.
Provide opportunity for expression of concerns, e.g., possible paralysis, effect on sexual ability, changes in employment/finances, altered role responsibilities.	Most patients have concerns that need to be expressed and responded to with accurate information to promote coping with situation.
Assess presence of secondary gains that may interfere with the wish to recover and may impede recovery.	The patient may unconsciously experience advantages such as relief from responsibilities; attention, and control of others. These need to be dealt with positively to promote recovery.
Note behaviors of SO that promote "sick role" for the patient.	SO may unconsciously enable patient to remain dependent by doing things that patient should do for self.
Collaborative	
Refer to community support groups, social services, financial/vocational counselor, marital therapy/psychotherapy.	Provides support for adapting to changes and provides resources to deal with problems.

ACTIONS/INTERVENTIONS	RATIONALE

Independent

Review disease/injury process and prognosis and activity restrictions/limitations; e.g., avoid riding in car for long periods, refrain from participation in aggressive sports.	Helpful in clarifying and developing understanding and acceptance of necessary lifestyle changes. Full knowledge base provides opportunity for patient to make informed choices. May enhance cooperation with treatment program and achievement of optimal recovery.
Give information about and instruct in proper body mechanics and exercises. Include information about proper posture/body mechanics for standing, sitting, lifting and use of supportive shoes.	Reduces risk of reinjuring back/neck area by using muscles of thighs/buttocks.
Discuss medications and side effects: e.g., some medications cause drowsiness (analgesics, muscle relaxants); others can aggravate ulcer disease (NSAIDs).	Reduces risk of complications/injury.
Recommend use of bedboards/firm mattress, small flat pillow under neck, sleeping on side with knees flexed, avoiding prone position.	May decrease muscle strain through structural support and prevention of hyperextension of spine.
Discuss dietary needs/goals.	High-fiber diet can reduce constipation; calorie restrictions promote weight control/reduction, which can decrease pressure on disc.
Avoid prolonged heat application.	Can increase local tissue congestion; decreased sensing of heat can result in thermal injury.
Review use of soft cervical collar.	Maintaining slight flexion of head (allows maximal opening of intervertebral foramina) may be useful for relieving pressure in mild to moderate cervical disc disease. Hyperextension should be avoided.
Encourage regular medical follow-up.	Evaluates resolution/progression of degenerative process; monitors development of side effects/complications of drug therapy; may indicate need for change in therapeutic regimen.
Provide information about what symptoms need to be reported for further evaluation, e.g., sharp pain, loss of sensation/ability to walk.	Progression of the process may necessitate further treatment/surgery.
Review treatment alternatives, e.g.:	
Chemonucleolysis;	As an alternative to surgery, the enzyme chymopapain may be injected into the disc (dissolves the mucoprotein disc material without effect on surrounding structure). Although many patients experience relief, the procedure is not widely done because of side effects including allergic reaction to the enzyme.
Surgical interventions.	Microdiscectomy may be performed to excise fragments of the disc with a comparatively lower risk than more invasive surgery. Laminectomy with/without spinal fusion may be performed when conservative treatment is ineffective or when neurologic deficits persist.

POTENTIAL CONSIDERATIONS following acute hospitalization (dependent on patient's age, physical condition/presence of complications, personal resources, and life responsibilities).

Adjustment, impaired—disability requiring change in lifestyle, assault to self-esteem, altered locus of control.

Pain, chronic—prolonged physical/psychosocial disability.

Therapeutic Regimen: Individual, ineffective management—complexity of therapeutic regimen, decisional conflicts, economic difficulties, perceived benefits, powerlessness.

Disuse Syndrome, risk for—severe pain, periods of immobility.

DISC SURGERY

Laminectomy is the excision of a vertebral posterior arch and is commonly performed for injury to the spinal column or to relieve pressure/pain in the presence of an HNP. The procedure may be done with or without fusion of vertebrae.

CARE SETTING

Inpatient surgical or orthopedic unit.

RELATED CONCERNS

Psychosocial Aspects of Care, p 783
Surgical Intervention, p 802

Patient Assessment Data Base

Refer to CP: Herniated Nucleus Pulposus (Ruptured Intervertebral Disc), p 259.

TEACHING/LEARNING

Discharge plan considerations: DRG projected mean length of inpatient stay: 10.8 days
May require assistance with ADLs, transportation, homemaker/maintenance tasks, vocational counseling, possible changes in layout of home

Refer to section at end of plan for postdischarge considerations.

DIAGNOSTIC STUDIES

Refer to CP: Herniated Nucleus Pulposus (Ruptured Intervertebral Disc), p 259.

NURSING PRIORITIES

1. Maintain tissue perfusion/neurologic function.
2. Promote comfort and healing.
3. Prevent/minimize complications.
4. Assist with return to normal mobility.
5. Provide information about condition/prognosis, treatment needs, and limitations.

DISCHARGE GOALS

1. Neurologic function maintained/improved.
2. Complications prevented.
3. Limited mobility achieved with potential for increasing mobility.
4. Condition/prognosis, therapeutic regimen, and behavior/lifestyle changes are understood.
5. Plan in place to meet needs after discharge.

NURSING DIAGNOSIS: Tissue Perfusion, altered [specify]

May be related to
Diminished/interrupted blood flow (e.g., edema of operative site, hematoma formation)
Hypovolemia

ACTIONS/INTERVENTIONS	RATIONALE
Independent	
Check neurologic signs periodically and compare with baseline. Assess movement/sensation of lower extremities and feet (lumbar) and hands/arms (cervical).	Although some degree of prior sensory impairment is usually present, deterioration/changes may reflect development/resolution of spinal cord edema, inflammation of the tissues secondary to damage to motor nerve roots from surgical manipulation; or tissue hemorrhage compressing the spinal cord requiring prompt medical evaluation.
Keep patient flat on back for several hours.	Pressure to operative site reduces risk of hematoma.
Monitor vital signs. Note color, warmth, capillary refill.	Hypotension (especially postural) with corresponding changes in pulse rate may reflect hypovolemia from blood loss, restriction of oral intake, nausea/vomiting.
Monitor intake/output and Hemovac drainage (if used).	Provides information about circulatory status and replacement needs.
Palpate operative site for swelling. Inspect dressing for excess drainage and test for glucose if indicated.	Change in contour of operative site suggests hematoma/edema formation. Inspection may reveal frank bleeding or dura leak of CSF (will test glucose-positive), requiring prompt intervention.
Measure Hemovac drainage each shift.	Excessive/prolonged blood loss requires further evaluation to determine appropriate intervention.
Collaborative	
Administer IV fluids/blood as indicated.	Fluid replacement is dependent on the degree of hypovolemia and duration of oozing/bleeding/spinal fluid leaking.
Monitor blood counts, e.g., Hb, Hct, and RBC.	Aids in establishing blood replacement needs and monitors effectiveness of therapy.

ACTIONS/INTERVENTIONS	RATIONALE
Independent	
Post sign at bedside regarding prescribed position.	Reduces risk of inadvertent strain/flexion of operative area.
Provide bedboard/firm mattress.	Aids in stabilizing back.
Maintain cervical collar postoperatively with cervical laminectomy procedure.	Decreases muscle spasm and supports the surrounding structures, allowing normal sensory stimulation to occur.
Limit activities when patient has had a spinal fusion.	Following surgery, spinal movement is restricted to promote healing of fusion, requiring a longer recuperation time.
Logroll patient from side to side. Have patient fold arms across chest, tighten long back muscles, keeping shoulders and pelvis straight. Use pillows between knees during position change and when on side. Use turning sheet and sufficient personnel when turning, especially on the 1st postoperative day.	Maintains body alignment while turning, preventing twisting motion, which may interfere with healing process.
Assist out of bed: logroll to side of bed, splint back, and raise to sitting position. Avoid prolonged sitting. Move to standing position in single smooth motion.	Avoids twisting and flexing of back while arising from bed/chair, protecting surgical area.
Avoid sudden stretching, twisting, flexing, or jarring of spine.	May cause vertebral collapse, shifting of bone graft, delayed hematoma formation, or subcutaneous wound dehiscence.
Check BP; note reports of dizziness or weakness. Change position slowly.	Presence of postural hypotension may result in fainting/fall and possible injury to surgical site.
Have patient wear firm/flat walking shoes when ambulating.	Reduces risk of falls.
Collaborative	
Apply lumbar brace/cervical collar as appropriate.	Brace/corset may be used in and/or out of bed during immediate postoperative phase to support spine and surrounding structures until muscle strength improves. Brace is applied while patient is supine in bed. Spinal fusion generally requires a lengthy recuperation period in a corset/collar.
Refer to physical therapy. Implement program as outlined.	Strengthening exercises may be indicated during the rehabilitative phase to decrease muscle spasm and strain on the vertebral disc area.

NURSING DIAGNOSIS: Breathing Pattern, ineffective/Airway Clearance, ineffective, risk for

Risk factors may include
Tracheal/bronchial obstruction/edema
Decreased lung expansion, pain

Possibly evidenced by
[Not applicable; presence of signs and symptoms establishes an *actual* diagnosis]

ACTIONS/INTERVENTIONS	RATIONALE
Independent	
Inspect for edema of face/neck (cervical laminectomy) especially first 24–48 hours after surgery.	Tracheal edema/compression or nerve injury can compromise respiratory function.
Listen for hoarseness. Encourage voice rest.	May indicate laryngeal nerve injury, which can negatively affect cough (ability to clear airway).
Auscultate breath sounds, note presence of wheezes/rhonchi.	Suggests accumulation of secretions/ineffective airway clearance.
Assist with coughing, turning, and deep breathing.	Facilitates movement of secretions and clearing of lungs; reduces risk of respiratory complications (pneumonia).
Collaborative	
Administer humidified supplemental oxygen, if indicated.	May be necessary for periods of respiratory distress or evidence of hypoxia.
Monitor/graph ABGs or pulse oximetry.	Monitors effectiveness of breathing pattern/therapy.

NURSING DIAGNOSIS: Pain [acute]

May be related to
Physical agent: surgical manipulation, edema, inflammation

Possibly evidenced by
Reports of pain
Autonomic responses: diaphoresis, changes in vital signs, pallor
Alteration in muscle tone
Guarding, distraction behaviors/restlessness

DESIRED OUTCOMES/EVALUATION CRITERIA—PATIENT WILL:
Report pain is relieved/controlled.
Verbalize methods that provide relief.
Demonstrate use of relaxation skills and diversional activities.

ACTIONS/INTERVENTIONS	RATIONALE
Independent	
Assess intensity, description, and location/radiation of pain, changes in sensation. Instruct in use of rating scale (e.g., 0–10).	May be mild to severe with radiation to shoulders/occipital area (cervical) or hips/buttocks (lumbar). If bone graft has been taken from the iliac crest, pain may be more severe at the donor site. Numbness/tingling discomfort may reflect return of sensation after nerve root decompression or result from developing edema of compressed nerve/operative site.

ACTIONS/INTERVENTIONS	RATIONALE
Independent	
Review expected manifestations/changes in intensity of pain.	Development/resolution of edema and inflammation in the immediate postoperative phase can affect pressure on various nerves and cause changes in degree of pain (especially 3 days after operation, when muscle spasms/improved nerve root sensation intensify pain).
Allow patient to assume position of comfort if indicated. Use logroll for position change.	Positioning is dictated by physical preference, type of operation (e.g., head of bed may be slightly elevated after cervical laminectomy). Readjustment of position aids in relieving muscle fatigue and discomfort. Logrolling avoids tension in the operative areas, maintains straight spinal alignment, and reduces risk of displacing epidural PCA when used.
Provide back rub/massage, avoiding operative site.	Relieves/reduces pain by alteration of sensory neurons, muscle relaxation.
Demonstrate/encourage use of relaxation skills, e.g., deep breathing, visualization.	Refocuses attention, reduces muscle tension, promotes sense of well-being, and controls/decreases discomfort.
Provide soft diet, room humidifier; encourage voice rest following cervical laminectomy.	Reduces discomfort associated with sore throat and difficulty swallowing.
Investigate patient reports of return of radicular pain.	Suggests complications (collapsing of disc space, shifting of bone graft or arachnoiditis with adhesions) requiring further medical evaluation and intervention. *Note:* Sciatica and muscle spasms often recur after laminectomy but should resolve within several days or weeks.
Collaborative	
Administer analgesics, as indicated:	
Narcotics, e.g., morphine, codeine, meperidine (Demerol), oxycodone (Tylox), hydrocodone (Vicodin), acetaminophen (Tylenol) with codeine;	Narcotics are used during the first few postoperative days, then non-narcotic agents are incorporated as intensity of pain diminishes. *Note:* Narcotics may be administered via epidural sites.
Muscle relaxants, e.g., cyclobenzaprine (Flexeril), diazepam (Valium).	May be used to relieve muscle spasms resulting from intraoperative nerve irritation.
Assist with PCA.	Gives patient control of medication administration (usually narcotics) to achieve a more constant level of comfort, which may enhance healing.
Provide throat sprays/lozenges, viscous xylocaine.	Sore throat may be a major complaint following cervical laminectomy.
Apply TENS unit as needed.	May be used for incisional pain or when nerve involvement continues after discharge. Decreases level of pain by blocking nerve transmission of pain.

ACTIONS/INTERVENTIONS	RATIONALE
Independent	
Schedule activity/procedures with rest periods. Encourage participation in ADLs within individual limitations.	Enhances healing and builds muscle strength and endurance. Patient participation promotes independence and sense of control.
Provide/assist with passive and active range of motion exercises dependent on surgical procedure.	Strengthens abdominal muscles and flexors of spine; promotes good body mechanics.
Assist with activity/progressive ambulation.	Until healing occurs, activity is limited and advanced slowly according to individual tolerance.

(Refer to CP: Herniated Nucleus Pulposus (Ruptured Intervertebral Disc), ND: Physical Mobility, impaired, p 259, for further considerations.)

ACTIONS/INTERVENTIONS	RATIONALE
Independent	
Note abdominal distention and auscultate bowel sounds.	Distention and absence of bowel sounds indicate that bowel is not functioning, possibly due to sudden loss of parasympathetic enervation of the bowel.
Use fracture or child-size bedpan until allowed out of bed.	Promotes comfort, reduces muscle tension.
Provide privacy.	Promotes psychologic comfort.
Encourage ambulation as able.	Stimulates peristalsis, facilitating passage of flatus.
Collaborative	
Begin progressive diet as tolerated.	Solid foods are not started until bowel sounds have returned/flatus passed and danger of ileus formation has abated.
Provide rectal tube, suppositories, and enemas as needed.	May be necessary to relieve abdominal distention, promote resumption of normal bowel habits.
Administer laxatives, stool softeners as indicated.	Softens stools, promotes normal bowel habits, decreases straining.

NURSING DIAGNOSIS: Urinary Retention, risk for

Risk factors may include
Pain and swelling in operative area
Need for remaining flat in bed

Possibly evidenced by
[Not applicable; presence of signs and symptoms establishes an *actual* diagnosis]

DESIRED OUTCOMES/EVALUATION CRITERIA—PATIENT WILL:
Empty bladder adequately according to individual need.

ACTIONS/INTERVENTIONS	RATIONALE
Independent	
Observe and record amount/time of voiding.	Determines whether bladder is being emptied and when interventions may be necessary.
Palpate for bladder distention.	May indicate urine retention.
Force fluids.	Maintains kidney function.
Stimulate bladder emptying by running water, pouring warm water over peritoneal area, putting hand in warm water as needed.	Promotes urination by relaxing urinary sphincter.
Collaborative	
Catheterize for bladder residual after voiding when indicated. Insert/maintain indwelling catheter as needed.	Intermittent or continuous catheterization may be necessary for several days postoperatively, until swelling is decreased.

273

ACTIONS/INTERVENTIONS	RATIONALE
Independent	
Review particular condition/prognosis.	Individual needs dictate tolerance levels/limitations of activity.
Discuss return to activities, stressing importance of increasing as tolerated.	Although the recuperative period may be lengthy, following prescribed activity program promotes muscle and tissue circulation, healing, and strengthening.
Encourage development of regular exercise program, e.g., walking.	Promotes healing, strengthens abdominal and erector muscles to provide support to the spinal column, and enhances general physical and emotional well-being.
Discuss importance of good posture and avoidance of prolonged standing/sitting. Recommend sitting in straight-backed chair with feet on a footstool or flat on the floor.	Prevents further injuries/stress by maintaining proper alignment of spine.
Stress importance of avoiding activities that increase the flexion of the spine, e.g., climbing stairs, automobile driving/riding, bending at the waist with knees straight, lifting more than 5 lb, engaging in strenuous exercise/sports. Discuss limitations on sexual relations/positions.	Flexing/twisting of the spine aggravates the healing process and increases risk of injury to spinal cord.
Encourage lying-down rest periods, balanced with activity.	Reduces general and spinal fatigue and assists in the healing/recuperative process.
Discuss possibility of unrelieved/renewed pain.	Some pain may continue for several months as activity level increases and scar tissue stretches. Pain relief from surgical procedure could be temporary if other discs have similar amount of degeneration.
Discuss use of heat, e.g., warm packs, heating pad, or showers.	Increased circulation to the back/surgical area transports nutrients for healing to the area and resolution of pathogens/exudates out of the area. Decreases muscle spasms that may result from nerve root irritation during healing process.

ACTIONS/INTERVENTIONS	RATIONALE
Independent	
Discuss judicious use of cold packs before/after stretching activity, if indicated.	May decrease muscle spasm in some instances more effectively than heat.
Avoid tub baths for 3–4 weeks, depending on physician recommendation.	Tub baths increase risk of flexing/twisting of spine as well as danger of falls.
Review dietary/fluid needs.	Should be tailored to reduce risk of constipation and avoid excess weight gain while meeting nutrient needs to facilitate healing.
Review/reinforce incisional care.	Correct care promotes healing, reduces risk of wound infection.
Identify signs/symptoms requiring notification of healthcare provider, e.g., fever, increased incisional pain, inflammation, wound drainage, decreased sensation/motor activity in extremities.	Prompt evaluation and intervention may prevent complications/permanent injury.
Discuss necessity of follow-up care.	Long-term medical supervision may be needed to manage problems/complications and to reincorporate individual into desired/altered lifestyle and activities.
Review need for/use of immobilization device, as indicated.	Correct application and wearing time is important to gaining the most benefit from the brace.
Assess current lifestyle/job, finances, activities at home and leisure.	Knowledge of current situation allows nurse to highlight areas for possible intervention, such as referral for occupational/vocational testing and counseling.
Listen/communicate with patient regarding alternatives and lifestyle changes. Be sensitive to patient's needs.	Laminectomy and low back pain are a frequent cause of chronic disability. Many patients may have to stop/modify work, creating marital/financial crises. Often the concern that the patient is a malingerer creates further problems in social relationships.
Note overt/covert expressions of concern about sexuality.	Although patient may not ask directly, there may be concerns about the effect of this surgery on not only ability to cope with usual role in the family/community but also ability to perform sexually.
Explore limitations/abilities.	Placing limitations into perspective with abilities allows the patient to understand own situation and exercise choice.
Provide written copy of all instructions.	Useful as a reference after discharge.
Refer to community resources as indicated, e.g., social services, rehabilitation/vocational counseling services.	A team effort can be helpful in providing support during recuperative period.
Refer for counseling, sex therapy, psychotherapy, as indicated.	Depression is common in conditions for which lengthy recuperative time (2–9 months) is expected. Therapy may alleviate further anxiety, assist patient to cope effectively, and enhance healing process. Presence of physical limitations, pain, and depression may negatively impact sexual desire/performance and add additional stress to relationship.

POTENTIAL CONSIDERATIONS following acute hospitalization (dependent on patient's age, physical condition/presence of complications, personal resources, and life responsibilities)

Physical Mobility, impaired—decreased strength/endurance, pain, immobilizing device.
Self Care deficit—decreased strength/endurance, pain, immobilizing device.
Trauma, risk for—weakness, balancing difficulties, decreased muscle coordination, reduced temperature/tactile sensation.
Family Coping: ineffective compromised—temporary family disorganization and role changes.

Sample CP: Cervical Laminectomy with Fusion. ELOS: 3 Days Orthopedic or Surgical Unit

ND and categories of care	Day 1 Day of surgery _____	Day 2 POD#1 _____	Day 3 POD#2 _____
Altered tissue perfusion, R/T to altered blood flow (operative site edema, hematoma formation, hypovolemia)	Goals: Maintain proper alignment of cervical spine Display stable/improved sensation in affected limbs	Display normal sensory/motor response Identify appropriate safety measures	
Diagnostic studies		Hb/Hct, RBC Electrolytes	C–spine–PA/lat
Additional assessments	VS q1hX4 then q4h	→ qid	→ q8h
	Neurovasc checks UE, q1hX4 then q4h	→ qid	→ q8h
	Dressings/drainage q4h	→	→ bid
	I & O q8h	→	→
	Hemovac (if used) q8h	→	→ D/C
	Palpate op site for swelling, inspect face/neck for edema qhX4	→ q8h	→ D/C
Medications	IV fluids/blood as indicated	→ D/C or convert to NS lock	→ D/C
Patient education	Purpose/necessity of cervical collar	Cessation of smoking if indicated	Use of heat Signs/symptoms to be reported to healthcare provider
	Protocol for position change		
Additional nursing actions	Position per protocol/HOB elevated 30°	→	→
	Log roll q2h	→ Chair X3	→ Ambulate as tol
	Cervical collar in place	→	
	BRP w/assist (tennis shoes–not slippers)	→	Per self as tol →
	Fluids as tol	→ Advance diet as tol	
Pain R/T to surgical intervention	Report pain controlled	→ Participate in activities to increase comfort	→ Verbalize understanding of → therapeutic interventions
Additional assessments	Pain characteristics/change	→	→
	Response to interventions		
Medications Allergies: _____	Analgesics–PCA or IM	→ D/C PCA	→ D/C IM
	Throat spray/lozenges	→ PO analgesics	→ D/C
Patient education	Orient to unit/room	Relaxation techniques	→ Use of TENS as indicated
	Reporting of pain/effects of interventions	Medication dose, frequency, purpose, side effects	Signs/symptoms to report to healthcare provider
	Proper use of PCA		
	Recovery/rehabilitation expectations		
	Limitations of movement (e.g., twisting, flexing, pulling)		
	Voice rest (anterior approach)		
Additional nursing actions	Provide firm mattress	→	→
	Comfort measures	→	→

Sample CP: Cervical Laminectomy with Fusion ELOS: 3 Days Orthopedic or Surgical Unit (*Continued*)

ND and categories of care	Day 1 Day of surgery _____	Day 2 POD#1 _____	Day 3 POD#2 _____
Impaired physical mobility R/T musculoskeletal impairment; pain and therapeutic restriction		Reestablish normal bowel/ bladder elimination	Verbalize understanding of activity program/restrictions Report plan in place to meet needs postdischarge
Referrals		Social Services Home care	
Additional assessments	General muscle tone/strength Level of functional ability Breath sounds q4h Bowel sounds q4h Amount/time of voids	→ Ability to perform ADLs independently → q8h → q8h → D/C Edema, pain lower extremities, Homans sign q8h	→ → →
Medications		Stool softener	→ Fleets if no BM
Patient Education	Activity level/progression Bed exercises Skin care needs	General wellness–diet, exercise, adequate rest Home exercise program Proper body mechanics Use of assistive devices as required	Activity restrictions e.g., shower instead of tub bath, no lifting, resumption of work, hobbies, sexual activity Provide written copy of instructions
Additional nursing actions	Assist w/passive and active ROM exercises Encourage particpation of ADLs w/in level of ability T, C, DB, q2h Incentive spirometry q4h Thigh-high TEDs Skin care per Risk Protocol	→ → → → → → q4 while awake → Remove q8h	→ → Per self → → → Per self → D/C → D/C

SPINAL CORD INJURY (ACUTE REHABILITATIVE PHASE)

Spinal cord lesions are classified as complete (total loss of sensation and voluntary motor function) and incomplete (mixed loss of sensation and voluntary motor function).

Physical findings will vary, depending on the level of injury, degree of spinal shock, and phase and degree of recovery:

C-1 to C-3: Quadriplegia with total loss of muscular/respiratory function.
C-4 to C-5: Quadriplegia with impairment, poor pulmonary capacity, complete dependency for ADLs.
C-6 to C-7: Quadriplegia with some arm/hand movement allowing some independence in ADLs.
C-7 to C-8: Quadriplegia with limited use of thumb/fingers, increasing independence.
T-1 to L-1: Paraplegia with intact arm function and varying function of intercostal and abdominal muscles.
L-1 to L-2 or below: Mixed motor-sensory loss; bowel and bladder dysfunction.

CARE SETTING

Inpatient medical/surgical and subacute/rehabilitation units.

RELATED CONCERNS

Fractures, p 659
Disc Surgery, p 267
Pneumonia: Microbial, p 130
Psychosocial Aspects of Care, p 783
Thrombophlebitis: Deep Vein Thrombosis, p 107
Total Nutritional Support: Parenteral/Enteral Feeding, p 491
Upper Gastrointestinal/Esophageal Bleeding, p 315
Ventilatory Assistance (Mechanical), p 176

Patient Assessment Data Base

ACTIVITY/REST

May exhibit: Paralysis of muscles (flaccid during spinal shock) at/below level of lesion
Muscle/generalized weakness (cord contusion and compression)

CIRCULATION

May report: Palpitations
Dizziness with position changes

May exhibit: Low BP, postural BP changes, bradycardia
Cool, pale extremities
Absence of perspiration in affected area

ELIMINATION

May exhibit: Incontinence of bladder and bowel
Urinary retention
Abdominal distention; loss of bowel sounds
Melena, coffee-ground emesis/hematemesis

EGO INTEGRITY

May report: Denial, disbelief, sadness, anger

May exhibit: Fear, anxiety, irritability, withdrawal

FOOD/FLUID

> **May exhibit:** Abdominal distention; loss of bowel sounds (paralytic ileus)

HYGIENE

> **May exhibit:** Variable level of dependence in ADLs

NEUROSENSORY

> **May report:** Numbness, tingling, burning, twitching of arms/legs
>
> **May exhibit:** Flaccid paralysis (spasticity may develop as spinal shock resolves, dependent on area of cord involvement)
> Loss of sensation (varying degrees may return after spinal shock resolves)
> Loss of muscle/vasomotor tone
> Loss of/asymmetric reflexes, including deep tendon reflexes
> Changes in pupil reaction, ptosis of upper eyelid
> Loss of sweating in affected area

PAIN/DISCOMFORT

> **May report:** Pain/tenderness in muscles
> Hyperesthesia immediately above level of injury
>
> **May exhibit:** Vertebral tenderness, deformity

RESPIRATION

> **May report:** Shortness of breath, "air hunger," inability to breathe
>
> **May exhibit:** Shallow/labored respirations; periods of apnea
> Diminished breath sounds, rhonchi
> Pallor, cyanosis

SAFETY

> **May exhibit:** Temperature fluctuations (taking on temperature of environment)

SEXUALITY

> **May report:** Expressions of concern about return to normal functioning
>
> **May exhibit:** Uncontrolled erection (priapism)
> Menstrual irregularities

TEACHING/LEARNING

> **Discharge plan considerations:** **DRG projected mean length of inpatient stay: 17.1 days (inclusive)**
> Will require varying degrees of assistance with transportation, shopping, food preparation, self-care, finances, medications/treatment, and homemaker/maintenance tasks.
> May require changes in physical layout of home and/or placement in a rehabilitative center.
>
> Refer to section at end of plan for postdischarge considerations.

DIAGNOSTIC STUDIES

Spinal x-rays: Locates level and type of bony injury (fracture, dislocation); determines alignment and reduction after traction or surgery.

CT scan: Locates injury, evaluates structural alterations. Useful for quick screening and providing addition information if x-rays questionable for fracture/cord status.

MRI: Identifies spinal cord lesions, edema, and compression.

Myelogram: May be done to visualize spinal column if pathology is unclear or if occlusion of spinal subarachnoid space is suspected (not usually done after penetrating injuries).

Somatosensory evoked potentials (SEP): Elicited by presenting a peripheral stimulus and measuring degree of latency in cortical response to evaluate spinal cord functioning/potential for recovery.

Chest x-ray: Demonstrates pulmonary status (e.g., changes in level of diaphragm, atelectasis).

Pulmonary function studies (vital capacity, tidal volume): Measures maximum volume of inspiration and expiration; especially important in patients with low cervical lesions or thoracic lesions with possible phrenic nerve and intercostal muscle involvement.

ABGs: Indicates effectiveness of gas exchange and ventilatory effort.

NURSING PRIORITIES

1. Maximize respiratory function.
2. Prevent further injury to spinal cord.
3. Promote mobility/independence.
4. Prevent or minimize complications.
5. Support psychologic adjustment of patient/SO.
6. Provide information about injury, prognosis and expectations, treatment needs, possible and preventable complications.

DISCHARGE GOALS

1. Ventilatory effort adequate for individual needs.
2. Spinal injury stabilized.
3. Complications prevented/controlled.
4. Self-care needs met by self/with assistance dependent on specific situation.
5. Beginning to cope with current situation and planning for future.
6. Condition/prognosis, therapeutic regimen, and possible complications understood.
7. Plan in place to meet needs after discharge.

NURSING DIAGNOSIS: Breathing Pattern, ineffective, risk for

Risk factors may include
Impairment of innervation of diaphragm (lesions at or above C-5)
Complete or mixed loss of intercostal muscle function
Reflex abdominal spasms; gastric distension

Possibly evidenced by
[Not applicable; presence of signs and symptoms establishes an *actual* diagnosis]

DESIRED OUTCOMES/EVALUATION CRITERIA—PATIENT WILL:
Maintain adequate ventilation as evidenced by absence of respiratory distress and ABGs within acceptable limits.
Demonstrate appropriate behaviors to support respiratory effort.

ACTIONS/INTERVENTIONS	RATIONALE
Independent	
Maintain patent airway: keep head in neutral position; elevate head of bed slightly if tolerated; use airway adjuncts as indicated.	Patients with high cervical injury and impaired gag/cough reflexes will require assistance in preventing aspiration/maintaining patent airway.
Suction as necessary. Document quality and quantity of secretions.	If cough is ineffective, suctioning may be needed to remove secretions, enhance gas distribution, and reduce risk of respiratory infections. *Note:* "Routine" suctioning increases risk of hypoxia, bradycardia (vagal response), tissue trauma. Therefore, suctioning needs are based on presence of/inability to move secretions.
Assess respiratory function by asking patient to take a deep breath. Note presence or absence of spontaneous effort and quality of respirations, e.g., labored, using accessory muscles.	C-1 to C-3 injuries result in complete loss of respiratory function. Injuries at C-4 or C-5 can result in variable loss of respiratory function, depending on phrenic nerve involvement and diaphragmatic function, but generally have decreased vital capacity and inspiratory effort. Injuries below C-6 or C-7 have respiratory muscle function preserved; however, weakness/impairment of intercostal muscles may impair effectiveness of cough, sigh, deep-breathing ability.
Auscultate breath sounds. Note areas of absent or decreased breath sounds or development of adventitious sounds (e.g., rhonchi).	Hypoventilation is common and leads to accumulation of secretions, atelectasis, and pneumonia (frequent complications).
Note strength/effectiveness of cough.	Level of injury determines function of intercostal muscles and ability to cough spontaneously/move secretions.
Assist with coughing (as indicated) by placing hands below diaphragm and pushing upward as patient exhales.	"Quad coughing" is performed to add volume to cough and to facilitate expectoration of secretions or to move them high enough to be suctioned out. *Note:* This procedure is usually performed only in stable persons some distance from acute injury.
Observe skin color for developing cyanosis, duskiness.	May reveal impending respiratory failure, need for immediate medical evaluation and intervention.
Assess for abdominal distention and muscle spasm.	Abdominal fullness may impede diaphragmatic excursion, reducing lung expansion and further compromising respiratory function.
Reposition/turn periodically. Avoid/limit prone position when indicated.	Enhances ventilation of all lung segments, mobilizes secretions, reducing risk of complications, e.g., atelectasis and pneumonia. *Note:* Prone position significantly decreases vital capacity, increasing risk of respiratory compromise, failure.
Encourage fluids (at least 2000 ml/d).	Aids in liquefying secretions, promoting mobilization/expectoration.
Monitor/limit visitors as indicated.	General debilitation and respiratory compromise place patient at increased risk for acquiring upper respiratory infections.
Elicit concerns/questions regarding mechanical ventilation devices.	Acknowledges reality of situation.

281

ACTIONS/INTERVENTIONS	RATIONALE
Independent	
Provide honest answers.	Future respiratory function/support needs will not be totally known until spinal shock resolves and acute rehabilitative phase is completed. Even though respiratory support may be required, alternative devices/techniques may be used to enhance mobility and promote independence.
Assist patient in "taking control" of respirations as indicated. Instruct in and encourage deep breathing, focusing attention on steps of breathing and so on.	Breathing may no longer be a totally voluntary activity but require conscious effort, depending on level of injury/involvement of respiratory muscles.
Monitor diaphragmatic movement when phrenic pacemaker is implanted.	Stimulation of phrenic nerve may enhance respiratory effort, decreasing dependency on mechanical ventilator.
Collaborative	
Measure/graph:	
Vital capacity, tidal volume, inspiratory force;	Determines level of respiratory muscle function. Serial measurements may be done to predict impending respiratory failure (acute injury) or determine level of function after spinal shock phase and/or while weaning from ventilatory support.
Serial ABGs and/or pulse oximetry.	Documents status of ventilation and oxygenation, identifies respiratory problems, e.g., hypoventilation (low PaO_2/elevated $PaCO_2$) and pulmonary complications.
Administer oxygen by appropriate method, e.g., nasal prongs, mask, intubation/ventilator.	Method is determined by level of injury, degree of respiratory insufficiency, and amount of recovery of respiratory muscle function after spinal shock phase.
Refer to/consult with respiratory and physical therapists.	Helpful in identifying exercises individually appropriate to stimulate and strengthen respiratory muscles/effort. For example, glossopharyngeal breathing uses muscles of mouth, pharynx, and larynx to swallow air into lungs, thereby enhancing vital capacity and chest expansion.
Assist with aggressive chest physiotherapy (e.g., chest percussion) and use of respiratory adjuncts (e.g., incentive spirometer, blow bottles).	Preventing retained secretions is essential to maximize gas diffusion and to reduce risk of pneumonia.

NURSING DIAGNOSIS: Trauma, risk for [additional spinal injury]

Risk factors may include
Temporary weakness/instability of spinal column

Possibly evidenced by
[Not applicable; presence of signs and symptoms establishes an *actual* diagnosis]

DESIRED OUTCOMES/EVALUATION CRITERIA—PATIENT WILL:
Maintain proper alignment of spine without further spinal cord damage.

ACTIONS/INTERVENTIONS	RATIONALE
Independent	
Maintain bed rest and immobilization device(s), e.g., sandbags, traction, halo, hard/soft cervical collars, brace.	Body rest prevents vertebral column instability and aids healing. *Note:* Traction is used *only* for cervical spine stabilization.
Check skeletal traction apparatus to ensure that frames are secure, pulleys aligned, weights hanging free.	Necessary for maintenance of specified traction for reduction and stabilization of vertebral column and prevention of further spinal cord injury.
Check weights for ordered traction pull (usually 10–20 lb).	Weight pull depends on patient's size and amount of reduction needed to maintain vertebral column alignment.
Elevate head of traction frame or bed as indicated.	Creates counterbalance to maintain both patient's position and traction pull.
Reposition at intervals, using adjuncts for turning and support, e.g., turn sheets, foam wedges, blanket rolls, pillows. Use several staff members when turning/logrolling patient. Follow special instructions for traction equipment, kinetic bed, and frames once halo is in place.	Maintains proper spinal column alignment reducing risk of further trauma. *Note:* Grasping the brace/halo vest to turn or reposition patient may cause additional injury.
Collaborative	
Maintain skeletal traction via tongs, calipers, halo/vest, as indicated.	Reduces vertebral fracture/dislocation.
Prepare for surgery, e.g., spinal laminectomy or fusion, if indicated.	Surgery may be indicated for spinal stabilization/cord decompression or removal of bony fragments.

NURSING DIAGNOSIS: Physical Mobility, impaired

May be related to
Neuromuscular impairment
Immobilization by traction

Possibly evidenced by
Inability to purposefully move; paralysis
Muscle atrophy; contractures

DESIRED OUTCOMES/EVALUATION CRITERIA—PATIENT WILL:
Maintain position of function as evidenced by absence of contractures, footdrop.
Increase strength of unaffected/compensatory body parts.
Demonstrate techniques/behaviors that enable resumption of activity.

ACTIONS/INTERVENTIONS	RATIONALE
Independent	
Continually assess motor function (as spinal shock/edema resolves) by requesting that patient perform actions, e.g., shrug shoulders, spread fingers, squeeze/release examiner's hands.	Evaluates status of individual situation (motor-sensory impairment may be mixed and/or not clear) for a specific level of injury affecting type and choice of interventions.

ACTIONS/INTERVENTIONS	RATIONALE
Independent	
Provide means to summon help, e.g., special sensitive call light.	Enables patient to have a sense of control and reduces fear of being left alone. *Note:* Quadriplegic on ventilator requires continuous observation in early management.
Perform/assist with full ROM exercises on all extremities and joints, using slow smooth movements. Hyperextend hips periodically.	Enhances circulation, restores/maintains muscle tone and joint mobility, and prevents disuse contractures and muscle atrophy.
Position arms at 90-degree angle at regular intervals.	Prevents frozen shoulder contractures.
Maintain ankles at 90 degrees with footboard, high-top tennis shoes, and so on. Use trochanter rolls along thighs when in bed.	Prevents footdrop and external rotation of hips.
Elevate lower extremities at intervals when in chair, or raise foot of bed when permitted in individual situation. Assess for edema of feet/ankles.	Loss of vascular tone and "muscle action" results in pooling of blood and venous stasis in the lower abdomen and lower extremities with increased risk of hypotension and thrombus formation.
Plan activities to provide uninterrupted rest periods. Encourage involvement within individual tolerance/ ability.	Prevents fatigue, allowing opportunity for maximal efforts/participation by patient.
Measure/monitor BP before and after activity in acute phases or until stable. Change position slowly. Use cardiac bed or tilt table/circoelectric bed as activity level is advanced.	Orthostatic hypotension may occur as a result of venous pooling (secondary to loss of vascular tone). Side-to-side movement or elevation of head can aggravate hypotension and cause syncope.
Reposition periodically even when sitting in chair. Teach patient how to employ weight-shifting techniques.	Reduces pressure areas, promotes peripheral circulation.
Prepare for weight-bearing activities, e.g., use of tilt table for upright position, strengthening/conditioning exercises for unaffected body parts.	Early weight bearing reduces osteoporotic changes in long bones and reduces incidence of urinary infections and kidney stones.
Encourage use of relaxation techniques.	Reduces muscle tension/fatigue, may help limit pain of muscle spasms, spasticity.
Inspect skin daily. Observe for pressure areas, and provide meticulous skin care. Teach patient to inspect skin surfaces and to use a mirror to look at hard-to-see areas.	Altered circulation, loss of sensation, and paralysis potentiate pressure sore formation. This is a life-long consideration. (Refer to ND: Skin Integrity, impaired, risk for, p 294.)
Assist with/encourage pulmonary hygiene, e.g., deep breathing, coughing, suctioning. (Refer to ND: Breathing Pattern, ineffective, risk for, p 280.)	Immobility/bed rest increases risk of pulmonary infection.
Assess for deep pain, redness, swelling/muscle tension of calf tissues. Record calf and thigh measurements if indicated.	In a high percentage of patients with cervical cord injury, thrombi develop because of altered peripheral circulation, immobilization, and flaccid paralysis.
Investigate sudden onset of dyspnea, cyanosis, and/or other signs of respiratory distress.	Development of pulmonary emboli may be "silent" because pain perception is altered and/or DVT is not readily recognized.

Collaborative

ACTIONS/INTERVENTIONS	RATIONALE
Place patient in kinetic therapy bed when appropriate.	Effectively immobilizes unstable spinal column, and improves systemic circulation, which is thought to decrease complications associated with immobility.
Apply antiembolic hose/leotard, sequential compression devices (SCD) to legs.	Limits pooling of blood in lower extremities or abdomen, thus improving vasomotor tone and reducing incidence of thrombus formation and pulmonary emboli.
Consult with physical/occupational therapists, rehabilitation team.	Helpful in planning and implementing individualized exercise program and identifying/developing assistive devices to maintain function, enhance mobility and independence.
Administer muscle relaxants as indicated, e.g., diazepam (Valium), baclofen (Lioresal), dantrolene (Dantrium).	May be useful in limiting or reducing pain associated with spasticity.

NURSING DIAGNOSIS: Sensory-Perceptual alterations (specify)

May be related to
Destruction of sensory tracts with altered sensory reception, transmission, and integration
Reduced environmental stimuli
Psychologic stress (narrowed perceptual fields caused by anxiety)

Possibly evidenced by
Measured change in sensory acuity, including position of body parts/proprioception
Change in usual response to stimuli
Motor incoordination
Anxiety, disorientation, bizarre thinking; exaggerated emotional responses

DESIRED OUTCOMES/EVALUATION CRITERIA—PATIENT WILL:
Recognize sensory impairments.
Identify behaviors to compensate for deficits.
Verbalize awareness of sensory needs and potential for deprivation/overload.

ACTIONS/INTERVENTIONS	RATIONALE
Independent	
Assess/document sensory function or deficit (by means of touch, pinprick, hot/cold, and so on), progressing from area of deficit to neurologically intact area.	Changes may not occur during acute phase, but as spinal shock resolves, changes should be documented by dermatome charts or anatomic landmarks, e.g., "2 inches above nipple line."
Protect from bodily harm, e.g., falls, burns, positioning of arm or objects.	Patient may not sense pain or be aware of body position.
Assist the patient to recognize and compensate for alterations in sensation.	May help reduce anxiety of the unknown and prevent injury.
Explain procedures prior to and during care, identifying the body part involved.	Enhances patient perception of "whole" body.

ACTIONS/INTERVENTIONS	RATIONALE

Independent

Provide tactile stimulation, touching patient in intact sensory areas, e.g., shoulders, face, head.	Touching conveys caring and fulfills a normal physiologic and psychologic need.
Position patient to see surroundings and activities. Provide prism glasses when prone on turning frame. Talk to patient frequently.	Provides sensory input, which may be severely limited, especially when patient is in prone position.
Provide diversional activities, e.g., television, radio, music, liberal visitation. Use clocks, calendars, pictures, bulletin boards, and so on. Encourage SO/family to discuss general and personal news.	Aids in maintaining reality orientation and provides some sense of normality in daily passage of time.
Provide uninterrupted sleep and rest periods.	Reduces sensory overload, enhances orientation and coping abilities, and aids in reestablishing natural sleep patterns.
Note presence of exaggerated emotional responses, altered thought processes, e.g., disorientation, bizarre thinking.	Indicative of damage to sensory tracts and/or psychologic stress, requiring further assessment and intervention.

NURSING DIAGNOSIS: Pain [acute]

May be related to
Physical injury
Traction apparatus

Possibly evidenced by
Hyperesthesia immediately above level of injury
Burning pain below level of injury (paraplegia)
Muscle spasm/spasticity
Phantom pain; headaches

DESIRED OUTCOMES/EVALUATION CRITERIA—PATIENT WILL:
Report relief or control of pain/discomfort.
Identify ways to manage pain.
Demonstrate use of relaxation skills and diversional activities as individually indicated.

ACTIONS/INTERVENTIONS	RATIONALE

Independent

Assess for presence of pain. Help patient identify and quantify pain, e.g., location, type of pain, intensity on scale of 0–10.	Patient usually reports pain above the level of injury, e.g., chest/back or headache possibly from stabilizer apparatus. After spinal shock phase, patient may report muscle spasms and phantom pain below level of injury.
Evaluate increased irritability, muscle tension, restlessness, unexplained vital sign changes.	Nonverbal cues indicative of pain/discomfort requiring intervention.
Assist patient in identifying precipitating factors.	Burning pain and muscle spasms can be precipitated/aggravated by multiple factors, e.g., anxiety, tension, external temperature extremes, sitting for long periods, bladder distention.

ACTIONS/INTERVENTIONS

Independent

Provide comfort measures, e.g., position changes, massage, ROM exercises warm/cold packs, as indicated.

Encourage use of relaxation techniques, e.g., guided imagery, visualization, deep-breathing exercises. Provide diversional activities, e.g., television, radio, telephone, unlimited visitors.

Collaborative

Administer medications as indicated: muscle relaxants, e.g., dantrolene (Dantrium), baclofen (Lioresal); analgesics; antianxiety agents, e.g., diazepam (Valium).

RATIONALE

Alternate measures for pain control are desirable for emotional benefit, in addition to reducing pain medication needs/undesirable effects on respiratory function.

Refocuses attention, promotes sense of control, and may enhance coping abilities.

May be desired to relieve muscle spasm/pain associated with spasticity or to alleviate anxiety and promote rest.

NURSING DIAGNOSIS: Grieving, anticipatory

May be related to
Perceived/actual loss of physiopsychosocial well-being

Possibly evidenced by
Altered communication patterns
Expression of distress, choked feelings, e.g., denial, guilt; fear, sadness; altered affect
Alterations in sleep patterns

DESIRED OUTCOMES/EVALUATION CRITERIA—PATIENT WILL:
Express feelings and begin to progress through recognized stages of grief, focusing on 1 day at a time.

ACTIONS/INTERVENTIONS

Independent

Identify signs of grieving (e.g., shock, denial, anger, depression).

Shock

Note lack of communication or emotional response, absence of questions.

Provide simple, accurate information to patient and SO regarding diagnosis and care. Be honest: do not give false reassurance while providing emotional support.

Encourage expressions of sadness, grief, guilt and fear among patient/SO/friends.

RATIONALE

Patient experiences many emotional reactions to the injury and its actual/potential impact on life. These stages are not static, and the rate at which the patient progresses through them is variable.

Shock is the initial reaction associated with overwhelming injury. Primary concern is to maintain life, and patient may be too ill to express feelings.

Patient's awareness of surroundings and activity may be blocked initially, and attention span may be limited. Little is actually known about the final outcome of the patient's injuries during acute phase, and knowledge may add to frustration and grief of family. Therefore, early focus of emotional support may be directed toward SO.

Knowledge that these are appropriate feelings that should be expressed may be very supportive to patient/SO.

ACTIONS/INTERVENTIONS	RATIONALE
Independent	
Incorporate SO into problem solving and planning for patient's care.	Assists in establishing therapeutic relationships. Provides some sense of control of situation of many losses/forced changes and promotes well-being of patient.
Denial	
Assist patient/SO to verbalize feelings about situation, avoiding judgment about what is expressed.	Important beginning step to deal with what has happened. Helpful in identifying patient's coping mechanisms.
Note comments indicating that patient expects to walk shortly and/or is making a bargain with God. Do not confront these comments in early phases of rehabilitation.	Patient may not deny entire disability but may deny its permanency. Situation is compounded by actual uncertainty of outcome, and denial may be useful for coping at this time.
Focus on present needs (e.g., ROM exercises, skin care).	Attention on "here and now" reduces frustration and hopelessness of uncertain future and may make dealing with today's problems more manageable.
Anger	
Identify use of manipulative behavior and reactions to caregivers.	Patient may express anger verbally or physically (e.g., spitting, biting). Patient may say that nothing is done right by caregivers/SO or may pit one caregiver against another.
Encourage patient to take control when possible, e.g., establishing care routines, dietary choices, diversional activities.	Helps reduce anger associated with powerlessness and provides patient with some sense of control and expectation of responsibility for own behavior.
Accept expressions of anger and hopelessness. Avoid arguing. Show concern for the patient.	Patient is acknowledged as a worthwhile individual, and nonjudgmental care is provided.
Set limits on acting-out and unacceptable behavior when necessary (e.g., abusive language, sexually aggressive or suggestive behavior).	Although it is important to express negative feelings, patient and staff need to be protected from violence and embarrassment. This phase is traumatic for all involved, and support of family is essential.
Depression	
Note loss of interest in living, sleep disturbance, suicidal thoughts, hopelessness. Listen to but do not confront these expressions. Let patient know nurse is available for support.	Phase may last weeks, months, or even years. Acceptance of these feelings and consistent support during this phase is important to a satisfactory resolution.
Arrange visit by individual similarly affected, as appropriate.	Talking with another person who has shared similar feelings/fears and survived may help patient reach acceptance of reality of condition and deal with perceived/actual losses.
Collaborative	
Consult with/refer to psychiatric nurse, social worker, psychiatrist, pastor.	Patient/SO will need assistance to work through feelings of alienation, guilt, and resentment concerning lifestyle and role changes. The family (required to make adaptive changes to a member who may be permanently "different") will benefit from supportive, long-term assistance and/or counseling in coping with these changes and the future. Patient and SO may suffer great spiritual distress, including feelings of guilt, deprivation of peace, and anger at God, which may interfere with resolution of grief process.

NURSING DIAGNOSIS: Self Esteem, situational low

May be related to

Traumatic injury; situational crisis; forced crisis

Possibly evidenced by

Verbalization of forced change in lifestyle

Fear of rejection/reaction by others

Focus on past strength, function, or appearance

Negative feelings about body

Feelings of helplessness, hopelessness, or powerlessness

Actual change in structure and/or function

Lack of eye contact

Change in physical capacity to resume role

Confusion about self, purpose, or direction of life

DESIRED OUTCOMES/EVALUATION CRITERIA—PATIENT WILL:

Verbalize acceptance of self in situation.

Recognize and incorporate changes into self-concept in accurate manner without negating self-esteem.

Develop realistic plans for adapting to new role/role changes.

ACTIONS/INTERVENTIONS	RATIONALE
Independent	
Acknowledge difficulty in determining degree of func7tional incapacity and/or chance of functional improvement.	During acute phase of injury, long-term effects are unknown, which delays the patient's ability to integrate situation into self-concept.
Listen to patient's comments and responses to situation.	Provides clues to view of self, role changes, and needs and is useful for providing information at patient's level of acceptance.
Assess dynamics of patient and SOs (e.g., patient's role in family, cultural factors).	Patient's previous role in family unit is disrupted or altered by injury, adding to difficulty in integrating self-concept. In addition, issues of independence/dependence need to be addressed.
Encourage SO to treat patient as normally as possible (e.g., discussing home situations, family news).	Involving patient in family unit reduces feelings of social isolation, helplessness, and uselessness and provides opportunity for SO to contribute to patient's welfare.
Provide accurate information. Discuss concerns about prognosis and treatment honestly at patient's level of acceptance.	Focus of information should be on present and immediate needs initially and incorporated into long-term rehabilitation goals. Information should be repeated until patient has assimilated or integrated information.
Discuss meaning of loss or change with patient/SO. Assess interactions between patient and SO.	Actual change in body image may be different from that perceived by patient. Distortions may be unconsciously reinforced by SO.

ACTIONS/INTERVENTIONS	RATIONALE
Independent	
Accept patient, show concern for individual as a person. Encourage patient, identify and build on strengths, give positive reinforcement for progress noted.	Establishes therapeutic atmosphere for patient to begin self-acceptance.
Include patient/SO in care, allowing patient to make decisions and to participate in self-care activities as possible.	Recognizes that patient is still responsible for own life and provides some sense of control over situation. Sets stage for future lifestyle, pattern, and interaction required in daily care. *Note:* Patient may reject all help or may be completely dependent during this phase.
Be alert to sexually oriented jokes/flirting or aggressive behavior. Elicit concerns, fears, feelings about current situation/future expectations.	Anxiety develops as a result of perceived loss/change in masculine/feminine self-image and role. Forced dependency is often devastating especially in light of change in function/appearance.
Be aware of own feelings/reaction to patient's sexual anxiety.	Behavior may be disruptive, creating conflict between patient/staff, further reinforcing negative feelings and possibly eliminating patient's desire to work through situation/participate in rehabilitation.
Arrange visit by similarly affected person if patient desires and/or situation allows.	May be helpful to patient by providing hope for the future/role model.
Collaborative	
Refer to counseling/psychotherapy as indicated, e.g., psychiatric nurse/clinical specialist, psychiatrist, social worker, sex therapist.	May need additional assistance to adjust to change in body image/life.

NURSING DIAGNOSIS: Bowel Incontinence/Constipation

May be related to
Disruption of innervation to bowel and rectum
Perceptual impairment
Altered dietary and fluid intake
Change in activity level

Possibly evidenced by
Loss of ability to evacuate bowel voluntarily
Constipation
Gastric dilatation, ileus

DESIRED OUTCOMES/EVALUATION CRITERIA—PATIENT WILL:
Verbalize behaviors/techniques for individual bowel program.
Reestablish satisfactory bowel elimination pattern.

ACTIONS/INTERVENTIONS	RATIONALE
Independent	
Auscultate bowel sounds, noting location and characteristics.	Bowel sounds may be absent during spinal shock phase. High tinkling sounds may indicate presence of ileus.

ACTIONS/INTERVENTIONS	RATIONALE

Independent

Observe for abdominal distention if bowel sounds are decreased or absent.

Loss of peristalsis (related to impaired innervation) paralyzes the bowel, creating ileus and bowel distention. *Note:* Overdistention of the bowel is a precipitator of autonomic dysreflexia once spinal shock subsides. (Refer to ND: Dysreflexia, risk for, p 293.)

Note reports of nausea, onset of vomiting. Check vomitus or gastric secretions (if tube in place) and stools for occult blood.

GI bleeding may occur in response to injury (Cushing's ulcer) or as a side effect of certain therapies (steroids or anticoagulants).

Record frequency, characteristics, and amount of stool.

Identifies degree of impairment/dysfunction and level of assistance required.

Recognize signs of/check for presence of impaction, e.g., no formed stool for several days, semiliquid stool, restlessness, increased feelings of fullness in abdomen.

Early intervention is necessary to effectively treat constipation/retained stool and reduce risk of complications.

Establish regular daily bowel program.

This lifelong program is necessary to routinely evacuate the bowel and usually includes digital stimulation, prune juice and/or warm beverage, and use of stool softeners/suppositories at set intervals. Ability to control bowel evacuation is important to the patient's physical independence and social acceptance. *Note:* Bowel movements in patient with upper motor neuron damage are generally regulated with suppositories or digital stimulation. Lower motor neurogenic bowel is more difficult to regulate and usually requires manual disimpaction.

Encourage well-balanced diet that includes bulk and roughage as well as increased fluid intake (at least 2000 ml/d), including fruit juices.

Improves consistency of stool for transit through the bowel.

Observe for incontinence and help patient relate incontinence to change in diet or routine.

Patient can eventually achieve fairly normal routine bowel habits, which enhance independence, self-esteem, and socialization.

Provide meticulous skin care.

Loss of sphincter control and innervation in the area potentiates risk of skin irritation/breakdown.

Collaborative

Insert/maintain nasogastric tube and attach to suction if appropriate.

May be used initially to reduce gastric distention and prevent vomiting (reduces risk of aspiration).

Consult with dietitian/nutritional support team.

Aids in creating dietary plan to meet individual nutritional needs with consideration of state of digestion/bowel function.

Insert rectal tube as needed.

Reduces bowel distention, which may precipitate autonomic responses.

Administer medications as indicated:

Stool softeners, laxatives, suppositories, enemas;

Stimulates peristalsis and routine bowel evacuation when necessary.

Antacids, cimetidine (Tagamet), ranitidine (Zantac).

Reduces or neutralizes gastric acid to lessen gastric irritation and risk of bleeding.

291

ACTIONS/INTERVENTIONS

Independent

Assess voiding pattern, e.g., frequency and amount. Compare urine output with fluid intake. Note specific gravity.

Palpate for bladder distention and observe for overflow.

Encourage fluid intake (2–4 L/d), including acid ash juices (e.g., cranberry).

Begin bladder retraining per protocol when appropriate e.g., fluids between certain hours, digital stimulation of trigger area, contraction of abdominal muscles, Credé's maneuver.

Observe for cloudy or bloody urine, foul odor.

Cleanse perineal area and keep dry. Provide catheter care as appropriate.

Collaborative

Keep bladder deflated by means of indwelling catheter initially. Begin intermittent catheterization program when appropriate.

RATIONALE

Identifies characteristics of bladder function (e.g., effectiveness of bladder emptying, renal function, and fluid balance).

Bladder dysfunction is variable but may include loss of bladder contraction/inability to relax urinary sphincter, resulting in urine retention and reflux incontinence. *Note:* Bladder distention can precipitate autonomic dysreflexia. (Refer to ND: Dysreflexia, risk for, following.)

Helps maintain renal function, prevents infection and formation of urinary stones. *Note:* Fluid may be restricted for a period during initiation of intermittent catheterization.

Timing and type of bladder program are dependent on type of injury (upper or lower neuron involvement). *Note:* Credé's maneuver should be used with caution because it may precipitate autonomic dysreflexia.

Signs of urinary tract or kidney infection that can potentiate sepsis.

Decreases risk of skin irritation/breakdown and development of ascending infection.

Indwelling catheter is used during acute phase for prevention of urinary retention and for monitoring output. Intermittent catheterization may be implemented to reduce complications usually associated with long-term use of indwelling catheters. A suprapubic catheter may also be inserted for long-term management.

ACTIONS/INTERVENTIONS

Collaborative

Monitor BUN, creatinine, WBC.

Administer medications as indicated, e.g., vitamin C, and/or urinary antiseptics, e.g., methenamine mandelate (Mandelamine).

RATIONALE

Reflects renal function, identifies complications.

Maintains acidic environment and discourages bacterial growth.

NURSING DIAGNOSIS: Dysreflexia, risk for

Risk factors may include
Altered nerve function (spinal cord injury at T-6 and above)
Bladder/bowel/skin stimulation (tactile, pain, thermal)

Possibly evidenced by
[Not applicable; presence of signs and symptoms establishes an *actual* diagnosis]

DESIRED OUTCOMES/EVALUATION CRITERIA—PATIENT WILL:
Recognize signs/symptoms of syndrome.
Identify preventive/corrective measures.
Experience no episodes of dysreflexia.

ACTIONS/INTERVENTIONS

Independent

Identify/monitor precipitating risk factors, e.g., bladder/bowel distention or manipulation; bladder spasms, stones, infection; skin/tissue pressure areas, prolonged sitting position; temperature extremes/drafts.

Observe for signs/symptoms of syndrome, e.g., changes in vital signs, paroxysmal hypertension, tachycardia, or bradycardia, autonomic responses: sweating, flushing above level of lesion, pallor below injury, chills, gooseflesh, nasal stuffiness, diffuse headache. Note associated symptoms, e.g., chest pains, blurred vision, nausea, metallic taste, Horner's syndrome.

Stay with patient during episode.

Monitor BP frequently (3–5 minutes) during acute autonomic dysreflexia, and take action to eliminate stimulus. Continue to monitor BP at intervals after symptoms subside.

Elevate head of bed to 45-degree angle or place in sitting position.

RATIONALE

Visceral distention is the most common cause of autonomic dysreflexia, which is considered an emergency. Treatment of acute episode must be carried out immediately (removing stimulus, treating unresolved symptoms), then interventions must be geared toward prevention.

Early detection and immediate intervention is essential to prevent serious consequences/complications.

This is a potentially fatal complication. Continuous monitoring/intervention may reduce patient's level of anxiety.

Aggressive therapy/removal of stimulus may drop BP rapidly resulting in a hypotensive crisis, especially in those patients who routinely have a low BP. In addition, autonomic dysreflexia may recur, particularly if stimulus is not eliminated.

Lowers BP to prevent intracranial hemorrhage, seizures, or even death. *Note:* Placing quadriplegic in sitting position automatically lowers BP.

ACTIONS/INTERVENTIONS	RATIONALE
Independent	
Correct/eliminate causative stimulus as able, e.g., bladder, bowel, skin pressure (including loosening tight leg bands/clothing), temperature extremes.	Removing noxious stimulus usually terminates episode and may prevent more serious autonomic dysreflexia, e.g., in the presence of sunburn, topical anesthetic should be applied. *Note:* Removal of bowel impaction must be delayed until cardiovascular condition is stabilized.
Inform patient/SO of warning signals and how to avoid onset of syndrome, e.g., gooseflesh, sweating, piloerection may indicate full bowel; sunburn may precipitate episode.	This lifelong problem can be largely controlled by the avoidance of pressure from overdistention of visceral organs or pressure on the skin.
Collaborative	
Administer medications as indicated and monitor response:	
Ganglion blockers, e.g., trimethaphan camsylate (Arfonad);	Blocks excessive autonomic nerve transmission.
Atropine sulfate;	Increases heart rate if bradycardia occurs.
Diazoxide (Hyperstat), hydralazine (Apresoline);	Reduces BP if severe/sustained hypertension occurs.
Nifedipine (Procardia);	Sublingual administration may be effective in absence of IV access for Hyperstat.
Adrenergic blockers, e.g., methysergide maleate (Sansert);	May be used prophylactically if problem persists/recurs frequently.
Antihypertensives, e.g., prazosin (Minipress), phe7noxybenzamine (Dibenzyline).	Long-term use may relax bladder neck/enhance bladder emptying, alleviating the most common cause of chronic autonomic dysreflexia.
Obtain urinary culture as indicated.	Presence of infection may trigger autonomic dysreflexia episode.
Apply local anesthetic ointment to rectum; remove impaction if indicated after symptoms subside.	Ointment blocks further autonomic stimulation and eases later removal of impaction without aggravating symptoms.
Prepare patient for pelvic/pudendal nerve block or posterior rhizotomy if indicated.	Procedures may be considered if autonomic dysreflexia does not respond to other therapies.

NURSING DIAGNOSIS: Skin Integrity, impaired, risk for

Risk factors may include
Altered/inadequate peripheral circulation; sensation
Presence of edema; pressure
Altered metabolic state
Immobility, traction apparatus

Possibly evidenced by
[Not applicable; presence of signs and symptoms establishes an *actual* diagnosis]

DESIRED OUTCOMES/EVALUATION CRITERIA—PATIENT WILL:
Identify individual risk factors.
Verbalize understanding of treatment needs.
Participate to level of ability to prevent skin breakdown.

ACTIONS/INTERVENTIONS	RATIONALE

Independent

Inspect all skin areas, noting capillary blanching/refill, redness, swelling. Pay particular attention to back of head, skin under halo frame or vest, and folds where skin continuously touches.

Skin is especially prone to breakdown because of changes in peripheral circulation, inability to sense pressure, immobility, altered temperature regulation.

Observe halo and tong insertion sites. Note swelling, redness, drainage. Cleanse routinely and apply antibiotic ointment per protocol.

These sites are prone to inflammation and infection and provide route for pathologic microorganisms to enter cranial cavity.

Massage and lubricate skin with bland lotion/oil. Protect pressure points by use of heel/elbow pads, lamb's wool, foam padding, egg-crate mattress. Use skin hardening agents, e.g., tincture of benzoin, Karaya, Sween cream.

Enhances circulation and protects skin surfaces, reducing risk of ulceration. Quadriplegic and paraplegic patients require lifelong protection from decubiti formation, which can cause extensive tissue necrosis and sepsis.

Reposition frequently, whether in bed or in sitting position. Place in prone position periodically.

Improves skin circulation and reduces pressure time on bony prominences.

Wash and dry skin, especially in high moisture areas such as perineum. Take care to avoid wetting lining of brace/halo vest.

Clean, dry skin is less prone to excoriation/breakdown.

Keep bedclothes dry and free of wrinkles, crumbs.

Reduces/prevents skin irritation.

Encourage continuation of regular exercise program.

Stimulates circulation, enhancing cellular nutrition/oxygenation to improve tissue health.

Elevate lower extremities periodically, if tolerated.

Enhances venous return. Reduces edema formation.

Avoid/limit injection of medication below the level of injury.

Reduced circulation and sensation increase risk of delayed absorption, local reaction, and tissue necrosis.

Collaborative

Provide kinetic therapy or alternating-pressure mattress as indicated.

Improves systemic and peripheral circulation and decreases pressure on skin, reducing risk of breakdown.

NURSING DIAGNOSIS: Knowledge deficit [learning need] regarding condition, prognosis, treatment, self care and discharge needs

May be related to
Lack of exposure
Information misinterpretation
Unfamiliarity with information resources

Possibly evidenced by
Questions; statement of misconception; request for information
Inadequate follow-through of instruction
Inappropriate or exaggerated behaviors, e.g., hostile, agitated, apathetic
Development of preventable complication(s)

DESIRED OUTCOMES/EVALUATION CRITERIA—PATIENT WILL:
Participate in learning process.
Verbalize understanding of condition, prognosis, and treatment.
Correctly perform necessary procedures and explain reasons for the actions.
Initiate necessary lifestyle changes and participate in treatment regimen.

ACTIONS/INTERVENTIONS	RATIONALE

Independent

Discuss injury process, current prognosis, and future expectations.

Provides common knowledge base necessary for making informed choices and commitment to the therapeutic regimen.

Provide information and demonstrate:

Positioning;

Promotes circulation; reduces tissue pressure and risk of complications.

Use of pillows/supports, splints.

Keeps spine aligned and prevents/limits contractures, thus improving function and independence.

Encourage continued participation in daily exercise and conditioning program and avoidance of fatigue/chills.

Reduces spasticity, risk of thromboemboli (common complication). Increases mobility, muscle strength and tone for improving organ/body function, e.g., squeezing rubber ball, arm exercises enhance upper body strength to increase independence in transfers/wheelchair mobility; tightening/contracting rectum or vaginal muscles improves bladder control; pushing abdomen up, bearing down, contracting abdomen strengthens trunk and improves GI function (paraplegic).

Have SO/caregivers participate in patient care and demonstrate proper procedures, e.g., applications of splints, braces, suctioning, positioning, skin care, transfers, bowel/bladder program, checking temperature of bath water and food.

Allows home caregivers to become adept and more comfortable with the care tasks they are called on to provide and reduces risk of injury/complications.

Recommend applying abdominal binder before arising (quadriplegic) and remind to change position slowly. Use safety belt and adequate number of people during bed-to-wheelchair transfers.

Reduces pooling of blood in abdomen/pelvis, minimizing postural hypotension. Protects the patient from falls and/or injury to caregivers.

Instruct in proper skin care, inspecting all skin areas daily, using adequate padding (foam, silicone gel, water pads) in bed and chair, and keeping skin dry.

Reduces skin irritation, decreasing incidence of decubitus (patient must manage this throughout life).

Discuss necessity of preventing excessive diaphoresis by using tepid bath water, providing comfortable environment (e.g., fans), removing excess clothes.

Reduces skin irritation/possible breakdown.

Review dietary needs including adequate bulk and roughage. Problem-solve solutions to alterations in muscular strength/tone and GI function.

Provides adequate nutrition to meet energy needs and promote healing, prevent complications (e.g., constipation, abdominal distention/gas formation).

Review medication regimen, including pain control techniques. Recommend avoidance of OTC drugs without approval of healthcare provider.

Enhances patient safety and may improve cooperation with specific regimen. *Note:* Pain often becomes chronic in patients with spinal cord injury. Dysesthetic pain (distal to site of injury) is extremely disabling (similar to phantom pain) and is usually treated with non-narcotic analgesics and TENS stimulator.

Discuss ways to identify and manage autonomic dysreflexia.

Patient may be able to recognize signs, but caregivers need to understand how to prevent precipitating factors and know what to do if autonomic dysreflexia occurs. (Refer to ND: Dysreflexia, risk for, p 293.)

Identify symptoms to report immediately to healthcare provider, e.g., infection of any kind, especially urinary, respiratory; skin breakdown; unresolved autonomic dysreflexia; suspected pregnancy.

Early identification allows for intervention to prevent/minimize complications.

ACTIONS/INTERVENTIONS	RATIONALE
Independent	
Stress importance of continuing with rehabilitation team to achieve specific functional goals as well as long-term monitoring of therapy needs.	No matter what the level of injury, individual may ultimately be able to exercise some independence, e.g., manipulate electric wheelchair with mouth stick (C-3/C-4); be independent for dressing, transfers to bed, car, toilet (C-7); total wheelchair independence (C-8 to T-4). Over time, new discoveries continue to modify equipment/therapy needs and patient's potential.
Evaluate home layout and make recommendations for necessary changes. Identify equipment/medical supply needs and resources.	Physical changes may be required to accommodate both patient and support equipment. Prior arrangements facilitate the transfer to the home setting.
Discuss sexual activity and reproductive concerns.	Concerns about individual sexuality/resumption of activity is frequently an *unspoken* concern that needs to be addressed. Spinal cord injury affects all areas of sexual functioning. In addition, choice of contraception is impacted by level of spinal cord injury and side effects/adverse complications of specific method. Finally, some female patients may develop autonomic dysreflexia during intercourse or labor/delivery.
Identify community resources/supports, e.g., health agencies, visiting nurse, financial counselor; service organizations, Spinal Cord Injury Foundation.	Enhances independence, assisting with home management, respite for caregivers.
Coordinate cooperation among community/rehabilitation resources.	Various agencies/therapists/individuals in community may be involved in the long-term care and safety of the patient, and coordination can ensure that needs are not overlooked and optimal level of rehabilitation is achieved.
Arrange for transmitter/emergency call system.	Provides for safety and access to emergency assistance and equipment.
Plan for alternate caregivers as needed.	May be needed to provide respite if regular caregivers are ill or other unplanned emergencies arise.

POTENTIAL CONSIDERATIONS following acute hospitalization (dependent on patient's age, physical condition/presence of complications, personal resources, and life responsibilities)

Disuse Syndrome, risk for—paralysis/mechanical immobilization.
Dysreflexia—bladder/bowel distention, skin irritation, lack of caregiver knowledge.
Self Care deficit—neuromuscular impairment, decreased strength/endurance, pain, depression.
Nutrition: altered, risk for (specify)—dysfunctional eating pattern, excessive/inadequate intake in relation to metabolic need.
Role Performance, altered/Sexual dysfunction—situational crisis and transition, altered body function.
Family Processes, altered—situational crisis and transition.
Caregiver Role Strain—discharge of family member with significant home care needs, situational stressors, such as significant loss, economic vulnerability; duration of caregiving required, lack of respite for caregiver, inexperience with caregiving, caregiver's competing role commitments.

MULTIPLE SCLEROSIS

Multiple sclerosis (MS) is the most common of the demyelinating disorders and the predominant CNS disease among young adults. It is a chronic disorder in which irregular demyelination of the central nervous system (brain and spinal cord) results in varying degrees of cognitive, motor and sensory dysfunction at the central and peripheral level, as well as emotional changes. MS is characterized by periods of exacerbations and remissions and is progressive in approximately 60% of patients. Individual prognosis is variable and unpredictable, presenting complex physical, psychosocial, and rehabilitative issues.

CARE SETTING

Community or long-term care with intermittent hospitalizations for disease-related complications.

RELATED CONCERNS

Long-Term Care, p 824
Pneumonia: Microbial, p 130
Psychosocial Aspects of Care, p 783
Sepsis/Septicemia, p 719

Patient Assessment Data Base

Degree of symptomatology is dependent on the stage of disease and extent, areas of neuronal involvement.

ACTIVITY/REST

May report: Extreme fatigue/weakness, exaggerated intolerance to activity, needing to rest after even simple activities such as shaving/showering; increased weakness/intolerance to temperature extremes, especially heat (i.e., summer weather, hot tubs)
Numbness, tingling in the extremities
Sleep disturbances, may awaken early or frequently for multiple reasons (e.g., nocturia, nocturnal spasticity, pain, worry, depression)

May exhibit: Absence of predictable pattern of symptoms
Generalized weakness, decreased muscle tone/mass (disuse), spasticity, tremors
Staggering, dragging of feet, ataxia
Intention tremors, decreased fine motor skills

CIRCULATION

May report: Dependent edema (steroid therapy or inactivity)

May exhibit: Blue/mottled, puffy extremities (inactivity)
Capillary fragility (especially on face)

EGO INTEGRITY

May report: Statements reflecting loss of self-esteem/body image
Expressions of grief
Anxiety/fear of exacerbations/progression of symptoms, pain, disability, rejection, pity
Keeping illness confidential
Feelings of helplessness, hopelessness, powerlessness (loss of control)
Personal tragedies (divorce, abandonment by SO/friends)
Difficult time with employment because of excessive fatigue/cognitive dysfunction, physical limitations

| **May exhibit:** | Denial, rejection |
| | Mood changes, irritability, restlessness, lethargy, euphoria, depression, anger |

ELIMINATION

May report: Nocturia
Incomplete bladder emptying, retention with overflow
Hesitancy or urgency (bowel/bladder)
Urinary/bowel incontinence of varying severity
Irregular bowel habits, constipation
Recurrent urinary tract infections

May exhibit: Loss of sphincter control
Kidney stone formation, kidney damage

FOOD/FLUID

May report: Difficulty chewing, swallowing (weak throat muscles), sense of food sticking in throat, coughing after swallowing
Problems getting food to mouth (related to intentional tremors of upper extremities)
Hiccups, possibly lasting extended periods

May exhibit: Difficulty feeding self
Weight loss
Decreased bowel sounds (slowed peristalsis)
Abdominal bloating

HYGIENE

May report: Difficulty with/dependence in some/all ADLs
Use of assistive devices/individual caregiver

May exhibit: Poor personal habits, disheveled appearance, signs of incontinence

NEUROSENSORY

May report: Weakness, nonsymmetric paralysis of muscles (may affect 1, 2, or 3 limbs, usually worse in lower extremities or may be unilateral), numbness, tingling (prickling sensations in parts of the body)
Change in visual acuity (diplopia), scotomas (holes in vision), eye pain (optic neuritis)
Moving head back and forth while watching television, difficulty driving (distorted visual field), blurred vision (difficulty focusing)
Memory loss, difficulty with incidental memory, retrieving/recalling, sorting out information (cerebral involvement)
Difficulty making decisions
Communication difficulties, such as coining words
Seizures

May exhibit: Mental status: Mood swings, depression, euphoria, irritability, apathy; lack of judgment; impairment of short-term memory; disorientation/confusion
Scanning speech, slow hesitant speech, poor articulation
Partial/total loss of vision in one eye; vision disturbances
Positional/vibration sense impaired or absent
Impaired touch/pain sensation
Facial/trigeminal nerve involvement, nystagmus, diplopia (brainstem involvement)
Loss of motor skills (major/fine), changes in muscle tone, spastic paresis/total immobility (advanced stages)

Ataxia, decreased coordination, tremors (may be originally misinterpreted as intoxication), intention tremor

Hyperreflexia, positive Babinski's sign, ankle clonus; absent superficial reflexes (especially abdominal).

PAIN/DISCOMFORT

May report: Painful spasms, burning pain along nerve path (some patients do not experience normal pain sensations)

Frequency: Varying, may be sporadic/intermittent (possibly once a day) or may be constant

Duration: Lightning-like, repetitive, intermittent; painful spasms of persistent long-term extremity or back pain

Facial neuralgia

Dull back pain

May exhibit: Distraction behaviors (restlessness, moaning), guarding

Self-focusing

SAFETY

May report: Uneasiness around small children or moving objects, fear of falling (weakness, decreased vision, slowed reflexes, loss of position sense, decreased judgment)

History of falls/accidental injuries

Use of ambulation devices

Vision impairment

Suicidal ideation

May exhibit: Wall/furniture walking

SEXUALITY

May report: Relationship stresses

Impotence/nocturnal erections or ejaculatory difficulties

Disturbances in sexual functioning (affected by nerve impairment, fatigue, bowel and bladder control, and vulnerability, and effects of medications)

Enhanced or decreased sexual desire

Problems with positioning

Genital anesthesia/hyperesthesia, decreased lubrication (female)

SOCIAL INTERACTION

May report: Lack of social activities/involvement

Withdrawal from interactions with others/isolation behaviors (e.g., stays at home/in room, watches TV all day)

Feelings of isolation (increased divorce rate/loss of friends)

May exhibit: Speech impairment

TEACHING/LEARNING

May report: Use of prescription/OTC medications, may forget to take regularly

Difficulty retaining information

Family history of disease (possibly due to common environmental/inherited factors)

Use of "holistic"/natural products/health care practices, "trying out cures"

DRG projected mean length of inpatient stay: 6.9 days.

| **Discharge plan considerations:** | May require assistance in any or all areas, depending on individual situation |
| | May eventually need total care/placement in assisted living/long-term care facility |

Refer to section at end of plan for postdischarge considerations.

DIAGNOSTIC STUDIES

MRI: Determines presence of plaques characteristic of MS that are due to the nerve sheaths demyelination (along with clinical symptoms, these findings are conclusive). *Note:* May be normal in up to 40% of patients during first year of disease process.

CT scan: Demonstrates brain lesions, ventricular enlargement or thinning.

Evoked potentials: Visual (VER), brainstem auditory (BAER), and somatosensory (SSER) may be abnormal early in disease process.

Lumbar puncture: CSF may show elevated levels of I_gG and I_gM. Protein level normal or only slightly elevated, oligoclonal bands present on electrophoresis; WBC slightly elevated; elevated concentration of myelin basic protein may be noted during active demyelination process.

EEG: May be mildly abnormal in some cases.

NURSING PRIORITIES

1. Maintain optimal functioning.
2. Assist with/provide for maintenance of ADLs.
3. Support acceptance of changes in body image/self-esteem and role performance.
4. Provide information about disease process/prognosis, therapeutic needs, and available resources.

DISCHARGE GOALS

1. Remains active within limits of individual situation.
2. ADLs are managed by patient/caregivers.
3. Changes in self-concept are acknowledged and being dealt with.
4. Disease process/prognosis, therapeutic regimen are understood and resources identified.
5. Plan in place to meet needs after discharge.

NURSING DIAGNOSIS: Fatigue

May be related to

Decreased energy production, increased energy requirements to perform activities

Psychologic/emotional demands

Pain/discomfort

Medication side effects

Possibly evidenced by

Verbalization of overwhelming lack of energy

Inability to maintain usual routines; decreased performance

Impaired ability to concentrate; disinterest in surroundings

Increase in physical complaints

DESIRED OUTCOMES/EVALUATION CRITERIA—PATIENT WILL:

Identify risk factors and individual actions affecting fatigue.

Identify alternatives to help maintain desired activity level.

Participate in recommended treatment program.

Report improved sense of energy.

ACTIONS/INTERVENTIONS	RATIONALE

Independent

Note and accept presence of fatigue.	The most common symptom of MS. Studies indicate that the fatigue encountered by patients with MS can be caused by expenditure of minimal energy, is more frequent and severe than "normal" fatigue, has a disproportionate impact on ADLs, has a slower recovery time, and may show no direct relationship between fatigue severity and neurologic status.
Identify/review factors affecting ability to be active, e.g., temperature extremes, inadequate food intake, insomnia, use of medications, time of day.	Provides opportunity to problem solve to maintain/improve mobility.
Accept when patient is unable to do activities.	Ability can vary from moment to moment. Nonjudgmental acceptance of the patient's evaluation of day-to-day variations in capabilities provides opportunity to promote independence while supporting fluctuations in level of required care.
Determine need for walking aids, e.g., Canadian canes, braces, walker, wheelchair, scooter; review safety considerations.	Mobility aids can decrease fatigue, enhancing independence and comfort, as well as safety. However, individual may display poor judgment about ability to safely engage in activity.
Schedule ADLs in AM as appropriate. Investigate use of cooling vest.	Fatigue commonly worsens in late afternoon (when body temperature rises). Some patients report lessening of fatigue with stabilization of body temperature.
Plan care with consistent rest periods between activities. Encourage afternoon nap.	Reduces fatigue, aggravation of muscle weakness.
Stress need for stopping exercise/activity just short of fatigue.	Pushing self beyond individual physical limits can result in excessive/prolonged fatigue and discouragement. Patient can become very adept at knowing where this limit is.

Collaborative

Recommend participation in groups involved in fitness/exercise and/or the Multiple Sclerosis Society.	Can help patient to stay motivated to remain active within the limits of the disability/condition. Group activities need to be selected carefully to meet the paetient's need(s) and prevent discouragement or anxiety.
Administer medications as indicated, e.g.:	
Amantadine (Symmetrel);	Positive antiviral drug effect in 30%–50% of patients. Use may be limited by side effects of increased spasticity, insomnia, paresthesias of hands/feet.
Pemoline (Cylert);	CNS stimulant may be effective when amatadine is ineffective/undesirable side effects develop.
Sertraline (Zoloft), fluoxetine (Prozac);	Antidepressants useful in lifting mood, "energizing" patient (especially when depression is a factor) and when patient is free of anticholinergic side effects.

ACTIONS/INTERVENTIONS

Collaborative

Tricyclic antidepressants, e.g., amitriptyline (Elavil), nortriptyline (Pamelor);

Tegretal (Carbamazepine);

Steroids, e.g., prednisone (Deltasone), dexamethasone (Decadron); pituitary hormones, (ACTH);

Vitamin B;

Immunosuppressives, e.g., cyclophosphamide (Cytoxin), azathioprine (Immuran), methotrexate (Mexate), interferon-β (Betaseron).

RATIONALE

Useful in treating emotional lability, neurogenic pain, and associated sleep disorders to enhance willingness to be more active.

Used to treat neurogenic pain as well as sudden intermittent spasms related to spinal cord irritation.

May be used during acute exacerbations to prevent edema at the sclerotic plaques; however, long-term therapy seems to have little effect on progression of symptoms. *Note:* Effects of ACTH are often unpredictable, limiting use.

Supports nerve-cell replication, enhances metabolic functions, and may increase sense of well-being/energy level (although reports are more anecdotal then research-based).

May be tried in effort to slow progression of disease, promote remission. Betaseron has been approved for use by ambulatory patients with remitting/relapsing MS and is the first drug found to alter the course of the disease.

NURSING DIAGNOSIS: Self Care deficit (specify)

May be related to
Neuromuscular/perceptual impairment; intolerance to activity; decreased strength and endurance; motor impairment, tremors
Pain, discomfort, fatigue
Memory loss
Depression

Possibly evidenced by
Frustration; inability to perform tasks of self-care

DESIRED OUTCOMES/EVALUATION CRITERIA—PATIENT WILL:
Identify individual areas of weakness/needs.
Demonstrate techniques/lifestyle changes to meet self-care needs.
Perform self-care activities within level of own ability.
Identify personal/community resources that provide assistance.

ACTIONS/INTERVENTIONS

Independent

Determine current activity level/physical condition. Assess degree of functional impairment using 0–4 scale.

Encourage patient to perform self-care to the maximum of ability as defined by the patient. Do not rush patient.

RATIONALE

Provides information to develop plan for care for rehabilitation. *Note:* Motor symptoms are less likely to improve than sensory ones.

Promotes independence and sense of control may decrease feelings of helplessness.

ACTIONS/INTERVENTIONS	RATIONALE

Independent

Assist according to degree of disability; allow as much autonomy as possible. Encourage patient input in planning schedule.	Participation in own care can ease the frustration over loss of independence. Patient's quality of life is enhanced when desires/likes are considered in daily activities.
Note presence of/accommodate for fatigue. Encourage scheduling activities earlier in the day.	Fatigue encountered by patients with MS can be very debilitating and greatly impact ability to participate in ADLs. The subjective nature of reports of fatigue can be misinterpreted by health care providers and family, leading to conflict and the belief that the patient is "manipulative" when in fact, this is not the case. Patients with MS expend more energy to complete ADLs, increasing the risk of fatigue, which often progresses through the day.
Allot sufficient time to perform task(s), and display patience when movements are slow.	Decreased motor skills/spasticity may interfere with ability to manage even simple activities.
Anticipate hygienic needs and assist as necessary with care of nails, skin, and hair; mouth care; shaving (use electric razor).	Example by caregiver can set a matter-of-fact tone for acceptance of handling mundane needs that may be embarrassing to patient/repugnant to SO.
Provide assistive devices/aids as indicated, e.g., shower chair, elevated toilet seat with arm supports.	Reduces fatigue, enhancing participation in self-care.
Reposition frequently when patient is immobile (bed/chairbound). Position/encourage to sleep prone as tolerated.	Reduces continued pressure on same areas, prevents skin breakdown. Minimizes flexor spasms at knees and hips.
Provide massage and active/passive range of motion exercises on a regular schedule. Encourage use of splints/footboards as indicated.	Prevents problems associated with muscle dysfunction and disuse. Helps to maintain muscle tone/strength and joint mobility and decreases risk of loss of calcium from bones.
Encourage stretching exercises and use of cold packs, splints when indicated.	Helps decrease spasticity.
Problem-solve ways to meet nutritional/fluid needs, e.g., wrap fork handle with tape, cut food, and show patient how to hold cup with both hands.	Provides for adequate intake and enhances patient's feelings of independence/self-esteem.

Collaborative

Consult with physical/occupational therapist.	Useful in identifying devices/equipment to relieve spastic muscles, improve motor functioning, prevent/reduce muscular atrophy and contractures; promoting independence and increasing sense of self-worth.
Administer medications as indicated, e.g.:	
Baclofen (Lioresal);	Drug of choice for spasticity, promoting muscle relaxation and inhibiting reflexes at the spinal nerve root level. Enhances mobility and maintenance of activity.
Diazepam (Valium); clonazepam (Klonopin);	Reduces spasticity by inhibiting spinal cord reflexes. *Note:* Used with caution because may exacerbate general weakness and produce CNS depression, further reducing mobility.

ACTIONS/INTERVENTIONS	RATIONALE
Collaborative	
Dantrolene (Dantrium);	Occasionally used for muscle relaxant properties to decrease spasticity; however, adverse effects may be increased muscle weakness, loss of muscle tone, and liver toxicity.
Meclizine (Antivert), scopolamine patches (TransdermScop);	Reduces dizziness, allowing patient to be more mobile.

NURSING DIAGNOSIS: Self Esteem (specify)

May be related to
Changes in structure/function
Disruption in how patient perceives own body
Role reversal; dependence

Possibly evidenced by
Confusion about sense of self, purpose, direction in life
Denial, withdrawal, anger
Negative/self-destructive behavior
Use of ineffective coping methods
Change in self/other's perception of role/physical capacity to resume role

DESIRED OUTCOMES/EVALUATION CRITERIA—PATIENT WILL:
Verbalize realistic view and acceptance of body as it is.
View self as a capable person.
Participate in and assume responsibility for meeting own needs.
Recognize and incorporate changes in self-concept/role without negating self-esteem.
Develop realistic plans for adapting to role changes.

ACTIONS/INTERVENTIONS	RATIONALE
Independent	
Establish/maintain a therapeutic nurse-patient relationship, discussing fears/concerns.	Conveys an attitude of caring and develops a sense of trust between patient and caregiver in which the patient is free to express fears of rejection, loss of previous functioning/appearance, feelings of helplessness, powerlessness about changes that may occur. Promotes a sense of well-being for the patient.
Note withdrawn behaviors/use of denial, or overconcern with body/disease process.	Initially may be a normal protective response, but if prolonged may prevent dealing appropriately with reality and may lead to ineffective coping.
Support use of defense mechanisms, allowing patient to deal with information in own time and way.	Confronting patient with reality of situation may result in increased anxiety and lessened ability to cope with changed self-concept/role.
Acknowledge reality of grieving process related to actual/perceived changes. Help patient deal realistically with feelings of anger and sadness.	Nature of the disease leads to ongoing losses and changes in all aspects of life, blocking resolution of grieving process.

ACTIONS/INTERVENTIONS	RATIONALE
Independent	
Review information about course of disease, possibility of remissions, prognosis.	When patient learns about disease, and becomes aware that own behavior (including maintaining a positive attitude) can significantly improve general well-being and daily functioning, the patient may feel more in control, enhancing sense of self-esteem. *Note:* Some patients may never have a remission.
Provide accurate verbal and written information about what is happening and discuss with patient/SO.	Helps patient to stay in the "here and now," reduces fear of the unknown, provides reference source for future use.
Explain that labile emotions are not unusual. Problem-solve ways to deal with these feelings.	Relieves anxiety and assists with efforts to manage unexpected emotional display.
Note presence of depression/impaired thought processes, expressions of suicidal ideation (evaluate on a scale of 1–10).	Adaptation to a long-term, progressively debilitating disease with a fatal outcome is a difficult emotional adjustment. In addition, brain damage may affect adaptation to these life changes. Individual may believe that suicide is the best way to deal with what is happening.
Assess interaction between patient and SO. Note changes in relationship.	SO may unconsciously/consciously reinforce negative attitudes and beliefs of the patient, or issues of secondary gain may interfere with progress and ability to manage situation.
Provide open environment for patient/SO to discuss concerns about sexuality.	Physical and psychologic changes often create stressors within the relationship, affecting usual roles/expectations, further impairing self-concept.
Collaborative	
Consult with occupational therapist/rehabilitation team.	Identifying assistive devices/equipment enhances level of function and participation in ADLs.
Refer to psychiatric clinical nurse specialist, social worker, psychologist as indicated.	May require more in-depth/supportive counseling to resolve conflicts, deal with life changes.

NURSING DIAGNOSIS: Caregiver Role Strain, risk for

Risk factors may include
Severity of illness of the care receiver, duration of caregiving required, complexity/amount of caregiving task
Caregiver is female, spouse
Care receiver exhibits deviant, bizarre behavior
Family/caregiver isolation; lack of respite and recreation

Possibly evidenced by
[Not applicable; presence of signs/symptoms establishes an *actual* diagnosis]

DESIRED OUTCOME/EVALUATION CRITERIA—CAREGIVER WILL:
Identify individual risk factors and appropriate interventions.
Demonstrate/initiate behaviors or lifestyle changes to prevent development of impaired function.
Use available resources appropriately.
Report satisfaction with plan and support available.

ACTIONS/INTERVENTIONS	RATIONALE
Independent	
Note physical/mental condition, therapeutic regimen of care receiver.	Determines individual needs for planning care. Identifies strengths and how much responsibility the patient may be expected to assume, as well as disabilities requiring accommodation.
Determine caregiver's level of commitment, responsibility, involvement in and anticipated length of care. Use assessment tool, such as Burden Interview, to further determine caregiver's abilities, when appropriate.	Progressive debilitation taxes caregiver and may alter ability to meet patient/own needs. (Refer to ND: Family Coping: ineffective compromised/disabling, p 310)
Discuss caregiver's view of and concerns about situation.	Allows ventilation and clarification of concerns, promoting understanding.
Determine available supports and resources currently used.	Provides information regarding adequacy of supports/current needs.
Facilitate family conference to share information and develop plan for involvement in care activities as appropriate.	When others are involved in care, the risk of one person becoming overloaded is lessened.
Identify additional resources to include financial, legal.	These areas of concern can add to burden of caregiving if not adequately resolved.
Identify equipment needs/resources, adaptive aids.	Enhances independence and safety of the care receiver.
Provide information and/or demonstrate techniques for dealing with acting-out/violent or disoriented behavior.	Helps caregiver to maintain sense of control and competency. Enhances safety for care receiver and giver.
Stress importance of self-nurturing, e.g., pursuing self-development interests, personal needs, hobbies, and social activities.	Taking time for self can lessen risk of "burnout"/being overwhelmed by situation.
Identify alternate care sources (such as sitter/day care facility), senior care services, e.g., meals on wheels/respite care, home care agency.	As patient's condition worsens, SO may need additional help from several sources to maintain patient at home even on a part-time basis.
Assist caregiver to plan for changes that may be necessary for the care receiver (e.g., eventual placement in long-term care facility).	Planning for this eventuality is important for the time when burden of care becomes too great.
Collaborative	
Refer to supportive services as need indicates.	Medical case manager or social services consultant may be needed to develop ongoing plan to meet changing needs of patient and SO/family.

NURSING DIAGNOSIS: Powerlessness [specify degree]/Hopelessness

May be related to

Illness-related regimen, unpredictability of disease

Lifestyle of helplessness

ACTIONS/INTERVENTIONS	RATIONALE
Independent	
Note behaviors indicative of powerlessness/hopelessness, e.g., statements of despair, "They don't care," "It won't make any difference."	The degree to which the patient believes own situation is hopeless, that he or she is powerless to change what is happening, affects how patient handles life situation.
Acknowledge reality of situation, at the same time expressing hope for the patient.	While the prognosis may be discouraging, remissions may occur; and because the future cannot be predicted, hope for some quality of life should be encouraged. Additionally, research is ongoing and new treatment options are being identified.
Determine degree of mastery patient has exhibited in life to the present. Note locus of control, i.e., internal/external.	The patient who has assumed responsibility in life previously will tend to do the same during difficult times of exacerbation of illness. However, if locus of control has been focused outward, patient may blame others and not take control over own circumstances.
Assist patient to identify factors that are under own control, e.g., list things that can or cannot be controlled.	Knowing and accepting what is beyond individual control can reduce helpless/acting out behaviors, promote focusing on areas individual can control.
Encourage patient to assume control over as much of own care as possible.	Even when unable to do much physical care, individual can help to plan care, having a voice in what is/is not desired.
Encourage/assist patient to identify activities he or she would like to be involved in (e.g., volunteer work) within the limits of his or her abilities.	Staying active and interacting with others counteracts feelings of helplessness.
Discuss needs openly with the patient/SO, setting up agreed-on routines for meeting identified needs.	Helps to deal with manipulative behavior, when patient feels powerless and not listened to.
Incorporate patient's daily routine into home care schedule/hospital stay, as possible.	Maintains sense of control/self-determination and independence.

ACTIONS/INTERVENTIONS

Independent

Discuss plans for the future. Suggest visiting alternate care facilities, taking a look at the possibilities for care as condition changes.

Collaborative

Refer to vocational rehabilitation as indicated.

Identify community resources e.g., adult day enrichment program.

RATIONALE

When options are considered and plans are made for any eventuality, patient has a sense of control over own circumstances.

Can assist patient to develop and impliment a vocational plan incorporating specific interests/abilities.

Participation in structured activities can reduce sense of isolation, and may enhance feeling of self-worth.

NURSING DIAGNOSIS: Coping, Individual, ineffective, risk for

Risk factors may include
Physiologic changes (cerebral and spinal lesions)
Psychologic conflicts; anxiety; fear
Impaired judgment, short-term memory loss; confusion; unrealistic perceptions/expectations, emotional lability
Personal vulnerability; inadequate support systems
Multiple life changes
Inadequate coping methods

Possibly evidenced by
[Not applicable; presence of signs and symptoms establishes an *actual* diagnosis]

DESIRED OUTCOMES/EVALUATION CRITERIA—PATIENT WILL:
Recognize relationship between disease process (cerebral lesions) and emotional responses, changes in thinking/behavior.
Verbalize awareness of own capabilities/strengths.
Display effective problem-solving skills.
Demonstrate behaviors/lifestyle changes to prevent/minimize changes in mentation and maintain reality orientation.

ACTIONS/INTERVENTIONS

Independent

Assess current functional capacity/limitations; note presence of distorted thinking processes, labile emotions, cognitive dissonance. Note how these affect the individual's coping abilities.

Determine patient's understanding of current situation and previous methods of dealing with life's problems.

Discuss ability to make decisions, care for children/dependent adults, handle finances, etc. Identify options available to individuals involved.

RATIONALE

Organic or psychologic effects may cause patient to be easily distracted; display difficulties with concentration; problem solving, dealing with what is happening, being responsible for own care.

Provides a clue to how the patient may deal with what is currently happening and helps identify individual resources and need for assistance.

Impaired judgment, confusion, inadequate support systems may interfere with ability to meet own needs/needs of others. Conservatorship, guardianship, or adult protective services may be required until (if ever) patient is able to manage own affairs.

ACTIONS/INTERVENTIONS

Independent

Maintain an honest, reality-oriented relationship.

Encourage verbalization of feelings/fears, accepting what patient says in a nonjudgmental manner. Note statements reflecting powerlessness, inability to cope. (Refer to ND: Powerlessness/Hopelessness, p 307–308.)

Observe nonverbal communication, e.g., posture, eye contact, movements, gestures, and use of touch. Compare with verbal content and verify meaning with patient as appropriate.

Provide clues for orientation, e.g., calendars, clocks, notecards, organizers/date book.

Encourage patient to tape-record important information and listen to it periodically.

Collaborative

Refer to cognitive retraining program.

Refer to counseling, psychiatric nurse clinical specialist/psychiatrist, as indicated.

RATIONALE

Reduces confusion and minimizes painful, frustrating struggles associated with adaptation to altered environment/lifestyle.

May diminish patient's fear, establish trust, and provide an opportunity to identify problems/begin the problem-solving process.

May provide significant information about what the patient is feeling; however, verification is important to ensure accuracy of communication. Discrepancy between feelings and what is being said can interfere with ability to cope, problem solve.

These serve as tangible reminders that aid recognition and permeate memory gaps and enable patient to cope with situation.

Repetition will put information in long-term memory, where it is more easily retrieved and can support decision-making/problem-solving process.

Improving cognitive abilities can enhance basic thinking skills when attention span is short; ability to process information is impaired; patient is unable to learn new tasks; or insight, judgment, and problem-solving skills are impaired.

May need additional help to resolve issues of self-esteem and regain effective coping skills.

NURSING DIAGNOSIS: Family Coping: ineffective compromised/disabling

May be related to

Situational crisis; temporary family disorganization and role changes

Highly ambivalent family relationships

Prolonged disease/disability progression that exhausts the supportive capacity of SO

Patient providing little support in turn for SO

SO with chronically unexpressed feelings of guilt, anxiety, hostility, despair

Possibly evidenced by

Patient expresses/confirms concern or complaint about SO response to patient's illness

SO withdraws or has limited personal communication with patient or displays protective behavior disproportionate to patient's abilities or need for autonomy

SO preoccupied with own personal reactions

Intolerance, abandonment

Neglectful care of the patient

Distortion of reality regarding patient's illness

DESIRED OUTCOMES/EVALUATION CRITERIA—FAMILY WILL:
Identify/verbalize resources within themselves to deal with the situation.
Express more realistic understanding and expectations of the patient.
Interact appropriately with the patient/staff, providing support and assistance as indicated.
Verbalize knowledge and understanding of disability/disease and community resources.

ACTIONS/INTERVENTIONS	RATIONALE
Independent	
Note length/severity of illness. Determine patient's role in family and how illness has changed the family organization.	Chronic/unresolved illness, accompanied by changes in role performance/responsibility, often exhausts supportive capacity and coping abilities of SO/family.
Determine SO's understanding of disease process and expectations for the future.	Inadequate information/misconception regarding disease process and/or unrealistic expectations affect ability to cope with current situation. *Note:* A particular area of misconception is the fatigue encountered by patients with MS. Family members may view the patient's inability to perform activities as manipulative behavior rather than an actual physiologic deficit.
Discuss with SO/family members their willingness to be involved in care. Identify other responsibilities/factors impacting participation.	Individuals may not have desire/time to assume responsibility for care. If several family members are available, they may be able to share tasks.
Assess other factors that are affecting abilities of family members to provide needed support, e.g., own emotional problems, work concerns.	Individual members' preoccupation with own needs/concerns can interfere with providing needed care/support for stresses of long-term illness. Additionally, caregiver(s) may incur ease of income/risk losing own health insurance if they alter their hours of work.
Discuss underlying reasons for patient's behaviors.	Helps SO understand and accept/deal with behaviors that may be triggered by emotional or physical effects of MS.
Encourage patient/SO to develop and strengthen problem-solving skills to deal with situation.	Family may/may not have handled conflict well before illness, and stress of long-term debilitating condition can create additional problems (including unresolved anger).
Encourage free expression of feelings, including frustration, anger, hostility, and hopelessness.	Individual members may be afraid to express "negative" feelings, believing it will discourage the patient. Free expression promotes awareness and can help with resolution of feelings and problems (especially when done in a caring manner).
Collaborative	
Identify community resources, e.g., local MS organization, support groups, home care agencies, respite programs.	Provides information, opportunities to share with others who are experiencing similar difficulties, and sources of assistance when needed.
Refer to social worker, financial adviser, psychiatric nurse specialist/psychiatrist as appropriate.	May need more in-depth assistance from professional sources.

311

ACTIONS/INTERVENTIONS

Independent

Note reports of frequency, urgency, burning, incontinence, nocturia, size of/force of urinary stream. Palpate bladder after voiding.

Institute bladder training program or timed voidings as appropriate.

Encourage adequate fluid intake, avoiding caffeine, and limiting intake during late evening and at bedtime. Recommend use of cranberry juice/vitamin C.

Promote continued mobility.

Recommend good hand-washing/perineal care.

Encourage patient to observe for sediment/blood in urine, foul odor, fever, or unexplained increase in MS symptoms (e.g., spasticity, dysarthia).

Collaborative

Catheterize as indicated.

Teach self-catheterization/instruct in use and care of indwelling catheter.

Obtain urine culture and sensitivity as indicated.

Administer medications as necessary, e.g.:

    Antimicrobial agent, nitrofurantoin macrocrystals (Macrodantin);

RATIONALE

Provides information about degree of interference with elimination or may indicate bladder infection. Fullness over bladder following void is indicative of inadequate emptying and requires intervention.

Helps to restore adequate bladder functioning; lessens occurrence of incontinence and bladder infection.

Sufficient hydration promotes urinary output and aids in preventing infection. *Note:* When patient is taking sulfa drugs, sufficient fluids are necessary to ensure adequate excretion of drug, reducing risk of cumulative effects.

Decreases risk of developing bladder and urinary tract infection.

Reduces skin irritation and risk of ascending infection.

Indicative of infection requiring further evaluation/treatment.

May be necessary if patient is unable to empty the bladder or retains urine.

Helps patient to maintain autonomy and encourages self-care. Indwelling catheter may be required dependent on patient's abilities and degree of urinary problem.

Colony count over 100,000 indicates presence of infection requiring treatment.

Bacteriostatic agent that inhibits bacterial growth. Prompt treatment of infection is necessary to prevent serious complications of sepsis/shock.

ACTIONS/INTERVENTIONS

Collaborative

Oxybutynin (Ditropan), propantheline (Pro-Banthine), hyoscyamine sulfate (Cytospaz), flavoxate hydrochloride (Urispaz).

RATIONALE

Reduce bladder spasticity and associated symptoms of frequency, urgency, incontinence, nocturia.

NURSING DIAGNOSIS: Knowledge deficit [learning need] regarding condition, prognosis, treatment, self care and discharge needs

May be related to
Lack of exposure; information misinterpretation
Unfamiliarity with information resources
Cognitive limitation, lack of recall

Possibly evidenced by
Statement of misconception
Request for information
Inaccurate follow-through of instruction
Inappropriate or exaggerated behaviors (e.g., hysterical, hostile, agitated, apathetic)

DESIRED OUTCOMES/EVALUATION CRITERIA—PATIENT WILL:
Participate in learning process.
Assume responsibility for own learning and begin to look for information and to ask questions.
Verbalize understanding of condition/disease process and treatment.
Initiate necessary lifestyle changes.
Participate in prescribed treatment regimen.

ACTIONS/INTERVENTIONS

Independent

Evaluate desire/readiness to learn.

Note signs of emotional lability or that patient is in dissociative state (loss of affect, inappropriate emotional responses).

Review disease process/prognosis, effects of climate, emotional stress, overexertion, fatigue.

Identify signs/symptoms requiring further evaluation.

Discuss importance of daily routine of rest, exercise, activity, eating, focusing on current capabilities. Instruct in use of appropriate devices to assist with ADLs, e.g., eating utensils, walking aids.

Discuss necessity of weight control.

Review possible problems that may arise such as decreased perception of heat and pain, susceptibility to skin breakdown, and infections, especially urinary tract infection.

RATIONALE

Determines amount/level of information to provide patient at any given moment.

Patient will not process/retain information and will have difficulty learning during this time.

Clarifies patient/SO understanding of individual situation.

Prompt intervention may help limit severity of exacerbation/complications.

Helps patient to maintain current level of physical independence and may limit fatigue.

Excess weight can interfere with balance and motor abilities and make care more difficult.

These effects of demyelination and associated complications may compromise patient's safety and/or precipitate an exacerbation of symptoms.

313

ACTIONS/INTERVENTIONS	RATIONALE
Independent	
Identify actions that can be taken to avoid injury: e.g., avoid hot baths, inspect skin regularly, take care with transfers and wheelchair/walker mobility, force fluids, and get adequate nutrition. Encourage avoidance of persons with upper respiratory infection.	Review of these factors can help patient take measures to maintain physical state at optimal level/prevent complications.
Identify bowel elimination concerns. Recommend adequate hydration and intake of fiber; use of stool softeners, bulking agents, suppositories, or possibly mild laxatives; bowel training program.	Constipation is common, and bowel urgency and/or accidents may occur as a result of dietary deficiencies or impaction.
Discuss/encourage options for enhancing/developing remaining skills, using diversional activities, continuing with usual interests as able.	Enables patient to maintain "active" quality of life.
Encourage patient to set goals for the future while focusing on the "here and now," what can be done today.	Having a plan for the future helps to retain hope as well as provide opportunity for patient to see that although today is to be lived, one can plan for tomorrow even in the worst of circumstances.
Identify financial concerns.	Loss or change of employment (for patient and/or SO) impacts income, insurance benefits, and level of independence, requiring additional family/social support.
Review specifics of individual medications. Recommend avoidance of OTC drugs.	Reduces likelihood of drug interactions/adverse effects and enhances cooperation with treatment regimen.
Discuss concerns regarding sexual relationships, contraception/reproduction, effects of pregnancy on affected woman. Identify alternate ways to meet individual needs; counsel regarding use of artificial lubrication (females), GU referral for males regarding available medications/sexual aids.	Pregnancy may be an issue for the young patient relative to issues of genetic predisposition and/or ability to manage pregnancy or parent offspring. Increased libido is not uncommon and may require adjustments within the existing relationship or in the absence of an acceptable partner. Information about different positions and techniques and/or other options for sexual fulfillment (e.g., fondling, cuddling) may enhance personal relationship and feelings of self-worth.
Refer for vocational rehabilitation as appropriate.	May need assessment of capabilities/job retraining as indicated by individual limitations/disease progression.
Recommend contacting local *and* national *MS* organizations.	Ongoing contact (e.g., mailings) inform patient of programs/services available, and can update patient's knowledge base.

POTENTIAL CONSIDERATIONS following acute hospitalization (dependent on patient's age, physical condition/presence of complications, personal resources, and life responsibilities)

Trauma, risk for—weakness, poor vision, balancing difficulties, reduced temperature/tactile sensation, reduced muscle, hand/eye coordination, cognitive or emotional difficulties, insufficient finances to purchase necessary equipment.

Home Maintenance Management, impaired—insufficient finances, unfamiliarity with neighborhood resources, inadequate support systems.

Disuse Syndrome, risk for [actual]—paralysis/immobilization, severe pain.

Therapeutic Regimen: Individual, ineffective management—economic difficulties, family conflict, social support deficits.

Gastrointestinal Disorders

UPPER GASTROINTESTINAL/ESOPHAGEAL BLEEDING

Bleeding duodenal ulcer is the most frequent cause of massive upper GI hemorrhage, but bleeding may also occur because of gastric ulcers, gastritis, and esophageal varices. Severe vomiting can precipitate gastric bleeding due to a tear of the mucosa at the gastroesophageal junction (Mallory-Weiss syndrome). Stress ulcer can occur owing to severe burns, major trauma/surgery, or severe systemic disease. Esophagitis, esophageal/gastric carcinoma, hiatal hernia, hemophilia, leukemia, and DIC are less common causes of upper GI bleeding.

CARE SETTING

Generally, a patient with severe, active bleeding will be admitted directly to the critical care unit; however, a patient may develop GI bleeding on the medical/surgical unit or be admitted there for evaluation/treatment of subacute bleeding.

RELATED CONCERNS

Cirrhosis of the Liver, p 466
Fluid and Electrolyte Imbalances, p 899
Psychosocial Aspects of Care, p 783
Renal Failure: Acute, p 555
Subtotal Gastrectomy/Gastric Resection, p 328

Patient Assessment Data Base

ACTIVITY/REST

May report:	Weakness, fatigue
May exhibit:	Tachycardia, tachypnea/hyperventilation (response to activity)

CIRCULATION

May report:	Palpitations Dizziness with position change
May exhibit:	Hypotension (including postural) Tachycardia, dysrhythmias (hypovolemia/hypoxemia) Weak/thready peripheral pulse

Capillary refill slow/delayed (vasoconstriction)
Skin color: pallor, cyanosis (depending on the amount of blood loss)
Skin/mucous membrane moisture: diaphoresis (reflecting shock state, acute pain, psychologic response)

EGO INTEGRITY

May report: Acute or chronic stress factors (financial, relationships, job-related)
Feelings of helplessness

May exhibit: Signs of anxiety, e.g., restlessness, pallor, diaphoresis, narrowed focus, trembling, quivering voice

ELIMINATION

May report: History of previous hospitalizations for GI bleeding or related GI problems, e.g., peptic/gastric ulcer, gastritis, gastric surgery, irradiation of gastric area
Change in usual bowel patterns/characteristics of stool

May exhibit: Abdominal tenderness, distention
Bowel sounds: often hyperactive during bleeding, hypoactive after bleeding subsides
Character of stool: diarrhea; dark bloody, tarry, or occasionally bright red stools; frothy, foul-smelling (steatorrhea); constipation may occur (changes in diet, antacid use)
Urine output: may be decreased, concentrated

FOOD/FLUID

May report: Anorexia, nausea, vomiting (protracted vomiting suggests pyloric outlet obstruction associated with duodenal ulcer)
Problems with swallowing; hiccups
Heartburn, burping with sour taste
Food intolerances, e.g., spicy food, chocolate; special diet for preexisting ulcer disease
Weight loss

May exhibit: Vomitus: coffee-ground or bright red, with or without clots
Mucous membranes dry, decreased mucus production, poor skin turgor (chronic bleeding)
Urine specific gravity may be elevated

NEUROSENSORY

May report: Fainting, dizziness/lightheadedness, weakness
Mental status: level of consciousness may be altered, ranging from slight drowsiness, disorientation/confusion, to stupor and coma (dependent on circulating volume/oxygenation)

PAIN/DISCOMFORT

May report: Pain, described as sharp, dull, burning, gnawing; sudden, excruciating pain can accompany perforation
Vague sensation of discomfort/distress following large meals and relieved by food (acute gastritis)
Left to mid-epigastric pain and/or pain radiating to back occurring 1–2 hours after eating and relieved by antacids (gastric ulcer)
Localized right epigastric pain occurring about 4 hours after meals when stomach is empty and relieved by food or antacids (duodenal ulcers)
Absence of pain (esophageal varices or gastritis)

Precipitating factors: may be foods, smoking, ingestion of alcohol, use of certain drugs (salicylates, reserpine, antibiotics, ibuprofen), psychologic stressors

May exhibit: Facial grimacing, guarding of affected area, pallor, diaphoresis, narrowed focus

SAFETY

May report: Drug allergies/sensitivities, e.g., ASA

May exhibit: Temperature elevation
Spider angiomas, palmar erythema (reflecting cirrhosis/portal hypertension)

TEACHING/LEARNING

May report: Recent use of prescription/OTC drugs containing ASA, alcohol, steroids
(NSAIDs are the leading cause of drug-induced GI bleeding)
Current complaint may reveal admission for related (e.g., anemia) or unrelated (e.g., head trauma) diagnosis; intestinal flu, or severe vomiting episode. Long-standing health problems, e.g., cirrhosis, alcoholism, hepatitis, eating disorders.

Discharge plan considerations: **DRG projected mean length of inpatient stay: 3.9–6.3 days**
May require changes in therapeutic/medication regimen.

Refer to section at end of plan for postdischarge considerations.

DIAGNOSTIC STUDIES

EGD (esophagogastroduodenoscopy): Key diagnostic test for upper GI bleeding, done to visualize site of bleeding/degree of tissue ulceration/injury.

Gastrointestinal nuclear scan: Radionuclide uptake at sites of bleeding identifies site (not cause) of bleeding. Test is considered to be more sensitive than EGD, upper GI studies with barium, or angiography in detecting sites of lower GI bleeding or persistent bleeding anywhere in GI tract.

Barium swallow with x-ray: Done after bleeding has ceased for differential diagnosis of cause/site of lesion, presence of structural defects such as strictures.

Gastric analysis: May be done in suspected peptic ulcer disease as indicated by low to normal pH and/or presence of blood; also in suspected gastric cancer (abnormal acidity, blood and/or abnormal cells on cytologic exam).

Gastric cultures: Helicobacter pylori (gram-negative urease-producing bacteria) recently discovered as organism responsible for 90% of duodenal and 70%–80% of gastric ulcers.

Angiography: GI vasculature may be reviewed if endoscopy is inconclusive or impractical. Demonstrates collateral circulation and possibly bleeding site.

Stools: Testing for blood will be positive.

Hb/Hct: Decreased levels occur within 6–24 hours after bleeding begins.

WBC: May elevate, reflecting body's response to injury.

BUN: Elevates within 24–48 hours as blood proteins are broken down in the GI tract and kidney filtration is decreased.

Creatinine: Usually not elevated if renal perfusion is maintained.

Ammonia: May be elevated when severe liver dysfunction disrupts the metabolism and proper excretion of urea or when massive whole blood transfusions have been given.

Coagulation profile: Increased platelets and decreased clotting times may be noted, reflecting the body's attempt to restore hemostasis. Severe abnormalities may reveal coagulopathy, e.g., DIC, as cause of bleeding.

ABGs: May reveal initial respiratory alkalosis (compensating for diminished blood flow through lungs). Later, metabolic acidosis develops in response to sluggish liver flow/accumulation of metabolic waste products.

Sodium: May be elevated as a hormonal compensation to conserve body fluid.

Potassium: May initially be depleted because of massive gastric emptying/vomiting or bloody diarrhea. Elevated potassium levels may occur after multiple transfusions of stored blood or with acute renal impairment.

Serum gastrin analysis: Elevated level suggests Zollinger-Ellison syndrome or possible presence of multiple poorly healed ulcers. Normal or low in type B gastritis.

Serum amylase: Elevated with posterior penetration of duodenal ulcer.

Pepsinogen level: Increased by duodenal ulcer; low level suggestive of gastritis.
Serum parietal cell antibodies: Presence suggestive of chronic gastritis.

NURSING PRIORITIES

1. Control hemorrhage.
2. Achieve/maintain hemodynamic stability.
3. Promote stress reduction.
4. Provide information about disease process/prognosis, treatment needs, and potential complications.

DISCHARGE GOALS

1. Hemorrhage curtailed.
2. Hemodynamically stable.
3. Anxiety/fear reduced to manageable level.
4. Disease process/prognosis, therapeutic regimen, and potential complications understood.
5. Plan in place to meet needs after discharge.

NURSING DIAGNOSIS: Fluid Volume deficit [active loss]

May be related to
Hemorrhage

Possibly evidenced by
Hypotension, tachycardia, delayed capillary refill
Changes in mentation, restlessness
Concentrated/decreased urine
Pallor, diaphoresis
Hemoconcentration

DESIRED OUTCOMES/EVALUATION CRITERIA—PATIENT WILL:
Demonstrate improved fluid balance as evidenced by individually adequate urinary output with normal specific gravity, stable vital signs, moist mucous membranes, good skin turgor, prompt capillary refill.

ACTIONS/INTERVENTIONS	RATIONALE
Independent	
Note characteristics of vomitus and/or drainage.	May be helpful in differentiating cause of gastric distress. Yellow-green bile content implies that the pylorus is open. Fecal content indicates bowel obstruction. Bright red blood signals recent or acute arterial bleeding, perhaps due to gastric ulceration; dark red blood may be old blood (retained in intestine) or venous bleeding from varices. Coffee-ground appearance is suggestive of partially digested blood from slowly oozing area. Undigested food indicates obstruction or gastric tumor.
Monitor vital signs; compare with patient's normal/previous readings. Take BP in sitting, lying, standing positions when possible.	Changes in BP and pulse may be used for rough estimate of blood loss, (e.g., BP <90 mm Hg, and pulse >110 suggests a 25% decrease in volume or approximately 1000 ml). Postural hypotension reflects a decrease in circulating volume.

ACTIONS/INTERVENTIONS	RATIONALE

Independent

Note patient's individual physiologic response to bleeding, e.g., changes in mentation, weakness, restlessness, anxiety; pallor, diaphoresis; tachypnea; temperature elevation.

Symptomatology may be useful in gauging severity/length of bleeding episode. Worsening of symptoms may reflect continued bleeding or inadequate fluid replacement.

Measure CVP, if available.

Reflects circulating volume and cardiac response to bleeding and fluid replacement; e.g., CVP values between 5 and 20 cm H_2O usually reflect adequate volume.

Monitor I&O, and correlate with weight changes. Measure blood/fluid losses via emesis, gastric suction/lavage, and stools.

Provides guidelines for fluid replacement.

Keep accurate record of subtotals of solutions/blood during replacement therapy.

Potential exists for overtransfusion of fluids, especially when volume expanders are given before blood transfusions.

Maintain bed rest; prevent vomiting and straining at stool. Schedule activities to provide undisturbed rest periods. Eliminate noxious stimuli.

Activity/vomiting increases intra-abdominal pressure and can predispose to further bleeding.

Elevate head of bed during antacid gavage.

Prevents gastric reflux and aspiration of antacids, which can cause serious pulmonary complications.

Note signs of renewed bleeding after cessation of initial bleeding.

Increased abdominal fullness/distention, nausea or renewed vomiting, and bloody diarrhea may indicate rebleeding.

Observe for secondary bleeding, e.g., nose/gums, oozing from puncture sites, appearance of ecchymotic areas following minimal trauma.

Loss of/inadequate replacement of clotting factors may precipitate development of DIC.

Provide clear/bland fluids when intake resumed. Avoid caffeinated and carbonated beverages.

Caffeine and carbonated beverages stimulate hydrochloric acid production, possibly potentiating rebleeding.

Collaborative

Administer fluids/volume expanders as indicated:

Fluid replacement is dependent on degree of hypovolemia and duration of bleeding (acute or chronic). Volume expanders (albumin) may be infused until type and cross-match can be completed and blood transfusions begun. Approximately 80%–90% of gastric bleeding is controlled by fluid resuscitation and medical management.

Fresh whole blood/packed red blood cells;

Fresh whole blood is indicated for acute bleeding (with shock), because stored blood may be deficient in clotting factors. Packed cells may be adequate for stable patients with subacute/chronic bleeding and are required for patients with HF to prevent fluid overload.

Fresh frozen plasma and/or platelets.

Clotting factors/components are depleted by 2 mechanisms: hemorrhagic loss and the clotting process at the site of bleeding. FFP is an excellent source of clotting factors. Platelet replacement may potentiate formation of platelet plug at injury sites.

ACTIONS/INTERVENTIONS	RATIONALE

Collaborative

Insert/maintain large-bore NG tube in acute bleeding.	Provides avenue for removing irritating gastric secretions, blood, and clots; reduces nausea/vomiting; and facilitates diagnostic endoscopy. *Note:* Blood remaining in the stomach/intestines will be broken down into ammonia, which can produce a toxic CNS effect, e.g., encephalopathy.
Perform gastric lavage with cool or room-temperature saline until aspirate is light pink or clear and free of clots. Simultaneous low gastric suctioning with continuous saline infusion through the air port of a salem sump tube may also be used.	Flushes out/breaks up clots and may reduce bleeding by local vasoconstriction. Facilitates visualization by endoscopy to locate bleeding source. *Note:* Research now suggests that iced saline is no more effective than room temperature solution in controlling bleeding, and it may actually damage gastric mucosa as well as lower the patient's core temperature, which could prolong bleeding by inhibiting platelet function.

Administer medications, as indicated:

Cimetidine (Tagamet), ranitidine (Zantac), famotidine (Pepcid), nizatidine (Axid);	Histamine H$_2$-blockers may be given parenterally during bleeding to reduce gastric acid production, increase gastric pH, and reduce irritation to gastric mucosa to aid in healing as well as prevention of lesion formation.
Sucralfate (Carafate);	Antiulcer agent decreases gastric acid secretion and increases the production of protective mucus useful in treating and preventing recurrence of duodenal ulcers. *Note:* Impairs absorption of some drugs, e.g., theophylline, digoxin, phenytoin, tetracycline, amitriptyline.
Omeprazole (Prilosec);	Classified as a gastric acid pump inhibitor or proton pump antagonist, which can completely inhibit acid secretion, has a long duration of action, and can heal duodenal ulcers in 2–4 weeks once severe bleeding is controlled.
Antacids: e.g., Amphojel, Maalox, Mylanta, Riopan;	Antacids (administered orally or by gavage) may be used as supplemental therapy to reduce pain or be given to maintain gastric pH level at 4.5 or higher to reduce risk of rebleeding. Antacids block the gastric absorption of oral histamine antagonists and therefore should not be administered within 1 hour after oral administration of histamine blockers.
Belladonna; atropine;	Anticholinergics may be used to decrease gastric motility, particularly in peptic ulcer disease after acute bleeding has subsided.
Vasopressin (Pitressin);	Administration of intra-arterial vasocontrictors may be needed in severe, prolonged bleeding (varices).
Vitamin K$_1$ (AquaMephyton);	Promotes hepatic synthesis of coagulation factors to support clotting. *Note:* Absorption of vitamin K may be decreased by use of sucralfate.

ACTIONS/INTERVENTIONS	RATIONALE
Collaborative	
Phenobarbital;	Mild sedatives may be given to promote rest, reduce intensity of bleeding, and alleviate pain. *Note:* Use with caution to avoid masking signs of developing hypovolemia.
Antiemetics, e.g., metoclopramide (Reglan), prochlorperazine (Compazine);	Alleviates nausea and prevents vomiting.
Supplemental vitamin B_{12};	In diffuse atrophic gastritis, the intrinsic factor necessary for B_{12} absorption from the GI tract is not secreted, and individual may develop pernicious anemia.
Anti-infectives, e.g., tetracycline (Achromycin), metronidazole (Flagyl), amoxicillin (Arnoxil).	Oral agents may be combined with antacids or histamine blockers to treat infections causing chronic gastritis *(Campylobacter pylori)* or PUD *(Helicobacter pylori)*. *Note:* Neomycin (Mycifradin) or lactulose (Cephulac) may be used in esophageal varices to block bacterial breakdown of shed blood in the gut to reduce the risk of encephalopathy.
Monitor laboratory studies, e.g.:	
Hb, Hct, RBC count;	Aids in establishing blood replacement needs and monitoring effectiveness of therapy, e.g., 1 U of whole blood should raise Hct 2–3 points. Levels may initially remain stable, due to loss of both plasma and RBCs.
BUN/creatinine levels.	BUN >40 with normal creatinine level indicates major bleeding. BUN should return to patient's normal level approximately 12 hours after bleeding has ceased.
Assist with/prepare for:	
Sclerotherapy;	Injection of an irritating (sclerosing) agent into esophageal varices (to create thrombosis) may be performed to prevent recurrence after initial bleeding is controlled.
Endoscopic variceal ligation (EVL);	This banding technique is used as an effective alternative to sclerotherapy. Active hemorrhage is controlled in a high percentage of patients with fewer complications than with sclerotherapy.
Electrocoagulation or photocoagulation (laser) therapy;	Provides direct coagulation of bleeding sites, e.g., gastritis, duodenal ulcer, tumor, esophageal (Mallory-Weiss) tear.
Surgical intervention.	Total/partial gastrectomy, pyloroplasty, and/or vagotomy may be required to control/prevent future gastric bleeding. Shunt procedures (portacaval, splenorenal, mesocaval, or distal splenorenal) may be done to divert blood flow and reduce pressure within esophageal vessels when other measures fail.

ACTIONS/INTERVENTIONS	RATIONALE
Independent	
Investigate changes in level of consciousness, reports of dizziness/headache.	Changes may reflect inadequate cerebral perfusion as a result of reduced arterial blood pressure. *Note:* Changes in sensorium may also reflect elevated ammonia levels/hepatic encephalophathy in patient with liver disease.
Investigate reports of chest pain. Note location, quality, duration, and what relieves pain.	May reflect cardiac ischemia related to decreased perfusion. *Note:* Impaired oxygenation status resulting from blood loss can bring on MI in patient with cardiac disease.
Auscultate apical pulse. Monitor cardiac rate/rhythm if continuous ECG available/indicated.	Dysrhythmias and ischemic changes can occur as a result of hypotension, hypoxia, acidosis, electrolyte imbalance, or cooling near the heart if cold saline lavage is used to control bleeding.
Assess skin for coolness, pallor, diaphoresis, delayed capillary refill, and weak, thready peripheral pulses.	Vasoconstriction is a sympathetic response to lowered circulating volume and/or may occur as a side effect of vasopressin administration.
Note urinary output and specific gravity.	Decreased systemic perfusion may cause kidney ischemia/failure manifested by decreased urine output. ATN may develop if hypovolemic state is prolonged.
Note reports of abdominal pain, especially sudden, severe pain or pain radiating to shoulder.	Pain caused by gastric ulcer is often relieved after acute bleeding because of buffering effects of blood. Continued severe or sudden pain may reflect ischemia due to vasoconstrictive therapy; bleeding into biliary tract (hematobilia); or perforation/onset of peritonitis.
Observe skin for pallor, redness. Massage with lotion. Change position frequently.	Compromised peripheral circulation increases risk of skin breakdown.
Collaborative	
Monitor ABGs/pulse oximetry.	Identifies hypoxemia, effectiveness of/need for therapy.
Provide supplemental oxygen if indicated.	Treats hypoxemia and lactic acidosis during acute bleed.

ACTIONS/INTERVENTIONS

Collaborative

Administer IV fluids as indicated.

RATIONALE

Maintains circulating volume and perfusion. *Note:* Use of lactated Ringer's solution may be contraindicated in presence of hepatic failure because metabolism of lactate is impaired, and lactic acidosis may develop.

NURSING DIAGNOSIS: Fear/Anxiety [specify level]

May be related to
Change in health status, threat of death

Possibly evidenced by
Increased tension, restlessness, irritability, fearfulness
Trembling, tachycardia, diaphoresis
Lack of eye contact, focus on self
Verbalization of specific concern
Withdrawal, panic or attack behavior

DESIRED OUTCOMES/EVALUATION CRITERIA—PATIENT WILL:
Discuss fears/concerns recognizing healthy versus unhealthy fears.
Verbalize appropriate range of feelings.
Appear relaxed and report anxiety is reduced to a manageable level.
Demonstrate problem solving and effective use of resources.

ACTIONS/INTERVENTIONS

Independent

Monitor physiologic responses, e.g., tachypnea, palpitations, dizziness, headache, tingling sensations.

Note behavioral cues, e.g., restlessness, irritability, lack of eye contact, combativeness/attack behavior.

Encourage verbalization of concerns. Assist patient in expressing feelings by active listening.

Acknowledge that this is a fearful situation and that others have expressed similar fears.

Provide accurate, concrete information about what is being done, e.g., sensations to expect, usual procedures undertaken.

Provide a calm, restful environment.

Encourage SO to stay with patient as able. Respond to call signal promptly. Use touch and eye contact as appropriate.

RATIONALE

May be indicative of the degree of fear patient is experiencing but may also be related to physical condition/shock state.

Indicators of degree of fear patient is experiencing; e.g., patient may feel out of control of the situation or reach a state of panic.

Establishes a therapeutic relationship. Assists the patient in dealing with feelings and provides opportunity to clarify misconceptions.

When patient is expressing own fear, the validation that these feelings are normal can help patient to feel less isolated.

Involves patient in plan of care and decreases unnecessary anxiety about unknowns.

Removing patient from outside stressors promotes relaxation, may enhance coping skills.

Helps reduce fear of going through a frightening experience alone.

ACTIONS/INTERVENTIONS	RATIONALE

Independent

Provide opportunity for SO to express feelings/concerns. Encourage SO to project positive, realistic attitude.

Helps SO to deal with own anxiety/fears that can be transmitted to the patient. Promotes a supportive attitude that can facilitate recovery.

Demonstrate/encourage relaxation techniques, e.g., visualization, deep-breathing exercises, guided imagery.

Learning ways to relax can be helpful in reducing fear and anxiety. As the patient with GI bleeding is often a person with type A personality who has difficulty relaxing, learning these skills can be important to recovery and prevention of recurrence.

Help the patient to identify and initiate positive coping behaviors used successfully in the past.

Successful behaviors can be fostered in dealing with current fear, enhancing patient's sense of self-control and providing reassurance.

Encourage and support patient in evaluation of lifestyle.

Changes may be necessary to avoid recurrence of ulcer condition.

Collaborative

Administer medications as indicated, e.g.:

Diazepam (Valium), clorazepate (Tranxene), alprazolam (Xanax).

Sedatives/antianxiety agents may be used on occasion to reduce anxiety and promote rest, particularly in the ulcer patient.

Refer to psychiatric nurse, social services, spiritual advisor.

May need additional assistance during recovery to deal with consequences of emergency situation/adjustments to required/desired changes in lifestyle.

NURSING DIAGNOSIS: Pain [acute]/chronic

May be related to
Chemical burn of gastric mucosa, oral cavity
Physical response, e.g., reflex muscle spasm in the stomach wall

Possibly evidenced by
Communication of pain descriptors
Abdominal guarding, rigid body posture, facial grimacing
Autonomic responses, e.g., changes in vital signs (acute pain)

DESIRED OUTCOMES/EVALUATION CRITERIA—PATIENT WILL:
Verbalize relief of pain.
Demonstrate relaxed body posture and be able to sleep/rest appropriately.

ACTIONS/INTERVENTIONS	RATIONALE

Independent

Note reports of pain, including location, duration, intensity (0–10 scale).

Pain is not always present, but if present should be compared with patient's previous pain symptoms. This comparison may assist in diagnosis of etiology of bleeding and development of complications.

Review factors that aggravate or alleviate pain.

Helpful in establishing diagnosis and treatment needs.

ACTIONS/INTERVENTIONS	RATIONALE

Independent

Note nonverbal pain cues, e.g., restlessness, reluctance to move, abdominal guarding, tachycardia, diaphoresis. Investigate discrepancies between verbal and nonverbal cues.

Nonverbal cues may be both physiologic and psychologic and may be used in conjunction with verbal cues to evaluate extent/severity of the problem.

Provide small, frequent meals as indicated for individual patient.

Food has an acid neutralizing effect, as well as diluting the gastric contents. Small meals prevent distention and the release of gastrin.

Identify and limit foods that create discomfort.

Specific foods that cause distress vary between individuals. Studies indicate pepper is harmful, and coffee (including decaffeinated) can precipitate dyspepsia.

Assist with active/passive ROM exercises.

Reduces joint stiffness, minimizing pain/discomfort.

Provide frequent oral care and comfort measures, e.g., back rub, position change.

Halitosis from stagnant oral secretions is unappetizing and can aggravate nausea. Gingivitis and dental problems may arise.

Collaborative

Provide and implement prescribed dietary modifications.

Patient may be NPO initially. When oral intake is allowed, food choices will depend on the diagnosis and etiology of the bleeding.

Use regular rather than skim milk, if milk is allowed.

Fat in regular milk may decrease gastric secretions; however, the calcium and protein content (especially in skim milk) increases them.

Administer medications, as indicated, e.g.:

Analgesics, e.g., morphine sulfate;

May be narcotic of choice to relieve acute/severe pain and reduce peristaltic activity. *Note:* Demerol has been associated with increased incidence of nausea/vomiting.

Acetaminophen (Tylenol);

Promotes comfort and rest.

Antacids;

Decreases gastric acidity by absorption or by chemical neutralization. Evaluate type of antacid in regard to total health picture, e.g., sodium restriction.

Anticholinergics, e.g., belladonna, atropine.

May be given at bedtime to decrease gastric motility, suppress acid production, delay gastric emptying, and alleviate nocturnal pain associated with gastric ulcer.

NURSING DIAGNOSIS: Knowledge deficit [learning need] regarding disease process, prognosis, treatment, self care and discharge needs

May be related to
Lack of information/recall
Unfamiliarity with information resources
Information misinterpretation

Possibly evidenced by
Verbalization of the problem, request for information, statement of misconceptions
Inaccurate follow-through of instructions
Development of preventable complications

ACTIONS/INTERVENTIONS	RATIONALE
Independent	
Determine patient perception of cause of bleeding.	Establishes knowledge base and provides some insight into how the teaching plan needs to be constructed for this individual.
Provide/review information regarding etiology of bleeding, cause/effect, relationship of lifestyle behaviors, and ways to reduce risk/contributing factors. Encourage questions.	Provides knowledge base on which patient can make informed choices/decisions about future and control of health problems.
Assist patient to identify relationship of food intake and precipitation of/or relief from epigastric pain, including avoidance of gastric irritants, e.g., pepper, caffeine, alcohol, fruit juices, carbonated beverages, and extremely hot, cold, fatty, or spicy foods.	Caffeine stimulates gastric acidity. Alcohol contributes to erosion of gastric mucosa. Although current research indicates that diet does not contribute to the development of PUD, individuals may find that certain foods/fluids increase gastric secretion and pain.
Recommend small, frequent meals/snacks, chewing food slowly, eating at regular time, and avoiding "skipping" meals.	Frequent eating keeps HCl neutralized, dilutes stomach contents to minimize action of acid on gastric mucosa. Small meals prevent gastric overdistention.
Stress importance of reading labels on OTC drugs and avoiding products containing aspirin or switching to enteric-coated aspirin.	Aspirin damages the protective mucosa, permitting gastric erosion, ulceration, and bleeding to occur.
Review significance of signs/symptoms such as coffee-ground emesis, tarry stools, abdominal distention, severe epigastric/abdominal pain radiating to shoulder/back.	Prompt medical evaluation/intervention is required to prevent more serious complications, e.g., perforation, Zollinger-Ellison syndrome.
Support use of stress management techniques, avoidance of emotional stress.	Decreases extrinsic stimulation of HCl, reducing risk of recurrence of bleeding.
Review drug regimen, possible side effects and interaction with other drugs as appropriate.	Helpful to patient's understanding of reason for taking drugs, and what symptoms are important to report to healthcare provider. *Note:* Aluminum-containing antacids inhibit the intestinal absorption of some drugs and affect scheduling of drug intake.
Encourage patient to inform all healthcare providers of bleeding history.	May affect drug choices and/or concomitant prescriptions, e.g., misoprostal (Cytotec) can be given with NSAIDs to inhibit gastric acid secretion and reduce risk of gastric irritability/lesions resulting from NSAID therapy.
Discuss importance of cessation of smoking.	Ulcer healing may be delayed in people who smoke, particularly in those treated with Tagamet. Smoking stimulates gastric acidity and is associated with increased risk of peptic ulcer development/recurrence.

ACTIONS/INTERVENTIONS	RATIONALE
Independent	
Refer to support groups/counseling for lifestyle/behavior changes/reduction of associated risk factors, e.g., substance abuse/stop-smoking clinics.	Alcohol users have a higher incidence of gastritis/esophageal varices, and cigarette smoking is associated with peptic ulcers and delayed healing.

POTENTIAL CONSIDERATIONS following acute hospitalization (dependent on patient's age, physical condition/presence of complications, personal resources, and life responsibilities)

Therapeutic Regimen: Individual, ineffective management—decisional conflicts (e.g., use of NSAIDs for arthritic/chronic pain condition, perceived benefits (e.g., cessation of smoking), economic difficulties (cost of medication).

SUBTOTAL GASTRECTOMY/GASTRIC RESECTION

Indicated for gastric hemorrhage/intractable ulcers, dysfunctional lower esophageal sphincter, pyloric obstruction, perforation, cancer.

CARE SETTING

Inpatient surgical unit.

RELATED CONCERNS

Cancer, p 875
Pancreatitis, p 481
Peritonitis, p 366
Psychosocial Aspects of Care, p 783
Surgical Intervention, p 802
Total Nutritional Support: Parenteral/Enteral Feeding, p 491
Upper Gastrointestinal/Esophageal Bleeding, p 315

Patient Assessment Data Base

The data is dependent on the underlying condition necessitating surgery.

TEACHING/LEARNING

Discharge plan considerations: **DRG projected mean length of inpatient stay: 3.5 days**
Assistance with administration of enteral feedings/TPN, (if required) and acquisition of supplies

Refer to section at end of plan for postdischarge considerations.

NURSING PRIORITIES

1. Promote healing and adequate nutritional intake.
2. Prevent complications.
3. Provide information about surgical procedure/prognosis, treatment needs, and concerns.

DISCHARGE GOALS

1. Nutritional intake adequate for individual needs.
2. Complications prevented/minimized.
3. Surgical procedure/prognosis, therapeutic regimen, and long-term needs understood.
4. Plan in place to meet needs after discharge.

(In addition to nursing diagnosis identified in this CP, refer to CP Surgical Intervention, p 802.)

NURSING DIAGNOSIS: Nutrition: altered, risk for less than body requirements

Risk factors may include
Restriction of fluids and food
Change in digestive process/absorption of nutrients

Possibly evidenced by
[Not applicable; presence of signs and symptoms establishes an *actual* diagnosis.]

DESIRED OUTCOMES/EVALUATION CRITERIA—PATIENT WILL:
Maintain stable weight/demonstrate progressive weight gain toward goal with normalization of laboratory values.
Be free of signs of malnutrition.
Verbalize understanding of functional changes.
Identify necessary interventions/behaviors to maintain appropriate weight.

ACTIONS/INTERVENTIONS	RATIONALE
Independent	
Maintain patency of NG tube. Do not reposition tube if it becomes dislodged.	Provides rest for GI tract during acute postoperative phase until return of normal function. *Note:* Even though gastric distention may cause stress on the sutures/possible rupture of stump (Billroth II), the tube needs to be repositioned by the physician to prevent injury to the operative area.
Note character and amount of gastric drainage.	Will be bloody for first 12 hours, and then should clear/turn greenish. Continued/recurrent bleeding suggests complications. Decline in output may reflect progression of fluid through the GI tract, suggesting return of function.
Caution the patient to limit the intake of ice chips.	Excessive intake of ice produces nausea and can wash out electrolytes via the NG tube.
Provide oral hygiene on a regular, frequent basis, including petroleum jelly for lips.	Prevents discomfort of dry mouth and cracked lips caused by fluid restriction and the NG tube.
Auscultate for bowel sounds and note passage of flatus.	Peristalsis can be expected to return about the 3rd postoperative day, signaling readiness to resume oral intake.
Monitor tolerance to fluid and food intake, noting abdominal distention, reports of increased pain/cramping, nausea/vomiting.	Complications of paralytic ileus, obstruction, delayed gastric emptying, and gastric dilatation may occur, possibly requiring reinsertion of NG tube.
Avoid milk and high carbohydrate foods in the diet.	May trigger dumping syndrome. (Refer to ND: Knowledge deficit [learning need], p 330.)
Note admission weight and compare with subsequent readings.	Provides information about adequacy of dietary intake/determination of nutritional needs.
Collaborative	
Administer IV fluids, TPN, and lipids as indicated.	Meets fluid/nutritional needs until oral intake can be resumed.
Monitor laboratory studies, e.g., Hb/Hct, electrolytes, and total protein/prealbumin.	Indicators of fluid/nutritional needs and effectiveness of therapy and detects developing complications.
Progress diet as tolerated, advancing from clear liquid to bland diet with several small feedings.	Usually NG tube is clamped for specified periods of time when peristalsis returns, to determine tolerance. After NG tube is removed, intake is advanced gradually to prevent gastric irritation/distention.

ACTIONS/INTERVENTIONS

Collaborative

Administer medications as indicated:

Anticholinergics, e.g., atropine, propantheline bromide (Pro-Banthine);

Fat-soluble vitamin supplements, including B_{12}; calcium;

Iron preparations;

Protein supplements;

Pancreatic enzymes, bile salts;

Medium-chain triglycerides (MCT).

RATIONALE

Controls dumping syndrome, enhancing digestion and absorption of nutrients.

Removal of the stomach prevents absorption of B_{12} (due to loss of intrinsic factor) and can lead to pernicious anemia. In addition, rapid emptying of the stomach reduces absorption of calcium.

Corrects/prevents iron deficiency anemia.

Additional protein may be helpful for tissue repair and healing.

Enhances digestive process.

Promotes absorption of fats and fat-soluble vitamins to prevent malabsorption problems.

NURSING DIAGNOSIS: Knowledge deficit [learning need] regarding procedure, prognosis, treatment, self care and discharge needs

May be related to
Lack of exposure/recall
Information misinterpretation
Unfamiliarity with information resources

Possibly evidenced by
Questions, statement of misconception
Inaccurate follow-through of instruction
Development of preventable complications

DESIRED OUTCOMES/EVALUATION CRITERIA—PATIENT WILL:
Verbalize understanding of procedure, disease process/prognosis, treatment.
Correctly perform necessary procedures, explaining reasons for actions.

ACTIONS/INTERVENTIONS

Independent

Review surgical procedure and long-term expectations.

Discuss and identify stress situations and how to avoid them. Investigate job-related issues.

RATIONALE

Provides knowledge base from which informed choices can be made. Recovery following gastric surgery is often slower than may be anticipated with similar types of surgery. Improved strength and partial normalization of dietary pattern may not be evident for at least 3 months, and full return to usual intake (3 "normal" meals/d) may take up to 12 months. This prolonged convalescence may be difficult for the patient/SO to deal with if he or she has not been prepared.

Can alter gastric motility, interfering with optimal digestion. *Note:* Patient may require vocational counseling if change in employment is indicated.

ACTIONS/INTERVENTIONS	RATIONALE
Independent	
Review dietary needs/regimen (e.g., low carbohydrate, low-fat, high-protein) and importance of maintaining vitamin supplementation.	May prevent deficiencies, enhance healing, and promote cooperation with therapy. *Note:* Low-fat diet may be required to reduce risk of alkaline reflux gastritis.
Discuss the importance of eating small, frequent meals slowly and in a relaxed atmosphere; resting after meals; avoiding extremely hot or cold food; restricting high-fiber foods, caffeine, milk products and alcohol, excess sugars and salt; and taking fluids between meals, rather than with food.	These measures can be helpful in avoiding gastric distention/irritation and/or stress on surgical repair, dumping syndrome, and reactive hypoglycemia. *Note:* Ice-cold fluids/foods can cause gastric spasms.
Instruct in avoiding certain fibrous foods and discuss the necessity of chewing food well.	Remaining gastric tissue may have reduced ability to digest such foods as citrus skins/seeds, which can collect, forming a mass (phytobezoar formation) that is not excreted.
Recommend foods containing pectin, e.g., citrus fruits, bananas, apples, yellow vegetables, and beans.	Increased intake of these foods may reduce incidence of dumping syndrome.
Identify foods that can cause gastric irritation and increase gastric acid, e.g., chocolate, spicy foods, whole grains, raw vegetables.	Limiting/avoiding these foods reduces risk of gastric bleeding/ulceration in some individuals. *Note:* Ingesting fresh fruits to reduce risk of dumping syndrome should be tempered with adverse effect of gastric irritation.
Identify symptoms that may indicate dumping syndrome, e.g., weakness, profuse perspiration, epigastric fullness, nausea/vomiting, abdominal cramping, faintness, flushing, explosive diarrhea, and palpitations occurring within 15 minutes–1 hour after eating.	Can cause severe discomfort or even shock, and reduces absorption of nutrients. Usually self-limiting (1–3 weeks after surgery) but can become chronic.
Discuss signs of hypoglycemia and corrective interventions, e.g., ingesting of cheese and crackers, orange/grape juice.	Awareness helps patient to take actions to prevent progression of symptoms.
Suggest patient weigh self on a regular basis.	Change in dietary pattern, early satiety, effort of avoiding dumping syndrome may limit intake, causing weight loss.
Review medication purpose, dosage, and schedule as well as possible side effects.	Understanding rationale/therapeutic needs can reduce risk of complications, e.g., anticholinergics/pectin powder may be given to reduce incidence of dumping syndrome; antacids/histamine antagonists reduce gastric irritation.
Caution patient to read labels and avoid products containing ASA, ibuprofen.	Can cause gastric irritation/bleeding.
Discuss reasons and importance of cessation of smoking.	Smoking stimulates gastric acid production and may cause vasoconstriction, compromising mucous membranes and increasing risk of gastric irritation/ulceration.
Identify signs/symptoms requiring medical evaluation, e.g., persistent nausea/vomiting or abdominal fullness, weight loss, diarrhea, foul-smelling fatty or tarry stools, bloody or coffee-ground vomitus/presence of bile, fever. Instruct patient to report changes in pain characteristics.	Prompt recognition and intervention may prevent serious consequences or potential complications such as pancreatitis, peritonitis, and afferent loop syndrome.

331

ACTIONS/INTERVENTIONS	RATIONALE
Independent	
Stress importance of regular checkup with healthcare provider.	Necessary to detect developing complications, e.g., anemia, problems with nutrition, and/or recurrence of disease.

POTENTIAL CONSIDERATIONS following acute hospitalization (dependent on patient's age, physical condition/presence of complications, personal resources, and life responsibilities)

Nutrition: altered, less than body requirements, risk for—change in digestive process/absorption of nutrients, early satiety, gastric irritation.

Fatigue—decreased energy production, states of discomfort, increased energy requirements to perform ADLs.

INFLAMMATORY BOWEL DISEASE (IBD): ULCERATIVE COLITIS, REGIONAL ENTERITIS (CROHN'S DISEASE, ILEOCOLITIS)

Inflammatory Bowel Disease: Researchers believe that IBD may result from a complex interplay between genetic and environmental factors. Similarities involve (1) chronic inflammation of the alimentary tract, (2) periods of remission interspersed with episodes of acute inflammation

Ulcerative colitis (UC): A chronic condition of unknown cause usually starting in the rectum and distal portions of the colon and possibly spreading upward to involve the sigmoid and descending colon or the entire colon. It is usually intermittent (acute exacerbation with long remissions), but some individuals (30%–40%) have continuous symptoms. Cure is effected only by total removal of colon and rectum/rectal mucosa.

Regional enteritis (Crohn's disease, ileocolitis): May be found in portions of the alimentary tract from the mouth to the anus but is most commonly found in the small intestine (terminal ileum). It is a slowly progressive chronic disease of unknown cause with intermittent acute episodes and no known cure.

UC and regional enteritis share common symptoms but differ in the segment and layer of intestine involved and the degree of severity and complications. Therefore, separate data bases are provided.

CARE SETTING

Usually handled at the community level; however, severe exacerbations requiring advanced pain control and rehydration may necessitate short stay in acute care medical unit.

RELATED CONCERNS

Fecal Diversions: Postoperative Care of Ileostomy and Colostomy, p 348
Fluid and Electrolyte Imbalances, p 899
Peritonitis, p 366
Psychosocial Aspects of Care, p 783
Total Nutritional Support: Parenteral/Enteral Feeding, p 491

Patient Assessment Data Base—Ulcerative Colitis

ACTIVITY/REST

May report: Weakness, fatigue, malaise, exhaustion
Insomnia, not sleeping through the night because of diarrhea
Feeling restless and anxious
Restriction of activities/work due to effects of disease process

CIRCULATION

May exhibit: Tachycardia (response to fever, dehydration, inflammatory process, and pain)
Bruising, ecchymotic areas (insufficient vitamin K)
BP: hypotension, including postural changes
Skin/mucous membranes: poor turgor; dry, cracking of tongue (dehydration/malnutrition)

EGO INTEGRITY

May report: Anxiety, apprehension, emotional upsets, e.g., feelings of helplessness/hopelessness
Acute/chronic stress factors, e.g., family/job-related, expense of treatment
Cultural factor—increased prevalence in Jewish population

May exhibit: Withdrawal, narrowed focus, depression

333

ELIMINATION

May report:
Stool texture varying from soft-formed to mushy or watery
Unpredictable, intermittent, frequent, uncontrollable episodes of bloody diarrhea (as many as 20–30 stools/d); sense of urgency/cramping (tenesmus); passing blood/pus/mucus with or without passing feces
Rectal bleeding
History of renal stones (dehydration)

May exhibit:
Diminished or hyperactive bowel sounds, absence of peristalsis or presence of visible peristaltic waves
Hemorrhoids, anal fissures (25%); perianal fistula (more frequently with Crohn's)
Oliguria

FOOD/FLUID

May report:
Anorexia; nausea/vomiting
Weight loss
Dietary intolerances/sensitivities, e.g., raw fruits/vegetables, dairy products, fatty foods

May exhibit:
Decreased subcutaneous fat/muscle mass
Weakness, poor muscle tone and skin turgor
Mucous membranes pale; sore, inflamed buccal cavity

HYGIENE

May report:
Inability to maintain self-care

May exhibit:
Stomatitis reflecting vitamin deficiency
Unkempt appearance; body odor

PAIN/DISCOMFORT

May report:
Mild cramping to severe pain/tenderness in lower-left quadrant (may be relieved with defecation)
Migratory joint pain, tenderness (arthritis)
Eye pain, photophobia (iritis)

May exhibit:
Abdominal tenderness, distention, rigidity

SAFETY

May report:
History of lupus erythematosus, hemolytic anemia, vasculitis
Arthritis (worsening of symptoms with exacerbations in bowel disease)
Temperature elevation 104–105°F (acute exacerbation)
Blurred vision
Allergies to foods/milk products (release of histamine into bowel has an inflammatory effect)

May exhibit:
Skin lesions may be present; e.g., erythema nodosum (raised, tender, red, and swollen) on arms, face; pyoderma gangrenosum (purulent pinpoint lesion/boil with a purple border) on trunk, legs, ankles
Ankylosing spondylitis
Uveitis, conjunctivitis/iritis

SEXUALITY

May report:
Reduced frequency/avoidance of sexual activity

SOCIAL INTERACTION

May report: Relationship/role problems related to condition
Inability to be active socially

TEACHING/LEARNING

May report: Family history of inflammatory bowel disease, immune disorders

Discharge plan considerations: **DRG projected mean length of inpatient stay: 6.6 days**
Assistance with dietary requirements, medication regimen, psychologic support

Refer to section at end of plan for postdischarge considerations.

DIAGNOSTIC STUDIES

Stool specimens (examinations are used in initial diagnosis and in following disease progression): Mainly composed of mucus, blood, pus, and intestinal organisms, especially *Entamoeba histolytica* (active stage).

Proctosigmoidoscopy: Visualizes ulcerations, edema, hyperemia, and inflammation (result of secondary infection of the mucosa and submucosa). Friability and hemorrhagic areas caused by necrosis and ulceration occur in 85% of these patients.

Cytology and rectal biopsy: Differentiates between infectious process and carcinoma (occurs 10–20 times more often than in general population). Neoplastic changes can be detected, as well as characteristic inflammatory infiltrates called crypt abscesses.

Barium enema: May be performed after visual examination has been done, although rarely done during acute, relapsing stage, because it can exacerbate condition.

Colonoscopy: Identifies adhesions, changes in luminal wall (narrowing/irregularity); rules out bowel obstruction.

Abdominal MRI/CT scan, ultrasound: Detects infections/inflammatory conditions.

CBC: May show hyperchromic anemia (active disease generally present due to blood loss and iron deficiency); leukocytosis may occur, especially in fulminating or complicated cases and in patients on steroid therapy.

Sedimentation rate (ESR): Increased according to severity of disease.

Serum iron level: Lowered due to blood loss.

Prothrombin time: Prolonged in severe cases from altered factors VII and X caused by vitamin K deficiency.

Thrombocytosis: May occur due to inflammatory disease process.

Electrolytes: Decreased potassium and magnesium are common in severe disease.

Prealbumin/Albumin level: Decreased because of loss of plasma proteins/disturbed liver function.

Alkaline phosphatase: Increased, along with serum cholesterol and hypoproteinemia, indicating disturbed liver function, (e.g., cholangitis, cirrhosis).

Bone marrow: A generalized depression is common in fulminating types/after a long inflammatory process.

Patient Assessment Data Base–Regional Enteritis

ACTIVITY/REST

May report: Weakness, fatigue, malaise, exhaustion
Feeling restless and anxious
Restriction of activities/work due to effects of disease process

EGO INTEGRITY

May report: Anxiety, apprehension, emotional upsets, feelings of helplessness/hopelessness
Acute/chronic stress factors, e.g., family/job-related, expense of treatment
Cultural factor—increased prevalence in Jewish population, frequency increasing in individuals of Northern European and Anglo-Saxon derivation

May exhibit: Withdrawal, narrowed focus, depression

ELIMINATION

May report: Unpredictable, intermittent, frequent, uncontrollable episodes of nonbloody diarrhea, soft or semiliquid with flatus; foul-smelling and fatty stools (steatorrhea)
Intermittent constipation
History of renal stones (increased oxalates in the urine)

May exhibit: Hyperactive bowel sounds with gurgling, splashing sound (borborygmus)
Visible peristalsis

FOOD/FLUID

May report: Anorexia; nausea/vomiting
Weight loss
Dietary intolerance/sensitivity, e.g., dairy products, fatty foods

May exhibit: Decreased subcutaneous fat/muscle mass
Weakness, poor muscle tone and skin turgor
Mucous membranes pale

HYGIENE

May report: Inability to maintain self-care

May exhibit: Unkempt appearance; body odor

PAIN/DISCOMFORT

May report: Tender abdomen with cramping pain in lower right quadrant (inflammation involving all layers of bowel wall and possibly the mesentary); pain in mid-lower abdomen (jejunal involvement)
Referred tenderness to periumbilical region
Perineal tenderness/pain
Migratory joint pain, tenderness (arthritis)
Eye pain, photophobia (iritis)

May exhibit: Abdominal tenderness/distention

SAFETY

May report: History of arthritis, lupus erythematosus, hemolytic anemia, vasculitis
Temperature elevation (low-grade fever)
Perianal fissures, anorectal fistula
Blurred vision

May exhibit: Skin lesions may be present: erythema nodosum (raised tender, red swelling) on face, arms; pyoderma gangrenosum (purulent pinpoint lesion/boil with a purple border) on trunk, legs, ankles; perineal lesions/fistulas
Ankylosing spondylitis
Uveitis, conjunctivitis/iritis

SOCIAL INTERACTION

May report: Relationship/role problems related to condition; inability to be active socially

TEACHING/LEARNING

May report: Family history of inflammatory bowel disease, immune disorders

Discharge plan considerations:	**DRG projected mean length of inpatient stay: 6.6 days** Assistance with dietary requirements, medication regimen, psychologic support

Refer to section at end of plan for postdischarge considerations.

DIAGNOSTIC STUDIES

Stool examination: Occult blood may be positive (mucosal erosion); steatorrhea and bile salts may be found.

X-rays: Barium swallow may demonstrate luminal narrowing in the terminal ileum, stiffening of the bowel wall, mucosal irritability or ulceration.

Barium enema: Small bowel is nearly always involved, but the rectal area is affected only 50% of the time. Fistulas are frequent and are usually found in the terminal ileum but may be present in segments throughout the GI tract.

Sigmoidoscopic examination: Can demonstrate edematous hyperemic colon mucosa, transverse fissures, or longitudinal ulcers.

Endoscopy: Provides visualization of involved areas.

Abdominal MRI/CT scan, ultrasound: Detects infections/inflammatory conditions.

CBC: Anemia (hypochromic, occasionally macrocytic) may occur due to malnutrition or malabsorption or depressed bone marrow function (chronic inflammatory process); increased WBCs.

Sedimentation rate (ESR): Increased reflecting inflammation.

Prealbumin/Albumin/total protein: Decreased.

Cholesterol: Elevated (may have gallstones).

Serum iron-binding folic acid capacity/transferin levels: Decreased due to chronic infection or secondary to blood loss.

Clotting studies: Alterations may occur due to poor vitamin B_{12} absorption.

Electrolytes: Decreased potassium, calcium, and magnesium, with increased sodium.

Urine: Hyperoxaluria (can cause kidney stones).

Urine culture: If *Escherichia coli* organisms are present, suspect fistula formation into the bladder.

NURSING PRIORITIES

1. Control diarrhea/promote optimal bowel function.
2. Minimize/prevent complications.
3. Promote optimal nutrition.
4. Minimize mental/emotional stress.
5. Provide information about disease process, treatment needs, and long-term aspects/potential complications of recurrent disease.

DISCHARGE GOALS

1. Bowel function stabilized.
2. Complications prevented/controlled.
3. Dealing positively with condition.
4. Disease process/prognosis, therapeutic regimen, and potential complications understood.
5. Plan in place to meet needs after discharge.

NURSING DIAGNOSIS: Diarrhea

May be related to
Inflammation, irritation, or malabsorption of the bowel
Presence of toxins
Segmental narrowing of the lumen

Possibly evidenced by
Increased bowel sounds/peristalsis
Frequent, and often severe, watery stools (acute phase)

Changes in stool color
Abdominal pain; urgency (sudden painful need to defecate), cramping

DESIRED OUTCOMES/EVALUATION CRITERIA—PATIENT WILL:
Report reduction in frequency of stools, return to more normal stool consistency.
Identify/avoid contributing factors.

ACTIONS/INTERVENTIONS	RATIONALE
Independent	
Observe and record stool frequency, characteristics, amount, and precipitating factors.	Helps differentiate individual disease and assesses severity of episode.
Promote bed rest, provide bedside commode.	Rest decreases intestinal motility as well as reducing the metabolic rate when infection or hemorrhage is a complication. Defecation urges may occur without warning and be uncontrollable, increasing risk of incontinence/falls if facilities are not close at hand.
Remove stool promptly. Provide room deodorizers.	Reduces noxious odors to avoid undue patient embarrassment.
Identify foods and fluids that precipitate diarrhea, e.g., raw vegetables and fruits, whole-grain cereals, condiments, carbonated drinks, milk products.	Avoidance of intestinal irritants promotes intestinal rest.
Restart oral fluid intake gradually. Offer clear liquids hourly; avoid cold fluids.	Provides colon rest by omitting or decreasing the stimulus of foods/fluids. Gradual resumption of liquids may prevent cramping and recurrence of diarrhea; however, cold fluids can increase intestinal motility.
Provide opportunity to vent frustrations related to disease process.	Presence of disease with unknown cause that is difficult to cure and that may require surgical intervention can lead to stress reactions that may aggravate condition.
Observe for fever, tachycardia, lethargy, leukocytosis, decreased serum protein, anxiety, and prostration.	May signify that toxic megacolon or perforation and peritonitis are imminent/have occurred necessitating immediate medical intervention.
Collaborative	
Administer medications as indicated:	
Anticholinergics, e.g., tincture of belladonna, atropine, diphenoxylate (Lomotil); anodyne suppositories;	Decreases GI motility/propulsion (peristalsis) and diminishes digestive secretions to relieve cramping and diarrhea. *Note:* Use with caution in UC as they may precipitate toxic megacolon.
Salicylate compounds: sulfasalazine (Azulfidine), mesalamine (5-ASA);	Useful in treating mild/moderate exacerbations because of their anti-inflammatory and anti-microbial properties. Long-term use may prolong remission. *Note:* Enteric-coated form is preferred.
Loperamide (Imodium); codeine;	May be required for intense/severe diarrhea. *Note:* Used with caution because toxic dilation may occur.

ACTIONS/INTERVENTIONS	RATIONALE
Collaborative	
Mesalamine (Rowasa);	May be given as an enema in place of Azulfidine for patients who are sensitive to oral sulfa drugs.
Psyllium (Metamucil);	Absorbs water to increase bulk in stools, thereby decreasing diarrhea.
Cholestyramine (Questran);	Binds bile salts, reducing diarrhea that results from excess bile acid.
Steroids, e.g., ACTH, hydrocortisone, prednisolone (Delta-Cortef), prednisone (Deltasone), or (Cortenema, Cortifoam);	Decreases acute inflammatory process. Steroid enemas may be given in mild/moderate disease to aid absorption of the drug (possibly with atropine sulfate or belladonna suppository). Current research suggests an 8-week course of timed-release steroids may effect remission in Crohn's disease; however, steroids are contraindicated if intra-abdominal abscesses are suspected.
Azathioprine (Imuran);	Immunosuppressant may be given to block inflammatory response, decrease steroid requirements, promote healing of fistulas. May be given in conjunction with sulfasalazine.
Antacids;	Decreases gastric irritation, preventing inflammation and reducing risk of infection in colitis.
Enema (hydrocortisone), with/without suppository;	Steroid enemas may be given in mild/moderate disease to aid absorption of the drug. May be given with atropine sulfate or belladonna suppository.
Anti-infectives e.g., metronidazole (Flagyl).	Treats local suppurative infections, or may be part of long-term treatment regimen.
Assist with/prepare for surgical intervention.	May be necessary if perforation or bowel obstruction occurs or disease is unresponsive to medical treatment.

NURSING DIAGNOSIS: Fluid Volume deficit, risk for

Risk factors may include
Excessive losses through normal routes (severe frequent diarrhea, vomiting)
Hypermetabolic state (inflammation, fever)
Restricted intake (nausea)

Possibly evidenced by
[Not applicable; presence of signs and symptoms establishes an *actual* diagnosis]

DESIRED OUTCOMES/EVALUATION CRITERIA—PATIENT WILL:
Maintain adequate fluid volume as evidenced by moist mucous membranes, good skin turgor, and capillary refill; stable vital signs; balanced I&O with urine of normal concentration/amount.

ACTIONS/INTERVENTIONS	RATIONALE
Independent	
Monitor I&O. Note number, character, and amount of stools; estimate insensible fluid losses, e.g., diaphoresis. Measure urine specific gravity; observe for oliguria.	Provides information about overall fluid balance, renal function, and bowel disease control, as well as guidelines for fluid replacement.
Assess vital signs (BP, pulse, temperature).	Hypotension (including postural), tachycardia, fever can indicate response to and/or effect of fluid loss.
Observe for excessively dry skin and mucous membranes, decreased skin turgor, slowed capillary refill.	Indicates excessive fluid loss/resultant dehydration.
Weight daily.	Indicator of overall fluid and nutritional status.
Maintain oral restrictions, bed rest; avoid exertion.	Colon is placed at rest for healing and to decrease intestinal fluid losses.
Observe for overt bleeding and test stool daily for occult blood.	Inadequate diet and decreased absorption may lead to vitamin K deficiency and defects in coagulation, potentiating risk of hemorrhage.
Note generalized muscle weakness or cardiac dysrhythmias.	Excessive intestinal loss may lead to electrolyte imbalance, e.g., potassium, which is necessary for proper skeletal and cardiac muscle function. Minor alterations in serum levels can result in profound and/or life-threatening symptoms.
Collaborative	
Administer parenteral fluids, blood transfusions as indicated.	Maintenance of bowel rest will require alternate fluid replacement to correct losses/anemia. *Note:* Fluids containing sodium may be restricted in presence of regional enteritis.
Monitor laboratory studies, e.g., electrolytes (especially potassium, magnesium) and ABGs (acid-base balance).	Determines replacement needs and effectiveness of therapy.
Administer medications as indicated:	
Antidiarrheal (Refer to ND: Diarrhea, p 337);	Reduces fluid losses from intestines.
Antiemetics, e.g., trimethobenzamide (Tigan), hydroxyzine (Vistaril), prochlorperazine (Compazine);	Used to control nausea/vomiting in acute exacerbations.
Antipyretics, e.g., acetaminophen (Tylenol);	Controls fever, reducing insensible losses.
Electrolytes, e.g., potassium supplement (KCl-IV; K-lyte, Slow-K);	Electrolytes are lost in large amounts, especially in bowel with denuded, ulcerated areas, and diarrhea can also lead to metabolic acidosis through loss of bicarbonate (HCO_3).
Vitamin K (Mephyton).	Stimulates hepatic formation of prothrombin, stabilizing coagulation and reducing risk of hemorrhage.

NURSING DIAGNOSIS: Nutrition: altered, less than body requirements
May be related to
Altered absorption of nutrients

Hypermetabolic state
Medically restricted intake; fear that eating may cause diarrhea
Possibly evidenced by
Weight loss; decreased subcutaneous fat/muscle mass; poor muscle tone
Hyperactive bowel sounds; steatorrhea
Pale conjunctiva and mucous membranes
Aversion to eating

DESIRED OUTCOMES/EVALUATION CRITERIA—PATIENT WILL:
Demonstrate stable weight or progressive gain toward goal with normalization of laboratory values and absence of signs of malnutrition.

ACTIONS/INTERVENTIONS

Independent

Weigh daily.

Encourage bed rest and/or limited activity during acute phase of illness.

Recommend rest before meals.

Provide oral hygiene.

Serve foods in well-ventilated, pleasant surroundings, with unhurried atmosphere, congenial company.

Limit foods that might cause/exacerbate abdominal cramping, flatulence (e.g., milk products, foods high in fiber or fat).

Record intake and changes in symptomatology.

Promote patient participation in dietary planning as possible.

Encourage patient to verbalize feelings concerning resumption of diet.

Collaborative

Keep patient NPO as indicated.

Resume/advance diet as indicated, e.g., clear liquids progressing to bland, low residue; then high-protein, high-calorie, and low-fiber as indicated.

RATIONALE

Provides information about dietary needs/effectiveness of therapy.

Decreasing metabolic needs aids in preventing caloric depletion and conserves energy.

Quiets peristalsis and increases available energy for eating.

A clean mouth can enhance the taste of food.

Pleasant environment aids in reducing stress and is more conducive to eating.

Individual tolerance varies depending on stage of disease and area of bowel affected.

Useful in identifying specific deficiencies and determining GI response to foods.

Provides sense of control for patient and opportunity to select food desired/enjoyed, which may increase intake.

Hesitation to eat may be result of fear that food will cause exacerbation of symptoms.

Resting the bowel decreases peristalsis and diarrhea, which causes malabsorption/loss of nutrients.

Allows the intestinal tract to readjust to the digestive process. Protein is necessary for tissue healing integrity. Low bulk decreases peristaltic response to meal. *Note:* Dietary measures depend on patient's condition, e.g., if disease is mild the patient may do well on low-residue, low-fat diet high in protein and calories with lactose restriction. In moderate disease, elemental enteral products may be given to provide nutrition without overstimulating the bowel. The patient with toxic colitis will be NPO and placed on parenteral nutrition.

341

Collaborative

Provide nutritional support, e.g.,

Enteral feedings via NG, PEG, or J tube;

Many clinical studies have shown benefit from early enteral feeding. Although elemental enteral solutions cannot provide all needed nutrients, they can prevent gut atrophy.

Intravenous TPN.

This regimen rests the GI tract completely while providing essential nutrients. Short-term TPN is indicated during periods of disease exacerbation when bowel rest is needed.

Administer medications as indicated, e.g.:

Donnatal, barbital sodium with belladonna (Butibel); propanthelene bromide (ProBanthine);

Anticholinergics given 15–30 minutes prior to eating provide relief from cramping pain and diarrhea, decreasing gastric motility and enhancing time for absorption of nutrients.

Iron (Imferon injectable);

Prevents/treats anemia. Oral route for iron supplement is ineffective because of intestinal alterations that severely reduce absorption.

Vitamin B_{12} (Crystimin, Rubisol);

Malabsorption of B_{12} is a result of marked loss of functional ileum. Replacement reverses bone marrow depression caused by prolonged inflammatory process, promoting RBC production/correction of anemia.

Folic acid (Folvite);

Folate deficiency is common in presence of Crohn's disease due to decreased intake/absorption, effect of drug therapy (Azulfidine).

Vitamin C (Ascorbicap).

Promotes tissue healing/regeneration.

NURSING DIAGNOSIS: Anxiety [specify level]

May be related to
Physiologic factors/sympathetic stimulation (inflammatory process)
Threat to self-concept (perceived or actual)
Threat to/change in health status, socioeconomic status, role functioning, interaction patterns

Possibly evidenced by
Exacerbation of acute stage of disease
Increased tension, distress, apprehension
Expressed concern regarding changes in life
Somatic complaints
Focus on self

DESIRED OUTCOMES/EVALUATION CRITERIA—PATIENT WILL:
Appear relaxed and report anxiety reduced to a manageable level.
Verbalize awareness of feelings of anxiety and healthy ways to deal with them.

ACTIONS/INTERVENTIONS	RATIONALE
Independent	
Note behavioral clues, e.g., restlessness, irritability, withdrawal, lack of eye contact, demanding behavior.	Indicators of degree of anxiety/stress, e.g., patient may feel out of control at home/work managing personal problems. Stress may develop as a result of physical symptoms of condition, as well as reaction of others.
Encourage verbalization of feelings. Provide feedback.	Establishes a therapeutic relationship. Assists the patient/SO in identifying problems causing stress. Patient with severe diarrhea may hesitate to ask for help for fear of becoming a burden to the staff.
Acknowledge that the anxiety and problems are similar to those expressed by others. Active-listen patient's concerns.	Validation that feelings are normal can help to reduce stress/isolation and belief that "I am the only one."
Provide accurate, concrete information about what is being done, e.g., reason for bed rest, restriction of oral intake, and procedures.	Involving patient in plan of care provides sense of control and helps to decrease anxiety.
Provide a calm, restful environment.	Removing patient from outside stressors promotes relaxation; helps to reduce anxiety.
Encourage staff/SO to project caring, concerned attitude.	A supportive manner can help the patient feel less stressed, allowing energy to be directed toward healing/recovery.
Help patient to identify/initiate positive coping behaviors used in the past.	Successful behaviors can be fostered in dealing with current problems/stress, enhancing patient's sense of self-control.
Assist patient to learn new coping mechanisms, e.g., stress management techniques, organizational skills.	Learning new ways to cope can be helpful in reducing stress and anxiety, enhancing disease control.
Collaborative	
Administer medications as indicated:	
Sedatives, e.g., barbiturates (Luminal); antianxiety agents, e.g., diazepam (Valium).	May be used to reduce anxiety and to facilitate rest, particularly in the patient with UC.
Refer to clinical specialist, psychiatric nurse, social services, spiritual advisor.	May require additional assistance in regaining control and coping with acute episodes/exacerbations, as well as learning to deal with the chronicity and consequences of the disease and therapeutic regimen.

NURSING DIAGNOSIS: Pain [acute]

May be related to

Hyperperistalsis, prolonged diarrhea, skin/tissue irritation, perirectal excoriation, fissures; fistulas

Possibly evidenced by

Reports of colicky/cramping abdominal pain/referred pain

Guarding/distraction behaviors, restlessness

Facial mask of pain; self-focusing

DESIRED OUTCOMES/EVALUATION CRITERIA—PATIENT WILL:
Report pain is relieved/controlled.
Appear relaxed and able to sleep/rest appropriately.

ACTIONS/INTERVENTIONS	RATIONALE
Independent	
Encourage patient to report pain.	May try to tolerate pain rather than request analgesics.
Assess reports of abdominal cramping or pain, noting location, duration, intensity (0–10 scale). Investigate and report changes in pain characteristics.	Colicky intermittent pain occurs with Crohn's. Predefecation pain frequently occurs in UC with urgency, which may be severe and continuous. Changes in pain characteristics may indicate spread of disease/developing complications, e.g., bladder fistula, perforation, toxic megacolon.
Note nonverbal cues, e.g., restlessness, reluctance to move, abdominal guarding, withdrawal, and depression. Investigate discrepancies between verbal and nonverbal cues.	Body language/nonverbal cues may be both physiologic and psychologic, and may be used in conjunction with verbal cues to identify extent/severity of the problem.
Review factors that aggravate or alleviate pain.	May pinpoint precipitating or aggravating factors (such as stressful events, food intolerance) or identify developing complications.
Permit patient to assume position of comfort, e.g., knees flexed.	Reduces abdominal tension and promotes sense of control.
Provide comfort measures (e.g., back rub, reposition) and diversional activities.	Promotes relaxation, refocuses attention, and may enhance coping abilities.
Cleanse rectal area with mild soap and water/wipes after each stool and provide skin care, e.g., A&D ointment, Sween ointment, karaya gel, Desitin, petroleum jelly.	Protects skin from bowel acids, preventing excoriation.
Provide sitz bath as appropriate.	Enhances cleanliness and comfort in the presence of perianal irritation/fissures.
Observe for ischiorectal and perianal fistulas.	Fistulas may develop from erosion and weakening of intestinal bowel wall.
Observe/record abdominal distention, increased temperature, decreased BP.	May indicate developing intestinal obstruction from inflammation, edema, and scarring.
Collaborative	
Implement prescribed dietary modifications, e.g., commence with liquids and increase to solid foods as tolerated.	Complete bowel rest can reduce pain, cramping.
Administer medications as indicated:	
Analgesics;	Pain varies from mild to severe and necessitates management to facilitate adequate rest and recovery. *Note:* Opiates should be used with caution because they may precipitate toxic megacolon.
Anticholinergics;	Relieves spasms of GI tract and resultant colicky pain.
Anodyne suppositories.	Relaxes rectal muscle, decreasing painful spasms.

NURSING DIAGNOSIS: Coping, Individual, ineffective

May be related to

Multiple stressors, repeated over period of time; situational crisis

Unpredictable nature of disease process

Personal vulnerability; inadequate coping method; lack of support systems

Severe pain

Lack of sleep, rest

Possibly evidenced by

Verbalization of inability to cope, discouragement, anxiety

Preoccupation with physical self, chronic worry, emotional tension, poor self-esteem

Depression and dependency

DESIRED OUTCOMES/EVALUATION CRITERIA—PATIENT WILL:

Assess the current situation accurately.

Identify ineffective coping behaviors and consequences.

Acknowledge own coping abilities.

Demonstrate necessary lifestyle changes to limit/prevent recurrent episodes.

ACTIONS/INTERVENTIONS	RATIONALE
Independent	
Assess patient/SO understanding and previous methods of dealing with disease process.	Enables the nurse to deal more realistically with current problems. Anxiety and other problems may have interfered with previous health teaching/patient learning.
Determine outside stresses, e.g., family, relationships, social or work environment.	Stress can alter autonomic nervous response and contribute to exacerbation of disease. Even the goal of independence in the dependent patient can be an added stressor.
Provide opportunity for patient to discuss how illness has affected relationship, including sexual concerns.	Stressors of illness affect all areas of life and patient may have difficulty coping with feelings of fatigue/pain in relation to relationship/sexual needs.
Help patient identify individually effective coping skills.	Use of previously successful behaviors can help patient deal with current situation/plan for future.
Provide emotional support:	
Active-listen in a nonjudgmental manner;	Aids in communication and understanding the patient's view-point. Adds to patient's feelings of self-worth.
Maintain nonjudgmental body language when caring for patient;	Prevents reinforcing patient's feelings of being a burden, e.g., frequent need to empty bedpan/commode.
Assign same staff as much as possible.	Provides a more therapeutic environment and lessens the stress of constant adjustments.
Provide uninterrupted sleep/rest periods.	Exhaustion brought on by the disease tends to magnify problems, interfering with ability to cope.
Encourage use of stress management skills, e.g., relaxation techniques, visualization, guided imagery, deep-breathing exercises.	Refocuses attention, promotes relaxation, and enhances coping abilities.

ACTIONS/INTERVENTIONS

Collaborative

Include patient/SO in team conferences to develop individualized program.

Administer medications as indicated: antipsychotics, e.g., thioridazine (Mellaril); antianxiety agents, e.g., lorazepam (Ativan), alprazolam (Xanax).

Refer to resources as indicated, e.g., social worker, psychiatric nurse, spiritual advisor.

RATIONALE

Promotes continuity of care and enables patient/SO to feel a part of the plan, imparting a sense of control and increasing cooperation with therapeutic regimen.

Aids in psychologic/physical rest. Conserves energy and may strengthen coping abilities.

Additional support and counseling can assist patient/SO in dealing with specific stress/problem areas.

NURSING DIAGNOSIS: Knowledge deficit [learning need] regarding condition, prognosis, treatment, self care and discharge needs

May be related to
Information misinterpretation, lack of recall
Unfamiliarity with resources

Possibly evidenced by
Questions, request for information, statements of misconceptions
Inaccurate follow-through of instructions
Development of preventable complications/exacerbations

DESIRED OUTCOMES/EVALUATION CRITERIA—PATIENT WILL:
Verbalize understanding of disease processes, treatment.
Identify stress situations and specific action(s) to deal with them.
Participate in treatment regimen.
Initiate necessary lifestyle changes.

ACTIONS/INTERVENTIONS

Independent

Determine patient's perception of disease process.

Review disease process, cause/effect relationship of factors that precipitate symptoms and identify ways to reduce contributing factors. Encourage questions.

Review medications, purpose, frequency, dosage, and possible side effects.

Remind patient to observe for side effects if steroids are given on a long-term basis, e.g., ulcers, facial edema, muscle weakness.

Stress importance of good skin care, e.g., proper handwashing techniques and perineal skin care.

RATIONALE

Establishes knowledge base and provides some insight into individual learning needs.

Precipitating/aggravating factors are individual; therefore, the patient needs to be aware of what foods, fluids, and lifestyle factors can precipitate symptoms. Accurate knowledge base provides opportunity for patient to make informed decisions/choices about future and control of chronic disease. Although most patients know about their own disease process, they may have outdated information or misconceptions.

Promotes understanding and may enhance cooperation with regimen.

Steroids may be used to control inflammation and to effect a remission of the disease; however, drug may lower resistance to infection and cause fluid retention.

Reduces spread of bacteria and risk of skin irritation/breakdown, infection.

ACTIONS/INTERVENTIONS	RATIONALE
Independent	
Recommend cessation of smoking.	Can increase intestinal motility, aggravating symptoms.
Emphasize need for long-term follow-up and periodic reevaluation.	Patients with inflammatory bowel disease are at increased risk for colon/rectal cancer, and regular diagnostic evaluations may be required.
Refer to appropriate community resources, e.g., Public Health Nurse, Ostomy Association, dietitian, support groups, and social services.	Patient may benefit from the services of these agencies in coping with chronicity of the disease and evaluating treatment options.

POTENTIAL CONSIDERATIONS following acute hospitalization (dependent on patient's age, physical condition/presence of complications, personal resources, and life responsibilities)

Pain [acute]—hyperperistalsis, prolonged diarrhea, skin/tissue irritation, perirectal excoriation, fissures, fistulas.

Coping, Individual, ineffective—multiple stressors, repeated over period of time; unpredictable nature of disease process; personal vulnerability; severe pain, situational crisis.

Infection, risk for—traumatized tissue, change in pH of secretions, altered peristalsis, suppressed inflammatory response, chronic disease, malnutrition.

Therapeutic Regimen: Individual, ineffective management—complexity of therapeutic regimen, perceived benefit, powerlessness.

FECAL DIVERSIONS: POSTOPERATIVE CARE OF ILEOSTOMY AND COLOSTOMY

An ileostomy is an opening in the ileum for the purpose of treating regional and ulcerative colitis and diverting intestinal contents in colon cancer, polyps, and trauma. It is usually permanent.

A colostomy is a diversion of the effluent of the colon, which may be temporary or permanent. Ascending, transverse, and sigmoid colostomies may be performed. Transverse colostomy is usually temporary. A sigmoid colostomy is the most common permanent stoma, usually performed for cancer.

CARE SETTING:

Inpatient acute care surgical unit.

RELATED CONCERNS

Cancer, p 875
Fluid and Electrolyte Imbalances, p 899
Inflammatory Bowel Disease (IBD): Ulcerative Colitis, Regional Enteritis, p 633
Psychosocial Aspects of Care, p 783
Surgical Interventions, p 802
Total Nutritional Support: Parenteral/Enteral Feeding, p 491

Patient Assessment Data Base

The data is dependent on the underlying problem, duration, and severity (e.g., obstruction, perforation, inflammation, congenital defects).

TEACHING/LEARNING

Discharge plan considerations:

DRG projected mean length of inpatient stay: 9.4 days
Assistance with dietary concerns, management of ostomy, and acquisition of supplies may be required

Refer to section at end of plan for postdischarge considerations.

NURSING PRIORITIES

1. Assist patient/SO in psychosocial adjustment.
2. Prevent complications.
3. Support independence in self-care.
4. Provide information about procedure/prognosis, treatment needs, potential complications, and community resources.

DISCHARGE GOALS

1. Adjusting to perceived/actual changes.
2. Complications prevented/minimized.
3. Self-care needs met by self/with assistance dependent on specific situation.
4. Procedure/prognosis, therapeutic regimen, potential complications understood and sources of support identified.
5. Plan in place to meet needs after discharge.

ACTIONS/INTERVENTIONS	RATIONALE
Independent	
Inspect stoma/peristomal skin area with each pouch change. Clean with water and pat dry. Note irritation, bruises (dark, bluish color), rashes.	Monitors healing process/effectiveness of appliances and identifies areas of concern, need for further evaluation/intervention. Maintaining a clean/dry area helps to prevent skin breakdown. Early identification of stomal necrosis/ischemia or fungal infection (from changes in normal bowel flora) provides for timely interventions to prevent serious complications. Stoma should be red and moist. Ulcerated areas on stoma may be from a pouch opening that is too small or a faceplate that cuts into stoma. In patients with an ileostomy, the effluent is rich in enzymes, increasing the likelihood of skin irritation. In the patient with a colostomy, skin care is not as great a concern, since the enzymes are no longer present in the effluent.
Measure stoma periodically, e.g., at each appliance change for first 6 weeks, then once a month for 6 months.	As postoperative edema resolves (during first 6 weeks) size of appliance must be altered to ensure proper fit so that effluent is collected as it flows from the ostomy and contact with the skin is prevented.
Verify that opening on adhesive backing of pouch is at least ⅛ inch larger than the base of the stoma, with adequate adhesiveness left to apply pouch.	Prevents trauma to the stoma tissue and protects the peristomal skin. Adequate adhesive area is important to maintain a seal. *Note:* Too tight a fit may cause stomal edema or stenosis.
Use a transparent, odor-proof drainable pouch.	A transparent appliance during first 4–6 weeks allows easy observation of stoma without necessity of removing pouch/irritating skin.
Apply appropriate skin barrier, e.g., stomahesive wafer, karaya gum, Reliaseal, or similar products.	Protects skin from pouch adhesive, enhances adhesiveness of pouch, and facilitates removal of pouch when necessary. *Note:* Sigmoid colostomy may not require use of a skin barrier once stool becomes formed and elimination is regulated through irrigation.

ACTIONS/INTERVENTIONS	RATIONALE
Independent	
Empty, irrigate, and cleanse ostomy pouch on a routine basis, using appropriate equipment.	Frequent pouch changes are irritating to the skin and should be avoided. Emptying and rinsing the pouch with the proper solution not only removes bacteria and odor-causing stool and flatus but also deodorizes the pouch.
Support surrounding skin when gently removing appliance. Apply adhesive removers as indicated, then wash thoroughly.	Prevents tissue irritation/destruction associated with "pulling" pouch off.
Investigate reports of burning/itching/blistering around stoma.	Indicative of effluent leakage with peristomal irritation, or possibly candida infection, requiring intervention.
Evaluate adhesive product and appliance fit on ongoing basis.	Provides opportunity for problem solving. Determines need for further intervention.
Collaborative	
Consult with enterostomal therapist/nurse.	Helpful in choosing products appropriate for patient's particular rehabilitation needs, including type of ostomy, physical/mental status, and financial resources.
Apply corticosteroid aerosol spray and nystatin powder as indicated.	Assists in healing if peristomal irritation persists/fungal infection develops. *Note:* These products can have potent side effects and should be used sparingly.

NURSING DIAGNOSIS: Body Image disturbance

May be related to
Biophysical: presence of stoma; loss of control of bowel elimination
Psychosocial: altered body structure
Disease process and associated treatment regimen, e.g., cancer, colitis

Possibly evidenced by
Verbalization of change in body image, fear of rejection/reaction of others, and negative feelings about body
Actual change in structure and/or function (ostomy)
Not touching/looking at stoma, refusal to participate in care

DESIRED OUTCOMES/EVALUATION CRITERIA—PATIENT WILL:
Verbalize acceptance of self in situation, incorporating change into self-concept without negating self-esteem.
Demonstrate beginning acceptance by viewing/touching stoma and participating in self-care.
Verbalize feelings about stoma/illness; begin to deal constructively with situation.

ACTIONS/INTERVENTIONS	RATIONALE
Independent	
Ascertain whether counseling was initiated when the possibility and/or necessity of ostomy was first discussed.	Provides information about patient's/SO's level of knowledge about individual situation and process of acceptance.

ACTIONS/INTERVENTIONS	RATIONALE
Independent	
Encourage patient/SO to verbalize feelings regarding the ostomy. Acknowledge normality of feelings of anger, depression, and grief over loss. Discuss daily "ups and downs" that can occur.	Helps the patient to realize that feelings are not unusual and that feeling guilty about them is not necessary/helpful. Patient needs to recognize feelings before they can be dealt with effectively.
Review reason for surgery and future expectations.	Patient may find it easier to accept/deal with an ostomy done to correct chronic/long-term disease than for traumatic injury, even if ostomy is only temporary. Also, the patient who will be undergoing a second procedure (to convert ostomy to a continent or anal reservoir) may possibly encounter less severe self-image problems because body function eventually will be "more normal".
Note behaviors of withdrawal, increased dependency, manipulation, or noninvolvement in care.	Suggestive of problems in adjustment that may require further evaluation and more extensive therapy.
Provide opportunities for patient/SO to view and touch stoma, using the moment to point out positive signs of healing, normal appearance, and so forth. Remind patient that it will take time to adjust, both physically and emotionally.	Although integration of stoma into body image can take months or even years, looking at the stoma and hearing comments (made in a normal, matter-of-fact manner) can help patient with this acceptance. Touching stoma reassures patient/SO that it is not fragile and that slight movements of stoma actually reflect normal peristalsis.
Provide opportunity for patient to deal with ostomy through participation in self-care.	Independence in self-care helps to improve self-confidence and acceptance of situation.
Plan/schedule care activities with patient.	Promotes sense of control and gives message that patient can handle this, enhancing self-esteem.
Maintain positive approach during care activities, avoiding expressions of disdain or revulsion. Do not take angry expressions personally.	Assists patient/SO to accept body changes and feel all right about self. Anger is most often directed at the situation and lack of control individual has over what has happened (powerlessness), not with the individual caregiver.
Discuss possibility of contacting ostomy visitor, and make arrangements for visit if desired.	Can provide a good support system. Helps to reinforce teaching (shared experiences) and facilitates acceptance of change as patient realizes "life does go on" and can be relatively normal.

NURSING DIAGNOSIS: Pain [acute]

May be related to
Physical factors: e.g., disruption of skin/tissues (incisions/drains)
Biologic: activity of disease process (cancer, trauma)
Psychologic factors: e.g., fear, anxiety

Possibly evidenced by
Reports of pain, self-focusing
Guarding/distraction behaviors, restlessness
Autonomic responses, e.g., changes in vital signs

ACTIONS/INTERVENTIONS	RATIONALE
Independent	
Assess pain, noting location, characteristics, intensity (0–10 scale).	Helps evaluate degree of discomfort and effectiveness of analgesia or may reveal developing complications; e.g., because abdominal pain usually subsides gradually by the 3rd or 4th postoperative day, continued or increasing pain may reflect delayed healing or peristomal skin irritation. *Note:* Pain in anal area associated with abdominal-perineal resection may persist for months.
Encourage patient to verbalize concerns. Active-listen these concerns, and provide support by acceptance, remaining with patient, and giving appropriate information.	Reduction of anxiety/fear can promote relaxation/comfort.
Provide comfort measures, e.g., mouth care, back rub, repositioning (use proper support measures as needed). Assure patient that position change will not injure stoma.	Prevents drying of oral mucosa and associated discomfort. Reduces muscle tension, promotes relaxation, and may enhance coping abilities.
Encourage use of relaxation techniques, e.g., guided imagery, visualization. Provide diversional activities.	Helps patient to rest more effectively and refocuses attention, thereby reducing pain and discomfort.
Assist with ROM exercises and encourage early ambulation. Avoid prolonged sitting position.	Reduces muscle/joint stiffness. Ambulation returns organs to normal position and promotes return of usual level of functioning. *Note:* Presence of edema, packing, and drains (if perineal resection has been done) increases discomfort and creates a sense of needing to defecate. Ambulation and frequent position changes reduce perineal pressure.
Investigate and report abdominal muscle rigidity, involuntary guarding, and rebound tenderness.	Suggestive of peritoneal inflammation, which requires prompt medical intervention.
Collaborative	
Administer medication as indicated, e.g., narcotics, analgesics, PCA.	Relieves pain, enhances comfort, and promotes rest. PCA may be more beneficial, especially following AP repair.
Provide sitz baths.	Relieves local discomfort, reduces edema, and promotes healing of perineal wound.
Apply/monitor effects of TENS unit.	Cutaneous stimulation may be used to block transmission of pain stimulus

NURSING DIAGNOSIS: Skin/Tissue Integrity, impaired

May be related to
Invasion of body structure (perineal resection)
Stasis of secretions/drainage
Altered circulation, edema; malnutrition

Possibly evidenced by
Disruption of skin/tissue: presence of incision, and sutures, drains

DESIRED OUTCOMES/EVALUATION CRITERIA—PATIENT WILL:
Achieve timely wound healing free of signs of infection.

ACTIONS/INTERVENTIONS	RATIONALE
Independent	
Observe wounds, note characteristics of drainage.	Postoperative hemorrhage is most likely to occur during first 48 hours, whereas infection may develop at any time. Dependent on type of wound closure (e.g., first or second intention), complete healing may take 6–8 months.
Change dressings as needed using aseptic technique.	Large amounts of serous drainage require that dressings be changed frequently to reduce skin irritation and potential for infection.
Encourage sidelying position with head elevated. Avoid prolonged sitting.	Promotes drainage from perineal wound/drains reducing risk of pooling. Prolonged sitting increases perineal pressure, reducing circulation to wound, and may delay healing.
Collaborative	
Irrigate wound as indicated, using normal saline, diluted hydrogen peroxide, or antibiotic solution.	May be required to treat preoperative inflammation/infection or intraoperative contamination.
Provide sitz baths.	Promotes cleanliness and facilitates healing especially after packing is removed (usually day 3–5).

NURSING DIAGNOSIS: Fluid Volume deficit, risk for

Risk factors may include
Excessive losses through normal routes, e.g., preoperative emesis and diarrhea
Losses through abnormal routes, e.g., NG/intestinal tube, perineal wound drainage tubes
High-volume ileostomy output
Medically restricted intake
Altered absorption of fluid, e.g., loss of colon function
Hypermetabolic states, e.g., inflammation, healing process

Possibly evidenced by
[Not applicable; presence of signs and symptoms establishes an *actual* diagnosis]

ACTIONS/INTERVENTIONS	RATIONALE
Independent	
Monitor I&O carefully, measure liquid stool. Weigh regularly.	Provides direct indicators of fluid balance. Greatest fluid losses occur with ileostomy, but they generally do not exceed 500–800 ml/d.
Monitor vital signs noting postural hypotension, tachycardia. Evaluate skin turgor, capillary refill, and mucous membranes.	Reflects hydration status/possible need for increased fluid replacement.
Limit intake of ice chips during period of gastric intubation.	Ice chips can stimulate gastric secretions and wash out electrolytes.
Collaborative	
Monitor laboratory results, e.g., Hct and electrolytes.	Detects homeostasis or imbalance and aids in determining replacement needs.
Administer IV fluid and electrolytes as indicated.	May be necessary to maintain adequate tissue perfusion/organ function.

NURSING DIAGNOSIS: Nutrition: altered, risk for less than body requirements

Risk factors may include
Prolonged anorexia/altered intake preoperatively
Hypermetabolic state (preoperative inflammatory disease; healing process)
Presence of diarrhea/altered absorption
Restriction of bulk and residue-containing foods

Possibly evidenced by
[Not applicable; presence of signs and symptoms establishes an *actual* diagnosis]

DESIRED OUTCOMES/EVALUATION CRITERIA—PATIENT WILL:
Maintain weight/demonstrate progressive weight gain toward goal with normalization of laboratory values and free of signs of malnutrition.
Plan diet to meet nutritional needs/limit GI disturbances.

ACTIONS/INTERVENTIONS	RATIONALE
Independent	
Obtain a thorough nutritional assessment.	Identifies deficiencies/needs to aid in choice of interventions.
Auscultate bowel sounds.	Return of intestinal function indicates readiness to resume oral intake.

ACTIONS/INTERVENTIONS

Independent

Resume solid foods slowly.

Identify odor-causing foods (e.g., cabbage, fish, beans) and temporarily restrict from diet. Gradually reintroduce 1 food at a time.

Recommend patient increase use of yogurt and buttermilk.

Suggest patient with ileostomy exercise caution in the use of prunes, dates, stewed apricots, strawberries, grapes, bananas, cabbage family, beans, and nuts and avoid cellulose products, e.g., peanuts.

Discuss mechanics of swallowed air as a factor in the formation of flatus and some ways the patient can exercise control.

Collaborative

Consult with dietician.

Advance diet from liquids to low-residue food when oral intake is resumed.

Administer enteral/parenteral feedings when indicated.

RATIONALE

Reduces incidence of abdominal cramps, nausea.

Sensitivity to certain foods is not uncommon following intestinal surgery. Patient can experiment with food several times before determining whether it is creating a problem.

May help decrease odor formation.

These products increase ileal effluent. Digestion of cellulose requires colon bacteria that are no longer present.

Drinking through a straw, snoring, anxiety, smoking, ill-fitting dentures, and gulping down food increase the production of flatus. Too much flatus not only necessitates frequent emptying, but can be a causative factor in leakage from too much pressure within the pouch.

Helpful in assessing patient's nutritional needs in light of changes in digestion and intestinal function including absorption of vitamins/minerals.

Low-residue diet may be maintained during first 6–8 weeks to provide adequate time for intestinal healing.

In the presence of severe debilitation/intolerance of oral intake, hyperalimentation may be used to supply needed components for healing and prevention of catabolic state.

NURSING DIAGNOSIS: Sleep Pattern disturbance

May be related to
External factors: necessity of ostomy care, excessive flatus/ostomy effluent
Internal factors: psychologic stress, fear of leakage of pouch/injury to stoma

Possibly evidenced by
Verbalizations of interrupted sleep, not feeling well rested
Changes in behavior, e.g., irritability, listlessness/lethargy

DESIRED OUTCOMES/EVALUATION CRITERIA—PATIENT WILL:
Sleep/rest between disturbances.
Report increased sense of well-being and feeling rested.

ACTIONS/INTERVENTIONS

Independent

Explain necessity to monitor intestinal function in early postoperative period.

RATIONALE

Patient is more apt to be tolerant of disturbances by staff if he or she understands the reasons for/importance of care.

ACTIONS/INTERVENTIONS

Independent

Provide adequate pouching system. Empty pouch before retiring and, if necessary, on a preagreed schedule.

Let patient know that stoma will not be injured when sleeping.

Restrict intake of caffeine-containing foods/fluids.

Support continuation of usual bedtime rituals.

Collaborative

Determine cause of excessive flatus or effluent, e.g., confer with dietitian regarding restriction of foods if diet-related.

Administer analgesics, sedatives at bedtime as indicated.

RATIONALE

Excessive flatus/effluent can occur despite interventions. Emptying on a regular schedule minimizes threat of leakage.

Patient will be able to rest better if feeling secure about stoma and ostomy function.

Caffeine may delay patient's falling asleep and interfere with REM sleep, resulting in patient not feeling well rested.

Promotes relaxation and readiness for sleep.

Identification of cause enables institution of corrective measures that may promote sleep/rest.

Pain can interfere with patient's ability to fall/remain asleep. Timely medication can enhance rest/sleep during initial postoperative period. *Note:* Pain pathways in the brain lie near the sleep center and may contribute to wakefulness.

NURSING DIAGNOSIS: Constipation/Diarrhea, risk for

Risk factors may include
Placement of ostomy in descending or sigmoid colon
Inadequate diet/fluid intake

Possibly evidenced by
[Not applicable; presence of signs and symptoms establishes an *actual* diagnosis]

DESIRED OUTCOMES/EVALUATION CRITERIA—PATIENT WILL:
Establish an elimination pattern suitable to physical needs and lifestyle with effluent of appropriate amount and consistency.

ACTIONS/INTERVENTIONS

Independent

Ascertain patient's previous bowel habits and lifestyle.

Investigate delayed onset/absence of effluent. Auscultate bowel sounds.

RATIONALE

Assists in formulation of an effective irrigating schedule for the patient with a colostomy.

Postoperative paralytic/adynamic ileus usually resolves within 48–72 hours and ileostomy should begin draining within 12–24 hours. Delay may indicate persistent ileus or stomal obstruction, which may occur postoperatively because of edema, improperly fitting pouch (too tight), prolapse, or stenosis of the stoma.

ACTIONS/INTERVENTIONS

Independent

Inform the patient with an ileostomy that initially the effluent will be liquid. If constipation occurs, it should be reported to enterostomal nurse or physician.

Review dietary pattern and amount/type of fluid intake.

Review physiology of the colon and discuss irrigation management of sigmoid ostomy, if appropriate.

Demonstrate use of irrigation equipment to inject normal saline per protocol until relief is obtained.

Instruct patient in the use of closed-end pouch or a patch, dressing/Band-Aid when irrigation is successful and the sigmoid colostomy effluent becomes more manageable, with stool expelled every 24 hours.

Involve the patient in care of the ostomy on an increasing basis.

Collaborative

Instruct in use of TENS unit if indicated.

RATIONALE

Although the small intestine eventually begins to take on water-absorbing functions to permit a more semisolid, pasty discharge, constipation may indicate an obstruction. Absence of stool requires emergency medical attention.

Adequate intake of fiber and roughage provides bulk, and fluid is an important factor in determining the consistency of the stool.

This knowledge helps the patient understand individual care needs.

Irrigations may be done on a daily basis or prior to special activities. There are differing views on the use of daily irrigations. Many believe cleaning the bowel on a regular basis is helpful. Others believe that this interferes with normal functioning. Most authorities agree that occasional irrigating is useful for emptying the bowel to avoid leakage when special events are planned.

Enables patient to feel more comfortable socially and is less expensive than regular ostomy pouches.

Rehabilitation can be facilitated by encouraging patient independence and control.

Electrical stimulation has been used in some patients to stimulate peristalsis and relieve postoperative ileus.

NURSING DIAGNOSIS: Sexual dysfunction, risk for

Risk factors may include
Altered body structure/function; radical resection/treatment procedures
Vulnerability/psychologic concern about response of SO
Disruption of sexual response pattern, e.g., erectile difficulty

Possibly evidenced by
[Not applicable; presence of signs and symptoms establishes an *actual* diagnosis]

DESIRED OUTCOMES/EVALUATION CRITERIA—PATIENT WILL:
Verbalize understanding of relationship of physical condition to sexual problems.
Identify satisfying/acceptable sexual practices and explore alternate methods.
Resume sexual relationship as appropriate.

ACTIONS/INTERVENTIONS	RATIONALE

Independent

Determine the patient/SO sexual relationship prior to the disease and/or surgery and whether they anticipate problems related to presence of ostomy.

Identify future expectations and desires. Mutilation and loss of privacy/control of a bodily function can affect patient's view of personal sexuality. When coupled with the fear of rejection by SO, the desired level of intimacy can be greatly impaired. Sexual needs are very basic, and the patient will be rehabilitated more successfully when a satisfying sexual relationship is continued/developed as desired.

Review with the patient/SO sexual functioning in relation to own situation.

Understanding if nerve damage has altered normal sexual functioning (e.g., erection) helps patient/SO to understand the need for exploring alternate methods of satisfaction.

Reinforce information given by the physician. Encourage questions. Provide additional information as needed.

Reiteration of data previously given assists the patient/SO to hear and process the knowledge again, moving toward acceptance of individual limitations/restrictions and prognosis (e.g., that it may take up to 2 years to regain potency after a radical procedure or that a penile prosthesis may be necessary).

Discuss resumption of sexual activity in approximately 6 weeks after discharge, beginning slowly and progressing (e.g., cuddling/caressing until both partners are comfortable with body image/function changes). Include alternate methods of stimulation as appropriate.

Knowing what to expect in progress of recovery helps patient avoid performance anxiety/reduce risk of "failure." If the couple is willing to try new ideas, this can assist with adjustment and may help to achieve sexual fulfillment.

Encourage dialogue between partners. Suggest wearing pouch cover, T-shirt, or shortie nightgown.

Disguising ostomy appliance may aid in reducing feelings of self-consciousness, embarrassment during sexual activity.

Stress awareness of factors that might be distracting (e.g., unpleasant odors and pouch leakage). Encourage use of sense of humor.

Promotes resolution of solvable problems. Laughter can help individuals to deal more effectively with difficult situation, promote positive sexual experience.

Problem-solve alternative positions for coitus.

Minimizing awkwardness of appliance and physical discomfort can enhance satisfaction.

Discuss/role-play possible interactions or approaches when dealing with new sexual partners.

Rehearsal is helpful in dealing with actual situations when they arise, preventing self-consciousness about "different" body image.

Provide birth control information as appropriate and stress that impotence does not mean the patient is sterile.

Confusion may exist that can lead to an unwanted pregnancy.

Collaborative

Arrange meeting with an ostomy visitor if appropriate.

Sharing of how these problems have been resolved by others can be helpful and reduce sense of isolation.

Refer to counseling/sex therapy as indicated.

If problems persist longer than several months after surgery, a trained therapist may be required to facilitate communication between patient and SO.

NURSING DIAGNOSIS: Knowledge deficit [learning need] regarding condition, prognosis, treatment, self care and discharge needs

May be related to

Lack of exposure/recall information misinterpretation

Unfamiliarity with information resources

Possibly evidenced by

Questions; statement of misconception/misinformation

Inaccurate follow-through of instruction/performance of ostomy care

Inappropriate or exaggerated behaviors (e.g., hostile, agitated, apathetic, withdrawal)

DESIRED OUTCOMES/EVALUATION CRITERIA—PATIENT WILL:

Verbalize understanding of condition/disease process, treatment and prognosis.

Correctly perform necessary procedures, explain reasons for the action.

Initiate necessary lifestyle changes.

ACTIONS/INTERVENTIONS	RATIONALE
Independent	
Evaluate patient's emotional and physical capabilities.	These factors affect patient's ability to master tasks and willingness to assume responsibility for ostomy care.
Review anatomy, physiology, and implications of surgical intervention. Discuss future expectations, including anticipated changes in character of effluent.	Provides knowledge base on which patient can make informed choices and an opportunity to clarify misconceptions regarding individual situation. (Temporary ileostomy may be converted to ileoanal reservoir at a future date; ileostomy and ascending colostomy cannot be regulated by diet, irrigations, or medications, and so on.)
Include written/picture resources.	Provides references after discharge to support patient efforts for independence in self-care.
Instruct patient/SO in stomal care. Allot time for return demonstrations and provide positive feedback for efforts.	Promotes positive management and reduces risk of improper ostomy care/development of complications.
Recommend increased fluid intake during warm weather months.	Loss of normal colon function of conserving water and electrolytes can lead to dehydration and constipation.
Discuss possible need to decrease salt intake.	Salt can increase ileal output, potentiating risk of dehydration and increasing frequency of ostomy care needs/patient's inconvenience.
Identify symptoms of electrolyte depletion, e.g., anorexia, abdominal muscle cramps, feelings of faintness or "cold" in arms/legs; general fatigue/weakness, bloating, decreased sensations in arms/legs.	Loss of colon function with altered fluid/electrolyte absorption may result in sodium/potassium deficits requiring dietary correction with foods/fluids high in sodium (e.g., bouillon, Gatorade) or potassium (e.g., orange juice, prunes, tomatoes, bananas, or Gatorade).
Discuss need for periodic evaluation/administration of supplemental vitamins and minerals as appropriate.	Depending on portion and amount of bowel resected, lack of absorption may cause deficiencies.
Stress importance of chewing food well, adequate intake of fluids with/following meals, and only moderate use of high-fiber foods; avoidance of cellulose.	Reduces risk of bowel obstruction, especially in patient with ileostomy.

ACTIONS/INTERVENTIONS	RATIONALE
Independent	
Review foods that are/may be a source of flatus (e.g., carbonated drinks, beer, beans, cabbage family, onions, fish, and highly seasoned foods) or odor (e.g., onions, cabbage family, eggs, fish, and beans).	These foods may be restricted or eliminated, based on individual reaction, for better ostomy control, or it may be necessary to empty the pouch more frequently if they are ingested.
Identify foods associated with diarrhea, such as green beans, broccoli, highly seasoned foods.	Promotes better bowel control.
Recommend foods used to manage constipation (e.g., bran, celery, raw fruits), as well as importance of increased fluid intake.	Proper management can prevent/minimize problems of constipation.
Discuss resumption of presurgery level of activity.	Patient should be able to manage same degree of activity as previously enjoyed and in some cases increase activity level.
Talk about the possibility of sleep disturbance, anorexia, loss of interest in usual activities.	"Homecoming depression" may occur, lasting for months after surgery, requiring patience/support and ongoing evaluation as the patient adjusts to living with a stoma.
Explain necessity of notifying healthcare providers and pharmacists of type of ostomy and avoidance of sustained-release medications.	Presence of ostomy may alter rate/extent of absorption of oral medications and increase risk of drug-related complications, e.g., diarrhea/constipation or peristomal excoriation. Liquid, chewable, or injectable forms of medication are preferred for patients with ileostomy to maximize absorption of drug.
Counsel patient concerning medication use and problems associated with altered bowel function. Refer to pharmacist for teaching/advice as appropriate.	The patient with an ostomy has 2 key problems, i.e., altered disintegration and absorption of oral drugs and unusual or pronounced adverse effects. Some of the medications, which these patients may respond to differently, include laxatives, salicylates, H_2 receptor antagonists, antibiotics, and diuretics.
Discuss effect of medications on effluent, i.e., changes in color, odor, consistency of stool; need to observe for drug residue indicating incomplete absorption.	Understanding decreases anxiety regarding intestinal function and enhances independence in self-care.
Stress necessity of close monitoring of chronic health conditions requiring routine oral medications.	Monitoring of clinical symptoms and serum blood levels is indicated, due to altered drug absorption requiring periodic dosage adjustments.
Identify community resources, e.g., United Ostomy Association, local ostomy support group, enterostomal therapist, visiting nurse, pharmacy/medical supply house.	Continued support after discharge is essential to facilitate the recovery process and patient's independence in care. Enterostomal nurse can be very helpful in solving appliance problems, identifying alternatives to meet individual patient needs.

POTENTIAL CONSIDERATIONS following acute hospitalization (dependent on patient's age, physical condition/presence of complications, personal resources, and life responsibilities)

Skin Integrity, impaired, risk for—absence of sphincter at stoma, character/flow of effluent and flatus from stoma.
Coping, Individual, ineffective—situational crises, vulnerability.
Social Interaction, impaired—self-concept disturbance, concern for loss of control of bodily functions.

APPENDECTOMY

Removal of an inflamed appendix may be performed using a laparoscopic approach. However, the presence of multiple adhesions, retroperitoneal positioning of the appendix or the likelihood of rupture necessitates an open (traditional) procedure.

CARE SETTING

Although many of the interventions included here are appropriate for the short-stay patient, this plan of care addresses the traditional appendectomy care provided on a surgical unit.

RELATED CONCERNS

Peritonitis, p 366
Psychosocial Aspects of Care, p 783
Surgical Intervention, p 802

Patient Assessment Data Base (Preoperative)

ACTIVITY/REST

May report: Malaise

CIRCULATION

May exhibit: Tachycardia

ELIMINATION

May report: Constipation of recent onset
Diarrhea (occasional)

May exhibit: Abdominal distention, tenderness/rebound tenderness, rigidity
Decreased or absent bowel sounds

FOOD/FLUID

May report: Anorexia
Nausea/vomiting

PAIN/DISCOMFORT

May report: Abdominal pain around the epigastrium and umbilicus, which becomes increasingly severe and localizes at McBurney's point (halfway between umbilicus and crest of right ileum), aggravated by walking, sneezing, coughing, or deep respiration (increasing severe and generalized pain or sudden cessation of pain suggests perforation or infarction of the appendix)
Varied reports of pain/vague symptoms (due to location of appendix, e.g., retrocecally or next to ureter, or due to onset of peritonitis)

May exhibit: Guarding behavior; lying on side or back with knees flexed; increased right lower quadrant (RLQ) pain with extension of right leg/upright position
Rebound tenderness on left side suggests peritoneal inflammation

SAFETY

May exhibit: Fever (usually low-grade)

RESPIRATION

May exhibit: Tachypnea; shallow respirations

TEACHING/LEARNING

May report: History of other conditions associated with abdominal pain, e.g., acute pyelitis, ureteral stone, acute salpingitis, regional ileitis

May occur at any age

Discharge plan considerations: **DRG projected mean length of inpatient stay: 4.2 days/short stay: 24 hours**

May need brief assistance with transportation, home maker tasks

Refer to section at end of plan for postdischarge considerations.

DIAGNOSTIC STUDIES

WBC: Leukocytosis above 12,000/mm^3, neutrophil count elevated to 75%.

Urinalysis: Normal, but erythrocytes/leukocytes may be present.

Abdominal x-rays: May reveal hardened bit of fecal material in appendix (fecalith), localized ileus.

CT scan: May be done for differentiation of appendicitis from other causes of abdominal pain, e.g., perforating ulcer, cholecystitis, reproductive organ infections.

NURSING PRIORITIES

1. Promote comfort.
2. Prevent complications.
3. Provide information about surgical procedure/prognosis, treatment needs, and potential complications.

DISCHARGE GOALS

1. Complications prevented/minimized.
2. Pain alleviated/controlled.
3. Surgical procedure/prognosis, therapeutic regimen, and possible complications understood.
4. Plan in place to meet needs after discharge.

NURSING DIAGNOSIS: Infection, risk for

Risk factors may include
Inadequate primary defenses; perforation/rupture of the appendix; peritonitis; abscess formation
Invasive procedures, surgical incision

Possibly evidenced by
[Not applicable; presence of signs and symptoms establishes an *actual* diagnosis]

DESIRED OUTCOMES/EVALUATION CRITERIA—PATIENT WILL:
Achieve timely wound healing; free of signs of infection/inflammation, purulent drainage, erythema, and fever.

ACTIONS/INTERVENTIONS

Independent

Monitor vital signs. Note onset of fever, chills, diaphoresis, changes in mentation, reports of increasing abdominal pain.

Practice good hand-washing and aseptic wound care. Encourage/provide pericare.

Inspect incision and dressings. Note characteristics of drainage from wound/drains (if inserted), presence of erythema.

Collaborative

Obtain drainage specimens if indicated.

Administer antibiotics as appropriate.

Prepare for/assist with I&D if indicated.

RATIONALE

Suggestive of presence of infection/developing sepsis, abscess, peritonitis.

Reduces risk of spread of bacteria.

Provides for early detection of developing infectious process, and/or monitors resolution of preexisting peritonitis.

Gram's stain, culture, and sensitivity are useful in identifying causative organism and choice of therapy.

May be given prophylactically or to reduce number of organisms (in preexisting infection) to decrease spread and seeding of the abdominal cavity.

May be necessary to drain contents of localized abscess.

NURSING DIAGNOSIS: Fluid Volume deficit, risk for

Risk factors may include
Preoperative vomiting
Postoperative restrictions (e.g., NPO)
Hypermetabolic state (e.g., fever, healing process)
Inflammation of peritoneum with sequestration of fluid

Possibly evidenced by
[Not applicable; presence of signs and symptoms establishes an *actual* diagnosis]

DESIRED OUTCOMES/EVALUATION CRITERIA—PATIENT WILL:
Maintain adequate fluid balance as evidenced by moist mucous membranes, good skin turgor, stable vital signs, and individually adequate urinary output.

ACTIONS/INTERVENTIONS

Independent

Monitor BP and pulse.

Inspect mucous membranes; assess skin turgor and capillary refill.

Monitor I&O; note urine color/concentration, specific gravity.

Auscultate bowel sounds. Note passing of flatus, bowel movement.

RATIONALE

Variations help identify fluctuating intravascular volumes.

Indicators of adequacy of peripheral circulation and cellular hydration.

Decreasing output of concentrated urine with increasing specific gravity suggests dehydration/need for increased fluids.

Indicators of return of peristalsis, readiness to begin oral intake.

ACTIONS/INTERVENTIONS	RATIONALE
Independent	
Provide clear liquids in small amounts when oral intake is resumed, and progress diet as tolerated.	Reduces risk of gastric irritation/vomiting to minimize fluid loss.
Give frequent mouth care with special attention to protection of the lips.	Dehydration results in drying and painful cracking of the lips and mouth.
Collaborative	
Maintain gastric/intestinal suction.	An NG tube may be inserted preoperatively and maintained in immediate postoperative phase to decompress the bowel, promote intestinal rest, prevent vomiting.
Administer IV fluids and electrolytes.	The peritoneum reacts to irritation/infection by producing large amounts of fluid that may reduce the circulating blood volume, resulting in hypovolemia. Dehydration and relative electrolyte imbalances may occur.

NURSING DIAGNOSIS: Pain [acute]

May be related to
Distention of intestinal tissues by inflammation
Presence of surgical incision

Possibly evidenced by
Reports of pain
Facial grimacing, muscle guarding; distraction behaviors
Autonomic responses

DESIRED OUTCOMES/EVALUATION CRITERIA—PATIENT WILL:
Report pain is relieved/controlled.
Appear relaxed, able to sleep/rest appropriately.

ACTIONS/INTERVENTIONS	RATIONALE
Independent	
Assess pain, noting location, characteristics, severity (0–10 scale). Investigate and report changes in pain as appropriate.	Useful in monitoring effectiveness of medication, progression of healing. Changes in characteristics of pain may indicate developing abscess/peritonitis, requiring prompt medical evaluation and intervention.
Provide accurate, honest information to patient/SO.	Being informed about progress of situation provides emotional support, helping to decrease anxiety.
Keep at rest in semi-Fowler's position.	Gravity localizes inflammatory exudate into lower abdomen or pelvis, relieving abdominal tension, which is accentuated by supine position.
Encourage early ambulation.	Promotes normalization of organ function, e.g., stimulates peristalsis and passing of flatus, reducing abdominal discomfort.
Provide diversional activities.	Refocuses attention, promotes relaxation, and may enhance coping abilities.

ACTIONS/INTERVENTIONS	RATIONALE
Collaborative	
Keep NPO/maintain NG suction initially.	Decreases discomfort of early intestinal peristalsis and gastric irritation/vomiting.
Administer analgesics as indicated.	Relief of pain facilitates cooperation with other therapeutic interventions, e.g., ambulation, pulmonary toilet.
Place ice bag on abdomen.	Soothes and relieves pain through desensitization of nerve endings. *Note:* Do not use heat, because it may cause tissue congestion.

NURSING DIAGNOSIS: Knowledge deficit [learning need] regarding condition, prognosis, treatment, self care and discharge needs

May be related to
Lack of exposure/recall; information misinterpretation
Unfamiliarity with information resources

Possibly evidenced by
Questions; request for information; verbalization of the problem/concerns
Statement of misconception
Inaccurate follow-through of instruction
Development of preventable complications

DESIRED OUTCOMES/EVALUATION CRITERIA—PATIENT WILL:
Verbalize understanding of disease process, treatment, and potential complications.
Participate in treatment regimen.

ACTIONS/INTERVENTIONS	RATIONALE
Independent	
Review postoperative activity restrictions, e.g., heavy lifting, exercise, sex, sports, driving.	Provides information for patient to plan for return to usual routines without untoward incidence.
Encourage progressive activities as tolerated with periodic rest periods.	Prevents fatigue, promotes healing and feeling of well-being, and facilitates resumption of normal activities.
Recommend use of mild laxative/stool softeners as necessary and avoidance of enemas.	Assists with return to usual bowel function; prevents undue straining for defecation.
Discuss care of incision, including dressing changes, bathing restrictions, and return to physician for suture/staple removal.	Understanding promotes cooperation with therapeutic regimen, enhancing healing and recovery process.
Identify symptoms requiring medical evaluation, e.g., increasing pain; edema/erythema of wound; presence of drainage, fever.	Prompt intervention reduces risk of serious complications, e.g., delayed wound healing, peritonitis.

POTENTIAL CONSIDERATIONS following acute hospitalization (dependent on patient's age, physical condition/presence of complications, personal resources, and life responsibilities).

Therapeutic Regimen: Individual, ineffective management—perceived seriousness/susceptibility, perceived benefit, demands made on individual (family, work).

365

PERITONITIS

Inflammation of the peritoneal cavity can be primary or secondary, acute or chronic, and results from contamination of the peritoneal cavity by either bacteria or chemicals. Primary peritonitis is a rare condition in which the peritoneum is infected via the blood/lymphatic circulation. Secondary sources of inflammation are from the GI tract, ovaries/uterus, urinary system, traumatic injuries, or surgical contaminants. Surgical intervention may be curative in localized peritonitis, e.g., appendicitis/appendectomy, ulcer plication, and bowel resection. If peritonitis is diffuse, medical management is necessary before or in place of surgical treatment.

CARE SETTING

Inpatient acute medical or surgical unit.

RELATED CONCERNS

Appendectomy, 361
Inflammatory bowel disease (IBD): Ulcerative Colitis, Regional Enteritis, p 333
Pancreatitis, p 481
Renal Dialysis: Peritoneal, p 591
Psychosocial Aspects of Care, p 783
Sepsis/Septicemia, p 719
Surgical Intervention, p 802
Total Nutritional Support: Parenteral/Enteral Feeding, p 491
Upper Gastrointestinal/Esophageal Bleeding, p 315

Patient Assessment Data Base

ACTIVITY/REST

May report: Weakness

May exhibit: Difficulty ambulating

CIRCULATION

May exhibit: Tachycardia, diaphoresis, pallor, hypotension (signs of shock)
Tissue edema

ELIMINATION

May report: Inability to pass stool or flatus
Diarrhea (occasionally)

May exhibit: Hiccups; abdominal distention; quiet abdomen
Decreased urinary output, dark color
Decreased/absent bowel sounds (ileus); intermittent loud, rushing bowel sounds (obstruction); abdominal rigidity, distention, rebound tenderness; hyperresonance/tympany (ileus); loss of dullness over liver (free air in abdomen)

FOOD/FLUID

May report: Anorexia, nausea/vomiting; thirst

May exhibit: Projectile vomiting
Dry mucous membranes, swollen tongue, poor skin turgor

PAIN/DISCOMFORT

May report: Sudden, severe abdominal pain, generalized or localized, referred to shoulder, intensified by movement

May exhibit: Distention, rigidity, rebound tenderness
Muscle guarding (abdomen); flexion of knees; distraction behaviors; restlessness; self-focus

RESPIRATION

May exhibit: Shallow respirations, tachypnea

SAFETY

May report: Fever, chills

SEXUALITY

May report: History of pelvic organ inflammation (salpingitis); puerperal infection; septic abortion; retroperitoneal abscess

TEACHING/LEARNING

May report: History of recent trauma with abdominal penetration, e.g., gunshot/stab wound or blunt trauma to the abdomen; bladder perforation/rupture; disease of GI tract, e.g., appendicitis with perforation, gangrenous/ruptured gall bladder, perforated carcinoma of the stomach, perforated gastric/duodenal ulcer, gangrenous obstruction of the bowel, perforation of diverticulum, UC, regional ileitis; strangulated hernia

Discharge plan considerations: **DRG projected length of inpatient stay: 5.1 days**
Assistance with homemaker/maintenance tasks

Refer to section at end of plan for postdischarge considerations.

DIAGNOSTIC STUDIES

CBC: WBCs elevated, sometimes greater than 20,000. RBC count may be increased, indicating hemoconcentration.
Serum protein/albumin: May be decreased owing to fluid shifts.
Serum amylase: Usually elevated.
Serum electrolytes: Hypokalemia may be present.
ABGs: Respiratory alkalosis and metabolic acidosis may be noted.
Cultures: Causative organism may be identified from blood, exudate/secretions or ascitic fluid.
Abdominal x-ray examination: May reveal gas distention of bowel/ileus. If a perforated viscera is the etiology, free air will be found in the abdomen.
Chest x-ray: May reveal elevation of diaphragm.
Paracentesis: Peritoneal fluid samples may contain blood, pus/exudate, amylase, bile, and creatinine.

NURSING PRIORITIES

1. Control infection.
2. Restore/maintain circulating volume.
3. Promote comfort.
4. Maintain nutrition.
5. Provide information about disease process, possible complications, and treatment needs.

DISCHARGE GOALS

1. Infection resolved.
2. Complications prevented/minimized.
3. Pain relieved.
4. Disease process, potential complications, and therapeutic regimen understood.
5. Plan in place to meet needs after discharge.

NURSING DIAGNOSIS: Infection, risk for [septicemia]

Risk factors may include
Inadequate primary defenses (broken skin, traumatized tissue, altered peristalsis)
Inadequate secondary defenses (immunosuppression)
Invasive procedures

Possibly evidenced by
[Not applicable; presence of signs and symptoms establishes an *actual* diagnosis]

DESIRED OUTCOMES/EVALUATION CRITERIA—PATIENT WILL:
Achieve timely healing; be free of purulent drainage or erythema; be afebrile.
Verbalize understanding of the individual causative/risk factor(s).

ACTIONS/INTERVENTIONS	RATIONALE
Independent	
Note individual risk factors, e.g., abdominal trauma, acute appendicitis, peritoneal dialysis.	Influences choice of interventions.
Assess vital signs frequently, noting unresolved or progressing hypotension, decreased pulse pressure, tachycardia, fever, tachypnea.	Signs of impending septic shock. Circulating endotoxins eventually produce vasodilation, shift of fluid from circulation, and a low cardiac output state.
Note changes in mental status (e.g., confusion, stupor).	Hypoxemia, hypotension, and acidosis can cause deteriorating mental status.
Note skin color, temperature, moisture.	Warm, flushed, dry skin is early sign of septicemia. Later manifestations include cool, clammy, pale skin and cyanosis as shock becomes refractory.
Monitor urine output.	Oliguria develops as a result of decreased renal perfusion, circulating toxins, effects of antibiotics.
Maintain strict aseptic technique in care of abdominal drains, incisions/open wounds, dressings, and invasive sites. Cleanse with Betadine or other appropriate solution.	Prevents access or limits spread of infecting organisms/cross-contamination.
Observe drainage from wounds/drains.	Provides information about status of infection.
Maintain sterile technique when catheterizing patient, and provide catheter care/perineal cleansing on a routine basis.	Prevents access, limits bacterial growth in urinary tract.
Monitor/restrict visitors and staff as appropriate. Provide protective isolation if indicated.	Reduces risk of exposure to/acquisition of secondary infection in immunosuppressed patient.
Collaborative	
Obtain specimens/monitor results of serial blood, urine, wound cultures.	Identifies causative microorganisms and helps in assessing effectiveness of antimicrobial regimen.

ACTIONS/INTERVENTIONS

Collaborative

Assist with peritoneal aspiration, if indicated.

Administer antimicrobials, e.g., gentamicin (Garamycin), amikacin (Amikin), clindamycin (Cleocin), via IV/peritoneal lavage.

Prepare for surgical intervention if indicated.

RATIONALE

May be done to remove fluid and to identify infecting organisms so appropriate antibiotic therapy can be instituted.

Therapy is directed at anaerobic bacteria and aerobic gram-negative bacilli. Lavage may be used to remove necrotic debris and treat inflammation that is poorly localized/diffuse.

May be treatment of choice (curative) in acute, localized peritonitis, e.g., to drain localized abscess; remove peritoneal exudates, ruptured appendix/gallbladder; plicate perforated ulcer, or resect bowel.

NURSING DIAGNOSIS: Fluid Volume deficit [active loss]

May be related to
Fluid shifts from extracellular, intravascular, and interstitial compartments into intestines and/or peritoneal space
Vomiting; NG/intestinal aspiration
Fever
Medically restricted intake

Possibly evidenced by
Dry mucous membranes, poor skin turgor, delayed capillary refill, weak peripheral pulses
Diminished urinary output, dark/concentrated urine
Hypotension, tachycardia

DESIRED OUTCOMES/EVALUATION CRITERIA—PATIENT WILL:
Demonstrate improved fluid balance as evidenced by adequate urinary output with normal specific gravity, stable vital signs, moist mucous membranes, good skin turgor, prompt capillary refill, and weight within acceptable range.

ACTIONS/INTERVENTIONS

Independent

Monitor vital signs, noting presence of hypotension (including postural changes), tachycardia, tachypnea, fever. Measure CVP if available.

Maintain accurate I&O and correlate with daily weights. Include measured/estimated losses, e.g., gastric suction, drains, dressings, hemovacs, diaphoresis, abdominal girth.

RATIONALE

Aids in evaluating degree of fluid deficit/effectiveness of fluid replacement therapy and response to medications.

Reflects overall hydration status. Urine output may be diminished owing to hypovolemia and decreased renal perfusion, but weight may still increase, reflecting tissue edema/ascites accumulation. Gastric suction losses may be large, and a great deal of fluid can be sequestered in the bowel and peritoneal space (ascites).

ACTIONS/INTERVENTIONS	RATIONALE
Independent	
Measure urine specific gravity.	Reflects hydration status and changes in renal function, which may warn of developing acute renal failure in response to hypovolemia, effect of toxins. *Note:* Many antibiotics also have nephrotoxic effects that may further affect kidney function/urine output.
Observe skin/mucous membrane dryness, turgor. Note peripheral/sacral edema.	Hypovolemia, fluid shifts, and nutritional deficits contribute to poor skin turgor, taut edematous tissues.
Eliminate noxious sights/smells from environment. Limit intake of ice chips.	Reduces gastric stimulation and vomiting response. *Note:* Excessive use of ice chips during gastric aspiration can increase gastric washout of electrolytes.
Change position frequently, provide frequent skin care, and maintain dry/wrinkle-free bedding.	Edematous tissue with compromised circulation is prone to breakdown.
Collaborative	
Monitor laboratory studies, e.g., Hb/Hct, electrolytes, protein, albumin, BUN, Cr.	Provides information about hydration, organ function. Varied alterations with significant consequences to systemic function are possible as a result of fluid shifts, hypovolemia, hypoxemia, circulating toxins, and necrotic tissue products.
Administer plasma/blood, fluids, electrolytes, diuretics as indicated.	Replenishes/maintains circulating volume and electrolyte balance. Colloids (plasma, blood) help move water back into intravascular compartment by increasing osmotic pressure gradient. Diuretics may be used to assist in excretion of toxins and to enhance renal function.
Maintain NPO with nasogastric/intestinal aspiration.	Reduces hyperactivity of bowel and diarrhea losses.

NURSING DIAGNOSIS: Pain [acute]

May be related to
Chemical irritation of the parietal peritoneum (toxins)
Trauma to tissues
Accumulation of fluid in abdominal/peritoneal cavity (abdominal distention)

Possibly evidenced by
Verbalizations of pain
Muscle guarding, rebound tenderness
Facial mask of pain, self-focus
Distraction behavior, autonomic/emotional responses (anxiety)

DESIRED OUTCOMES/EVALUATION CRITERIA—PATIENT WILL:
Report pain is relieved/controlled.
Demonstrate use of relaxation skills, other methods to promote comfort.

ACTIONS/INTERVENTIONS

Independent

Investigate pain reports, noting location, duration, intensity (0–10 scale), and characteristics (dull, sharp, constant).

Maintain semi-Fowler's position as indicated.

Move patient slowly and deliberately, splinting painful area.

Provide comfort measures, e.g., massage, back rubs; deep breathing, relaxation/visualization exercises.

Provide frequent oral care. Remove noxious environmental stimuli.

Collaborative

Administer medications as indicated:

Analgesics, narcotics;

Antiemetics, e.g., hydroxyzine (Vistaril);

Antipyretics, e.g., acetaminophen (Tylenol).

RATIONALE

Changes in location/intensity are not uncommon but may reflect developing complications. Pain tends to become constant, more intense, and diffuse over the entire abdomen as inflammatory process accelerates; pain may localize if an abscess develops.

Facilitates fluid/wound drainage by gravity, reducing diaphragmatic irritation/abdominal tension, and thereby reducing pain.

Reduces muscle tension/guarding, which may help minimize pain of movement.

Promotes relaxation and may enhance patient's coping abilities by refocusing attention.

Reduces nausea/vomiting, which can increase intra-abdominal pressure/pain.

Reduces metabolic rate and intestinal irritation from circulating/local toxins, which aids in pain relief and promotes healing. *Note:* Pain is usually severe and may require narcotic pain control. Analgesics may be withheld during diagnostic process as they can mask signs/symptoms.

Reduces n/v, which can increase abdominal pain

Reduces discomfort associated with fever/chills.

NURSING DIAGNOSIS: Nutrition: altered, risk for less than body requirements

Risk factors may include
Nausea/vomiting, intestinal dysfunction
Metabolic abnormalities
Increased metabolic needs

Possibly evidenced by
[Not applicable; presence of signs and symptoms establishes an *actual* diagnosis]

DESIRED OUTCOMES/EVALUATION CRITERIA—PATIENT WILL:
Maintain usual weight and positive nitrogen balance.

ACTIONS/INTERVENTIONS

Independent

Monitor NG tube output. Note presence of vomiting/diarrhea.

RATIONALE

Large amounts of gastric aspirant and vomiting/diarrhea suggest bowel obstruction, requiring further evaluation.

371

ACTIONS/INTERVENTIONS	RATIONALE
Independent	
Auscultate bowel sounds, noting absent/hyperactive sounds.	Although bowel sounds are frequently absent, inflammation/irritation of the intestine may be accompanied by intestinal hyperactivity, diminished water absorption, and diarrhea.
Measure abdominal girth.	Provides quantitative evidence of changes in gastric/intestinal distention and/or accumulation of ascites.
Weigh regularly.	Initial losses/gains reflect changes in hydration, but sustained losses suggest nutritional deficit.
Assess abdomen frequently for return to softness, reappearance of normal bowel sounds, and passage of flatus.	Indicates return of normal bowel function and ability to resume oral intake.
Collaborative	
Monitor BUN, protein, prealbumin/albumin, glucose, nitrogen balance as indicated.	Reflects organ function and nutritional status/needs.
Advance diet as tolerated, e.g., clear liquids to soft food.	Careful progression of diet when intake is resumed reduces risk of gastric irritation.
Administer hyperalimentation (TPN) as indicated.	Promotes nutrient utilization and positive nitrogen balance in patients who are unable to assimilate nutrients in a normal fashion.

NURSING DIAGNOSIS: Anxiety [specify level]/Fear

May be related to
Situational crisis
Threat of death/change in health status
Physiologic factors, hypermetabolic state

Possibly evidenced by
Increased tension/helplessness
Apprehension, uncertainty, worry
Sense of impending doom
Sympathetic stimulation; restlessness; focus on self

DESIRED OUTCOMES/EVALUATION CRITERIA—PATIENT WILL:
Verbalize awareness of feelings and healthy ways to deal with them.
Report anxiety is reduced to a manageable level.
Appear relaxed.

ACTIONS/INTERVENTIONS	RATIONALE
Independent	
Evaluate anxiety level, noting patient's verbal and nonverbal response. Encourage free expression of emotions.	Apprehension may be escalated by severe pain, increasingly ill feeling, urgency of diagnostic procedures, and possibility of surgery.
Provide information regarding disease process and anticipated treatment.	Knowing what to expect can reduce anxiety.

ACTIONS/INTERVENTIONS

RATIONALE

Independent

Schedule adequate rest and uninterrupted periods for sleep.

Limits fatigue, conserves energy, and can enhance coping ability.

Refer to CP: Psychosocial Aspects of Care, p 783 for additional interventions.

NURSING DIAGNOSIS: Knowledge deficit [learning need] regarding condition, prognosis, treatment, self-care and discharge needs

May be related to
Lack of exposure/recall
Information misinterpretation
Unfamiliarity with information resources

Possibly evidenced by
Questions; request for information
Statement of misconception
Inaccurate follow-through of instruction

DESIRED OUTCOMES/EVALUATION CRITERIA—PATIENT WILL:
Verbalize understanding of disease process and treatment.
Identify relationship of signs/symptoms to the disease process and correlate symptoms with causative factors.
Correctly perform necessary procedures and explain reasons for actions.

ACTIONS/INTERVENTIONS

RATIONALE

Independent

Review underlying disease process and recovery expectations.

Provides knowledge base on which patient can make informed choices.

Discuss medication regimen, schedule, and possible side effects.

Antibiotics may be continued after discharge, dependent on length of stay.

Recommend gradual resumption of usual activities as tolerated, allowing for adequate rest.

Prevents fatigue, enhances feeling of well-being.

Review activity restrictions/limitations, e.g., avoid heavy lifting, constipation.

Avoids unnecessary increase of intra-abdominal pressure and muscle tension.

Demonstrate aseptic dressing change, wound care.

Reduces risk of contamination. Provides opportunity to evaluate healing process.

Identify signs/symptoms requiring medical evaluation, e.g., recurrent abdominal pain/distention, vomiting, fever, chills, or presence of purulent drainage, swelling/erythema of surgical incision (if present).

Early recognition and treatment of developing complications may prevent more serious illness/injury.

POTENTIAL CONSIDERATIONS following acute hospitalization (dependent on patient's age, physical condition/presence of complications, personal resources, and life responsibilities)

Fatigue–decreased metabolic energy production, increased energy requirements to perform ADLs, states of discomfort.
Pain [acute]–chemical irritation of the peritoneum, prolonged healing process.

373

CHOLECYSTITIS WITH CHOLELITHIASIS

Cholecysititis is an acute or chronic inflammation of the gallbladder, usually associated with gallstone(s) impacted in the cystic duct, causing distention of the gallbladder. Stones (calculi) are made up of cholesterol, calcium bilirubinate, or a mixture, caused by changes in the bile composition. Gallstones can develop in the common bile duct, the cystic duct, hepatic duct, small bile duct, and pancreatic duct. Crystals can also form in the submucosa of the gallbladder causing widespread inflammation. Acute cholecystitis with cholelithiasis is usually treated by surgery, although several other treatment methods (fragmentation and dissolution of stones) are now being used.

CARE SETTING

Severe acute attacks may require brief hospitalization on a medical unit. This plan of care deals with the acutely ill, hospitalized patient.

RELATED CONCERNS

Cholecystectomy, p 382
Fluid and Electrolyte Imbalances, p 899
Psychosocial Aspects of Care, p 783
Total Nutritional Support: Parenteral/Enteral Feeding, p 491

Patient Assessment Data Base

ACTIVITY/REST

May report:	Fatigue
May exhibit:	Restlessness

CIRCULATION

May exhibit:	Tachycardia, diaphoresis

ELIMINATION

May report:	Change in color of urine and stools
May exhibit:	Abdominal distention Palpable mass in upper right quadrant Dark, concentrated urine Clay-colored stool, steatorrhea

FOOD/FLUID

May report:	Anorexia, nausea/vomiting Intolerance of fatty and "gas-forming" foods; recurrent regurgitation, heartburn, indigestion, flatulence, bloating (dyspepsia) Belching (eructation)
May exhibit:	Obesity; recent weight loss Normal to hypoactive bowel sounds

PAIN/DISCOMFORT

May report:	Severe epigastric and right upper abdominal pain, may radiate to back or right shoulder Midepigastric colicky pain associated with eating

Pain starting suddenly and usually peaking in 30 minutes
Recurring episodes of similar pain

May exhibit: Rebound tenderness, muscle guarding or rigidity when RUQ is palpated; positive Murphy's sign

RESPIRATION

May exhibit: Increased respiratory rate
Splinted respiration marked by short, shallow breathing

SAFETY

May exhibit: Fever, chills
Jaundice, with dry, itching skin (pruritus)
Bleeding tendencies (vitamin K deficiency)

TEACHING/LEARNING

May report: Familial tendency for gallstones
Recent pregnancy/delivery; history of DM, inflammatory bowel disease, blood dyscrasias

Discharge plan considerations: **DRG projected mean length of inpatient stay: 3.4 days**
May require support with dietary changes/weight reduction

Refer to section at end of plan for postdischarge considerations.

DIAGNOSTIC STUDIES

CBC: Moderate leukocytosis (acute).

Serum bilirubin and amylase: Elevated.

Serum liver enzymes—AST; ALT; LDH: Slight elevation; alkaline phosphatase and 5-nucleotidase: markedly elevated in biliary obstruction.

Prothrombin levels: Reduced when obstruction to the flow of bile into the intestine decreases absorption of vitamin K.

Biliary ultrasound: Reveals calculi, with gallbladder and/or bile duct distention (frequently the initial diagnostic procedure).

Oral cholecystography (OCG): Preferred method of visualizing general appearance and function of gallbladder, including presence of filling defects, structural defects, and/or stone in ducts/biliary tree. Can be done IV (IVC) when nausea/vomiting prevent oral intake; with failure to visualize the gallbladder following OCG; and with a persistence of symptoms following cholecystectomy. IVC may also be done perioperatively to assess structure and function of ducts; detect remaining stones after lithotripsy or cholecystectomy, and/or to detect surgical complications. Dye can also be injected via T-tube drain postoperatively.

Endoscopic retrograde cholangiopancreatography (ERCP): Visualizes biliary tree by cannulation of the common bile duct through the duodenum.

Percutaneous transhepatic cholangiography (PTC): Fluoroscopic imaging distinguishes between gallbladder disease and cancer of the pancreas (when jaundice is present).

Cholecystograms (for chronic cholecystitis): Reveals stones in the biliary system. *Note:* contraindicated in acute cholecystitis because the patient is too ill to take the dye by mouth.

Non-nuclear CT scan: May reveal gallbladder cysts, dilation of bile ducts, and distinguish between obstructive/nonobstructive jaundice.

Hepatobiliary (HIDA, PIPIDA) scan: May be done to confirm diagnosis of cholecystitis, especially when barium studies are contraindicated. Scan may be combined with cholecystokinin injection to demonstrate abnormal gallbladder ejection.

Abdominal x-ray films (multipositional): Reveal radiopaque (calcified) gallstones, calcification of the wall or enlargement of the gallbladder.

Chest x-ray: Rule out respiratory causes of referred pain.

NURSING PRIORITIES

1. Relieve pain and promote rest.
2. Maintain fluid and electrolyte balance.
3. Prevent complications.
4. Provide information about disease process, prognosis, and treatment needs.

DISCHARGE GOALS

1. Pain relieved.
2. Homeostasis achieved.
3. Complications prevented/minimized.
4. Disease process, prognosis, and therapeutic regimen understood.
5. Plan in place to meet needs after discharge.

NURSING DIAGNOSIS: Pain [acute]

May be related to

Biologic injuring agents: obstruction/ductal spasm, inflammatory process, tissue ischemia/necrosis

Possibly evidenced by

Reports of pain, biliary colic (waves of pain)
Facial mask of pain; guarding behavior
Autonomic responses (changes in BP, pulse)
Self-focusing; narrowed focus

DESIRED OUTCOMES/EVALUATION CRITERIA—PATIENT WILL:

Report pain is relieved/controlled.
Demonstrate use of relaxation skills and diversional activities as indicated for individual situation.

ACTIONS/INTERVENTIONS	RATIONALE
Independent	
Observe and document location, severity (0–10 scale), and character of pain (steady, intermittent, colicky).	Assists in differentiating cause of pain and provides information about disease progression/resolution, development of complications, and effectiveness of interventions.
Note response to medication, and report to physician if pain is not being relieved.	Severe pain not relieved by routine measures may indicate developing complications/need for further intervention.
Promote bed rest, allowing patient to assume position of comfort.	Bed rest in low-Fowler's position reduces intra-abdominal pressure; however, patient will naturally assume least painful position.
Use soft/cotton linens; calamine lotion, oil (Alpha-Keri) bath; cool/moist compresses as indicated.	Reduces irritation/dryness of the skin and itching sensation.
Control environmental temperature.	Cool surroundings aid in minimizing dermal discomfort.

ACTIONS/INTERVENTIONS	RATIONALE
Independent	
Encourage use of relaxation techniques, e.g., guided imagery, visualization, deep-breathing exercises. Provide diversional activities.	Promotes rest, redirects attention, may enhance coping.
Make time to listen to and maintain frequent contact with patient.	Helpful in alleviating anxiety and refocusing attention, which can relieve pain.
Collaborative	
Maintain NPO status, insert/maintain NG suction as indicated.	Removes gastric secretions that stimulate release of cholecystokinin and gallbladder contractions.
Administer medications as indicated:	
Anticholinergics, e.g., atropine, propantheline (Pro-Banthine);	Relieves reflex spasm/smooth muscle contraction and assists with pain management.
Sedatives, e.g., phenobarbital;	Promotes rest and relaxes smooth muscle, relieving pain.
Narcotics, e.g., meperidine hydrochloride (Demerol), morphine sulfate;	Given to reduce severe pain. Morphine is used with caution because it may increase spasms of the sphincter of Oddi, although nitroglycerin may be given to reduce morphine-induced spasms if they occur.
Monoctanoin (Moctanin);	This medication may be tried after a cholecystectomy for retained stones, or for newly formed large stones in the bile duct. It is a lengthy treatment (1–3 weeks) and is administered via a nasal-biliary tube. A cholangiogram is done periodically to monitor stone dissolution.
Smooth muscle relaxants, e.g., papaverine (Pavabid), nitroglycerin, amyl nitrate;	Relieves ductal spasm.
Chenodeoxycholic acid (Chenix), ursodeoxycholic acid (UCDA, Actigall);	These natural bile acids decrease cholesterol synthesis, dissolving gallstones. Success of this treatment depends on the number and size of gallstone (3 or fewer stones under 20 mm in diameter).
Antibiotics.	To treat infectious process, reducing inflammation.
Prepare for procedures, e.g.:	
Endoscopic papillotomy (removal of ductal stone);	Choice of procedure is dictated by individual situation.
Extracorporeal shock wave lithotripsy (ESWL);	Shock wave treatment indicated when patient has mild or moderate symptoms, cholesterol stones in gallbladder are 0.5 mm or larger, and there is no biliary tract obstruction. Depending on the machine being used, the patient may sit in a tank of water or lie prone on a water-filled cushion. Treatment takes about 1–2 hours and is 75%–95% successful.
Endoscopic sphincterotomy;	Procedure done to widen the mouth of the common bile duct where it empties into the duodenum. This procedure may also include the manual retrieval of stones from the duct by means of a tiny basket or balloon on the end of the endoscope. Stones must be smaller than 15 mm.

ACTIONS/INTERVENTIONS

Collaborative

Surgical intervention.

RATIONALE

Cholecystectomy may be indicated due to size of stones and degree of tissue involvement/presence of necrosis.

NURSING DIAGNOSIS: Fluid Volume deficit, risk for

Risk factors may include
Excessive losses through gastric suction; vomiting, distention, and gastric hypermotility
Medically restricted intake
Altered clotting process

Possibly evidenced by
[Not applicable; presence of signs and symptoms establishes an *actual* diagnosis]

DESIRED OUTCOMES/EVALUATION CRITERIA—PATIENT WILL:
Demonstrate adequate fluid balance evidenced by stable vital signs, moist mucous membranes, good skin turgor, capillary refill, individually appropriate urinary output, absence of vomiting.

ACTIONS/INTERVENTIONS

Independent

Maintain accurate I&O, noting output less than intake, increased urine specific gravity. Assess skin/mucous membranes, peripheral pulses, and capillary refill.

Monitor for signs/symptoms of increased/continued n/v, abdominal cramps, weakness, twitching, seizures, irregular heart rate, paresthesia, hypoactive or absent bowel sounds, depressed respirations.

Eliminate noxious sights/smells from environment.

Perform frequent oral hygiene with alcohol-free mouthwash; apply lubricants.

Use small-gauge needles for injections and apply firm pressure for longer than usual after venipuncture.

Assess for unusual bleeding, e.g., oozing from injection sites, epistaxis, bleeding gums, ecchymosis, petechiae, hematemesis/melena.

Collaborative

Keep patient NPO as necessary.

Insert NG tube, connect to suction, and maintain patency as indicated.

Administer antiemetics, e.g., prochlorperazine (Compazine).

RATIONALE

Provides information about fluid status/circulating volume and replacement needs.

Prolonged vomiting, gastric aspiration, and restricted oral intake can lead to deficits in sodium, potassium, and chloride.

Reduces stimulation of vomiting center.

Decreases dryness of oral mucous membranes; reduces risk of oral bleeding.

Reduces trauma, risk of bleeding/hematoma formation.

Blood prothrombin is reduced and coagulation time prolonged when bile flow is obstructed, increasing risk of bleeding/hemorrhage.

Decreases GI secretions and motility.

Provides rest for GI tract.

Reduces nausea and prevents vomiting.

ACTIONS/INTERVENTIONS	RATIONALE
Collaborative	
Review laboratory studies, e.g., Hb/Hct; electrolytes; ABGs (pH); clotting times.	Aids in evaluating circulating volume, identifies deficits, and influences choice of intervention for replacement/correction.
Administer IV fluids, electrolytes, and vitamin K.	Maintains circulating volume and corrects imbalances.

NURSING DIAGNOSIS: Nutrition: altered, risk for less than body requirements

Risk factors may include
Self-imposed or prescribed dietary restrictions; nausea/vomiting, dyspepsia, pain
Loss of nutrients; impaired fat digestion due to obstruction of bile flow

Possibly evidenced by
[Not applicable; presence of signs and symptoms establishes an *actual* diagnosis]

DESIRED OUTCOMES/EVALUATION CRITERIA—PATIENT WILL:
Report relief of nausea/vomiting.
Demonstrate progression toward desired weight gain or maintain weight as individually appropriate.

ACTIONS/INTERVENTIONS	RATIONALE
Independent	
Assess for abdominal distention, frequent belching, guarding, reluctance to move.	Nonverbal signs of discomfort associated with impaired digestion, gas pain.
Estimate/calculate caloric intake. Keep comments about appetite to a minimum.	Identifies nutritional deficiencies/needs. Focusing on problem creates a negative atmosphere and may interfere with intake.
Weigh as indicated.	Monitors effectiveness of dietary plan.
Consult with patient about likes/dislikes, foods that cause distress, and preferred meal schedule.	Involving patient in planning enables patient to have a sense of control and encourages eating.
Provide a pleasant atmosphere at mealtime; remove noxious stimuli.	Useful in promoting appetite/reducing nausea.
Provide oral hygiene before meals.	A clean mouth enhances appetite.
Offer effervescent drinks with meals, if tolerated.	May lessen nausea and relieve gas. *Note:* May be contraindicated if beverage causes gas formation/gastric discomfort.
Ambulate and increase activity as tolerated.	Helpful in expulsion of flatus, reduction of abdominal distention. Contributes to overall recovery and sense of well-being and decreases possibility of secondary problems related to immobility (e.g., pneumonia, thrombophlebitis).
Collaborative	
Consult with dietician/nutritional support team as indicated.	Useful in establishing individual nutritional needs and most appropriate route.

ACTIONS/INTERVENTIONS	RATIONALE

Collaborative

Begin low-fat liquid diet after NG tube is removed.

Limiting fat content reduces stimulation of gall-bladder and pain associated with incomplete fat digestion and is helpful in preventing recurrence.

Advance diet as tolerated, usually low-fat, high-fiber. Restrict gas-producing foods (e.g., onions, cabbage, popcorn) and foods/fluids high in fats (e.g., butter, fried foods, nuts).

Meets nutritional requirements while minimizing stimulation of the gallbladder.

Administer bile salts, e.g., Bilron, Zanchol, dehydrocholic acid (Decholin), as indicated.

Promotes digestion and absorption of fats, fat-soluble vitamins, cholesterol. Useful in chronic cholecystitis.

Monitor laboratory studies, e.g., BUN, prealbumin, albumin, total protein, transferrin levels.

Provides information about nutritional deficits/effectiveness of therapy.

Provide TPN as needed.

Alternate feeding may be required dependent on degree of disability/gallbladder involvement and need for prolonged gastric rest.

NURSING DIAGNOSIS: Knowledge deficit [learning need] regarding condition, prognosis, treatment, self care and discharge needs

May be related to
Lack of knowledge/recall
Information misinterpretation
Unfamiliarity with information resources

Possibly evidenced by
Questions; request for information
Statement of misconception
Inaccurate follow-through of instruction
Development of preventable complications

DESIRED OUTCOMES/EVALUATION CRITERIA—PATIENT WILL:
Verbalize understanding of disease process, treatment, prognosis.
Initiate necessary lifestyle changes and participate in treatment regimen.

ACTIONS/INTERVENTIONS	RATIONALE

Independent

Provide explanations of/reasons for test procedures and preparation needed.

Information can decrease anxiety, thereby reducing sympathetic stimulation.

Review disease process/prognosis. Discuss hospitalization and prospective treatment as indicated. Encourage questions, expression of concern.

Provides knowledge base on which patient can make informed choices. Effective communication and support at this time can diminish anxiety and promote healing.

Review drug regimen, possible side effects.

Gallstones often recur, necessitating long-term therapy. Development of diarrhea/cramps during chenodiol therapy may be dose related/correctable. *Note:* Women of childbearing age should be counseled regarding birth control to prevent pregnancy and risk of fetal hepatic damage.

ACTIONS/INTERVENTIONS	RATIONALE

Independent

Discuss weight reduction programs if indicated.	Obesity is a risk factor associated with cholecystitis, and weight loss is beneficial in medical management of chronic condition.
Instruct patient to avoid food/fluids high in fats (e.g., whole milk, ice cream, butter, fried foods, nuts, gravies, pork); gas producers (e.g., cabbage, beans, onions, carbonated beverages); or gastric irritants (e.g., spicy foods, caffeine, citrus).	Prevents/limits recurrence of gallbladder attacks.
Review signs/symptoms requiring medical intervention, e.g., recurrent fever; persistent n/v, or pain; jaundice of skin or eyes, itching; dark urine; clay-colored stools; blood in urine, stools; vomitus; or bleeding from mucous membranes.	Indicative of progression of disease process/development of complications requiring further intervention.
Recommend resting in semi-Fowler's position after meals.	Promotes flow of bile and general relaxation during initial digestive process.
Suggest patient limit gum chewing, sucking on straw/ hard candy, or smoking.	Promotes gas formation, which can increase gastric distention/discomfort.
Discuss avoidance of aspirin-containing products, forceful blowing of nose, straining for bowel movement, contact sports. Recommend use of soft toothbrush, electric razor.	Reduces risk of bleeding related to changes in coagulation time, mucosal irritation, and trauma.

POTENTIAL CONSIDERATIONS following acute hospitalization (dependent on patient's age, physical condition/presence of complications, personal resources, and life responsibilities)

Pain [acute]—recurrence of obstruction/ductal spasm, inflammation, tissue ischemia.

CHOLECYSTECTOMY

Cholecystectomy is the treatment of choice for many patients with multiple/large gallstones either because of acute symptomatology or to prevent recurrence of stones. Cholecystectomy can now be performed by laser through laparoscopic incisions.

CARE SETTING

This procedure is usually done on a short-stay basis; however, in the presence of suspected complications, e.g., empyema, gangrene, or perforation, an inpatient stay on a surgical unit is indicated.

RELATED CONCERNS

Cholecystitis with Cholelithiasis, p 374
Pancreatitis, p 481
Peritonitis, p 366
Psychosocial Aspects of Care, p 783
Surgical Intervention, p 802

Patient Assessment Data Base/Diagnostic Studies

Refer to CP: Cholecystitis with Cholelithiasis, p 374

TEACHING/LEARNING

Discharge plan considerations: **DRG projected mean length of inpatient stay: 1.8 (laparoscopic)–8.2 days**
May require assistance with wound care/supplies, homemaker tasks

Refer to section at end of plan for postdischarge considerations.

NURSING PRIORITIES

1. Promote respiratory function.
2. Prevent complications.
3. Provide information about disease, procedure(s), prognosis, and treatment needs.

DISCHARGE GOALS

1. Ventilation/oxygenation adequate for individual needs.
2. Complications prevented/minimized.
3. Disease process, surgical procedure, prognosis, and therapeutic regimen understood.
4. Plan in place to meet needs after discharge.

NURSING DIAGNOSIS: Breathing Pattern, ineffective

May be related to
Pain
Muscular impairment
Decreased energy/fatigue

Possibly evidenced by
Tachypnea
Respiratory depth changes, reduced vital capacity
Holding breath; reluctance to cough

ACTIONS/INTERVENTIONS

RATIONALE

Independent

Observe respiratory rate/depth.

Shallow breathing, splinting with respirations, holding breath may result in hypoventilation/atelectasis.

Auscultate breath sounds.

Areas of decreased/absent breath sounds suggest atelectasis, whereas adventitious sounds (wheezes, rhonchi) reflect congestion.

Assist patient to turn, cough, and deep breathe periodically. Show patient how to splint incision. Instruct in effective breathing techniques.

Promotes ventilation of all lung segments and mobilization and expectoration of secretions.

Elevate head of bed, maintain low-Fowler's position. Support abdomen when coughing, ambulating.

Facilitates lung expansion. Splinting provides incisional support/decreases muscle tension to promote cooperation with therapeutic regimen.

Collaborative

Assist with respiratory treatments, e.g., incentive spirometer.

Maximizes expansion of lungs to prevent/resolve atelectasis.

Administer analgesics before breathing treatments/therapeutic activities.

Facilitates more effective coughing, deep breathing, and activity.

NURSING DIAGNOSIS: Fluid Volume deficit, risk for

Risk factors may include
Losses from NG aspiration, vomiting
Medically restricted intake
Altered coagulation, e.g., reduced prothrombin, prolonged coagulation time

Possibly evidenced by
[Not applicable; presence of signs and symptoms establishes an *actual* diagnosis]

DESIRED OUTCOMES/EVALUATION CRITERIA—PATIENT WILL:
Display adequate fluid balance as evidenced by stable vital signs, moist mucous membranes, good skin turgor/capillary refill, and individually appropriate urinary output.

ACTIONS/INTERVENTIONS

RATIONALE

Independent

Monitor I&O, including drainage from NG tube, T tube, and wound. Weigh patient periodically.

Provides information about replacement needs and organ function. Initially, 200–500 ml of bile drainage is to be expected, decreasing as more bile enters the intestine. Continuing large amounts of bile drainage may be an indication of obstruction or, occasionally, a biliary fistula.

ACTIONS/INTERVENTIONS	RATIONALE
Independent	
Monitor vital signs. Assess mucous membranes, skin turgor, peripheral pulses, and capillary refill.	Indicators of adequacy of circulating volume/perfusion.
Observe for signs of bleeding, e.g., hematemesis, melena; petechiae, ecchymosis.	Prothrombin is reduced and coagulation time prolonged when bile flow is obstructed, increasing risk of bleeding/hemorrhage.
Use small-gauge needles for injections, and apply firm pressure for longer than usual after venipuncture.	Reduces trauma, risk of bleeding/hematoma.
Have the patient use cotton/sponge swabs and mouthwash instead of a toothbrush.	Avoids trauma and bleeding of the gums.
Collaborative	
Monitor laboratory studies, e.g., Hb/Hct, electrolytes, prothrombin level/clotting time.	Provides information about circulating volume, electrolyte balance, and adequacy of clotting factors.
Administer IV fluids, blood products, as indicated;	Maintains adequate circulating volume and aids in replacement of clotting factors.
Electrolytes;	Corrects imbalances resulting from excessive gastric/wound losses.
Vitamin K.	Provides replacement of factors necessary for clotting process.

NURSING DIAGNOSIS: Skin/Tissue Integrity, impaired

May be related to
Chemical substance (bile), stasis of secretions
Altered nutritional state (obesity)/metabolic state
Invasion of body structure (T tube)

Possibly evidenced by
Disruption of skin/subcutaneous tissues

DESIRED OUTCOMES/EVALUATION CRITERIA—PATIENT WILL:
Achieve timely wound healing without complications.
Demonstrate behaviors to promote healing/prevent skin breakdown.

ACTIONS/INTERVENTIONS	RATIONALE
Independent	
Observe the color and character of the drainage.	Initially, drainage may contain blood and blood-stained fluid, normally changing to greenish brown (bile color) after the first several hours.
Change dressings as often as necessary. Clean the skin with soap and water. Use sterile petroleum jelly gauze, zinc oxide, or karaya powder around the incision.	Keeps the skin around the incision clean and provides a barrier to protect skin from excoriation.
Apply Montgomery straps.	Facilitates frequent dressing changes and minimizes skin trauma.

ACTIONS/INTERVENTIONS	RATIONALE
Independent	
Use a disposable ostomy bag over a stab wound drain.	Ostomy appliance may be used to collect heavy drainage for more accurate measurement of output and protection of the skin.
Place patient in low- or semi-Fowler's position.	Facilitates drainage of bile.
Monitor endoscopic puncture sites (3–5) if endoscopic procedure is done.	These areas may bleed, or staples and steristrips may loosen at puncture wound sites.
Check the T tube and incisional drains; make sure they are free flowing.	T tube may remain in common bile duct for 7–10 days to remove retained stones. Incision site drains are used to remove any accumulated fluid and bile. Correct positioning prevents backup of the bile in the operative area.
Maintain T tube in closed collection system.	Prevents skin irritation and facilitates measurement of output. Reduces risk of contamination.
Anchor drainage tube, allowing sufficient tubing to permit free turning, and avoid kinks and twists.	Avoids dislodging tube and/or occlusion of the lumen.
Observe for hiccups, abdominal distention, or signs of peritonitis, pancreatitis.	Dislodgment of the T tube can result in diaphragmatic irritation or more serious complications if bile drains into abdomen or pancreatic duct is obstructed.
Observe skin, sclerae, urine for change in color.	Developing jaundice may indicate obstruction of bile flow.
Note color and consistency of stools.	Clay-colored stools result when bile is not present in the intestines.
Investigate reports of increased/unrelenting RUQ pain; development of fever, tachycardia; leakage of bile drainage around tube/from wound.	Signs suggestive of abscess or fistula formation, requiring medical intervention.
Collaborative	
Administer antibiotics as indicated.	Necessary for treatment of abscess/infection.
Clamp the T tube per schedule.	Tests the patency of the common bile duct before tube is removed.
Prepare for surgical interventions as indicated.	I&D or fistulectomy may be required to treat abscess/fistula.
Monitor laboratory studies, e.g., WBC.	Leukocytosis reflects inflammatory process, e.g., abcess formation or development of peritonitis/pancreatitis.

NURSING DIAGNOSIS: Knowledge deficit [learning need] regarding condition, prognosis, treatment, self care and discharge needs

May be related to

Lack of exposure; information misinterpretation

Unfamiliarity with information resources

Lack of recall

Possibly evidenced by

Questions; statement of misconception

ACTIONS/INTERVENTIONS	RATIONALE
Independent	
Review disease process, surgical procedure/prognosis.	Provides knowledge base on which patient can make informed choices.
Demonstrate care of incisions/dressings and drains.	Promotes independence in care and reduces risk of complications (e.g., infection, biliary obstruction).
Recommend periodic drainage of T-tube collection bag and recording of output.	Reduces risk of reflux, strain on tube/appliance seal. Provides information about resolution of ductal edema/return of ductal function.
Stress importance of maintaining low-fat diet, eating frequent small meals, gradual reintroduction of foods/fluids containing fats over a 4–6 month period.	During initial 6 months after surgery, low-fat diet limits need for bile and reduces discomfort associated with inadequate digestion of fats.
Discuss use of florantyrone (Sancho) or dehydrocholic acid (Decholin).	Oral replacement of bile salts may be required to facilitate fat absorption.
Avoid alcoholic beverages.	Minimizes risk of pancreatic involvement.
Inform patient that loose stools may occur for several months.	Intestines require time to adjust to stimulus of continuous output of bile.
Advise patient to note and avoid foods that seem to aggravate the diarrhea.	Although dietary changes are not usually necessary, certain restrictions may be helpful; e.g., fats in small amounts are usually tolerated. After a period of adjustment, patient usually will not have problems with most foods.
Identify signs/symptoms requiring notification of healthcare provider, e.g., dark urine, jaundiced color of eyes/skin, clay-colored stools, excessive stools; or recurrent heartburn, bloating.	Indicators of obstruction of bile flow/altered digestion, requiring further evaluation and intervention.
Review activity limitations dependent on individual situation.	Resumption of usual activities is normally accomplished within 4–6 weeks.

POTENTIAL CONSIDERATIONS following acute hospitalization (dependent on patient's age, physical conditon/presence of complications, personal resources, and life responsibilities)

Diarrhea—continuous excretion of bile into bowel, changes in digestive process.
Infection, risk for—invasive procedure (discharge with T tube in place).

Metabolic and Endocrine Disorders

EATING DISORDERS: ANOREXIA NERVOSA/BULIMIA NERVOSA

Anorexia nervosa is an illness of starvation, brought on by severe disturbance of body image and a morbid fear of obesity.

Bulimia nervosa is an eating disorder (binge-purge syndrome) characterized by extreme overeating followed by self-induced vomiting. It may include abuse of laxatives and diuretics.

Although these disorders affect women primarily, approximately 5%–10% of those afflicted are men, and both disorders can be present in the same individual.

CARE SETTING

Acute care is provided through inpatient stay on medical or behavioral unit and for correction of severe nutritional deficits/electrolyte imbalances or initial psychiatric stabilization. Long-term care is provided in outpatient/day treatment program (partial hospitalization) or in the community.

RELATED CONCERNS

Dysrhythmias, p 85
Fluid and Electrolyte Imbalances, p 899
Metabolic Alkalosis (Primary Base Bicarbonate Excess), p 510
Total Nutritional Support: Parenteral/Enteral Feeding, p 491
Psychosocial Aspects of Care, p 783

Patient Assessment Data Base

ACTIVITY/REST

May report: Disturbed sleep patterns, e.g., early morning insomnia; fatigue
Feeling "hyper" and/or anxious
Increased activity/participation in high-energy sports

May exhibit: Periods of hyperactivity, constant vigorous exercising

CIRCULATION

May report: Feeling cold even when room is warm

May exhibit: Low BP
Tachycardia, bradycardia, dysrhythmias

EGO INTEGRITY

May report: Powerlessness/helplessness (lack of control over eating, e.g., cannot stop eating/control what or how much is eaten [bulimia])
Distorted (unrealistic) body image—reports self as fat regardless of weight (denial), and sees thin body as fat; persistent overconcern with body shape and weight—fears gaining weight
High self-expectations
Stress factors, e.g., family move/divorce, onset of puberty
Suppression of anger

May exhibit: Emotional states of depression, withdrawal, anger, anxiety, pessimistic outlook

ELIMINATION

May report: Diarrhea/constipation
Vague abdominal pain and distress, bloating
Laxative/diuretic abuse

FOOD/FLUID

May report: Constant hunger or denial of hunger; normal or exaggerated appetite (rarely vanishes until late in the disorder)
Intense fear of gaining weight; may have prior history of being overweight
Preoccupation with food, e.g., calorie counting, gourmet cooking
An unrealistic pleasure in weight loss, while denying self pleasure in other areas
Refusal to maintain body weight over minimal norm for age/height
Recurrent episodes of binge eating; a feeling of lack of control over behavior during eating binges; a minimum average of 2 binge eating episodes a week for at least 3 months
Regularly engaging in either self-induced vomiting or strict dieting or fasting

May exhibit: Weight loss/maintenance of body weight 15% or more below that expected (anorexia), or weight may be normal or slightly below normal (bulimia)
No medical illness evident to account for weight loss
Cachectic appearance; skin may be dry, yellowish/pale, with poor turgor
Hiding food, cutting food into small pieces, rearranging food on plate
Irrational thinking about eating, food, and weight
Binge-purge syndrome (bulimia) independently or as a complication of anorexia
Peripheral edema
Swollen salivary glands; sore, inflamed buccal cavity; continuous sore throat
Vomiting, bloody vomitus (may indicate esophageal tearing, Mallory-Weiss syndrome)
Excessive gum chewing

HYGIENE

May exhibit: Increased hair growth on body (lanugo); hair loss (axillary/pubic)
Hair is dull/not shiny
Brittle nails
Signs of erosion of tooth enamel; gums in poor condition

NEUROSENSORY

May exhibit:
Appropriate affect, except in regard to body and eating, or depressive affect

Mental changes (apathy, confusion, memory impairment) brought on by malnutrition/starvation

Hysterical or obsessive personality style; no other psychiatric illness or evidence of a psychiatric thought disorder present (although a significant number may show evidence of an affective disorder)

PAIN/DISCOMFORT

May report:
Headaches, sore throat, generalized vague complaints

SAFETY

May exhibit:
Body temperature below normal

Recurrent infectious processes (indicative of depressed immune system)

Eczema/other skin problems

SOCIAL INTERACTION

May report:
Middle-class or upper-class family background

History of being a quiet, cooperative child

Problems of control issues in relationships, difficult communications with others/authority figures

Engagement in power struggles

An emotional crisis of some sort, such as the onset of puberty or a family move

Altered relationships or problems with relationships (not married/divorced), withdrawal from friends/social contacts

Sexual abuse, abusive family relationships

Sense of helplessness

History of legal difficulties, e.g., shoplifting

May exhibit:
Poor communications within family of origin

Passive father/dominant mother, family members closely fused, togetherness prized, personal boundaries not respected

SEXUALITY

May report:
Absence of at least three consecutive menstrual cycles

Promiscuity or denial/loss of sexual interest

May exhibit:
Breast atrophy, amenorrhea

TEACHING/LEARNING

May report:
Family history of higher than normal incidence of depression, other family members with eating disorders (genetic predisposition)

Onset of the illness usually between the ages of 10 and 22

Health beliefs/practice, e.g., certain foods have "too many" calories, use of "health" foods

High academic achievement

Discharge plan considerations:
DRG projected mean length of inpatient stay: 6.4 days

Assistance with maintenance of treatment plan

Refer to section at end of plan for postdischarge considerations.

DIAGNOSTIC STUDIES

CBC with differential: Determines presence of anemia, leukopenia, lymphocytosis. Blood platelets show significantly less than normal activity by the enzyme monoamine oxidase (thought to be a marker for depression).

Electrolytes: Imbalances may include decreased potassium, sodium, chloride, and magnesium.

Endocrine studies:

Thyroid function: Thyroxine (T$_4$) levels usually normal; however, circulating triiodothyronine (T$_3$) levels may be low.

Pituitary function: TSH response to TRF is abnormal in anorexia nervosa. Propranolol-glucagon stimulation test (studies the response of human GH): depressed level of GH in anorexia nervosa. Gonadotropic hypofunction is noted.

Cortisol metabolism: May be elevated.

DST: (Evaluates hypothalamic-pituitary function) dexamethasone resistance indicates cortisol suppression, suggesting malnutrition and/or depression.

Luteinizing hormone secretions test: Pattern often resembles those of prepubertal girls.

Estrogen: Decreased.

Blood sugar and BMR: May be low.

Other chemistries: AST elevated. Hypercarotenemia, hypoproteinemia, hypocholesterolemia.

MHP 6 levels: Decreased, suggestive of malnutrition/depression.

Urinalysis and renal function: BUN may be elevated; ketones present reflecting starvation; decreased urinary 17-ketosteroids.

ECG: Abnormal tracing with low voltage, T-wave inversion, dysrhythmias.

NURSING PRIORITIES

1. Reestablish adequate/appropriate nutritional intake.
2. Correct fluid and electrolyte imbalance.
3. Assist patient to develop realistic body image/improve self-esteem.
4. Provide support/involve SO, if available, in treatment program.
5. Coordinate total treatment program with other disciplines.
6. Provide information about disease, prognosis, and treatment to patient/SO.

DISCHARGE GOALS

1. Adequate nutrition and fluid intake maintained.
2. Maladaptive coping behaviors and stressors that precipitate anxiety recognized.
3. Adaptive coping strategies and techniques for anxiety reduction and self-control implemented.
4. Self-esteem increased.
5. Disease process, prognosis, and treatment regimen understood.
6. Plan in place to meet needs after discharge.

NURSING DIAGNOSIS: Nutrition: altered, less than body requirements

May be related to

Inadequate food intake; self-induced vomiting
Chronic/excessive laxative use

Possibly evidenced by

Body weight 15% (or more) below expected, or may be within normal range (bulimia)
Pale conjunctiva and mucous membranes; poor skin turgor/muscle tone; edema
Excessive loss of hair; increased growth of hair on body (lanugo)
Amenorrhea
Electrolyte imbalances
Hypothermia
Bradycardia; cardiac irregularities; hypotension

ACTIONS/INTERVENTIONS	RATIONALE
Independent	
Establish a minimum weight goal and daily nutritional requirements.	Malnutrition is a mood-altering condition leading to depression and agitation and affecting cognitive function/decision making. Improved nutritional status enhances thinking ability, and psychologic work can begin.
Use a consistent approach. Sit with patient while eating; present and remove food without persuasion and/or comment. Promote pleasant environment and record intake.	Patient detects urgency and may react to pressure. Any comment that might be seen as coercion provides focus on food. When staff responds in a consistent manner, patient can begin to trust staff responses. The single area in which the patient has exercised power and control is food/eating, and he or she may experience guilt or rebellion if forced to eat. Structuring meals and decreasing discussions about food will decrease power struggles with patient and avoid manipulative games.
Provide smaller meals and supplemental snacks, as appropriate.	Gastric dilation may occur if refeeding is too rapid following a period of starvation dieting.
Make selective menu available, and allow patient to control choices as much as possible.	Patient who gains confidence in self and feels in control of environment is more likely to eat preferred foods.
Be alert to choices of low-calorie foods/beverages; hoarding food; disposing of food in various places such as pockets or wastebaskets.	Patient will try to avoid taking in what is viewed as excessive calories and may go to great lengths to avoid eating.
Maintain a regular weighing schedule, such as Monday, Wednesday, and Friday before breakfast in same attire, and graph results.	Provides accurate ongoing record of weight loss/gain. Also diminishes obsessing about changes in weight.
Weigh with back to scale (dependent on program protocols).	Although some programs prefer patient see the results of the weighing, this can force the issue of trust in patient who usually does not trust others.
Avoid room checks and other control devices whenever possible.	Reinforces feelings of powerlessness and are usually not helpful.
Provide 1-to-1 supervision and have the patient with bulimia remain in the day-room area with no bathroom privileges for a specified period (e.g., 2 hours) following eating, if contracting is unsuccessful.	Prevents vomiting during/after eating. Patient may desire food and use a binge-purge syndrome to maintain weight. *Note:* Purging may occur for the first time in a patient as a response to establishment of a weight gain program.
Monitor exercise program and set limits on physical activities. Chart activity/level of work (pacing and so on).	Moderate exercise helps in maintaining muscle tone/weight and combatting depression; however, patient may exercise excessively to burn calories.

ACTIONS/INTERVENTIONS	RATIONALE
Independent	
Maintain matter-of-fact, nonjudgmental attitude if giving tube feedings, hyperalimentation, and so on.	Perception of punishment is counterproductive to patient's self-confidence and faith in own ability to control destiny.
Be alert to possibility of patient disconnecting tube and emptying hyperalimentation if used. Check measurements, and tape tubing snugly.	Sabotage behavior is common in attempt to prevent weight gain.
Collaborative	
Provide nutritional therapy within a hospital treatment program as indicated when condition is life-threatening.	Cure of the underlying problem cannot happen without improved nutritional status. Hospitalization provides a controlled environment in which food intake, vomiting/elimination, medications, and activities can be monitored. It also separates the patient from SO (who may be contributing factor) and provides exposure to others with the same problem, creating an atmosphere for sharing.
Involve patient in setting up/carrying out program of behavior modification. Provide reward for weight gain as individually determined; ignore loss.	Provides structured eating situation while allowing patient some control in choices. Behavior modification may be effective in mild cases or for short-term weight gain.
Provide diet and snacks with substitutions of preferred foods when available.	Having a variety of foods available will enable the patient to have a choice of potentially enjoyable foods.
Administer liquid diet and/or tube feedings/hyperalimentation if needed.	When caloric intake is insufficient to sustain metabolic needs, nutritional support can be used to prevent malnutrition/death while therapy is continuing. High-calorie liquid feedings may be given as medication, at preset times separate from meals, as an alternative means of increasing caloric intake.
Blenderize and tube-feed anything left on the tray after a given period of time if indicated.	May be used as part of behavior modification program to provide total intake of needed calories.
Administer supplemental nutrition as appropriate.	TPN may be required for life-threatening situations; however, enteral feedings are preferred as they preserve GI function and reduce atrophy of the gut.
Avoid giving laxatives.	Use is counterproductive because they may be used by patient to rid body of food/calories.
Administer medications as indicated:	
Cypropheptadine (Periactin);	A serotonin and histamine antagonist that may be used in high doses to stimulate the appetite, decrease preoccupation with food, and combat depression. Does not appear to have serious side effects, although decreased mental alertness may occur.
Tricyclic antidepressants, e.g., amitriptyline (Elavil, Endep);	Lifts depression and stimulates appetite.
Antianxiety agents, e.g., alprazolam (Xanax);	Reduces tension, anxiety/nervousness and may help patient to participate in treatment.
Antipsychotic drugs, e.g., chlorpromazine (Thorazine).	Promotes weight gain and cooperation with psychotherapeutic program; however, used only when absolutely necessary, because of extrapyramidal side effects.

ACTIONS/INTERVENTIONS

Collaborative

MAO inhibitors, e.g., tranylcypromine sulfate (Parnate).

Prepare for/assist with ECT if indicated. Help patient understand this is not punishment.

RATIONALE

May be used to treat depression when other drug therapy is ineffective, decreases urge to binge in bulimia.

In rare and difficult cases in which malnutrition is severe/life-threatening, a short-term ECT series may enable the patient to begin eating and become accessible to psychotherapy.

NURSING DIAGNOSIS: Fluid Volume deficit, risk for or actual

May be related to
Inadequate intake of food and liquids
Consistent self-induced vomiting
Chronic/excessive laxative/diuretic use

Possibly evidenced by: (actual)
Dry skin and mucous membranes, decreased skin turgor
Increased pulse rate, body temperature, decreased BP
Output greater than input (diuretic use); concentrated urine/decreased urine output (dehydration)
Weakness
Change in mental state
Hemoconcentration, altered electrolyte balance

DESIRED OUTCOMES/EVALUATION CRITERIA—
Maintain/demonstrate improved fluid balance, as evidenced by adequate urine output, stable vital signs, moist mucous membranes, good skin turgor.
Verbalize understanding of causative factors and behaviors necessary to correct fluid deficit.

ACTIONS/INTERVENTIONS

Independent

Monitor vital signs, capillary refill, status of mucous membranes, skin turgor.

Monitor amount and types of fluid intake. Measure urine output accurately.

Discuss strategies to stop vomiting and laxative/diuretic use.

Identify actions necessary to regain/maintain optimal fluid balance, e.g., specific fluid intake schedule.

Collaborative

Review electrolyte/renal function test results.

RATIONALE

Indicators of adequacy of circulating volume. Orthostatic hypotension may occur with risk of falls/injury following sudden changes in position.

Patient may abstain from all intake, with resulting dehydration; or substitute fluids for caloric intake, disturbing electrolyte balance.

Helping patient deal with the feelings that lead to vomiting and/or laxative/diuretic use will prevent continued fluid loss. *Note:* The patient with bulimia has learned that vomiting provides a release of anxiety.

Involving patient in plan to correct fluid imbalances improves chances for success.

Fluid/electrolyte shifts, decreased renal function can adversely affect patient's recovery/prognosis and may require additional intervention.

ACTIONS/INTERVENTIONS

Collaborative

Administer/monitor IV, FPN;

Potassium supplements, oral or IV as indicated.

RATIONALE

Used as an emergency measure to correct fluid/electrolyte imbalance.

May be required to prevent cardiac dysrhythmias.

NURSING DIAGNOSIS: Thought Processes, altered

May be related to
Severe malnutrition/electrolyte imbalance
Psychologic conflicts, e.g., sense of low self-worth, perceived lack of control

Possibly evidenced by
Impaired ability to make decisions, problem-solve
Non-reality-based verbalizations
Ideas of reference
Altered sleep patterns, e.g., may go to bed late (stay up to binge/purge) and get up early
Altered attention span/distractibility
Perceptual disturbances with failure to recognize hunger; fatigue, anxiety, and depression

DESIRED OUTCOMES/EVALUATION CRITERIA—PATIENT WILL:
Verbalize understanding of causative factors and awareness of impairment.
Demonstrate behaviors to change/prevent malnutrition.
Display improved ability to make decisions, problem-solve.

ACTIONS/INTERVENTIONS

Independent

Be aware of patient's distorted thinking ability.

Listen to and do not challenge irrational, illogical thinking. Present reality concisely and briefly.

Adhere strictly to nutritional regimen.

Collaborative

Review electrolyte/renal function tests.

RATIONALE

Allows the caregiver to have more realistic expectations of the patient and provide appropriate information and support.

It is not possible to respond logically when thinking ability is physiologically impaired. The patient needs to hear reality, but challenging the patient leads to distrust and frustration.

Improved nutrition is essential to improved brain functioning. (Refer to ND: Nutrition: altered, less than body requirements, p 390.)

Imbalances negatively affect cerebral functioning and may require correction before therapeutic interventions can begin.

NURSING DIAGNOSIS: Body Image disturbance/Self Esteem, chronic low

May be related to
Morbid fear of obesity; perceived loss of control in some aspect of life
Personal vulnerability; unmet dependency needs
Dysfunctional family system
Continual negative evaluation of self

Possibly evidenced by
Distorted body image (views self as fat even in the presence of normal body weight or severe emaciation)
Expresses little concern, uses denial as a defense mechanism, and feels powerless to prevent/make changes
Expressions of shame/guilt
Overly conforming, dependent on others' opinions

DESIRED OUTCOMES/EVALUATION CRITERIA—PATIENT WILL:
Establish a more realistic body image.
Acknowledge self as an individual.
Accept responsibility for own actions.

ACTIONS/INTERVENTIONS

Independent

Establish a therapeutic nurse/patient relationship.

Promote self-concept without moral judgment.

Have patient draw picture of self.

State rules clearly regarding weighing schedule, remaining in sight during medication and eating times, and consequences of not following the rules. Without undue comment, be consistent in carrying out rules.

Respond (confront) with reality when patient makes unrealistic statements such as "I'm gaining weight; so there's nothing really wrong with me."

Be aware of own reaction to patient's behavior. Avoid arguing.

RATIONALE

Within a helping relationship, patient can begin to trust and try out new thinking and behaviors.

Patient sees self as weak-willed, even though part of person may feel sense of power and control (e.g., dieting/weight loss).

Provides opportunity to discuss patient's perception of self/body image and realities of individual situation.

Consistency is important in establishing trust. As part of the behavior modification program, patient knows risks involved in not following established rules (e.g., decrease in privileges). Failure to follow rules is viewed as the patient's choice and accepted by staff in matter-of-fact manner so as not to provide reinforcement for the undesirable behavior.

Patient may be denying the psychologic aspects of own situation and is often expressing a sense of inadequacy and depression.

Feelings of disgust, hostility, and infuriation are not uncommon when caring for these patients. Prognosis often remains poor even with a gain in weight, because other problems may remain. Many patients continue to see themselves as fat, and there is also a high incidence of affective disorders, social phobias, obsessive-compulsive symptoms, drug abuse, and psychosexual dysfunction. Nurse needs to deal with own response/feelings so they do not interfere with care of patient.

395

ACTIONS/INTERVENTIONS	RATIONALE
Independent	
Assist the patient to assume control in areas other than dieting/weight loss, e.g., management of own daily activities, work/leisure choices.	Feelings of personal ineffectiveness, low self-esteem, and perfectionism are often part of the problem. Patient feels helpless to change and requires assistance to problem-solve methods of control in life situations.
Help the patient formulate goals for self (not related to eating) and create a manageable plan to reach those goals, one at a time, progressing from simple to more complex.	Patient needs to recognize ability to control other areas in life and may need to learn problem-solving skills to achieve this control. Setting realistic goals fosters success.
Assist patient to confront sexual fears. Provide sex education as necessary.	Major physical/psychologic changes in adolescence can contribute to development of eating disorders. Feelings of powerlessness and loss of control of feelings (in particular sexual sensations) lead to an unconscious desire to desexualize themselves. Patient often believes that these fears can be overcome by taking control of bodily appearance/development/function.
Note patient's withdrawal from and/or discomfort in social settings.	May indicate feelings of isolation and fear of rejection/judgment by other's. Avoidance of social situations and contact with others can compound feelings of worthlessness.
Encourage patient to take charge of own life in a more healthful way by making own decisions and accepting self as she or he is at this moment. Encourage acceptance of inadequacies as well as strengths. Let patient know that it is acceptable to be different from family, particularly mother.	Patient often does not know what he or she may want for self. Parents (mother) often make decisions for patient. Patient may also believe he or she has to be the best in everything and holds self responsible for being perfect. Developing a sense of identity separate from family and maintaining sense of control in other ways besides dieting and weight loss is a desirable goal of therapy/program.
Involve in personal development program, preferably in a group setting. Provide information about proper application of makeup and grooming.	Learning about methods of enhancing personal appearance may be helpful to long-range sense of self-esteem/image. Feedback from others can promote feelings of self-worth.
Suggest disposing of "thin" clothes as weight gain occurs. Recommend consultation with an image consultant.	Provides incentive to at least maintain and not lose weight. Removes visual reminder of thinner self. Positive image enhances sense of self-esteem.
Use interpersonal psychotherapy approach, rather than interpretive therapy.	Interaction between persons is more helpful for the patient to discover feelings/impulses/needs from within own self. Patient has not learned this internal control as a child and may not be able to interpret or attach meaning to behavior.
Encourage patient to express anger and acknowledge when it is verbalized.	Important to know that anger is part of self and as such is acceptable. Expressing anger may need to be taught to patient, because anger is generally considered unacceptable in the family, and therefore patient does not express it.
Assist patient to learn strategies other than eating for dealing with feelings. Have patient keep a diary of feelings, particularly when thinking about food.	Feelings are the underlying issue, and patient often uses food instead of dealing with feelings appropriately. Patient needs to learn to recognize feelings and how to express them clearly.

ACTIONS/INTERVENTIONS	RATIONALE
Independent	
Assess feelings of helplessness/hopelessness.	Lack of control is a common/underlying problem for this patient and may be accompanied by more serious emotional disorders. *Note:* 54% of patients with anorexia have a history of major affective disorder, and 33% have a history of minor affective disorder.
Be alert to suicidal ideation/behavior.	Intense anxiety/panic about weight gain, depression, hopeless feelings may lead to suicidal attempts, particularly if patient is impulsive.
Collaborative	
Involve in group therapy.	Provides an opportunity to talk about feelings and try out new behaviors.
Refer to occupational/recreational therapy.	Can develop interests and skills to fill time that has been occupied by obsession with eating. Involvement in recreational activities encourages social interactions with others and promotes fun and relaxation.
Encourage participation in directed activities, e.g., bicycle tours and wilderness adventures, such as Outward Bound Program.	While exercise is often used negatively by these patients, participation in these directed activities provides an opportunity to learn self-reliance, enhance self-esteem, as well as realize that food is the fuel required by the body to do its work.
Refer to therapist trained in dealing with sexuality.	May need professional assistance to deal with sexuality issues and accept self as a sexual adult.

NURSING DIAGNOSIS: Skin Integrity, impaired, risk for or actual

May be related to
Altered nutritional/metabolic state; edema
Dehydration/cachectic changes (skeletal prominence)

Possibly evidenced by (actual)
Dry/scaly skin with poor turgor
Tissue fragility
Brittle/dry hair
Reports of itching

DESIRED OUTCOMES/EVALUATION CRITERIA—PATIENT WILL:
Verbalize understanding of causative factors and relief of itching.
Identify and demonstrate behaviors to maintain soft, supple, intact skin.

ACTIONS/INTERVENTIONS	RATIONALE
Independent	
Observe for reddened, blanched, excoriated areas.	These areas are at increased risk of breakdown and require more intense treatment.
Encourage bathing every other day instead of daily.	Frequent baths contribute to dryness of the skin.
Use skin cream twice a day and after bathing.	Lubricates skin and decreases itching.

397

ACTIONS/INTERVENTIONS	RATIONALE

Independent

Massage skin gently, especially over bony prominences.	Improves circulation to the skin, enhances skin tone.
Discuss importance of frequent position changes, need for remaining active.	Enhances circulation and perfusion to skin by preventing prolonged pressure on tissues.
Stress importance of adequate nutrition/fluid intake. (Refer to ND: Nutrition: altered, less than body requirements, p 390.)	Improved nutrition and hydration will improve skin condition.

NURSING DIAGNOSIS: Family Processes, altered

May be related to
Issues of control in family
Situational/maturational crises
History of inadequate coping methods

Possibly evidenced by
Dissonance among family members
Family developmental tasks not being met
Focus on ''Identified Patient'' (IP)
Family needs not being met
Family member(s) acting as ''enablers'' for IP
Ill-defined family rules, function, and roles

DESIRED OUTCOMES/EVALUATION CRITERIA—FAMILY WILL:
Demonstrate individual involvement in problem-solving process directed at encouraging patient toward independence.
Express feelings freely and appropriately.
Demonstrate more autonomous coping behaviors with individual family boundaries more clearly defined.
Recognize and resolve conflict appropriately with the individuals involved.

ACTIONS/INTERVENTIONS	RATIONALE

Independent

Identify patterns of interaction. Encourage each family member to speak for self. Do not allow 2 members to discuss a third without that member's participation.	Helpful information for planning interventions. The enmeshed, overinvolved family members often speak for each other and need to learn to be responsible for their own words and actions.
Discourage members from asking for approval from each other. Be alert to verbal or nonverbal checking with others for approval. Acknowledge competent actions of patient.	Each individual needs to develop own internal sense of self-esteem. Individual often is living up to others' (family's) expectations rather than making own choices. Acknowledgment provides recognition of self in positive ways.
Listen with regard when the patient speaks.	Sets an example and provides a sense of competence and self-worth, in that the patient has been heard and attended to.
Encourage individuals not to answer to everything.	Reinforces individualization and return to privacy.

ACTIONS/INTERVENTIONS

Independent

Communicate message of separation, that it is acceptable for family members to be different from each other.

Encourage and allow expression of feelings (e.g., crying, anger) by individuals.

Prevent intrusion in dyads by other members of the family.

Reinforce importance of parents as a couple who have rights of their own.

Prevent patient from intervening in conflicts between parents. Assist parents in identifying and solving their marital differences.

Be aware and confront sabotage behavior on the part of family members.

Collaborative

Refer to community resources such as family therapy groups, parents' groups as indicated, and parent effectiveness classes.

RATIONALE

Individuation needs reinforcement. Such a message confronts rigidity and opens options for different behaviors.

Often these families have not allowed free expression of feelings and will need help and permission to learn and accept this.

Inappropriate interventions in family subsystems prevent individuals from working out problems successfully.

The focus on the child with anorexia is very intense and often is the only area around which the couple interact. The couple needs to explore their own relationship and restore the balance within it to prevent its disintegration.

Triangulation occurs in which a parent-child coalition exists. Sometimes the child is openly pressed to ally self with one parent against the other. The symptom (anorexia) is the regulator in the family system, and the parents deny their own conflicts.

Feelings of blame, shame, and helplessness may lead to unconscious behavior designed to maintain the status quo.

May help reduce overprotectiveness, support/facilitate the process of dealing with unresolved conflicts and change.

NURSING DIAGNOSIS: Knowledge deficit [learning need] regarding condition, prognosis, treatment, self care and discharge needs

May be related to
Lack of exposure to/unfamiliarity with information about condition
Learned maladaptive coping skills

Possibly evidenced by
Verbalization of misconception of relationship of current situation and behaviors
Preoccupation with extreme fear of obesity and distortion of own body image
Refusal to eat; binging and purging
Abuse of laxatives and diuretics
Excessive exercising
Verbalization of need for new information
Expressions of desire to learn more adaptive ways of coping with stressors

DESIRED OUTCOMES/EVALUATION CRITERIA—PATIENT WILL:
Verbalize awareness of and plan for lifestyle changes to maintain normal weight.
Identify relationship of signs/symptoms (weight loss, tooth decay) to behaviors of not eating/binging-purging.
Assume responsibility for own learning.
Seek out sources/resources to assist with making identified changes.

ACTIONS/INTERVENTIONS	RATIONALE
Independent	
Determine level of knowledge and readiness to learn.	Learning is easier when it begins where the learner is.
Note blocks to learning, e.g., physical/intellectual/emotional.	Malnutrition, family problems, drug abuse, affective disorders, and obsessive-compulsive symptoms can be blocks to learning requiring resolution before effective learning can occur.
Review dietary needs, answering questions as indicated. Encourage inclusion of high-fiber foods and adequate fluid intake.	Patient/family may need assistance with planning for new way of eating. Constipation may occur when laxative use is curtailed.
Encourage the use of relaxation and other stress-management techniques, e.g., visualization, guided imagery, biofeedback.	New ways of coping with feelings of anxiety and fear will help patient to manage these feelings in more effective ways, assisting in giving up maladaptive behaviors of not eating/binging-purging.
Assist with establishing a sensible exercise program. Caution regarding overexercise.	Exercise can assist with developing a positive body image and combats depression (release of endorphins in the brain enhances sense of well-being). Patient may use excessive exercise as a way of controlling weight.
Provide written information for patient/SO(s).	Helpful as reminder of and reinforcement for learning.
Discuss need for information about sex and sexuality.	Because avoidance of own sexuality is an issue for this patient, realistic information can be helpful in beginning to deal with self as a sexual being.
Refer to National Association of Anorexia Nervosa and Associated Disorders, Overeaters Anonymous, and other local resources.	May be a helpful source of support and information for patient/SO.

POTENTIAL CONSIDERATIONS following acute hospitalization (dependent on patient's age, physical condition/presence of complications, personal resources, and life responsibilities)

Nutrition: altered, less than body requirements, risk for—inadequate food intake, self-induced vomiting, history of chronic laxative use

Therapeutic Regimen: Individual, ineffective management—complexity of therapeutic regimen, perceived seriousness/benefits, mistrust of regimen and/or health care personnel, excessive demands made on individual, family conflict

Sample CP: Eating Disorders Program. ELOS: 28 Days Behavioral Unit

ND and categories of care	Time dimension	Goals/actions	Time dimension	Goals/actions	Time dimension	Goals/actions
Altered nutrition: less than body requirements R/T inadequate intake, self induced vomiting, laxative use	Ongoing	Gain 3 lb/wk as indicated	Day 2–28	Consume at least 75% of food provided at each meal	Day 15–28	Demonstrate ability to select foods to meet at least 80% of nutritional needs
Risk for fluid volume deficit	Ongoing	Be free of signs/symptoms of dehydration	Day 2–28	Ingest at least 1500 ml fluid/day	Day 22–28	Refrain from self-induced vomiting
			Day 3	Vital signs WNL	Day 28	

ND and categories of care	Time dimension	Goals/actions	Time dimension	Goals/actions	Time dimension	Goals/actions
Risk for fluid volume deficit—*cont'd*		Display balanced I&O				Be free of signs/symptoms of malnutrition with all laboratory results WNL
Referral	Day 1 & PRN	Dietician				
Diagnostic studies	Day 1	Electrolytes, CBC, BUN/Cr, Thyroid Function UA ECG as indicated	Day 14	Repeat selected studies		
Additional assessments	Day 1–2	Vital signs/I&O q shift	Day 3–7 q AM		Day 8–28	As indicated
	Day 1	Weight	Day 7, 14	7:30 AM/same clothes		
	Day 1–28	Types and amount of food/fluid intake Behavior/purging following meals Level of activity				
Medications Allergies: _____ _____	Day 1–28	Periactin Tricyclic Antidepressant Vitamin supplement				
Patient education	Day 1 & PRN	Orient to unit and schedule Behavior modification program Minimum weight goal and initial nutritional needs	Day 7–14	Principles of nutrition; foods for maintenance of wellness	Day 21–28	Incorporating nutritional plan into lifestyle and home setting
Additional nursing actions	Day 1–3	Assist pt with formulation of behavioral contract and monitoring of cooperation	Day 7–28	Involve mother/SO as appropriate in nutritional counseling and planning for future		
	Day 1–7	Administer tube feeding/blenderized food as indicated				
	Day 1–21	Bathroom locked for 1 hr following meals				
	Day 1–28	Provide social setting for meals				
Ineffective denial R/T presence of overwhelming anxiety-producing feelings, learned response pattern, personal/family value system	Ongoing	Participate in behavior modification program and adhere to unit policies	Day 8–28	Attend and contribute to group sessions	Day 18–28	Verbalize acceptance of reality that eating behaviors are maladaptive
	Day 2–28	Cooperate with therapy to restore nutritional well-being	Day 14	Develop trusting relationship with at least one staff member on each shift		Demonstrate ability to cope more adaptively
					Day 28	Identify ways to gain control in life situation Refrain from use of manipulation of others to achieve control Plan in place to meet needs post-discharge

ND and categories of care	Time dimension	Goals/actions	Time dimension	Goals/actions	Time dimension	Goals/actions
Referrals	Day 5 (or when physical condition stable)	Psychologist Social worker Psychodramatist	Day 8–28	Group psychotherapy sessions	Day 25	Community resource contact person(s)
Additional assessments	Day 1/ ongoing	Degree and stage of denial Perception of situation	Day 5–7	Readiness to participate in group sessions		
	Day 1–17	Ability to trust Use of manipulation to achieve control	Day 7–28	Congruence betwen verbalizations and behaviors (insight)		
			Day 8–28	Degree/quality of involvement in group sessions		
Patient education	Day 1 and prn	Privileges and responsibilities of behavior modification Consequences of behaviors	Day 3/ ongoing	Eating disorder and consequences of eating behavior	Day 21	Role of support groups/community resources
Additional nursing actions	Day 1/ ongoing	Encourage expression of feelings Avoid agreeing with inaccurate statements/perceptions Provide positive feedback for desired insight/behaviors Set limits on maladaptive behavior	Day 5–28	Promote involvement in unit activities Support interactions with family members	Day 21–28	Involve family (as appropriate) in long range planning for meeting individual needs
			Day 8–28	Encourage interactions in group sessions		
Body image disturbance/chronic low self-esteem R/T perceived loss of control, unmet dependency needs, personal vulnerability, negative evaluation of self	Day 7	Acknowledge that attention will not be given to discussion of body image and food	Day 21	Acknowledge misperception of body image as fat Verbalize positive self attributes	Day 28	Demonstrate realistic body image and self-awareness Verbalize acceptane of self, including "imperfections" Acknowledge self as sexual assault
Referrals	Day 1 (or when physical condition stable)	Therapists: Occupational, recreational, music, art	Day 14	Image consultant	Day 28	Therapist to address issues of sexuality postdischarge as indicated
Additional assessments	Day 1–7	Suicidal ideation/ behaviors	Day 8	Individual strengths/ weaknesses		
	Day 3	Sexual history including abuse	Day 8–28	Congruency of feelings/perceptions with actions		
	Day 3–28	Perceptions of body image Family patterns of interaction				
Patient education	Day 1–28	Responsibility for self in family setting	Day 8–10	General wellness needs	Day 21–28	Sex education reflecting individual sexuality and needs
	Day 7–28	Clarify misconceptions of body image	Day 8-28	Human behavior and interactions with family/others–transactional analysis (TA)		

ND and categories of care	Time dimension	Goals/actions	Time dimension	Goals/actions	Time dimension	Goals/actions
Patient education—*cont'd*			Day 14	Personal appearance and grooming		
			Day 14–28	Alternative coping strategies for dealing with feelings		
Additional nursing actions	Day 1	Develop therapeutic relationship	Day 7	Compare actual measurements of pt's body with pt's perceptions	Day 14–28	Have pt keep diary of feelings, especially when thinking of food
	Day 1–28	Provide positive feedback for participation and independent decision making	Day 7–9	Assist with planning to meet individual goals		Role-play new behaviors for dealing with feelings and conflicts
	Day 3–5	Confront sabotoge behavior by family members	Day 8–28	Involve in physical activity/exercise program		
		Encourage control in areas other than diet				
	Day 4-6	Support development of goals not related to eating				

EATING DISORDERS: OBESITY

Obesity is defined as an excess accumulation of body fat at least 20% over average weight for age, sex, and height. The general prognosis for achieving and maintaining weight loss is poor; however, the desire for a healthier lifestyle and reduction of risk factors associated with life-threatening illnesses motivates many people toward diets and weight-loss programs.

CARE SETTING

Community level

RELATED CONCERNS

Cerebrovascular Accident/Stroke, p 243
Cholecystitis with Cholelithiasis, p 374
Cirrhosis of the Liver, p 466
Heart Failure: Chronic, p 41
Diabetes Mellitus/Diabetic Ketoacidosis, p 422
Hypertension: Severe, p 32
Myocardial Infarction, p 711
Obesity: Surgical Interventions (Gastric Partitioning/Gastroplasty, Gastric Bypass), p 412
Psychosocial Aspects of Care, p 783
Thrombophlebitis: Deep Vein Thrombosis, p 107

Patient Assessment Data Base

ACTIVITY/REST

May report: Fatigue, constant drowsiness
Inability/lack of desire to be active or engage in regular exercise
Dyspnea with exertion

May exhibit: Increased heart rate/respirations with activity

CIRCULATION

May exhibit: Hypertension, edema

EGO INTEGRITY

May report: History of cultural/lifestyle factors affecting food choices
Weight may/may not be perceived as a problem
Eating relieves unpleasant feelings, e.g., loneliness, frustration, boredom
Perception of body image as undesirable
SOs resistant to weight loss (may sabotage patient's efforts)

FOOD/FLUID

May report: Normal/excessive ingestion of food
Experimentation with numerous types of diets ("yo-yo" dieting) with varied/short-lived
results
History of recurrent weight loss and gain

May exhibit: Weight disproportionate to height
Endomorphic body type (soft/round)
Failure to adjust food intake to diminishing requirements (e.g., change in lifestyle from
active to sedentary, aging)

PAIN/DISCOMFORT

May report: Pain/discomfort on weight-bearing joints or spine

RESPIRATION

May report: Dyspnea

May exhibit: Cyanosis, respiratory distress (Pickwickian syndrome)

SEXUALITY

May report: Menstrual disturbances, amenorrhea

TEACHING/LEARNING

May report: Problem may be lifelong or related to life event
Family history of obesity
Concomitant health problems may include hypertension, diabetes, gallbladder and cardiovascular disease, hypothyroidism

Discharge plan considerations: **DRG projected mean length of inpatient stay: 5.1 days**
May require support with therapeutic regimen

Refer to section at end of plan for postdischarge considerations.

DIAGNOSTIC STUDIES

Metabolic/endocrine studies: May reveal abnormalities, e.g., hypothyroidism, hypopituitarism, hypogonadism, Cushing's syndrome (increased insulin levels), hyperglycemia, hyperlipidemia, hyperuricemia, hyperbilirubinemia. It is also suggested that the cause of these disorders may arise out of neuroendocrine abnormalities within the hypothalamus, which result in various chemical disturbances.

Anthropometric measurements: Measures fat-to-muscle ratio.

NURSING PRIORITIES

1. Assist patient to identify a workable method of weight control incorporating healthful foods.
2. Promote improved self-concept, including body image, self-esteem.
3. Encourage health practices to provide for weight control throughout life.

DISCHARGE GOALS

1. Healthy patterns for eating and weight control identified.
2. Weight loss toward desired goal established.
3. Positive perception of self verbalized.
4. Plans developed for future weight control.
5. Plan in place to meet needs after discharge.

NURSING DIAGNOSIS: Nutrition: altered, more than body requirements

May be related to
Food intake that exceeds body needs
Psychosocial factors
Socioeconomic status

ACTIONS/INTERVENTIONS	RATIONALE
Independent	
Review individual cause for obesity, e.g., organic or nonorganic.	Identifies/influences choice of interventions.
Implement/review daily food diary, e.g., caloric intake, types of food, eating habits.	Provides the opportunity for the individual to focus on/internalize a realistic picture of the amount of food ingested and corresponding eating habits/feelings. Identifies patterns requiring change and/or a base on which to tailor the dietary program.
Discuss emotions/events associated with eating.	Helps to identify when patient is eating to satisfy an emotional need, rather than physiologic hunger.
Formulate an eating plan with the patient.	While there is no basis for recommending one diet over another, a good reducing diet should contain foods from all basic food groups with a focus on low-fat intake. It is helpful to keep the plan as similar to patient's usual eating pattern as possible. A plan developed with and agreed to by the patient is more apt to be successful. *Note:* It is important to maintain adequate protein intake to prevent loss of lean muscle mass.
Use knowledge of individual's height, body build, age, gender, and individual patterns of eating, energy, and nutrient requirements.	Standard tables are subject to error when applied to individual situations, and circadian rhythms/lifestyle patterns need to be considered.
Stress the importance of avoiding fad diets.	Elimination of needed components can lead to metabolic imbalances, e.g., excessive reduction of carbohydrates can lead to fatigue, headache, instability/weakness, and metabolic acidosis (ketosis) interfering with effectiveness of weight loss program.
Discuss realistic increment goals for weekly weight loss.	Reasonable weight loss (1–2 lb/wk) results in more lasting effects. Excessive/rapid loss may result in fatigue and irritability and ultimately lead to failure in meeting goals for weight loss. Motivation is more easily sustained by meeting ''stair-step'' goals.

ACTIONS/INTERVENTIONS

Independent

Weigh periodically as individually indicated, and obtain appropriate body measurements.

Determine current activity levels and plan progressive exercise program (e.g., walking) tailored to the individual's goals and choice.

Develop an appetite reeducation plan with patient.

Stress the importance of avoiding tension at mealtimes and not eating too quickly.

Encourage patient to eat only at a table or designated eating place and to avoid standing while eating.

Discuss restriction of salt intake and diuretic drugs if used.

Collaborative

Consult with dietitian to determine caloric/nutrient requirements for individual weight loss.

Provide medications as indicated:

Appetite-suppressant drugs, e.g., diethylpropion (Tenuate), mazindol (Sanorex);

Hormonal therapy, e.g., thyroid (Euthroid);

Vitamin, mineral supplements.

Maintain fasting regimen and/or stabilization of medical problems, when indicated.

RATIONALE

Provides information about effectiveness of therapeutic regimen and visual evidence of success of patient's efforts. During hospitalization for controlled fasting, daily weighing may be required. Weekly weighing is more appropriate after discharge.

Exercise furthers weight loss by reducing appetite, increasing energy, toning muscles, and enhancing sense of well-being and accomplishment. Commitment on the part of the patient enables the setting of more realistic goals and adherence to the plan.

Signals of hunger and fullness often are not recognized, have become distorted, or are ignored.

Reducing tension provides a more relaxed eating atmosphere and encourages more leisurely eating patterns. This is important because a period of time is required for the appestat mechanism to know the stomach is full.

Techniques that modify behavior may be helpful in avoiding diet failure.

Water retention may be a problem because of increased fluid intake, as well as the result of fat metabolism.

Individual intake can be calculated by several different formulas, but weight reduction is based on the basal caloric requirement for 24 hours, depending on patient's sex, age, current/desired weight, and length of time estimated to achieve desired weight.

May be used with caution/supervision at the beginning of a weight loss program to support patient during stress of behavioral/lifestyle changes. They are only effective for a few weeks and may cause problems of addiction in some people.

May be necessary when hypothyroidism is present. When no deficiency is present, replacement therapy is not helpful and may actually be harmful. *Note:* Other hormonal treatments, such as HCG, although widely publicized, have no documented evidence of value.

Obese individuals have large fuel reserves but are often deficient in vitamins and minerals.

Aggressive therapy/support may be necessary to initiate weight loss, although fasting is not generally a treatment of choice. Patient can be monitored more effectively in a controlled setting, to minimize complications such as postural hypotension, anemia, cardiac irregularities, and decreased uric acid excretion with hyperuricemia.

407

ACTIONS/INTERVENTIONS

Independent

Prepare for surgical interventions, e.g., gastric bypass, partitioning, if indicated.

RATIONALE

These interventions may be necessary to help the patient lose weight when obesity is life-threatening.

NURSING DIAGNOSIS: Body Image disturbance/Self Esteem, chronic low

May be related to

Biophysical/psychosocial factors such as patient's view of self (slimness is valued in this society, and mixed messages are received when thinness is stressed)

Family/subculture encouragement of overeating

Control, sex, and love issues

Possibly evidenced by

Verbalization of negative feelings about body (mental image often does not match physical reality)

Fear of rejection/reaction by others

Feelings of hopelessness/powerlessness

Preoccupation with change (attempts to lose weight)

Lack of follow-through with diet plan

Verbalization of powerlessness to change eating habits

DESIRED OUTCOMES/EVALUATION CRITERIA—PATIENT WILL:

Verbalize a more realistic self-image.

Demonstrate some acceptance of self as is, rather than an idealized image.

Acknowledge self as an individual who has responsibility for self.

Seek information and actively pursue appropriate weight loss.

ACTIONS/INTERVENTIONS

Independent

Discuss with the patient view of being fat and what it does for the individual. Be sure to provide privacy during care activities.

Have patient recall coping patterns related to food in family of origin and explore how these may affect current situation.

Determine relationship history and possibility of sexual abuse.

Determine the patient's motivation for weight loss and assist with goal setting.

RATIONALE

Mental image includes our ideal and is usually not up to date. Fat and compulsive eating behaviors may have deep-rooted psychologic implications, e.g., compensating for lack of love and nurturing, or be a defense against intimacy. Individual usually is sensitive/self-conscious about body.

Parents act as role models for the child. Maladaptive coping patterns (overeating) are learned within the family system and are supported through positive reinforcement. Food may be substituted by the parent for affection and love, and eating is associated with a feeling of satisfaction, becoming the primary defense.

May contribute to current issues of self-esteem/patterns of coping.

The individual may harbor repressed feelings of hostility, which may be expressed inward on the self. Because of a poor self-concept, the person often has difficulty with relationships. *Note:* When losing weight for someone else, the patient is less likely to be successful/maintain weight loss.

ACTIONS/INTERVENTIONS	RATIONALE
Independent	
Be alert to myths the patient/SO may have about weight and weight loss.	Beliefs about what an ideal body looks like or unconscious motivations can sabotage efforts at weight loss. Some of these include the feminine thought of "If I become thin, men will pursue me or rape me"; the masculine counterpart, "I don't trust myself to stay in control of my sexual feelings"; as well as issues of strength, power, or the "good cook" image.
Assist patient to identify feelings that lead to compulsive eating. Develop strategies for doing something besides eating for dealing with these feelings, e.g., talking with a friend.	Awareness of emotions that lead to overeating can be the first step in behavior change, e.g., people often eat because of depression, anger, and guilt.
Graph weight on a weekly basis.	Provides ongoing visual evidence of weight changes (reality orientation).
Promote open communication avoiding criticism/judgment about patient's behavior.	Supports patient's own responsibility for weight loss; enhances sense of control, and promotes willingness to discuss difficulties/setbacks and problem-solve. *Note:* Distrust and accusations of "cheating" on caloric intake are not helpful.
Outline and clearly state responsibilities of patient and nurse.	It is helpful for each individual to understand area of own responsibility in the program so that misunderstandings do not arise.
Be alert to binge eating and develop strategies for dealing with these episodes, e.g., substituting other actions for eating.	The patient who binges experiences guilt about it, which is also counterproductive because negative feelings may sabotage further weight loss efforts.
Encourage patient to use imagery to visualize self at desired weight and to practice handling of new behaviors.	Mental rehearsal is very useful to help the patient plan for and deal with anticipated change in self-image or deal with occasions that may arise (family gatherings, special dinners) where confrontations with food will occur.
Provide information about the use of make-up, hairstyles, and ways of dressing to maximize figure assets.	Enhances feelings of self-esteem; promotes improved body image.
Encourage buying clothes as a reward for weight loss instead of food treats.	Properly fitting clothes enhance the body image as small losses are made and the individual feels more positive. Waiting until the desired weight loss is reached can become discouraging.
Suggest the patient dispose of "fat clothes."	Removes the "safety valve" of having clothes available "in case" the weight is regained. Retaining fat clothes can convey the message that the weight loss will not occur/be maintained.
Help staff be aware of and deal with own feelings when caring for patient.	Judgmental attitudes, feelings of disgust, anger, and weariness can interfere with care/be transmitted to patient, reinforcing negative self-concept/image.
Collaborative	
Refer to support and/or therapy group.	Support groups can provide companionship, enhance motivation, decrease loneliness and social ostracism, and give practical solutions to common problems. Group therapy can be helpful in dealing with underlying psychologic concerns.

ACTIONS/INTERVENTIONS	RATIONALE
Independent	
Review family patterns of relating and social behaviors.	Social interaction is primarily learned within the family of origin. When inadequate patterns are identified, actions for change can be instituted.
Encourage patient to express feelings and perceptions of problems.	Helps to identify and clarify reasons for difficulties in interacting with others, e.g., may feel unloved/unlovable or insecure about sexuality.
Assess patient's use of coping skills and defense mechanisms.	May have coping skills that will be useful in the process of weight loss. Defense mechanisms used to protect the individual may contribute to feelings of aloneness/isolation.
Have patient list behaviors that cause discomfort.	Identifies specific concerns and suggests actions that can be taken to effect change.
Involve in role-playing new ways to deal with identified behaviors/situations.	Practicing these new behaviors enables the individual to become comfortable with them in a safe situation.
Discuss negative self-concepts and self-talk, e.g., "No one wants to be with a fat person," "Who would be interested in talking to me?"	May be impeding positive social interactions.
Encourage use of positive self-talk such as telling oneself "I am OK," or "I can enjoy social activities and do not need to be controlled by what others think or say."	Positive strategies enhance feelings of comfort and support efforts for change.
Collaborative	
Refer for ongoing family or individual therapy as indicated.	Patient benefits from involvement of SO to provide support and encouragement.

ACTIONS/INTERVENTIONS

Independent

Determine level of nutritional knowledge and what patient believes is most urgent need.

Provide information about ways to maintain satisfactory food intake in settings away from home.

Identify other sources of information, e.g., books, tapes, community classes, groups.

Stress necessity of continued follow-up care/counseling, especially when plateaus occur.

Reassess caloric requirements every 2–4 weeks.

Identify alternatives to chosen activity program to accommodate weather, travel, and so on. Discuss use of mechanical devices/equipment for reducing.

Discuss necessity of good skin care, especially during summer months.

Identify alternative ways to "reward" self/family for accomplishments or to provide solace.

Encourage involvement in social activities that are not centered around food, e.g., bike ride/nature hike, attending musical event, group sporting activities.

RATIONALE

Necessary to know what additional information to provide. When patient's views are listened to, trust is enhanced.

"Smart" eating when dining out or when traveling helps individual to manage weight while still enjoying social outlets.

Using different avenues of accessing information will further patient's learning. Involvement with others who are also losing weight can provide support.

As weight is lost, changes in metabolism occur, interfering with further loss by creating a plateau as the body activates a survival mechanism, attempting to prevent "starvation." This requires new strategies and aggressive support to continue weight loss.

Changes in weight and exercise may necessitate changes in reducing diet.

Promotes continuation of program. *Note:* Fat loss occurs on a generalized overall basis, and there is no evidence that spot reducing or mechanical devices aid in weight loss in specific areas; however, specific types of exercise or equipment may be useful in *toning* specific body parts.

Prevents skin breakdown in moist skinfolds.

Reduces likelihood of relying on food to deal with feelings.

Provides opportunity for pleasure and relaxation without "temptation." Activities/exercise may also use calories to help maintain desired weight.

POTENTIAL CONSIDERATIONS following acute hospitalization (dependent on patient's age, physical condition/presence of complications, personal resources and life responsibilities)

Therapeutic Regimen: Individual, ineffective management—complexity of therapeutic regimen, perceived seriousness/benefits, mistrust of regimen and/or health care personnel, excessive demands made on individual, family conflict

OBESITY: SURGICAL INTERVENTIONS (GASTRIC PARTITIONING/GASTROPLASTY, GASTRIC BYPASS)

A number of surgical treatments for morbid obesity have been tried and discarded because of ineffectiveness or complications. Two procedures now dominate and have advanced beyond the experimental stage. The procedure of choice is vertical-banded gastroplasty. On occasion, gastric bypass may be performed. Weight reduction surgery has been reported to improve several co-morbid conditions such as sleep apnea, glucose intolerance and frank diabetes, hypertension, and hyperlipidemia.

Gastroplasty (gastric stapling): A small pouch with a restricted outlet is created across the stomach just distal to the gastroesophageal junction. A small opening is left, through which food passes into stomach.

Gastric bypass: Anastomosis of jejunum to upper portion of stomach, bypassing rest of stomach. Use has been generally abandoned due to complications, particularly hepatic failure.

CARE SETTING

Inpatient acute surgical unit

RELATED CONCERNS

Eating Disorders: Obesity, p 404
Peritonitis, p 366
Psychosocial Aspects of Care, p 783
Surgical Intervention, p 802
Thrombophlebitis: Deep Vein Thrombosis, p 107

Patient Assessment Data Base

ACTIVITY/REST

May report: Difficulty sleeping
Exertional discomfort, inability to participate in desired activity/sports

EGO INTEGRITY

May report: Motivated to lose weight for oneself (or for gratification of others)
Repressed feelings of hostility toward authority figures
History of psychiatric illness/treatment

May exhibit: Symptoms of emotional/psychiatric illness

FOOD/FLUID

May report: Adequate trials and failure of other treatment approaches
Desire to lose weight

May exhibit: Weight exceeding ideal body weight by 100% or more (morbid obesity)

TEACHING/LEARNING

May report: Presence of chronic conditions (hypertension, diabetes, arthritis, sleep apnea, Pickwickian syndrome, infertility)

Discharge plan considerations: **DRG projected mean length of inpatient stay: 7.4 days**
May require support with therapeutic regimen/weight loss, assistance with self-care, homemaker/maintenance tasks

Refer to section at end of plan for postdischarge considerations.

DIAGNOSTIC STUDIES

Studies are dependent on individual situation, to rule out underlying disease in addition to preoperative workup including psychiatric evaluation.

NURSING PRIORITIES

1. Support respiratory function.
2. Prevent/minimize complications.
3. Provide appropriate nutritional intake.
4. Provide information regarding surgical procedure, postoperative expectations, and treatment needs.

DISCHARGE GOALS

1. Ventilation and oxygenation adequate for individual needs.
2. Complications prevented/controlled.
3. Nutritional intake modified for specific procedure.
4. Procedure, prognosis, and therapeutic regimen understood.
5. Plan in place to meet needs after discharge.

NURSING DIAGNOSIS: Breathing Pattern, ineffective

May be related to
Decreased lung expansion
Pain, anxiety
Decreased energy, fatigue
Tracheobronchial obstruction

Possibly evidenced by
Shortness of breath, dyspnea
Tachypnea, respiratory depth changes, reduced vital capacity
Wheezes, rhonchi
Abnormal ABGs

DESIRED OUTCOMES/EVALUATION CRITERIA—PATIENT WILL:
Maintain adequate ventilation.
Experience no cyanosis or other signs of hypoxia, with ABGs within acceptable range.

ACTIONS/INTERVENTIONS	RATIONALE
Independent	
Monitor respiratory rate/depth. Auscultate breath sounds. Investigate presence of pallor/cyanosis, increased restlessness, or confusion.	Shallow respirations/effects of anesthesia decrease ventilation, potentiate atelectasis, and may result in hypoxia. *Note:* Many anesthetic agents are fat-soluble, so that postoperative sedation and respiratory complications are increased.
Elevate head of bed 30 degrees.	Encourages optimal diaphragmatic excursion/lung expansion and minimizes pressure of abdominal contents on the thoracic cavity. *Note:* When kept recumbent, obese patients are at high risk for severe hypoventilation postoperatively.
Encourage deep-breathing exercises. Assist with coughing and splint incision.	Promotes maximal lung expansion and aids in clearing airways, thus reducing risk of atelectasis, pneumonia.

413

ACTIONS/INTERVENTIONS

Independent

Turn periodically and ambulate as early as possible.

Pad side rails and teach patient to use them as armrests.

Use small pillow under head when indicated.

Avoid use of abdominal binders.

Collaborative

Administer supplemental O_2.

Assist in use of IPPB and/or respiratory adjuncts, e.g., incentive spirometer, blow bottles.

Monitor/graph serial ABGs/pulse oximetry when indicated.

Monitor PCA/administer analgesics as appropriate.

RATIONALE

Promotes aeration of all segments of the lung, mobilizing and aiding in expectoration of secretions.

Using the side rail as an armrest allows for greater chest expansion.

Many obese patients have large, thick necks, and use of large, fluffy pillows may obstruct the airway.

Can restrict lung expansion.

Maximizes available O_2 for exchange and reduces work of breathing.

Enhances lung expansion; reduces potential for atelectasis.

Reflects ventilation/oxygenation and acid-base status. Used as a basis for evaluating need for/effectiveness of respiratory therapies.

Maintenance of comfort level enhances participation in respiratory therapy, as well as promoting increased lung expansion.

NURSING DIAGNOSIS: Tissue Perfusion, altered: peripheral, risk for

Risk factors may include
Diminished blood flow, hypovolemia
Immobility/bed rest
Interruption of venous blood flow (thrombosis)

Possibly evidenced by
[Not applicable; presence of signs and symptoms establishes an *actual* diagnosis]

DESIRED OUTCOMES/EVALUATION CRITERIA—PATIENT WILL:
Maintain perfusion as individually appropriate, e.g., skin warm/dry, peripheral pulses present/strong, vital signs within acceptable range.
Identify causative/risk factors.
Demonstrate behaviors to improve/maintain circulation.

ACTIONS/INTERVENTIONS

Independent

Monitor vital signs. Palpate peripheral pulses routinely; evaluate capillary refill and changes in mentation. Note 24-hour fluid balance.

Encourage frequent ROM exercises for legs and ankles.

Assess for Homans' sign, redness, and edema of calf.

RATIONALE

Indicators of circulatory adequacy. (Refer to ND: Fluid Volume deficit, risk for, p 415.)

Stimulates circulation in the lower extremities; reduces venous stasis.

Indicators of thrombus formation but may not always be present, particularly in obese individuals.

ACTIONS/INTERVENTIONS

Independent

Encourage early ambulation; discourage sitting and/or dangling at the bedside.

Provide adequate/appropriate equipment and sufficient staff for handling patient.

Collaborative

Administer heparin therapy, as indicated.

Monitor Hb/Hct and coagulation studies.

RATIONALE

Sitting constricts venous flow, whereas walking encourages venous return.

Helpful in dealing with the bulky patient for moving, bowel care, and ambulating. Reduces risk of traumatic injury to patient and caregivers.

May be used prophylactically to reduce risk of thrombus formation or to treat thromboemboli.

Provides information about circulatory volume/alterations in coagulation and indicates therapy needs/effectiveness.

NURSING DIAGNOSIS: Fluid Volume deficit, risk for

Risk factors may include
Excessive gastric losses: nasogastric suction, diarrhea
Reduced intake

Possibly evidenced by
[Not applicable; presence of signs and symptoms establishes an *actual* diagnosis]

DESIRED OUTCOMES/EVALUATION CRITERIA—PATIENT WILL:
Maintain adequate fluid volume with balanced I&O and be free of signs reflecting dehydration.

ACTIONS/INTERVENTIONS

Independent

Assess vital signs, noting changes in BP (postural), tachycardia, fever. Assess skin turgor, capillary refill, and moisture of mucous membranes.

Monitor I&O, noting/measuring diarrhea and NG suction losses.

Evaluate muscle strength/tone. Observe for muscle tremors.

Establish individual needs/replacement schedule.

Encourage increased oral intake when able.

RATIONALE

Indicators of dehydration/hypovolemia, adequacy of current fluid replacement. *Note:* Adequate sized cuff must be used to ensure factual measurement of BP. If cuff is too small, reading will be falsely elevated.

Changes in gastric capacity/intestinal motility and nausea greatly influence intake and fluid needs, increasing risk of dehydration.

Large gastric losses may result in decreased magnesium and calcium, leading to neuromuscular weakness/tetany.

Determined by amount of measured losses/estimated insensible losses and dependent on gastric capacity.

Permits discontinuation of invasive fluid support measures and contributes to return of normal bowel functioning.

415

ACTIONS/INTERVENTIONS

Collaborative

Administer supplemental IV fluids as indicated.

Monitor electrolytes and replace as indicated.

RATIONALE

Replaces fluid losses and restores fluid balance in immediate postoperative phase and/or until patient is able to take sufficient oral fluids.

Use of NG tube, and/or vomiting, onset of diarrhea can deplete electrolytes, affecting organ function.

NURSING DIAGNOSIS: Nutrition: altered, risk for less than body requirements

Risk factors may include
Decreased intake, dietary restrictions, early satiety
Increased metabolic rate/healing
Malabsorption of nutrients/impaired absorption of vitamins

Possibly evidenced by
[Not applicable; presence of signs and symptoms establishes an *actual* diagnosis]

DESIRED OUTCOMES/EVALUATION CRITERIA—PATIENT WILL:
Identify individual nutritional needs.
Demonstrate appropriate weight loss with normalization of laboratory values.
Display behaviors to maintain adequate nutritional intake.

ACTIONS/INTERVENTIONS

Independent

Establish hourly intake schedule. Instruct in measuring fluids/foods and sipping or eating slowly.

Weigh daily. Establish regular schedule after discharge.

Provide food and fluids in amount specified following gastric stapling.

Stress importance of being aware of satiety and stopping intake.

Require that patient sit up to drink/eat.

Determine foods that are gas-forming.

Discuss food preferences with patient and include in pureed diet.

Collaborative

Provide liquid diet, advancing to soft, high in protein and bulk, and low in fat, with liquid supplements as needed.

RATIONALE

After partitioning, gastric capacity is reduced to approximately 50 ml, necessitating frequent/small feedings.

Monitors losses and aids in assessing nutritional needs/effectiveness of therapy.

Management of optimal nutrition is dependent on reducing the amount of food/fluid (e.g., 1 oz of fluid or 300 calories) passing through the GI system at one time. Constant sipping of fluid increases satiety and reduces risk of dehydration.

Overeating may cause nausea/vomiting or damage partitioning.

Reduces possibility of aspiration.

May interfere with appetite/digestion and restrict nutritional intake.

May enhance intake, promote sense of participation/control.

Provides nutrients without exceeding calorie limits *Note:* Liquid diet is usually maintained for 8 weeks after partitioning procedure.

ACTIONS/INTERVENTIONS

Collaborative

Refer to dietician.

Administer vitamin supplements as well as B_{12} injections, folate, and calcium as indicated.

RATIONALE

May need assistance in planning a diet that meets nutritional needs.

Supplements may be needed to prevent anemia as absorption is impaired. Increased intestinal motility following bypass procedure lowers calcium level and increases absorption of oxalates, which can lead to urinary stone formation.

NURSING DIAGNOSIS: Skin Integrity, impaired: actual and risk for

May be related to
Trauma/surgery; difficulty in approximation of suture line of fatty tissue
Reduced vascularity, altered circulation
Altered nutritional state: obesity

Possibly evidenced by (actual)
Disruption of skin surface, altered healing

DESIRED OUTCOMES/EVALUATION CRITERIA—PATIENT WILL:
Display timely wound healing without complication.
Demonstrate behaviors to reduce tension on suture line.

ACTIONS/INTERVENTIONS

Independent

Support incision when turning, coughing, deep-breathing, and ambulating.

Observe incisions periodically, noting approximation of wound edges, hematoma formation and resolution, bleeding/drainage.

Provide routine incisional care, being careful to keep dressings dry and sterile. Assess patency of drains.

Encourage frequent position change, inspect pressure points, and massage gently as indicated. Apply transparent skin barrier to elbows/heels.

Provide meticulous skin care; pay particular attention to skin folds.

Provide foam/air mattress or kinetic therapy as indicated.

RATIONALE

Reduces possibility of dehiscence and later incisional hernia.

Influences choice of interventions.

Promotes healing. Accumulation of serosanguinous drainage in subcutaneous layers increases tension on suture line, may delay wound healing, and serves as a medium for bacterial growth.

Reduces pressure on skin, promoting peripheral circulation and reducing risk of skin breakdown. Skin barrier reduces risk of shearing injury.

Moisture or excoriation enhances growth of bacteria that can lead to postoperative infection.

Reduces skin pressure and enhances circulation.

ACTIONS/INTERVENTIONS	RATIONALE
Independent	
Stress proper hand-washing technique.	Prevents spread of bacteria, cross-contamination.
Maintain aseptic technique in dressing changes, invasive procedures.	Reduces risk of nosocomial infection.
Inspect surgical incisions/invasive sites for erythema, purulent drainage.	Early detection of developing infection provides for prevention of more serious complications.
Encourage frequent position changes; deep breathing, coughing, use of respiratory adjuncts, e.g., incentive spirometer.	Promotes mobilization of secretions, reducing risk of pneumonia.
Provide routine catheter care/encourage good perineal care.	Prevents ascending bladder infections.
Encourage patient to drink acid-ash juices, such as cranberry.	Maintains urine acidity to retard bacterial growth.
Observe for reports of abdominal pain (especially after 3rd postoperative day), elevated temperature, increased white count.	Suggests possibility of developing peritonitis.
Collaborative	
Apply topical antimicrobials/antibiotics as indicated.	Reduces bacterial or fungal colonization on skin; prevents infection in wound.
Administer IV antibiotics as indicated.	A prophylactic antibiotic regimen is usually standard in these patients to reduce risk of perioperative contamination and/or peritonitis.

ACTIONS/INTERVENTIONS	RATIONALE
Independent	
Observe/record stool frequency, characteristics, and amount.	Diarrhea often develops after resumption of diet.
Encourage diet high in fiber/bulk within dietary limitations, with moderate fluid intake as diet resumes.	Increases consistency of the effluent. Although fluid is necessary for optimal body function, excessive amounts contribute to diarrhea.
Restrict fat intake as indicated.	Low-fat diet reduces risk of steatorrhea and limits laxative effect of decreased fat absorption.
Observe for signs of "dumping syndrome," e.g., instant diarrhea, sweating, nausea, and weakness after eating.	Rapid emptying of food from the stomach may result in gastric distress and alter bowel function.
Assist with frequent perianal care, using ointments as indicated. Provide whirlpool bath.	Anal irritation, excoriation, and pruritus occur because of diarrhea. The patient often cannot reach the area for proper cleansing and may be embarrassed to ask for help.
Collaborative	
Administer medications as indicated, e.g., diphenoxylate with atropine (Lomotil).	May be necessary to control frequency of stools until body adjusts to changes in function brought about by surgery.
Monitor serum electrolytes.	Increased gastric losses potentiate the risk of electrolyte imbalance, which can lead to more serious/life-threatening complications.

NURSING DIAGNOSIS: Knowledge deficit [learning need] regarding condition, prognosis, treatment, self care and discharge needs

May be related to
Lack of exposure, unfamiliarity with resources
Information misinterpretation
Lack of recall

Possibly evidenced by
Questions, request for information
Statement of misconceptions
Inaccurate follow-through of instructions
Development of preventable complications

DESIRED OUTCOMES/EVALUATION CRITERIA—PATIENT WILL:
Verbalize understanding of surgical procedure, potential complications, treatment regimen, and postoperative expectations.
Initiate necessary lifestyle changes and participate in treatment regimen.

ACTIONS/INTERVENTIONS	RATIONALE

Independent

Review specific surgical procedure and postoperative expectations.

Provides knowledge base on which informed choices can be made and goals formulated. Initial weight loss is rapid, with patient often losing half of the total weight loss during the first 6 months. Weight loss then gradually slows over a 2-year period.

Address concerns about altered body size/image.

Anticipation of problems can be helpful in dealing with situations that arise. (Refer to CP: Eating Disorders: Obesity, ND: Body Image disturbance/Self-Esteem, chronic low, p 408.) *Note:* Feelings that often occur during more conventional weight loss therapies generally are not encountered in the surgically treated patient.

Review medication regimen, dosage, and side effects.

Knowledge may enhance cooperation with therapeutic regimen and in maintenance of schedule.

Recommend avoidance of alcohol.

May contribute to liver/pancreatic dysfunction.

Discuss responsibility for self-care with patient/SO.

Full cooperation is important for successful outcome after procedure.

Stress importance of regular medical follow-up, including laboratory studies, and discuss possible health problems.

Periodic assessment/evaluation (e.g., over 3–12 months) promotes early recognition/prevention of such complications as liver dysfunction, malnutrition, electrolyte imbalances, and kidney stones, which may develop after bypass procedure.

Encourage progressive exercise/activity program balanced with adequate rest periods.

Promotes weight loss, enhances muscle tone, and minimizes postoperative complications while preventing undue fatigue.

Review proper eating habits, e.g., eat small amounts of food slowly and chew well, sit at table in calm/relaxed environment, eat only at prescribed times, avoid between-meal snacking, do not "make up" skipped feedings.

Focuses attention on eating, increasing awareness of intake and feelings of satiety.

Avoid fluid intake ½ hour before/after meals and use of carbonated beverages.

May cause gastric fullness/gaseous distention, limiting intake.

Identify signs of hypokalemia, e.g., diarrhea, muscle cramps/weakness of lower extremities, weak/irregular pulse, dizziness with position changes.

Increasing dietary intake of potassium (e.g., milk, coffee, potatoes, carrots, bananas, oranges) may correct deficit, preventing serious respiratory/cardiac complications.

Discuss symptoms that may indicate dumping syndrome, e.g., weakness, profuse perspiration, nausea, vomiting, faintness, flushing, and epigastric discomfort or palpitations, occurring during or immediately following meals. Problem-solve solutions.

Generally occurring in early postoperative period (1–3 weeks), syndrome is usually self-limiting but may become chronic and require medical intervention.

Review symptoms requiring medical evaluation, e.g., persistent n/v, abdominal distention, abdominal tenderness, change in pattern of bowel elimination, fever, purulent wound drainage, excessive weight loss or plateauing/weight gain.

Early recognition of developing complications allows for prompt intervention, preventing serious outcome.

ACTIONS/INTERVENTIONS	RATIONALE
Independent	
Refer to community support groups.	Involvement with others who have dealt with same problems enhances coping; may promote cooperation with therapeutic regimen and long-term positive recovery.

POTENTIAL CONSIDERATIONS following acute hospitalization (dependent on patient's age, physical condition/presence of complications, personal resources and life responsibilities)

Refer to Potential Considerations in Surgical Intervention plan of care (p 802)
Nutrition: altered, risk for more than body requirements—dysfunctional eating patterns, observed use of food as reward/comfort measure, history of morbid obesity

DIABETES MELLITUS/DIABETIC KETOACIDOSIS

Diabetic ketoacidosis (DKA) is a life-threatening emergency caused by a relative or absolute deficiency of insulin. DKA occurs in patients with IDDM (also called type I diabetes). Conditions or situations known to exacerbate glucose/insulin imbalance include: (1) previously undiagnosed or newly diagnosed type I diabetes; (2) food intake in excess of available insulin, (3) adolescence and puberty; (4) exercise in uncontrolled diabetes; and (5) stress associated with illness, infection, trauma, or emotional distress.

CARE SETTING

Although DKA may be encountered in any setting, mild DKA may be managed at the community level; however, severe metabolic imbalance requires inpatient acute care on a medical unit.

RELATED CONCERNS

Metabolic Acidosis (Primary Base Bicarbonate Deficit), p 506
Fluid and Electrolyte Imbalances, p 899
Psychosocial Aspects of Care, p 783

Patient Assessment Data Base

Data depend on the severity and duration of metabolic imbalance, length/stage of diabetic process, and effects on other organ function.

ACTIVITY/REST

May report:
Sleep/rest disturbances
Weakness, exhaustion, difficulty walking/moving
Muscle cramps, decreased muscle strength

May exhibit:
Tachycardia and tachypnea at rest or with activity
Lethargy/disorientation, coma
Decreased muscle strength/tone

CIRCULATION

May report:
History of hypertension; acute MI
Claudication, numbness, tingling of extremities (long-term effects)
Leg ulcers, slow healing

May exhibit:
Tachycardia
Postural BP changes; hypertension
Decreased/absent pulses
Dysrhythmias
Crackles; JVD (HF)
Hot, dry, flushed skin; sunken eyeballs

EGO INTEGRITY

May report:
Stress; dependence on others
Life stressors including financial concerns related to condition

May exhibit:
Anxiety, irritability

ELIMINATION

May report:
Change in usual voiding pattern (polyuria), nocturia
Pain/burning, difficulty voiding (infection), recent/recurrent UTI

Abdominal tenderness, bloating
Diarrhea

May exhibit: Pale, yellow, dilute urine; polyuria (may progress to oliguria/anuria if severe hypovolemia occurs)
Cloudy, odorous urine (infection)
Abdomen firm, distended
Bowel sounds diminished or hyperactive (diarrhea)

FOOD/FLUID

May report: Loss of appetite
Nausea/vomiting
Not following diet; increased intake of glucose/carbohydrates
Weight loss over a period of days/weeks
Thirst
Use of medications exacerbating dehydration, such as diuretics (thiazides)

May exhibit: Dry/cracked skin, poor skin turgor
Abdominal rigidity/distention, vomiting
Thyroid may be enlarged (increased metabolic needs with increased blood sugar)
Halitosis/sweet, fruity odor (acetone breath)

NEUROSENSORY

May report: Fainting spells/dizziness
Headaches
Tingling, numbness, weakness in muscles
Visual disturbances

May exhibit: Confusion/disorientation; drowsiness, lethargy, stupor/coma (later stages)
Memory impairment (recent, remote)
DTRs decreased (coma)
Seizure activity (late stages of DKA or hypoglycemia)

PAIN/DISCOMFORT

May report: Abdominal bloating/pain (mild/severe)

May exhibit: Facial grimacing with palpation; guarding

RESPIRATION

May report: Air hunger (late stages of DKA)
Cough, with/without purulent sputum (infection)

May exhibit: Increased respiratory rate (tachypnea); deep, rapid (Kussmaul's) respirations (metabolic acidosis)
Rhonchi, wheezes
Yellow or green sputum (infection)

SAFETY

May report: Dry, itching skin; skin ulcerations
Paresthesia (diabetic neuropathy)

May exhibit: Fever, diaphoresis
Skin breakdown, lesions/ulcerations
Decreased general strength/ROM
Weakness/paralysis of muscles including respiratory musculature (if potassium levels are markedly decreased)

423

May report: Vaginal discharge (prone to infection)
Problems with impotence (men); orgasmic difficulty (women)

TEACHING/LEARNING

May report: Familial risk factors; DM, heart disease, strokes, hypertension
Slow/delayed healing
Use of drugs, e.g., steroids, thiazide diuretics, Dilantin, and phenobarbital (can increase glucose levels)
May/may not be taking diabetic medications as ordered

Discharge plan considerations: **DRG projected mean length of inpatient stay: 5.9 days**
May need assistance with dietary regimen, medication administration/supplies, self-care, glucose monitoring

Refer to section at end of plan for postdischarge considerations.

DIAGNOSTIC STUDIES

Serum glucose: Increased 200–1000 mg/dL, or more.

Serum acetone (ketones): Strongly positive.

Fatty acids: Lipids, triglycerides, and cholesterol level elevated.

Serum osmolality: Elevated but usually less than 330 mOsm/L.

Glucagon: Elevated level is associated with conditions that produce (1) actual hypoglycemia, (2) relative lack of glucose (e.g., trauma, infection), or (3) insulin lack. Therefore, glucagon may be elevated with severe DKA despite hyperglycemia.

Electrolytes:
 Sodium: May be normal, elevated, or decreased.
 Potassium: Normal or falsely elevated (cellular shifts), then decreased.
 Phosphorus: Frequently decreased.

Glycosylated hemoglobin: Levels 2 to 4 times normal reflect poor control of DM during past 3–5 weeks (life span of RBCs) and is therefore useful in differentiating inadequate control versus incident-related DKA (e.g., current URI).

ABGs: Usually reflects low pH and decreased HCO_3^- (metabolic acidosis) with compensatory respiratory alkalosis.

CBC: Hct may be elevated (dehydration); leukocytosis suggests hemoconcentration, response to stress, or infection.

BUN: May be normal or elevated (dehydration/decreased renal perfusion).

Serum amylase: May be elevated, indicating acute pancreatitis as cause of DKA.

Serum insulin: May be decreased/absent (type I) or normal to high (type II), indicating insulin insufficiency/improper utilization (endogenous/exogenous). Insulin resistance may develop secondary to formation of antibodies.

Thyroid function tests: Increased thyroid activity can increase blood glucose and insulin needs.

Urine: Positive for glucose and ketones; specific gravity and osmolality may be elevated.

Cultures and sensitivities: Possible UTI, respiratory, or wound infections.

NURSING PRIORITIES

1. Restore fluid/electrolyte, and acid/base balance.
2. Correct/reverse metabolic abnormalities.
3. Identify/assist with management of underlying cause/disease process.
4. Prevent complications.
5. Provide information about disease process/prognosis, self-care, and treatment needs.

DISCHARGE GOALS

1. Homeostasis achieved.
2. Causative/precipitating factors corrected/controlled.

3. Complications prevented/minimized.
4. Disease process/prognosis, self-care needs, and therapeutic regimen understood.
5. Plan in place to meet needs after discharge.

NURSING DIAGNOSIS: Fluid Volume deficit [regulatory failure]

May be related to
Osmotic diuresis (from hyperglycemia)
Excessive gastric losses: Diarrhea, vomiting
Restricted intake: Nausea, confusion

Possibly evidenced by
Increased urinary output, dilute urine
Weakness; thirst; sudden weight loss
Dry skin/mucous membranes, poor skin turgor
Hypotension, tachycardia, delayed capillary refill

DESIRED OUTCOMES/EVALUATION CRITERIA—PATIENT WILL:
Demonstrate adequate hydration as evidenced by stable vital signs, palpable peripheral pulses, good skin turgor and capillary refill, individually appropriate urinary output, and electrolyte levels within normal range.

ACTIONS/INTERVENTIONS

Independent

Obtain history from patient/SO related to duration/intensity of symptoms such as vomiting, excessive urination.

Monitor vital signs; note orthostatic BP changes;

Respiratory pattern, e.g., Kussmaul's respirations; acetone breath;

Respiratory rate and quality; use of accessory muscles, periods of apnea, and appearance of cyanosis;

Temperature, skin color/moisture.

RATIONALE

Assists in estimation of total volume depletion. Symptoms may have been present for varying amounts of time (hours–days). Presence of infectious process results in fever and hypermetabolic state, increasing insensible fluid losses.

Hypovolemia may be manifested by hypotension and tachycardia. Estimates of severity of hypovolemia may be made when patient's systolic BP drops more than 10 mm Hg from a recumbent to a sitting/standing position. *Note:* Cardiac neuropathy may block reflexes that normally increase heart rate.

Lungs remove carbonic acid through respirations, producing a compensatory respiratory alkalosis for ketoacidosis. Acetone breath is due to breakdown of acetoacetic acid and should diminish as ketosis is corrected.

Correction of hyperglycemia and acidosis will cause the respiratory rate and pattern to approach normal. In contrast, increased work of breathing; shallow, rapid respirations; and presence of cyanosis may indicate respiratory fatigue and/or that patient is losing ability to compensate for acidosis.

Although fever, chills, and diaphoresis are common with infectious process, fever with flushed, dry skin may reflect dehydration.

ACTIONS/INTERVENTIONS	RATIONALE
Independent	
Assess peripheral pulses, capillary refill, skin turgor, and mucous membranes.	Indicators of level of hydration, adequacy of circulating volume.
Monitor I&O; note urine specific gravity.	Provides ongoing estimate of volume replacement needs, kidney function, and effectiveness of therapy.
Weigh daily.	Provides the best assessment of current fluid status and adequacy of fluid replacement.
Maintain fluid intake of at least 2500 ml/d within cardiac tolerance when oral intake is resumed.	Maintains hydration/circulating volume.
Promote comfortable environment. Cover patient with light sheets.	Avoids overheating of patient, which could promote further fluid loss.
Investigate changes in mentation/sensorium.	Changes in mentation can be due to abnormally high or low glucose, electrolyte abnormalities, acidosis, decreased cerebral perfusion, or developing hypoxia. Regardless of the cause, impaired consciousness can predispose the patient to aspiration.
Note reports of nausea, abdominal pain; presence of vomiting and gastric distention.	Fluid and electrolyte deficits alter gastric motility, frequently resulting in vomiting and potentiating the fluid/electrolyte losses.
Observe for increased fatigue, crackles, edema, increased weight, bounding pulse, vascular distention.	Rapid fluid replacement may potentiate overload and HF.
Collaborative	
Administer fluids as indicated:	
Normal or half-normal saline with/without dextrose;	Type and amount of fluid are dependent on degree of deficit and individual patient response. *Note:* Patients with DKA are often severely dehydrated and commonly need 5–10 L of isotonic saline (2–3 L within first 2 hours of treatment).
Albumin, plasma, dextran.	Plasma expanders may occasionally be needed if the deficit is life-threatening/BP does not normalize with rehydration efforts.
Insert/maintain urinary catheter.	Provides for accurate/ongoing measurement of urinary output, especially if autonomic neuropathies result in neurogenic bladder (urinary retention/overflow incontinence). May be removed when patient is stable to reduce risk of infection.
Monitor laboratory studies, e.g.:	
Hct;	Assesses level of hydration and is often elevated because of hemoconcentration that occurs after osmotic diuresis.
BUN/Cr;	Elevated values may reflect cellular breakdown from dehydration or signal the onset of renal failure.
Serum osmolality;	Elevated due to hyperglycemia and dehydration.

ACTIONS/INTERVENTIONS	RATIONALE
Collaborative	
Sodium;	May be decreased reflecting shift of fluids from the intracellular compartment (osmotic diuresis). High sodium values reflect severe fluid loss/dehydration, or sodium reabsorption in response to aldosterone secretion.
Potassium.	Initially, intravascular hyperkalemia occurs in response to acidosis, but as this potassium is lost in the urine, the absolute potassium level in the body is depleted. As insulin is replaced and acidosis is corrected, serum potassium deficit becomes apparent.
Administer potassium and other electrolytes via IV and/or by oral route as indicated.	Potassium should be added to the IV (as soon as urinary flow is adequate) to prevent hypokalemia. *Note:* Potassium phosphate may be given if IV fluids contain sodium chloride in order to prevent chloride overload.
Administer bicarbonate if pH is less than 7.0.	Given with caution to help correct acidosis in the presence of hypotension or shock.
Insert NG tube and attach to suction as indicated.	Decompresses stomach and may relieve vomiting.

NURSING DIAGNOSIS: Nutrition: altered, less than body requirements

May be related to

Insulin deficiency (decreased uptake and utilization of glucose by the tissues resulting in increased protein/fat metabolism)

Decreased oral intake: Anorexia, nausea, gastric fullness, abdominal pain; altered consciousness

Hypermetabolic state: Release of stress hormones (e.g., epinephrine, cortisol, and growth hormone), infectious process

Possibly evidenced by

Reported inadequate food intake, lack of interest in food

Recent weight loss; weakness, fatigue, poor muscle tone

Diarrhea

Increased ketones (end products of fat metabolism)

DESIRED OUTCOMES/EVALUATION CRITERIA—PATIENT WILL:

Ingest appropriate amounts of calories/nutrients.

Display usual energy level.

Demonstrate stabilized weight or gain toward usual/desired range with normal laboratory values.

ACTIONS/INTERVENTIONS	RATIONALE
Independent	
Weigh daily or as indicated.	Assesses adequacy of nutritional intake (absorption and utilization).
Ascertain patient's dietary program and usual pattern; compare with recent intake.	Identifies deficits and deviations from therapeutic needs.

427

ACTIONS/INTERVENTIONS	RATIONALE

Independent

Auscultate bowel sounds. Note reports of abdominal pain/bloating, nausea, vomiting of undigested food. Maintain NPO status as indicated.	Hyperglycemia and fluid and electrolyte disturbances can decrease gastric motility/function (distention or ileus) affecting choice of interventions. *Note:* Long-term difficulties with decreased gastric emptying and poor intestinal motility suggest autonomic neuropathies affecting the GI tract and requiring symptomatic treatment.
Provide liquids containing nutrients and electrolytes as soon as patient can tolerate oral fluids; progress to more solid food as tolerated.	Oral route is preferred when patient is alert and bowel function is restored.
Identify food preferences, including ethnic/cultural needs.	If patient's food preferences can be incorporated into the meal plan, cooperation may be facilitated after discharge.
Include SO in meal planning as indicated.	Promotes sense of involvement; provides information for SO to understand nutritional needs of the patient. *Note:* Various methods available for dietary planning include exchange list, point system, glycemic index, or preselected menus.
Observe for signs of hypoglycemia, e.g., changes in level of consciousness, cool/clammy skin, rapid pulse, hunger, irritability, anxiety, headache, light-headedness, shakiness.	Once carbohydrate metabolism begins (blood glucose level reduced), and as insulin is being given, hypoglycemia can occur. If patient is comatose, hypoglycemia may occur without notable change in level of consciousness. This potentially life-threatening emergency should be assessed and treated quickly per protocol. *Note:* Type I diabetics of long standing may not display usual signs of hypoglycemia because normal response to low blood sugar may be diminished.

Collaborative

Perform fingerstick glucose testing.	Bedside analysis of serum glucose is more accurate (displays current levels) than monitoring urine sugar, which is not sensitive enough to detect fluctuations in serum levels and can be affected by patient's individual renal threshold or the presence of urinary retention/renal failure. *Note:* Some studies have found that a urine glucose of 20% may be correlated to a blood glucose of 140–360 mg/dl.
Monitor laboratory studies, e.g., serum glucose, acetone, pH, HCO_3^-.	Blood sugar will decrease slowly with controlled fluid replacement and insulin therapy. With the administration of optimal insulin dosages, glucose can then enter the cells and be used for energy. When this happens, acetone levels decrease and acidosis is corrected.
Administer regular insulin by intermittent or continuous IV method, e.g., IV bolus followed by a continuous drip via pump of approximately 5–10 U/h so that glucose is maintained at 200–300 mg/dl.	Regular insulin has a rapid onset and thus will quickly help move glucose into cells. The IV route is the initial route of choice, because absorption from subcutaneous tissues may be erratic. Many believe the continuous method is the optimal way to facilitate transition to carbohydrate metabolism and reduce incidence of hypoglycemia.

ACTIONS/INTERVENTIONS

Collaborative

Administer glucose solutions, e.g., dextrose and half-normal saline.

Consult with dietician.

Provide diet of approximately 60% carbohydrates, 20% proteins, 20% fats in designated number of meals/snacks.

Administer metoclopramide (Reglan); tetracycline.

RATIONALE

Glucose solutions are added after insulin and fluids have brought the blood glucose to approximately 250 mg/dL. As carbohydrate metabolism approaches normal, care must be taken to avoid hypoglycemia.

Useful in calculating and adjusting diet to meet patient's needs; answers questions and can assist patient/ SO in developing meal plans.

Complex carbohydrates (e.g., corn, peas, carrots, broccoli, dried beans, oats, apples) decrease glucose levels/insulin needs, reduce serum cholesterol levels, and promote satiation. Food intake will be scheduled according to specific insulin characteristics (e.g., peak effect) and individual patient response. *Note:* HS snack of complex carbohydrates is especially important (if insulin is given in divided doses) to prevent hypoglycemia during sleep and potential Somogyi response.

May be useful in treating symptoms related to autonomic neuropathies affecting GI tract, thus enhancing oral intake and absorption of nutrients.

NURSING DIAGNOSIS: Infection, risk for [sepsis]

Risk factors may include
High glucose levels, decreased leukocyte function, alterations in circulation
Preexisting respiratory infection, or UTI

Possibly evidenced by
[Not applicable; presence of signs and symptoms establishes an *actual* diagnosis]

DESIRED OUTCOMES/EVALUATION CRITERIA—PATIENT WILL:
Identify interventions to prevent/reduce risk of infection.
Demonstrate techniques, lifestyle changes to prevent development of infection.

ACTIONS/INTERVENTIONS

Independent

Observe for signs of infection and inflammation, e.g., fever, flushed appearance, wound drainage, purulent sputum, cloudy urine.

Promote good hand-washing by staff and patient.

Maintain aseptic technique for IV insertion procedure, administration of medications, and providing maintenance care. Rotate IV sites as indicated.

Provide catheter/perineal care. Teach the female patient to clean from front to back after elimination.

RATIONALE

Patient may be admitted with infection, which could have precipitated the ketoacidotic state, or may develop a nosocomial infection.

Reduces risk of cross-contamination.

High glucose in the blood creates an excellent medium for bacterial growth.

Minimizes risk of UTI. Comatose patient may be at particular risk if urinary retention occurred prior to hospitalization. *Note:* Elderly female diabetic patients are especially prone to urinary tract/vaginal yeast infections.

ACTIONS/INTERVENTIONS	RATIONALE
Independent	
Provide conscientious skin care; massage bony areas. Keep the skin dry, linens dry and wrinkle-free.	Peripheral circulation may be impaired, placing the patient at increased risk for skin irritation/breakdown and infection.
Auscultate breath sounds.	Rhonchi indicates accumulation of secretions possibly related to pneumonia/bronchitis (may have precipitated the DKA). Pulmonary congestion/edema (crackles) may result from rapid fluid replacement/ HF.
Place in semi-Fowler's position.	Facilitates lung expansion; reduces risk of aspiration.
Reposition and encourage coughing/deep breathing if patient is alert and cooperative. Otherwise, suction airway, using sterile technique, as needed.	Aids in ventilating all lung areas and mobilization of secretions. Prevents stasis of secretions with increased risk of infection.
Provide tissues and trash bag in a convenient location for sputum and other secretions.	Minimizes spread of infection.
Assist with oral hygiene.	Reduces risk of oral/gum disease.
Encourage adequate dietary and fluid intake (approximately 3000 ml/d if not contraindicated).	Decreases susceptibility to infection. Increased urinary flow prevents stasis, and aids in maintaining urine pH/ acidity, reducing bacteria growth and flushing organisms out of system.
Collaborative	
Obtain specimens for culture and sensitivities as indicated.	Identifies organism(s) so that most appropriate drug therapy can be instituted.
Administer antibiotics as appropriate.	Early treatment may help prevent sepsis.

NURSING DIAGNOSIS: Sensory/Perceptual alterations: (specify), risk for

Risk factors may include
Endogenous chemical alteration: Glucose/insulin and/or electrolyte imbalance

Possibly evidenced by
[Not applicable; presence of signs and symptoms establishes an *actual* diagnosis]

DESIRED OUTCOMES/EVALUATION CRITERIA—PATIENT WILL:
Maintain usual level of mentation.
Recognize and compensate for existing sensory impairments.

ACTIONS/INTERVENTIONS	RATIONALE
Independent	
Monitor vital signs and mental status.	Baseline from which to compare abnormal findings; e.g., high temperature may affect mentation.
Address patient by name; reorient as needed to place, person, and time. Give short explanations, speaking slowly and enunciating clearly.	Decreases confusion and helps to maintain contact with reality.

ACTIONS/INTERVENTIONS	RATIONALE
Independent	
Schedule nursing time to provide for uninterrupted rest periods.	Promotes restful sleep, reduces fatigue, and may improve cognition.
Keep patient's routine as consistent as possible. Encourage participation in ADLs as able.	Helps keep the patient in touch with reality and maintain orientation to the environment.
Protect patient from injury (use of restraints) when level of consciousness is impaired. Pad bed rails and provide soft airway if patient is prone to seizures.	Disoriented patient is prone to injury, especially at night, and precautions need to be taken as indicated. Seizure precautions need to be taken to prevent physical injury, aspiration, and so forth.
Evaluate visual acuity as indicated.	Retinal edema/detachment, hemorrhage, presence of cataracts or temporary paralysis of extraocular muscles may impair vision, requiring corrective therapy and/or supportive care.
Investigate reports of hyperesthesia, pain, or sensory loss in the feet/legs. Look for ulcers, reddened areas, pressure points, loss of pedal pulses.	Peripheral neuropathies may result in severe discomfort, lack of/distortion of tactile sensation potentiating risk of dermal injury and impaired balance. *Note:* Mononeuropathy affects a single nerve (most often femoral or cranial), causing sudden pain and loss of motor/sensory function along affected nerve path.
Provide bed cradle. Keep hands/feet warm, avoiding exposure to cool drafts/hot water or use of heating pad.	Reduces discomfort and potential for dermal injury. *Note:* Sudden development of cold hands/feet may reflect hypoglycemia, suggesting need to evaluate serum glucose level.
Assist with ambulation/position changes.	Promotes patient safety, especially when sense of balance is affected.
Collaborative	
Carry out prescribed regimen for correcting DKA as indicated.	Alteration in thought processes/potential for seizure activity is usually alleviated once hyperosmolar state is corrected.
Monitor laboratory values, e.g., blood glucose, serum osmolality, Hb/Hct, BUN/Cr.	Imbalances can impair mentation. *Note:* If fluid is replaced too quickly, excess water may enter brain cells and cause alteration in the level of consciousness (water intoxication).

NURSING DIAGNOSIS: Fatigue

May be related to
Decreased metabolic energy production
Altered body chemistry: Insufficient insulin
Increased energy demands: Hypermetabolic state/infection

Possibly evidenced by
Overwhelming lack of energy, inability to maintain usual routines, decreased performance, accident-prone
Impaired ability to concentrate, listlessness, disinterest in surroundings

DESIRED OUTCOMES/EVALUATION CRITERIA—PATIENT WILL:
Verbalize increase in energy level.
Display improved ability to participate in desired activities.

ACTIONS/INTERVENTIONS

Independent

Discuss with patient the need for activity. Plan schedule with patient and identify activities that lead to fatigue.

Alternate activity with periods of rest/uninterrupted sleep.

Monitor pulse, respiratory rate, and BP before/after activity.

Discuss ways of conserving energy while bathing, transferring, and so on.

Increase patient participation in ADLs as tolerated.

RATIONALE

Education may provide motivation to increase activity level even though patient may feel too weak initially.

Prevents excessive fatigue.

Indicates physiologic levels of tolerance.

Patient will be able to accomplish more with a decreased expenditure of energy.

Increases confidence level/self-esteem as well as tolerance level.

NURSING DIAGNOSIS: Powerlessness

May be related to
Long-term/progressive illness that is not curable
Dependence on others

Possibly evidenced by
Reluctance to express true feelings; expressions of having no control/influence over situation
Apathy, withdrawal, anger
Does not monitor progress, nonparticipation in care/decision making
Depression over physical deterioration/complications despite patient cooperation with regimen

DESIRED OUTCOMES/EVALUATION CRITERIA—PATIENT WILL:
Acknowledge feelings of helplessness.
Identify healthy ways to deal with feelings.
Assist in planning own care and independently take responsibility for self-care activities.

ACTIONS/INTERVENTIONS

Independent

Encourage patient/SO to express feelings about hospitalization and disease in general.

Acknowledge normality of feelings.

RATIONALE

Identifies concerns and facilitates problem solving.

Recognition that reactions are normal can help the patient to problem-solve and seek help as needed. Diabetic control is a full-time job that serves as a constant reminder of both presence of disease and threat to patient's health/life.

ACTIONS/INTERVENTIONS	RATIONALE
Independent	
Assess how patient has handled problems in the past. Identify locus of control.	Knowledge of individual's style helps to determine needs for treatment goals. Patient whose locus of control is internal usually looks at ways to gain control over own treatment program. Patient who operates with an external locus of control wants to be cared for by others and may project blame for circumstances onto external factors.
Provide opportunity for SO to express concerns and discuss ways in which they can be helpful to the patient.	Enhances sense of being involved and gives SO a chance to problem-solve solutions to help patient prevent recurrence.
Ascertain expectations/goals of patient and SO.	Unrealistic expectations/pressure from others or self may result in feelings of frustration/loss of control and may impair coping abilities. *Note:* Even with rigid adherence to medical regimen, complications/setbacks may occur.
Determine whether a change in relationship with SO has occurred.	Constant energy and thought required for diabetic control often shifts the focus of a relationship. Development of psychologic concerns/visceral neuropathies affecting self-concept (especially sexual role function) may add further stress.
Encourage patient to make decisions related to care, e.g., ambulation, time for activities, and so forth.	Communicates to patient that some control can be exercised over care.
Support participation in self-care and give positive feedback for efforts.	Promotes feeling of control over situation.

NURSING DIAGNOSIS: Knowledge deficit [learning need] regarding disease, prognosis, treatment, self care and discharge needs

May be related to
Lack of exposure/recall, information misinterpretation
Unfamiliarity with information resources

Possibly evidenced by
Questions/request for information, verbalization of the problem
Inaccurate follow-through of instructions, development of preventable complications

DESIRED OUTCOMES/EVALUATION CRITERIA—PATIENT WILL:
Verbalize understanding of disease process.
Identify relationship of signs/symptoms to the disease process and correlate symptoms with causative factors.
Correctly perform necessary procedures and explain reasons for the actions.
Initiate necessary lifestyle changes and participate in treatment regimen.

ACTIONS/INTERVENTIONS	RATIONALE
Independent	
Create an environment of trust by listening to concerns, being available.	Rapport and respect need to be established before patient will be willing to take part in the learning process.

ACTIONS/INTERVENTIONS	RATIONALE

Independent

Work with patient in setting mutual goals for learning.	Participation in the planning promotes enthusiasm and cooperation with the principles learned.
Select a variety of teaching strategies, e.g., demonstrate needed skills and have patient do return demonstration, incorporate new skills into the hospital routine.	Use of different means of accessing information promotes learner retention.
Discuss essential elements, e.g.:	
What is a normal glucose blood level and how it compares with the patient's level, the type of DM the patient has, the relationship between insulin deficiency and a high glucose level.	Provides knowledge base on which patient can make informed lifestyle choices.
Reasons for the ketoacidotic episode.	Knowledge of the precipitating factors may help to avoid recurrences.
Acute and chronic complications of the disease, including visual disturbances, neurosensory and cardiovascular changes, renal impairment/hypertension.	Awareness helps patient to be more consistent with care and may prevent/delay onset of complications.
Demonstrate fingerstick testing and have patient return demonstration. Instruct patient to check urine ketones if glucose is greater than 250 mg/dL.	Self-monitoring of blood glucose 4 or more times a day allows flexibility in self-care, promotes tighter control of serum levels (e.g., 60–150 mg/dL) and may prevent/delay development of long-term complications.
Discuss dietary plan, use of high-fiber foods, and ways to deal with meals outside the home.	Awareness of importance of dietary control will aid patient in planning meals/sticking to regimen. Fiber can slow glucose absorption, decreasing fluctuations in serum levels, but may cause GI discomfort, increase flatus, and affect vitamin/mineral absorption.
Review medication regimen, including onset, peak, and duration of prescribed insulin, as applicable, with patient/SO.	Understanding all aspects of drug usage promotes proper use. Dose algorithms are created, taking into account drug dosages established during inpatient evaluation, usual amount and schedule of physical activity, and meal plan. Including SO provides additional support/resource for patient.
Review self-administration of insulin and care of equipment. Have patient demonstrate procedure (e.g., drawing up and injection or use of continuous pump).	Verifies understanding and correctness of procedure. Identifies potential problems (e.g., vision, memory, and so on) so that alternate solutions can be found for insulin administration. *Note:* If multiple daily injections are required, combinations of regular, intermediate, and long-acting insulin will be used. If the pump method is used, only regular insulin is administered, with a basal dose throughout the day and bolus doses before meals and as needed.
Stress importance and necessity of maintaining diary of glucose testing, medication dose/time, dietary intake, activity, feelings/sensations, life events.	Aids in creating overall picture of patient situation to achieve better disease control and promotes self-care/independence.

ACTIONS/INTERVENTIONS	RATIONALE

Independent

Discuss factors that play a part in diabetic control, e.g., exercise (aerobic versus isometric), stress, surgery, and illness. Review "sick day" rules.

This information promotes diabetic control and can greatly reduce the occurrence of ketoacidosis. *Note:* Aerobic exercise (e.g., walking, swimming) promotes effective use of insulin, lowering glucose levels, and strengthens the cardiovascular system. A "sick day" management plan helps maintain equilibrium during illness, minor surgery, severe emotional stress, or any condition that might send glucose spiraling upward.

Review effects of smoking on insulin use. Encourage cessation of smoking.

Nicotine constricts the small blood vessels, and insulin absorption is delayed for as long as these vessels remain constricted. *Note:* Insulin absorption may be reduced by as much as 30% below normal in the first 30 minutes after smoking.

Establish regular exercise/activity schedule and identify corresponding insulin concerns.

Exercise times should not coincide with the peak action of insulin. A snack should be ingested before or during exercise as needed, and rotation of injection sites should avoid the muscle group that will be used in the activity (e.g., abdominal site is preferred over thigh/arm before jogging or swimming) to prevent accelerated uptake of insulin.

Identify the symptoms of hypoglycemia (e.g., weakness, dizziness, lethargy, hunger, irritability, diaphoresis, pallor, tachycardia, tremors, headache, changes in mentation) and explain causes.

May promote early detection and treatment, preventing/limiting occurrence. *Note:* Early morning hyperglycemia may reflect the dawn phenomenon (indicating need for additional insulin) or a rebound response to hypoglycemia during sleep (Somogyi effect), requiring a decrease in insulin dosage/change in diet (e.g., HS snack). Testing serum levels at 3 AM aids in identifying the specific problem.

Instruct in importance of routine examination of the feet and proper foot care. Demonstrate ways to examine feet; inspect shoes for fit; and care for toenails, calluses, and corns. Encourage use of natural fiber stockings.

Prevents/delays complications associated with peripheral neuropathies and/or circulatory impairment, especially cellulitis, gangrene, and amputation.

Demonstrate/discuss proper use of TENS unit. Identify safety concerns following local nerve block.

May provide relief of discomfort associated with neuropathies.

Stress importance of regular eye examinations, especially for patients who have had type I diabetes for 5 years or more.

Changes in vision may be gradual and are more pronounced in persons with poorly controlled DM. Problems include changes in visual acuity and may progress to retinopathy and blindness.

Arrange for vision aids when needed, e.g., magnifying sleeve for insulin syringe, large-print instructions, one-touch glucose meters.

Adaptive aids have been developed in recent years to help the visually impaired manage their own DM more effectively.

Discuss sexual functioning and answer questions patient/SO may have.

Not infrequently, impotence occurs (may be first symptom of onset of DM). *Note:* Counseling and/or use of penile prosthesis may be of benefit.

Stress importance of use of identification bracelet.

Can promote quick entry into the health system and appropriate care with fewer resultant complications in the event of an emergency.

435

Independent

ACTIONS/INTERVENTIONS	RATIONALE
Recommend avoidance of OTC drugs without prior approval of healthcare provider.	These products may contain sugars/interact with prescribed medications.
Discuss importance of follow-up care.	Helps to maintain tighter control of disease process and may prevent exacerbations of DM, retarding development of systemic complications.
Review signs/symptoms requiring medical evaluation, e.g., fever; cold or flu symptoms; cloudy, odorous urine, painful urination; delayed healing of cuts/sores; sensory changes (pain or tingling) of lower extremities; changes in blood sugar level, presence of ketones in urine.	Prompt intervention may prevent development of more serious/life-threatening complications.
Demonstrate stress management techniques, e.g., deep-breathing exercises, guided imagery, visualization.	Promotes relaxation and control of stress response, which may help to limit incidence of glucose/insulin imbalances.
Identify community resources, e.g., American Diabetic Association, visiting nurse, weight-loss/stop-smoking clinic, contact person/diabetic instructor.	Continued support is usually necessary to sustain lifestyle changes and promote well-being.

POTENTIAL CONSIDERATIONS following acute hospitalization (dependent on patient's age, physical condition/presence of complications, personal resources, and life responsibilities)

Therapeutic Regimen: Individual, ineffective management—complexity of therapeutic regimen, economic concerns, perceived susceptibility (recurrence of problem)

Sensory-Perceptual alterations (diabetic neuropathy/visual changes)—endogenous chemical alterations (elevated glucose level)

HYPERTHYROIDISM (THYROTOXICOSIS, GRAVES' DISEASE)

Hyperthyroidism is a metabolic imbalance that results from overproduction of thyroid hormone. The most common form is Graves' disease, but other forms of hyperthyroidism include toxic adenoma, TSH-secreting pituitary tumor, subacute or silent thyroiditis, and some forms of thyroid cancer.

Thyroid storm is a rarely encountered manifestation of hyperthyroidism, which can be precipitated by such events as thyroid ablation (surgical or radioiodine), medication overdosage, and trauma. This condition constitutes a medical emergency.

CARE SETTING

Most people with classic hyperthyroidism rarely need hospitalization. Critically ill patients, those with extreme manifestations of thyrotoxicosis plus a significant concurrent illness, require inpatient acute care on a medical unit.

RELATED CONCERNS

Heart Failure: Chronic, p 41
Psychosocial Aspects of Care, p 783
Thyroidectomy, p 449

Patient Assessment Data Base

Data depend on the severity/duration of hormone imbalance and involvement of other organs.

ACTIVITY/REST

May report: Nervousness, increased irritability, insomnia
Muscle weakness, incoordination
Extreme fatigue

May exhibit: Muscle atrophy

CIRCULATION

May report: Palpitations
Chest pain (angina)

May exhibit: Dysrhythmias (atrial fibrillation); gallop rhythm, murmurs
Elevated BP with widened pulse pressure
Tachycardia at rest
Circulatory collapse, shock (thyrotoxic crisis)

ELIMINATION

May report: Urinating in large amounts
Stool changes; diarrhea

EGO INTEGRITY

May report: Recent stressful experience, e.g., emotional/physical

May exhibit: Emotional lability (mild euphoria to delirium); anxiety/depression.

FOOD/FLUID

May report: Recent/sudden weight loss
Increased appetite; large meals, frequent meals; thirst
Nausea/vomiting

May exhibit: Enlarged thyroid; goiter
Nonpitting edema, especially in pretibial area

NEUROSENSORY

May exhibit: Rapid and hoarse speech
Mental status and behavior alterations, e.g., confusion, disorientation, nervousness, irritability, delirium, frank psychosis, stupor, coma
Fine tremor in hands; purposeless, quick, jerky movements of body parts
Hyperactive DTRs

PAIN/DISCOMFORT

May report: Orbital pain, photophobia (eye involvement)

RESPIRATION

May exhibit: Increased respiratory rate, tachypnea
Dyspnea
Pulmonary edema (thyrotoxic crisis)

SAFETY

May report: Heat intolerance, excessive sweating
Allergy to iodine (may be used in testing)

May exhibit: Elevated temperature (above 100°F), diaphoresis
Skin smooth, warm, and flushed; hair fine, silky, straight
Exophthalmia, lid retraction; conjunctival irritation, tearing
Pruritic, erythematous lesions (often in pretibial area) that become brawny

SEXUALITY

May report: Decreased libido
Hypomenorrhea, amenorrhea
Impotence

TEACHING/LEARNING

May report: Family history of thyroid problems
History of hypothyroidism, thyroid hormone replacement therapy or antithyroid therapy, premature withdrawal of antithyroid drugs, recent partial thyroidectomy
History of insulin-induced hypoglycemia, cardiac disorders or surgery, recent illness (pneumonia), trauma; x-ray contrast studies

Discharge plan considerations: **DRG projected mean length of inpatient stay: 4.3 days**
May require assistance with treatment regimen, self-care activities, homemaker/maintenance tasks

Refer to section at end of plan for postdischarge considerations.

DIAGNOSTIC STUDIES

RAI uptake test: High in Graves' disease and toxic nodular goiter; low in thyroiditis.

Serum T₄ and free T₄: Increased in hyperthyroidism. Normal level with T₃ elevated indicates thyrotoxicosis.

TSH: Suppressed and does not respond to thyrotropin-releasing hormone (TRH).

Thyroglobulin: Increased.

TRH stimulation: Hyperthyroidism is indicated if TSH fails to rise after administration of TRH.

Thyroid ¹³¹I uptake: Increased.

Protein-bound iodine: Increased.

Blood glucose: Elevated (related to adrenal involvement).

Plasma cortisol: Low levels (less adrenal reserve).

Alkaline phosphatase and serum calcium: Increased.

Liver function tests: Abnormal.

Electrolytes: Hyponatremia may reflect adrenal response or dilutional effect in fluid replacement therapy. Hypokalemia occurs owing to GI losses and diuresis.

Serum catecholamines: Decreased.

Urine creatinine: Increased.

ECG: Atrial fibrillations; shorter systole time; cardiomegaly, heart enlarged with fibrosis and necrosis (late signs or in elderly with masked hyperthyroidism).

NURSING PRIORITIES

1. Reduce metabolic demands and support cardiovascular function.
2. Provide psychologic support.
3. Prevent complications.
4. Provide information about disease process/prognosis and therapy needs.

DISCHARGE GOALS

1. Homeostasis achieved.
2. Patient dealing with current situation.
3. Complications prevented/minimized.
4. Disease process/prognosis and therapeutic regimen understood.
5. Plan in place to meet needs after discharge.

NURSING DIAGNOSIS: Cardiac output, decreased, risk for

Risk factors may include

Uncontrolled hyperthyroidism, hypermetabolic state

Increasing cardiac workload

Changes in venous return and systemic vascular resistance

Alterations in rate, rhythm, conduction

Possibly evidenced by

[Not applicable; presence of signs and symptoms establishes an *actual* diagnosis]

DESIRED OUTCOMES/EVALUATION CRITERIA—PATIENT WILL:

Maintain adequate cardiac output for tissue needs as evidenced by stable vital signs, palpable peripheral pulses, good capillary refill, usual mentation, and absence of dysrhythmias.

Independent

ACTIONS/INTERVENTIONS	RATIONALE
Monitor BP lying/sitting and standing, if able. Note widened pulse pressure.	General/orthostatic hypotension may occur as a result of excessive peripheral vasodilation and decreased circulating volume. Widened pulse pressure reflects compensatory increase in stroke volume and decreased systemic vascular resistance.
Monitor CVP if available.	Provides more direct measure of circulating volume and cardiac function.
Investigate reports of chest pain/angina.	May reflect increased myocardial oxygen demands/ischemia.
Assess pulse/heart rate while patient is sleeping.	Provides a more accurate assessment of tachycardia.
Auscultate heart sounds, noting extra heart sounds, development of gallops and systolic murmurs.	Prominent S_1 and murmurs are associated with forceful cardiac output of hypermetabolic state; development of S_3 may warn of impending cardiac failure.
Monitor ECG, noting rate/rhythm. Document dysrhythmias.	Tachycardia (greater than normally expected with fever/increased circulatory demand) may reflect direct myocardial stimulation by thyroid hormone. Dysrhythmias often occur and may compromise cardiac function/output.
Auscultate breath sounds, noting adventitious sounds (e.g., crackles).	Early sign of pulmonary congestion, reflecting developing cardiac failure.
Monitor temperature; provide cool environment, limit bed linens/clothes, administer tepid sponge baths.	Fever (may exceed 104°F) may occur as a result of excessive hormone levels and can aggravate diuresis/dehydration and cause increased peripheral vasodilation, venous pooling, and hypotension.
Observe signs/symptoms of severe thirst, dry mucous membranes, weak/thready pulse, poor capillary refill, decreased urinary output, and hypotension.	Rapid dehydration can occur, which reduces circulating volume and compromises cardiac output.
Record I&O. Note urine specific gravity.	Significant fluid losses (through vomiting, diarrhea, diuresis, diaphoresis) can lead to profound dehydration, concentrated urine, and weight loss.
Weigh daily. Encourage chair/bed rest; limit non-essential activity.	Activity increases metabolic/circulatory demands, which may potentiate cardiac failure.
Note history of asthma/bronchoconstrictive disease, pregnancy, sinus bradycardia/heart blocks, advanced heart failure.	Presence of these conditions affects choice of therapy; e.g., use of β-adrenergic blocking agents is contraindicated.
Observe for adverse side effects of adrenergic antagonists, e.g., severe decrease in pulse, BP; signs of vascular congestion/HF; cardiac arrest.	Indicates need for reduction/discontinuation of therapy.

Collaborative

ACTIONS/INTERVENTIONS	RATIONALE
Administer IV fluids as indicated.	Rapid fluid replacement may be necessary to improve circulating volume but must be balanced against signs of cardiac failure/need for inotropic support.

ACTIONS/INTERVENTIONS	RATIONALE
Collaborative	
Administer medications as indicated:	
β-blockers, e.g., propranolol (Inderal), atenolol (Tenormin), nadolol (Corgard);	Given to control thyrotoxic effects of tachycardia, tremors, and nervousness and is first drug of choice for acute storm. Decreases heart rate/cardiac work by blocking β-adrenergic receptor sites and blocking conversion of T_4 to T_3. *Note:* If severe bradycardia develops, atropine may be required.
Thyroid hormone antagonists, e.g., propylthiouracil (PTU), methimazole (Tapazole);	Blocks thyroid hormone synthesis and inhibits peripheral conversion of T_4 to T_3. May be definitive treatment or used to prepare patient for surgery; but effect is slow and so may not relieve thyroid storm. *Note:* Once PTU therapy is begun, abrupt withdrawal may precipitate thyroid crisis.
Sodium iodine (Lugol's solution) or supersaturated potassium iodide (SSKI) po.	Temporarily acts to prevent release of thyroid hormone into circulation by increasing the amount of thyroid hormone stored within the gland. May interfere with RAI treatment and may exacerbate the disease in some people. May be used as surgical preparation to decrease size and vascularity of the gland or to treat thyroid storm. *Note:* Should be started 1–3 hours after initiation of antithyroid drug therapy to minimize hormone formation from the iodine.
RAI ($Na^{131}I$ or $Na^{125}I$);	Destroys functioning gland tissue. Peak results take 6–12 weeks (several treatments may be necessary); however, a single dose controls hyperthyroidism in about 90% of patients. *Note:* This therapy is contraindicated during pregnancy.
Corticosteroids, e.g., dexamethasone (Decadron);	Provides glucocorticol support. Decreases hyperthermia; relieves relative adrenal insufficiency; inhibits calcium absorption; and reduces peripheral conversion of T_3 from T_4.
Digoxin (Lanoxin);	Digitalization may be required in patients with HF before β-adrenergic blocking therapy can be considered/safely initiated.
Furosemide (Lasix);	Diuresis may be necessary if HF occurs. *Note:* It also may be effective in reducing calcium level if neuromuscular function is impaired.
Acetaminophen (Tylenol);	Drug of choice to reduce temperature and associated metabolic demands. Aspirin is contraindicated because it actually increases level of circulating thyroid hormones by blocking binding of T_3 and T_4 with thyroid-binding proteins.
Sedative, barbiturates;	Promotes rest, thereby reducing metabolic demands/cardiac workload.
Muscle relaxants.	Reduces shivering associated with hyperthermia, which can further increase metabolic demands.

ACTIONS/INTERVENTIONS	RATIONALE
Collaborative	
Monitor laboratory studies, as indicated, e.g.:	
Serum potassium (replace as indicated);	Hypokalemia resulting from intestinal losses, altered intake, or diuretic therapy may cause dysrhythmias and compromise cardiac function/output.
Serum calcium;	Elevation may alter cardiac contractility.
Sputum culture.	Pulmonary infection is most frequent precipitating factor of crisis.
Review serial ECGs;	May demonstrate effects of electrolyte imbalance or ischemic changes reflecting inadequate myocardial oxygen supply in presence of increased metabolic demands.
Chest x-rays.	Cardiac enlargement may occur in response to increased circulatory demands. Pulmonary congestion may be noted with cardiac decompensation.
Provide supplemental O_2 as indicated.	May be necessary to support increased metabolic demands/O_2 consumption.
Provide hypothermia blanket as indicated.	Occasionally used to lower uncontrolled hyperthermia (104°F and greater) to reduce metabolic demands/O_2 consumption, and cardiac workload.
Administer transfusions; assist with plasmapheresis, hemoperfusion, dialysis.	May be done to achieve rapid depletion of extrathyroidal hormone pool in desperately ill/comatose patient.
Prepare for surgery.	Subtotal thyroidectomy (removal of five sixths of the gland) may be treatment of choice for hyperthyroidism once euthyroid state is achieved.

NURSING DIAGNOSIS: Fatigue

May be related to
Hypermetabolic state with increased energy requirements
Irritability of CNS; altered body chemistry

Possibly evidenced by
Verbalization of overwhelming lack of energy to maintain usual routine, decreased performance
Emotional lability/irritability; nervousness, tension
Jittery behavior
Impaired ability to concentrate

DESIRED OUTCOMES/EVALUATION CRITERIA—PATIENT WILL:
Verbalize increase in level of energy.
Display improved ability to participate in desired activities.

ACTIONS/INTERVENTIONS

Independent

Monitor vital signs, noting pulse rate at rest as well as when active.

Note development of tachypnea, dyspnea, pallor, and cyanosis.

Provide for quiet environment; cool room, decreased sensory stimuli, soothing colors, quiet music.

Encourage patient to restrict activity and rest in bed as much as possible.

Provide comfort measures, e.g., judicious touch/massage, cool showers.

Provide for diversional activities that are calming, e.g., reading, radio, television.

Avoid topics that irritate or upset the patient. Discuss ways to respond to these feelings.

Discuss with SO reasons for fatigue and emotional lability.

Collaborative

Administer medications as indicated:

Sedatives, e.g., phenobarbital (Luminal); antianxiety agents, e.g., chlordiazepoxide (Librium).

RATIONALE

Pulse is typically elevated and, even at rest, tachycardia (up to 160 bpm) may be noted.

O_2 demand and consumption are increased in hypermetabolic state, potentiating risk of hypoxia with activity.

Reduces stimuli that may aggravate agitation, hyperactivity, and insomnia.

Helps counteract effects of increased metabolism.

May decrease nervous energy, promoting relaxation.

Allows for use of nervous energy in a constructive manner and may reduce anxiety.

Increased irritability of the CNS may cause patient to be easily excited, agitated, and prone to emotional outbursts.

Understanding that the behavior is physically based may enhance coping with current situation and encourage SO to respond positively and provide support for the patient.

Combats nervousness, hyperactivity, and insomnia.

NURSING DIAGNOSIS: Nutrition: altered, risk for less than body requirements

Risk factors may include
Increased metabolism (increased appetite/intake with loss of weight)
Nausea/vomiting, diarrhea
Relative insulin insufficiency; hyperglycemia

Possibly evidenced by
[Not applicable; presence of signs and symptoms establishes an *actual* diagnosis]

DESIRED OUTCOMES/EVALUATION CRITERIA—PATIENT WILL:
Demonstrate stable weight with normal laboratory values and be free of signs of malnutrition.

Independent

Auscultate bowel sounds.

Hyperactive bowel sounds reflect increased gastric motility, which can reduce/alter absorption.

Note reports of anorexia, generalized weakness/aches, abdominal pain; presence of nausea/vomiting.

Increased adrenergic activity can cause impaired insulin secretion/resistance, resulting in hyperglycemia, polydipsia, polyuria; changes in respiratory rate/depth.

Monitor daily food intake. Weigh daily and report losses.

Continued weight loss in face of adequate caloric intake may indicate failure of antithyroid therapy.

Encourage patient to eat and increase number of meals and snacks, using high-calorie foods that are easily digested.

Aids in keeping caloric intake high enough to keep up with rapid expenditure of calories caused by hypermetabolic state.

Avoid foods that increase peristalsis (e.g., tea, coffee, fibrous and highly seasoned foods) and fluids that cause diarrhea (e.g., apple/prune juice).

Increased motility of GI tract may result in diarrhea and impair absorption of needed nutrients.

Collaborative

Consult with dietician to provide diet high in calories, protein, carbohydrates, and vitamins.

May need assistance to ensure adequate intake of nutrients, identify appropriate supplements.

Administer medications as indicated:

    Glucose, vitamin B complex.

Given to meet energy requirements and prevent or correct hypoglycemia.

    Insulin (small doses).

Aids in controlling serum glucose if elevated.

NURSING DIAGNOSIS: Anxiety [specify level]

May be related to
Physiologic factors: Hypermetabolic state (CNS stimulation), pseudocatecholamine effect of thyroid hormones

Possibly evidenced by
Increased feelings of apprehension, shakiness, loss of control, panic
Changes in cognition, distortion of environmental stimuli
Extraneous movements, restlessness, tremors

DESIRED OUTCOMES/EVALUATION CRITERIA—PATIENT WILL:
Appear relaxed.
Report anxiety reduced to a manageable level.
Identify healthy ways to deal with feelings.

| ACTIONS/INTERVENTIONS | RATIONALE |

Independent

Observe behavior indicative of level of anxiety.

Mild anxiety may be displayed by irritability and insomnia. Severe anxiety progressing to panic state may produce feelings of impending doom, terror, inability to speak or move, shouting/swearing.

ACTIONS/INTERVENTIONS

Independent

Monitor physical responses, noting palpitations, repetitive movements, hyperventilation, insomnia.

Stay with patient, maintaining calm manner. Acknowledge fear and allow patient's behavior to belong to the patient.

Describe/explain procedures, surrounding environment or sounds that may be heard by the patient.

Speak in brief statements, using simple words.

Reduce external stimuli: Place in quiet room; provide soft, soothing music; reduce bright lights; reduce number of persons contacting patient.

Discuss with patient/SO reasons for emotional lability/psychotic reaction. (Refer to ND: Thought Processes, altered, risk for, following.)

Reinforce expectation that emotional control should return as drug therapy progresses.

Collaborative

Administer antianxiety agents or sedatives and monitor effects.

Refer to support systems as needed, e.g., counseling, social services, pastoral care.

RATIONALE

Increased number of β-adrenergic receptor sites, coupled with effects of excess thyroid hormones, produces clinical manifestations of catecholamine excess even when normal levels of norepinephrine/epinephrine exist.

Affirms to patient/SO that although patient feels out of control, environment is safe. Avoiding personal responses to inappropriate remarks or actions prevents conflicts/overreaction to stressful situation.

Provides accurate information, which reduces distortions/misinterpretations, that can contribute to anxiety/fear reactions.

Attention span may be shortened, concentration reduced, limiting ability to assimilate information.

Creates a therapeutic environment; shows recognition that unit activity/personnel may increase patient's anxiety.

Understanding that behavior is physically based can allow for different responses/approaches, acceptance of situation.

Provides information and reassures patient that the situation is temporary and will improve with treatment.

May be used in conjunction with medical regimen to reduce effects of hyperthyroid secretion.

Ongoing therapy support may be desired/required by patient/SO if crisis precipitates lifestyle alterations.

NURSING DIAGNOSIS: Thought Processes, altered, risk for

Risk factors may include
Physiologic changes: Increased CNS stimulation/accelerated mental activity
Altered sleep patterns

Possibly evidenced by
[Not applicable; presence of signs and symptoms establishes an *actual* diagnosis]

DESIRED OUTCOMES/EVALUATION CRITERIA—PATIENT WILL:
Maintain usual reality orientation.
Recognize changes in thinking/behavior and causative factors.

ACTIONS/INTERVENTIONS

Independent

Assess thinking processes, e.g., memory, attention span, orientation to person/place/time.

RATIONALE

Determines extent of interference with sensory processing.

ACTIONS/INTERVENTIONS

Independent

Note changes in behavior.

Assess level of anxiety. (Refer to ND: Anxiety, p 444.)

Provide quiet environment; decreased stimuli, cool room, dim lights. Limit procedures/personnel.

Reorient to person/place/time.

Present reality concisely and briefly without challenging illogical thinking.

Provide clock, calendar, room with outside window; alter level of lighting to simulate day/night

Provide safety measures, e.g., padded side rails, soft restraints, close supervision.

Encourage visits by family/SO. Provide support as needed.

Collaborative

Administer medications as indicated, e.g., sedatives/antianxiety agents/antipsychotic drugs.

RATIONALE

May be hypervigilant, restless, extremely sensitive, or crying or may develop frank psychosis.

Anxiety may alter thought processes.

Reduction of external stimuli may decrease hyperactivity/reflexia, CNS irritability, auditory/visual hallucinations.

Helps to establish and maintain awareness of reality/environment.

Limits defensive reaction.

Promotes continual orientation cues to assist patient in maintaining sense of normality.

Prevents injury to patient who may be hallucinating/disoriented.

Aids in maintaining socialization and orientation. *Note:* Patient's agitation/psychotic behavior may precipitate family quarrels/conflicts.

Promotes relaxation, reduces CNS hyperactivity/agitation to enhance thought processes.

NURSING DIAGNOSIS: Tissue integrity, impaired, risk for

Risk factors may include
Alterations of protective mechanisms of eye: Impaired closure of eyelid/exophthalmos

Possibly evidenced by
[Not applicable; presence of signs and symptoms establishes an *actual* diagnosis]

DESIRED OUTCOMES/EVALUATION CRITERIA—PATIENT WILL:
Maintain moist eye membranes, free of ulcerations.
Identify measures to provide protection for eyes and prevent complications.

ACTIONS/INTERVENTIONS

Independent

Observe for periorbital edema, lid lag, wide-eyed stare, excessive tearing. Note reports of photophobia, feeling of foreign object in eye; eye pain.

Evaluate visual acuity; note reports of blurred or double vision.

RATIONALE

Common manifestations of excessive adrenergic stimulation related to thyrotoxicosis, requiring supportive interventions until therapeutic resolution of crisis state relieves symptomatology.

Infiltrative ophthalmopathy (Graves' disease) is the result of increased retro-orbital tissue, creating exophthalmos and lymphocytic infiltration of extraocular muscles, which causes weakness. Corresponding visual impairment may worsen or improve independent of therapy and clinical course of disease.

ACTIONS/INTERVENTIONS	RATIONALE
Independent	
Encourage use of dark glasses when awake and taping the eyelids shut during sleep as needed.	Protects exposed cornea if patient is unable to close eyelids completely due to edema/fibrosis of fat pads.
Elevate the head of the bed and restrict salt intake if indicated.	Decreases tissue edema when appropriate, e.g., HF, which can aggravate existing exophthalmos.
Instruct the patient in extraocular muscle exercises if appropriate.	Improves circulation and maintains mobility of the eyelids.
Provide opportunity for patient to discuss feelings about altered appearance and measures to enhance self-image.	Protruding eyes may be viewed as unattractive. Appearance can be enhanced with proper use of makeup, overall grooming, and use of shaded glasses.
Collaborative	
Administer medications as indicated:	
Methylcellulose drops;	Lubricates the eyes.
ACTH, prednisone;	Given to decrease rapidly progressive and marked inflammation.
Antithyroid drugs;	May decrease signs/symptoms or prevent worsening of the condition.
Diuretics.	Can decrease edema in mild involvement.
Prepare for surgery as indicated.	Eyelids may need to be sutured shut temporarily to protect the corneas until edema resolves (rare); or increasing space within sinus cavity and adjusting musculature may return eye to a more normal position.

NURSING DIAGNOSIS: Knowledge deficit [learning need] regarding condition, prognosis, treatment, self care and discharge needs

May be related to
Lack of exposure/recall
Information misinterpretation
Unfamiliarity with information resources

Possibly evidenced by
Questions; request for information; statement of misconception
Inaccurate follow-through of instructions/development of preventable complications

DESIRED OUTCOMES/EVALUATION CRITERIA—PATIENT WILL:
Verbalize understanding of disease process and treatment.
Identify relationship of signs/symptoms to the disease process and correlate symptoms with causative factors.
Initiate necessary lifestyle changes and participate in treatment regimen.

ACTIONS/INTERVENTIONS	RATIONALE
Independent	
Review disease process and future expectations.	Provides knowledge base on which patient can make informed choices.

ACTIONS/INTERVENTIONS	RATIONALE
Independent	
Provide information appropriate to individual situation.	Severity of condition, cause, age, and concurrent complications determines course of treatment.
Identify stressors, and discuss precipitators of thyroid crises, e.g., personal/social and job concerns, infection, pregnancy.	Psychogenic factors are often of prime importance in the occurrence/exacerbation of this disease.
Provide information about signs/symptoms of hypothyroidism and the need for continuing follow-up care.	The patient who has been treated for hyperthyroidism needs to be aware of possible development of hypothyroidism, which can occur immediately after treatment or as long as 5 years later.
Discuss drug therapy, including need for adhering to regimen, and expected therapeutic and side effects.	Antithyroid medication (either as primary therapy or in preparation for thyroidectomy), requires adherence to a medical regimen over an extended period to inhibit hormone production. Agranulocytosis is the most serious side effect that can occur, and alternative drugs may be given when problems arise.
Identify signs/symptoms requiring medical evaluation, e.g., fever, sore throat, and skin eruptions.	Early identification of toxic reactions (thiourea therapy) and intervention are important in preventing development of agranulocytosis.
Explain need to check with physician/pharmacist before taking other prescribed or OTC drugs.	Antithyroid medications can affect or be affected by numerous other medications, requiring monitoring of medication levels, side effects, and interactions.
Emphasize importance of planned rest periods.	Prevents undue fatigue; reduces metabolic demands. As euthyroid state is achieved, stamina and activity level will increase.
Review need for nutritious diet and periodic review of nutrient needs; avoid caffeine, red/yellow food dyes, artificial preservatives.	Provides adequate nutrients to support hypermetabolic state. As hormonal imbalance is corrected, diet will need to be readjusted to prevent excessive weight gain. Irritants and stimulants should be limited to avoid cumulative systemic effects.
Stress necessity of continued medical follow-up.	Necessary for monitoring effectiveness of therapy and prevention of potentially fatal complications.

POTENTIAL CONSIDERATIONS following acute hospitalization (dependent on patient's age, physical condition/presence of complications, personal resources, and life responsibilities)

Fatigue—hypermetabolic state diminishing body energy reserves, prolonged recovery.
Nutrition: altered, risk for more than body requirements—change in BMR and metabolic needs

THYROIDECTOMY

Thyroidectomy, although rare, may be performed for patients with thyroid cancer, hyperthyroidism and drug reactions to antithyroid agents, pregnant women who cannot be managed with drugs, patients who do not want radiation therapy, and patients with large goiters who do not respond to antithyroid drugs. The two types of thyroidectomy include:

Total thyroidectomy: The gland is removed completely. Usually done in the case of malignancy. Thyroid replacement therapy is necessary for life.

Subtotal thyroidectomy: Up to ⅚ of the gland is removed when antithyroid drugs do not correct hyperthyroidism or RAI therapy is contraindicated.

CARE SETTING

Inpatient acute surgical unit

RELATED CONCERNS

Cancer, p 875
Hyperthyroidism (Thyrotoxicosis, Graves' Disease), p 437
Psychosocial Aspects of Care, p 783
Surgical Intervention, p 802

Patient Assessment Data Base

Refer to CP: Hyperthyroidism (Thyrotoxicosis, Graves' Disease), p 437 for assessment information.

Discharge plan considerations: **DRG projected mean length of inpatient stay: 3.0 days.**

Refer to section at end of plan for postdischarge considerations.

NURSING PRIORITIES

1. Reverse hyperthyroid state preoperatively.
2. Prevent complications.
3. Relieve pain.
4. Provide information about surgical procedure, prognosis, and treatment needs.

DISCHARGE GOALS

1. Complications prevented/minimized.
2. Pain alleviated.
3. Surgical procedure/prognosis and therapeutic regimen understood.
4. Plan in place to meet needs after discharge.

NURSING DIAGNOSIS: Airway Clearance, ineffective, risk for

Risk factors may include
Tracheal obstruction; swelling, bleeding, laryngeal spasms

Possibly evidenced by
[Not applicable; presence of signs and symptoms establishes an *actual* diagnosis]

DESIRED OUTCOMES/EVALUATION CRITERIA—PATIENT WILL:
Maintain patent airway, with aspiration prevented.

ACTIONS/INTERVENTIONS	RATIONALE

Independent

Monitor respiratory rate, depth and work of breathing.	Respirations may remain somewhat rapid, but development of respiratory distress is indicative of tracheal compression from edema or hemorrhage.
Auscultate breath sounds, noting presence of rhonchi.	Rhonchi may indicate airway obstruction/accumulation of copious thick secretions.
Assess for dyspnea, stridor, "crowing," and cyanosis. Note quality of voice.	Indicators of tracheal obstruction/laryngeal spasm, requiring prompt evaluation and intervention.
Caution patient to avoid bending neck; support head with pillows.	Reduces likelihood of tension on surgical wound.
Assist with repositioning, deep-breathing exercises and/or coughing as indicated.	Maintains clear airway and ventilation. Although coughing is not encouraged and may be painful, it may be needed to clear secretions.
Suction mouth and trachea as indicated, noting color and characteristics of sputum.	Edema/pain may impair patient's ability to clear own airway.
Check dressing frequently, especially posterior portion.	If bleeding occurs, anterior dressing may appear dry as blood pools dependently.
Investigate reports of difficulty swallowing, drooling of oral secretions.	May indicate edema/sequestered bleeding in tissues surrounding operative site.
Keep tracheostomy tray at bedside.	Compromised airway may create a life-threatening situation requiring emergency procedure.

Collaborative

Provide steam inhalation; humidify room air.	Reduces discomfort of sore throat and tissue edema and promotes expectoration of secretions.
Assist with/prepare for procedures, e.g.;	
Tracheostomy;	May be necessary to maintain airway if obstructed by edema of glottis or hemorrhage.
Return to surgery.	May require ligation of bleeding vessels.

NURSING DIAGNOSIS: Communication, impaired verbal

May be related to
Vocal cord injury/laryngeal nerve damage
Tissue edema; pain
Discomfort

Possibly evidenced by
Impaired articulation, does not/cannot speak; use of nonverbal cues such as gestures

DESIRED OUTCOMES/EVALUATION CRITERIA—PATIENT WILL:
Establish method of communication in which needs can be understood.

ACTIONS/INTERVENTIONS

Independent

Assess speech periodically; encourage voice rest.

Keep communication simple; ask yes/no questions.

Provide alternate methods of communication as appropriate, e.g., slate board, letter/picture board. Place IV line to minimize interference with written communication.

Anticipate needs as possible. Visit patient frequently.

Post notice of patient's voice limitations at central station and answer call bell promptly.

Maintain quiet environment.

RATIONALE

Hoarseness and sore throat may occur secondary to tissue edema or surgical damage to recurrent laryngeal nerve and may last several days. Permanent nerve damage can occur (rare) that causes paralysis of vocal cords and/or compression of the trachea.

Reduces demand for response; promotes voice rest.

Facilitates expression of needs.

Reduces anxiety and patient's need to communicate.

Prevents patient from straining voice to make needs known/summon assistance.

Enhances ability to hear whispered communication and reduces necessity for patient to raise/strain voice to be heard.

NURSING DIAGNOSIS: Injury, risk for [tetany]

Risk factors may include
Chemical imbalance: Excessive CNS stimulation

Possibly evidenced by
[Not applicable; presence of signs and symptoms establishes an *actual* diagnosis]

DESIRED OUTCOMES/EVALUATION CRITERIA—PATIENT WILL:
Demonstrate absence of injury with complications minimized/controlled.

ACTIONS/INTERVENTIONS

Independent

Monitor vital signs noting elevating temperature, tachycardia (140–200/min), dysrhythmias, respiratory distress, cyanosis (developing pulmonary edema/HF).

Evaluate reflexes periodically. Observe for neuromuscular irritability, e.g., twitching, numbness, paresthesias, positive Chvostek's and Trousseau's signs, seizure activity.

Keep side rails raised/padded, bed in low position, and airway at bedside. Avoid use of restraints.

Collaborative

Monitor serum calcium levels.

RATIONALE

Manipulation of gland during subtotal thyroidectomy may result in increased hormone release, causing thyroid storm.

Hypocalcemia with tetany (usually transient) may occur 1–7 days postoperatively and indicates hypoparathyroidism, which can occur as a result of inadvertent trauma to/partial-to-total removal of parathyroid gland(s) during surgery.

Reduces potential for injury if seizures occur.

Patients with levels less than 7.5 mg/100 ml generally require replacement therapy.

ACTIONS/INTERVENTIONS

Collaborative

Administer medications as indicated:

Calcium (gluconate, lactate);

Phosphate-binding agents;

Sedatives;

Anticonvulsants.

RATIONALE

Corrects deficiency, which is usually temporary but may be permanent. *Note:* Use with caution in digitalized patient, as calcium increases cardiac sensitivity to digitalis, potentiating risk of toxicity.

Helpful in lowering elevated phosphorus levels associated with hypocalcemia.

Promotes rest, reducing exogenous stimulation.

Controls seizures until corrective therapy is successful.

NURSING DIAGNOSIS: Pain [acute]

May be related to
Surgical interruption/manipulation of tissues/muscles
Postoperative edema

Possibly evidenced by
Reports of pain
Narrowed focus; guarding behavior; restlessness
Autonomic responses

DESIRED OUTCOMES/EVALUATION CRITERIA—PATIENT WILL:
Report pain is relieved/controlled.
Demonstrate use of relaxation skills and diversional activities appropriate to situation.

ACTIONS/INTERVENTIONS

Independent

Assess verbal/nonverbal reports of pain, noting location, intensity (0–10 scale), and duration.

Place in semi-Fowler's position and support head/neck with sandbags or small pillows.

Maintain head/neck in neutral position and support during position changes. Instruct patient to use hands to support neck during movement and to avoid hyperextension of neck.

Keep call bell and frequently needed items within easy reach.

Give cool liquids po or soft foods, such as ice cream or popsicles.

Encourage patient to use relaxation techniques, e.g., guided imagery, soft music, progressive relaxation.

RATIONALE

Useful in evaluating pain, choice of interventions, effectiveness of therapy.

Prevents hyperextension of the neck and protects integrity of the suture line.

Prevents stress on the suture line and reduces muscle tension.

Limits stretching, muscle strain in operative area.

Soothing to sore throat but soft foods may be tolerated better than liquids if patient experiences difficulty swallowing.

Helps to refocus attention and assists patient to manage pain/discomfort more effectively.

ACTIONS/INTERVENTIONS

Collaborative

Administer analgesics and/or analgesic throat sprays/lozenges as necessary.

Provide ice collar if indicated.

RATIONALE

Reduces pain and discomfort; enhances rest.

Reduces tissue edema and decreases perception of pain.

NURSING DIAGNOSIS: Knowledge deficit [learning need] regarding condition, prognosis, treatment, self care and discharge needs

May be related to
Lack of exposure/recall, misinterpretation
Unfamiliarity with information resources

Possibly evidenced by
Questions; request for information; statement of misconception
Inaccurate follow-through of instructions/development of preventable complications

DESIRED OUTCOMES/EVALUATION CRITERIA—PATIENT WILL:
Verbalize understanding of surgical procedure and treatment.
Participate in treatment regimen.
Initiate necessary lifestyle changes.

ACTIONS/INTERVENTIONS

Independent

Review surgical procedure and future expectations.

Discuss need for well-balanced, nutritious diet and when appropriate, inclusion of iodized salt.

Recommend avoidance of goitrogenic foods, e.g., excessive ingestion of seafood, soybeans, turnips.

Identify foods high in calcium (e.g., dairy products) and vitamin D (e.g., fortified dairy products, egg yolks, liver).

Encourage progressive general exercise program.

Review postoperative exercises to be instituted after incision heals, e.g., flexion, extension, rotation, and lateral movement of head and neck.

Review importance of rest and relaxation, avoiding stressful situations and emotional outbursts.

Instruct in incisional care, e.g., cleansing, dressing application.

RATIONALE

Provides knowledge base on which patient can make informed decisions.

Promotes healing and helps patient to regain/maintain appropriate weight. Use of iodized salt is often sufficient to meet iodine needs unless salt is restricted for other health care problems, e.g., HF.

Contraindicated after partial thyroidectomy because these foods inhibit thyroid activity.

Maximizes supply and absorption of calcium if parathyroid function is impaired.

In patients with subtotal thyroidectomy, exercise can stimulate the thyroid gland and production of hormones, facilitating recovery of general well-being.

Regular ROM exercises strengthen neck muscles, enhance circulation and healing process.

Effects of hyperthyroidism usually subside completely, but it takes some time for the body to recover.

Enables patient to provide competent self-care.

ACTIONS/INTERVENTIONS	RATIONALE
Independent	
Give information about the use of loose-fitting scarves to cover scar. Avoid the use of jewelry.	Covers the incision without aggravating healing or precipitating infections of suture line.
Apply cold cream after sutures have been removed.	Softens tissues and may help to minimize scarring.
Discuss possibility of change in voice.	Alteration in vocal cord function may cause changes in pitch and quality of voice, which may be temporary or permanent.
Review drug therapy and the necessity of continuing even when feeling well.	If thyroid replacement is needed because of surgical removal of gland, patient needs to understand rationale for replacement therapy and consequences of failure to routinely take medication.
Identify signs/symptoms requiring medical evaluation, e.g., fever, chills, continued/purulent wound drainage, erythema, gaps in wound edges; sudden weight loss, intolerance to heat, n/v, diarrhea, insomnia, weight gain, fatigue, intolerance to cold, constipation, drowsiness.	Early recognition of developing complications such as infection, hyperthyroidism, or hypothyroidism may prevent progression to life-threatening situation. *Note:* As many as 43% of patients with subtotal thyroidectomy will develop hypothyroidism in time.
Stress necessity of continued medical follow-up.	Provides opportunity for evaluating effectiveness of therapy and prevention of complications.

POTENTIAL CONSIDERATIONS following acute hospitalization (dependent on patient's age, physical condition/presence of complications, personal resources, and life responsibilities)

Refer to Potential Considerations in Surgical Intervention plan of care (p 802)
Fatigue—decreased metabolic energy production, altered body chemistry, (hypothyroidism)

HEPATITIS

Inflammation of the liver can be due to bacterial invasion, injury by physical or chemical agents (nonviral, including autoimmune), or viral infections (Hepatitis A, B, C, D, E, and so forth).

CARE SETTING

Usually community level, although brief inpatient acute care on a medical unit may be required, especially in toxic states.

RELATED CONCERNS:

Alcoholism [Acute]: Intoxication/Overdose, p 847
Substance Dependence/Abuse Rehabilitation, p 862
Cirrhosis of the Liver, p 466
Psychosocial Aspects of Care, p 783
Renal Dialysis, p 580
Total Nutritional Support: Parenteral/Enteral Feeding, p 491

Patient Assessment Data Base

Data are dependent on the cause and severity of liver involvement/damage.

ACTIVITY/REST

May report: Fatigue, weakness, general malaise

CIRCULATION

May exhibit: Bradycardia (severe hyperbilirubinemia)
Jaundiced sclera, skin, mucous membranes

ELIMINATION

May report: Dark urine
Diarrhea/constipation; clay-colored stools
Current/recent hemodialysis

FOOD/FLUID

May report: Loss of appetite (anorexia), weight loss or gain (edema)
Nausea/vomiting

May exhibit: Ascites

NEUROSENSORY

May exhibit: Irritability, drowsiness, lethargy, asterixis

PAIN/DISCOMFORT

May report: Abdominal cramping, RUQ tenderness
Myalgias, arthralgias; headache
Itching (pruritus)

May exhibit: Muscle guarding, restlessness

455

RESPIRATION

May report: Distaste for/aversion to cigarettes (smokers)

SAFETY

May report: Recent transfusion of blood/blood products

May exhibit: Fever
Urticaria, maculopapular lesions, irregular patches of erythema
Exacerbation of acne
Spider angiomas, palmar erythema, gynecomastia in men (sometimes present in alcoholic hepatitis)
Splenomegaly, posterior cervical node enlargement

SEXUALITY

May report: Lifestyle/behaviors increasing risk of exposure (e.g., sexual promiscuity, sexually active homosexual/bisexual male)

TEACHING/LEARNING

May report: History of known/possible exposure to virus, bacteria, or toxins (contaminated food, water, needles, surgical equipment or blood); carriers (symptomatic or asymptomatic); recent surgical procedure with halothane anesthesia; exposure to toxic chemicals (e.g., carbon tetrachloride, vinyl chloride); prescription drug use (e.g., sulfonamides, phenothiazines, isoniazid)
Travel to/immigration from China, Africa, Southeast Asia, Middle East (hepatitis B [HB] is endemic in these areas)
Street (IV) drug or alcohol use
Concurrent diabetes, HF, malignancy or renal disease
Recent flulike upper respiratory infection

Discharge plan considerations: **DRG projected mean length of inpatient stay: 6.7 days**
May require assistance with homemaker/maintenance tasks

Refer to section at end of plan for postdischarge considerations.

DIAGNOSTIC STUDIES

Liver enzymes/isoenzymes: Abnormal (4–10 times normal values). *Note:* Of limited value in differentiating viral from nonviral hepatitis.

> *AST (SGOT)/ALT (SGPT):* Initially elevated. May rise 1–2 weeks before jaundice is apparent, then declines.
> *Alkaline phosphatase:* Slight elevation (unless severe cholestasis present).

Hepatitis A, B, C, D, E panels (antibody/antigen tests): Specify type and stage of disease and determine possible carriers.

CBC: RBCs decreased due to decreased life of RBCs (liver enzyme alterations) or result of hemorrhage.

WBCs: Leukopenia reflecting thrombocytopenia may be present (splenomegaly).

Differential WBC: Leukocytosis, monocytosis, atypical lymphocytes, and plasma cells.

Serum albumin: Decreased.

Blood glucose: Transient hyperglycemia/hypoglycemia (altered liver function).

Prothrombin time: May be prolonged (liver dysfunction).

Serum bilirubin: Above 2.5 mg/100 ml. (If above 200 mg/100 ml, poor prognosis is probable due to increased cellular necrosis.)

Stools: Clay-colored, steatorrhea (decreased hepatic function).

BSP excretion test: Blood level elevated.

Liver biopsy: Defines diagnosis and extent of inflammation/fatty necrosis.

Liver scan: Aids in estimation of severity of parenchymal damage.

Urinalysis: Elevated bilirubin levels; protein/hematuria may occur.

NURSING PRIORITIES

1. Reduce demands on liver while promoting physical well-being.
2. Prevent complications.
3. Enhance self-concept, acceptance of situation.
4. Provide information about disease process, prognosis, and treatment needs.

DISCHARGE GOALS

1. Meeting basic self-care needs.
2. Complications prevented/minimized.
3. Dealing with reality of current situation.
4. Disease process, prognosis, and therapeutic regimen understood.
5. Plan in place to meet needs after discharge.

NURSING DIAGNOSIS: Fatigue

May be related to
Decreased metabolic energy production
States of discomfort
Altered body chemistry (e.g., changes in liver function, effect on target organs)

Possibly evidenced by
Reports of lack of energy/inability to maintain usual routines
Decreased performance
Increase in physical complaints

DESIRED OUTCOMES/EVALUATION CRITERIA—PATIENT WILL:
Report improved sense of energy.
Perform ADLs and participate in desired activities at level of ability.

ACTIONS/INTERVENTIONS	RATIONALE
Independent	
Promote bed/chair rest. Provide quiet environment; limit visitors as needed.	Promotes rest and relaxation. Available energy is used for healing. Activity and an upright position are believed to decrease hepatic blood flow, which prevents optimal circulation to the liver cells.
Recommend changing position frequently. Provide/instruct caregiver in good skin care.	Promotes optimal respiratory function and minimizes pressure areas to reduce risk of tissue breakdown.
Do necessary tasks quickly and at one time as tolerated.	Allows for extended periods of uninterrupted rest.
Determine and prioritize role responsibilities and alternate providers/possible community resources available, e.g., meals on wheels, homemaker/housekeeper services.	Promotes problem-solving of most pressing needs of individual/family.
Identify energy-conserving techniques, e.g., sitting to shower and brush teeth, planning steps of activity so that all needed materials are at hand, scheduling of rest periods.	Helps to lessen progression of fatigue, allowing patient to accomplish more and feel better about self.

457

ACTIONS/INTERVENTIONS

Independent

Increase activity as tolerated, demonstrate with passive/active ROM exercises.

Encourage use of stress management techniques, e.g., progressive relaxation, visualization, guided imagery. Discuss appropriate diversional activities, e.g., radio, TV, reading.

Monitor for recurrence of anorexia and liver tenderness/enlargement.

Collaborative

Administer medications as indicated: sedatives, antianxiety agents, e.g., diazepam (Valium), lorazepam (Ativan).

Monitor serial liver enzyme levels.

Administer antidote or assist with inpatient procedures as indicated (e.g.: lavage, catharsis, hyperventilation) dependent on route of exposure.

RATIONALE

Prolonged bedrest can be debilitating. This can be offset by limited activity alternating with rest periods.

Promotes relaxation and conserves energy, redirects attention, and may enhance coping.

Indicates lack of resolution/exacerbation of the disease, requiring further rest, change in therapeutic regimen.

Assists in managing required rest. *Note:* Use of barbiturates and antianxiety agents, such as Compazine and Thorazine, is contraindicated due to hepatotoxic effects.

Aids in determining appropriate levels of activity, as premature increase in activity potentiates risk of replapse.

Removal of causative agent in toxic hepatitis may limit degree of tissue involvement/damage.

NURSING DIAGNOSIS: Nutrition: altered, less than body requirements

May be related to
Insufficient intake to meet metabolic demands: anorexia, nausea/vomiting
Altered absorption and metabolism of ingested foods: reduced peristalsis (visceral reflexes), bile stasis
Increased calorie needs/hypermetabolic state

Possibly evidenced by
Aversion to eating/lack of interest in food
Altered taste sensation
Abdominal pain/cramping
Loss of weight; poor muscle tone

DESIRED OUTCOMES/EVALUATION CRITERIA—PATIENT WILL:
Initiate behaviors, lifestyle changes to regain/maintain appropriate weight.
Demonstrate progressive weight gain toward goal with normalization of laboratory values and free of signs of malnutrition.

ACTIONS/INTERVENTIONS

Independent

Monitor dietary intake/calorie count. Suggest several small feedings and offer largest meal at breakfast.

Encourage mouth care before meals.

RATIONALE

Large meals are difficult to manage when patient is anorexic. Anorexia may also worsen during the day, making intake of food difficult later in the day.

Eliminating unpleasant taste may enhance appetite.

ACTIONS/INTERVENTIONS	RATIONALE
Independent	
Recommend eating in upright position.	Reduces sensation of abdominal fullness and may enhance intake.
Encourage intake of fruit juices, carbonated beverages, and hard candy throughout the day.	These supply extra calories and may be more easily digested/tolerated when other foods are not.
Collaborative	
Consult with dietitian, nutritional support team to provide diet according to patient's needs, with fat and protein intake as tolerated.	Useful in formulating dietary program to meet individual needs. Fat metabolism varies according to bile production and excretion and may necessitate restriction of fat intake if diarrhea develops. If tolerated, a normal or increased protein intake will help with liver regeneration. Protein restriction may be indicated in severe disease (e.g., fulminating hepatitis) because the accumulation of the end products of protein metabolism can potentiate hepatic encephalopathy.
Monitor blood glucose as indicated.	Hyperglycemia/hypoglycemia may develop, necessitating dietary changes/insulin administration. Fingerstick monitoring may be done by patient on a regular schedule to determine therapy needs.
Administer medications as indicated:	
Antiemetics, e.g., metalopramide (Reglan), trimethobenzamide (Tigan);	Given ½ hour before meals, may reduce nausea and increase food tolerance. *Note:* Compazine is contraindicated in hepatic disease.
Antacids, e.g., Mylanta, Titralac;	Counteracts gastric acidity reducing irritation/risk of bleeding.
Vitamins, e.g., B complex, C, other dietary supplements as indicated;	Corrects deficiencies and aids in the healing process.
Steroid therapy, e.g., prednisone (Deltasone), alone or in combination with azathioprine (Imuran).	Steroids may be contraindicated as they can increase risk of relapse/development of chronic hepatitis in patients with viral hepatitis; however, antiinflammatory effect may be useful in chronic active hepatitis (especially idiopathic) to reduce n/v and enable patient to retain food and fluids. Steroids may decrease serum aminotransferase and bilirubin levels, but they do not affect liver necrosis or regeneration. Combination therapy has fewer steroid-related side effects.
Provide supplemental feedings/TPN if needed.	May be necessary to meet caloric requirements if marked deficits are present/symptoms are prolonged.

NURSING DIAGNOSIS: Fluid Volume deficit, risk for

Risk factors may include
Excessive losses through vomiting and diarrhea, third-space shift (ascites)
Altered clotting process

Possibly evidenced by
[Not applicable; presence of signs and symptoms establishes an *actual* diagnosis]

459

ACTIONS/INTERVENTIONS	RATIONALE
Independent	
Monitor I&O, compare with periodic weight. Note enteric losses, e.g., vomiting and diarrhea.	Provides information about replacement needs/effects of therapy. *Note:* Diarrhea may be due to transient flulike response to viral infection or may represent a more serious problem of obstructed portal blood flow with vascular congestion in the GI tract or be the intended result of medication use (neomycin, lactulose) to decrease serum ammonia levels in the presence of hepatic encephalopathy.
Assess vital signs, peripheral pulses, capillary refill, skin turgor, and mucous membranes.	Indicators of circulating volume/perfusion.
Check for ascites or edema formation. Measure abdominal girth as indicated.	Useful in monitoring progression/resolution of fluid shifts (edema/ascites).
Use small-gauge needles for injections, applying pressure for longer than usual after venipuncture.	Reduces possibility of bleeding into tissues.
Have patient use cotton/sponge swabs and mouthwash instead of toothbrush.	Avoids trauma and bleeding of the gums.
Observe for signs of bleeding, e.g., hematuria/melena, ecchymosis, oozing from gums/puncture sites.	Prothrombin levels are reduced and coagulation times prolonged when vitamin K absorption is altered in GI tract and synthesis of prothrombin is decreased in affected liver.
Collaborative	
Monitor periodic laboratory values, e.g., Hb/Hct, Na$^+$, albumin, and clotting times.	Reflects hydration and identifies sodium retention/protein deficits, which may lead to edema formation. Deficits in clotting potentiate risk of bleeding/hemorrhage.
Administer medications as indicated e.g.,	
vitamin K;	Because absorption is altered, supplementation may prevent coagulation problems, which may occur if clotting factors/prothrombin time is depressed.
Antacids or H$_2$-receptor antagonists, e.g., cimetadine (Tagamet);	Neutralizes/reduces gastric secretions to lower risk of gastric irritation/bleeding.
Antidiarrheal agents, e.g., diphenoxylate and atropine (Lomotil).	Reduces fluid/electrolyte loss from GI tract.
Provide IV fluids (usually glucose), electrolytes;	Provides fluid and electrolyte replacement in acute toxic state.
Protein hydrolysates;	Correction of albumin/protein deficits can aid in return of fluid from tissues to the circulatory system.
Fresh frozen plasma.	May be required to replace clotting factors in the presence of coagulation defects.

NURSING DIAGNOSIS: Self Esteem, situational low

May be related to

Annoying/debilitating symptoms, confinement/isolation, length of illness/recovery period

Possibly evidenced by

Verbalization of change in lifestyle; fear of rejection/reaction of others, negative feelings about body; feelings of helplessness

Depression; lack of follow-through; self-destructive behavior

DESIRED OUTCOMES/EVALUATION CRITERIA—PATIENT WILL:

Identify feelings and methods for coping with negative perception of self.

Verbalize acceptance of self in situation, including length of recovery/need for isolation.

Acknowledge self as worthwhile; be responsible for self.

ACTIONS/INTERVENTIONS	RATIONALE
Independent	
Contract with patient regarding time for listening. Encourage discussion of feelings/concerns.	Establishing time enhances trusting relationship. Providing opportunity to express feelings allows patient to feel more in control of the situation. Verbalization decreases anxiety and depression and facilitates positive coping behaviors. Patient may need to express feelings about being ill; length and cost of illness; possibility of infecting others; and in severe illness, fear of death. May have concerns regarding the stigma of the disease.
Avoid making moral judgments regarding lifestyle (alcohol use/sexual practices).	Patient may already feel upset/angry, and condemn self; judgments from others will further damage self-esteem.
Discuss recovery expectations.	Recovery period may be prolonged (up to 6 months), potentiating family/situational stress and necessitating need for planning, support, and follow-up.
Assess effect of illness on economic factors of patient/SO.	Financial problems may exist because of loss of patient's role functioning in the family/prolonged recovery.
Offer diversional activities based on energy levels.	Enables patient to use time and energy in constructive ways that enhance self-esteem and minimize anxiety and depression.
Suggest patient wear bright reds or blues/blacks instead of yellows or greens.	Enhances appearance, because yellow skin tones are intensified by yellow/green colors. Jaundice usually peaks within 1–2 weeks, then gradually resolves over 2–4 weeks.
Collaborative	
Make appropriate referrals for help, as needed, e.g., case manager/discharge planner, social services, and/or other community agencies.	Can facilitate problem-solving and help involved individuals to cope more effectively with situation.

461

ACTIONS/INTERVENTIONS	RATIONALE
Independent	
Establish isolation techniques for enteric and respiratory infections according to infection guidelines/policy; include effective hand-washing.	Prevents transmission of viral disease to others. Thorough hand-washing is effective in preventing virus transmission. Type A (infectious) is transmitted by oral-fecal route, contaminated water, and milk and food, especially inadequately cooked shellfish. Type B (serum) is transmitted by contaminated blood/blood products; needle punctures; open wounds; and contact with saliva, urine, stool, and semen. Type C is also transmitted by exposure to blood/blood products. Incidence of both HBV and HCV has increased among healthcare providers and high-risk patients. *Note:* Toxic and alcoholic hepatitis are not communicable and do not require special measures/isolation.
Stress need to monitor/restrict visitors as indicated.	Patient exposure to infectious processes (especially respiratory) potentiates risk of secondary complications.
Explain isolation procedures to patient/SO.	Understanding of reasons for safeguarding themselves and others can lessen feelings of isolation and stigmatization. Isolation may last 2–3 weeks from onset of illness, depending on type/duration of symptoms.
Give information regarding availability of γ-globulin, ISG, H-BIG, hepatitis B vaccine (Recombivax HB, Engerix-B) through health department or family physician.	Immune globulins may be effective in preventing viral hepatitis in those who have been exposed, depending on type of hepatitis and period of incubation.
Administer medications as indicated:	
Antiviral drugs: vidaralune (Vira-A), acyclovir (Zovirax);	Useful in treating chronic active hepatitis.
Interferon alfa-2b (Intron-A);	Effective in treating liver disease related to HCV.
Antibiotics appropriate to causative agents (e.g., gram-negative, anaerobic bacteria) or secondary process.	Treatment of bacterial hepatitis, or to prevent/limit secondary infections.

NURSING DIAGNOSIS: Skin/Tissue Integrity, impaired, risk for

Risk factors may include
Chemical substance: Bile salt accumulation in the tissues

Possibly evidenced by
[Not applicable; presence of signs and symptoms establishes an *actual* diagnosis]

DESIRED OUTCOMES/EVALUATION CRITERIA—PATIENT WILL:
Display intact skin/tissues, free of excoriation.
Report absence/decrease of pruritus/scratching.

ACTIONS/INTERVENTIONS	RATIONALE
Independent	
Use cool showers and baking soda or starch baths. Avoid use of alkaline soaps. Apply calamine lotion as indicated.	Prevents excessive dryness of skin. Provides relief from itching.
Provide diversional activities.	Aids in refocusing attention, reducing tendency to scratch.
Suggest use of knuckles if desire to scratch is uncontrollable. Keep fingernails cut short, apply gloves on comatose patient or during hours of sleep. Recommend loose-fitting clothing. Provide soft cotton linens.	Reduces potential for dermal injury.
Provide a soothing massage at bedtime.	May be helpful in promoting sleep by reducing skin irritation.
Avoid comments regarding patient's appearance.	Minimizes psychologic stress associated with skin changes.
Collaborative	
Administer medications as indicated:	
Antihistamines, e.g., methdilazine (Tacaryl), diphenhydramine (Benadryl);	Relieves itching. *Note:* Use cautiously in severe hepatic disease.
Antilipemics, e.g., cholestyramine (Questran).	May be used to bind bile acids in the intestine and prevent their absorption. Note side effects of nausea and constipation.

NURSING DIAGNOSIS: Knowledge deficit [learning need] regarding condition, prognosis, treatment, self care and discharge needs

May be related to
Lack of exposure/recall; information misinterpretation
Unfamiliarity with resources

Possibly evidenced by
Questions or statements of misconception
Request for information
Inaccurate follow-through of instructions

ACTIONS/INTERVENTIONS	RATIONALE
Independent	
Assess level of understanding of the disease process, expectations/prognosis, possible treatment options.	Identifies areas of lack of knowledge/misinformation and provides opportunity to give additional information as necessary. *Note:* Liver transplantation may be required in the presence of fulminating disease with liver failure.
Provide specific information regarding prevention/transmission of disease, e.g., contacts may require γ-globulin; personal items should not be shared; strict hand-washing and sanitizing of clothes, dishes, and toilet facilities while liver enzymes are elevated. Avoid intimate contact, such as kissing and sexual contact and exposure to infections, especially URI.	Needs/recommendations vary with type of hepatitis (causative agent) and individual situation.
Plan resumption of activity as tolerated with adequate periods of rest. Discuss restriction of heavy lifting, strenuous exercise/contact sports.	It is not necessary to wait until serum bilirubin levels return to normal to resume activity (may take as long as 2 months), but strenuous activity needs to be limited until the liver returns to normal size. When patient begins to feel better, he or she needs to understand the importance of continued adequate rest in preventing relapse or recurrence. (Relapse occurs in 5%–25% of adults.) *Note:* Energy level may take up to 3–6 months to return to normal.
Help patient identify appropriate diversional activities.	Enjoyable activities will help patient avoid focusing on prolonged convalescence.
Encourage continuation of balanced diet.	Promotes general well-being and enhances energy for healing process/tissue regeneration.
Identify ways to maintain usual bowel function, e.g., adequate intake of fluids/dietary roughage, moderate activity/exercise to tolerance.	Decreased level of activity, changes in food/fluid intake, and slowed bowel motility may result in constipation.
Discuss the side effects and dangers of taking OTC/prescribed drugs (e.g., acetaminophen, aspirin, sulfonamides, some anesthetics) and necessity of notifying future healthcare providers of diagnosis.	Some drugs are toxic to the liver; many others are metabolized by the liver and should be avoided in severe liver diseases because they may cause cumulative toxic effects/chronic hepatitis.
Discuss restrictions on donating blood.	Prevents spread of infectious disease. Most state laws prevent accepting as donors those who have a history of any type of hepatitis.
Emphasize importance of follow-up physical examination and laboratory evaluation.	Disease process may take several months to resolve. If symptoms persist longer than 6 months, liver biopsy may be required to verify presence of chronic hepatitis.

ACTIONS/INTERVENTIONS	RATIONALE
Independent	
Review necessity of avoidance of alcohol for a minimum of 6–12 months or longer based on individual tolerance.	Increases hepatic irritation and may interfere with recovery.
Refer to community resources, drug/alcohol treatment program as indicated.	May need additional assistance to withdraw from substance and maintain abstinence to avoid further liver damage.

POTENTIAL CONSIDERATIONS following acute hospitalization (dependent on patient's age, physical condition/presence of complications, personal resources, and life responsibilities)

Fatigue—generalized weakness, decreased strength/endurance, pain, imposed activity restrictions, depression

Home Maintenance Management, impaired—prolonged recovery/chronic condition, insufficient finances, inadequate support systems, unfamiliarity with neighborhood resources

Nutrition: altered, less than body requirements—insufficient intake to meet metabolic demands; anorexia, nausea/vomiting; altered absorption and metabolism of ingested foods; increased calorie needs/hypermetabolic state

Infection, risk for—inadequate secondary defenses; malnutrition; insufficient knowledge to avoid exposure to pathogens

CIRRHOSIS OF THE LIVER

Cirrhosis is a chronic disease of the liver characterized by alteration in structure and degenerative changes, impairing cellular function and impeding blood flow through the liver. Causes include malnutrition, inflammation (bacterial or viral), and poisons (e.g., alcohol, carbon tetrachloride, acetaminophen).

CARE SETTING

May be hospitalized on a medical unit during initial or recurrent acute episodes with potentially life-threatening complications. Otherwise, this condition is handled at the community level.

RELATED CONCERNS

Alcoholism (Acute): Intoxication/Overdose, p 847
Substance Dependence/Abuse Rehabilitation, p 862
Fluid and Electrolyte Imbalances, p 899
Psychosocial Aspects of Care, p 783
Renal Dialysis, p 580
Renal Failure: Acute, p 555
Total Nutritional Support: Parenteral/Enteral Feeding, p 491
Upper Gastrointestinal/Esophageal Bleeding, p 315

Patient Assessment Data Base

Data are dependent on underlying cause of the condition.

ACTIVITY/REST

May report:	Weakness, fatigue, exhaustion
May exhibit:	Lethargy Decreased muscle mass/tone

CIRCULATION

May report:	History of chronic HF, pericarditis, rheumatic heart disease, cancer (liver malfunction leading to liver failure)
May exhibit:	Hypertension or hypotension (fluid shifts) Dysrhythmias, extra heart sounds (S_3, S_4) JVD; distended abdominal veins

ELIMINATION

May report:	Flatulence Diarrhea or constipation; gradual abdominal enlargement
May exhibit:	Abdominal distention (hepatomegaly, splenomegaly, ascites) Decreased/absent bowel sounds Clay-colored stools, melena Dark, concentrated urine

FOOD/FLUID

May report:	Anorexia, food intolerance/indigestion Nausea/vomiting

May exhibit: Weight loss or gain (fluid)
Tissue wasting
Edema generalized in tissues
Dry skin, poor turgor
Jaundice; spider angiomas
Halitosis/fetor hepaticus, bleeding gums

NEUROSENSORY

May report: SO(s) may report personality changes, depressed mentation

May exhibit: Changes in mentation, confusion, hallucinations, coma
Slowed/slurred speech
Asterixis (hepatic encephalopathy)

PAIN/DISCOMFORT

May report: Abdominal tenderness/RUQ pain
Pruritus
Peripheral neuritis

May exhibit: Guarding/distraction behaviors
Self-focus

RESPIRATION

May report: Dyspnea

May exhibit: Tachypnea, shallow respiration, adventitious breath sounds
Limited thoracic expansion (ascites)
Hypoxia

SAFETY

May report: Pruritus

May exhibit: Fever (more common in alcoholic cirrhosis)
Jaundice, ecchymosis, petechiae
Spider angiomas/telangiectasis, palmar erythema

SEXUALITY

May report: Menstrual disorders (women), impotence (men)

May exhibit: Testicular atrophy, gynecomastia, loss of hair (chest, underarm, pubic)

TEACHING/LEARNING

May report: History of long-term alcohol use/abuse, alcoholic liver disease
History of biliary disease, hepatitis, exposure to toxins; liver trauma; upper GI bleeding; episodes of bleeding esophageal varices; use of drugs affecting liver function

Discharge plan considerations: **DRG projected mean length of inpatient stay: 7.2 days**
May need assistance with homemaker/management tasks

Refer to section at end of plan for postdischarge considerations.

DIAGNOSTIC STUDIES

Liver scans/biopsy: Detects fatty infiltrates, fibrosis, destruction of hepatic tissues, tumors (primary or metastatic), associated ascites.

467

Percutaneous transhepatic cholangiography (PTHC): May be done to rule out/differentiate causes of jaundice or to perform biopsy of liver.

Esophagogastroduodenoscopy (EGD): May demonstrate presence of esophageal varices.

Percutaneous transhepatic portal angiography (PTPA): Visualizes portal venous system circulation.

Serum bilirubin: Elevated because of cellular disruption, inability of liver to conjugate, or biliary obstruction.

Liver enzymes:

    AST/ALT, LDH and isoenzymes (LDH$_5$): Increased owing to cellular damage and release of enzymes.

    Alkaline phosphatase (ALP) and isoenzyme (LAP$_1$): Elevated owing to reduced excretion.

Gamma glutamyl transpeptidase (GTT): Elevated.

Serum albumin: Decreased owing to depressed synthesis.

Globulins (I$_g$A and I$_g$G): Increased synthesis.

CBC: Hb/Hct and RBCs may be decreased because of bleeding. RBC destruction and anemia is seen with hypersplenism and iron deficiency. Leukopenia may be present as a result of hypersplenism.

Prothrombin time/aPTT: Prolonged (decreased synthesis of prothrombin).

Fibrinogen: Decreased.

BUN: Elevation indicates breakdown of blood/protein.

Serum ammonia: Elevated owing to inability to convert ammonia to urea.

Serum glucose: Hypoglycemia suggests impaired glycogenesis.

Electrolytes: Hypokalemia may reflect increased aldosterone, although various imbalances may occur.

Calcium: May be decreased due to impaired absorption of vitamin D.

Nutrient studies: Deficiency of vitamins A, B$_{12}$, C, K; folic acid, and iron may be noted.

Urine urobilinogen: May/may not be present. Serves as guide for differentiating liver disease, hemolytic disease, and biliary obstruction.

Fecal urobilinogen: Decreased.

NURSING PRIORITIES

1. Maintain adequate nutrition.
2. Prevent complications.
3. Enhance self-concept, acceptance of situation.
4. Provide information about disease process/prognosis, potential complications, and treatment needs.

DISCHARGE GOALS

1. Nutritional intake adequate for individual needs.
2. Complications prevented/minimized.
3. Dealing with current reality.
4. Disease process, prognosis, potential complications, and therapeutic regimen understood.
5. Plan in place to meet needs after discharge.

NURSING DIAGNOSIS: Nutrition: altered, less than body requirements

May be related to
Inadequate diet; inability to process/digest nutrients
Anorexia, nausea/vomiting, indigestion, early satiety (ascites)
Abnormal bowel function

Possibly evidenced by
Weight loss
Changes in bowel sounds and function
Poor muscle tone/wasting
Imbalances in nutritional studies

ACTIONS/INTERVENTIONS	RATIONALE
Independent	
Measure dietary intake by calorie count.	Provides information about intake, needs/deficiencies.
Weigh as indicated. Compare changes in fluid status, recent weight history, triceps skin measurement.	It may be difficult to use weight as a direct indicator of nutritional status in view of edema/ascites. Triceps skinfold measurement is useful in assessing changes in muscle mass and subcutaneous fat reserves.
Assist/encourage patient to eat; explain reasons for the type of diet. Feed patient if tiring easily, or have SO assist patient. Consider preferences in food choices.	Proper diet is vital to recovery. Patient may eat better if family is involved and preferred food is included as much as possible.
Encourage patient to eat all meals/supplementary feedings.	Patient may pick at food or eat only a few bites because of loss of interest in food and experience nausea, generalized weakness, malaise.
Recommend/provide small, frequent meals.	Poor tolerance to larger meals may be due to increased intra-abdominal pressure/ascites.
Provide salt substitutes if allowed; avoid those containing ammonium.	Salt substitutes enhance the flavor of food and aid in increasing appetite; ammonia potentiates risk of encephalopathy.
Restrict intake of caffeine, gas-producing or spicy and excessively hot or cold foods.	Aids in reducing gastric irritation/diarrhea and abdominal discomfort that may impair oral intake/digestion.
Suggest soft foods, avoiding roughage if indicated.	Hemorrhage from esophageal varices may occur in advanced cirrhosis.
Encourage mouth care frequently and prior to meals.	Patient is prone to sore and/or bleeding gums and bad taste in mouth, which adds to anorexia.
Promote undisturbed rest periods, especially before meals.	Conserving energy reduces metabolic demands on the liver and promotes cellular regeneration.
Recommend cessation of smoking.	Reduces excessive gastric stimulation and risk of irritation/bleeding.
Collaborative	
Monitor laboratory studies, e.g., serum glucose, prealbumin/albumin, total protein, ammonia.	Glucose may be decreased because of impaired glycogenesis, depleted glycogen stores, or inadequate intake. Protein may be low because of impaired metabolism, decreased hepatic synthesis, or loss into peritoneal cavity (ascites). Elevation of ammonia level may require restriction of protein intake to prevent serious complications.

469

ACTIONS/INTERVENTIONS	RATIONALE
Collaborative	
Maintain NPO status when indicated.	Initially, GI rest may be required in acutely ill patients to reduce demands on the liver and production of GI ammonia/urea.
Consult with dietician to provide diet that is high in calories and simple carbohydrates, low in fat, and moderate to high in protein; limit sodium and fluid as necessary. Provide liquid supplements as indicated.	High-calorie foods are desired inasmuch as patient intake is usually limited. Carbohydrates supply readily available energy. Fats are poorly absorbed because of liver dysfunction and may contribute to abdominal discomfort. Proteins are needed to improve serum protein levels to reduce edema and to promote liver cell regeneration. *Note:* Protein and foods high in ammonia (e.g., gelatin) are restricted if ammonia level is elevated or if patient has clinical signs of hepatic encephalopathy. In addition, these individuals may tolerate vegetable protein better than meat protein.
Provide tube feedings, TPN, lipids if indicated.	May be required to supplement diet or to provide nutrients when patient is too nauseated or anorexic to eat, or when esophageal varices interfere with oral intake.
Administer medications as indicated, e.g.:	
Vitamin supplements, thiamine, iron, folic acid;	Patient may be vitamin-deficient because of previous poor diet. Also, the injured liver is unable to store vitamins A, B complex, D, and K. Anemia due to iron and folic acid deficiencies may also exist.
Zinc;	Enhances sense of taste/smell, which may stimulate appetite.
Digestive enzymes, e.g., pancreatin (Viokase);	Promotes digestion of fats and may reduce steatorrhea/diarrhea.
Antiemetics, e.g., trimethobenzamide (Tigan).	Used with caution to reduce nausea/vomiting and increase oral intake.

NURSING DIAGNOSIS: Fluid Volume excess

May be related to

Compromised regulatory mechanism (e.g., SIADH, decreased plasma proteins, malnutrition)

Excess sodium/fluid intake

Possibly evidenced by

Edema, anasarca, weight gain

Intake greater than output, oliguria, changes in urine specific gravity

Dyspnea, adventitious breath sounds, pleural effusion

BP changes, including CVP

JVD, positive hepatojugular reflex

Altered electrolytes

Change in mental status

DESIRED OUTCOMES/EVALUATION CRITERIA—PATIENT WILL:

Demonstrate stabilized fluid volume, with balanced I&O, stable weight, vital signs within patient's normal range, and absence of edema.

ACTIONS/INTERVENTIONS	RATIONALE
Independent	
Measure I&O, noting positive balance (intake in excess of output). Weigh daily, and note gain greater than 0.5 kg/d.	Reflects circulating volume status, developing/resolution of fluid shifts, and response to therapy. Positive balance/weight gain often reflects continuing fluid retention. *Note:* Decreased circulating volume (fluid shifts) may directly affect renal function/urine output, resulting in hepatorenal syndrome.
Monitor BP (and CVP if available). Note JVD/abdominal vein distention.	BP elevations are usually associated with fluid volume excess but may not occur because of fluid shifts out of the vascular space. Distention of external jugular and abdominal veins is associated with vascular congestion.
Assess respiratory status, noting increased respiratory rate, dyspnea.	Indicative of pulmonary congestion/edema.
Auscultate lungs, noting diminished/absent breath sounds and developing adventitious sounds (e.g., crackles).	Increasing pulmonary congestion may result in consolidation, impaired gas exchange, and complications, e.g., pulmonary edema.
Monitor for cardiac dysrhythmias. Auscultate heart sounds, noting development of S_3/S_4 gallop rhythm.	May be caused by HF, decreased coronary arterial perfusion, and electrolyte imbalance.
Assess degree of peripheral/dependent edema.	Fluids shift into tissues as a result of sodium and water retention, decreased albumin, and increased ADH.
Measure abdominal girth.	Reflects accumulation of fluid (ascites) resulting from loss of plasma proteins/fluid into peritoneal space. *Note:* Excessive fluid accumulation can reduce circulating volume creating a deficit (signs of dehydration).
Encourage bed rest when ascites is present.	May promote recumbency-induced diuresis.
Provide frequent mouth care; occasional ice chips (if NPO).	Decreases sensation of thirst.
Collaborative	
Monitor serum albumin and electrolytes (particularly potassium and sodium).	Decreased serum albumin affects plasma colloid osmotic pressure, resulting in edema formation. Reduced renal blood flow accompanied by elevated ADH and aldosterone levels and the use of diuretics (to reduce total body water) may cause various electrolyte shifts/imbalances.
Monitor serial chest x-rays.	Vascular congestion, pulmonary edema, and pleural effusions frequently occur.
Restrict sodium and fluids as indicated.	Sodium may be restricted to minimize fluid retention in extravascular spaces. Fluid restriction may be necessary to correct/prevent dilutional hyponatremia.
Administer salt-free albumin/plasma expanders as indicated.	Albumin may be used to increase the colloid osmotic pressure in the vascular compartment (pulling fluid into vascular space), thereby increasing effective circulating volume and decreasing formation of ascites.

ACTIONS/INTERVENTIONS

RATIONALE

Collaborative

Administer medications as indicated:

Diuretics, e.g., spironolactone (Aldactone), furosemide (Lasix);

Used with caution to control edema and ascites, block effect of aldosterone, and increase water excretion while sparing potassium, when conservative therapy with bed rest and sodium restriction do not alleviate problem.

Potassium;

Serum and cellular potassium are usually depleted because of liver disease as well as urinary losses.

Positive inotropic drugs and arterial vasodilators.

Given to increase cardiac output/improve renal blood flow and function, thereby reducing excess fluid.

NURSING DIAGNOSIS: Skin Integrity, impaired, risk for

Risk factors may include
Altered circulation/metabolic state
Accumulation of bile salts in skin
Poor skin turgor, skeletal prominence, presence of edema, ascites

Possibly evidenced by
[Not applicable; presence of signs and symptoms establishes an *actual* diagnosis]

DESIRED OUTCOMES/EVALUATION CRITERIA—PATIENT WILL:
Maintain skin integrity.
Identify individual risk factors and demonstrate behaviors/techniques to prevent skin breakdown.

ACTIONS/INTERVENTIONS

RATIONALE

Independent

Inspect skin surfaces/pressure points routinely. Gently massage bony prominences or areas of continued stress. Use emollient lotions; limit use of soap for bathing.

Edematous tissues are more prone to breakdown and to the formation of decubiti. Ascites may stretch the skin to the point of tearing in severe cirrhosis.

Encourage/assist with repositioning on a regular schedule, while in bed/chair; and active/passive ROM exercises as appropriate.

Repositioning reduces pressure on edematous tissues to improve circulation. Exercises enhance circulation and improve/maintain joint mobility.

Recommend elevating lower extremities.

Enhances venous return and reduces edema formation in extremities.

Keep linens dry and free of wrinkles.

Moisture aggravates pruritus and increases risk of skin breakdown.

Suggest clipping fingernails short; provide mittens/gloves if indicated.

Prevents the patient from inadvertently injuring the skin, especially while sleeping.

Encourage/provide perineal care following urination and bowel movement.

Prevents skin excoriation breakdown from bile salts.

ACTIONS/INTERVENTIONS	RATIONALE
Collaborative	
Use alternating pressure mattress, egg carton mattress, waterbed, sheepskins, as indicated.	Reduces dermal pressure, increases circulation, and diminishes risk of tissue ischemia/breakdown.
Apply calamine lotion, provide baking soda baths. Administer medications such as cholestyramine (Questran), hydroxyzine (Atarax), diphenhydramine (Benadryl) if indicated.	May be soothing/provide for itching associated with jaundice, bile salts in skin.

NURSING DIAGNOSIS: Breathing Pattern, ineffective, risk for

Risk factors may include
Intra-abdominal fluid collection (ascites)
Decreased lung expansion, accumulated secretions
Decreased energy, fatigue

Possibly evidenced by
[Not applicable; presence of signs and symptoms establishes an *actual* diagnosis]

DESIRED OUTCOMES/EVALUATION CRITERIA—PATIENT WILL:
Maintain effective respiratory pattern; be free of dyspnea and cyanosis, with ABGs and vital capacity within acceptable range.

ACTIONS/INTERVENTIONS	RATIONALE
Independent	
Monitor respiratory rate, depth, and effort.	Rapid shallow respirations/dyspnea may be present due to hypoxia and/or fluid accumulation in abdomen.
Auscultate breath sounds, noting crackles, wheezes, rhonchi.	Indicates developing complications, (e.g., presence of adventitious sounds reflects accumulation of fluid/secretions; absent/diminished sounds suggest atelectasis) increasing risk of infection.
Investigate changes in level of consciousness.	Changes in mentation may reflect hypoxemia and respiratory failure, which often accompany hepatic coma.
Keep head of bed elevated. Position on sides.	Facilitates breathing by reducing pressure on the diaphragm and minimizes risk of aspiration of secretions.
Encourage frequent repositioning; and deep-breathing exercises/coughing as appropriate.	Aids in lung expansion and mobilizing secretions.
Monitor temperature. Note presence of chills, increased coughing, changes in color/character of sputum.	Indicative of onset of infection, e.g., pneumonia.
Collaborative	
Monitor serial ABGs, pulse oximetry, vital capacity measurements, chest x-rays.	Reveals changes in respiratory status, developing pulmonary complications.

ACTIONS/INTERVENTIONS

Collaborative

Provide supplemental O$_2$ as indicated.

Demonstrate/assist with respiratory adjuncts, e.g., incentive spirometer, blow bottles.

Prepare for/assist with acute care procedure, e.g.:

    Paracentesis;

    Peritoneovenous shunt.

RATIONALE

May be necessary to treat/prevent hypoxia. If respirations/oxygenation inadequate, mechanical ventilation may be required.

Reduces incidence of atelectasis, enhances mobilization of secretions.

Occasionally done to remove ascites fluid when respiratory embarrassment is not corrected by other measures.

Surgical implant of a catheter to return accumulated fluid in the abdominal cavity to systemic circulation via the vena cava, providing long-term relief of ascites and improvement in respiratory function.

NURSING DIAGNOSIS: Injury, risk for [hemorrhage]

Risk factors may include
Abnormal blood profile: altered clotting factors (decreased production of prothrombin, fibrinogen, and factors VIII, IX, and X; impaired vitamin K absorption; and release of thromboplastin)
Portal hypertension, development of esophageal varices

Possibly evidenced by
[Not applicable; presence of signs and symptoms establishes an *actual* diagnosis]

DESIRED OUTCOMES/EVALUATION CRITERIA—PATIENT WILL:
Maintain homeostasis with absence of bleeding.
Demonstrate behaviors to reduce risk of bleeding.

ACTIONS/INTERVENTIONS

Independent

Assess for signs/symptoms of GI bleeding; e.g., check all secretions for frank or occult blood. Observe color and consistency of stools, NG drainage, or vomitus.

Observe for presence of petechiae, ecchymosis, bleeding from one or more sites.

Monitor pulse, BP (and CVP if available).

Note changes in mentation/level of consciousness.

Avoid rectal temperature; be gentle with GI tube insertions.

RATIONALE

The GI tract (esophagus and rectum) is the most usual source of bleeding due to mucosal fragility and alterations in hemostasis associated with cirrhosis.

Subacute DIC may develop secondary to altered clotting factors.

An increased pulse with decreased BP and CVP can indicate loss of circulating blood volume, requiring further evaluation.

Changes may indicate decreased cerebral perfusion secondary to hypovolemia, hypoxemia.

Rectal and esophageal vessels are most vulnerable to rupture.

ACTIONS/INTERVENTIONS	RATIONALE
Independent	
Encourage use of soft toothbrush, electric razor, avoiding straining for stool, forceful nose blowing, and so forth.	In the presence of clotting factor disturbances, minimal trauma can cause mucosal bleeding.
Use small needles for injections. Apply pressure to small bleeding/venipuncture sites for longer than usual.	Minimizes damage to tissues, reducing risk of bleeding/hematoma.
Recommend avoidance of aspirin-containing products.	Prolongs coagulation, potentiating risk of hemorrhage.
Collaborative	
Monitor Hb/Hct and clotting factors.	Indicators of anemia, active bleeding or impending complications (e.g., DIC).
Administer medications as indicated:	
Supplemental vitamins (e.g., vitamins K, D, and C);	Promotes prothrombin synthesis and coagulation if liver is functional. Vitamin C deficiencies increase susceptibility of GI system to irritation/bleeding.
Stool softeners.	Prevents straining for stool with resultant increase in intra-abdominal pressure and risk of vascular rupture/hemorrhage.
Provide gastric lavage with room temperature/cool saline solution or water as indicated.	In presence of acute bleeding, evacuation of blood from GI tract reduces ammonia production and risk of hepatic encephalopathy.
Assist with insertion/maintenance of GI/esophageal tube (e.g., Sengstaken-Blakemore tube).	Temporarily controls bleeding of esophageal varices when control by other means (e.g., lavage) and hemodynamic stability cannot be achieved.
Prepare for surgical procedures, e.g., direct ligation (banding) of varices, esophagogastric resection, splenorenalportacaval anastomosis.	May be needed to control active hemorrhage or to decrease portal and collateral blood vessel pressure to minimize risk of recurrence of bleeding.

NURSING DIAGNOSIS: Confusion, acute, risk for

Risk factors may include
Alcohol abuse
Inability of liver to detoxify certain enzymes/drugs

Possibly evidenced by
[Not applicable; presence of signs and symptoms establishes an *actual* diagnosis]

DESIRED OUTCOMES/EVALUATION CRITERIA—PATIENT WILL:
Maintain usual level of mentation/reality orientation.
Initiate behaviors/lifestyle changes to prevent or minimize recurrence of problem.

ACTIONS/INTERVENTIONS	RATIONALE

Independent

Observe for changes in behavior and mentation, e.g., lethargy, confusion, drowsiness, slowing/slurring of speech, and irritability (may be intermittent). Arouse patient at intervals as indicated.	Ongoing assessment of behavior and mental status is important because of fluctuating nature of impending hepatic coma.
Review current medication regimen/schedules.	Adverse drug reactions or interactions (e.g., cimetidine plus antacids), may potential/exacerbate confusion.
Evaluate sleep/rest schedule.	Difficulty falling/staying asleep leads to sleep deprivation, resulting in diminished cognition and lethargy.
Note development/presence of asterixis, fetor hepaticus, seizure activity.	Suggests elevating serum ammonia levels; increased risk of progression to encephalopathy.
Consult with SO about patient's usual behavior and mentation.	Provides baseline for comparison of current status.
Have patient write name periodically and keep this record for comparison. Report deterioration of ability. Have patient do simple arithmetic computations.	Easy test of neurologic status and muscle coordination.
Reorient to time, place, person as needed.	Assists in maintaining reality orientation, reducing confusion/anxiety.
Maintain a pleasant, quiet environment and approach in a slow, calm manner. Encourage uninterrupted rest periods.	Reduces excessive stimulation/sensory overload, promotes relaxation, and may enhance coping.
Provide continuity of care. If possible, assign same nurse over a period of time.	Familiarity provides reassurance, aids in reducing anxiety, and provides a more accurate documentation of subtle changes.
Reduce provocative stimuli, confrontation. Refrain from forcing activities. Assess potential for violent behavior.	Avoids triggering agitated, violent responses; promotes patient safety.
Discuss current situation, future expectation.	Patient/SO may be reassured that intellectual (as well as emotional) function may improve as liver involvement resolves.
Maintain bed rest, assist with self-care activities.	Reduces metabolic demands on liver, prevents fatigue, and promotes healing, lowering risk of ammonia buildup.
Identify/provide safety needs, e.g., supervision during smoking, side rails up and pad if necessary. Provide close supervision.	Reduces risk of injury when confusion, seizures, or violent behavior occurs.
Investigate temperature elevations. Monitor for signs of infection.	Infection may precipitate hepatic encephalopathy owing to tissue catabolism and release of nitrogen.
Recommend avoidance of narcotics or sedatives, antianxiety agents, and limiting/restricting use of medications metabolized by the liver.	Certain drugs are toxic to the liver, while other drugs may not be metabolized because of cirrhosis, causing cumulative effects that affect mentation, mask signs of developing encephalopathy, or precipitate coma.

ACTIONS/INTERVENTIONS	RATIONALE
Collaborative	
Monitor laboratory studies, e.g., ammonia, electrolytes, pH, BUN, glucose, CBC with differential.	Elevated ammonia levels, hypokalemia, metabolic alkalosis, hypoglycemia, anemia, and infection can precipitate or potentiate development of hepatic coma.
Eliminate or restrict protein in diet. Provide glucose supplements, adequate hydration.	Ammonia (product of the breakdown of protein in the GI tract) is responsible for mental changes in hepatic encephalopathy. Dietary changes may result in constipation, which also increases bacterial action and formation of ammonia. Glucose provides a source of energy, reducing need for protein catabolism. *Note:* Vegetable protein may be better tolerated than meat protein.
Administer medications as indicated:	
Electrolytes;	Corrects imbalances and may improve cerebral function/metabolism of ammonia.
Stool softeners, colonic purges (e.g., magnesium sulfate), enemas, Lactulose;	Removes protein and blood from intestines. Acidifying the intestine produces diarrhea and decreases production of nitrogenous substances, reducing risk/severity of encephalopathy. *Note:* Long-term use of Lactulose may be required for patients with hepatic encephalopathy to reduce ammonia on a daily/regular basis.
Bactericidal agents, e.g., neomycin (Neobiotic), kanamycin (Kantrex).	Destroys intestinal bacteria, reducing production of ammonia, to prevent encephalopathy.
Administer supplemental O_2.	Mentation is affected by O_2 concentration and utilization in the brain.
Assist with procedures as indicated, e.g., dialysis, plasmapheresis, or extracorporeal liver perfusion.	May be used to reduce serum ammonia levels if encephalopathy develops/other measures are not successful.

NURSING DIAGNOSIS: Self Esteem/Body Image disturbance

May be related to
Biophysical changes/altered physical appearance
Uncertainty of prognosis, changes in role function
Personal vulnerability
Self-destructive behavior (alcohol-induced disease)

Possibly evidenced by
Verbalization of change/restriction in lifestyle
Fear of rejection or reaction by others
Negative feelings about body/abilities
Feelings of helplessness, hopelessness, or powerlessness

DESIRED OUTCOMES/EVALUATION CRITERIA—PATIENT WILL:
Verbalize understanding of changes and acceptance of self in the present situation.
Identify feelings and methods for coping with negative perception of self.

ACTIONS/INTERVENTIONS	RATIONALE

Independent

Discuss situation/encourage verbalization of fears and concerns. Explain relationship between nature of disease and symptoms.

The patient is very sensitive to body changes and may also experience feelings of guilt when cause is related to alcohol (80%) or other drug use.

Support and encourage patient; provide care with a positive, friendly attitude.

Caregivers sometimes allow judgmental feelings to affect the care of the patient and need to make every effort to help the patient feel valued as a person.

Encourage family/SO to verbalize feelings, visit freely/participate in care.

Family members may feel guilty about the patient's condition and may be fearful of impending death. They need nonjudgmental emotional support and free access to the patient. Participation in care helps them feel useful and promotes trust between staff, patient, and SO.

Assist patient/SO to cope with change in appearance; suggest clothing that does not emphasize altered appearance, e.g., use of red, blue, or black clothing.

Patient may present unattractive appearance due to jaundice, ascites, ecchymotic areas. Providing support can enhance self-esteem and promote patient sense of control.

Collaborative

Refer to support services, e.g., counselors, psychiatric resources, social service, clergy, and/or alcohol treatment program.

Increased vulnerability/concerns associated with this illness may require services of additional professional resources.

NURSING DIAGNOSIS: Knowledge deficit [learning need] regarding condition, prognosis, treatment, self care and discharge needs

May be related to
Lack of exposure/recall; information misinterpretation
Unfamiliarity with information resources

Possibly evidenced by
Questions; request for information
Statement of misconception
Inaccurate follow-through of instructions/development of preventable complications

DESIRED OUTCOMES/EVALUATION CRITERIA—PATIENT WILL:
Verbalize understanding of disease process/prognosis.
Correlate symptoms with causative factors.
Initiate necessary lifestyle changes and participate in care.

ACTIONS/INTERVENTIONS	RATIONALE

Independent

Review disease process/prognosis and future expectations.

Provides knowledge base on which patient can make informed choices.

Stress importance of avoiding alcohol. Give information about community services available to aid in alcohol rehabilitation if indicated.

Alcohol is the leading cause in the development of cirrhosis.

ACTIONS/INTERVENTIONS	RATIONALE

Independent

Inform the patient of altered effects of medications with cirrhosis and the importance of using only drugs prescribed or cleared by a physician who is familiar with patient's history.	Some drugs are hepatotoxic (especially narcotics, sedatives, and hypnotics). In addition, the damaged liver has a decreased ability to metabolize all drugs, potentiating cumulative effect and/or aggravation of bleeding tendencies.
Review procedure for maintaining function of peritoneovenous shunt when present.	Insertion of a Denver shunt requires the patient to periodically pump the chamber to maintain patency of the device. Patients with a LeVeen shunt may wear an abdominal binder and/or engage in a Valsalva maneuver to maintain shunt function.
Assist patient in identifying support person(s).	Because of length of recovery, potential for relapses, and slow convalescence, support systems are extremely important in maintaining behavior modifications.
Emphasize the importance of good nutrition. Recommend avoidance of high-protein/salty foods, onions, and strong cheeses. Provide written dietary instructions.	Proper dietary maintenance and avoidance of foods high in sodium and protein aids in remission of symptoms and helps prevent ammonia buildup and further liver damage. Written instructions will be helpful for patient to refer to at home.
Stress necessity of follow-up care and adherence to therapeutic regimen.	Chronic nature of disease has potential for life-threatening complications. Provides opportunity for evaluation of effectiveness of regimen including patency of shunt if used.
Discuss sodium and salt substitute restrictions and necessity of reading food/OTC drug labels.	Minimizes ascites and edema formation. Overuse of substitutes may result in other electrolyte imbalances. Food, OTC/personal care products (e.g., antacids, some mouthwashes) may contain sodium or alcohol.
Encourage scheduling activities with adequate rest periods.	Adequate rest decreases metabolic demands on the body and increases energy available for tissue regeneration.
Promote diversional activities that are enjoyable to the patient.	Prevents boredom and minimizes anxiety and depression.
Recommend avoidance of persons with infections, especially URI.	Decreased resistance, altered nutritional status, and immune response (e.g., leukopenia may occur with splenomegaly) potentiate risk of infection.
Identify environmental dangers, e.g., carbon tetrachloride-type cleaning agents, exposure to hepatitis.	Can precipitate recurrence.
Instruct patient/SO of signs and symptoms that warrant notification of healthcare provider, e.g., increased abdominal girth; rapid weight loss/gain; increased peripheral edema; increased dyspnea, fever; blood in stool or urine; excess bleeding of any kind, jaundice.	Prompt reporting of symptoms reduces risk of further hepatic damage and provides opportunity to treat complications before they become life-threatening.
Instruct SO to notify healthcare providers of any confusion, untidiness, night wandering, tremors, or personality change.	Changes (reflecting deterioration) may be more apparent to SO, although insidious changes may be noted by others with less frequent contact with patient.

POTENTIAL CONSIDERATIONS following acute hospitalization (dependent on patient's age, physical condition/presence of complications, personal resources, and life responsibilities)

Fatigue—decreased metabolic energy production, states of discomfort, altered body chemistry (e.g., changes in liver function, effect on target organs, alcohol withdrawal)

Nutrition: altered, less than body requirements—inadequate diet; inability to process/digest nutrients; anorexia, nausea/vomiting, indigestion, early satiety (ascites); abnormal bowel function

Family Process, altered: alcoholism—abuse of alcohol, resistance to treatment, inadequate coping/lack of problem-solving skills, addictive personality/codependency

Caregiver Role Strain, risk for—addiction or codependency, family dysfunction prior to caregiving situation, presence of situational stressors, such as economic vulnerability, hospitalization, changes in employment

PANCREATITIS

Pancreatitis is a painful inflammatory condition in which the pancreatic enzymes are prematurely activated resulting in autodigestion of the pancreas. Pancreatitis may be acute or chronic, with symptoms mild to severe.

CARE SETTING

Inpatient acute medical unit for initial incident or exacerbations with serious complications; otherwise condition is managed at the community level.

RELATED CONCERNS

Alcoholism (Acute): Intoxication/Overdose, p 847
Substance Dependence/Abuse Rehabilitation, p 862
Diabetes Mellitus/Diabetic Ketoacidosis, p 422
Peritonitis, p 366
Psychosocial Aspects of Care, p 783
Renal Failure: Acute, p 555
Sepsis/Septicemia, p 719
Total Nutritional Support: Parenteral/Enteral Feeding, p 491

Patient Assessment Data Base

CIRCULATION

May exhibit: Hypertension (acute pain); hypotension and tachycardia (hypovolemic shock or toxemia)
Edema, ascites
Skin pale, cold, mottled with diaphoresis (vasoconstriction/fluid shifts); jaundiced (inflammation/obstruction of common duct); blue-green-brown discoloration around umbilicus (Cullen's sign) from accumulation of blood (hemorrhagic pancreatitis)

EGO INTEGRITY

May exhibit: Agitation, restlessness, distress, apprehension

ELIMINATION

May report: Diarrhea, vomiting

May exhibit: Abdominal guarding, distention, and rebound tenderness; rigidity
Bowel sounds decreased/absent (reduced peristalsis/ileus)
Dark amber or brown, foamy urine (bile)
Frothy, foul-smelling, grayish, greasy, nonformed stool (steatorrhea)
Polyuria (developing DM)

FOOD/FLUID

May report: Food intolerance, anorexia; frequent/persistent vomiting, retching, dry heaves
Weight loss

May exhibit: Diffuse epigastric/abdominal tenderness to palpation, abdominal rigidity
Hypoactive bowel sounds
Urine positive for glucose

NEUROSENSORY

May exhibit: Confusion, agitation
Coarse tremors of extremities (hypocalcemia)

PAIN/DISCOMFORT

May report: Unrelenting severe deep abdominal pain, usually located in the epigastrium and peri-umbilical regions but may radiate to the back. Onset may be sudden and is often associated with heavy drinking or a large meal
Radiation to chest and back, may increase in supine position

May exhibit: May curl up on left side with both arms over abdomen and knees/hips flexed
Abdominal rigidity

RESPIRATION

May exhibit: Tachypnea, with/without dyspnea
Decreased depth of respiration with splinting/guarding actions
Bibasilar crackles (pleural effusion)

SAFETY

May exhibit: Fever

SEXUALITY

May exhibit: Current pregnancy (3rd trimester) with shifting of abdominal contents and compression of biliary tract

TEACHING/LEARNING

May report: Family history of pancreatitis
History of cholelithiasis with partial or complete common bile duct obstruction; gastritis, duodenal ulcer, duodenitis; diverticulitis; Crohn's disease; recent abdominal surgery (e.g., procedures on the pancreas, biliary tract, stomach, or duodenum), external abdominal trauma
Excessive alcohol intake
Use of medications, e.g., salicylates, pentamidine, antihypertensives, opiates, thiazides, steroids, some antibiotics, estrogens

Discharge plan considerations: **DRG projected mean length of inpatient stay: 6.1 days**
May require assistance with dietary program, homemaker/maintenance tasks.

Refer to section at end of plan for postdischarge considerations.

DIAGNOSTIC STUDIES

CT scan: Determines extent of edema and necrosis.

Ultrasound of abdomen: May be used to identify pancreatic inflammation, abscess, pseudocysts, carcinoma, or obstruction of biliary tract.

Endoscopy: Visualization of pancreatic ducts is useful to diagnose fistulas, obstructive biliary disease, and pancreatic duct strictures/anomalies. *Note:* This procedure is contraindicated in acute phase.

CT-guided needle aspiration: Done to determine if infection is present.

Abdominal x-rays: May demonstrate dilated loop of small bowel adjacent to pancreas or other intra-abdominal precipitator of pancreatitis, presence of free intraperitoneal air caused by perforation or abscess formation, pancreatic calcification.

Upper GI series: Frequently exhibits evidence of pancreatic enlargement/inflammation.

Serum amylase: Increased due to obstruction of normal outflow of pancreatic enzymes (normal level does not rule out disease). May be 5 or more times normal level in acute pancreatitis.

Serum lipase: Usually elevates along with amylase, but stays elevated longer.

Serum bilirubin: Increase is common (may be caused by alcoholic liver disease or compression of common bile duct).

Alkaline phosphatase: Usually elevated if pancreatitis is accompanied by biliary disease.

Serum albumin and protein: May be decreased (increased capillary permeability and transudation of fluid into extracellular space).

Serum calcium: Hypocalcemia may appear 2–3 days after onset of illness (usually indicates fat necrosis and may accompany pancreatic necrosis).

Potassium: Hypokalemia may occur because of gastric losses; hyperkalemia may develop secondary to tissue necrosis, acidosis, renal insufficiency.

Triglycerides: Levels may exceed 1700 mg/dL and may be causative agent in acute pancreatitis.

LDH/AST (SGOT): May be elevated up to 15 times normal because of biliary and liver involvement.

CBC: WBC of 10,000–25,000 is present in 80% of patients. Hb may be lowered because of bleeding. Hct is usually elevated (hemoconcentration associated with vomiting or from effusion of fluid into pancreas or retroperitoneal area).

Serum glucose: Transient elevations are common, especially during initial/acute attacks. Sustained hyperglycemia reflects widespread β cell damage and pancreatic necrosis and is a poor prognostic sign.

PTT: Prolonged if coagulopathy develops due to liver involvement and fat necrosis.

Urinalysis: Amylase, myoglobin, hematuria, and proteinuria may be present (glomerular damage).

Urine amylase: Increased within 2–3 days after onset of attack.

Stool: Increased fat content (steatorrhea) indicative of insufficient digestion of fats and protein.

NURSING PRIORITIES

1. Control pain and promote comfort.
2. Prevent/treat fluid and electrolyte imbalance.
3. Reduce pancreatic stimulation while maintaining adequate nutrition.
4. Prevent complications.
5. Provide information about disease process/prognosis and treatment needs.

DISCHARGE GOALS

1. Pain relieved/controlled.
2. Hemodynamically stable.
3. Complications prevented/minimized.
4. Disease process/prognosis, potential complications, and therapeutic regimen understood.
5. Plan in place to meet needs after discharge.

NURSING DIAGNOSIS: Pain [acute]

May be related to
Obstruction of pancreatic, biliary ducts
Chemical contamination of peritoneal surfaces by pancreatic exudate/autodigestion of pancreas
Extension of inflammation to the retroperitoneal nerve plexus

Possibly evidenced by
Reports of pain
Self-focusing, grimacing, distraction/guarding behaviors
Autonomic responses, alteration in muscle tone

DESIRED OUTCOMES/EVALUATION CRITERIA—PATIENT WILL:
Report pain is relieved/controlled.
Follow prescribed therapeutic regimen.
Demonstrate use of methods that provide relief.

ACTIONS/INTERVENTIONS	RATIONALE
Independent	
Investigate verbal reports of pain, noting specific location and intensity (0–10 scale). Note factors that aggravate and relieve pain.	Pain is often diffuse, severe, and unrelenting in acute or hemorrhagic pancreatitis. Severe pain is often the major symptom in patients with chronic pancreatitis. Isolated pain in the RUQ reflects involvement of the head of the pancreas. Pain in the LUQ suggests involvement of the pancreatic tail. Localized pain may indicate development of pseudocysts or abscesses.
Maintain bed rest during acute attack. Provide quiet, restful environment.	Decreases metabolic rate and GI stimulation/secretions, thereby reducing pancreatic activity.
Promote position of comfort, e.g., on one side with knees flexed, sitting up and leaning forward.	Reduces abdominal pressure/tension, providing some measure of comfort and pain relief. *Note:* Supine position often increases pain.
Provide alternate comfort measures (e.g., back rub); encourage relaxation techniques (e.g., guided imagery, visualization); quiet diversional activities (e.g., TV, radio).	Promotes relaxation and enables patient to refocus attention; may enhance coping.
Keep environment free of food odors.	Sensory stimulation can activate pancreatic enzymes, increasing pain.
Administer analgesics in timely manner (smaller, more frequent doses).	Severe/prolonged pain can aggravate shock and is more difficult to relieve, requiring larger doses of medication, which can mask underlying problems/complications and may contribute to respiratory depression.
Maintain meticulous skin care, especially in presence of draining abdominal wall fistulas.	Pancreatic enzymes can digest the skin and tissues of the abdominal wall, creating a chemical burn.
Collaborative	
Administer medications as indicated:	
Narcotic analgesics, e.g., meperidine (Demerol);	Meperidine is usually effective in relieving pain and may be preferred over morphine, which can display side effect of biliary-pancreatic spasms. Paravertebral block has been used to achieve prolonged pain control. *Note:* Patients who have recurrent or chronic pancreatitis episodes may be difficult to manage because they may become addicted to the narcotics given for pain control.
Sedatives, e.g., diazepam (Valium); antispasmodics, e.g., atropine;	Potentiates action of narcotic to promote rest and to reduce muscular/ductal spasm, thereby reducing metabolic needs, enzyme secretions.
Antacids, e.g., Mylanta, Maalox, Amphojel, Riopan;	Neutralizes gastric acid to reduce production of pancreatic enzymes and to reduce incidence of upper GI bleeding.
Cimetidine (Tagamet), ranitidine (Zantac).	Decreasing secretion of HCl reduces stimulation of the pancreas and associated pain.
Withhold food and fluid as indicated.	Limits/reduces release of pancreatic enzymes and resultant pain.

ACTIONS/INTERVENTIONS

Collaborative

Maintain gastric suction when used.

Prepare for surgical intervention if indicated.

RATIONALE

Prevents accumulation of gastric secretions, which can stimulate pancreatic enzyme activity.

Surgical exploration may be required in presence of intractable pain/complications involving the biliary tract.

NURSING DIAGNOSIS: Fluid Volume deficit, risk for

Risk factors may include
Excessive losses: vomiting, gastric suctioning
Increase in size of vascular bed (vasodilation, effects of kinins)
Third-space fluid transudation, ascites formation
Alteration of clotting process, hemorrhage

Possibly evidenced by
[Not applicable; presence of signs and symptoms establishes an *actual* diagnosis]

DESIRED OUTCOMES/EVALUATION CRITERIA—PATIENT WILL:
Maintain adequate hydration as evidenced by stable vital signs, good skin turgor, prompt capillary refill, strong peripheral pulses, and individually appropriate urinary output.

ACTIONS/INTERVENTIONS

Independent

Monitor BP and measure CVP if available.

Measure I&O including vomiting/gastric aspirate, diarrhea. Calculate 24-hour fluid balance.

Note decrease in urine output (less than 400 ml/24 hours).

Record color and character of gastric drainage as well as noting pH and presence of occult blood.

Weigh as indicated. Correlate with calculated fluid balance.

Note poor skin turgor, dry skin/mucous membranes, reports of thirst.

RATIONALE

Fluid sequestration (shifts into third space,) bleeding, and release of vasodilators (kinins) and cardiac depressant factor triggered by pancreatic ischemia may result in profound hypotension. Reduced cardiac output/poor organ perfusion secondary to a hypotensive episode can precipitate widespread systemic complications.

Indicators of replacement needs/effectiveness of therapy.

Oliguria may occur, signaling renal impairment/ATN, related to increase in renal vascular resistance or reduced/altered renal blood flow.

Risk of gastric bleeding/hemorrhage is high.

Weight loss may suggest hypovolemia; however, edema, fluid retention, and ascites may be reflected by increased or stable weight, even in the presence of muscle wasting.

Further physiologic indicators of dehydration.

485

ACTIONS/INTERVENTIONS	RATIONALE
Independent	
Observe/record peripheral and dependent edema. Measure abdominal girth if ascites present.	Edema/fluid shifts occur as a result of increased vascular permeability, sodium retention, and decreased colloid osmotic pressure in the intravascular compartment. *Note:* Fluid loss (sequestration) of greater than 6 L/48 h is considered a poor prognostic sign.
Investigate changes in sensorium, e.g., confusion, slowed responses.	Changes may be related to hypovolemia, hypoxia, electrolyte imbalance, or impending delirium tremens (in the patient with acute pancreatitis secondary to excessive alcohol intake). Severe pancreatic disease may cause toxic psychosis.
Auscultate heart sounds; note rate and rhythm. Monitor/document rhythm changes.	Cardiac changes/dysrhythmias may reflect hypovolemia and/or electrolyte imbalance, commonly hypokalemia/hypocalcemia. Hyperkalemia may occur related to tissue necrosis, acidosis, and renal insufficiency and may precipitate lethal dysrhythmias if uncorrected. S_3 gallop in conjunction with JVD and crackles suggest heart failure/pulmonary edema. *Note:* Cardiovascular complications are common and include MI, pericarditis, and pericardial effusion with/without tamponade.
Inspect skin for petechiae, hematomas, and unusual wound or venipuncture bleeding. Note hematuria, mucous membrane bleeding, and bloody gastric contents.	DIC may be initiated by release of active pancreatic proteases into the circulation. The most frequently affected organs are the kidneys, skin, and lungs.
Observe/report coarse muscle tremors, twitching, positive Chvostek's or Trousseau's sign.	Symptoms of calcium imbalance. Calcium binds with free fats in the intestine and is lost by secretion in the stool.
Collaborative	
Administer fluid replacement as indicated, e.g., saline solutions, albumin, blood/blood products, dextran.	Choice of replacement solution may be less important than rapidity and adequacy of volume restoration. Saline solutions and albumin may be used to promote mobilization of fluid back into vascular space. Low-molecular-weight dextran is sometimes used to reduce risk of renal dysfunction and pulmonary edema associated with pancreatitis.
Monitor laboratory studies, e.g., Hb/Hct, protein, albumin, electrolytes, BUN, creatinine, urine osmolality and sodium/potassium, coagulation studies.	Identifies deficits/replacement needs and developing complications, e.g., ATN, DIC.
Replace electrolytes, e.g., sodium, potassium, chloride, calcium as indicated.	Decreased oral intake and excessive losses greatly affect electrolyte/acid base balance, which is necessary to maintain optimal cellular/organ function.
Prepare for/assist with peritoneal lavage, hemoperitoneal dialysis.	Removes toxic chemicals/pancreatic enzymes and allows for more rapid correction of metabolic abnormalities in severe/unresponsive cases of acute pancreatitis.

NURSING DIAGNOSIS: Nutrition: altered, less than body requirements

May be related to

Vomiting, decreased oral intake; prescribed dietary restrictions

Loss of digestive enzymes and insulin (related to pancreatic outflow obstruction or necrosis/autodigestion)

Possibly evidenced by

Reported inadequate food intake

Aversion to eating, reported altered taste sensation, lack of interest in food

Weight loss

Poor muscle tone

DESIRED OUTCOMES/EVALUATION CRITERIA—PATIENT WILL:

Demonstrate progressive weight gain toward goal with normalization of laboratory values.

Experience no signs of malnutrition.

Demonstrate behaviors, lifestyle changes to regain and/or maintain appropriate weight.

ACTIONS/INTERVENTIONS	RATIONALE
Independent	
Assess abdomen, noting presence/character of bowel sounds, abdominal distention, and reports of nausea.	Gastric distention and intestinal atony are frequently present, resulting in reduced/absent bowel sounds. Return of bowel sounds and relief of symptoms signal readiness for discontinuation of gastric aspiration (NG tube).
Provide frequent oral care.	Decreases vomiting stimulus and inflammation/irritation of dry mucous membranes associated with dehydration and mouth breathing when NG is in place.
Assist patient in selecting food/fluids that meet nutritional needs and restrictions when diet is resumed.	Previous dietary habits may be unsatisfactory in meeting current needs for tissue regeneration and healing. Use of gastric stimulants, e.g., caffeine, alcohol, cigarettes, gas-producing foods or ingestion of large meals may result in excessive stimulation of the pancreas/recurrence of symptoms.
Observe color/consistency/amount of stools. Note frothy consistency/foul odor.	Steatorrhea may develop from incomplete digestion of fats.
Note signs of increased thirst and urination or changes in mentation and visual acuity.	May warn of developing hyperglycemia associated with increased release of glucagon (damage to α cells) or decreased release of insulin (damage to β cells).
Test urine for sugar and acetone.	Early detection of inadequate glucose utilization may prevent development of ketoacidosis.
Collaborative	
Maintain NPO status and gastric suctioning in acute phase.	Prevents stimulation and release of pancreatic enzymes (secretin), released when chyme and HCl acid enter the duodenum.

487

ACTIONS/INTERVENTIONS	RATIONALE
Collaborative	
Monitor serum glucose.	Indicator of insulin needs because hyperglycemia is frequently present, although not usually in levels high enough to produce ketoacidosis.
Administer hyperalimentation and lipids, if indicated.	IV administration of calories, lipids, and amino acids should be instituted before nutrition/nitrogen depletion is advanced.
Resume oral intake with clear liquids and advance diet slowly to provide high-protein, high-carbohydrate diet, when indicated.	Oral feedings given too early in the course of illness may exacerbate symptoms. Loss of pancreatic function/reduced insulin production may require initiation of a diabetic diet.
Provide medium-chain triglycerides (e.g., MCT, Portagen).	MCTs are elements of enteral feedings (NG or J-tube) that provide supplemental calories/nutrients that do not require pancreatic enzymes for digestion/absorption.
Administer medications as indicated:	
Vitamins, e.g., A, D, E, K;	Replacement required as fat metabolism is altered, reducing absorption/storage of fat-soluble vitamins.
Replacement enzymes, e.g., pancreatin (Viokase), pancrelipase (Cotazym);	Used in chronic pancreatitis to correct deficiencies to promote digestion and absorption of nutrients.
Insulin.	Corrects persistent hyperglycemia caused by injury to β cells and increased release of glucocorticoids. Insulin therapy is usually short-term unless permanent damage to pancreas occurs.

NURSING DIAGNOSIS: Infection, risk for

Risk factors may include
Inadequate primary defenses: stasis of body fluids, altered peristalsis, change in pH secretions
Immunosuppression
Nutritional deficiencies
Tissue destruction, chronic disease

Possibly evidenced by:
[Not applicable; presence of signs and symptoms establishes an *actual* diagnosis]

DESIRED OUTCOMES/EVALUATION CRITERIA—PATIENT WILL:
Achieve timely healing, free of signs of infection.
Be afebrile.
Participate in activities to reduce risk of infection.

ACTIONS/INTERVENTIONS	RATIONALE
Independent	
Use strict aseptic technique when changing surgical dressings or working with IV lines, indwelling catheters/tubes, drains. Change soiled dressings promptly.	Limits sources of infection, which can lead to sepsis in a compromised patient. *Note:* Studies indicate that infectious complications are responsible for about 80% of deaths associated with pancreatitis.

ACTIONS/INTERVENTIONS

Independent

Stress importance of good hand-washing.

Observe rate and characteristics of respirations, breath sounds. Note occurrence of cough and sputum production.

Encourage frequent position changes, deep-breathing and coughing. Assist with ambulation as soon as stable.

Observe for signs of infection, e.g.:

Fever and respiratory distress in conjunction with jaundice;

Increased abdominal pain, rigidity/rebound tenderness, diminished/absent bowel sounds;

Increased abdominal pain/tenderness, recurrent fever (greater than 101°F), leukocytosis, hypotension, tachycardia, and chills.

Collaborative

Obtain culture specimens, e.g., blood, wound, urine, sputum, or pancreatic aspirate.

Administer antibiotic therapy as indicated:

Cephalosporins, e.g., cefoxitin sodium (Mefoxin); plus aminoglycosides, e.g., gentamicin (Garamycin), tobramycin (Nebcin).

Prepare for surgical intervention as necessary.

RATIONALE

Reduces risk of cross-contamination.

Fluid accumulation and limited mobility predisposes to respiratory infections and atelectasis. Accumulation of ascites fluid may cause elevated diaphragm and shallow abdominal breathing.

Enhances ventilation of all lung segments and promotes mobilization of secretions.

Cholestatic jaundice and decreased pulmonary function may be first sign of sepsis involving gram-negative organisms.

Suggestive of peritonitis.

Abscesses can occur 2 or more weeks after the onset of pancreatitis (mortality can exceed 50%) and should be suspected whenever the patient is deteriorating despite supportive measures.

Identifies presence of infection and causative organism.

Broad-spectrum antibiotics are generally recommended for sepsis; however, therapy will be based on the specific organisms cultured.

Abscesses may be surgically drained with resection of necrotic tissue. Sump tubes may be inserted for antibiotic irrigation and drainage of pancreatic debris. Pseudocysts (persisting for several weeks) may be drained because of the risk and incidence of infection/rupture.

NURSING DIAGNOSIS: Knowledge deficit [learning need] regarding condition, prognosis, treatment, self care and discharge needs

May be related to
Lack of exposure/recall
Information misinterpretation, unfamiliarity with information resources

Possibly evidenced by
Questions, request for information
Statement of misconception
Inaccurate follow-through of instructions/development of preventable complication

DESIRED OUTCOMES/EVALUATION CRITERIA—PATIENT WILL:
Verbalize understanding of condition/disease process and treatment.
Correctly perform necessary procedures and explain reasons for the actions.
Initiate necessary lifestyle changes and participate in treatment regimen.

ACTIONS/INTERVENTIONS	RATIONALE

Independent

Review specific cause of current episode and prognosis.

Provides knowledge base on which patient can make informed choices.

Discuss other causative/associated factors, e.g., excessive alcohol intake, gallbladder disease, duodenal ulcer, hyperlipoproteinenemias, some drugs (e.g., oral contraceptives, thiazides, Lasix, INH, glucocorticoids, sulfonamides).

Avoidance may help to limit damage and prevent development of a chronic condition.

Explore availability of treatment programs/rehabilitation of chemical dependency if indicated.

Alcohol abuse is currently the most common cause of recurrence of chronic pancreatitis. Usage of other drugs, whether prescribed or illicit, is increasing as a factor. Note: Pain of pancreatitis can be severe and prolonged and may lead to narcotic dependence, requiring need for referral to pain clinic.

Stress the importance of follow-up care, and review symptoms that need to be reported immediately to physician, e.g., recurrence of pain, persistent fever, n/v, abdominal distention, frothy/foul-smelling stools, general intolerance of food.

Prolonged recovery period requires close monitoring to prevent recurrence/complications, e.g., infection, pancreatic pseudocysts.

Review importance of initially continuing bland, low-fat diet with frequent small feedings and restricted caffeine, with gradual resumption of a normal diet within individual tolerance.

Understanding the purpose of the diet in maximizing the use of available enzymes while avoiding overstimulation of the pancreas may enhance patient involvement in self-monitoring of dietary needs and responses to foods.

Instruct in use of pancreatic enzyme replacements and bile salt therapy as indicated, avoiding concomitant ingestion of hot foods/fluids.

If permanent damage to the pancreas has occurred, exocrine deficiencies will occur, requiring long-term replacement. Hot foods/fluids can inactivate enzymes.

Recommend cessation of smoking.

Nicotine stimulates gastric secretions and unnecessary pancreatic activity.

Discuss signs/symptoms of DM, i.e., polydipsia, polyuria, weakness, weight loss.

Damage to the β cells may result in a temporary or permanent alteration of insulin production.

POTENTIAL CONSIDERATIONS following acute hospitalization (dependent on patient's age, physical condition/presence of complications, personal resources, and life responsibilities)

Nutrition: altered, less than body requirements—preexisting malnutrition, prescribed dietary restrictions, persistent nausea/vomiting, imbalances in digestive enzymes

Pain—chemical irritation of peritoneal surfaces by pancreatic enzymes, spasms of biliary ducts, general inflammatory process

Family Process, altered: alcoholism—abuse of alcohol, resistance to treatment, inadequate coping/lack of problem-solving skills, addictive personality/codependency

Therapeutic Regimen: Individual, ineffective management—complexity of therapeutic regimen, economic difficulties, mistrust of regimen, perceived benefit, social support deficits

TOTAL NUTRITIONAL SUPPORT: PARENTERAL/ENTERAL FEEDING

Specifically designed nutritional therapy can be administered by the parenteral or enteral route when the use of standard diets via the oral route is inadequate or not possible, to prevent/correct protein-calorie malnutrition.

Enteral nutrition is preferred for the patient who has a functional GI tract but is unable to consume an adequate nutritional intake, or for whom oral intake is contraindicated/impossible. Feeding may be done via NG or orogastric tube, esophagostomy, gastrostomy, duodenostomy, or jejunostomy.

Parenteral nutrition may be chosen because of altered metabolic states or when mechanical or functional abnormalities of the GI tract prevent enteral feeding. Amino acids, fat, carbohydrates, trace elements, vitamins, and electrolytes may be infused via a central or peripheral vein.

CARE SETTING

May be acute care—any unit, or community level

RELATED CONCERNS

Burns: Thermal/Chemical/Electrical (Acute and Convalescent Phases), p 698
Cancer, p 875
Fluid and Electrolyte Imbalances, p 899
Psychosocial Aspects of Care, p 783
Surgical Intervention, p 802

Patient Assessment Data Base

Clinical signs listed below are dependent on the degree and duration of malnutrition and include observations indicative of vitamin and mineral as well as protein/calorie deficiency.

ACTIVITY/REST

May exhibit: Muscle wasting (temporal, intercostal, gastrocnemius, dorsum of hand); thin extremities, flaccid muscles, decreased activity tolerance

CIRCULATION

May exhibit: Tachycardia, bradycardia
Diaphoresis, cyanosis

ELIMINATION

May report: Diarrhea or constipation; flatulence associated with food intake

May exhibit: Abdominal distention/increased girth, ascites; tenderness on palpation.
Stools may be loose, hard-formed, fatty, or clay-colored.

FOOD/FLUID

May report: Weight loss of 10% or more of body weight within previous 6 months
Problems with chewing, swallowing, choking, or saliva production
Changes in the taste of food; anorexia, nausea/vomiting; inadequate oral intake (NPO) status for 7–10 days, long-term use of 5% dextrose intravenously

May exhibit: Actual weight (measured) as compared with usual or pre-illness weight is less than 90% of ideal body weight for height, sex, and age or equal to or greater than 120% of ideal body weight (patient risk in obesity is a tendency to overlook protein and calorie requirements). A distorted actual weight may occur due to the presence of edema, ascites, organomegaly, tumor bulk, anasarca, amputation

Edentulous or with ill-fitting dentures

Bowel sounds diminished, hyperactive, or absent

Thyroid, parotid enlargement

Lips dry, cracked, red, swollen; angular stomatitis

Tongue may be smooth, pale, slick, coated. Color often magenta, beefy red. Lingual papillae atrophy/swelling

Gums swollen/bleeding, multiple caries

Mucous membranes dry, pale, red, swollen

NEUROSENSORY

May exhibit: Lethargy, apathy, listlessness, irritability, disorientation, coma

Gag/swallow reflex may be decreased/absent, e.g., CVA, head trauma, nerve injury

RESPIRATION

May exhibit: Increased respiratory rate; respiratory distress

Dyspnea, increased sputum production

Breath sounds: crackles (protein deficiency/related fluid shifts)

SAFETY

May report: Recent course of radiation therapy (radiation enteritis)

May exhibit: Hair may be fragile, coarse, lackluster. Alopecia, decreased pigmentation may be present.

Skin dry, scaly, tented; "flaky paint" dermatosis; edema; draining or unhealed wounds, pressure sores; ecchymoses, perifollicular petechiae, subcutaneous fat loss

Eyes sunken, dull, dry, with pale conjunctiva; Bitot's spots (triangular, shiny, gray spots on the conjunctiva seen in vitamin A deficiency), or scleral icterus

Nails may be brittle, thin, flattened, ridged, spoon-shaped

SEXUALITY

May report: Loss of libido

Amenorrhea

TEACHING/LEARNING

May report: History of conditions causing protracted protein losses, e.g., malabsorption or short-gut syndrome with increased diarrhea, acute pancreatitis, renal dialysis, fistulas, draining wounds, thermal injuries

Presence of factors known to alter nutritional requirements/increase energy demands, e.g., single or multiorgan failure; sepsis; fever; trauma; extensive burns; use of steroids, antitumor agents, immunosuppressants

Use of medications that cause untoward drug/nutrient interactions, e.g., laxatives, anticonvulsants, diuretics, antacids, narcotics, immunosuppressants, high-dose chemotherapy

Illness of psychiatric origin, e.g., anorexia nervosa/bulimia

Educational/social factors, e.g., lack of nutrition knowledge, kitchen facilities, reduced/limited financial resources

Discharge plan considerations: **DRG projected mean length of inpatient stay: 6.1 days,** depending on underlying disease process necessitating therapy.

May require assistance with solution preparation, therapy supplies, and maintenance of feeding device for home nutritional care.

Refer to section at end of plan for postdischarge considerations.

DIAGNOSTIC STUDIES

Anthropometrics: Includes measurement of weight-to-height ratio, osseometry, and ratios of lean-to-fat weight:

Triceps skin fold measurement: Estimates subcutaneous fat stores; fat reserves less than 10th percentile suggest advanced depletion; levels less than the 30th percentile suggest mild-to-moderate depletion.

Midarm muscle circumference: Measures somatic muscle mass and is used in combination with triceps skinfold measurement; a decrease of 15–20 percentiles from the expected value suggests a significant reduction.

Visceral proteins:

Serum albumin (the classic marker measured): Values of 2.7–3.4 g/dl indicate mild depletion; 2.1–2.7 g/dl, moderate depletion; and less than 2.1 g/dl, severe depletion. (Decreased levels are due to poor protein intake, nephrotic syndrome, sepsis, burns, HF, cirrhosis, eclampsia, protein-losing enteropathy. Above-normal values [greater than 4.5 g/dl] are seen in dehydration.) *Note:* Serum prealbumin has a shorter half-life than albumin, so body stores turn over quickly, making it a more sensitive indicator of improvement/change in protein status.

Serum transferrin: More sensitive to changes in visceral protein stores than albumin; levels of 150–200 mg/dl reflect mild depletion; 100–150 mg/dl, moderate depletion; and 100 mg/dl, severe depletion. (Elevated values are seen with iron deficiency, pregnancy, hypoxia, and chronic blood loss. Decreased values are seen with pernicious anemia, chronic infection, liver disease, iron overload, and protein-losing enteropathy.)

Thyroxine-binding prealbumin: Reflects rapid changes in hepatic protein synthesis and thus is a more sensitive indicator of visceral protein depletion. (Decreased levels less than 200 mEq/ml are noted with cirrhosis, inflammation, and surgical trauma.)

Amino acid profile: Alterations reflect an imbalance of plasma proteins with depressed levels of branched-chain amino acids (common with hepatic encephalopathy or sepsis).

Tests of immune system:

Total lymphocyte count: Less than 1500 cells/mm indicates leukopenia and results from decreased generation of T cells, which are very sensitive to malnutrition. (Levels are also altered by infection and administration of immunosuppressants.)

Tests of micronutrients:

Potassium: Deficiency occurs with inadequate intake and with loss of potassium-containing fluids (e.g., urine, diarrhea, vomiting, fistula drainage, continuous NG suctioning). Potassium is also lost from cells during muscle wasting and is excreted by the kidneys.

Sodium: Levels are dependent on state of hydration/presence of active loss as may exist in excessive diuresis, GI suctioning, burns.

Phosphorus: May be decreased reflecting inadequate intake or increased cellular uptake; may be elevated in renal failure.

Magnesium: Deficiency is common in alcoholics, chronic vomiting, diarrhea; may be elevated in renal failure.

Calcium: Levels are decreased with conditions associated with hypoalbuminemia, e.g., renal failure (majority of calcium is bound to albumin). Absorption is decreased by fat malabsorption and low-protein diet.

Zinc: Deficiency is seen in alcoholic cirrhosis; or may be secondary to hypoalbuminemia and GI losses (diarrhea).

Tests reflecting protein (nitrogen) loss:

Nitrogen balance studies: Nitrogen (protein) excretion via urine, stool and insensible losses often exceed nitrogen intake in the acutely ill, reflecting catabolic response to stress and use of endogenous protein stores for energy production (gluconeogenesis). BUN may be severely decreased as a result of chronic malnutrition and depletion of skeletal protein stores.

24-hour creatinine excretion: Because Cr is concentrated in muscle mass, there is a good correlation between lean body mass and 24-hour Cr excretion. Actual values are compared with ideal values (based on height and weight) times 100, known as the Cr height index: 60%–80% indicates moderate depletion; less than 60%, severe depletion.

Tests of GI function (Include Schilling test, D-xylose test, 72-hour stool fat, GI series): Determine malabsorption.

Chest x-ray: May be normal or show evidence of pleural effusion; small heart silhouette.

ECG: May be normal or demonstrate low voltage, dysrhythmias/patterns reflective of electrolyte imbalances.

NURSING PRIORITIES

1. Promote consistent intake of estimated calorie and protein requirements.
2. Prevent complications.
3. Minimize energy losses/needs.
4. Provide information about condition, prognosis, and treatment needs.

DISCHARGE GOALS

1. Nutritional intake adequate for individual needs.
2. Complications prevented/minimized.
3. Fatigue alleviated.
4. Condition, prognosis, and therapeutic regimen understood.
5. Plan in place to meet needs after discharge.

NURSING DIAGNOSIS: Nutrition: altered, less than body requirements

May be related to

Conditions that interfere with nutrient intake or increase nutrient need/metabolic demand, e.g., cancer and associated treatments, anorexia, surgical procedures, dysphagia/difficulty swallowing, depressed mental status/level of consciousness.

Possibly evidenced by

Body weight 10% or more under ideal

Decreased subcutaneous fat/muscle mass, poor muscle tone

Changes in gastric motility and stool characteristics

DESIRED OUTCOMES/EVALUATION CRITERIA—PATIENT WILL:

Demonstrate stable weight or progressive weight gain toward goal with normalization of laboratory values and be free of signs of malnutrition.

ACTIONS/INTERVENTIONS	RATIONALE
Independent	
General	
Assess nutritional status continually, during daily nursing care, noting energy level; condition of skin, nails, hair, oral cavity; desire to eat/anorexia.	Provides the opportunity to observe deviations from normals/patient baseline and influences choice of interventions.
Weigh daily and compare with admission weight.	Establishes baseline, aids in monitoring effectiveness of therapeutic regimen, and alerts nurse to inappropriate trends in weight loss/gain.

ACTIONS/INTERVENTIONS	RATIONALE

Independent

Document oral intake by use of 24-hour recall, food history, calorie counts as appropriate.

Identifies imbalance between estimated nutritional requirements and actual intake.

Ensure accurate collection of specimens (urine, stool, drainage) for nitrogen balance studies.

Inaccurate collection can alter test results, leading to improper interpretation of patient's current status and needs.

Administer nutritional solutions at prescribed rate via infusion control device as needed. Adjust rate to deliver prescribed hourly rate. Do not increase rate to "catch up."

Nutrition support prescriptions are based on individually estimated caloric and protein requirements. A consistent rate of nutrient administration will assure proper utilization with fewer side effects, such as hyperglycemia or dumping syndrome. *Note:* Continuous and cyclic infusion of enteral formulas are generally better tolerated than bolus feedings and result in improved absorption.

Be familiar with electrolyte content of nutritional solutions.

Metabolic complications of nutritional support often result from a lack of appreciation of changes that can occur as a result of refeeding, e.g., hyperglycemic, hyperosmotic nonketotic coma, electrolyte imbalances.

Schedule activities with adequate rest periods. Promote relaxation techniques.

Conserves energy/reduces calorie needs. (Refer to ND: Fatigue, p 502.)

Parenteral

Observe appropriate "hang" time of parenteral solutions per protocol.

Effectiveness of IV vitamins diminishes and solution degrades after 24 hours.

Monitor fingerstick glucose per protocol (e.g., qid during initiation of therapy).

High glucose content of solutions may lead to pancreatic fatigue, requiring use of supplemental insulin to prevent HHNC. *Note:* Fingerstick determination of glucose level is more accurate/may be preferred over urine testing because of variations in renal glucose threshold.

Enteral

Assess GI function and tolerance to enteral feedings: note bowel sounds; reports of nausea/vomiting, abdominal discomfort; presence of diarrhea/constipation; development of weakness, lightheadedness, diaphoresis, tachycardia, abdominal cramping.

Because protein turnover of the GI mucosa occurs approximately every 3 days, the GI tract is at great risk for early dysfunction and atrophy from disease and malnutrition. Intolerance of formula/presence of dumping syndrome may require alteration of rate of administration/concentration or type of formula, or possibly change to parenteral administration.

Check gastric residuals if bolus feedings are done, and as otherwise indicated; hold feeding/return aspirate per protocol for type/rate of feeding used if residual is greater than predetermined level.

Delayed gastric emptying can be caused by a specific disease process, e.g., paralytic ileus/surgery, shock; by drug therapy (especially narcotics); or the protein/fat content of the individual formula. *Note:* Replacement of gastric aspirate reduces loss of gastric acid/electrolytes.

Maintain patency of enteral feeding tubes by flushing with warm water after feeding and as indicated.

Enteral formulas contain protein that can clog feeding tubes (more likely with silicone than with polyurethane tubes) necessitating removal/replacement of tube. *Note:* Cranberry juice or colas are not recommended. Pancrelipase (a pancreatic enzyme) may be effective in clearing tubing of persistent clog.

495

ACTIONS/INTERVENTIONS	RATIONALE

Independent

Transitional

Stress importance of transition to oral feedings as appropriate.

Although patient may have little interest in food or desire to eat, transition to oral feedings is preferred in view of potential side effects/complications of nutritional support therapy.

Assess gag reflex, ability to chew/swallow, and motor skills when progressing to transitional feedings.

May require additional interventions, e.g., retraining by dysphagia expert (speech therapist) or long-term nutritional support.

Provide self-help utensils as indicated, e.g., plate guard, utensils with built-up handles, lidded cups.

Patients with neuromuscular deficits, e.g., post-CVA, brain injury, may require use of special aids developed for feeding.

Create optimal environment, e.g., remove noxious stimuli, bedpans, soiled linens. Provide cheerful, attractive tray/table, soft music, companionship.

Encourages patient's attempts to eat, reduces anorexia, and introduces some of the social pleasures usually associated with mealtime.

Allow adequate time for chewing, swallowing, savoring food; provide socialization and feeding assistance as indicated.

Patients need encouragement/assistance to overcome underlying problems such as anorexia, fatigue, muscular weakness.

Offer small, frequent feedings; incorporate patient likes/dislikes in meal planning as much as possible, and include "home foods" as appropriate.

May enhance patient's desire for food and amount of intake.

Provide calorie-containing beverages when oral intake is possible, e.g., juices/jello water, dietary supplements (Sustacal, Ensure, Polycase) to beverages/water.

Maximizes calorie intake when oral intake is limited/restricted.

Collaborative

Refer to nutritional team/registered dietician.

Aids in identification of nutrient deficits and need for parenteral/enteral nutritional intervention.

Calculate basal energy expenditure (BEE) using formula based on sex, height, weight, age, and estimated energy requirements.

Provides an estimation of calorie and protein needs.

Review results of indirect calorimetry test if available.

Measures O_2 consumption at basal or resting metabolic rate, to aid in estimating calorie/protein requirements.

Assist with insertion and confirm proper placement of infusion/feeding line (e.g., chest x-ray for central venous catheter or aspiration of gastric contents from feeding tube) prior to administration of solutions.

Reduces risk of feeding-induced complications, including pneumothorax/hemothorax, hydrothorax, air embolus, arterial puncture (central venous line), or aspiration (NG tube).

Administer dextrose-electrolyte or dextrose-amino acid and lipid emulsions (3-in-1) solutions as indicated.

Solutions provide calories, essential amino acids, and micronutrients, usually combined with lipids for complete nutrition known as total nutrient admixtures (TNA). Solutions are modified to meet specific needs, e.g., renal and liver failure (lower protein), respiratory failure (higher fat). *Note:* 3-in-1 solution bags are larger (2–3 L) and can infuse over 24 hours, eliminating the need for frequent bag changes and reducing line manipulation/risk of contamination.

ACTIONS/INTERVENTIONS	RATIONALE
Collaborative	
Co-infuse lipid emulsions if 3-in-1 solutions not used.	Useful in meeting excessive calorie requirements (e.g., burns) or as a source of essential fatty acids during long-term hyperalimentation. *Note:* Lipid solutions may be contraindicated in patients with alterations in fat metabolism or in the presence of pancreatitis, liver damage, anemia, coagulation disorders, pulmonary disease.
Administer medications, as indicated, e.g.:	
Multivitamin preparations;	Water-soluble vitamins will be added to parenteral solutions. Other vitamins may be given for identified deficiencies.
Insulin;	High glucose content of solutions may require exogenous insulin for metabolism especially in presence of pancreatic insufficiency or disease. *Note:* Insulin is usually now added directly to parenteral solution.
Diphenoxylate with atropine (Lomotil), camphorated tincture of opium (Paregoric), and metoclopramide (Reglan).	GI side effects of enteral feeding may need to be controlled with antidiarrheal agents (Lomotil/Paregoric) or peristaltic stimulants (Reglan) if more conservative measures such as alteration of rate/strength or type of formula are not successful.
Monitor laboratory studies, e.g., serum glucose, electrolytes, transferrin, prealbumin/albumin, total protein, phosphate, BUN/Cr, liver enzymes, CBC, ABGs.	Serum chemistries, blood counts, and lipid profiles are performed prior to initiation of therapy, providing a baseline for comparison with repeat (monitoring) studies to determine therapy needs/complications. Untoward metabolic effects of TPN include: hypokalemia, hyponatremia and fluid retention, hyperglycemia, hypophosphatemia, increased CO_2 production resulting in respiratory compromise, elevation of liver function tests, renal dysfunction.

NURSING DIAGNOSIS: Infection, risk for

Risk factors may include
Invasive procedures: Insertion of venous catheter; surgically placed gastrostomy/jejunostomy feeding tube
Malnutrition; chronic disease
Environmental exposure: Access devices in place for extended periods, improper preparation/handling/contamination of the feeding solution

Possibly evidenced by
[Not applicable; presence of signs and symptoms establishes an *actual* diagnosis]

DESIRED OUTCOMES/EVALUATION CRITERIA—PATIENT WILL:
Experience no fever or chills.
Demonstrate clean catheter insertion sites, free of drainage and erythema/edema.

ACTIONS/INTERVENTIONS	RATIONALE

Independent

Parenteral

Maintain an optimal aseptic environment during bedside insertion of central venous catheters and during changes of TPN bottles and administration tubing.

Catheter-related sepsis may result from entry of pathogenic microorganisms through skin insertion tract, or from touch contamination during manipulations of TPN system.

Secure external portion of catheter/administration tubing to dressing with tape. Note intactness of skin suture.

Manipulation of catheter in/out of insertion site can result in tissue trauma (coring) and potentiate entry of skin organisms into catheter tract.

Maintain a sterile occlusive dressing over catheter insertion site. Perform central/peripheral venous catheter dressing care per protocol.

Protects catheter insertion sites from potential sources of contamination. *Note:* Central venous catheter sites can easily become contaminated from tracheostomy or endotracheal secretions or from wounds of the head, neck, and chest.

Inspect insertion site of catheter for erythema, induration, drainage, tenderness.

The catheter is a potential irritant to the surrounding skin and subcutaneous skin tract, and extended use may result in insertion site irritation and infection.

Refrigerate premixed solutions prior to use; observe a 24-hour hang time for amino acid or total nutrient admixture solutions and a 12-hour hang time for individual IV fat emulsions.

TPN solutions and fat emulsions have been shown to support the growth of a variety of pathogenic organisms once contaminated.

Monitor temperature and glucose.

A rise in temperature or loss of glucose tolerance (glycosuria, hyperglycemia) are early indications of possible catheter-related sepsis.

Enteral

Keep manipulations of enteral feeding system to a minimum and wash hands before opening system.

Touch contamination by caregiver during enteral formula administration has been shown to cause contamination of formula.

Alternate nares for tube placement in long-term NG feedings.

Reduces risk of trauma/infection of paranasal tissue (especially important in facial trauma/burns).

Provide daily/prn site care to abdominally placed feeding tubes.

GI secretions leaking through or around gastrostomy/jejunostomy tube tracts can cause skin breakdown severe enough to require removal of the feeding tube.

Refrigerate reconstituted enteral formulas before use; observe a hang time of 4–8 hours; discard unused formula after 24 hours.

Enteral formulas easily support bacterial growth and can be contaminated during formula preparation. For example, bacterial growth has been shown to occur within 4 hours after contamination.

Collaborative

Aseptically prepare parenteral solutions/enteral formulas for administration.

TPN solutions should be prepared under a laminar flow hood in the department of pharmacy. Enteral formulas should be mixed in a clean environment in the dietary or pharmacy department, although with the advent of canned/modular formulas, this may not be necessary. *Note:* Additives to TPN solutions, as a rule, should not be made on the unit because of the potential for contamination and drug incompatibilities.

ACTIONS/INTERVENTIONS

Collaborative

Notify physician if signs of infection present. Follow protocol for obtaining appropriate culture specimens, e.g., blood, solutions. Change bottle/tubing as indicated.

Administer antibiotics as indicated.

RATIONALE

Necessary to identify source of infection and initiate appropriate therapy. May require removal of TPN line and culture of catheter tip.

May be given prophylactically or for specifically identified organism.

NURSING DIAGNOSIS: Injury, risk for [multifactor]

Risk factors may include

External environment: Catheter-related complications (air emboli and septic thrombophlebitis)
Internal factors: Aspiration; effects of therapy/drug interactions

Possibly evidenced by

[Not applicable; presence of signs and symptoms establishes an *actual* diagnosis]

DESIRED OUTCOMES/EVALUATION CRITERIA—PATIENT WILL:

Be free of complications associated with nutritional support.
Modify environment/correct hazards to enhance safety for in-home therapy.

ACTIONS/INTERVENTIONS

Independent

Parenteral

Maintain a closed central IV system using Luer-Lok connections/taping of all connections.

Administer appropriate TPN solution via peripheral or central venous route (including PICC lines and tunneled catheters).

Monitor for potential drug/nutrient interactions.

Assess catheter for signs of displacement out of central venous position, i.e., extended length of catheter on skin surface; leaking of IV solution onto dressing; patient complaints of neck/arm pain, tenderness at catheter site, or swelling of extremity on side of catheter insertion.

Inspect peripheral TPN catheter site routinely and change sites at least every 3 days or per protocol.

RATIONALE

Inadvertent disconnection of central IV system can result in lethal air emboli.

Solutions containing high concentrations of dextrose (greater than 10%) must be delivered via a central vein because they will result in chemical phlebitis when delivered through small peripheral veins.

Various interactions are possible, for example, digoxin (in conjunction with diuretic therapy) can cause hypomagnesemia; hypokalemia may result from chronic use of laxatives, mineralocortico-steroids, diuretics, or amphotericin.

Central venous catheter tip may slip out of superior vena cava and migrate into smaller innominate and jugular veins, causing a chemical thrombophlebitis. Incidence of subclavian or superior vena cava thrombosis is increased with extended use of central venous catheters.

Peripheral TPN solutions (although less hyperosmolar) can still irritate small veins and cause phlebitis. Peripheral venous access is often limited in malnourished patients, but site should still be changed if signs of irritation develop.

ACTIONS/INTERVENTIONS

Independent

Investigate reports of severe chest pain/coughing in patients with central line. Turn patient to left side in Trendelenburg position if indicated and notify physician.

Maintain an occlusive dressing on catheter insertion sites for 24 hours after subclavian catheter is removed.

Enteral

Assess gastrostomy or jejunostomy tube sites for evidence of malposition.

Collaborative

Review chest x-ray as indicated.

Consult with pharmacist in regard to site/time of delivery of drugs that might have action adversely affected by enteral formula.

RATIONALE

Suggests presence of air embolus requiring immediate intervention to displace air into apex of heart away from the pulmonary artery.

Extended catheter use may result in development of catheter skin tract. Once the catheter is removed, air embolus is still a potential risk until skin tract has sealed.

Indwelling and mushroom catheters are still frequently used for feeding tubes inserted via the abdomen. Migration of the catheter balloon can result in duodenal or jejunal obstruction. Improperly sutured gastrostomy tubes may easily fall out.

Central parenteral line placement is routinely confirmed by x-ray.

Absorption of vitamin D is impaired by administration of mineral oil (inhibits micelle formation of bile salts) and by neomycin (inactivates bile salts). Aluminum-containing antacids bind with the phosphorus in the feeding solution, potentiating hypophosphatemia.

NURSING DIAGNOSIS: Aspiration, risk for

Risk factors may include
Presence of the GI tube, bolus tube feedings, medication administration
Increased intragastric pressure, delayed gastric emptying

Possibly evidenced by
[Not applicable; presence of signs and symptoms establishes an *actual* diagnosis]

DESIRED OUTCOMES/EVALUATION CRITERIA—PATIENT WILL:
Maintain clear airway, be free of signs of aspiration.

ACTIONS/INTERVENTIONS

Independent

Confirm placement of nasoenteral feeding tubes. Determine feeding tube position in stomach by x-ray, confirmation of pH of 2 or 3 of the gastric fluid withdrawn through tube, or auscultation of injected air prior to intermittent feedings. Observe for ability to speak/cough.

RATIONALE

Malplacement of nasoenteral feeding tubes may result in aspiration of enteral formula. Patients at particular risk include those who are intubated or obtunded, following CVA, or surgery of the head/neck and upper GI system.

ACTIONS/INTERVENTIONS	RATIONALE
Independent	
Maintain aspiration precautions during enteral feedings, e.g.:	
Keep head of bed elevated at 30–45 degrees during feeding and at least 1 hour after feeding;	Aspiration of enteral formulas is irritating to the lung parenchyma and may result in pneumonia and respiratory compromise.
Inflate tracheostomy cuff during and for 1 hour after intermittent feeding. Interrupt feeding when patient is in prone position;	
Add blue food coloring to enteral formula as indicated.	Helps identify aspiration of enteral formula and/or tracheal esophageal fistula, if discovered in sputum/lung secretions. *Note:* Avoid use of methylene blue dye, which may cause false-positive guaiac test when assessing for GI bleeding.
Monitor gastric residuals after bolus feedings (as previously noted in ND: Nutrition: altered, less than body requirements, p 494.)	Presence of large gastric residuals may potentiate an incompetent esophageal sphincter, leading to vomiting and aspiration.
Note characteristics of sputum/tracheal aspirate. Investigate development of dyspnea, cough, tachypnea, cyanosis. Auscultate breath sounds.	Presence of formula in tracheal secretions or signs/symptoms reflecting respiratory distress suggests aspiration.
Note indicators of NG tube intolerance, e.g., absence of gag reflex, high risk of aspiration, frequent removal of NG feeding tubes.	May require consideration of surgically placed feeding tubes PEG (percutaneous endoscopic gastrostomy, jejunostomy) for patient safety and consistency of enteral formula delivery.
Collaborative	
Review abdominal x-ray if done.	Confirmation of placement of gastric feeding tube may be obtained by x-ray.

NURSING DIAGNOSIS: Fluid Volume [fluctuation], risk for

May be related to

Active loss and/or failure of regulatory mechanisms (specific to underlying disease process/trauma); complications of nutrition therapy, e.g., high glucose solutions, hyperglycemia (hyperosmolar nonketotic coma and severe dehydration)
Inability to obtain/ingest fluids

Possibly evidenced by

[Not applicable; presence of signs and symptoms establishes an *actual* diagnosis]

DESIRED OUTCOMES/EVALUATION CRITERIA—PATIENT WILL:

Display moist skin/mucous membranes, stable vital signs, individually adequate urinary output; be free of edema and excessive weight loss/inappropriate gain.

ACTIONS/INTERVENTIONS	RATIONALE

Independent

Assess for clinical signs of dehydration (e.g., thirst, dry skin/mucous membranes, hypotension); or fluid excess (e.g., peripheral edema, tachycardia, adventitious breath sounds).

Early detection and intervention may prevent occurrence/excessive fluctuation in fluid balance. *Note:* Severely malnourished patients have an increased risk of developing refeeding syndrome, e.g., life-threatening fluid overload, intracellular electrolyte shifts, and cardiac strain occurring during initial 3–5 days of therapy.

Incorporate knowledge of caloric density of enteral formulas into assessment of fluid balance.

Enteric solutions are usually concentrated and do not meet free water needs.

Provide additional water/flush tubing as indicated.

With higher calorie formula, additional water is needed to prevent dehydration/HHNC.

Record I&O; calculate fluid balance. Measure urine specific gravity.

Excessive urinary losses may reflect developing HHNC. Specific gravity is an indicator of hydration and renal function.

Weigh daily or as indicated; evaluate changes.

Rapid weight gain (reflecting fluid retention) can predispose/potentiate HF or pulmonary edema. Gain of greater than 0.5 lb/d indicates fluid retention and not deposition of lean body mass.

Collaborative

Monitor laboratory studies, e.g.:
  Serum potassium/phosphorus;

Hypokalemia/phosphatemia can occur due to intracellular shifts during initial refeeding and may compromise cardiac function if not corrected.

  Hct;

Reflects hydration/circulating volume.

  Serum albumin.

Hypoalbuminemia/decreased colloidal osmotic pressure leads to third spacing of fluid (edema).

Dilute formula or change from hypertonic to isotonic formula as indicated.

May decrease gastric intolerance, reducing occurrence of diarrhea and associated fluid losses.

NURSING DIAGNOSIS: Fatigue

May be related to
Decreased metabolic energy production; increased energy requirements (hypermetabolic states, healing process)
Altered body chemistry: Medications, chemotherapy

Possibly evidenced by
Overwhelming lack of energy, inability to maintain usual routines/accomplish routine tasks
Lethargy, impaired ability to concentrate

DESIRED OUTCOMES/EVALUATION CRITERIA—PATIENT WILL:
Report increased sense of well-being/energy level.
Demonstrate measurable increase in physical activity.

ACTIONS/INTERVENTIONS	RATIONALE
Independent	
Monitor physiologic response to activity, e.g., changes in BP, or heart/respiratory rate.	Tolerance varies greatly, depending on the stage of the disease process, nutritional state, and fluid balance.
Establish realistic activity goals with patient.	Provides for a sense of control and feelings of accomplishment.
Plan care to allow for rest periods. Schedule activities for periods when patient has most energy. Involve patient/SO in schedule planning.	Frequent rest periods are needed to restore/conserve energy. Planning will allow patient to be active during times when energy level is higher, which may restore a feeling of well-being and a sense of control.
Encourage patient to do whatever possible, e.g., self-care, sitting up in chair, walking. Increase activity level as indicated.	Increases strength/stamina and enables patient to become more active without undue fatigue.
Provide passive/active ROM exercises to bedridden patients.	The development of healthy lean muscle mass is dependent on the provision of both isotonic and isometric exercises.
Keep bed in low position, pathways clear of furniture; assist with ambulation.	Protects patient from injury during activities.
Assist with self-care needs as necessary.	Weakness may make ADLs almost impossible for the patient to complete.
Collaborative	
Provide supplemental O_2 as indicated.	Presence of anemia/hypoxemia reduces O_2 available for cellular uptake and contributes to fatigue.
Refer to physical/occupational therapy.	Programmed daily exercises and activities help patient to maintain/increase strength and muscle tone and enhance sense of well-being.

NURSING DIAGNOSIS: Knowledge deficit [learning need] regarding condition, prognosis, treatment, self care and discharge needs

May be related to
Lack of exposure/recall, information misinterpretation
Cognitive limitation

Possibly evidenced by
Request for information, questions/statement of misconception
Inaccurate follow-through of instructions/development of preventable complications

DESIRED OUTCOMES/EVALUATION CRITERIA—PATIENT WILL:
Verbalize understanding of condition/disease process and individual nutritional needs.
Correctly perform necessary procedures and explain reasons for the actions.

ACTIONS/INTERVENTIONS	RATIONALE

Independent

Assess patient/SO knowledge of nutritional state. Review individual situation, signs/symptoms of malnutrition, future expectations, transitional feeding needs.

Provides information on which the patient/SO can base informed choices. Knowledge of the interaction between malnutrition and illness is helpful to understanding need for special therapy.

Discuss reasons for use of parenteral/enteral nutrition support.

May experience anxiety regarding inability to eat and may not comprehend the nutritional value of the prescribed TPN/tube feedings.

Provide adequate time for patient/SO teaching when patient is going home on enteral/parenteral feedings. Document patient/SO understanding and ability/competence to deliver safe home therapy.

Generally, 3–4 days is sufficient for patient/SO to become proficient with tube feedings. Parenteral therapy is more complex and may require a week or longer for patient/SO to feel ready for home management and requires follow-up in the home.

Discuss proper handling, storage, preparation of nutritional solutions or blenderized feedings; also discuss aseptic or clean techniques for care of insertion sites and use of dressings.

Reduces risk of formula-/solution-related problems, metabolic complications, and infection.

Review use/care of nutritional support devices.

Patient understanding and cooperation are key to the safe insertion and maintenance of nutritional support access devices as well as prevention of complications.

Review specific precautions dependent on type of feeding, e.g., checking placement of tube, sitting upright for enteral feeding, maintaining patency of tube, anchoring of tubing.

Promotes safe self-care and reduces risk of complications.

Discuss/demonstrate reinsertion of enterostomal feeding tube if appropriate.

Tube may be changed routinely or inserted only for feedings. Intermittent feedings enhance patient mobility and aid in transition to regular feeding pattern.

Identify signs and symptoms requiring medical evaluation, e.g., nausea/vomiting, abdominal cramping or bloating, diarrhea, rapid weight changes; erythema, drainage, foul odor at tube insertion site, fever/chills; coughing/choking or difficulty breathing during enteral feeding.

Early evaluation and treatment of problems (e.g., feeding intolerance, infection, aspiration) may prevent progression to more serious complications.

Instruct patient/SO in glucose monitoring if indicated.

Timely recognition of changes in blood sugar levels reduces risk of hypoglycemic reactions in patient on hyperalimentation.

Discuss signs/symptoms and treatment of hyperglycemia/hypoglycemia.

Hyperglycemia is more common for patients receiving parenteral feedings and those who have pancreas or liver disease or are on large doses of corticosteroids. Rebound hypoglycemia can occur when feedings are intentionally/accidentally discontinued.

Encourage use of diary for recording test results, physical feelings/reactions, activity level, oral intake if any, I&O, weekly weight.

Provides resource for review by healthcare providers for optimal management of individual situation.

Recommend daily exercise/activity to tolerance, scheduling of adequate rest periods.

Enhances gastric motility for enteral/transition feedings, promotes feelings of general well-being, and prevents undue fatigue.

ACTIONS/INTERVENTIONS	RATIONALE
Independent	
Ascertain that all supplies are in place in the home prior to discharge; make arrangements as needed with suppliers, e.g., hospital, pharmacy, medical equipment company, laboratory.	Provides for successful and competent home therapy.
Refer to nutritional support team, home healthcare agency, and counseling resources. Provide with immediate access phone numbers.	Patient/SO need readily available support persons to assist with nutrition therapy, equipment problems, and emotional adjustments in long-term/home-based therapy.

POTENTIAL CONSIDERATIONS following acute hospitalization (dependent on patient's age, physical condition/presence of complications, personal resources, and life responsibilities)

Fatigue—decreased metabolic energy production; increased energy requirements (hypermetabolic states, healing process); altered body chemistry, e.g., medications, chemotherapy.

Injury, risk for—catheter-related complications (catheter breaks, dislodgement, occlusion), effects of therapy (e.g., electrolyte/fluid shifts, diarrhea)/drug interactions, aspiration.

Infection, risk for—invasive tubes, environmental exposure, malnutrition, chronic disease.

Family Processes, altered—situational crises.

METABOLIC ACID/BASE IMBALANCES

The body has the remarkable ability to maintain plasma pH within the narrow range of 7.35–7.45. It does so by means of chemical buffering mechanisms by the kidneys and the lungs. Although single acid/base (e.g., metabolic acidosis) imbalances do occur, mixed acid/base imbalances are more common (e.g., metabolic acidosis/respiratory acidosis as occurs with cardiac arrest).

METABOLIC ACIDOSIS
(PRIMARY BASE BICARBONATE DEFICIT)

Reflects an excess of acid (hydrogen) and a deficit of base (bicarbonate) resulting from acid overproduction, loss of intestinal bicarbonate, inadequate conservation of bicarbonate, and excretion of acid, or anaerobic metabolism. Metabolic acidosis is characterized by normal or high anion gap situations. If the primary problem is direct loss of bicarbonate, gain of chloride, or decreased ammonia production, the anion gap will be within normal limits. If the primary problem is the accumulation of organic anions (such as ketones or lactic acid), the condition is known as high anion gap acidosis. Compensatory mechanisms to correct this imbalance include an increase in respirations to blow off excess CO_2, an increase in ammonia formation, and acid excretion (H^+) by the kidneys, with retention of bicarbonate and sodium.

High anion gap acidosis occurs in diabetic ketoacidosis; starvational or alcoholic lactic acidosis; renal failure; high-fat diets/lipid administration; poisoning, e.g., salicylate intoxication (after initial stage); paraldehyde intoxication; and drug therapy, e.g., Diamox, NH_4Cl.

Normal anion gap acidosis is associated with loss of bicarbonate from the body, as may occur in renal tubular acidosis, hyperalimentation, vomiting/diarrhea, small-bowel/pancreatic fistulas, and ileostomy and use of IV sodium chloride in presence of preexisting kidney dysfunction.

CARE SETTING

This condition does not occur in isolation but rather is a complication of a broader problem that may require inpatient care in a medical/surgical or subacute unit.

RELATED CONCERNS

Plans of care specific to predisposing factors
Fluid and Electrolyte Imbalances, p 899
Renal Dialysis, p 580
Respiratory Acidosis (Primary Carbonic Acid Excess), p 200
Respiratory Alkalosis (Primary Carbonic Acid Deficit), p 204

Patient Assessment Data Base (Dependent on underlying cause)

ACTIVITY/REST

May report: Lethargy, fatigue; muscle weakness

CIRCULATION

May exhibit: Hypotension, wide pulse pressure
Pulse may be weak, irregular (dysrhythmias)
Jaundiced sclera, skin, mucous membranes (liver failure)

ELIMINATION

May report: Diarrhea

May exhibit: Dark/concentrated urine

FOOD/FLUID

May report: Anorexia, nausea/vomiting

May exhibit: Poor skin turgor, dry mucous membranes

NEUROSENSORY

May report: Headache, drowsiness, decreased mental function

May exhibit: Changes in sensorium, e.g., stupor, confusion, lethargy, depression, delirium, coma

RESPIRATION

May report: Dyspnea on exertion

May exhibit: Hyperventilation, Kussmaul's respirations (deep, rapid breathing)

SAFETY

May report: Transfusion of blood/blood products
Exposure to hepatitis virus

May exhibit: Fever, signs of sepsis

TEACHING/LEARNING

History of alcohol abuse
Use of carbonic anhydrase inhibitors or anion-exchange resins, e.g., cholestyramine (Questran)

Discharge plan considerations: **DRG projected mean length of inpatient stay dependent on underlying cause**
May require change in therapies for underlying disease process/condition.

Refer to section at end of plan for postdischarge considerations.

DIAGNOSTIC STUDIES

Arterial pH: Decreased, less than 7.35.
Bicarbonate: Decreased, less than 22 mEq/L.
PaCO$_2$: Less than 35–40 mm Hg.
Base excess: Decreased or absent.
Anion gap: Greater than 14 mEq/L (high anion gap) or range of 10 to 14 mEq/L (normal anion gap).
Serum potassium: Increased.
Serum chloride: Increased.
Serum glucose: May be decreased or increased dependent on etiology.
Serum ketones: Increased in DM, starvation, alcohol intoxication.
Plasma lactic acid: Elevated in lactic acidosis.
Urine pH: Decreased, less than 4.5 (in absence of renal disease).
ECG: Cardiac dysrhythmias (bradycardia) and pattern changes associated with hyperkalemia, e.g., tall T wave.

NURSING PRIORITIES

1. Achieve homeostasis.
2. Prevent/minimize complications.
3. Provide information about condition/prognosis and treatment needs as appropriate.

DISCHARGE GOALS

1. Physiologic balance restored.
2. Free of complications.

3. Condition, prognosis, and treatment needs understood.
4. Plan in place to meet needs after discharge.

As no current nursing diagnosis speaks clearly to metabolic imbalances, the following interventions are presented in a general format for inclusion in the primary plan of care.

ACTIONS/INTERVENTIONS	RATIONALE
Independent	
Monitor BP.	Arteriolar dilation/decreased cardiac contractility, (e.g., sepsis) and hypovolemia (e.g., ketoacidosis) occurs, resulting in systemic shock, evidenced by hypotension, and tissue hypoxia.
Assess level of consciousness and note progressive changes in neuromuscular status, e.g., strength, tone, movement.	Decreased mental function, confusion, seizures, weakness, flaccid paralysis can occur due to hypoxia, hyperkalemia, and decreased pH of CNS fluid.
Provide seizure/coma precautions, e.g., bed in low position, use of side rails, frequent observation.	Protects patient from injury resulting from decreased mentation/convulsions.
Monitor heart rate/rhythm.	Acidemia may be manifested by changes in ECG configuration and presence of bradydysrhythmias as well as increased ventricular irritability such as fibrillation (signs of hyperkalemia). Life-threatening cardiovascular collapse may also occur due to vasodilation and decreased cardiac contractility. *Note:* Hypokalemia can occur as acidosis is corrected, resulting in PVCs/ventricular tachycardia.
Observe for altered respiratory excursion, rate, and depth.	Deep, rapid respirations (Kussmaul's) may be noted as a compensatory mechanism to eliminate excess acid; however, as potassium shifts out of cell in an attempt to correct acidosis, respirations may become depressed. Transient respiratory depression may be the result of overcorrection of metabolic acidosis with sodium bicarbonate.
Assess skin temperature, color, capillary refill.	Evaluates circulatory status, tissue perfusion, effects of hypotension.
Auscultate bowel sounds; measure abdominal girth as indicated.	In the presence of coexisting hyperkalemia, GI distress (e.g., distention, diarrhea, and colic) may occur.
Monitor I&O closely and weigh daily.	Marked dehydration may be present due to vomiting, diarrhea. Therapy needs are based on underlying cause and fluid balance.
Test/monitor urine pH.	Kidneys attempt to compensate for acidosis by excreting excess hydrogen in the form of weak acids and ammonia. Maximum urine acidity is pH of 4.0.
Provide oral hygiene with sodium bicarbonate washes, lemon/glycerine swabs.	Neutralizes mouth acids and provides protective lubrication.
Collaborative	
Assist with identification/treatment of underlying cause.	Treatment of disorder is directed at mild correction of acidosis until organ(s) function is improved. Addressing the primary condition (e.g., DKA, liver/renal failure, drug poisoning, sepsis) promotes correction of the acid/base disorder.

ACTIONS/INTERVENTIONS	RATIONALE
Collaborative	
Monitor/graph serial ABGs.	Evaluates therapy needs/effectiveness. Blood bicarbonate and pH should slowly increase toward normal levels.
Monitor serum electrolytes, e.g., potassium.	As acidosis is corrected, serum potassium deficit may occur as potassium shifts back into the cells.
Replace fluids, as indicated depending on underlying etiology, e.g., D5W/saline solutions.	Choice of solution varies with cause of acidosis, e.g., DKA. *Note:* Lactate-containing solutions may be contraindicated in the presence of lactic acidosis.
Administer medications as indicated, e.g.:	
Sodium bicarbonate/lactate or saline IV;	Corrects bicarbonate deficit, but is used cautiously to correct severe acidosis (pH less than 7.2) because sodium bicarbonate can cause rebound metabolic alkalosis.
Potassium chloride;	May be required as potassium reenters the cell, causing a serum deficit.
Phosphate;	May be administered to enhance acid excretion in presence of chronic acidosis with hypophosphatemia.
Calcium.	May be given to improve neuromuscular conduction/function.
Modify diet as indicated, e.g., low-protein, high-carbohydrate diet in presence of renal failure or ADA diet for diabetic.	Restriction of protein may be necessary to decrease production of acid waste products, whereas addition of complex carbohydrates will correct acid production from the metabolism of fats in the diabetic.
Administer exchange resins and/or assist with dialysis as indicated.	May be desired to reduce acidosis by decreasing excess potassium and acid waste products if pH less than 7.1 and other therapies are ineffective, or HF develops.

POTENTIAL CONSIDERATIONS: Refer to Potential Considerations relative to underlying cause of acid/base disorder.

METABOLIC ALKALOSIS
(PRIMARY BASE BICARBONATE EXCESS)

Metabolic alkalosis is characterized by a high pH (loss of hydrogen ions) and high plasma bicarbonate caused by excessive intake of sodium bicarbonate, gastric/intestinal loss of acid, renal excretion of hydrogen and chloride, prolonged hypercalcemia, hypokalemia, and hyperaldosteronism. Compensatory mechanisms include slow, shallow respirations to increase CO_2 level and an increase of bicarbonate excretion and hydrogen reabsorption by the kidneys.

CARE SETTING

This condition does not occur in isolation but rather is a complication of a broader problem that may require inpatient care in a medical/surgical or subacute unit.

RELATED CONCERNS

Plans of care specific to predisposing factors
Fluid and Electrolye Imbalances, p 899
Renal Dialysis, p 580
Respiratory Acidosis (Primary Carbonic Acid Excess), p 200
Respiratory Alkalosis (Primary Carbonic Acid Deficit), p 204

Patient Assessment Data Base (Dependent on underlying cause)

CIRCULATION

May exhibit: Tachycardia, irregularities/dysrhythmias
Cyanosis

ELIMINATION

May report: Diarrhea (with high chloride content)
Use of diuretics (thazides, Lasix, ethacrynic acid)
Laxative abuse

FOOD/FLUID

May report: Nausea/prolonged vomiting
High salt intake; excessive ingestion of licorice
Frequent use of antacids/baking soda

NEUROSENSORY

May report: Tingling of fingers and toes; circumoral paresthesia
Dizziness

May exhibit: Hypertonicity of muscles, tetany, tremors, convulsions
Confusion, irritability, restlessness, belligerence, apathy, coma
Picking at bedclothes

SAFETY

May report: Recent blood transfusions (citrated blood)

510

RESPIRATION

May exhibit: Hypoventilation (increases Pco_2 and conserves carbonic acid), periods of apnea

TEACHING/LEARNING

History of Cushing's syndrome; corticosteroid therapy

Discharge plan considerations: **DRG projected mean length of inpatient stay dependent on underlying cause**

May require change in therapy for underlying disease process/condition.

Refer to section at end of plan for postdischarge considerations.

DIAGNOSTIC STUDIES

Arterial pH: Increased, greater than 7.45.
Bicarbonate: Increased, greater than 26 mEq/L (primary).
Paco$_2$: Slightly increased, greater than 45 mm Hg (compensatory).
Base excess: Increased.
Serum chloride: Decreased, less than 98 mEq/L (if alkalosis is hypochloremia) disproportionately to serum sodium decreases.
Serum potassium: Decreased.
Serum calcium: Usually decreased. Prolonged hypercalcemia (nonparathyroid) may be a predisposing factor.
Urine pH: Increased, greater than 7.0.
Urine chloride: Less than 10 mEq/L suggests chloride responsive alkalosis, whereas levels greater than 20 mEq/L suggest chloride resistance.
ECG: May show hypokalemic changes including peaked P waves, flat T waves, depressed ST segment, low T wave merging to P wave, and elevated U waves.

NURSING PRIORITIES

1. Achieve homeostasis.
2. Prevent/minimize complications.
3. Provide information about condition/prognosis and treatment needs as appropriate.

DISCHARGE GOALS

1. Physiologic balance restored.
2. Free of complications.
3. Condition, prognosis, and treatment needs understood.
4. Plan in place to meet needs after discharge.

As no current nursing diagnosis speaks clearly to metabolic imbalances, the following interventions are presented in a general format for inclusion in the primary plan of care.

ACTIONS/INTERVENTIONS

Independent

Monitor respiratory rate, rhythm, and depth.

Assess level of consciousness and neuromuscular status, e.g., strength, tone, movement; note presence of Chvostek's/Trousseau's signs.

RATIONALE

Hypoventilation is a compensatory mechanism to conserve carbonic acid and represents definite risks to the individual, e.g., hypoxemia and respiratory failure.

The CNS may be hyperirritable (increased pH of CNS fluid), resulting in tingling, numbness, dizziness, restlessness, or apathy and confusion. Hypocalcemia may contribute to tetany (although occurrence is rare).

511

ACTIONS/INTERVENTIONS	RATIONALE
Independent	
Monitor heart rate/rhythm.	Atrial/ventricular ectopics and tachydysrhythmias may develop.
Record amount and source of output. Monitor intake and daily weight.	Helpful in identifying source of ion loss; e.g., potassium and HCl are lost in vomiting and GI suctioning.
Restrict oral intake and reduce noxious environmental stimuli; use intermittent/low suction during NG suctioning; irrigate gastric tube with isotonic solutions rather than water.	Limits gastric losses of hydrochloric acid, potassium, and calcium.
Provide seizure/safety precautions as indicated, e.g., padded side rails, airway protection, bed in low position, frequent observation.	Changes in mentation and CNS/neuromuscular hyperirritability may result in patient harm, especially if tetany/convulsions occur.
Encourage intake of foods and fluids high in potassium and possibly calcium (dependent on blood level), e.g., canned grapefruit and apple juices, bananas, cauliflower, dried peaches, figs, and wheat germ.	Useful in replacing potassium losses when oral intake permitted.
Review medication regimen for use of diuretics (thiazides, Lasix, ethacrynic acid); and cathartics.	Discontinuation of these potassium-losing drugs may prevent recurrence of imbalance.
Instruct patient to avoid use of excessive amounts of sodium bicarbonate.	Ulcer patients can cause alkalosis by taking baking soda and milk of magnesia in addition to prescribed alkaline antacids.
Collaborative	
Assist with identification/treatment of underlying disorder.	Addressing the primary condition (e.g., prolonged vomiting/diarrhea, hyperaldosteronism, Cushing's syndrome) promotes correction of the acid/base disorder.
Monitor laboratory studies as indicated, e.g., ABGs/pH, serum electrolytes (especially potassium), and BUN.	Evaluates therapy needs/effectiveness and monitors renal function.
Administer medications as indicated, e.g.;	
Sodium chloride PO/Ringer's solution IV unless contraindicated;	Correcting sodium, water, and chloride defects may be all that is needed to permit kidneys to excrete bicarbonate and correct alkalosis but must be used with caution in patients with HF or renal insufficiency.
Potassium chloride;	Hypokalemia is frequently present. Chloride is needed so kidney can absorb sodium with chloride, enhancing excretion of bicarbonate.
Ammonium chloride or arginine hydrochloride;	Increases amount of circulating hydrogen ions. Monitor administration closely to prevent too rapid a decrease in pH, hemolysis of RBCs. *Note:* May cause rebound metabolic acidosis and is usually contraindicated in patients with renal/hepatic failure.
Acetazolamide (Diamox);	A carbonic anhydrase inhibitor that increases renal excretion of bicarbonate.
Spironolactone (Aldactone).	Effective in treating chloride-resistant alkalosis, e.g., Cushing's syndrome.

ACTIONS/INTERVENTIONS	RATIONALE
Collaborative	
Avoid/limit use of sedatives or hypnotics.	If respirations are depressed, may cause hypoxia/respiratory failure.
Encourage fluids IV/PO.	Replaces extracellular fluid losses, and adequate hydration facilitates removal of pulmonary secretions to improve ventilation.
Administer supplemental O_2 as indicated and respiratory treatments to improve ventilation.	Respiratory compensation for metabolic alkalosis is hypoventilation, which may cause decreased PaO_2 levels/hypoxia.
Assist with dialysis as needed.	Useful when renal dysfunction prevents clearance of bicarbonate.

POTENTIAL CONSIDERATIONS Refer to Potential Considerations relative to underlying cause of acid/base disorder.

Diseases of The Blood/Blood-Forming Organs

ANEMIAS (IRON DEFICIENCY, PERNICIOUS, APLASTIC, HEMOLYTIC)

Anemia is a symptom of an underlying condition, such as loss of blood components, inadequate elements, or lack of required nutrients for the formation of blood cells, that results in decreased oxygen-carrying capacity of the blood. There are numerous types of anemias with various causes. The following types of anemia are discussed here: Iron deficiency (ID), the result of inadequate absorption or excessive loss of iron; *pernicious* (PA), the result of a lack of the intrinsic factor essential for the absorption of vitamin B_{12}; *aplastic,* due to failure of bone marrow; and *hemolytic,* due to RBC destruction. Nursing care for the anemic patient has a common theme even though the medical treatments vary widely.

CARE SETTING

Treated at the community level, except in the presence of severe cardiovascular/immune compromise.

RELATED CONCERNS

AIDS, p 739
Burns: Thermal/Chemical/Electrical (Acute and Convalescent Phases), p 698
Cancer, p 875
Cirrhosis of the Liver, p 466
Heart Failure: Chronic, p 41
Psychosocial Aspects of Care, p 783
Renal Failure: Acute, p 555
Renal Failure: Chronic, p 568
Rheumatoid Arthritis, p 764
Pulmonary Tuberculosis (TB), p 190
Upper Gastrointestinal/Esophageal Bleeding, p 315

Patient Assessment Data Base

ACTIVITY/REST

May report: Fatigue, weakness, general malaise
Loss of productivity; diminished enthusiasm for work

Low exercise tolerance
Greater need for rest and sleep

May exhibit: Tachycardia/tachypnea; dyspnea on exertion or at rest (severe anemia)
Lethargy, withdrawal, apathy, lassitude, and lack of interest in surroundings
Muscle weakness and decreased strength
Ataxia, unsteady gait
Slumping of shoulders, drooping posture, slow walk, and other cues indicative of fatigue

CIRCULATION

May report: History of chronic blood loss, e.g., chronic GI bleeding, heavy menses (ID); angina, HF (due to increased workload of the heart)
History of chronic infective endocarditis
Palpitations (compensatory tachycardia)

May exhibit: BP: Increased systolic with stable diastolic and a widened pulse pressure; postural hypotension
Dysrhythmias: ECG abnormalities, e.g., ST-segment depression and flattening or depression of the T wave; tachycardia
Throbbing carotid pulsations (compensatory mechanism to provide oxygen/nutrients to cells)
Heart sounds: Systolic murmur (ID)
Extremities (color): Pallor of the skin and mucous membranes (conjunctiva, mouth, pharynx, lips) and nail beds. (*Note:* In black patients, pallor may appear as a grayish cast); waxy, pale skin (aplastic, PA) or bright lemon yellow (PA)
Sclera: Blue or pearl white (ID)
Capillary refill delayed (diminished blood flow to the periphery and compensatory vasoconstriction)
Nails: Brittle, spoon-shaped (koilonychia) (ID)
Hair: Dry, brittle, thinning; premature graying (PA)

EGO INTEGRITY

May report: Negative feelings about self, ability to handle situation/events

May exhibit: Depression

ELIMINATION

May report: History of pyelonephritis, renal failure
Flatulence, malabsorption syndrome (ID)
Hematemesis, fresh blood in stool, melena
Diarrhea or constipation
Diminished urine output

May exhibit: Abdominal distention

FOOD/FLUID

May report: Decreased dietary intake, low intake of animal protein/high intake of cereal products (ID)
Mouth or tongue pain, difficulty swallowing (ulcerations in pharynx)
Nausea/vomiting, dyspepsia, anorexia
Recent weight loss
Insatiable craving or pica for ice, dirt, cornstarch, paint, clay, and so forth (ID)

May exhibit: Beefy red/smooth appearance of tongue (PA; folic acid and vitamin B_{12} deficiencies)
Dry, pale mucous membranes

Skin turgor: Poor, with dry, shriveled appearance/loss of elasticity (ID)
Stomatitis and glossitis (deficiency states)
Lips: cheilitis, i.e., inflammation of the lips with cracking at the corners of the mouth (ID)

HYGIENE

May report: Difficulty maintaining ADLs

May exhibit: Unkempt appearance, poor personal hygiene

NEUROSENSORY

May report: Headaches, fainting, dizziness, vertigo, tinnitus, inability to concentrate
Insomnia, dimness of vision, and spots before eyes
Weakness, poor balance, wobbly legs; paresthesias of hands/feet (PA); claudication
Sensation of being cold

May exhibit: Irritability, restlessness, depression, drowsiness, apathy
Mentation: Notable slowing and dullness in response
Ophthalmic: Retinal hemorrhages (aplastic, PA)
Epistaxis, bleeding from other orifices (aplastic)
Disturbed coordination, ataxia: Decreased vibratory and position sense, positive Romberg's sign, paralysis (PA)

PAIN/DISCOMFORT

May report: Vague abdominal pains; headache (ID)
Oral pain

RESPIRATION

May report: History of TB, lung abscesses
Shortness of breath at rest and with activity

May exhibit: Tachypnea, orthopnea, and dyspnea

SAFETY

May report: History of occupational exposure to chemicals, e.g., benzene, lead, insecticides, phenylbutazone, naphthalene
History of exposure to radiation either as a treatment modality or by accident
History of cancer, cancer therapies
Cold and/or heat intolerance
Previous blood transfusions
Impaired vision
Poor wound healing, frequent infections

May exhibit: Low-grade fever, chills, night sweats
Generalized lymphadenopathy
Petechiae and ecchymosis (aplastic)

SEXUALITY

May report: Changes in menstrual flow, e.g., menorrhagia or amenorrhea in women (ID)
Loss of libido (men and women)
Impotence in men

May exhibit: Pale cervix and vaginal walls in women

May report: Family tendency for anemia (ID/PA)

Past/present use of anticonvulsants, antibiotics, chemotherapeutic agents (bone marrow failure), aspirin, anti-inflammatory drugs, or anticoagulants

Chronic use of alcohol

Religious/cultural beliefs affecting treatment choices, e.g., refusal of blood transfusions

Recent/current episode of active bleeding (ID)

History of liver, renal disease; hematologic problems; celiac or other malabsorption disease; regional enteritis; tapeworm manifestations; polyendocrinopathies; autoimmune problem (e.g., antibodies to parietal cells, intrinsic factor, thyroid and T-cell antibodies)

Prior surgeries, e.g., splenectomy; tumor excision; prosthetic valve replacement; surgical excision of duodenum or gastric resection, partial/total gastrectomy (ID/PA)

History of problems with wound healing or bleeding; chronic infections, (RA), chronic granulomatous disease, or cancer (secondary anemias)

Discharge plan
considerations: **DRG projected mean length of inpatient stay:** dependent on type/cause of anemia and severity of complications

May require assistance with treatment (injections); self-care activities and/or homemaker/maintenance tasks; changes in dietary plan

Refer to section at end of plan for postdischarge considerations.

DIAGNOSTIC STUDIES

CBC:

Hemoglobin and hematocrit: Decreased.

Erythrocyte count: Decreased (PA), severely decreased (aplastic); MCV and MCH decreased and microcytic with hypochromic erythrocytes (ID), elevated (PA); pancytopenia (aplastic).

Reticulocyte count: Varies, e.g., decreased (PA); elevated (bone marrow response to blood loss/hemolysis).

Stained RBC examination: Detects changes in color and shape (may indicate particular type of anemia).

Sedimentation rate (ESR): Elevation indicates presence of inflammatory reaction, e.g., increased RBC destruction or malignant disease.

RBC survival time: Useful in the differential diagnosis of the anemias, e.g., in certain types of anemias, RBCs have shortened life spans.

Erythrocyte fragility test: Decreased (ID); increased fragility confirms hemolytic and autoimmune anemias.

WBCs: Total cell count as well as specific WBCs (differential) may be increased (hemolytic) or decreased (aplastic).

Hemoglobin electrophoresis: Identifies type of hemoglobin structure, aids in determining source of hemolytic anemia.

Platelet count: Decreased (aplastic); elevated (ID); normal or high (hemolytic).

Serum bilirubin (unconjugated): Elevated (PA, hemolytic).

Serum folate and vitamin B_{12}: Aids in diagnosing anemias related to deficiencies in dietary intake/malabsorption.

Serum iron: Absent (ID); elevated (hemolytic, aplastic).

Serum TIBC: Increased (ID); normal or slightly reduced (AP).

Serum ferritin: Decreased (ID).

Bleeding time: Prolonged (aplastic).

Serum LDH: May be elevated (PA).

Schilling test: Decreased urinary excretion of vitamin B_{12} (PA).

Guaiac: May be positive for occult blood in urine, stools, and gastric contents, reflecting acute/chronic bleeding (ID).

Gastric analysis: Decreased secretions with elevated pH and absence of free hydrochloric acid (PA).

Bone marrow aspiration/biopsy examination: Cells may show changes in number, size and shape, helping to differentiate type of anemia, e.g., increased megaloblasts (PA); fatty marrow with diminished or absence of blood cells at several sites (aplastic).

Endoscopic and radiographic studies: Checks for bleeding sites, e.g., acute/chronic GI bleeding.

NURSING PRIORITIES

1. Enhance tissue perfusion.
2. Provide nutritional/fluid needs.
3. Prevent complications.
4. Provide information about disease process, prognosis, and treatment regimen.

DISCHARGE GOALS

1. ADLs met by self or with assistance of others.
2. Complications prevented/minimized.
3. Disease process/prognosis and therapeutic regimen understood.
4. Plan in place to meet needs after discharge.

NURSING DIAGNOSIS: Activity intolerance

May be related to
Imbalance between oxygen supply (delivery) and demand

Possibly evidenced by
Weakness and fatigue
Reports of decreased exercise/activity tolerance
Greater need for sleep/rest
Palpitations, tachycardia, increased BP/respiratory response with minor exertion

DESIRED OUTCOMES/EVALUATION CRITERIA—PATIENT WILL:
Report an increase in activity tolerance (including ADLs).
Demonstrate a decrease in physiologic signs of intolerance, e.g., pulse, respirations, and BP remain within patient's normal range.

ACTIONS/INTERVENTIONS	RATIONALE
Independent	
Assess patient's ability to perform normal tasks/ADLs, noting reports of weakness, fatigue, and difficulty accomplishing tasks.	Influences choice of interventions/needed assistance.
Note changes in balance/gait disturbance, muscle weakness.	May indicate neurologic changes associated with vitamin B_{12} deficiency, affecting patient safety/risk of injury.
Monitor BP, pulse, respirations during and after activity. Note adverse responses to increased levels of activity (e.g., increased HR/BP, dysrhythmias, dizziness, dyspnea, tachypnea, cyanosis of mucous membranes/nail beds.	Cardiopulmonary manifestations result from attempts by the heart and lungs to bring adequate amounts of oxygen to the tissues.
Recommend quiet atmosphere; bedrest if indicated. Stress need to monitor and limit visitors, phone calls, and repeated unplanned interruptions.	Enhances rest to lower body's oxygen requirements and reduces strain on the heart and lungs.
Elevate head of bed as tolerated.	Enhances lung expansion to maximize oxygenation for cellular uptake. *Note:* May be contraindicated if hypotension is present.

ACTIONS/INTERVENTIONS	RATIONALE

Independent

Suggest patient change position slowly and monitor for dizziness.

Postural hypotension or cerebral hypoxia may cause dizziness, fainting, and increased risk of injury.

Assist patient to prioritize ADLs/desired activities. Alternate rest periods with activity periods. Write out schedule for patient to refer to.

Promotes adequate rest, maintains energy level and alleviates strain on the cardiac and respiratory systems.

Provide assistance with activities/ambulation as necessary, allowing patient to do as much as possible.

While help may be necessary, self-esteem is enhanced when patient does some things for self.

Plan activity progression with patient, including activities that the patient views as essential. Increase activity levels as tolerated.

Promotes gradual return to normal activity level and improved muscle tone/stamina without undue fatigue. Increases self-esteem and sense of control.

Identify energy-saving techniques, e.g., shower chair, sitting to perform tasks.

Encourages patient to do as much as possible, while conserving limited energy and preventing fatigue.

Instruct patient to stop activity if palpitations, chest pain, shortness of breath, weakness, or dizziness occur.

Cellular ischemia potentiates risk of infarction and excessive cardiopulmonary strain/stress may lead to decompensation/failure.

Discuss importance of maintaining environmental temperature and body warmth as indicated.

Vasoconstriction (shunting of blood to vital organs) decreases peripheral circulation, impairing tissue perfusion. Patient's comfort/need for warmth must be balanced with need to avoid excessive heat with resultant vasodilation (reduces organ perfusion).

Collaborative

Monitor laboratory studies, e.g., HB/Hct and RBC count, ABGs.

Identifies deficiencies in RBC components affecting oxygen transport, and treatment needs/response to therapy.

Provide supplemental oxygen as indicated.

Maximizing oxygen transport to tissues improves ability to function.

Administer as indicated:

Colony-stimulating factors, e.g., Interleukin-2 (Aldesleukin);

CSFs may be given to stimulate growth of specific blood elements.

Whole blood/packed RBCs, blood products as indicated. Monitor closely for transfusion reactions.

Increases number of oxygen-carrying cells; corrects deficiencies to reduce risk of hemorrhage in acutely compromised individuals. *Note:* Transfusions are reserved for emergency blood loss anemias/cardiovascular compromise; after other therapies have failed to restore homeostasis.

Prepare for surgical intervention if indicated.

Bone marrow transplant may be done in presence of bone marrow failure/aplastic anemia.

NURSING DIAGNOSIS: Nutrition: altered, less than body requirements

May be related to
Failure to ingest or inability to digest food/absorb nutrients necessary for formation of normal RBCs

Possibly evidenced by
Weight loss/weight below normal for age, height, and build
Decreased triceps skinfold measurement

ACTIONS/INTERVENTIONS	RATIONALE
Independent	
Review nutritional history, including food preferences.	Identifies deficiencies, suggests possible interventions.
Observe and record patient's food intake.	Monitors caloric intake or insufficient quality of food consumption.
Weigh periodically as appropriate (e.g., weekly).	Monitors weight loss and effectiveness of nutritional interventions.
Recommend small, frequent meals and/or between-meal nourishments.	May reduce fatigue and thus enhance intake, while preventing gastric distension. Use of Ensure/Isomil, or similar product provides additional protein and calories.
Suggest bland diet, low in roughage, avoiding hot, spicy, or very acidic foods as indicated.	When oral lesions are present, pain may restrict type of foods patient can tolerate.
Have patient record and report occurrence of nausea/vomiting, flatus, and other related symptoms, such as irritability or impaired memory.	May reflect effects of anemias (hypoxia, vitamin B_{12} deficiency) on organs.
Encourage/assist with good oral hygiene; before and after meals, use soft-bristled toothbrush for gentle brushing. Provide dilute, alcohol-free mouthwash if oral mucosa is ulcerated.	Enhances appetite and oral intake. Diminishes bacterial growth, minimizing possibility of infection. Special mouth-care techniques may be needed if tissue is fragile/ulcerated/bleeding and pain are severe.
Collaborative	
Consult with dietician.	Aids in establishing dietary plan to meet individual needs.
Monitor laboratory studies, e.g., Hb/Hct, BUN, prealbumin/albumin, protein, transferrin, serum iron, B_{12}, folic acid, TIBC, serum electrolytes.	Evaluates effectiveness of treatment regimen, including dietary sources of needed nutrients.
Administer medications as indicated, e.g.:	
Vitamin and mineral supplements, e.g., cyanocobalamin (vitamin B_{12}), folic acid (Folvite); ascorbic acid (vitamin C);	Replacements needed depend on type of anemia and/or presence of poor oral intake and identified deficiencies.

ACTIONS/INTERVENTIONS	RATIONALE
Collaborative	
Iron dextran (Infed) IM/IV;	Administered until estimated deficit is corrected. Reserved for those who cannot absorb or comply with oral iron therapy, or when blood loss is too rapid for oral replacement to be effective.
Oral iron supplements, e.g., ferrous sulfate (Feosol), ferrous gluconate (Fergon);	May be useful in some types of iron deficiency anemias. Oral preparations are taken between meals to enhance absorption and will usually correct anemia and replace iron stores over a period of several months.
Antifungal or anesthetic mouthwash if indicated.	May be needed in the presence of stomatitis/glossitis to promote oral tissue healing and facilitate intake.

NURSING DIAGNOSIS: Constipation/Diarrhea

May be related to
Decreased dietary intake; changes in digestive processes
Drug therapy side effects

Possibly evidenced by
Changes in frequency, characteristics, and amount of stool
Nausea/vomiting, decreased appetite
Reports of abdominal pain, urgency, cramping
Altered bowel sounds

DESIRED OUTCOMES/EVALUATION CRITERIA—PATIENT WILL:
Establish/return to normal patterns of bowel functioning.
Demonstrate changes in behaviors/lifestyle, as necessitated by causative, contributing factors.

ACTIONS/INTERVENTIONS	RATIONALE
Independent	
Determine stool color, consistency, frequency, and amount.	Assists in identifying causative/contributing factors and appropriate interventions.
Auscultate bowel sounds.	Bowel sounds are generally increased in diarrhea and decreased in constipation.
Monitor intake and output with specific attention to food/fluid intake.	May identify dehydration, excessive loss of fluids or aid in identifying dietary deficiencies.
Encourage fluid intake of 2500–3000 ml/d within cardiac tolerance.	Assists in improving stool consistency if constipated. Will help to maintain hydration status if diarrhea is present.
Recommend avoiding foods that are gas-forming.	Decreases gastric distress and abdominal distention.
Assess perianal skin condition frequently, noting changes or beginning breakdown. Encourage/assist with pericare after each BM if diarrhea is present.	Prevents skin excoriation and breakdown.
Discuss use of stool softeners, mild stimulants, bulk-forming laxatives, or enemas as indicated. Monitor effectiveness.	Facilitates defecation when constipation is present.

ACTIONS/INTERVENTIONS

Collaborative

Consult with dietitian to provide well-balanced diet high in fiber and bulk.

Administer antidiarrheal medications, e.g., diphenoxylate hydrochloride with atropine (Lomotil) and water-absorbing drugs, e.g., Metamucil.

RATIONALE

Fiber resists enzymatic digestion and absorbs liquids in its passage along the intestinal tract and thereby produces bulk, which acts as a stimulant to defecation.

Decreases intestinal motility when diarrhea is present.

NURSING DIAGNOSIS: Infection, risk for

Risk factors may include

Inadequate secondary defenses, e.g., decreased hemoglobin, leukopenia, or decreased granulocytes (suppressed inflammatory response)

Inadequate primary defenses, e.g., broken skin, stasis of body fluids; invasive procedures; chronic disease, malnutrition

Possibly evidenced by

[Not applicable; presence of signs and symptoms establishes an *actual* diagnosis]

DESIRED OUTCOMES/EVALUATION CRITERIA—PATIENT WILL:

Identify behaviors to prevent/reduce risk of infection.

Achieve timely wound healing, free of purulent drainage or erythema, and be afebrile.

ACTIONS/INTERVENTIONS

Independent

Perform/promote meticulous hand-washing by caregivers and patient.

Maintain strict aseptic techniques with procedures/wound care.

Provide meticulous skin, oral, and perianal care.

Encourage frequent position changes/ambulation, coughing, and deep-breathing exercises.

Promote adequate fluid intake.

Stress need to monitor/limit visitors. Provide protective isolation if appropriate. Restrict live plants/cut flowers.

Monitor temperature. Note presence of chills and tachycardia with/without fever.

Observe for wound erythema/drainage.

RATIONALE

Prevents cross-contamination/bacterial colonization. *Note:* Patient with severe/aplastic anemia may be at risk from normal skin flora.

Reduces risk of bacterial colonization/infection.

Reduces risk of skin/tissue breakdown and infection.

Promotes ventilation of all lung segments and aids in mobilizing secretions to prevent pneumonia.

Assists in liquefying respiratory secretions to facilitate expectoration and prevent stasis of body fluids (e.g., respiratory and renal).

Limits exposure to bacteria/infections. Protective isolation may be required in aplastic anemia, when immune response is most compromised.

Reflective of inflammatory process/infection requiring evaluation and treatment. *Note:* With bone marrow suppression, leukocytic failure may lead to fulminating infections.

Indicators of local infection. *Note:* Pus formation may be absent if granulocytes are depressed.

ACTIONS/INTERVENTIONS	RATIONALE
Collaborative	
Obtain specimens for culture/sensitivity as indicated.	Verifies presence of infection, identifies specific pathogen and influences choice of treatment.
Administer topical antiseptics; systemic antibiotics.	May be used prophylactically to reduce colonization or used to treat specific infectious process.

NURSING DIAGNOSIS: Knowledge deficit [learning need] regarding condition, prognosis, treatment, self care and discharge needs

May be related to
Lack of exposure/recall
Information misinterpretation
Unfamiliarity with information resources

Possibly evidenced by
Questions; request for information
Statement of misconception
Inaccurate follow-through of instructions/development of preventable complications

DESIRED OUTCOMES/EVALUATION CRITERIA—PATIENT WILL:
Verbalize understanding of the nature of the disease process, diagnostic procedures, and treatment plan.
Identify causative factors.
Initiate necessary behaviors/lifestyle changes.

ACTIONS/INTERVENTIONS	RATIONALE
Independent	
Provide information about specific anemia and explain that therapy depends on the type and severity of the anemia.	Provides knowledge base on which patient can make informed choices. Allays anxiety and may promote cooperation with therapeutic regimen.
Discuss effects of anemias on preexisting conditions.	Anemias aggravate heart, lung, and cerebrovascular disease.
Review purpose and preparations for diagnostic studies.	Anxiety/fear of the unknown increases stress level, which in turn increases the cardiac workload. Knowledge of what to expect can diminish anxiety.
Explain that blood taken for laboratory studies will not worsen anemia.	This is often an unspoken concern that can potentiate patient's anxiety.
Review required diet alterations to meet specific dietary needs (determined by type of anemia/deficiency).	Red meat, liver, egg yolks, green leafy vegetables, whole wheat bread, and dried fruits are sources of iron. Green vegetables, whole grains, liver, and citrus fruits are sources of folic acid and vitamin C (enhances absorption of iron).
Assess resources (e.g., financial and cooking).	Inadequate resources may affect ability to purchase/prepare appropriate food items.
Encourage cessation of smoking.	Smoking decreases available oxygen and causes vasonstriction.

523

ACTIONS/INTERVENTIONS	RATIONALE

Independent

Provide information about purpose, dosage, schedule, precautions and potential side effects, interactions, and adverse reactions to all prescribed medications.	Information enhances cooperation with regimen. Recovery from anemias can be slow, requiring lengthy treatment and prevention of secondary complications.
Stress importance of reporting signs of fatigue, weakness, paresthesias, irritability, impaired memory.	Indicates that anemia is progressing or failing to resolve, necessitating further evaluation/treatment changes.
Instruct and demonstrate self-administration of oral iron preparations:	Iron replacement usually takes 3–6 months, whereas vitamin B_{12} injections may be necessary for the rest of the patient's life.
Discuss importance of taking only prescribed dosages;	Overdose of iron medication can be toxic.
Advise taking with meals or immediately after meals;	Iron is best absorbed on an empty stomach. However, iron salts are gastric irritants and may cause dyspepsia, diarrhea, and abdominal discomfort if taken on an empty stomach.
Dilute liquid preparations (preferably with orange juice) and administer through a straw;	Undiluted liquid iron preparations may stain the teeth. Ascorbic acid promotes iron absorption.
Caution that BM may appear greenish black/tarry;	Excretion of excessive iron will change stool color.
Stress importance of good oral hygiene measures.	Certain iron supplements (e.g., Feosol) may leave deposits on teeth and gums.
Instruct patient/SO about parenteral iron administration:	
Z-track administration of medication;	Prevents extravasation (leaking) with accompanying pain.
Use separate needles for withdrawing and injecting the medication;	Medication may stain the skin.
Caution regarding possible systemic reaction, (e.g., flushing, vomiting, nausea, myalgia) and discuss importance of reporting symptoms.	Possible side effects of therapy requiring reevaluation of drug choice and dosage.
Discuss increased susceptibility to infections, signs/symptoms requiring medical intervention, e.g., fever, sore throat; erythema/draining wound; cloudy urine, burning with urination.	Decreased leukocyte production potentiates risk of infection. *Note:* Purulent drainage may not form in absence of granulocytes (aplastic).
Identify safety concerns, e.g., avoidance of forceful blowing of nose, contact sports, constipation/straining for stool; use of electric razors, soft toothbrush.	Reduces risk of hemorrhage from fragile tissues and general decrease of coagulation factors.
Recommend avoiding use of heating pads or hot water bottles; measuring temperature of bath water with a thermometer.	Thermoreceptors in the dermal tissues may be dulled due to oxygen deprivation, thus increasing the risk of thermal injury.
Recommend routine observation of skin, noting changes in turgor, altered color, local warmth, erythema, excoriation.	Condition of the skin is affected by circulation, nutrition, and immobility. Tissues may become fragile and prone to infection and breakdown.
Identify measures for healthy skin, e.g.:	
Reposition periodically and gently massage bony surfaces when sedentary or in bed;	Increases circulation to all skin areas limiting tissue ischemia/effects of cellular hypoxia.

ACTIONS/INTERVENTIONS	RATIONALE
Independent	
Keep skin surfaces dry and clean. Limit use of soap;	Moist, contaminated areas provide excellent media for growth of pathogenic organisms. Soap may dry skin excessively and increase irritation.
Engage regularly in ROM exercises;	Promotes circulation to tissues, prevents stasis.
Suggest use of protective devices, e.g., sheepskin, egg-crate, alternating air pressure/water mattress, heel/elbow protectors, and pillows as indicated.	Avoids skin breakdown by preventing/reducing pressure against skin surfaces.
Review good oral hygiene, necessity for regular dental care.	Effects of anemia (oral lesions) and/or iron supplements increase risk of infection/bacteremia.
Instruct to avoid use of aspirin products.	Increases bleeding tendencies.
Refer to appropriate community resources when indicated, e.g., social services for food stamps, meals on wheels.	May need assistance with groceries/meal preparation.

POTENTIAL CONSIDERATIONS following acute hospitalization (dependent on patient's age, physical condition/presence of complications, personal resources, and life responsibilities)

Activity intolerance—imbalance between oxygen supply (delivery) and demand

Nutrition: altered, less than body requirements—failure to ingest or inability to digest food/absorb nutrients necessary for formation of normal RBCs

Infection, risk for—inadequate secondary defenses, e.g., decreased hemoglobin, leukopenia, or decreased granulocytes (suppressed inflammatory response); inadequate primary defenses, e.g., broken skin, stasis of body fluids; invasive procedures; chronic disease, malnutrition

Therapeutic Regimen: Individual, ineffective management—economic difficulties, perceived benefits

SICKLE CELL CRISIS

Sickle cell anemia is a genetic disease that primarily affects black populations and people of Mediterranean descent. It renders the individual vulnerable to repeated painful crises that can progressively destroy vital organs. These crises are:

Vaso-occlusive/thrombocytic crisis: Related to infection, dehydration, fever, hypoxia, and characterized by multiple infarcts of bones, joints, and other target organs, with tissue pain and necrosis caused by plugs of sickled cells in the microcirculation.

Hypoplastic/aplastic crisis: May be secondary to severe (usually viral) infection or folic acid deficiency, resulting in cessation of production of RBCs and bone marrow.

Hyperhemolytic crisis: Reticulocytes are increased in peripheral blood; and bone marrow is hyperplastic. Characterized by anemia and jaundice (effects of hemolysis).

Sequestration crisis: Massive, sudden erythrostasis with pooling of blood in the viscera (splenomegaly), resulting in hypovolemic shock/possible death. This crisis occurs in patients with intact splenic function.

CARE SETTING

Sickle cell disease is generally managed at the community level, with many of the interventions included here being appropriate for this focus; however, this plan of care speaks to sickle cell crisis, which usually requires hospitalization during the acute phase.

RELATED CONCERNS

Patient Assessment Data Base

ACTIVITY/REST

May report: Lethargy, fatigue, weakness, general malaise
Loss of productivity; decreased exercise tolerance; greater need for sleep and rest

May exhibit: Listlessness; severe weakness and increasing pallor (aplastic crisis)
Gait disturbances (pain, kyphosis, lordosis); inability to walk (pain)
Poor body posture (slumping of shoulders indicative of fatigue)
Decreased ROM (swollen, inflamed joints); joint, bone deformities
Generalized retarded growth; tower-shaped skull with frontal bossing; disproportionately long arms and legs, short trunk, narrowed shoulders/hips, and long, tapered fingers

CIRCULATION

May report: Palpitations or anginal chest pain (concomitant CAD/myocardial ischemia)
Intermittent claudication

May exhibit: Apical pulse: PMI may be displaced to the left (cardiomegaly)
Tachycardia, dysrhythmias (hypoxia), systolic murmurs
BP: widened pulse pressure
Generalized symptoms of shock, e.g., hypotension, rapid thready pulse, and shallow respirations (sequestration crisis)

Peripheral pulses: Throbbing on palpation

Bruits (reflects compensatory mechanisms of anemia; may also be auscultated over the spleen due to multiple splenic infarcts)

Capillary refill delayed (anemia or hypovolemia)

Skin color: Pallor or cyanosis of skin, mucous membranes, and conjunctiva. *Note:* Pallor may appear as yellowish brown color in brown-skinned patients, and as ashen gray in black-skinned patients. Jaundice: Scleral icterus, generalized icteric coloring (excessive RBC hemolysis)

Dry skin/mucous membranes

Diaphoresis (either sequestration or vaso-occlusive crisis; acute pain or shock)

ELIMINATION

May report: Frequent voiding, voiding in large amounts, nocturia

May exhibit: RUQ abdominal tenderness, enlargement/distention (hepatomegaly); ascites

LUQ fullness (enlarged spleen or may be atrophic and nonfunctional from repeated splenic infarcts and fibrosis)

Dilute, pale, straw-colored urine; hematuria or smoky appearance (multiple renal infarcts)

Urine specific gravity decreased (may be fixed with progressive renal disease)

EGO INTEGRITY

May report: Resentment and frustration with disease, fear of rejection from others

Negative feelings about self, ability to deal with life/situation

Concern regarding being a burden to SOs; financial concerns, possible loss of insurance/benefits; lost time at work/school, fear of genetic transmission of disease

May exhibit: Anxiety, restlessness, irritability, apprehension, withdrawal, narrowed focus, self-focusing, unresponsiveness to questions, regression; depression, decreased self-concept

Dependent relationship with whomever can offer security and protection.

FOOD/FLUID

May report: Thirst

Anorexia, nausea/vomiting

May exhibit: Height/weight usually in the lower percentiles

Poor skin turgor with visible tenting (crisis, infection, and dehydration)

Dry skin, mucous membranes

JVD and general peripheral edema (concomitant HF)

HYGIENE

May report: Difficulty maintaining ADLs (pain or severe anemia)

May exhibit: Unkempt appearance, poor personal hygiene

NEUROSENSORY

May report: Headaches or dizziness

Transient visual disturbances (e.g., hemianopsia, nystagmus)

Tingling in the extremities

Disturbances in pain and position sense

May exhibit: Mental status: Usually unaffected except in cases of severe sickling (cerebral infarction/intracranial hemorrhage)

527

Weakness of the mouth, tongue, and facial muscles; aphasia (in cerebral infarction when dominant hemisphere infarcted)

Abnormal reflexes, decreased muscle strength/tone; abnormal involuntary movements; hemiplegia or sudden hemiparesis, quadriplegia

Ataxia, seizures

Meningeal irritation (intracranial hemorrhage), e.g., decreasing level of consciousness, nuchal rigidity, focal neurologic deficits, vomiting, severe headache

PAIN/DISCOMFORT

May report: Pain as severe, throbbing, gnawing of varied location (localized, migratory, or generalized)

Recurrent, sharp, transient headaches

Back pain (changes in vertebral column from recurrent infarctions); joint/bone pain accompanied by warmth, tenderness, erythema, and occasional effusions (vaso-occlusive crisis). *Note:* Deep bone infarctions may have no apparent signs of irritation

Gallbladder tenderness and pain (excessive accumulation of bilirubin due to increased erythrocyte destruction)

May exhibit: Sensitivity to palpation over affected areas

Holding joints in position of comfort; decreased ROM (result of pain and swollen joints)

Maladaptive pain behaviors, e.g., guilt for being ill, denial of any aspect of disease, indulgence in precipitating factors (overwork, strenuous exercise)

RESPIRATION

May report: Dyspnea on exertion or at rest

History of repeated pulmonary infections/infarctions, pulmonary fibrosis, pulmonary hypertension or cor pulmonale

May exhibit: Acute respiratory distress, e.g., dyspnea, chest pain, and cyanosis (especially in crisis)

Bronchial/bronchovesicular sounds in lung periphery; diminished breath sounds (pulmonary fibrosis)

Crackles, rhonchi, wheezes, diminished breath sounds (HF)

Increased AP diameter of the chest (barrel chest)

SAFETY

May report: History of transfusions

May exhibit: Low-grade fever

Impaired vision (sickle retinopathy), decreased visual acuity (temporary/permanent blindness)

Leg ulcers (common in adult patients, especially found on the internal and external malleoli and the medial aspect of the tibia)

Lymphadenopathy

SEXUALITY

May report: Loss of libido; amenorrhea; priapism, impotence

May exhibit: Delayed sexual maturity

Pale cervix and vaginal walls (anemia)

TEACHING/LEARNING

May report: History of HF (chronic anemic state); pulmonary hypertension or cor pulmonale (multiple pulmonary infections/infarctions); chronic leg ulcers, delayed healing

| **Discharge plan considerations:** | **DRG projected mean length of inpatient stay: 4.6 days** |
| | May need assistance with shopping, transportation, self-care, homemaker/maintenance tasks |

Refer to section at end of plan for postdischarge considerations.

DIAGNOSTIC STUDIES

CBC: Reticulocytosis (count may vary from 30%–50%); leukocytosis (especially in vaso-occlusive crisis), decreased Hb/Hct and total RBCs, thrombocytosis, and a normal to decreased MCV.

Stained RBC examination: Demonstrates partially or completely sickled, crescent-shaped cells, anisocytosis, poikilocytosis, polychromasia, target cells, Howell-Jolly bodies, basophilic stippling, occasional nucleated RBCs (normoblasts).

Sickle-turbidity tube test (Sickledex): Routine screening test that determines the presence of hemoglobin S but does not differentiate between sickle cell anemia and trait.

Hemoglobin electrophoresis: Identifies any abnormal hemoglobin types and differentiates between sickle cell trait and sickle cell anemia. Results may be inaccurate if patient has received a blood transfusion within 3–4 months prior to testing.

Sedimentation rate (ESR): Elevated.

Erythrocyte fragility: Decreased (osmotic fragility or RBC fragility). RBC survival time decreased (accelerated breakdown).

ABGs: May reflect decreased Po_2 (defects in gas exchange at the alveolar capillary level); acidosis (hypoxemia and acidic states in vaso-occlusive crisis).

Serum bilirubin (total and indirect): Elevated (increased RBC hemolysis).

Acid phosphatase: Elevated (release of erythrocytic ACP into the serum).

Alkaline phosphatase: Elevated during vaso-occlusive crisis (bone and liver damage).

LDH: Elevated (RBC hemolysis).

Serum potassium and uric acid: Elevated during vaso-occlusive crisis (RBC hemolysis).

Serum iron: May be elevated or normal (increased iron absorption due to excessive RBC destruction).

TIBC: Normal or decreased.

Urine/fecal urobilinogen: Increased (more sensitive indicators of RBC destruction than serum levels).

IVP: May be done to evaluate kidney damage.

Bone radiographs: May demonstrate skeletal changes, e.g., osteoporosis, osteosclerosis, osteomyelitis, or avascular necrosis.

X-rays: May indicate bone thinning, osteoporosis.

NURSING PRIORITIES

1. Promote adequate cellular oxygenation/perfusion.
2. Alleviate pain.
3. Prevent complications.
4. Provide information about disease, process/prognosis, and treatment needs.

DISCHARGE GOALS

1. Oxygenation/perfusion adequate to meet cellular needs.
2. Pain relieved/controlled.
3. Complications prevented/minimized.
4. Disease process, future expectations, potential complications, and therapeutic regimen understood.
5. Plan in place to meet needs after discharge.

NURSING DIAGNOSIS: Gas Exchange, impaired

May be related to

Decreased oxygen-carrying capacity of the blood, reduced RBC life span/premature destruction, abnormal RBC structure; sensitivity to low oxygen tension (strenuous exercise, increase in altitude).

Increased blood viscosity (occlusions created by sickled cells packing together within the capillaries) and pulmonary congestion (impairment of surface phagocytosis). Predisposition to bacterial pneumonia, pulmonary infarcts.

Possibly evidenced by
Dyspnea, use of accessory muscles
Restlessness, confusion
Tachycardia
Cyanosis (hypoxia)

DESIRED OUTCOMES/EVALUATION CRITERIA—PATIENT WILL:
Demonstrate improved ventilation/oxygenation as evidenced by respiratory rate within normal limits, absence of cyanosis and use of accessory muscles; clear breath sounds.
Participate in ADLs without weakness and fatigue.
Display improved/normal pulmonary function tests.

ACTIONS/INTERVENTIONS	RATIONALE
Independent	
Monitor respiratory rate/depth, use of accessory muscles, areas of cyanosis.	Indicators of adequacy of respiratory function or degree of compromise, and therapy needs/effectiveness.
Auscultate breath sounds, noting presence/absence, and adventitious sounds.	Development of atelectasis and stasis of secretions can impair gas exchange.
Monitor vital signs; note changes in cardiac rhythm.	Compensatory changes in vital signs and development of dysrhythmias reflect effects of hypoxia on cardiovascular system.
Investigate reports of chest pain and increasing fatigue. Observe for signs of increased fever, cough, adventitious breath sounds.	Reflective of developing respiratory infection, which increases the workload of the heart and oxygen demand.
Assist in turning, coughing, and deep breathing exercises.	Promotes optimal chest expansion, mobilization of secretions, and aeration of all lung fields; reduces risk of stasis of secretions/pneumonia.
Assess level of consciousness/mentation regularly.	Brain tissue is very sensitive to decreases in oxygen and may be an early indicator of developing hypoxia.
Evaluate activity tolerance; limit activities to those within patient tolerance or place patient on bed rest. Assist with ADLs and mobility as needed.	Reduction of the metabolic requirements of the body reduces the oxygen requirements/degree of hypoxia.
Encourage patient to alternate periods of rest and activity. Schedule rest periods as indicated.	Protects from excessive fatigue, reduces oxygen demands/degree of hypoxia.
Demonstrate and encourage use of relaxation techniques, e.g., guided imagery and visualization.	Relaxation decreases muscle tension and anxiety and hence the metabolic demand for oxygen.
Promote adequate fluid intake, e.g., 2–3 L/d within cardiac tolerance.	Sufficient intake is necessary to provide for mobilization of secretions and to prevent hyperviscosity of blood/capillary occlusion.
Screen health status of visitors/staff.	Protects from potential sources of respiratory infection.

ACTIONS/INTERVENTIONS	RATIONALE
Collaborative	
Administer supplemental humidified oxygen as indicated.	Maximizes oxygen transport to tissues, particularly in presence of pulmonary insults/pneumonia.
Monitor laboratory studies, e.g., CBC, cultures, ABGs/pulse oximetry, chest x-ray, pulmonary function tests.	Patients are particularly prone to pneumonia, which is potentially fatal due to its hypoxemic effect of increasing sickling.
Perform/assist with chest physiotherapy, IPPB, and incentive spirometer.	Done to mobilize secretions and increase aeration of lung fields.
Administer packed RBCs or exchange transfusions as indicated.	Increases number of oxygen-carrying cells, dilutes the percentage of hemoglobin S (to prevent sickling), improves circulation, and dislodges sickled cells. Packed RBCs are usually used because they are less likely to create circulatory overload. *Note:* Partial transfusions are sometimes used prophylactically in high-risk situations, e.g., chronic, severe leg ulcers, preparation for general anesthesia, third trimester of pregnancy.
Administer medications as indicated:	
Antipyretics, e.g., acetaminophen (Tylenol);	Maintains normothermia to reduce metabolic oxygen demands without affecting serum pH, which may occur with aspirin.
Antibiotics.	A broad-spectrum antibiotic is started immediately pending culture results of suspected infections, then may be changed when the specific pathogen is identified.

NURSING DIAGNOSIS: Tissue Perfusion, altered (specify)

May be related to
Vaso-occlusive nature of sickling, inflammatory response
AV shunts in both pulmonary and peripheral circulation
Myocardial damage from small infarcts, iron deposits, and fibrosis

Possibly evidenced by
Changes in vital signs; diminished peripheral pulses/capillary refill; general pallor
Decreased mentation, restlessness
Angina, palpitations
Tingling in extremities, intermittent claudication, bone pain
Transient visual disturbances
Ulcerations of lower extremities, delayed healing

DESIRED OUTCOMES/EVALUATION CRITERIA—PATIENT WILL:
Demonstrate improved tissue perfusion as evidenced by stabilized vital signs, strong/palpable peripheral pulses, adequate urine output, absence of pain; usual mentation; normal capillary refill; skin warm/dry; nail beds, lips, and ear lobes of natural pale, pink color; absence of paresthesias.

Independent

Monitor vital signs carefully. Assess pulses for rate, rhythm, and volume. Note hypotension; rapid, weak, thready pulse; and increased/shallow respirations.

Sludging and sickling in peripheral vessels may lead to complete or partial obliteration of a vessel with diminished perfusion to surrounding tissues. Sudden massive splenic sequestration of cells can lead to shock.

Assess skin for coolness, pallor, cyanosis, diaphoresis, delayed capillary refill.

Changes reflect diminished circulation/hypoxia potentiating capillary occlusion. (Refer to ND: Gas Exchange, impaired, p 529.)

Note changes in level of consciousness; reports of headaches, dizziness; development of sensory/motor deficits (e.g., hemiparesis or paralysis), seizure activity.

Changes may reflect diminished perfusion to the CNS due to ischemia or infarction. Stagnant cells must be mobilized immediately to reduce further ischemia/infarction.

Maintain adequate fluid intake. (Refer to ND: Fluid Volume deficit, risk for, p 533.) Monitor urine output.

Dehydration not only causes hypovolemia but increases sickling and occlusion of capillaries. Decreased renal perfusion/failure may occur due to vascular occlusion.

Assess lower extremities for skin texture, edema, ulcerations (especially of internal and external malleoli).

Reduced peripheral circulation often leads to dermal changes and delayed healing.

Investigate reports of change in character of pain, or development of bone pain, angina, tingling of extremities, eye pain/vision disturbances.

Changes may reflect increased sickling of cells/diminished circulation with further involvement of organs, e.g., MI or pulmonary infarction, occlusion of vasculature of the eye.

Maintain environmental temperature and body warmth.

Prevents vasoconstriction; aids in maintaining circulation and perfusion.

Evaluate for developing edema (including genitals in men).

Vaso-occlusion/circulatory stasis may lead to edema of extremities (and priapism in men), potentiating risk of tissue ischemia/necrosis.

Collaborative

Monitor laboratory studies, e.g.:

ABGs, CBC, LDH, AST/ALT, CPK, BUN;

Decreased tissue perfusion may lead to gradual infarction of organ tissues such as the brain, liver, spleen, kidney, skeletal muscle, and so forth with consequent release of intracellular enzymes.

Serum electrolytes. Provide replacements as indicated.

Electrolyte losses (especially sodium) are increased during crisis because of fever, diarrhea, vomiting, diaphoresis.

Administer hypo-osmolar solutions (e.g., 0.45 NS) via an infusion pump.

Hydration lowers the hemoglobin S concentration within the RBCs, which decreases the sickling tendency, and also reduces blood viscosity, which helps to maintain perfusion. Infusion pump may prevent circulatory overload. *Note:* D5W or LR may cause RBC hemolysis and potentiate thrombus formation.

ACTIONS/INTERVENTIONS

Collaborative

Administer experimental antisickling agents (e.g., sodium cyanate) or antineoplastic agents, carefully (e.g., hydroxyurea [Hydrea]) observing for possible lethal side effects.

Assist with/prepare for surgical diathermy or photocoagulation.

Assist with/prepare for needle aspiration of blood from corpora cavernosa;

Surgical intervention.

RATIONALE

Antisickling agents (currently under investigational use) are aimed at prolonging erythrocyte survival and preventing sickling by affecting cell membrane changes. Research indicates that hydroxyurea dramatically decreases the number of sickle cell episodes, and reduces the severity of complications such as fever and severe chest pain. The drug has been approved for use in polycythemia vera, and thus it is now available (although not specifically approved for use in sickle cell disease). *Note:* Use of anticoagulants, plasma expanders, nitrates, vasodilators, and alkylating agents have proven essentially unsuccessful in the management of the vaso-occlusive crisis.

Direct coagulation of bleeding sites in the eye (resulting from vascular stasis/edema) may prevent progression of proliferative changes if initiated early.

Sickling within the penis can cause sustained erection (priapism) and edema. Removal of sludged sickled cells can improve circulation, decreasing psychologic trauma and risk of necrosis/infection.

Direct incision and ligation of the dorsal arteries of the penis and saphenocavernous shunting may be necessary in severe cases of priapism to prevent tissue necrosis.

NURSING DIAGNOSIS: Fluid Volume deficit, risk for

Risk factors may include
Increased fluid needs, e.g., hypermetabolic state/fever, inflammatory processes
Renal parenchymal damage/infarctions limiting the kidney's ability to concentrate urine (hyposthenuria)

Possibly evidenced by
[Not applicable; presence of signs and symptoms establishes an *actual* diagnosis]

DESIRED OUTCOMES/EVALUATION CRITERIA—PATIENT WILL:
Maintain adequate fluid balance as evidenced by individually appropriate urine output with a near-normal specific gravity, stable vital signs, moist mucous membranes, good skin turgor, and prompt capillary refill.

ACTIONS/INTERVENTIONS

Independent

Maintain accurate I&O. Weigh daily.

RATIONALE

Patient may reduce fluid intake during periods of crisis because of malaise, anorexia, and so on. Dehydration from vomiting, diarrhea, fever, may reduce urine output and precipitate a vaso-occlusive crisis.

ACTIONS/INTERVENTIONS

Independent

Note urine characteristics and specific gravity.

Monitor vital signs, comparing with patient's normal/previous readings. Take BP in lying, sitting, and standing positions if possible.

Observe for fever, changes in level of consciousness, poor skin turgor, dryness of skin and mucous membranes, pain.

Monitor vital signs closely during blood transfusions and note presence of dyspnea, crackles, rhonchi, wheezes, JVD, diminished breath sounds, cough, frothy sputum, and cyanosis.

Collaborative

Administer fluids as indicated.

Monitor laboratory studies, e.g., Hb/Hct, serum and urine electrolytes.

RATIONALE

Kidney can lose its ability to concentrate urine, resulting in excessive losses of dilute urine.

Reduction of circulating blood volume can occur from increased fluid loss resulting in hypotension and tachycardia.

Symptoms reflective of dehydration/hemoconcentration with consequent vaso-occlusive state.

Patient's heart may already be weakened and prone to failure due to chronic demands placed on it by the anemic state. Heart may be unable to tolerate the added fluid volume from transfusions or rapid IV fluid administered to treat crisis/shock.

Replaces losses/deficits; may reverse renal concentration of RBCs/presence of failure. Fluids must be given immediately (especially in CNS involvement) to decrease hemoconcentration and prevent further infarction.

Elevations may indicate hemoconcentration. Kidneys' loss of ability to concentrate urine may result in serum depletions of Na^+, K^+, and CI^-.

NURSING DIAGNOSIS: Pain [acute]/chronic

May be related to
Intravascular sickling with localized stasis, occlusion, and infarction/necrosis
Activation of pain fibers due to deprivation of oxygen and nutrients, accumulation of noxious metabolites

Possibly evidenced by
Localized, migratory, or more generalized pain, described as throbbing, gnawing, or severe and incapacitating; affecting peripheral extremities, bones, joints, back, abdomen, or head (headaches recurrent/transient)
Decreased ROM, guarding of the affected areas
Facial grimacing, narrowed/self-focus

DESIRED OUTCOMES/EVALUATION CRITERIA—PATIENT WILL:
Verbalize relief/control of pain.
Demonstrate relaxed body posture, have freedom of movement, be able to sleep/rest appropriately.

ACTIONS/INTERVENTIONS

Independent

Assess reports of pain, including location, duration, and intensity (scale of 0–10).

RATIONALE

Sickling of cells potentiates cellular hypoxia and may lead to infarction of tissues without resultant pain.

ACTIONS/INTERVENTIONS	RATIONALE
Independent	
Observe nonverbal pain cues, e.g., gait disturbances, body positioning, reluctance to move, facial expressions, and physiologic manifestations of pain (e.g., elevated BP, tachycardia, increased respiratory rate). Explore discrepancies between verbal and nonverbal cues.	Pain is very unique to each patient; therefore, one may encounter varying descriptions due to individualized perceptions. Nonverbal cues may aid in evaluation of pain and effectiveness of therapy.
Discuss with the patient/SO what pain relief measures were effective in the past.	Involves patient/SO in care and allows for identification of remedies that have already been found to relieve pain. Helpful in establishing individualized treatment needs.
Explore alternate pain relief measures, e.g., relaxation techniques, biofeedback, yoga, meditation, progressive relaxation techniques, distraction (e.g., visual auditory, tactile kinesthetic, guided imagery, and breathing techniques).	May reduce reliance on pharmacologic therapy and enhance patient's sense of control.
Provide support for and carefully position affected extremities.	Reduces edema, discomfort, and risk of injury, especially if osteomyelitis is present.
Apply local massage gently to affected areas.	Helps to reduce muscle tension.
Encourage ROM exercises.	Prevents joint stiffness and possible contracture formation.
Plan activities during peak analgesic effect.	Maximizes movement of joints, enhancing mobility.
Maintain adequate fluid intake.	Dehydration increases sickling/vaso-occlusion and corresponding pain.
Collaborative	
Apply warm, moist compresses to affected joints or other painful areas. Avoid use of ice or cold compresses.	Warmth causes vasodilation and increases circulation to hypoxic areas. Cold causes vasoconstriction and compounds the crisis.
Administer medications as indicated: narcotics, e.g., meperidine (Demerol), morphine; nonnarcotic analgesics, e.g., acetaminophen (Tylenol) or sedatives, e.g., hydroxyzine (Vistaril).	Reduces pain and promotes rest and comfort. *Note:* Tylenol can be used for control of headache, pain, and fever. Aspirin should be avoided because it alters blood pH and can make cells sickle more easily.
Administer/monitor RBC transfusion.	Frequency of painful crises may be reduced by routine partial exchange transfusions to maintain population of normal RBCs.

NURSING DIAGNOSIS: Physical Mobility, impaired

May be related to
Multiple/recurrent bone infarctions or infections (weight-bearing bones)
Pain/discomfort: Kyphosis of upper back/lordosis of lower back, possible joint effusions
Osteoporosis with fragmentation/collapse of femoral head or vertebra (compression deformities)
Bacterial infections (osteomyelitis)

Possibly evidenced by
Reports of pain
Limited joint ROM, reluctance to move, inability to walk/perform ADLs, guarding of
joints, gait disturbances
Generalized weakness, therapeutic restrictions (e.g., bed rest)

DESIRED OUTCOMES/EVALUATION CRITERIA—PATIENT WILL:
Maintain/increase strength and function of affected body parts.
Participate in activities with absence of or improvement in gait disturbances, increased
joint ROM, and absence of inflammatory signs.

Refer to CP: Long-Term Care, ND: Physical Mobility, impaired, p 852.

NURSING DIAGNOSIS: Skin Integrity, impaired, risk for

Risk factors may include
Impaired circulation (venous stasis and vaso-occlusion); altered sensation
Decreased mobility/bed rest

Possibly evidenced by:
[Not applicable; presence of signs and symptoms establishes an *actual* diagnosis]

DESIRED OUTCOMES/EVALUATION CRITERIA—PATIENT WILL:
Prevent dermal ischemic injury.
Participate in behaviors to reduce risk factors/skin breakdown.
Observe improvement in wound/lesion healing if present.

ACTIONS/INTERVENTIONS	RATIONALE
Independent	
Reposition frequently, even when sitting in chair.	Prevents prolonged tissue pressure where circulation is already compromised, reducing risk of tissue trauma/ischemia.
Inspect skin/pressure points regularly for redness, provide gentle massage.	Poor circulation may predispose to rapid skin breakdown.
Protect bony prominences with sheepskin, heel/elbow protectors, pillows, as indicated.	Decreases pressure on tissues, preventing skin breakdown.
Keep skin surfaces dry and clean; linens dry/wrinkle-free.	Moist, contaminated areas provide excellent media for growth of pathogenic organisms.
Monitor leg bruises, cuts, bumps closely for ulcer formation.	Potential entry sites for pathogenic organisms. In presence of altered immune system, this increases risk of infection/delayed healing.
Elevate lower extremities when sitting.	Enhances venous return reducing venous stasis/edema formation.
Collaborative	
Provide egg-crate, alternating air pressure, or water mattresses.	Reduces tissue pressure and aids in maximizing cellular perfusion to prevent dermal injury.

ACTIONS/INTERVENTIONS

Collaborative

Monitor status of ischemic areas, ulcer. Note distribution, size, depth, character, and drainage. Cleanse with hydrogen peroxide, boric acid, or povidone-iodine (Betadine) solutions as indicated.

Prepare for/assist with hyperbaric oxygenation to ulcer sites.

RATIONALE

Improvement or delayed healing reflects status of tissue perfusion and effectiveness of interventions. *Note:* These patients are at increased risk of serious complications because of lowered resistance to infection, and decreased nutrients for healing.

Maximizes oxygen delivery to tissues, enhancing healing.

NURSING DIAGNOSIS: Infection, risk for

Risk factors may include

Chronic disease process, tissue destruction, e.g., infarction, fibrosis, loss of spleen (autosplenectomy)

Inadequate primary defenses (broken skin, stasis of body fluids, decreased ciliary action)

Possibly evidenced by

[Not applicable; presence of signs and symptoms establishes an *actual* diagnosis]

DESIRED OUTCOMES/EVALUATION CRITERIA—PATIENT WILL:

Verbalize understanding of individual causative/risk factors.

Identify interventions to prevent/reduce risk of infection.

Refer to CPs: Pneumonia: Microbial, p 130; Sepsis/Septicemia, p 719; Fractures, ND: Infection, risk for, p 671.

NURSING DIAGNOSIS: Knowledge deficit [learning need] regarding condition, prognosis, treatment, self-care and discharge needs

May be related to

Lack of exposure/recall

Information misinterpretation

Unfamiliarity with resources

Possibly evidenced by

Questions; request for information

Statement of misconceptions

Inaccurate follow-through of instructions; development of preventable complications

Verbal/nonverbal cues of anxiety

DESIRED OUTCOMES/EVALUATION CRITERIA—PATIENT WILL:

Verbalize understanding of disease process, including symptoms of crisis.

Initiate necessary behaviors/lifestyle changes to prevent complications.

Participate in continued medical follow-up; genetic counseling/family planning services.

ACTIONS/INTERVENTIONS

Independent

Review disease process and treatment needs.

RATIONALE

Provides knowledge base on which patient can make informed choices.

537

Independent

Assess patient's knowledge of precipitating factors, e.g.:

    Cold environmental temperatures, failure to dress warmly when engaging in winter activities; wearing tight, restrictive clothing; stressful situations.

Causes peripheral vasoconstriction, which may result in sludging of the circulation, increased sickling, and may precipitate a vaso-occlusive crisis.

    Strenuous physical activity/contact type sports, and extremely warm temperatures;

Increases metabolic demand for oxygen and increases insensible fluid losses (evaporation and perspiration), which may increase blood viscosity and tendency to sickle.

    Travel to places more than 7000 ft above sea level or flying in unpressurized aircraft;

Decreased oxygen tension present at higher altitudes causes hypoxia and potentiates sickling of cells.

Encourage consumption of at least 4–6 qt of fluid daily, during a steady state of the disease. Increase the amount to 6–8 qt during a painful crisis or while engaging in activities that might precipitate dehydration.

Prevents dehydration and consequent hyperviscosity that can potentiate sickling/crisis.

Encourage ROM exercise and regular physical activity with a balance between rest and activity.

Prevents bone demineralization and may reduce risk of fractures. Aids in maintaining level of resistance and decreases oxygen needs.

Review patient's current diet, reinforcing the importance of diet including liver, green leafy vegetables, citrus fruits, and wheat germ. Provide necessary instruction regarding supplementary vitamins such as folic acid.

Sound nutrition is essential because of increased demands placed on bone marrow (e.g., folate and vitamin B_{12} are used in greater quantities than usual), and folic acid supplements are frequently ordered to prevent aplastic crisis.

Discourage smoking and alcohol consumption; identify community support groups.

Nicotine induces peripheral vasoconstriction and decreases oxygen tension, which may contribute to cellular hypoxia and sickling. Alcohol increases the possibility of dehydration (precipitating sickling). Maintaining these changes in behavior/lifestyle may require prolonged support.

Discuss principles of skin/extremity care and protection from injury. Encourage prompt treatment of cuts, insect bites, sores.

Due to impaired tissue perfusion, especially in the periphery, distal extremities are especially susceptible to altered skin integrity/infection.

    Include instructions on care of any leg ulcers that might develop.

Fosters independence and maintenance of self-care at home.

Instruct patient to avoid persons with infections such as URI.

Altered immune response places patient at risk for infections, especially bacterial pneumonia.

Recommend patient avoid cold remedies and decongestants containing ephedrine. Stress the importance of reading labels on OTC drugs and consulting healthcare provider prior to consuming any drugs.

Those remedies containing vasoconstrictors may decrease peripheral tissue perfusion and cause sludging of sickled cells.

Discuss conditions for which medical attention should be sought, e.g.:

    Urine that appears blood tinged or smoky;

Symptoms suggestive of sickling in the renal medulla.

    Indigestion, persistent vomiting, diarrhea, high fever, excessive thirst;

Dehydration may trigger a vaso-occlusive crisis.

    Severe joint or bone pain;

May signify a vaso-occlusive crisis due to sickling in the bones or spleen (ischemia or infarction) or onset of osteomyelitis.

ACTIONS/INTERVENTIONS	RATIONALE
Independent	
Severe chest pain, with or without cough;	May reflect angina, impending MI, or pneumonia.
Abdominal pain; gastric distress following meals;	High incidence of gallbladder disease/stone formation.
Fever, swelling, redness, increasing fatigue/pallor, leg ulcers, dizziness, drowsiness.	Suggestive of infections that may precipitate a vaso-occlusive crisis if dehydration develops. *Note:* Severe infections are the most frequent cause of aplastic crisis.
Assist patient to strengthen coping abilities, e.g., deal appropriately with anxiety, get adequate information, use relaxation techniques.	Promotes patient's sense of control, may avert a crisis.
Suggest wearing a medical alert bracelet or carrying a wallet card.	May prevent inappropriate treatment in emergency situation.
Discuss genetic implications of the condition. Encourage SO/family members to seek testing to determine presence of hemoglobin S.	Screening may identify other family members with sickle cell trait. Hereditary nature of the disease with the possibility of transmitting the mutation may have a bearing on the decision to have children.
Explore concerns regarding childbearing/family planning and refer to community resources as indicated.	Provides opportunity to correct misconceptions/present information necessary to make informed decisions. Pregnancy can precipitate a vaso-occlusive crisis because the placenta's tortuous blood supply and low oxygen tension potentiate sickling, which in turn can lead to fetal hypoxia.
Encourage patient to have routine follow-ups, e.g.:	
Periodic laboratory studies, e.g., CBC;	Monitors changes in blood components; identifies need for changes in treatment regimen.
Biannual dental examination;	Sound oral hygiene limits opportunity for bacterial invasion/sepsis.
Annual ophthalmologic examination.	May develop sickle retinopathy with either proliferative or nonproliferative ocular changes.
Determine need for vocational/career guidance.	Sedentary career may be necessary because of the decreased oxygen-carrying capacity and diminished exercise tolerance.
Encourage participation in community support groups available to sickle cell patients/SO, such as the National Association for Sickle Cell Anemia, March of Dimes, Public Health/visiting nurse.	Helpful in adjustment to long-term situation; reduces feelings of isolation and enhances problem solving through sharing of common experiences. *Note:* Failure to resolve concerns/deal with situation may require more intensive therapy/psychologic support.

POTENTIAL CONSIDERATIONS following acute hospitalization (dependent on patient's age, physical condition/presence of complications, personal resources, and life responsibilities)

Pain [acute]/chronic—intravascular sickling with localized stasis, occlusion, and infarction/necrosis; activation of pain fibers due to deprivation of oxygen and nutrients, accumulation of noxious metabolites

Fluid Volume deficit, risk for—increased fluid needs, e.g., hypermetabolic state/fever, inflammatory processes; renal parenchymal damage/infarctions limiting the kidney's ability to concentrate urine (hyposthenuria)

Infection, risk for—chronic disease process, tissue destruction, e.g., infarction, fibrosis, loss of spleen (autosplenectomy); inadequate primary defenses (broken skin, stasis of body fluids, decreased ciliary action)

LEUKEMIAS

The term leukemia describes a variety of cancers that arise in the blood-forming organs of the body (spleen, lymphatic system, bone marrow). They are differentiated according to the leukocytic system that is involved. The common trait of all leukemias is the unregulated proliferation of WBCs in the bone marrow that replaces the normal elements. There is an apparent abnormality in the hematopoietic stem cell, which results in its inability to differentiate into normal cells. As the normal cells are replaced by leukemic cells, anemia, neutropenia, and thrombocytopenia occur. In adults, the most common of the acute leukemias is acute myelocytic leukemia, which involves neutrophils, a type of granulocyte. The most common of the chronic leukemias is chronic lymphocytic leukemia, which is characterized by an abnormal increase in lymphocytes.

CARE SETTING

Acute inpatient care on medical unit for initial evaluation and treatment, then at the community level.

RELATED CONCERNS

Cancer, p 875
Psychosocial Aspects of Care, p 783

Patient Assessment Data Base

The data are dependent on degree/duration of the disease and other organ involvement.

ACTIVITY/REST

May report: Fatigue, malaise, weakness; inability to engage in usual activities

May exhibit: Muscle wasting
Increased need for sleep, somnolence

CIRCULATION

May report: Palpitations

May exhibit: Tachycardia, heart murmurs
Pallor of skin, mucous membranes
Cranial nerve deficits and/or signs of cerebral hemorrhage

ELIMINATION

May report: Diarrhea; perianal tenderness, pain
Bright red blood on tissue paper, tarry stools
Blood in urine, decreased urine output

May exhibit: Perianal abscess; hematuria

EGO INTEGRITY

May report: Feelings of helplessness/hopelessness

May exhibit: Depression, withdrawal, anxiety, fear, anger, irritability
Mood changes, confusion

FOOD/FLUID

May report: Loss of appetite, anorexia, vomiting
Change in taste/taste distortions

Weight loss
Pharyngitis, dysphagia

May exhibit: Abdominal distention, decreased bowel sounds
Splenomegaly, hepatomegaly; jaundice
Stomatitis, oral ulcerations
Gum hypertrophy (gum infiltration may be indicative of acute monocytic leukemia)

NEUROSENSORY

May report: Lack of coordination/decreased coordination
Mood changes, confusion, disorientation, lack of concentration
Dizziness; numbness, tingling, paresthesias

May exhibit: Muscle irritability, seizure activity

PAIN/DISCOMFORT

May report: Abdominal pain, headaches, bone/joint pain; sternal tenderness, muscle cramping

May exhibit: Guarding/distraction behaviors, restlessness; self-focus

RESPIRATION

May report: Shortness of breath with minimal exertion

May exhibit: Dyspnea, tachypnea
Cough
Crackles, rhonchi
Decreased breath sounds

SAFETY

May report: History of recent/recurrent infections; falls
Visual disturbances/impairment
Spontaneous uncontrollable bleeding with minimal trauma

May exhibit: Fever, infections
Bruises, purpura, retinal hemorrhages, gum bleeding, or epistaxis
Enlarged lymph nodes, spleen, or liver (due to tissue invasion)
Papilledema and exophthalmos
Leukemic infiltrates in the dermis

SEXUALITY

May report: Changes in libido
Changes in menstrual flow, menorrhagia
Impotence

TEACHING/LEARNING

May report: History of exposure to chemicals, e.g., benzene, phenylbutazone, and chloramphenicol; excessive levels of ionizing radiation; previous treatment with chemotherapy, especially alkalating agents
Chromosomal disorder, e.g., Down syndrome or Fanconi's aplastic anemia

Discharge plan
considerations: **DRG projected mean length of inpatient stay: 3.9–10.0 days**
May need assistance with therapy and treatment needs/supplies, shopping, food preparation, self-care activities, homemaker/maintenance tasks, transportation

Refer to section at end of plan for postdischarge considerations.

CEA (carcinoembryonic antigen): May be elevated.

Cold agglutinins: May be elevated (greater than 1:16) in lymphatic leukemia.

Cryoglobulins: Positive cryoglobulin findings may be present in patients with lymphocytic leukemia.

CBC: Indicates a normocytic, normochromic anemia.

> *Hemoglobin:* May be less than 10 g/100 ml.
>
> *Reticulocytes:* Count is usually low.
>
> *Platelet count:* May be very low (<50,000/mm).
>
> *WBC:* May be more than 50,000/cm with increased immature WBCs ("shift to left"). Leukemic blast cells may be present.

PT/aPTT: Prolonged.

LDH: May be elevated.

Serum/urine uric acid: May be elevated.

Serum muramidase (a lysozyme): Elevated in acute monocytic and myelomonocytic leukemias.

Serum copper: Elevated.

Serum zinc: Decreased.

Bence-Jones protein (urine): Increased.

Bone marrow biopsy: Abnormal WBCs usually make up 50% or more of the WBCs in the bone marrow. Often 60%–90% of the cells are blast cells, with erythroid precursors, mature cells, and megakaryocytes reduced.

Chest x-ray and lymph node biopsies: May indicate degree of involvement.

NURSING PRIORITIES

1. Prevent infection during acute phases of disease/treatment.
2. Maintain circulating blood volume.
3. Alleviate pain.
4. Promote optimal physical functioning.
5. Provide psychologic support.
6. Provide information about disease process/prognosis and treatment needs.

DISCHARGE GOALS

1. Complications prevented/minimized.
2. Pain relieved/controlled.
3. ADLs met by self or with assistance.
4. Dealing with disease realistically.
5. Disease process/prognosis and therapeutic regimen understood.
6. Plan in place to meet needs after discharge.

Refer to CP: Cancer, p 875, for further discussion/expansion of interventions related to cancer care and for patient teaching.

NURSING DIAGNOSIS: Infection, risk for

Risk factors may include

Inadequate secondary defenses: Alterations in mature WBC (low granulocyte and abnormal lymphocyte count), increased number of immature lymphocytes; immunosuppression, bone marrow suppression (effects of therapy/transplant)

Inadequate primary defenses (stasis of body fluids, traumatized tissue)

Invasive procedures

Malnutrition; chronic disease

Possibly evidenced by

[Not applicable; presence of signs and symptoms establishes an *actual* diagnosis]

DESIRED OUTCOMES/EVALUATION CRITERIA—PATIENT WILL:
Identify actions to prevent/reduce risk of infection.
Demonstrate techniques, lifestyle changes to promote safe environment, achieve timely healing.

ACTIONS/INTERVENTIONS	RATIONALE
Independent	
Place in private room. Screen/limit visitors as indicated. Prohibit use of live plants/cut flowers. Restrict fresh fruits and vegetables.	Protects patient from potential sources of pathogens/infection. *Note:* Profound bone marrow suppression, neutropenia, and chemotherapy place the patient at great risk for infection.
Require good hand-washing protocol for all personnel and visitors.	Prevents cross-contamination/reduces risk of infection.
Monitor temperature. Note correlation between temperature elevations and chemotherapy treatments. Observe for fever associated with tachycardia, hypotension, subtle mental changes.	Although fever may accompany some forms of chemotherapy, progressive hyperthermia occurs in some types of infections, and fever (unrelated to drugs or blood products) occurs in most leukemia patients. *Note:* Septicemia may occur without fever.
Prevent chilling. Force fluids, administer tepid sponge bath.	Helps reduce fever, which contributes to fluid imbalance, discomfort, and CNS complications.
Encourage frequent turning and deep breathing.	Prevents stasis of respiratory secretions, reducing risk of atelectasis/pneumonia.
Auscultate breath sounds, noting crackles, rhonchi; inspect secretions for changes in characteristics, e.g., increased sputum production or cloudy, foul-smelling urine with urgency or burning.	Early intervention is essential to prevent sepsis/septicemia in immunosuppressed person.
Handle patient gently. Keep linens dry/wrinkle-free.	Prevents sheet burn/skin excoriation.
Inspect skin for tender, erythematous areas; open wounds. Cleanse skin with antibacterial solutions.	May indicate local infection. *Note:* Open wounds may not produce pus because of insufficient number of granulocytes.
Inspect oral mucous membranes. Provide good oral hygiene. Use a soft toothbrush, sponge or swabs for frequent mouth care.	The oral cavity is an excellent medium for growth of organisms.
Promote good perianal hygiene. Provide sitz baths, using Betadine or Hibiclens if indicated. Avoid rectal temperatures, use of suppositories.	Promotes cleanliness, reducing risk of perianal abscess; enhances circulation and healing.
Provide uninterrupted rest periods.	Conserves energy for healing, cellular regeneration.
Encourage increased intake of foods high in protein and fluids with adequate fiber.	Enhances antibody formation and prevents dehydration. *Note:* Constipation potentiates retention of toxins and risk of rectal irritation/tissue injury.
Avoid/limit invasive procedures (e.g., venipuncture and injections) as possible.	Break in skin could provide an entry for pathogenic/potentially lethal organisms. Use of central venous lines (e.g., tunneled catheter or implanted port) can effectively reduce need for invasive procedure and risk of infection. *Note:* Myelosuppression may be cumulative in nature especially when multiple drug therapy (including steroids) is prescribed.

543

ACTIONS/INTERVENTIONS	RATIONALE
Collaborative	
Monitor laboratory studies, e.g.:	
CBC, noting whether WBC falls or sudden changes occur in neutrophils;	Decreased numbers of normal/mature WBCs can result from the disease process or chemotherapy, compromising the immune response and increasing risk of infection.
Gram stain cultures/sensitivity.	Verifies presence of infections; identifies specific organisms and appropriate therapy.
Review serial chest x-rays.	Indicator of development/resolution of respiratory complications.
Administer medications as indicated, e.g., antibiotics.	May be given prophylactically or to treat specific infection.
Avoid use of aspirin-containing antipyretics.	Aspirin can cause gastric bleeding and further decrease platelet count.
Provide low-bacteria diet, e.g., cooked, processed foods, single servings in sealed containers.	Minimizes potential sources of bacterial contamination.

NURSING DIAGNOSIS: Fluid Volume deficit, risk for

Risk factors may include

Excessive losses, e.g., vomiting, hemorrhage, diarrhea

Decreased fluid intake, e.g., nausea, anorexia

Increased fluid need, e.g., hypermetabolic state, fever; predisposition for kidney stone formation/tumor lysis syndrome

Possibly evidenced by

[Not applicable; presence of signs and symptoms establishes an *actual* diagnosis]

DESIRED OUTCOMES/EVALUATION CRITERIA—PATIENT WILL:

Demonstrate adequate fluid volume, as evidenced by stable vital signs; palpable pulses; urine output, specific gravity, and pH within normal limits.

Identify individual risk factors and appropriate interventions.

Initiate behaviors/lifestyle changes to prevent development of fluid volume deficit.

ACTIONS/INTERVENTIONS	RATIONALE
Independent	
Monitor intake/output. Calculate insensible losses and fluid balance. Note decreased urine in presence of adequate intake. Measure specific gravity and urine pH.	Decreased circulation secondary to destruction of RBCs and their precipitation in the kidney tubules and/or development of kidney stones (related to elevated uric acid levels) may lead to urinary retention or renal failure.
Weigh daily.	Measure of adequacy of fluid replacement as well as kidney function. Continued intake greater than output may indicate renal insult/obstruction.
Monitor BP and heart rate.	Changes may reflect effects of hypovolemia (bleeding/dehydration).

ACTIONS/INTERVENTIONS	RATIONALE

Independent

Evaluate skin turgor, capillary refill, and general condition of mucous membranes.	Indirect indicators of fluid status/hydration.
Note presence of nausea, fever.	Affects intake, fluid needs, and route of replacement.
Encourage fluids of up to 3–4 L/d when oral intake is resumed.	Promotes urine flow, prevents uric acid precipitation, and enhances clearance of antineoplastic drugs.
Inspect skin/mucous membranes for petechiae, ecchymotic areas; note bleeding gums, frank or occult blood in stools and urine; oozing from invasive-line sites.	Suppression of bone marrow and platelet production places the patient at risk for spontaneous/uncontrolled bleeding.
Implement measures to prevent tissue injury/bleeding, e.g., gentle brushing of teeth or gums with soft toothbrush, cotton swab, or sponge-tipped applicator; using electric razor and avoiding sharp razors when shaving; avoid forceful nose blowing, and needle sticks when possible; use sustained pressure on oozing puncture sites.	Fragile tissues and altered clotting mechanisms increase the risk of hemorrhage following even minor trauma.
Limit oral care to mouthwash if indicated (a mixture of ¼ tsp baking soda in 4–8 oz water or hydrogen peroxide in water). Avoid mouthwashes with alcohol.	When bleeding is present even gentle brushing may cause more tissue damage. Alcohol has a drying effect and may be painful to irritated tissues.
Provide soft diet.	May help reduce gum irritation.

Collaborative

Administer IV fluids as indicated.	Maintains fluid/electrolyte balance in the absence of oral intake; reduces risk of renal complications.
Monitor laboratory studies, e.g., platelets, Hb/Hct, clotting.	When the platelet count is less than 20,000/mm (due to proliferation of WBCs and/or bone marrow suppression secondary to antineoplastic drugs), the patient is prone to spontaneous life-threatening bleeding. Decreasing Hb/Hct is indicative of bleeding (may be occult).
Administer RBCs, platelets, clotting factors.	Restores/normalizes RBC count and oxygen-carrying capacity to correct anemia. Used to prevent/treat hemorrhage.
Maintain external central vascular access device (subclavian or tunneled catheter or implanted port).	Eliminates peripheral venipuncture as source of bleeding.
Administer medications as indicated, e.g.:	
Antiemetics: $5\text{-}HT_3$ receptor antagonist drugs such as ondansetron (Zofran) or granisetron (Kytril);	Relieves nausea/vomiting associated with administration of chemotherapy agents.
Allopurinol (Zyloprim);	May be given to reduce the chances of nephropathy as a result of uric acid production.
Potassium acetate or citrate, sodium bicarbonate;	May be used to alkalinize the urine preventing formation of kidney stones.
Stool softeners.	Helpful in reducing straining at stool with trauma to rectal tissues.

545

NURSING DIAGNOSIS: Pain [acute]

May be related to

Physical agents, e.g., enlarged organs/lymph nodes, bone marrow packed with leukemic cells

Chemical agents, e.g., antileukemic treatments

Psychologic manifestations, e.g., anxiety, fear

Possibly evidenced by

Reports of pain (bone, nerve, headaches, and so forth)

Guarding/distraction behaviors, facial grimacing, alteration in muscle tone

Autonomic responses

DESIRED OUTCOMES/EVALUATION CRITERIA—PATIENT WILL:

Report pain is relieved/controlled.

Demonstrate behaviors to manage pain.

Appear relaxed and able to sleep/rest appropriately.

ACTIONS/INTERVENTIONS	RATIONALE
Independent	
Investigate reports of pain. Note changes in degree and site (use scale of 0–10).	Helpful in assessing need for intervention; may indicate developing complications.
Monitor vital signs, note nonverbal cues, e.g., muscle tension, restlessness.	May be useful in evaluating verbal comments and effectiveness of interventions.
Provide quiet environment and reduce stressful stimuli, e.g., noise, lighting, constant interruptions.	Promotes rest and enhances coping abilities.
Place in position of comfort and support joints, extremities with pillows/padding.	May decrease associated bone/joint discomfort.
Reposition periodically and provide/assist with gentle ROM exercises.	Improves tissue circulation and joint mobility.
Provide comfort measures (e.g., massage, cool packs), and psychologic support (e.g., encouragement, presence).	Minimizes need for/enhances effects of medication.
Review/promote patient's own comfort interventions, position, physical activity/nonactivity, and so forth.	Successful management of pain requires patient involvement. Use of effective techniques provides positive reinforcement, promotes sense of control, and prepares patient for interventions to be used after discharge.
Evaluate and support patient's coping mechanisms.	Using own learned perceptions/behaviors to manage pain can help the patient to cope more effectively.
Encourage use of stress management techniques, e.g., relaxation/deep-breathing exercises, guided imagery, visualization; therapeutic touch.	Facilitates relaxation, augments pharmacologic therapy, and enhances coping abilities.
Assist with/provide diversional activities, relaxation techniques.	Helps with pain management by redirecting attention.

ACTIONS/INTERVENTIONS

Collaborative

Monitor uric acid level.

Administer medications as indicated:

Analgesics, e.g., acetaminophen (Tylenol);

Narcotics, e.g., codeine, meperidine (Demerol), morphine, hydromorphone (Dilaudid);

Antianxiety agents, e.g., diazepam (Valium), lorazepam (Ativan).

RATIONALE

Rapid turnover and destruction of leukemic cells during chemotherapy elevates uric acid, causing swollen, painful joints.

Given for mild pain not relieved by comfort measures. *Note:* Avoid aspirin-containing products as they may potentiate hemorrhage.

Used when pain is severe. Use of PCA may be beneficial in preventing peaks and valleys associated with intermittent drug administration.

May be given to enhance the action of analgesics/narcotics.

NURSING DIAGNOSIS: Activity intolerance

May be related to
Generalized weakness; reduced energy stores, increased metabolic rate from massive production of leukocytes
Imbalance between oxygen supply and demand (anemia/hypoxia)
Therapeutic restrictions (isolation/bed rest); effect of drug therapy

Possibly evidenced by:
Verbal report of fatigue or weakness
Exertional discomfort or dyspnea
Abnormal heart rate or BP response

DESIRED OUTCOMES/EVALUATION CRITERIA—PATIENT WILL:
Report a measurable increase in activity tolerance.
Participate in ADLs to level of ability.
Demonstrate a decrease in physiologic signs of intolerance; e.g., pulse, respiration, and BP remain within patient's normal range.

ACTIONS/INTERVENTIONS

Independent

Evaluate reports of fatigue, noting inability to participate in activities or ADLs.

Encourage patient to keep a diary of daily routines and energy levels, noting activities that increase fatigue.

Provide quiet environment and uninterrupted rest periods. Encourage rest periods before meals.

Implement energy-saving techniques, e.g., sitting, rather than standing, use of shower chair. Assist with ambulation/other activities as indicated.

RATIONALE

Effects of leukemia, anemia, and chemotherapy may be cumulative (especially during acute and active treatment phase), necessitating assistance.

Helps patient prioritize activities and arrange them around fatigue pattern.

Restores energy needed for activity and cellular regeneration/tissue healing.

Maximizes available energy for self-care tasks.

547

ACTIONS/INTERVENTIONS	RATIONALE
Independent	
Schedule meals around chemotherapy. Give oral hygiene before meals and administer antimetics as indicated.	May enhance intake by reducing nausea. (Refer to CP: Cancer, ND: Nutrition: altered, less than body requirements, p 885.)
Recommend small nutritious, high-protein meals and snacks throughout the day.	Smaller meals require less energy for digestion than larger meals. Increased intake provides fuel for energy.
Collaborative	
Provide supplemental oxygen.	Maximizes oxygen available for cellular uptake, improving tolerance of activity.

NURSING DIAGNOSIS: Knowledge deficit [learning need] regarding disease, prognosis, treatment, self care and discharge needs

May be related to
Lack of exposure to resources
Information misinterpretation/lack of recall

Possibly evidenced by
Verbalization of problem/request for information
Statement of misconception

DESIRED OUTCOMES/EVALUATION CRITERIA—PATIENT WILL:
Verbalize understanding of condition/disease process and treatment.
Initiate necessary lifestyle changes.
Participate in treatment regimen.

ACTIONS/INTERVENTIONS	RATIONALE
Independent	
Review pathology of specific form of leukemia and various treatment options.	Treatments can include various antineoplastic drugs, whole body or liver/spleen radiation, transfusions, peripheral progenitor cell transplant, and bone marrow transplant.

For additional interventions refer to CP: Cancer, ND: Knowledge deficit, p 896.

POTENTIAL CONSIDERATIONS following acute hospitalization (dependent on patient's age, physical condition/presence of complications, personal resources, and life responsibilities)

Infection, risk for—inadequate secondary defenses: alterations in mature WBC (low granulocyte and abnormal lymphocyte count), increased number of immature lymphocytes; immunosuppression, bone marrow suppression (effects of therapy/transplant)

Role Performance, altered—situational crisis; health-illness, change in physical capacity

Therapeutic Regimen: Individual, ineffective management—complexity of therapeutic regimen, decisional conflicts, economic difficulties, excessive demands made on individual or family, perceived benefits, powerlessness

Family Processes, altered—situational crisis (illness, disabling/expensive treatments)

LYMPHOMAS

Malignant lymphomas are cancers of the lymphoid tissue, classified according to four primary features: cell type, degree of differentiation, type of reaction elicited by tumor cells, and growth patterns. If a nodular growth pattern is observed, the term *nodular* is used after the cell type. If no mention of growth pattern is made, the lymphoma is of a *diffuse* type.

HODGKIN'S DISEASE:

The malignant cell of origin for Hodgkin's is not known, but it is thought to be derived from a B-lymphocyte, T-lymphocyte, or macrophage cell line.

Hodgkin's disease is divided into four different categories: lymphocyte-predominant, mixed cellularity, lymphocyte-depleted, and nodular sclerosing. The lymphocyte-predominant and nodular sclerosing types usually have a more favorable prognosis than the other two types. Stages I–IV of Hodgkin's disease range from one lymph node region to involvement of multiple systems in the body. Treatment for Hodgkin's disease includes extensive radiotherapy, a combination of radiotherapy and chemotherapy, or chemotherapy alone. Bone marrow transplant or peripheral progenitor cell transplants with high-dose chemotherapy are also treatment modalities showing promise.

NON-HODGKIN'S DISEASE:

Non-Hodgkin's lymphoma is a malignancy of the B-lymphocyte and T-lymphocyte cell systems. Most patients with non-Hodgkin's lymphoma fall into two broad categories related to their clinical features: the nodular, indolent type and the diffuse, aggressive lymphomas. For treatment purposes, they may also be classified as low-, intermediate-, or high-grade lymphomas. Treatment for non-Hodgkin's lymphomas includes radiotherapy or chemotherapy (usually multiple combinations of antineoplastic agents), and/or peripheral progenitor cell transplant.

CARE SETTING

Acute inpatient care on a medical unit for initial evaluation and treatment, then at community level. This plan of care addresses respiratory complications that may be encountered in acute care or hospice settings.

RELATED CONCERNS

Anemias (Iron Deficiency, Pernicious, Aplastic, Hemolytic), p 514
Cancer, p 875
Leukemias, p 540
Psychosocial Aspects of Care, p 783
Spinal Cord Injury (Acute Rehabilitative Phase), p 278

Patient Assessment Data Base

ACTIVITY/REST

May report:	Fatigue, weakness, or general malaise Loss of productivity and decreased exercise tolerance Need for more sleep and rest
May exhibit:	Diminished strength, slumping of the shoulders, slow walk, and other cues indicative of fatigue Night sweats

CIRCULATION

May report:	Palpitations, angina/chest pain
May exhibit:	Tachycardia, dysrhythmias Cyanosis of the face and neck (superior vena cava syndrome—obstruction of venous drainage from enlarged lymph nodes is a rare occurrence)

549

Scleral icterus and a generalized icteric coloring related to liver damage and consequent obstruction of bile ducts by enlarged lymph nodes (may be a late sign)

Pallor (anemia), diaphoresis, night sweats

EGO INTEGRITY

May report: Stress factors, e.g., school, job, family

Fear related to diagnosis and possibity of dying

Anxiety related to diagnostic testing and treatment modalities (chemotherapy and radiation therapy)

Financial concerns: Hospital costs, treatment expenses, fear of losing job-related benefits due to lost time from work

Relationship status: Fear and anxiety related to being a burden on the family

May exhibit: Varied behaviors, e.g., angry, withdrawn, passive

ELIMINATION

May report: Changes in characteristics of urine and/or stool

History of intestinal obstruction, e.g., intussusception, or malabsorption syndrome (infiltration from retroperitoneal lymph nodes)

May exhibit: RUQ tenderness and enlargement on palpation (hepatomegaly); LUQ tenderness and enlargement on palpation (splenomegaly)

Decreased output, dark/concentrated urine, anuria (ureteral obstruction/renal failure)

Bowel and bladder dysfunction (spinal cord compression occurs late)

FOOD/FLUID

May report: Anorexia/loss of appetite

Dysphagia (pressure on the esophagus)

Recent unexplained weight loss equivalent to 10% or more of body weight in previous 6 months with no attempt at dieting

May exhibit: Swelling of the face, neck, jaw, or right arm (secondary to superior vena cava compression by enlarged lymph nodes)

Extremities: Edema of the lower extremities related to inferior vena cava obstruction from intra-abdominal lymph node enlargement (non-Hodgkin's)

Ascites (inferior vena cava obstruction related to intra-abdominal lymph node enlargement)

NEUROSENSORY

May report: Nerve pain (neuralgias) reflecting compression of nerve roots by enlarged lymph nodes in the brachial, lumbar, and sacral plexuses

Muscle weakness, paresthesia

May exhibit: Mental status: lethargy, withdrawal, general lack of interest in surroundings.

Paraplegia (tumor involvement-spinal cord compression from collapse of vertebral body, disc involvement with compression/degeneration, or compromised blood supply to the spinal cord).

PAIN/DISCOMFORT

May report: Tenderness/pain over involved lymph nodes, e.g., in or around the mediastinum; chest pain, back pain (vertebral compression); generalized bone pain (lymphomatous bone involvement)

Immediate pain in involved areas following ingestion of alcohol

May exhibit: Self-focusing; guarding behaviors

RESPIRATION

May report:	Dyspnea on exertion or at rest; chest pain
May exhibit:	Dyspnea; tachypnea
	Dry, nonproductive cough
	Signs of respiratory distress, e.g., increased respiratory rate and depth, use of accessory muscles, stridor, cyanosis
	Hoarseness/laryngeal paralysis (pressure from enlarged nodes on the laryngeal nerve)

SAFETY

May report:	History of frequent/recurrent infections (abnormalities in cellular immunity predispose the patient to systemic herpes virus infections, TB, toxoplasmosis, or bacterial infections)
	History of mononucleosis (higher risk of Hodgkin's disease in patient with high titers of Epstein-Barr virus); history of ulcers/perforation, gastric bleeding
	Waxing and waning pattern of lymph node size
	Cyclical pattern of evening temperature elevations lasting a few days to weeks (Pel-Ebstein fever) followed by alternate afebrile periods; drenching night sweats without chills
	Generalized rash/pruritus
May exhibit:	Unexplained, persistent fever greater than 38°C (100.4°F) without symptoms of infection
	Asymmetric, painless, yet swollen/enlarged lymph nodes (cervical nodes most commonly involved, left side more than right; then axillary and mediastinal nodes)
	Nodes may feel rubbery and hard, discrete and movable
	Tonsilar enlargement
	Generalized pruritus
	Patchy areas of loss of melanin pigmentation (vitiligo)

SEXUALITY

May report:	Concern about fertility/pregnancy (while disease does not affect either, treatment does)
	Decreased libido

TEACHING/LEARNING

May report:	Familial risk factors (higher incidence among families of Hodgkin's patients than in general population)
	Occupational exposure to herbicides (woodworkers/chemists).
Discharge plan considerations:	**DRG projected mean length of inpatient stay: 3.9 days; with surgical intervention 9.2 days**
	May need assistance with medical therapies/supplies, self-care activities and/or homemaker/maintenance tasks, transportation, shopping.

Refer to section at end of plan for postdischarge considerations.

DIAGNOSTIC STUDIES

These diseases are staged according to the microscopic appearance of involved lymph nodes and the extent and severity of the disorder. Accurate staging is most important in deciding on subsequent treatment regimens and prognosis.

Blood studies may vary from completely normal to marked abnormalities. In stage I, few patients have abnormal blood findings.

CBC:

WBC: Variable, may be normal, decreased, or markedly elevated.

Differential WBC: Neutrophilia, monocytosis, basophilia, and eosinophilia may be found. Complete lymphopenia (late symptom).

RBC and Hb/Hct: Decreased.

Erythrocytes:
> *Stained RBC examination:* May demonstrate mild to moderate normocytic, normochromic anemia (hypersplenism).
> *Sedimentation rate (ESR):* Elevated during active stages and indicates inflammatory or malignant disease. Useful to monitor patients in remission and to detect early evidence of recurrence of disease.
> *Erythrocyte osmotic fragility:* Increased.
> *Platelets:* Decreased (may be severely depleted; bone marrow replacement by the lymphoma and by hypersplenism).

Coombs' test: Positive reaction (hemolytic anemia) may occur; however, a negative result usually occurs in advanced disease.

C-reactive protein (CRP) serum titer: May be positive in patients with Hodgkin's disease.

Serum cryoglobulins: May be positive in patients with Hodgkin's disease.

Serum haptoglobin: May be elevated in patient's with Hodgkin's disease, as well as those with cancer of the lung, large intestine, stomach, breast, and liver.

Serum iron and TIBC: Decreased.

Serum alkaline phosphatase: Elevation may indicate either liver or bone involvement.

Serum copper: Elevation may be seen in exacerbations.

Serum calcium: May be elevated when bone is involved.

Serum uric acid: Elevated related to increased destruction of nucleoproteins, and liver and kidney involvement.

BUN: May be elevated when kidney involvement is present. Serum creatinine, bilirubin, ASL, creatinine clearance, and so forth may be done to detect organ involvement.

Gammaglobulin: Hypergammaglobulinemia is common; hypogammaglobulinemia may occur in advanced disease.

Chest x-ray: May reveal mediastinal or hilar adenopathy, nodular infiltrates, or pleural effusions.

X-rays of thoracic, lumbar vertebrae, proximal extremities, pelvis, or areas of bone tenderness: Determine areas of involvement and assist in staging.

IVP: May be done to detect renal involvement or ureteral deviation by involved nodes.

Whole lung tomography or chest CT scan: Done if hilar adenopathy is present. Reveals possible involvement of mediastinal lymph nodes.

Abdominal CT scan: May be done to rule out diseased nodes in the abdomen and pelvis and associated organs.

Abdominal ultrasound: Evaluates extent of involvement of retroperitoneal lymph nodes.

Bone scans: Done to detect bone involvement.

Gallium-67 scintigraphy: Proven useful for detecting recurrent nodal disease, especially above the diaphragm.

Bone marrow biopsy: Determines bone marrow involvement. Bone marrow invasion is seen in advanced stages.

Lymph node biopsy: Establishes the diagnosis of Hodgkin's disease based on the presence of the Reed-Sternberg cell.

Mediastinoscopy: May be performed to establish mediastinal node involvement.

Staging laparotomy: May be done to obtain specimens of retroperitoneal nodes, of both lobes of the liver, and/or to remove the spleen. (Splenectomy is controversial because it may increase the risk of infection and is currently not usually implemented unless the patient has clinical manifestations of stage IV disease. Laparoscopy sometimes done as an alternative approach to obtain specimens).

NURSING PRIORITIES

1. Provide physical and psychologic support during extensive diagnostic testing and treatment regimen.
2. Prevent complications.
3. Alleviate pain.
4. Provide information about disease process/prognosis and treatment needs.

DISCHARGE GOALS

1. Complications prevented/diminished.
2. Dealing with situation realistically.
3. Pain relieved/controlled.
4. Disease process/prognosis, possible complications, and therapeutic regimen understood.
5. Plan in place to meet needs after discharge.

Refer to CPs: Cancer, p 875, Leukemias, p 540, for general nursing diagnoses and interventions.

NURSING DIAGNOSIS: Breathing Pattern/Airway Clearance, ineffective, risk for

Risk factors may include:

Tracheobronchial obstruction: Enlarged mediastinal nodes and/or airway edema (Hodgkin's and non-Hodgkin's); superior vena cava syndrome (non-Hodgkin's)

Possibly evidenced by:

[Not applicable; presence of signs and symptoms establishes an *actual* diagnosis]

DESIRED OUTCOMES/EVALUATION CRITERIA—PATIENT WILL:

Maintain a normal/effective respiratory pattern, free of dyspnea, cyanosis, or other signs of respiratory distress.

ACTIONS/INTERVENTIONS	RATIONALE
Independent	
Assess/monitor respiratory rate, depth, rhythm. Note reports of dyspnea and/or use of accessory muscles, nasal flaring, altered chest excursion.	Changes (such as tachypnea, dyspnea, use of accessory muscles) may indicate progression of respiratory involvement/compromise requiring prompt intervention.
Place patient in position of comfort, usually with head of bed elevated or sitting upright leaning forward (weight supported on arms), feet dangling.	Maximizes lung expansion, decreases work of breathing, and reduces risk of aspiration.
Reposition and assist with turning periodically.	Promotes aeration of all lung segments and mobilizes secretions.
Instruct in/assist with deep-breathing techniques and/or pursed lip or abdominal diaphragmatic breathing if indicated.	Helps promote gas diffusion and expansion of small airways. Provides patient with some control over respiration, helping to reduce anxiety.
Monitor/evaluate skin color, noting pallor, development of cyanosis (particularly in nail beds, ear-lobes, and lips).	Proliferation of WBCs can reduce oxygen-carrying capacity of the blood, leading to hypoxemia.
Assess respiratory response to activity. Note reports of dyspnea/"air hunger," increased fatigue. Schedule rest periods between activities.	Decreased cellular oxygenation reduces activity tolerance. Rest reduces oxygen demands and prevents fatigue and dyspnea.
Identify/encourage energy-saving techniques, e.g., rest periods before and after meals, use of shower chair, sitting for care.	Aids in reducing fatigue and dyspnea and conserves energy for cellular regeneration and respiratory function.
Promote bed rest and provide care as indicated during acute/prolonged exacerbation.	Worsening respiratory involvement/hypoxia may necessitate cessation of activity to prevent more serious respiratory compromise.
Encourage expression of feelings. Acknowledge reality of situation and normality of feelings.	Anxiety increases oxygen demand and hypoxemia potentiates respiratory distress/cardiac symptoms, which in turn escalates anxiety.
Provide calm, quiet environment.	Promotes relaxation, conserving energy and reducing oxygen demand.
Observe for neck vein distention, headache, dizziness, periorbital/facial edema, dyspnea, and stridor.	Non-Hodgkin's patients are at risk for superior vena cava syndrome, which may result in tracheal deviation and airway obstruction, representing an oncologic emergency.

553

ACTIONS/INTERVENTIONS	RATIONALE
Collaborative	
Provide supplemental oxygen.	Maximizes oxygen available for circulatory uptake; aids in reducing hypoxemia.
Monitor laboratory studies, e.g., ABGs, oximetry.	Measures adequacy of respiratory function and effectiveness of therapy.
Administer analgesics and tranquilizers as indicated.	Reducing physiologic responses to pain/anxiety decreases oxygen demands and may limit respiratory compromise.
Assist with respiratory treatments/adjuncts, e.g., IPPB, incentive spirometer if appropriate.	Promotes maximal aeration of all lung segments, preventing atelectasis.
Assist with intubation and mechanical ventilation.	May be necessary to support respiratory function until airway edema is resolved in acutely ill hospitalized patient.
Prepare for emergency radiation therapy when indicated.	Treatment of choice for superior vena cava syndrome.

POTENTIAL CONSIDERATIONS following acute hospitalization (dependent on patient's age, physical condition/presence of complications, personal resources, and life responsibilities)

Fatigue—decreased metabolic energy production, overwhelming psychologic or emotional demands, states of discomfort, altered body chemistry, e.g., chemotherapy

Family Processes, altered—situational crisis (illness, disabling/expensive treatments)

Renal and Urinary Tract

RENAL FAILURE: ACUTE

Acute renal failure (ARF) has four well-defined stages: onset, oliguric or anuric, diuretic, and convalescent. Treatment depends on stage and severity of renal compromise. ARF can be divided into three major classifications, dependent on site:

Prerenal: Interference with renal perfusion (e.g., blood volume depletion, volume shifts ("third-space" sequestration of fluid), or excessive/too-rapid volume expansion); manifested by decreased glomerular filtration rate (GFR).

Renal (or intrarenal): Parenchymal changes caused by ischemia or nephrotoxic substances. Acute tubular necrosis (ATN) accounts for 90% of cases of acute oliguria. Destruction of tubular epithelial cells results from (1) ischemia/hypoperfusion (similar to prerenal hypoperfusion except that correction of the causative factor may be followed by continued oliguria for up to 30 days) and/or (2) direct damage from nephrotoxins.

Postrenal: Occurs as the result of an obstruction in the urinary tract anywhere from the tubules to the urethral meatus.

Note: Iatrogenically induced ARF should be considered when failure develops during or shortly after hospitalization. The most common causative factors are administration of potentially nephrotoxic agents.

CARE SETTING

Inpatient acute medical or surgical unit

RELATED CONCERNS

Metabolic Acidosis (Primary Base Bicarbonate Deficit), p 506
Fluid and Electrolyte Imbalances, p 899
Psychosocial Aspects of Care, p 783
Renal Dialysis, p 580
Renal Failure: Chronic, p 568
Sepsis/Septicemia, p 719
Total Nutritional Support: Parenteral/Enteral Feeding, p 491
Upper Gastrointestinal/Esophageal Bleeding, p 315

Patient Assessment Data Base

ACTIVITY/REST

May report:	Fatigue, weakness, malaise
May exhibit:	Muscle weakness, loss of tone

CIRCULATION

May exhibit: Hypotension or hypertension (including malignant hypertension, eclampsia/pregnancy-
      induced hypertension)
Cardiac dysrhythmias
Weak/thready pulses, orthostatic hypotension (hypovolemia)
JVD, full/bounding pulses (hypervolemia)
Generalized tissue edema (including periorbital area, ankles, sacrum)
Pallor (anemia); bleeding tendencies

ELIMINATION

May report: Change in usual urination pattern: Increased frequency, polyuria (early failure), or de-
      creased frequency/oliguria (later phase)
Dysuria, hesitancy, urgency, and retention (inflammation/obstruction/infection)
Abdominal bloating, diarrhea, or constipation
History of BPH, or kidney/bladder stones/calculi

May exhibit: Change in urinary color, e.g., deep yellow, red, brown, cloudy
Oliguria (usually 12–21 days); polyuria (2–6 L/d)

FOOD/FLUID

May report: Weight gain (edema), weight loss (dehydration)
Nausea, anorexia, heartburn, vomiting
Use of diuretics

May exhibit: Changes in skin turgor/moisture
Edema (generalized, dependent)

NEUROSENSORY

May report: Headache, blurred vision
Muscle cramps/twitching; ''restless leg'' syndrome

May exhibit: Altered mental state, e.g., decreased attention span, inability to concentrate, loss of mem-
      ory, confusion, decreasing level of consciousness (azotemia, electrolyte/acid/base
      imbalance)
Twitching, muscle fasciculations, seizure activity

PAIN/DISCOMFORT

May report: Flank pain, headache

May exhibit: Guarding/distraction behaviors, restlessness

RESPIRATION

May report: Shortness of breath

May exhibit: Tachypnea, dyspnea, increased rate/depth (Kussmaul's respiration); ammonia breath
Cough productive of pink-tinged sputum (pulmonary edema)

SAFETY

May report: Recent transfusion reaction

May exhibit: Fever (sepsis, dehydration)
Petechiae, ecchymotic areas on skin
Pruritus, dry skin

TEACHING/LEARNING

May report: Family history of polycystic disease, hereditary nephritis, urinary calculus, malignancy

History of exposure to toxins, e.g., drugs, environmental poisons

Current/recent use of nephrotoxic drugs, e.g., aminoglycosides antibiotics, amphotericin B; anesthetics; vasodilators

Recent diagnostic testing with radiographic contrast media

Concurrent conditions: Tumors in the urinary tract, gram-negative sepsis; trauma/crush injuries, hemorrhage, DIC, burns, electrocution injury; autoimmune disorders (e.g., scleroderma, vasculitis), vascular occlusion/surgery, DM, cardiac/liver failure

Discharge plan considerations: **DRG projected mean length of inpatient stay: 6.4 days**

May require alteration/assistance with medications, treatments, supplies; transportation, homemaker/maintenance tasks

Refer to section at end of plan for postdischarge considerations.

DIAGNOSTIC STUDIES

Urine:

Volume: Usually less than 400 ml/24 h (oliguric phase), which occurs within 24–48 hours after renal insult.

Color: Dirty, brown sediment indicates presence of RBCs, hemoglobin, myoglobin, porphyrins.

Specific gravity: Less than 1.020 reflects kidney disease, e.g., glomerulonephritis, pyelonephritis with loss of ability to concentrate; fixed at 1.010 reflects severe renal damage.

pH: Greater than 7 found in UTIs, renal tubular necrosis, and chronic renal failure (CRF).

Osmolality: Less than 350 mOsm/kg is indicative of tubular damage, and urine/serum ratio is often 1:1.

Creatinine clearance: May be significantly decreased before BUN and serum creatinine show significant elevation.

Sodium: Usually decreased but may be greater than 40 mEq/L if kidney is not able to resorb sodium.

Bicarbonate: Elevated if metabolic acidosis is present.

RBCs: May be present because of infection, stones, trauma, tumor, or altered GF.

Protein: High-grade proteinuria (3–4+) strongly indicates glomerular damage when RBCs and casts are also present. Low-grade proteinuria (1–2+) and WBCs may be indicative of infection or interstitial nephritis. In ATN, there is usually minimal proteinuria.

Casts: Usually signal renal disease or infection. Cellular casts with brownish pigments and numerous renal tubular epithelial cells are diagnostic of ATN. Red casts suggest acute glomerular nephritis.

Blood:

BUN/Cr: Elevated and usually rise in proportion with ratio of 10:1 or greater.

CBC: Hb: Decreased in presence of anemia. RBCs often decreased owing to increased fragility/decreased survival.

ABGs: pH: Metabolic acidosis (less than 7.2) may develop because of decreased renal ability to excrete hydrogen and end products of metabolism. Bicarbonate decreased.

Sodium: Usually increased, but may vary.

Potassium: Elevated related to retention as well as cellular shifts (acidosis) or tissue release (red cell hemolysis).

Chloride, phosphorus, and magnesium: Usually elevated.

Calcium: Decreased.

Serum osmolality: Greater than 285 mOsm/kg; often equal to urine.

Protein: Decreased serum level may reflect protein loss via urine, fluid shifts, decreased intake, or decreased synthesis owing to lack of essential amino acids.

Radionuclide imaging: May reveal calicectasis, hydronephrosis, narrowing, and delayed filling or emptying as a cause of ARF.

KUB x-ray: Demonstrates size of kidneys/ureters/bladder, presence of cysts, tumors, and kidney displacement or obstruction (stones).

Retrograde pyelogram: Outlines abnormalities of renal pelvis and ureters.

Renal arteriogram: Assesses renal circulation and identifies extravascularities, masses.

Voiding cystoureterogram: Shows bladder size, reflux into ureters, retention.

Renal ultrasound: Determines kidney size and presence of masses, cysts, obstruction in upper urinary tract.

Non-nuclear CT scan: Cross-sectional view of kidney and urinary tract detects presence/extent of disease.

MRI: Provides information about soft tissue.

Excretory urography (intravenous urogram or pyelogram): Radiopaque contrast concentrates in urine and facilitates visualization of kidneys, ureters and bladder.

Endourology: Direct visualization may be done of urethra, bladder, ureters, and kidney to diagnose problems, biopsy, and remove small lesions and/or calculi.

ECG: May be abnormal reflecting electrolyte and acid/base imbalances.

NURSING PRIORITIES

1. Reestablish/maintain Fluid and electrolyte balance.
2. Prevent complications.
3. Provide emotional support for patient/SO.
4. Provide information about disease process/prognosis and treatment needs.

DISCHARGE GOALS

1. Homeostasis achieved.
2. Complications prevented/minimized.
3. Dealing realistically with current situation.
4. Disease process/prognosis and therapeutic regimen understood.
5. Plan in place to meet needs after discharge.

NURSING DIAGNOSIS: Fluid Volume excess

May be related to
Compromised regulatory mechanism (renal failure)

Possibly evidenced by
Intake greater than output, oliguria; changes in urine specific gravity
Venous distention; BP/CVP changes
Generalized tissue edema, weight gain
Changes in mental status, restlessness
Decreased Hb/Hct, altered electrolytes; pulmonary congestion on x-ray

DESIRED OUTCOMES/EVALUATION CRITERIA—PATIENT WILL:
Display appropriate urinary output with specific gravity/laboratory studies near normal; stable weight, vital signs within patient's normal range; and absence of edema.

ACTIONS/INTERVENTIONS	RATIONALE
Independent	
Record accurate I&O. Include "hidden" fluids such as IV antibiotic additives. Measure GI losses, and estimate insensible losses, e.g., diaphoresis.	Low output (less than 400 ml/24 hours) may be first indicator of acute failure, especially in a high-risk patient. Accurate I&O is necessary for determining renal function, fluid replacement needs, and reducing risk of fluid overload. *Note:* Hypervolemia occurs in the anuric phase of ARF.
Monitor urine specific gravity.	Measures the kidney's ability to concentrate urine. In intrarenal failure, specific gravity is usually equal to/less than 1.010, indicating loss of ability to concentrate the urine.

ACTIONS/INTERVENTIONS	RATIONALE

Independent

Weigh daily on same scale with same equipment and clothing.

Daily body weight is best monitor of fluid status. A weight gain of more than 0.5 kg/d suggests fluid retention.

Assess skin, face, dependent areas for edema. Evaluate degree of edema (on scale of +1 to +4).

Edema occurs primarily in dependent tissues of the body, e.g., hands, feet, lumbosacral area. Patient can gain up to 10 lb (4.5 kg) of fluid before pitting edema is detected. Periorbital edema may be a presenting sign of this fluid shift, because these fragile tissues are easily distended by even minimal fluid accumulation.

Monitor HR, BP, and JVD/CVP.

Tachycardia and hypertension can occur because of (1) failure of the kidneys to excrete urine, (2) excessive fluid resuscitation during efforts to treat hypovolemia/hypotension or convert oliguric phase of renal failure, and/or (3) changes in the renin-angiotensin system. *Note:* Invasive monitoring may be needed for assessing intravascular volume, especially in patients with poor cardiac function.

Auscultate lung and heart sounds.

Fluid overload may lead to pulmonary edema and HF evidenced by development of adventitious breath sounds, extra heart sounds. (Refer to ND: Cardiac Output, decreased, risk for, p 560.)

Assess level of consciousness; investigate changes in mentation, presence of restlessness.

May reflect fluid shifts, accumulation of toxins, acidosis, electrolyte imbalances, or developing hypoxia.

Plan oral fluid replacement with patient, within multiple restrictions. Space desired beverages throughout 24 hours. Vary offerings, e.g., hot, cold, frozen.

Helps avoid periods without fluids; minimizes boredom of limited choices and reduces sense of deprivation and thirst.

Collaborative

Correct any reversible cause of ARF, e.g., replace blood loss, maximize cardiac output, discontinue nephrotopic drug, relieve obstruction via surgery.

Kidneys may be able to return to normal functioning, preventing or limiting residual effects.

Monitor laboratory/diagnostic studies, e.g.:

   BUN, Cr;

Assesses progression and management of renal dysfunction/failure. Although both values may be increased, creatinine is a better indicator of renal function because it is not affected by hydration, diet, and tissue catabolism. *Note:* Dialysis is indicated if ratio is greater than 10:1 or if therapy fails to correct fluid overload or metabolic acidosis.

   Urine sodium and creatinine;

In ATN, tubular functional integrity is lost and sodium resorption is impaired, resulting in increased sodium excretion. Urine creatinine is usually decreased as serum creatinine elevates.

   Serum sodium;

Hyponatremia may result from fluid overload (dilutional) or inability of kidney to conserve sodium. Hypernatremia indicates deficit of total body water.

   Serum potassium;

Lack of renal excretion and/or selective retention of potassium to excrete excess hydrogen ions leads to hyperkalemia, requiring prompt intervention.

559

ACTIONS/INTERVENTIONS	RATIONALE
Collaborative	
Hb/Hct;	Decreased values may indicate hemodilution (hypervolemia); however, during prolonged failure, anemia frequently develops as a result of RBC loss/decreased production. Other possible causes (active or occult hemorrhage) should also be evaluated.
Serial chest x-rays.	Increased cardiac size, prominent pulmonary vascular markings, pleural effusion, infiltrates/congestion indicate acute responses to fluid overload, or chronic changes associated with renal and heart failure.
Administer/restrict fluids as indicated.	Fluid management is usually calculated to replace output from all sources plus estimated insensible losses (metabolism, diaphoresis). Prerenal failure (azotemia) is treated with volume replacement and/or vasopressors. The oliguric patient with adequate circulating volume or fluid overload who is unresponsive to fluid restriction and diuretics requires dialysis.
Administer medications as indicated:	
Diuretics, e.g., furosemide (Lasix), mannitol (Osmitrol);	Given early in oliguric phase of ARF in an effort to convert to nonoliguric phase, to flush the tubular lumen of debris, reduce hyperkalemia, and promote adequate urine volume.
Antihypertensives, e.g., clonidine (Catapres), methyldopa (Aldomet), prazosin (Minipress).	May be given to treat hypertension by counteracting effects of decreased renal blood flow, and/or circulating volume overload.
Insert/maintain indwelling catheter, as indicated.	Catheterization excludes lower tract obstruction and provides means of accurate monitoring of urine output during acute phase; however, indwelling catheterization may be contraindicated due to increased risk of infection.
Prepare for dialysis as indicated.	Done to correct volume overload, electrolyte and acid/base imbalances, and to remove toxins.

NURSING DIAGNOSIS: Cardiac Output, decreased, risk for

Risk factors may include
Fluid overload (kidney dysfunction/failure, overzealous fluid replacement)
Fluid shifts, fluid deficit (excessive losses)
Electrolyte imbalance (potassium, calcium); severe acidosis
Uremic effects on cardiac muscle/oxygenation

Possibly evidenced by
[Not applicable; presence of signs and symptoms establishes an *actual* diagnosis]

DESIRED OUTCOMES/EVALUATION CRITERIA—PATIENT WILL:
Maintain cardiac output as evidenced by BP and HR/rhythm within patient's normal limits; peripheral pulses strong and equal with adequate capillary refill time.

ACTIONS/INTERVENTIONS	RATIONALE

Independent

Monitor BP and heart rate.

Fluid volume excess, combined with hypertension (often occurs in renal failure) and effects of uremia, increases cardiac workload and can lead to cardiac failure. In ARF, cardiac failure is usually reversible.

Observe ECG or telemetry for changes in rhythm.

Changes in electromechanical function may become evident in response to progressing renal failure/accumulation of toxins and electrolyte imbalance. For example, hyperkalemia is associated with peaked T wave, wide QRS, prolonged P-R interval, flattened/absent P wave. Hypokalemia is associated with flat T wave, peaked P wave, and appearance of U waves. Prolonged Q-T interval may reflect calcium deficit.

Auscultate heart sounds.

Development of S_3/S_4 are indicative of failure. Pericardial friction rub may be only manifestation of uremic pericarditis, requiring prompt intervention/possibly acute dialysis.

Assess color of skin, mucous membranes, and nail beds. Note capillary refill time.

Pallor may reflect vasoconstriction or anemia. Cyanosis is a late sign and is related to pulmonary congestion and/or cardiac failure.

Note occurrence of slow pulse, hypotension, flushing, nausea/vomiting, and depressed level of consciousness (CNS depression).

Using drugs (e.g., antacids) containing magnesium can result in hypermagnesmia, potentiating neuromuscular dysfunction and risk of respiratory/cardiac arrest.

Investigate reports of muscle cramps, numbness/tingling of fingers, with muscle twitching, hyperreflexia.

Neuromuscular indicators of hypocalcemia, which can also affect cardiac contractility and function.

Maintain bed rest or encourage adequate rest and provide assistance with care and desired activities.

Reduces oxygen consumption/cardiac workload.

Collaborative

Monitor laboratory studies, e.g.:

  Potassium;

During oliguric phase, hyperkalemia will be present but often shifts to hypokalemia in diuretic or recovery phase. Any potassium value associated with ECG changes requires intervention. *Note:* A serum level of 6.5 mEq or greater constitutes a medical emergency.

  Calcium;

In addition to its own cardiac effects, calcium deficit enhances the toxic effects of potassium.

  Magnesium.

Dialysis or calcium administration may be necessary to combat the CNS-depressive effects of an elevated serum magnesium level.

Administer/restrict fluids as indicated (Refer to NDs: Fluid Volume excess, p 558 and Fluid Volume deficit, risk for, pp 564–565.)

Cardiac output is dependent on circulating volume (affected by both fluid excess and deficit) and myocardial muscle function.

Provide supplemental oxygen if indicated.

Maximizes available oxygen for myocardial uptake to reduce cardiac workload and cellular hypoxia.

Collaborative

Administer medications as indicated:

Inotropic agents, e.g., digoxin (Lanoxin);

May be used to improve cardiac output by increasing myocardial contractility and stroke volume. Dosage is dependent on renal function and potassium balance to obtain therapeutic effect without toxicity.

Calcium gluconate;

Serum calcium is often low but usually does not require specific treatment in ARF. Calcium gluconate may be given to treat hypocalcemia and to offset the effects of hyperkalemia by modifying cardiac irritability.

Aluminum hydroxide gels (Amphojel, Basalgel);

Increased phosphate levels may occur as a result of failure of glomerular filtration and require use of phosphate-binding antacids to limit phosphate absorption from the GI tract.

Glucose/insulin solution;

Temporary measure to lower serum potassium by driving potassium into cells when cardiac rhythm is endangered.

Sodium bicarbonate or sodium citrate;

May be used to correct acidosis or hyperkalemia (by increasing serum pH) if patient is severely acidotic and not suffering from fluid overload.

Sodium polystyrene sulfonate (Kayexalate) with/without sorbitol.

Exchange resin that trades sodium for potassium in the GI tract to lower serum potassium level. Sorbitol may be included to cause osmotic diarrhea to help excrete potassium.

Prepare for/assist with dialysis as necessary.

May be indicated for persistent dysrhythmias, progressive heart failure unresponsive to other therapies.

NURSING DIAGNOSIS: Nutrition: altered, risk for less than body requirements

Risk factors may include
Protein catabolism; dietary restrictions to reduce nitrogenous waste products
Increased metabolic needs
Anorexia, nausea/vomiting; ulcerations of oral mucosa

Possibly evidenced by
[Not applicable; presence of signs and symptoms establishes an *actual* diagnosis]

DESIRED OUTCOMES/EVALUATION CRITERIA—PATIENT WILL:
Maintain/regain weight as indicated by individual situation, free of edema.

Independent

Assess/document dietary intake.

Aids in identifying deficiencies and dietary needs. General physical condition, uremic symptoms (e.g., nausea, anorexia, altered taste), and multiple dietary restrictions affect food intake.

ACTIONS/INTERVENTIONS	RATIONALE

Independent

Provide frequent, small feedings.

Minimizes anorexia and nausea associated with uremic state/diminished peristalsis.

Give patient/SO a list of permitted foods/fluids and encourage involvement in menu choices.

Provides patient with a measure of control within dietary restrictions. Food from home may enhance appetite.

Offer frequent mouth care/rinse with dilute (0.25%) acetic acid solution; provide gum, hard candy, breath mints between meals.

Mucous membranes may become dry and cracked. Mouth care soothes, lubricates, and helps freshen mouth taste, which is often unpleasant owing to uremia and restricted oral intake. Rinsing with acetic acid helps neutralize ammonia formed by conversion of urea.

Weigh daily.

The fasting/catabolic patient will normally lose 0.2–0.5 kg/d. Changes in excess of 0.5 kg may reflect shifts in fluid balance.

Collaborative

Monitor laboratory studies, e.g., BUN, prealbumin/albumin, transferrin, sodium, and potassium.

Indicators of nutritional needs, restrictions, and necessity for/effectiveness of therapy.

Consult with dietitian/nutritional support team.

Determines individual calorie and nutrient needs within the restrictions, and identifies most effective route and product, e.g., oral supplements, enteral or parenteral nutrition.

Provide high-calorie, low-/moderate-protein diet. Include complex carbohydrates and fat sources to meet caloric needs (avoiding concentrated sugar sources) and essential amino acids.

The amount of needed exogenous protein is less than normal unless the patient is on dialysis. Carbohydrates meet energy needs and limit tissue catabolism, preventing ketoacid formation from protein and fat oxidation. Carbohydrate intolerance mimicking DM may occur in severe renal failure. Essential amino acids improve nitrogen balance and nutritional status.

Restrict potassium, sodium, and phosphorus intake as indicated.

Restriction of these electrolytes may be needed to prevent further renal damage, especially if dialysis is not part of treatment, and/or during recovery phase of ARF.

Administer medications as indicated:

Iron preparations;

Iron deficiency may occur if protein is restricted, patient is anemic, or GI function is impaired.

Calcium carbonate;

Restores normal serum levels to improve cardiac and neuromuscular function, blood clotting, and bone metabolism. *Note:* Low serum calcium is often corrected as phosphate absorption is decreased in the GI system. Calcium may be substituted as a phosphate binder.

Vitamin D;

Necessary to facilitate absorption of calcium from the GI tract.

B complex vitamins;

Vital as coenzyme in cell growth and actions. Intake is decreased owing to protein restrictions.

Antiemetics, e.g., prochlorperazine (Compazine), trimethobenzamide (Tigan).

Given to relieve nausea/vomiting and may enhance oral intake.

ACTIONS/INTERVENTIONS

Independent

Promote good hand-washing by patient and staff.

Avoid invasive procedures, instrumentation, and manipulation of indwelling catheters whenever possible. Use aseptic technique when caring for/manipulating IV/invasive lines. Change site/dressings per protocol. Note edema, purulent drainage.

Provide routine catheter care and promote meticulous perianal care. Keep urinary drainage system closed and remove indwelling catheter as soon as possible.

Encourage deep breathing, coughing, frequent position changes.

Assess skin integrity. (Refer to CP: Renal Failure: Chronic; ND: Skin Integrity, impaired, risk for, p 575.)

Monitor vital signs.

Collaborative

Monitor laboratory studies, e.g., WBC with differential.

Obtain specimen(s) for culture and sensitivity and administer appropriate antibiotics as indicated.

RATIONALE

Reduces risk of cross-contamination.

Limits introduction of bacteria into body. Early detection/treatment of developing infection may prevent sepsis.

Reduces bacterial colonization and risk of ascending UTI.

Prevents atelectasis and mobilizes secretions to reduce risk of pulmonary infections.

Excoriations from scratching may become secondarily infected.

Fever with increased pulse and respirations is typical of increased metabolic rate resulting from inflammatory process, although sepsis can occur without a febrile response.

Although elevated WBCs may indicate generalized infection, leukocytosis is commonly seen in ARF and may reflect inflammation/injury within the kidney. A shifting of the differential to the left is indicative of infection.

Verification of infection and identification of specific organism aids in choice of the most effective treatment. *Note:* A number of anti-infective agents require adjustments of dose and/or time while renal clearance is impaired.

Possibly evidenced by
[Not applicable; presence of signs and symptoms establishes an *actual* diagnosis]

DESIRED OUTCOMES/EVALUATION CRITERIA—PATIENT WILL:
Display I&O near balance; good skin turgor, moist mucous membranes, palpable peripheral pulses, stable weight and vital signs, electrolytes within normal range.

ACTIONS/INTERVENTIONS	RATIONALE
Independent	
Measure I&O accurately. Weigh daily. Calculate insensible fluid losses.	Helps estimate fluid replacement needs. Fluid intake should approximate losses through urine, nasogastric/wound drainage, and insensible losses (e.g., diaphoresis and metabolism). *Note:* Some sources believe that fluid replacement should not exceed two thirds of the previous day's output to prevent prolonging the diuresis.
Provide allowed fluids throughout 24-hour period.	Diuretic phase of ARF may revert to oliguric phase if fluid intake is not maintained or nocturnal dehydration occurs.
Monitor BP (noting postural changes) and heart rate.	Orthostatic hypotension and tachycardia suggests hypovolemia.
Note signs/symptoms of dehydration, e.g., dry mucous membranes, thirst, dulled sensorium, peripheral vasoconstriction.	In diuretic or postobstructive phase of renal failure, urine output can exceed 3 L/d. Extracellular fluid volume depletion activates the thirst center, and sodium depletion causes persistent thirst, unrelieved by drinking water. Continued fluid losses/inadequate replacement may lead to hypovolemic state.
Control environmental temperature; limit bed linens as indicated.	May reduce diaphoresis, which contributes to overall fluid losses.
Collaborative	
Monitor laboratory studies, e.g., sodium.	In nonoliguric ARF or in diuretic phase of ARF, large urine losses may result in sodium wasting while elevated urinary sodium acts osmotically to increase fluid losses. Restriction of sodium may be indicated to break the cycle.

NURSING DIAGNOSIS: Knowledge deficit [learning need] regarding condition, prognosis, treatment, self care and discharge needs
May be related to
Lack of exposure/recall
Information misinterpretation
Unfamiliarity with information resources
Possibly evidenced by
Questions/request for information, statement of misconception
Inaccurate follow-through of instructions/development of preventable complications

ACTIONS/INTERVENTIONS	RATIONALE
Independent	
Review disease process, prognosis, and precipitating factors if known.	Provides knowledge base on which patient can make informed choices.
Explain level of renal function after acute episode is over.	Patient may experience residual defects in kidney function, which may/may not be permanent.
Discuss renal dialysis or transplantation if these are likely options for the future.	Although these options would have been previously presented by the physician, the patient may now be at a point when decisions must be made and may desire additional input.
Review dietary plan/restrictions. Include fact sheet listing food restrictions.	Adequate nutrition is necessary to promote healing/tissue regeneration while adherence to restrictions may prevent complications.
Encourage patient to observe characteristics of urine and amount/frequency of output.	Changes may reflect alterations in renal function/need for dialysis.
Establish regular schedule for weighing.	Useful tool for monitoring fluid and dietary status/needs.
Review fluid intake/restriction. Remind patient to spread fluids over entire day and to include all fluids (e.g., ice) in daily fluid counts.	Depending on the cause of ARF, patient may need to either restrict or increase intake of fluids.
Discuss activity restriction and gradual resumption of desired activity. Encourage use of energy-saving, relaxation, and diversional techniques.	Patient with severe ARF may need to restrict activity and/or may feel weak for an extended period during lengthy recovery phase, requiring measures to conserve energy and reduce boredom/depression.
Discuss reality of continued presence of fatigue.	Decreased metabolic energy production, presence of anemia, and states of discomfort commonly result in fatigue.
Determine/prioritize ADLs and personal responsibilities. Identify available resources/support systems.	Helps patient to manage lifestyle changes and meet personal/family needs.
Recommend scheduling activities with adequate rest periods.	Prevents excessive fatigue and conserves energy for healing, tissue regeneration.
Discuss/review medication use. Encourage patient to discuss all medications (including OTC drugs) with physician.	Medications that are concentrated in/excreted by the kidneys can cause toxic cumulative reactions and/or permanent damage to kidneys.
Stress necessity of follow-up care, laboratory studies.	Renal function may be slow to return following acute failure (up to 12 months) and deficits may persist, requiring changes in therapy to avoid recurrence/complications.

ACTIONS/INTERVENTIONS	RATIONALE
Independent	
Identify symptoms requiring medical intervention, e.g., decreased urinary output, sudden weight gain, presence of edema, lethargy, bleeding, signs of infection; altered mentation.	Prompt evaluation and intervention may prevent serious complications/progression to CRF.

POTENTIAL CONSIDERATIONS following acute hospitalization (dependent on patient's age, physical condition/presence of complications, personal resources, and life responsibilities)

Fluid Volume deficit (specify)—dependent on cause, duration, and stage of recovery

Fatigue—decreased metabolic energy production/dietary restriction, anemia, increased energy requirements, e.g., fever/inflammation, tissue regeneration

Infection, risk for—depression of immunologic defenses (secondary to uremia), changes in dietary intake/malnutrition, increased environmental exposure

Therapeutic Regimen: Individual, ineffective management—complexity of therapeutic regimen, economic difficulties, perceived benefit

RENAL FAILURE: CHRONIC

Chronic renal failure (CRF) is usually the end result of a gradual, progressive loss of kidney function. Causes include chronic glomerulonephritis, chronic infections, vascular diseases (nephrosclerosis), obstructive processes (calculi), collagen diseases (systemic lupus), nephrotoxic agents (aminoglycosides), endocrine diseases (diabetes).

This syndrome is generally progressive and produces major changes in all body systems.

CARE SETTING

Primary focus is at the community level, although inpatient acute hospitalization may be required for life-threatening complications.

RELATED CONCERNS

Metabolic Acidosis (Primary Base Bicarbonate Deficit), p 506
Fluid and Electrolyte Imbalances, p 899
Heart Failure: Chronic, p 45
Hypertension: Severe, p 32
Psychosocial Aspects of Care, p 783
Anemias (Iron Deficiency, Pernicious, Aplastic, Hemolytic), p 514
Upper Gastrointestinal/Esophageal Bleeding, p 315
Additional associated nursing diagnoses are found in:
Renal Dialysis, p 580
Renal Failure: Acute, p 555
Seizure Disorders/Epilepsy, p 214

Patient Assessment Data Base

ACTIVITY/REST

May report:	Extreme fatigue, weakness, malaise
	Sleep disturbances (insomnia/restlessness or somnolence)
May exhibit:	Muscle weakness, loss of tone, decreased ROM

CIRCULATION

May report:	History of prolonged or severe hypertension
	Palpitations; chest pain (angina)
May exhibit:	Hypertension; JVD, full/bounding pulses, generalized tissue and pitting edema of feet, legs, hands
	Cardiac dysrhythmias
	Weak thready pulses, orthostatic hypotension reflects hypovolemia, which is rare in end-stage disease
	Pericardial friction rub (response to accumulated wastes)
	Pallor; bronze-gray, yellow skin
	Bleeding tendencies

EGO INTEGRITY

May report:	Stress factors, e.g., financial, relationship, and so on
	Feelings of helplessness, hopelessness, powerlessness
May exhibit:	Denial, anxiety, fear, anger, irritability, personality changes

ELIMINATION

May report: Decreased urinary frequency; oliguria, anuria (advanced failure)
Abdominal bloating, diarrhea, or constipation

May exhibit: Change in urine color, e.g., deep yellow, red, brown, cloudy
Oliguria, may become anuric

FOOD/FLUID

May report: Rapid weight gain (edema), weight loss (malnutrition)
Anorexia, heartburn, n/v; unpleasant metallic taste in the mouth (ammonia breath)
Use of diuretics

May exhibit: Abdominal distention/ascites, liver enlargement (end-stage)
Changes in skin turgor/moisture
Edema (generalized, dependent)
Gum ulcerations, bleeding of gums/tongue
Muscle wasting, decreased subcutaneous fat, debilitated appearance

NEUROSENSORY

May report: Headache, blurred vision
Muscle cramps/twitching, "restless leg" syndrome; burning numbness of soles of feet
Numbness/tingling and weakness, especially of lower extremities (peripheral neuropathy)

May exhibit: Altered mental state, e.g., decreased attention span, inability to concentrate, loss of memory, confusion, decreasing level of consciousness, stupor, coma
Diminished DTRs
Positive Chvostek's and Trousseau's signs
Twitching, muscle fasciculations, seizure activity
Thin, brittle nails; thin hair

PAIN/DISCOMFORT

May report: Flank pain; headache; muscle cramps/leg pain (worse at night)

May exhibit: Guarding/distraction behaviors, restlessness

RESPIRATION

May report: Shortness of breath; paroxysmal nocturnal dyspnea; cough with/without thick, tenacious sputum

May exhibit: Tachypnea, dyspnea, increased rate/depth (Kussmaul's respiration)
Cough productive of pink-tinged sputum (pulmonary edema)

SAFETY

May report: Itching skin
Recent/recurrent infections

May exhibit: Pruritus
Fever (sepsis, dehydration); normothermia may actually represent an elevation in the patient who has developed a lower-than-normal body temperature (effect of CRF/depressed immune response)
Petechiae, ecchymotic areas on skin
Bone fractures; calcium phosphate deposits (metastatic calcifications) in skin, soft tissues, joints; limited joint movement

SEXUALITY

May report: Decreased libido; amenorrhea; infertility

SOCIAL INTERACTION

May report: Difficulties imposed by condition, e.g., unable to work, maintain social contacts or usual role function in family

TEACHING/LEARNING

May report: Family history of DM (high risk for renal failure), polycystic disease, hereditary nephritis, urinary calculus, malignancy

History of exposure to toxins, e.g., drugs, environmental poisons

Current/recent use of nephrotoxic antibiotics

Discharge plan considerations: **DRG projected mean length of inpatient stay: 6.4 days**

May require alteration/assistance with medications, treatments, supplies; transportation, homemaker/maintenance tasks

Refer to section at end of plan for postdischarge considerations.

DIAGNOSTIC STUDIES

Urine:

   Volume: Usually less than 400 ml/24 h (oliguria) or urine is absent (anuria).

   Color: Abnormally cloudy urine may be caused from pus, bacteria, fat, colloidal particles, phosphates, or urates. Dirty, brown sediment indicates presence of RBCs, hemoglobin, myoglobin, porphyrins.

   Specific gravity: Less than 1.015 (fixed at 1.010 reflects severe renal damage).

   Osmolality: Less than 350 mOsm/kg is indicative of tubular damage, and urine/serum ratio is often 1:1.

   Creatinine clearance: May be significantly decreased.

   Sodium: Greater than 40 mEq/L because kidney is not able to reabsorb sodium.

   Protein: High-grade proteinuria (3–4+) strongly indicates glomerular damage when RBCs and casts are also present.

Blood:

   BUN/Cr: Elevated, usually in proportion. Creatinine level of 10 mg/dL suggests end stage (may be as low as 5).

   CBC: Hb: Decreased in presence of anemia, usually less than 7–8 g/dL. *RBCs:* Life span decreased owing to erythropoietin deficiency, as well as azotemia.

   ABGs: pH: Decreased. Metabolic acidosis (less than 7.2) occurs because of loss of renal ability to excrete hydrogen and ammonia or end products of protein catabolism. Bicarbonate decreased. PCO_2 decreased.

   Serum sodium: May be low (if kidney "wastes sodium") or normal (reflecting dilutional state of hypernatremia).

   Potassium: Elevated related to retention as well as cellular shifts (acidosis) or tissue release (RBC hemolysis). In end-stage disease, ECG changes may not occur until potassium is 6.5 mEq or greater.

   Magnesium, phosphorus: Elevated.

   Calcium: Decreased.

   Proteins (especially albumin): Decreased serum level may reflect protein loss via urine, fluid shifts, decreased intake, or decreased synthesis owing to lack of essential amino acids.

   Serum osmolality: Greater than 285 mOsm/kg; often equal to urine.

KUB x-rays: Demonstrates size of kidneys/ureters/bladder and presence of obstruction (stones).

Retrograde pyelogram: Outlines abnormalities of renal pelvis and ureters.

Renal arteriogram: Assesses renal circulation and identifies extravascularities, masses.

Voiding cystourethrogram: Shows bladder size, reflux into ureters, retention.

Renal ultrasound: Determines kidney size and presence of masses, cysts, obstruction in upper urinary tract.

Renal biopsy: May be done endoscopically to examine tissue cells for histologic diagnosis.

Renal endoscopy, nephroscopy: Done to examine renal pelvis; flush out calculi, hematuria; and remove selected tumors.

ECG: May be abnormal, reflecting electrolyte and acid/base imbalances.

X-ray of feet, skull, spinal column, and hands: May reveal demineralization/calcifications resulting from electrolyte shifts associated with CRF.

NURSING PRIORITIES

1. Maintain homeostasis.
2. Prevent complications.
3. Provide information about disease process/prognosis and treatment needs.
4. Support adjustment to lifestyle changes.

DISCHARGE GOALS

1. Fluid/electrolyte balance stabilized.
2. Complications prevented/minimized.
3. Disease process/prognosis and therapeutic regimen understood.
4. Dealing realistically with situation; initiating necessary lifestyle changes.
5. Plan in place to meet needs after discharge.

NURSING DIAGNOSIS: Cardiac Output, decreased, risk for

Risk factors may include

Fluid imbalances affecting circulating volume, myocardial workload, and systemic vascular resistance

Alterations in rate, rhythm, cardiac conduction (electrolyte imbalances, hypoxia)

Accumulation of toxins (urea), soft-tissue calcification (deposition of Ca phosphate)

Possibly evidenced by

[Not applicable; presence of signs and symptoms establishes an *actual* diagnosis]

DESIRED OUTCOMES/EVALUATION CRITERIA—PATIENT WILL:

Maintain cardiac output as evidenced by BP and heart rate within patient's normal range; peripheral pulses strong and equal with prompt capillary refill time.

ACTIONS/INTERVENTIONS	RATIONALE

(In addition to those in CP: Renal Failure: Acute; ND: Cardiac Output, decreased, risk for, p 560.)

Independent

Auscultate heart and lung sounds. Evaluate presence of peripheral edema/vascular congestion and reports of dyspnea.	S_3/S_4 heart sounds with muffled tones, tachycardia, irregular heart rate, tachypnea, dyspnea, crackles, wheezes, and edema/jugular distention suggest HF.
Assess presence/degree of hypertension: monitor BP; note postural changes, e.g., sitting, lying, standing.	Significant hypertension can occur because of disturbances in the renin-angiotensin-aldosterone system (caused by renal dysfunction). Although hypertension is common, orthostatic hypotension may occur due to intravascular fluid deficit, response to effects of antihypertensive medications, or uremic pericardial tamponade.
Investigate reports of chest pain, noting location, radiation, severity (0–10 scale), and whether or not it is intensified by deep inspiration and supine position.	While hypertension and chronic HF may cause MI, approximately half of CRF patients on dialysis develop pericarditis, potentiating risk of pericardial effusion/tamponade.

571

ACTIONS/INTERVENTIONS

Independent

Evaluate heart sounds (note friction rub), BP, peripheral pulses, capillary refill, vascular congestion, temperature, and sensorium/mentation.

Assess activity level, response to activity.

Collaborative

Monitor laboratory/diagnostic studies, e.g.:

Electrolytes (potassium, sodium, calcium, magnesium), BUN/Cr;

Chest x-rays.

Administer antihypertensive drugs, e.g., prazosin (Minipress), captopril (Capoten), clonidine (Catapres), hydralazine (Apresoline).

Prepare for dialysis.

Assist with pericardiocentesis as indicated.

RATIONALE

Presence of sudden hypotension, paradoxic pulse, narrow pulse pressure, diminished/absent peripheral pulses, marked jugular distention, pallor, and a rapid mental deterioration indicate tamponade, which is a medical emergency.

Weakness can be attributed to HF as well as anemia.

Imbalances can alter electrical conduction and cardiac function.

Useful in identifying developing cardiac failure or soft-tissue calcification.

Reduces systemic vascular resistance and/or renin release to decrease myocardial workload and aid in prevention of HF and/or MI.

Reduction of uremic toxins and correction of electrolyte imbalances and fluid overload may limit/prevent cardiac manifestations, including hypertension and pericardial effusion.

Accumulation of fluid within pericardial sac can compromise cardiac filling and myocardial contractility, impairing cardiac output and potentiating risk of cardiac arrest.

NURSING DIAGNOSIS: Injury, risk for (abnormal blood profile)

Risk factors may include
Suppressed erythropoietin production/secretion; decreased RBC production and survival; altered clotting factors; increased capillary fragility

Possibly evidenced by
[Not applicable; presence of signs and symptoms establishes an *actual* diagnosis]

DESIRED OUTCOMES/EVALUATION CRITERIA—PATIENT WILL:
Experience no signs/symptoms of bleeding/hemorrhage.
Maintain/demonstrate improvement in laboratory values.

ACTIONS/INTERVENTIONS

Independent

Note reports of increasing fatigue, weakness. Observe for tachycardia, pallor of skin/mucous membranes, dyspnea, and chest pain. Plan patient activities to avoid fatigue.

RATIONALE

May reflect effects of anemia, and cardiac response necessary to keep cells oxygenated.

ACTIONS/INTERVENTIONS	RATIONALE
Independent	
Monitor level of consciousness and behavior.	Anemia may cause cerebral hypoxia manifested by changes in mentation, orientation, and behavioral responses.
Evaluate response to activity, ability to perform tasks. Assist as needed and develop schedule for rest.	Anemia decreases tissue oxygenation and increases fatigue, which may require intervention, changes in activity, and rest.
Limit vascular sampling, combine laboratory tests when possible.	Recurrent/excessive blood sampling can worsen anemia.
Observe for oozing from venipuncture sites, bleeding/ecchymotic areas following slight trauma, petechiae; joint swelling or mucous membrane involvement, e.g., bleeding gums, recurrent epistaxis, hematemesis, melena, and hazy/red urine.	Bleeding can occur easily because of capillary fragility/altered clotting functions and may worsen anemia.
Hematest GI secretions/stool for blood.	Mucosal changes and altered platelet function due to uremia may result in GI hemorrhage.
Provide soft toothbrush, electric razor; use smallest needle possible and apply prolonged pressure following injections/vascular punctures.	Reduces risk of bleeding/hematoma formation.
Collaborative	
Monitor laboratory studies, e.g.:	
CBC: RBCs, Hb/Hct;	Uremia (e.g., elevated ammonia, urea, other toxins) decreases production of erythropoietin and depresses RBC production and survival time. In chronic renal failure, hemoglobin and hematocrit are usually low but tolerated; e.g., patient may not be symptomatic until Hb is below 7.
Platelet count, clotting factors;	Suppression of platelet formation and inadequate levels of factors III and VIII impair clotting and potentiate risk of bleeding. *Note:* Bleeding may become intractable in end-stage disease.
PT level.	Abnormal prothrombin consumption lowers serum levels and impairs clotting.
Administer fresh blood, packed RBCs as indicated.	May be necessary when patient is symptomatic with anemia. Packed RBCs are usually given when patient is fluid overloaded or being dialyzed. Washed RBCs are used to prevent hyperkalemia associated with stored blood.
Administer medications, as indicated, e.g.:	
Erythropoietin preparations, (Epogen, EPO);	Corrects many of the symptoms of CRF that are the result of anemia by stimulating the production and maintenance of RBCs, thus decreasing the need for transfusion.
Iron preparations: folic acid (Folvite), cyanocobalamin (Betalin);	Useful in correcting symptomatic anemia related to nutritional/dialysis-induced deficits. *Note:* Iron should not be given with phosphate binders because they may decrease iron absorption.

ACTIONS/INTERVENTIONS

Collaborative

Cimetidine (Tagamet), ranitidine (Zantac); antacids;

Hemastatics/fibrinolysis inhibitors, e.g., aminocaproic acid (Amicar);

Stool softeners (Colace); bulk laxative (Metamucil).

RATIONALE

May be given prophylactically to reduce/neutralize gastric acid and thereby reduce the risk of GI hemorrhage.

Inhibits bleeding that does not subside spontaneously/respond to usual treatment.

Straining to pass hard-formed stool increases likelihood of mucosal/rectal bleeding.

NURSING DIAGNOSIS: Thought Processes, altered

May be related to
Physiologic changes: Accumulation of toxins (e.g., urea, ammonia), metabolic acidosis, hypoxia; electrolyte imbalances, calcifications in the brain

Possibly evidenced by
Disorientation to person, place, time
Memory deficit; altered attention span, decreased ability to grasp ideas
Impaired ability to make decisions, problem solve
Changes in sensorium: somnolence, stupor, coma
Changes in behavior: irritability, withdrawal, depression, psychosis

DESIRED OUTCOMES/EVALUATION CRITERIA—PATIENT WILL:
Regain/maintain optimal level of mentation.
Identify ways to compensate for cognitive impairment/memory deficits.

ACTIONS/INTERVENTIONS

Independent

Assess extent of impairment in thinking ability, memory, and orientation. Note attention span.

Ascertain from SO patient's usual level of mentation.

Provide SO with information about patient's status.

Provide quiet/calm environment and judicious use of television, radio, and visitation.

Reorient to surroundings, person, and so forth. Provide calendars, clocks, outside window.

Present reality concisely, briefly, and do not challenge illogical thinking.

RATIONALE

Uremic syndrome's effect can begin with minor confusion/irritability and progress to altered personality or inability to assimilate information and participate in care. Awareness of changes provides opportunity for evaluation and intervention.

Provides comparison to evaluate progression/resolution of impairment.

Some improvement in mentation may be expected with restoration of more normal levels of BUN, electrolytes, and serum pH.

Minimizes environmental stimuli to reduce sensory overload/increased confusion while preventing sensory deprivation.

Provides clues to aid in recognition of reality.

Confrontation potentiates defensive reactions and may lead to patient mistrust and heightened denial of reality.

ACTIONS/INTERVENTIONS

Independent

Communicate information/instructions in simple, short sentences. Ask direct, yes/no questions. Repeat explanations as necessary.

Establish a regular schedule for expected activities.

Promote adequate rest and undisturbed periods for sleep.

Collaborative

Monitor laboratory studies, e.g., BUN/creatinine, serum electrolytes, glucose level, and ABGs (Po_2, pH).

Provide supplemental O_2 as indicated.

Avoid use of barbiturates and opiates.

Prepare for dialysis.

RATIONALE

May aid in reducing confusion and increases possibility that communications will be understood/remembered.

Aids in maintaining reality orientation and may reduce fear/confusion.

Sleep deprivation may further impair cognitive abilities.

Correction of elevations/imbalances can have profound effects on cognition/mentation.

Correction of hypoxia alone can improve cognition.

Drugs normally detoxified in the kidneys will have increased half-life/cumulative effects, worsening confusion.

Marked deterioration of thought processes may indicate worsening of azotemia and general condition, requiring prompt intervention to regain homeostasis.

NURSING DIAGNOSIS: Skin Integrity, impaired, risk for

Risk factors may include
Altered metabolic state, circulation (anemia with tissue ischemia), and sensation (peripheral neuropathy)
Alterations in skin turgor (edema/dehydration)
Reduced activity/immobility
Accumulation of toxins in the skin

Possibly evidenced by
[Not applicable; presence of signs and symptoms establishes an *actual* diagnosis]

DESIRED OUTCOMES/EVALUATION CRITERIA—PATIENT WILL:
Maintain intact skin.
Demonstrate behaviors/techniques to prevent skin breakdown/injury.

ACTIONS/INTERVENTIONS

Independent

Inspect skin for changes in color, turgor, vascularity. Note redness, excoriation. Observe for ecchymosis, purpura.

Monitor fluid intake and hydration of skin and mucous membranes.

Inspect dependent areas for edema. Elevate legs as indicated.

RATIONALE

Indicates areas of poor circulation/breakdown that may lead to decubitus formation/infection.

Detects presence of dehydration or overhydration that affect circulation and tissue integrity at the cellular level.

Edematous tissues are more prone to breakdown. Elevation promotes venous return limiting venous stasis/edema formation.

ACTIONS/INTERVENTIONS

Independent

Change position frequently; move patient carefully; pad bony prominences with sheepskin, elbow/heel protectors.

Provide soothing skin care. Restrict use of soaps. Apply ointments or creams (e.g., lanolin, Aquaphor).

Keep linens dry, wrinkle-free.

Investigate reports of itching.

Recommend patient use cool, moist compresses to apply pressure (rather than scratch) pruritic areas. Keep fingernails short; encourage use of gloves during sleep if needed.

Suggest wearing loose-fitting cotton garments.

Collaborative

Provide foam/flotation mattress.

RATIONALE

Decreases pressure on edematous, poorly perfused tissues to reduce ischemia.

Baking soda, cornstarch baths decrease itching and are less drying than soaps. Lotions and ointments may be desired to relieve dry, cracked skin.

Reduces dermal irritation and risk of skin breakdown.

Although dialysis has largely eliminated skin problems associated with uremic frost, itching can occur because the skin is an excretory route for waste products, e.g., phosphate crystals (associated with hyperparathyroidism in end-stage disease).

Alleviates discomfort and reduces risk of dermal injury.

Prevents direct dermal irritation and promotes evaporation of moisture on the skin.

Reduces prolonged pressure on tissues, which can limit cellular perfusion potentiating ischemia/necrosis.

NURSING DIAGNOSIS: Oral Mucous Membrane, altered, risk for

Risk factors may include
Lack of/or decreased salivation, fluid restrictions
Chemical irritation, conversion of urea in saliva to ammonia

Possibly evidenced by
[Not applicable; presence of signs and symptoms establishes an *actual* diagnosis]

DESIRED OUTCOMES/EVALUATION CRITERIA—PATIENT WILL:
Maintain integrity of mucous membranes.
Identify/initiate specific interventions to promote healthy oral mucosa.

ACTIONS/INTERVENTIONS

Independent

Inspect oral cavity; note moistness, character of saliva, presence of inflammation, ulcerations, leukoplakia.

Provide fluids throughout 24-hour period within prescribed limit.

RATIONALE

Provides opportunity for prompt intervention and prevention of infection.

Prevents excessive oral dryness from prolonged period without oral intake.

ACTIONS/INTERVENTIONS

Independent

Offer frequent mouth care/rinse with 0.25% acetic acid solution; provide gum, hard candy, breath mints between meals.

Encourage good dental hygiene after meals and at bedtime. Recommend avoidance of dental floss.

Recommend patient stop smoking and avoid lemon/glycerine products or mouthwash containing alcohol.

Provide artificial saliva as needed, e.g., Ora-Lube.

Collaborative

Administer medications as indicated, e.g., antihistamines: cyproheptadine (Periactin).

RATIONALE

Mucous membranes may become dry and cracked. Mouth care soothes, lubricates, and helps freshen mouth taste, which is often unpleasant owing to uremia and restricted oral intake. Rinsing with acetic acid helps neutralize ammonia formed by conversion of urea.

Reduces bacterial growth and potential for infection. Dental floss may cut gums, potentiating bleeding.

These substances are irritating to the mucosa and have a drying effect, potentiating discomfort.

Prevents dryness, buffers acids, and promotes comfort.

May be given for relief of itching.

NURSING DIAGNOSIS: Knowledge deficit [learning need] regarding condition, prognosis, treatment, self care and discharge needs

May be related to
Lack of exposure/recall, information misinterpretation
Cognitive limitation

Possibly evidenced by
Questions/request for information, statement of misconception
Inaccurate follow-through of instructions/development of preventable complications

DESIRED OUTCOMES/EVALUATION CRITERIA—PATIENT WILL:
Verbalize understanding of condition/disease process and treatment.
Correctly perform necessary procedures and explain reasons for the actions.
Demonstrate/initiate necessary lifestyle changes.
Participate in treatment regimen.

ACTIONS/INTERVENTIONS

(In addition to interventions outlined in CP: Renal Failure: Acute; Knowledge deficit, pp 565–566.)

Independent

Review disease process/prognosis and future expectations.

Review dietary restrictions, including phosphorus (e.g., milk products, poultry, corn, peanuts) and magnesium. (e.g., whole grain products, legumes).

Discuss other nutritional concerns, e.g., regulating protein intake according to level of renal function.

RATIONALE

Provides knowledge base on which patient can make informed choices.

Retention of phosphorus stimulates the parathyroid glands to shift calcium from bones (renal osteodystrophy), and accumulation of magnesium can impair neuromuscular function and mentation.

Metabolites that accumulate in blood derive almost entirely from protein catabolism; as renal function declines proteins may be restricted proportionately.

ACTIONS/INTERVENTIONS	RATIONALE

Independent

Encourage high calorie intake, especially from carbohydrates.	Spares protein, prevents wasting, and provides energy.
Discuss drug therapy, including use of calcium supplements and phosphate binders, e.g., aluminum hydroxide antacids (Amphojel, Basalgel) and avoidance of magnesium antacids (Mylanta, Maalox, Gelusil).	Prevents serious complications, e.g., reducing phosphate absorption from the GI tract and supplying calcium to maintain normal serum levels, reducing risk of bone demineralization/fractures, tetany; however, use of aluminum-containing products should be monitored, because accumulation in the bones potentiates osteodystrophy. Magnesium products potentiate risk of hypermagnesemia.
Stress importance of reading all product labels (drugs and food) and not taking medications without prior approval of healthcare provider.	It is difficult to maintain electrolyte balance when exogenous intake is not factored into dietary restrictions, e.g., hypercalcemia can result from routine supplement use in combination with increased dietary intake of calcium-fortified foods and medications containing calcium.
Review measures to prevent bleeding/hemorrhage, e.g., use of soft toothbrush, electric razor; avoidance of constipation, forceful blowing of nose, strenuous exercise/contact sports.	Reduces risks related to alteration of clotting factors/decreased platelet count.
Instruct in self-observation and self-monitoring of BP, including scheduling rest period before taking BP, using same arm/position.	Incidence of hypertension is increased in CRF, often requiring management with antihypertensive drugs, necessitating close observation of treatment effects, e.g., vascular response to medication.
Caution against exposure to external temperature extremes, e.g., heating pad/snow.	Peripheral neuropathy may develop, especially in lower extremities (effects of uremia, electrolyte/acid/base imbalances), impairing peripheral sensation and potentiating risk of tissue injury.
Establish routine exercise program, within individual ability; intersperse adequate rest periods with activities.	Aids in maintaining muscle tone and joint flexibility. Reduces risks associated with immobility (including bone demineralization), while preventing fatigue.
Address sexual concerns.	Physiologic effects of uremia/antihypertensive therapy may impair sexual desire/performance.
Identify available resources as indicated. Stress necessity of medical and laboratory follow-up.	Close monitoring of renal function and electrolyte balance is necessary to readjust treatment and/or make decisions about dialysis/transplantation.
Identify signs/symptoms requiring immediate medical evaluation, e.g.:	
Low-grade fever, chills, changes in characteristics of urine/sputum, tissue swelling/drainage, oral ulcerations;	Depressed immune system, anemia, malnutrition all contribute to increased risk of infection.
Numbness/tingling of digits, abdominal/muscle cramps, carpopedal spasms;	Uremia and decreased absorption of calcium may lead to peripheral neuropathies.

ACTIONS/INTERVENTIONS	RATIONALE
Independent	
Joint swelling/tenderness, decreased ROM, reduced muscle strength;	Hyperphosphatemia with corresponding calcium shifts from the bone may result in deposition of the excess calcium phosphate as calcifications in joints and soft tissues. Symptoms of skeletal involvement are often noted before impairment in organ function is evident.
Headaches, blurred vision, periorbital/sacral edema, "red eyes."	Suggestive of development/poor control of hypertension, and/or changes in eyes caused by calcium.
Review strategies to prevent constipation, including stool softeners (Colace) and bulk laxatives (Metamucil) but avoiding magnesium products (Milk of Magnesia).	Reduced fluid intake, changes in dietary pattern and use of phosphate-binding products often result in constipation that is not responsive to nonmedical interventions. Use of products containing magnesium increases risk of hypermagnesemia.

POTENTIAL CONSIDERATIONS following acute hospitalization (dependent on patient's age, physical condition/presence of complications, personal resources, and life responsibilities)

Fluid Volume, excess—compromised regulatory mechanism

Fatigue—decreased metabolic energy production/dietary restriction, anemia, increased energy requirements, e.g., fever/inflammation, tissue regeneration

Therapeutic Regimen: Individual, ineffective management—complexity of therapeutic regimen, decisional conflicts: patient value system; health beliefs, cultural influences; powerlessness; economic difficulties; family conflict; lack of/refusal of support systems

Hopelessness—deteriorating physiologic condition, long-term stress, prolonged activity limitations

RENAL DIALYSIS

Dialysis is a process that substitutes for renal function by removing excess fluid and/or accumulated endogenous or exogenous toxins. Dialysis is most often used for patients with acute or chronic (end-stage) renal disease. The two most common types are hemodialysis and peritoneal dialysis.

CARE SETTING

Community level/dialysis center, although inpatient acute stay may be required during initiation of therapy.

RELATED CONCERNS

Anemias (Iron Deficiency, Pernicious, Aplastic, Hemolytic), p 514
Heart Failure: Chronic, p 45
Peritonitis, p 366
Psychosocial Aspects of Care, p 783
Sepsis/Septicemia, p 719
Total Nutritional Support: Parenteral/Enteral Feeding, p 491

Patient Assessment Data Base

Refer to CPs: Renal Failure: Acute, p 555; Renal Failure: Chronic, p 568 for assessment information.

Discharge plan considerations: **DRG projected mean length of inpatient stay: 2.2 days to initiate therapy**
May require assistance with treatment regimen, transportation, ADLs, homemaker/maintenance tasks

Refer to section at end of plan for postdischarge considerations.

DIAGNOSTIC STUDIES

Studies and results are variable, depending on reason for dialysis (e.g., removal of excess fluid or toxins/drugs), degree of renal involvement, and patient considerations (e.g., distance from treatment center, cognition, available support).

NURSING PRIORITIES

1. Promote homeostasis.
2. Maintain comfort.
3. Prevent complications.
4. Support patient independence/self-care.
5. Provide information about disease process/prognosis and treatment needs.

DISCHARGE GOALS

1. Fluid and electrolyte balance maximized.
2. Complications prevented/minimized.
3. Discomfort alleviated.
4. Dealing realistically with current situation; independent within limits of condition.
5. Disease process/prognosis and therapeutic regimen understood.
6. Plan in place to meet needs after discharge.

GENERAL CONSIDERATIONS

This section addresses the general nursing management issues of the patient receiving some form of dialysis.

NURSING DIAGNOSIS: Nutrition: altered, less than body requirements

May be related to

GI disturbances (result of uremia/medication side effects): anorexia, n/v and stomatitis

Sensation of feeling full (abdominal distention during CAPD)

Dietary restrictions (bland, tasteless food); lack of interest in food

Loss of peptides and amino acids (building blocks for proteins) during dialysis

Possibly evidenced by

Inadequate food intake, aversion to eating, altered taste sensation

Poor muscle tone/weakness

Sore, inflamed buccal cavity; pale conjunctiva/mucous membranes

DESIRED OUTCOMES/EVALUATION CRITERIA—PATIENT WILL:

Demonstrate stable weight/gain toward goal with normalization of laboratory values and no signs of malnutrition.

ACTIONS/INTERVENTIONS	RATIONALE
Independent	
Monitor food/fluid ingested and calculate daily caloric intake.	Identifies nutritional deficits/therapy needs.
Recommend patient keep a food diary, including estimation of ingested calories, electrolytes (of individual concern, e.g., sodium, potassium, chloride, magnesium), and protein.	Helps patient to realize "big picture" and allows opportunity to alter dietary choices to meet individual desires within identified restriction.
Measure muscle mass via triceps skinfold or similar procedure. Determine muscle-to-fat ratio.	Assesses adequacy of nutrient utilization by measuring changes in fat deposits that may suggest presence/absence of tissue catabolism.
Note presence of nausea/anorexia.	Symptoms accompany accumulation of endogenous toxins that can alter/reduce intake and require intervention.
Encourage patient to participate in menu planning.	May enhance oral intake and promote sense of control/responsibility.
Recommend small, frequent meals. Schedule meals according to dialysis needs.	Smaller portions may enhance intake. Type of dialysis influences meal patterns, e.g., patients receiving hemodialysis might not be fed directly before/during procedure, because this can alter fluid removal; and patients undergoing peritoneal dialysis may be unable to ingest food while abdomen is distended with dialysate.
Suggest socialization during meals.	Provides diversion and promotes social aspects of eating.
Encourage frequent mouth care.	Reduces discomfort of oral stomatitis and undesirable/metallic taste in mouth, which can interfere with food intake.
Collaborative	
Refer to dietitian.	Useful for individualizing dietary program to meet cultural/lifestyle needs enhancing patient cooperation.

ACTIONS/INTERVENTIONS	RATIONALE
Collaborative	
Provide a high-carbohydrate diet that includes ordered amount of high-quality protein and essential amino acids with restriction of sodium/potassium as indicated.	Provides sufficient nutrients to improve energy and prevent muscle wasting (catabolism); promotes tissue regeneration/healing, and electrolyte balance. *Note:* 50% of protein intake should be derived from protein sources with high biologic value, such as red meat, poultry, fish.
Administer multivitamins, including ascorbic acid, folic acid, vitamin D, and iron supplements, as indicated.	Replaces vitamin/mineral deficits (malnutrition/anemia or lost during dialysis).
Administer parenteral supplements as indicated.	Hyperalimentation may be needed to enhance renal tubular regeneration/resolution of underlying disease process and to provide nutrients if oral/enteral feeding is contraindicated.
Monitor laboratory studies e.g.,	
Serum protein, prealbumin/albumin levels;	Indicator of protein needs. *Note:* Peritoneal dialysis is associated with significant protein loss.
Hb, RBC and iron levels.	Anemia is the most pervasive complication affecting energy levels in end-stage renal disease.
Administer medications as appropriate:	
Antiemetics, e.g., prochlorperazine (Compazine);	Reduces stimulation of the vomiting center.
Histamine blockers, e.g., famotidine (Pepcid);	Gastric distress is common and may be a neuropathy-induced gastric paresis. Hypersecretion can cause persistent gastric distress and digestive dysfunction.
Hormones and supplements as indicated, e.g., erythropoietin (EPO, Epogen) and iron supplement (Niferex).	While EPO is given to increase numbers of RBCs, it is not effective without iron supplementation. Nifrex is preferred as it can be given once daily and has fewer side effects than many iron preparations.
Insert/maintain nasogastric tube if indicated.	May be necessary when persistent vomiting occurs or when enteral feeding is desired.

NURSING DIAGNOSIS: Physical Mobility, impaired

May be related to
Restrictive therapies, e.g., lengthy dialysis procedure
Fear of/real danger of dislodging dialysis lines/catheter
Decreased strength/endurance; musculoskeletal impairment
Perceptual/cognitive impairment

Possibly evidenced by
Reluctance to attempt movement
Inability to move within physical environment
Decreased muscle mass/tone and strength
Impaired coordination
Pain, discomfort

DESIRED OUTCOMES/EVALUATION CRITERIA—PATIENT WILL:
Maintain optimal mobility/function.
Display increased strength and be free of associated complications (contractures, decubiti).

ACTIONS/INTERVENTIONS	RATIONALE

Independent

Assess activity limitations, noting presence/degree of restriction/ability.

Influences choice of interventions.

Encourage frequent change of position when on bed/chair rest; support affected body parts/joints with pillows, rolls, sheepskin, elbow/heel pads as indicated.

Decreases discomfort, maintains muscle strength/joint mobility, enhances circulation, and prevents skin breakdown.

Provide gentle massage. Keep skin clean and dry. Keep linens dry and wrinkle-free.

Stimulates circulation; prevents skin irritation.

Encourage deep breathing and coughing. Elevate head of bed as appropriate.

Mobilizes secretions, improves lung expansion, and reduces risk of respiratory complications, e.g., atelectasis, pneumonia.

Suggest diversion as appropriate to patient's condition, e.g., visitors, radio/television, books.

Decreases boredom; promotes relaxation.

Instruct in and assist with active/passive ROM exercises.

Maintains joint flexibility, prevents contractures, and aids in reducing muscle tension.

Institute a planned activity/exercise program as appropriate, with patient's input.

Increases patient's energy and sense of well-being/control. Studies have shown that regular exercise programs have benefitted end-stage renal disease patients both physically and emotionally, and, in stable patients, have not been shown to have adverse effects.

Collaborative

Provide foam/flotation mattress.

Reduces tissue pressure and may enhance circulation, thereby reducing risk of dermal ischemia/breakdown.

NURSING DIAGNOSIS: Self Care deficit (specify)

May be related to
Perceptual/cognitive impairment (accumulated toxins)
Intolerance to activity; decreased strength and endurance; pain/discomfort

Possibly evidenced by
Reported inability to carry out ADLs
Disheveled/unkempt appearance, strong body odor

DESIRED OUTCOMES/EVALUATION CRITERIA—PATIENT WILL:
Participate in ADLs within level of own ability/constraints of the illness.

ACTIONS/INTERVENTIONS	RATIONALE

Independent

Determine patient's ability to participate in self-care activities (scale of 0–4).

Underlying condition will dictate level of deficit/needs.

Provide assistance with activities as necessary.

Meets needs while supporting patient participation and independence.

ACTIONS/INTERVENTIONS

Independent

Encourage/use energy-saving techniques, e.g., sitting, not standing; shower chair; doing tasks in small increments.

Recommend scheduling activities to allow patient sufficient time to accomplish tasks to fullest extent of ability.

RATIONALE

Conserves energy, reduces fatigue, and enhances patient ability to perform tasks.

Unhurried approach reduces frustration, promotes patient participation, enhancing self-esteem.

NURSING DIAGNOSIS: Constipation, risk for

Risk factors may include
Decreased fluid intake, altered dietary pattern
Reduced intestinal motility, compression of bowel (peritoneal dialysate); electrolyte imbalances; decreased mobility

Possibly evidenced by
[Not applicable; presence of signs and symptoms establishes an *actual* diagnosis]

DESIRED OUTCOMES/EVALUATION CRITERIA—PATIENT WILL:
Maintain usual/improved bowel function.

ACTIONS/INTERVENTIONS

Independent

Auscultate bowel sounds. Note consistency/frequency of BMs, presence of abdominal distention.

Review current medication regimen.

Ascertain usual dietary pattern/food choices.

Suggest adding fresh fruits, vegetables, and fiber to diet (within restrictions) when indicated.

Encourage/assist with ambulation when able.

Provide privacy at bedside commode/bathroom.

Collaborative

Administer stool softeners (e.g., Colace), bulk-forming laxatives (e.g., Metamucil) as indicated.

Keep patient NPO; insert NG tube as indicated.

RATIONALE

Decreased bowel sounds, passage of hard-formed/dry stools suggests constipation and requires ongoing intervention to manage.

Side effects of some drugs (e.g., iron products, some antacids) may compound problem.

Although restrictions may be present, thoughtful consideration of menu choices can aid in controlling problem.

Provides bulk, which improves stool consistency.

Activity may stimulate peristalsis, promoting return to normal bowel activity.

Promotes psychologic comfort needed for elimination.

Produces a softer/more easily evacuated stool.

Decompresses stomach when recurrent episodes of unrelieved vomiting occur. Large gastric output suggests ileus (common early complication of peritoneal dialysis) with accumulation of gas and intestinal fluid that cannot be passed rectally.

> **NURSING DIAGNOSIS: Thought Processes, altered**
>
> **May be related to**
>
> Physiologic changes, e.g., presence of uremic toxins, electrolyte imbalances, hypervolemia/fluid shifts; hyperglycemia (infusion of a dialysate with a high-glucose concentration)
>
> **Possibly evidenced by**
>
> Changes in mentation/behavior, e.g., decreased concentration, memory; disorientation; altered sleep patterns; lethargy, confusion, stupor, dementia
>
> **DESIRED OUTCOMES/EVALUATION CRITERIA—PATIENT WILL:**
>
> Regain usual/improved level of mentation.
>
> Recognize changes in thinking/behavior and demonstrate behaviors to prevent/minimize changes.

ACTIONS/INTERVENTIONS	RATIONALE
Independent	
Assess for behavioral change/change in level of consciousness, e.g., orientation to time, place, and person.	May indicate level of uremic toxicity, response to or developing complication of dialysis, and requires further assessment/intervention.
Keep explanations simple, reorient frequently. Provide "normal" day/night lighting patterns, clock, calendar.	Improves reality orientation.
Provide a safe environment, restrain as indicated, pad side rails during procedure as appropriate.	Prevents patient trauma and/or inadvertent removal of dialysis lines/catheter.
Drain peritoneal dialysate promptly at end of specified equilibration period.	Prompt outflow will decrease risk of hyperglycemia/hyperosmolar fluid shifts affecting cerebral function.
Investigate reports of headache, associated with onset of nausea/vomiting, confusion/agitation, hypertension, tremors, or seizure activity.	May reflect development of disequilibrium syndrome, which can occur near completion of/following hemodialysis and is thought to be caused by ultrafiltration or by the too rapid removal of urea from the bloodstream not accompanied by equivalent removal from brain tissue. The hypertonic CSF causes a fluid shift into the brain, resulting in cerebral edema.
Monitor changes in speech pattern, development of dementia, myoclonus activity during hemodialysis.	Occasionally, accumulation of aluminum may cause dialysis dementia, progressing to death if untreated.
Collaborative	
Monitor BUN/Cr, serum glucose; alternate/change dialysate concentrations or add insulin as indicated.	Follows progression/resolution of azotemia. Hyperglycemia may develop secondary to glucose crossing peritoneal membrane and entering circulation. May require initiation of insulin therapy.
Obtain aluminum level as indicated.	Elevation may warn of impending cerebral involvement/dialysis dementia.
Administer medication, as indicated, e.g., phenytoin (Dilantin).	If disequilibrium syndrome occurs during dialysis, medication may be needed to control seizures in addition to a change in dialysis prescription or discontinuation of therapy.

May be related to

Situational crisis, threat to self-concept; change in health status/role functioning, socioeconomic status

Threat of death, unknown consequences/outcome

Possibly evidenced by

Increased tension, apprehension, uncertainty, fear

Expressed concerns

Sympathetic stimulation; focus on self

DESIRED OUTCOMES/EVALUATION CRITERIA—PATIENT WILL:

Verbalize awareness of feelings and reduction of anxiety/fear to a manageable level.

Demonstrate problem-solving skills and effective use of resources.

Appear relaxed, able to rest/sleep appropriately.

ACTIONS/INTERVENTIONS	RATIONALE
Independent	
Assess level of fear of both patient and SO. Note signs of denial, depression, or narrowed focus of attention.	Helps determine the kind of interventions required.
Explain procedures/care as delivered. Repeat explanations frequently/as needed. Provide information in multiple formats, including pamphlets and films.	Fear of unknown is lessened by information/knowledge and may enhance acceptance of dialysis. Alteration in thought processes and high levels of anxiety/fear may reduce comprehension, requiring repetition of important information. *Note:* Uremia can impair short-term memory, requiring repetition/reinforcement of information provided.
Acknowledge normalcy of feelings in this situation.	Knowing feelings are normal can allay fear that patient is losing control.
Provide opportunities for patient/SO to ask questions and verbalize concerns.	Creates feeling of openness and cooperation and provides information that will assist in problem identification/solving.
Encourage SO to participate in care, as indicated.	Involvement promotes sense of sharing, strengthens feelings of usefulness, provides opportunity to acknowledge individual capabilities, and may lessen fear of the unknown.
Acknowledge concerns of patient/SO.	Prognosis/possibility of need for long-term dialysis and resultant lifestyle changes are a major concern for this patient and those who may be involved in future care.
Point out positive indicators of treatment, e.g., improvement in laboratory values, stable BP, lessened fatigue.	Promotes sense of success/progress.
Collaborative	
Arrange for visit to dialysis center/meeting with another dialysis patient as appropriate.	Interaction with others who have encountered similar problems may assist patient/SO to work toward acceptance of chronic condition/focus on problem-solving activities.

NURSING DIAGNOSIS: Body Image disturbance/Self Esteem, situational low

May be related to
Situational crisis, chronic illness with changes in usual roles/body image

Possibly evidenced by
Verbalization of changes in lifestyle; focus on past function, negative feelings about body; feelings of helplessness, powerlessness

Extension of body boundary to incorporate environmental objects (e.g., dialysis machine)

Change in social involvement

Overdependence on others for care, not taking responsibility for self-care/lack of follow-through, self-destructive behavior

DESIRED OUTCOMES/EVALUATION CRITERIA—PATIENT WILL:
Identify feelings and methods for coping with negative perception of self.

Verbalize acceptance of self in situation.

Demonstrate adaptation to changes/events that have occurred, as evidenced by setting realistic goals and active participation in care/life.

ACTIONS/INTERVENTIONS	RATIONALE
Independent	
Assess level of patient's knowledge about condition and treatment, and anxiety related to current situation.	Identifies extent of problem/concern and necessary interventions.
Discuss meaning of loss/change to the patient.	Some patients may view situation as a challenge, though many have difficulty dealing with changes in life/role performance and loss of ability to control own body.
Note withdrawn behavior, ineffective use of denial or behaviors indicative of overconcern with body and its functions.	Indicators of developing difficulty handling stress of what is happening.
Assess use of addictive substances (e.g., alcohol), self-destructive/suicidal behavior.	May reflect dysfunctional coping and attempt to handle problems in an ineffective manner.
Determine stage of grieving. Note signs of severe/prolonged depression.	Identification of stage patient is experiencing provides guide to recognizing and dealing appropriately with behavior. Prolonged depression may indicate need for further intervention.
Acknowledge normalcy of feelings.	Recognition that feelings are to be expected helps patient to accept and deal with them more effectively.
Encourage verbalization of personal and work conflicts that may arise. Active-listen concerns.	Helps patient to identify problems and problem-solve solutions.
Determine patient's role in family constellation and patient's perception of expectation of self and others.	Long-term/permanent illness and disability alter patient's ability to fulfill usual role(s) in family/work setting. Unrealistic expectations can undermine self-esteem and affect outcome of illness.
Recommend SO treat patient normally and not as an invalid.	Conveys expectation that patient is able to manage situation and helps to maintain sense of self-esteem and purpose in life.

587

ACTIONS/INTERVENTIONS

Independent

Assist patient to incorporate disease management into lifestyle.

Identify strengths, past successes, previous methods patient has used to deal with life stressors.

Help patient identify areas over which they have some measure of control. Provide opportunity to participate in decision-making process.

Collaborative

Recommend participation in local support group.

Refer to healthcare/community resources, e.g., social service, vocational counselor, psychiatric nurse specialist.

RATIONALE

Necessities of treatment assume a more normal aspect when they are a part of the daily routine.

Focusing on these reminders of own ability to deal with problems can help patient to deal with current situation.

Provides sense of control over uncontrollable situation, fostering independence.

Reduces sense of isolation as patient learns that others have been where patient is now. Provides role models for dealing with situation, problem solving. Reinforces that therapeutic regimen can be beneficial.

Provides additional assistance for long-term management of chronic illness/change in lifestyle.

NURSING DIAGNOSIS: Knowledge deficit [learning need] regarding condition, prognosis, treatment, self care and discharge needs

May be related to
Lack of exposure/recall
Unfamiliarity with information resources
Cognitive limitations

Possibly evidenced by
Questions/request for information; statement of misconception
Inaccurate follow-through of instruction/development of preventable complications

DESIRED OUTCOMES/EVALUATION CRITERIA—PATIENT WILL:
Verbalize understanding of condition and relationship of signs/symptoms of the disease process.
Correctly perform necessary procedures and explain reasons for actions.

ACTIONS/INTERVENTIONS

Independent

Note level of anxiety/fear and alteration of thought processes.

Review particular disease process, procedures, and purpose of dialysis in terms understandable to the patient. Repeat explanations as required.

RATIONALE

These factors directly affect ability to participate/access and use knowledge. In addition, studies indicate that during the dialysis procedure, the patient's cognitive function may be impaired and that patients themselves state that they feel "fuzzy." Therefore, learning may not be optimal during this time.

Providing information at the level of the patient/SO understanding will reduce anxiety and misconceptions about what the patient is experiencing.

ACTIONS/INTERVENTIONS	RATIONALE
Independent	
Acknowledge that certain feelings/patterns of response are normal during course of therapy.	Patient/SO may initially be hopeful and positive about the future, but as treatment continues and progress is less dramatic, they can become discouraged/depressed, and conflicts of dependence/independence may develop.
Encourage and provide opportunity for questions.	Enhances learning process, promotes informed decision making, and reduces anxiety associated with the unknown.
Stress necessity of reading all product labels (food/beverage and OTC drugs) and not taking medications without prior approval of healthcare provider.	It is difficult to maintain electrolyte balance when exogenous intake is not factored into dietary restriction, e.g., hypercalcemia can result from routine supplement use in combination with increased dietary intake of calcium-fortified foods and medicines.
Discuss significance of maintaining nutritious eating habits; preventing wide fluctuation of fluid/electrolyte balance; avoidance of crowds/people with infectious processes.	Depressed immune system, presence of anemia, invasive procedures, and malnutrition potentiate risk of infection.
Instruct patient/SO in home dialysis as indicated:	
Purpose of dialysis;	Provides knowledge base on which patient can make informed observations/choices.
Operation and maintenance of equipment (including vascular shunt); sources of supplies;	Information diminishes anxiety of the unknown and provides opportunity for patient to be knowledgeable about own care.
Aseptic/clean technique;	Prevents contamination and reduces risk of infection.
Self-monitoring of effectiveness of procedure;	Provides information necessary to evaluate effects of therapy/need for change.
Management of potential complications;	Reduces concerns regarding personal well-being; supports efforts at self-care.
Contact person.	Readily available support person can answer questions, troubleshoot problems, and facilitate timely medical intervention when indicated.
Instruct patient about Epoetin alpha when indicated. Have patient/SO demonstrate ability to self-administer and state adverse side effects and healthcare practices associated with this therapy.	Epogen was recently approved by the Food and Drug Administration for the management of the anemia associated with CRF. The drug is given to increase and maintain RBC production, which can allow the patient to feel better and stronger. Contraindications may include adverse side effects such as polycythemia/increased clotting, failure to administer correctly or have appropriate follow-up.
Identify healthcare/community resources, e.g., dialysis support group, social services, mental health clinic.	Knowledge and use of these resources assist patient/SO to manage care more effectively. Interaction with others in similar situation provides opportunity for discussion of options and in making informed choices, e.g., stopping dialysis, renal transplantation.

(Refer to Renal Dialysis: Peritoneal, following, or Acute Hemodialysis, p 596, to complete the plan of care.)

POTENTIAL CONSIDERATIONS following acute hospitalization (dependent on patient's age, physical condition/presence of complications, personal resources, and life responsibilities)

Fatigue—decreased metabolic energy production, states of discomfort, overwhelming psychologic or emotional demands, altered body chemistry

Fluid Volume excess—fluid retention/excessive intake, inadequate therapeutic regimen

Infection, risk for—invasive procedures, decreased hemoglobin, chronic disease, malnutrition

Caregiver Role Strain, risk for—severity of illness of care receiver, discharge of family member with significant home care needs, caregiver is female/spouse, presence of situational stressors

RENAL DIALYSIS: PERITONEAL

The peritoneum serves as the semipermeable membrane permitting transfer of nitrogenous wastes/toxins and fluid from the blood into a dialysate solution. Peritoneal dialysis is sometimes preferred because it uses a simpler technique and provides more gradual physiologic changes than hemodialysis.

The manual single-bag method is usually done as an inpatient procedure with short dwell times of only 30–60 minutes, and is repeated until desired effects are achieved.

Continuous ambulatory peritoneal dialysis (CAPD) permits the patient to manage procedure at home with bag and gravity flow, using a prolonged dwell time at night and a total of 3–5 cycles daily, 7 days a week.

Continuous cycling peritoneal dialysis (CCPD) mechanically cycles shorter dwell times during night, with a longer dwell time during daylight hours, increasing the patient's independence.

NURSING DIAGNOSIS: Fluid Volume excess, risk for

Risk factors may include
Inadequate osmotic gradient of dialysate
Fluid retention (malpositioned or kinked/clotted catheter, bowel distention; peritonitis, scarring of peritoneum)
Excessive PO/IV intake

Possibly evidenced by
[Not applicable; presence of signs and symptoms establishes an *actual* diagnosis]

DESIRED OUTCOMES/EVALUATION CRITERIA—PATIENT WILL:
Demonstrate dialysate outflow exceeding/approximating infusion.
Experience no rapid weight gain, edema, or pulmonary congestion.

ACTIONS/INTERVENTIONS

Independent

Maintain a record of inflow/outflow volumes, and cumulative fluid balance.

Record serial weights, compare with I&O balance. Weigh patient when abdomen is empty of dialysate (consistent reference point).

Assess patency of catheter, noting difficulty in draining. Note presence of fibrin strings/plugs.

Check tubing for kinks; note placement of bottles/bags. Anchor catheter so that adequate inflow/outflow is achieved.

Turn from side to side, elevate the head of the bed, apply gentle pressure to the abdomen.

Note abdominal distention associated with decreased bowel sounds, changes in stool consistency, reports of constipation.

Monitor BP and pulse, noting hypertension, bounding pulses, neck vein distention, peripheral edema; measure CVP if available.

RATIONALE

In most cases, the amount drained should equal or exceed the amount instilled. A positive balance indicates need of further evaluation.

Serial body weights are an accurate indicator of fluid volume status. A positive fluid balance with an increase in weight indicates fluid retention.

Slowing of flow rate/presence of fibrin suggests partial catheter occlusion requiring further evaluation/intervention.

Improper functioning of equipment may result in retained fluid in abdomen and insufficient clearance of toxins.

May enhance outflow of fluid when catheter is malpositioned/obstructed by the omentum.

Bowel distention/constipation may impede outflow of effluent. (Refer to CP: Renal Dialysis; ND: Constipation, risk for, p 584.)

Elevations indicate hypervolemia. Assess heart and breath sounds, noting S_3 and/or crackles, rhonchi. Fluid overload may potentiate HF/pulmonary edema.

591

ACTIONS/INTERVENTIONS

Independent

Evaluate development of tachypnea, dyspnea, increased respiratory effort. Drain dialysate, and notify physician.

Assess for headache, muscle cramps, mental confusion, disorientation.

Collaborative

Alter dialysate regimen as indicated.

Monitor serum sodium.

Add heparin to initial dialysis runs, assist with irrigation of catheter with heparinized saline.

Maintain fluid restriction as indicated.

RATIONALE

Abdominal distention/diaphragmatic compression may cause respiratory distress.

Symptoms suggest hyponatremia or water intoxication.

Changes may be needed in the glucose or sodium concentration to facilitate efficient dialysis.

Hypernatremia may be present, although serum levels may reflect dilutional effect of fluid volume overload.

May be useful in preventing fibrin clot formation, which can obstruct peritoneal catheter.

Fluid restrictions may have to be continued to decrease fluid volume overload.

NURSING DIAGNOSIS: Fluid Volume deficit, risk for

Risk factors may include
Use of hypertonic dialysate with excessive removal of fluid from circulating volume.

Possibly evidenced by
[Not applicable; presence of signs and symptoms establishes an *actual* diagnosis]

DESIRED OUTCOMES/EVALUATION CRITERIA—PATIENT WILL:
Achieve desired alteration in fluid volume and weight with BP electrolyte levels within acceptable range.
Experience no symptoms of dehydration.

ACTIONS/INTERVENTIONS

Independent

Maintain record of inflow/outflow volumes and individual/cumulative fluid balance.

Adhere to schedule for draining dialysate from abdomen.

Weigh when abdomen is empty, following initial 6–10 runs, then as indicated.

Monitor BP (lying and sitting) and pulse. Note level of jugular pulsation.

Note reports of dizziness, nausea, increasing thirst.

Inspect mucous membranes, evaluate skin turgor, peripheral pulses, capillary refill.

RATIONALE

Provides information about the status of the patient's loss or gain at the end of each exchange.

Prolonged dwell times, especially when 4.5% glucose solution is used, may cause excessive fluid loss.

Detects rate of fluid removal by comparison with baseline body weights.

Decreased BP, postural hypotension, and tachycardia are early signs of hypovolemia.

May indicate hypovolemia/hyperosmolar syndrome.

Dry mucous membranes, poor skin turgor and diminished pulses/capillary refill are indicators of dehydration and need for increased intake/changes in strength of dialysate.

ACTIONS/INTERVENTIONS

Collaborative

Monitor laboratory studies as indicated, e.g.:

Serum sodium and glucose levels;

Serum potassium levels.

RATIONALE

Hypertonic solutions may cause hypernatremia by removing more water than sodium. In addition, dextrose may be absorbed from the dialysate, thereby elevating serum glucose.

Hypokalemia may occur and can cause cardiac dysrhythmias.

NURSING DIAGNOSIS: Trauma, risk for

Risk factors may include
Catheter inserted into peritoneal cavity
Site near the bowel/bladder with potential for perforation during insertion or by manipulation of the catheter

Possibly evidenced by
[Not applicable; presence of signs and symptoms establishes an *actual* diagnosis]

DESIRED OUTCOMES/EVALUATION CRITERIA—PATIENT WILL:
Experience no injury to bowel or bladder.

ACTIONS/INTERVENTIONS

Independent

Have patient empty bladder prior to peritoneal catheter insertion if indwelling catheter not present.

Anchor catheter/tubing with tape. Stress importance of patient avoiding pulling/pushing on catheter. Restrain hands if indicated.

Note presence of fecal material in dialysate effluent, or strong urge to defecate, accompanied by severe, watery diarrhea.

Note reports of intense urge to void, or large urine output following initiation of dialysis run. Test urine for sugar as indicated.

Stop dialysis if there is evidence of bowel/bladder perforation, leaving peritoneal catheter in place.

RATIONALE

An empty bladder is more distant from insertion site and reduces likelihood of being punctured during catheter insertion.

Reduces risk of trauma by manipulation of the catheter.

Suggests bowel perforation with mixing of dialysate and bowel contents.

Suggests bladder perforation with dialysate leaking into bladder. Presence of glucose-containing dialysate in the bladder, will elevate glucose level of urine.

Prompt action will prevent further injury. Immediate surgical repair may be required. Leaving catheter in place facilitates diagnosing/locating the perforation.

NURSING DIAGNOSIS: Pain [acute]

May be related to
Insertion of catheter through abdominal wall/catheter irritation, improper catheter placement
Irritation/infection within the peritoneal cavity
Infusion of cold or acidic dialysate, abdominal distention, rapid infusion of dialysate

ACTIONS/INTERVENTIONS	RATIONALE
Independent	
Investigate patient's reports of pain; note intensity (0–10), location, and precipitating factors.	Assists in identification of source of pain and appropriate interventions.
Explain that initial discomfort usually subsides after the first few exchanges.	Explanation may reduce anxiety and promote relaxation during procedure.
Monitor for pain that begins during inflow and continues during equilibration phase. Slow infusion rate as indicated.	Pain will occur at these times if acidic dialysate causes chemical irritation of peritoneal membrane.
Note reports of discomfort that is most pronounced near the end of inflow and instill no more than 2000 ml of solution at a single time.	Likely the result of abdominal distention from dialysate. Amount of infusion may have to be decreased initially.
Prevent air from entering peritoneal cavity during infusion. Note report of pain in area of shoulder blade.	Inadvertent introduction of air into the abdomen irritates the diaphragm and results in referred pain to shoulder blade. This type of discomfort may also be reported during initiation of therapy/during infusions and usually is related to stretching/irritation of the diaphragm with abdominal distention. Smaller exchange volumes may be required until patient adjusts.
Elevate head of bed at intervals. Turn patient from side to side. Provide back care and tissue massage.	Position changes and gentle massage may relieve abdominal and general muscle discomfort.
Warm dialysate to body temperature before infusing.	Warming the solution increases the rate of urea removal by dilating peritoneal vessels. Cold dialysate causes vasoconstriction, which can cause discomfort and/or excessively lower the core body temperature, precipitating cardiac arrest.
Monitor for severe/continuous abdominal pain, and temperature elevation (especially after dialysis has been discontinued).	May indicate developing peritonitis. (Refer to ND: Infection, risk for [peritonitis], following.)
Encourage use of relaxation techniques, e.g., deep-breathing exercises, guided imagery, visualization. Provide diversional activities.	Redirects attention, promotes sense of control.
Collaborative	
Administer analgesics.	Relieves pain and discomfort.
Add sodium hydroxide to dialysate, if indicated.	Occasionally used to alter pH if patient is not tolerating acidic dialysate.

NURSING DIAGNOSIS: Infection, risk for [peritonitis]

Risk factors may include
Contamination of the catheter during insertion, periodic changing of tubings/bags
Skin contaminants at catheter insertion site
Sterile peritonitis (response to the composition of dialysate)

Possibly evidenced by
[Not applicable; presence of signs and symptoms establishes an *actual* diagnosis]

DESIRED OUTCOMES/EVALUATION CRITERIA—PATIENT WILL:
Identify interventions to prevent/reduce risk of infection.
Experience no signs/symptoms of infection.

ACTIONS/INTERVENTIONS	RATIONALE
Independent	
Observe meticulous aseptic techniques and wear masks during catheter insertion, dressing changes and whenever the system is opened. Change tubings per protocol.	Prevents the introduction of organisms and airborne contamination that may cause infection.
Change dressings as indicated, being careful not to dislodge the catheter. Note character, color, odor or drainage from around insertion site.	Moist environment promotes bacterial growth. Purulent drainage at insertion site suggests presence of local infection. *Note:* Polyurethane adhesive film (e.g., Blister film) dressings have been found to decrease amount of pressure on catheter and exit site, as well as incidence of site infections.
Observe color and clarity of effluent.	Cloudy effluent is suggestive of peritoneal infection.
Apply povidone-iodine (Betadine) barrier in distal, clamped portion of catheter when intermittent dialysis therapy used.	Reduces risk of bacterial entry through catheter between dialysis treatments when catheter is disconnected from closed system.
Investigate reports of nausea/vomiting, increased/severe abdominal pain; rebound tenderness, fever, and leukocytosis.	Signs/symptoms suggesting peritonitis, requiring prompt intervention.
Collaborative	
Monitor WBC count of effluent.	Presence of WBCs initially may reflect normal response to a foreign substance; however, continued/new elevation suggests developing infection.
Obtain specimens of blood, effluent, and/or drainage from insertion site as indicated for culture/sensitivity.	Identifies types of organism(s) present, choice of interventions.
Monitor renal clearance/BUN, Cr.	Choice and dosage of antibiotics will be influenced by renal function.
Administer antibiotics systemically or in dialysate as indicated.	Treats infection, prevents sepsis.

ACTIONS/INTERVENTIONS	RATIONALE
Independent	
Monitor respiratory rate/effort. Reduce infusion rate if dyspnea is present.	Tachypnea, dyspnea, shortness of breath, and shallow breathing during dialysis suggests diaphragmatic pressure from distended peritoneal cavity or may indicate developing complications.
Auscultate lungs, noting decreased, absent, or adventitious breath sounds, e.g., crackles/wheezes/rhonchi.	Decreased areas of ventilation suggest presence of atelectasis, whereas adventitious sounds may suggest fluid overload, retained secretions, or infection.
Note character, amount, and color of secretions.	Patient is susceptible to pulmonary infections as a result of depressed cough reflex and respiratory effort, increased viscosity of secretions, as well as altered immune response and chronic/debilitating disease.
Elevate head of bed. Promote deep-breathing exercises and coughing.	Facilitates chest expansion/ventilation and mobilization of secretions.
Collaborative	
Review ABGs/pulse oximetry and serial chest x-rays.	Changes in Pao_2/$Paco_2$ and appearance of infiltrates/congestion on chest x-ray suggests developing pulmonary problems.
Administer supplemental O_2 as indicated.	Maximizes oxygen for vascular uptake, preventing/lessening hypoxia.
Administer analgesics as indicated.	Alleviates pain, promotes comfortable breathing, maximal cough effort.

ACUTE HEMODIALYSIS

Blood is shunted through an artificial kidney (dialyzer) for removal of toxins/excess fluid and then returned to the venous circulation. Hemodialysis is a faster and more efficient method than peritoneal dialysis for removing urea and other toxic products, but requires permanent arteriovenous access. Procedure is usually performed 2–3 times per week.

ACTIONS/INTERVENTIONS	RATIONALE
Independent	
Clotting	
Monitor internal AV shunt patency at frequent intervals:	
Palpate for distal thrill;	Thrill is caused by turbulence of high-pressure arterial blood flow entering low-pressure venous system and should be palpable above venous exit site.
Auscultate for a bruit;	Bruit is the sound caused by the turbulence of arterial blood entering venous system and should be audible by stethoscope, although may be very faint.
Note color of blood and/or obvious separation of cells and serum;	Change of color from uniform medium red to dark purplish red suggests sluggish blood flow/early clotting. Separation in tubing is indicative of clotting. Very dark reddish-black blood next to clear yellow fluid indicates full clot formation.
Palpate skin around shunt for warmth.	Diminished blood flow will result in "coolness" of shunt.
Notify physician and/or initiate declotting procedure if there is evidence of loss of shunt patency.	Rapid intervention may save access; however, declotting must be done by experienced personnel.
Evaluate reports of pain, numbness/tingling; note extremity swelling distal to access.	May indicate inadequate blood supply.
Avoid trauma to shunt; e.g., handle tubing gently, maintain cannula alignment. Limit activity of extremity. Avoid taking BP or drawing blood samples in shunt extremity. Instruct patient not to sleep or carry packages, books, purse on affected extremity.	Decreases risk of clotting/disconnection.
Hemorrhage	
Attach two cannula clamps to shunt dressing. Have tourniquet available. If cannulas separate, clamp first the arterial then the venous cannula. If tubing comes out of vessel, clamp cannula that is still in place and apply direct pressure to bleeding site. Place tourniquet above site or inflate BP cuff to pressure just above patient's systolic BP.	Prevents massive blood loss while awaiting medical assistance if cannula separates or shunt is dislodged.

ACTIONS/INTERVENTIONS	RATIONALE

Independent

Infection

Assess skin around vascular access, noting redness, swelling, local warmth, exudate, tenderness.	Signs of local infection, which can progress to sepsis if untreated.
Avoid contamination of access site. Use aseptic technique and masks when giving shunt care, applying/changing dressings, and when starting/completing dialysis process.	Prevents introduction of organisms that can cause infection.
Monitor temperature. Note presence of fever, chills, hypotension.	Signs of infection/sepsis requiring prompt medical intervention.

Collaborative

Culture the site/obtain blood samples as indicated.	Determines presence of pathogens.
Monitor PT, aPTT as appropriate.	Identifies treatment needs and evaluates effectiveness.
Administer medications as indicated, e.g.:	
Heparin (low-dose);	Infused on arterial side of filter to prevent clotting in the filter without systemic side effects.
Antibiotics (systemic and/or topical).	Prompt treatment of infection may save access, prevent sepsis.
Discuss use of ASA, Coumadin as appropriate.	Ongoing low-dose anticoagulation may be useful in maintaining patency of shunt.

NURSING DIAGNOSIS: Fluid Volume deficit, risk for

Risk factors may include
Ultrafiltration
Fluid restrictions; actual blood loss (systemic heparinization or disconnection of the shunt)

Possibly evidenced by
[Not applicable; presence of signs and symptoms establishes an *actual* diagnosis]

DESIRED OUTCOMES/EVALUATION CRITERIA—PATIENT WILL:
Maintain fluid balance as evidenced by stable/appropriate weight and vital signs, good skin turgor, moist mucous membranes, absence of bleeding.

ACTIONS/INTERVENTIONS	RATIONALE

Independent

Measure all sources of I&O. Have patient keep diary.	Aids in evaluating fluid status, especially when compared with weights. *Note:* Urine output is an inaccurate evaluation of renal function in dialysis patients. Some individuals have water output with little renal clearance of toxins while others have oliguria or anuria.
Weigh daily before/after dialysis run.	Weight loss over precisely measured time is a measure of ultrafiltration and fluid removal.

ACTIONS/INTERVENTIONS	RATIONALE
Independent	
Monitor BP, pulse, and hemodynamic pressures if available during dialysis.	Hypotension, tachycardia, falling hemodynamic pressures suggest volume depletion.
Note/ascertain whether diuretics and/or antihypertensives are to be withheld.	Dialysis potentiates hypotensive effects if these drugs have been administered.
Verify continuity of shunt/access catheter.	Disconnected shunt/open access will permit exsanguination.
Apply external shunt dressing. Permit no puncture of shunt.	Minimizes stress on cannula insertion site to reduce inadvertent dislodgement and bleeding from site.
Place patient in a supine/Trendelenburg's position as necessary.	Maximizes venous return if hypotension occurs.
Assess for oozing or frank bleeding at access site or mucous membranes, incisions/wounds. Hematest/guaiac stools, gastric drainage.	Systemic heparinization during dialysis increases clotting times and places patient at risk for bleeding, especially during the first 4 hours after procedure.
Collaborative	
Monitor laboratory studies as indicated:	
Hb/Hct;	May be reduced because of anemia, hemodilution, or actual blood loss.
Serum electrolytes and pH;	Imbalances may require changes in the dialysate solution or supplemental replacement to achieve balance.
Clotting times, e.g., PT/aPTT, and platelet count.	Use of heparin to prevent clotting in blood lines and hemofilter alters coagulation and potentiates active bleeding.
Administer IV solutions (e.g., normal saline)/volume expanders (e.g., albumin) during dialysis as indicated;	Saline/dextrose solutions, electrolytes, and $NaHCO_3$ may be infused in the venous side of CAV hemofilter when high ultrafiltration rates are used for removal of extracellular fluid and toxic solutes. Volume expanders may be required during/following hemodialysis if sudden/marked hypotension occurs.
Blood/packed RBCs if needed.	Destruction of RBCs (hemolysis) by mechanical dialysis, hemorrhagic losses, decreased RBC production may result in profound/progressive anemia.
Reduce rate of ultrafiltration during dialysis as indicated.	Reduces the amount of water being removed and may correct hypotension/hypovolemia.
Administer protamine sulfate if indicated.	May be needed to return clotting times to normal or if heparin rebound occurs (up to 16 hours after hemodialysis).

> **NURSING DIAGNOSIS: Fluid Volume excess, risk for**
>
> **Risk factors may include**
> Rapid/excessive fluid intake; IV, blood, plasma expanders, saline given to support BP during dialysis
>
> **Possibly evidenced by**
> [Not applicable; presence of signs and symptoms establishes an *actual* diagnosis]

599

ACTIONS/INTERVENTIONS	RATIONALE
Independent	
Measure all sources of I&O. Weigh routinely.	Aids in evaluating fluid status especially when compared with weight. Weight gain between treatments should not exceed 0.5 kg/d.
Monitor BP, pulse.	Hypertension and tachycardia between hemodialysis runs may result from fluid overload and/or heart failure.
Note presence of peripheral/sacral edema, respiratory rales, dyspnea, orthopnea, distended neck veins, ECG changes indicative of ventricular hypertrophy.	Fluid volume excess because of inefficient dialysis or repeated hypervolemia between dialysis treatments may cause/exacerbate heart failure, as indicated by signs/symptoms of respiratory and/or systemic venous congestion.
Note changes in mentation. (Refer to CP: Renal Dialysis; ND: Thought Processes, altered, p 585.)	Fluid overload/hypervolemia, may potentiate cerebral edema (disequilibrium syndrome).
Collaborative	
Monitor serum sodium levels. Restrict sodium intake as indicated.	High sodium levels are associated with fluid overload, edema, hypertension, and cardiac complications.
Restrict po/IV fluid intake as indicated, spacing allowed fluids through 24-hour period.	The intermittent nature of hemodialysis results in fluid retention/overload between procedures and may require fluid restriction. Spacing fluids helps reduce thirst.

URINARY DIVERSIONS/UROSTOMY (POSTOPERATIVE CARE)

Ileal conduit: Ureters are anastomosed to a segment of ileum resected with the blood supply intact (usually 15–20 cm long). The proximal section is closed, and the distal end brought to skin opening to form a stoma (a passageway, not a storage reservoir).

Colonic conduit: This is a similar procedure using a segment of colon.

Ureterostomy: The ureter(s) is brought directly through the abdominal wall to form its own stoma.

Continent diversion: A section of intestine is used to form a pouch inside the patient's abdomen creating a reservoir that the patient periodically drains by inserting a catheter through the stoma, thus negating the need for an external collecting device. In some male patients, with a Kock pouch (reservoir using small intestine), drainage may be achieved through the urethra using the valsalva maneuver at timed intervals.

CARE SETTING:

Inpatient acute surgical unit.

RELATED CONCERNS

Surgical Intervention, p 802
Peritonitis, p 366
Psychosocial Aspects of Care, p 783

Patient Assessment Data Base

Data is dependent on underlying problem, duration, and severity, e.g., malignant bladder tumor, congenital malformations, trauma, chronic infections, or intractable incontinence due to injury/disease of other body systems (e.g., multiple sclerosis). (Refer to appropriate CP.)

TEACHING/LEARNING

Discharge plan considerations: DRG projected mean length of inpatient stay: 5.5 days
May require assistance with management of ostomy and acquisition of supplies.

Refer to section at end of plan for postdischarge considerations.

DIAGNOSTIC STUDIES

IVP: Visualizes size/location of kidneys and ureters and rules out presence of tumors elsewhere in urinary tract.

Cystoscopy with biopsy: Determines tumor location/degree of malignancy. Ultraviolet cystoscopy outlines bladder lesion.

Bone scan: Determines presence of metastatic disease.

Bilateral pedal lymphangiogram: Determines involvement of pelvic nodes, where bladder tumor easily seeds because of close proximity.

CT scan: Defines size of tumor mass, degree of pelvic spread.

Urine cystoscopy: Detects tumor cells in urine (for determining presence and type of tumor).

Endoscopy: Evaluates intestines for use as conduit.

Conduitogram: Assesses length and emptying ability of the conduit and presence of stricture, obstruction, reflux, angulation, calculi, or tumor (may complicate or contraindicate use as a urinary diversion).

NURSING PRIORITIES

1. Prevent complications.
2. Assist patient/SO in physical and psychosocial adjustment.
3. Support independence in self-care.
4. Provide information about procedure/prognosis, treatment needs, potential complications, and resources.

601

DISCHARGE GOALS

1. Complications prevented/minimized.
2. Adjusting to perceived/actual changes.
3. Self-care needs met by self/with assistance as necessary.
4. Procedure/prognosis, therapeutic regimen, potential complications understood and sources of support identified.
5. Plan in place to meet needs after discharge.

NURSING DIAGNOSIS: Skin Integrity, impaired, risk for

Risk factors may include
Absence of sphincter at stoma [actual]
Character/flow of urine from stoma
Reaction to product/chemicals; improper fitting of appliance or removal of adhesive

Possibly evidenced by
[Not applicable; presence of signs and symptoms establishes an *actual* diagnosis]

DESIRED OUTCOMES/EVALUATION CRITERIA—PATIENT WILL:
Maintain skin integrity.
Identify individual risk factors.
Demonstrate behaviors/techniques to promote healing/prevent skin breakdown.

ACTIONS/INTERVENTIONS	RATIONALE
Independent	
Inspect stoma/peristomal skin. Note irritation, bruises (dark, bluish color), rashes, status of sutures.	Monitors healing process/effectiveness of appliances, and identifies areas of concern, need for further evaluation/intervention. Stoma should be pink or reddish, similar to mucous membranes. Color changes may be temporary, but persistent changes may require surgical intervention. Early identification of stomal necrosis/ischemia or fungal infection provides for timely interventions to prevent skin necrosis.
Clean with water and pat dry (or use hair dryer on cool setting).	Maintaining a clean/dry area helps to prevent skin breakdown.
Handle stoma gently to prevent irritation.	Mucosa has good blood supply and bleeds easily with rubbing or trauma.
Measure stoma periodically, e.g., each appliance change for first 6 weeks, then monthly times 6.	As postoperative edema resolves (during first 6 weeks), size of appliance must be altered to ensure proper fit so that urine is collected as it flows from the stoma, and contact with the skin is prevented.
Apply effective sealant barrier, e.g., Skin Prep or similar products.	Protects skin from pouch adhesive, enhances adhesives of pouch, and facilitates removal of pouch when necessary.
Make sure opening for adhesive backing of pouch is at least ⅛ in larger than the base of the stoma, with adequate adhesiveness left to apply pouch.	Prevents trauma to the stoma tissue and protects the peristomal skin. Adequate adhesive area is important to maintain a seal. *Note:* Too tight a fit may cause stomal edema or stenosis.

ACTIONS/INTERVENTIONS	RATIONALE
Independent	
Use a transparent, odor-proof drainable pouch. Keep gauze square/wick over stoma while cleansing area, and have patient cough or strain before applying pouch.	A transparent appliance during first 4–6 weeks allows easy observation of stoma and stents (when used) without necessity of removing pouch and irritating skin. Covering stoma prevents urine from wetting the peristomal area during pouch changes. Coughing empties distal portion of conduit, followed by a brief pause in drainage to facilitate application of pouch.
Avoid use of karaya-type appliances.	Will not protect skin as urine melts karaya.
Apply waterproof tape around pouch edges if desired.	Reinforces anchoring.
Connect collecting pouch to continuous bedside drainage system, when necessary.	May be needed during times when rate of urine formation is increased, e.g., while IV fluids are administered. Weight of the urine can cause pouch to pull loose/leak when pouch becomes more than half full.
Cleanse ostomy pouch on a routine basis, using vinegar solution.	Frequent pouch changes are irritating to the skin and should be avoided. Emptying and rinsing the pouch with vinegar not only removes bacteria but also deodorizes the pouch.
Change pouch every 3–5 days or as needed for leakage. Remove appliance gently while supporting skin. Use adhesive removers as indicated and wash off completely.	Prevents tissue irritation/destruction associated with "pulling" pouch off.
Investigate reports of burning/itching around stoma.	Suggests peristomal irritation or possibly Candida infections, both requiring intervention. *Note:* Continuous exposure of skin to urine can cause hyperplasia around stoma, affecting pouch fit and increasing risk of infection.
Evaluate adhesive product and appliance fit on ongoing basis.	Provides opportunity for problem solving. Determines need for further intervention.
Monitor for distention of lower abdomen (with ileal conduit); assess bowel sounds.	Intestinal distention can cause tension on new suture lines with possibility of rupture.
Collaborative	
Consult with enterostomal nurse.	Helpful in problem solving and choosing products appropriate for patient needs, considering stoma characteristics, patient's physical/mental status, and financial resources. In the presence of persistent or recurring problems, the ostomy nurse has a wider range of knowledge and resources.
Apply antifungal spray or powder, as indicated.	Assists in healing if peristomal irritation is caused by fungal infection. *Note:* These products can have potent side effects and should be used sparingly. Creams/ointments are to be avoided, because they interfere with adhesion of the appliance.

603

ACTIONS/INTERVENTIONS	RATIONALE
Independent	
Review reason for surgery and future expectations.	Patient may find it easier to accept/deal with an ostomy done for chronic/long-term disease (e.g., intractable incontinence, infections) than for traumatic injury.
Ascertain whether counseling was initiated when the possibility and/or necessity of urinary diversion was first discussed.	Provides information about patient's/SO's level of knowledge about individual situation and process of acceptance.
Answer all questions concerning urostomy and its function.	Establishes rapport and conveys interest/concern of caregiver. Provides additional information for patient to consider.
Encourage the patient/SO to verbalize feelings. Acknowledge normality of feelings of anger, depression, and grief over loss. Discuss daily "ups and downs" that can occur after discharge.	Provides opportunity to deal with issues/misconceptions. Helps the patient/SO to realize that feelings experienced are not unusual and that feeling guilty for them is not necessary/helpful. Patient needs to recognize feelings before they can be dealt with effectively.
Note behaviors of withdrawal, increased dependency, manipulation, or noninvolvement in care.	Suggestive of problems in adjustment that may require further evaluation and more extensive therapy. May reflect grief response to loss of body part/function and worry over acceptance by others as well as fear of further disability/loss of life from cancer.
Provide opportunities for patient/SO to view and touch stoma, using the moment to point out positive signs of healing, normal appearance, and so forth.	Although integration of stoma into body image can take months or even years, looking at the stoma and hearing comments (made in a normal, matter-of-fact manner) can help patient with this acceptance. Touching stoma reassures patient/SO that it is not fragile and that slight movements of stoma actually reflect normal peristalsis.

ACTIONS/INTERVENTIONS

Independent

Provide opportunity for patient to deal with ostomy through participation in self-care.

Maintain positive approach, during care activities, avoiding expressions of disdain or revulsion. Do not take patient's angry expressions personally.

Plan/schedule care activities with patient.

Discuss possibility of contacting ostomy/urostomy visitor and make arrangements for visit if desired.

Discuss sexual functioning and penile implant, if applicable, and alternate ways for sexual pleasuring. (Refer to ND: Sexual dysfunction, risk for, p 609.)

RATIONALE

Independence in self-care helps to improve self-esteem.

Assists patient/SO to accept body changes and feel all right about self. Anger is most often directed at the situation and lack of control individual has over what has happened (powerlessness), not the individual caregiver.

Promotes sense of control, and gives message that the patient can handle this, enhancing self-esteem.

Can provide a good support system. Helps to reinforce teaching (shared experiences) and facilitates acceptance of change as patient realizes "life does go on" and can be relatively normal.

Patient may experience anticipatory anxiety, fear of failure in relation to sex after surgery, usually because of ignorance, lack of knowledge. Surgery that removes the bladder and prostate (removed with the bladder) may disrupt parasympathetic nerve fibers that control erection in men, although newer techniques are available that may be used in individual cases to preserve these nerves.

NURSING DIAGNOSIS: Pain [acute]

May be related to
Physical factors, e.g., disruption of skin/tissues (incisions/drains)
Biologic: Activity of disease process (cancer, trauma)
Psychologic factors, e.g., fear, anxiety

Possibly evidenced by
Reports of pain, self-focusing
Guarding/distraction behaviors, restlessness
Autonomic responses, e.g., changes in vital signs

DESIRED OUTCOMES/EVALUATION CRITERIA—PATIENT WILL:
Verbalize/display relief of pain.
Demonstrate ability to assist with general comfort measures and able to sleep/rest appropriately.

ACTIONS/INTERVENTIONS

Independent

Assess pain, noting location, characteristics, intensity (0–10 scale).

RATIONALE

Helps evaluate degree of discomfort and effectiveness of analgesia or may reveal developing complications, e.g., because abdominal pain usually subsides gradually by the 3rd or 4th postoperative day, continued or increasing pain may reflect delayed healing, peristomal skin irritation, infection, intestinal obstruction.

605

ACTIONS/INTERVENTIONS	RATIONALE
Independent	
Auscultate bowel sounds; note passage of flatus.	Indicates reestablishment of bowel function. Lack of return of bowel sounds/function within 72 hours may indicate presence of complication, e.g., peritonitis, hypokalemia, mechanical obstruction.
Note urine flow and characteristics.	Decreased flow may reflect urinary retention (due to edema) with increased pressure in upper urinary tract or leakage into peritoneal cavity (failure of anastomosis). Cloudy urine may be normal (presence of mucus) or indicate infectious process.
Encourage patient to verbalize concerns. Active-listen these concerns and provide support by acceptance, remaining with patient and giving appropriate information.	Reduction of anxiety/fear can promote relaxation and comfort.
Provide comfort measures, e.g., back rub, repositioning (using body support measures as needed). Assure patient that position change will not injure stoma.	Reduces muscle tension, promotes relaxation, and may enhance coping abilities.
Encourage use of relaxation techniques, e.g., guided imagery, visualization, diversional activities.	Helps patient to rest more effectively and refocuses attention, which may enhance coping ability, reducing pain and discomfort.
Assist with ROM exercises and encourage early ambulation.	Reduces muscle/joint stiffness. Ambulation returns organs to normal position and promotes return of peristalsis/passage of flatus and feelings of general well-being.
Investigate and report abdominal muscle rigidity, involuntary guarding, and rebound tenderness.	Suggestive of peritoneal inflammation, requiring prompt medical intervention.
Collaborative	
Administer medications as indicated, e.g., narcotics, analgesics; PCA.	Relieves pain, enhances comfort, and promotes rest. PCA may be more beneficial than intermittent analgesia, especially following radical resection.
Provide sitz baths, if indicated.	Relieves local discomfort, reduces edema, and promotes healing of perineal wound associated with radical procedure.
Apply/monitor effects of TENS unit.	Cutaneous stimulation may be used to block transmission of pain stimulus.
Maintain patency of NG tube.	Decompresses stomach/intestines; prevents abdominal distention when intestinal function is impaired.

NURSING DIAGNOSIS: Infection, risk for

Risk factors may include

Inadequate primary defenses (e.g., break in skin/incision; reflux of urine into urinary tract)

Possibly evidenced by

[Not applicable; presence of signs and symptoms establishes an *actual* diagnosis]

DESIRED OUTCOMES/EVALUATION CRITERIA—PATIENT WILL:
Achieve timely wound healing, be free of purulent drainage or erythema, and be afebrile.
Verbalize understanding of individual causative/risk factors.
Demonstrate techniques, lifestyle changes to reduce risk.

ACTIONS/INTERVENTIONS	RATIONALE
Independent	
Empty ostomy pouch when it becomes one third full, once IV fluids and continuous pouch drainage have been discontinued.	Reduces risk of urinary reflux and maintains integrity of appliance seal if pouch does not have an antireflux valve.
Document urine characteristics, and note whether changes are associated with reports of flank pain.	Cloudy odorous urine indicates infection (possibly pyelonephritis); however, urine normally contains mucus after a conduit procedure.
Test urine pH with Nitrazine paper (use fresh specimen, not from pouch); notify physician if greater than 6.5.	Urine is normally acidic, which discourages bacterial growth/UTIs. *Note:* Presence of alkaline urine also creates favorable environment for stone formation in presence of hypercalciuria.
Report sudden cessation of urethral drainage.	Constant drainage usually subsides within 10 days; however, abrupt cessation may indicate plugging and lead to abscess formation.
Note red rash around stoma.	Rash is most commonly caused by yeast. Urine leakage or allergy to appliance or products may also cause red, irritated areas.
Inspect incision line around stoma. Observe and document wound drainage, signs of incisional inflammation, systemic indicators of sepsis.	Provides baseline reference. Complications may include interrupted anastomosis of intestine/bowel or ureteral conduit, with leakage of bowel contents into abdomen or urine into peritoneal cavity.
Change dressings as indicated when used.	Moist dressings act as a wick to the wound and provide media for bacterial growth.
Assess skinfold areas in groin, perineum, under arms and breasts.	Use of antibiotics and trapping of moisture in skinfold areas increases risk of monilial infections.
Monitor vital signs.	Elevation of temperature suggests incisional or UTI and/or respiratory complications.
Auscultate breath sounds.	Patient is at high risk for development of respiratory complications because of length of time under anesthesia. Often this patient is older and may already have a compromised immune system. Also, painful abdominal incisions cause patient to breathe more shallowly than normal and to limit coughing. Accumulation of secretions in respiratory system predisposes to atelectasis and infections.
Collaborative	
Use pouch with antireflux valve, if available.	Prevents backflow of urine into stoma, reducing risk of infection.

607

ACTIONS/INTERVENTIONS	RATIONALE
Collaborative	

ACTIONS/INTERVENTIONS	RATIONALE
Obtain specimens of exudates, urine, sputum, blood as indicated.	Identifies source of infection/most effective treatment. Infected urine may cause pyelonephritis. *Note:* Urine specimen must be obtained from the conduit because the pouch is considered contaminated.
Administer medications as indicated:	
Cephalosporins, e.g., cefoxitin (Mefoxin), cefazolin (Ancef);	Given to treat identified infection or may be given prophylactically, especially with history of recurrent pyelonephritis.
Antifungal powder;	Used to treat yeast infections around stoma.
Ascorbic acid/vitamin C.	Given to acidify urine, reduce bacterial growth/risk of infection. *Note:* Large doses of vitamin C can impair GI absorption of B_{12}, potentiating pernicious anemia.
Assist with injection of IV methylene blue.	Dye appearing in wound drainage signifies urine leakage into peritoneal cavity and need for surgical repair.

NURSING DIAGNOSIS: Urinary Elimination, altered

May be related to
Surgical diversion; tissue trauma, postoperative edema

Possibly evidenced by
Loss of continence
Changes in amount, character of urine; urinary retention

DESIRED OUTCOMES/EVALUATION CRITERIA—PATIENT WILL:
Display continuous flow of urine, with output adequate for individual situation.

ACTIONS/INTERVENTIONS	RATIONALE
Independent	
Assess for presence of stents/ureteral catheters. Label "right" and "left" and observe urine flow through each.	Maintains patency of ureters and assists in healing of anastomosis by keeping it urine-free.
Record urinary output; investigate sudden reduction/cessation of urine flow.	Sudden decrease in urine flow may indicate obstruction/dysfunction, (e.g., blockage by edema or mucus) or dehydration. *Note:* Reduced urinary output (not related to hypovolemia) associated with abdominal distention, fever, and clear/watery discharge from incision suggests urinary fistula, also requiring prompt intervention.
Observe and record color of urine. Note hematuria and/or bleeding from stoma.	Urine may be slightly pink, which should clear up in 2–3 days. Rubbing/washing stoma may cause temporary oozing due to vascular nature of tissues. Continued bleeding, frank blood in the pouch, or oozing around the base of stoma requires medical evaluation/intervention.

ACTIONS/INTERVENTIONS	RATIONALE

Independent

Position tubing and drainage pouch so that it allows unimpeded flow of urine. Monitor/protect placement of stents.

Blocked drainage allows pressure to build within urinary tract, risking anastomosis leakage and damage to renal parenchyma. *Note:* Stents inserted to maintain patency of ureters during period of postoperative edema may be inadvertently dislodged, compromising urine flow.

Demonstrate self-catheterization techniques and reservoir irrigations as appropriate.

Patients with continent diversions do not require an external collection device. Periodic catheterization empties the internal reservoir. Daily irrigations remove accumulated mucus from the reservoir. *Note:* Patients with Kock pouches connected to the urethra are instructed to void every 2 hours during the day and every 3 hours during the night. This is done by bearing down and applying hand pressure on the lower abdomen to aid in emptying the reservoir.

Encourage increased fluids and maintain accurate intake.

Maintains hydration and good urine flow.

Monitor vital signs. Assess peripheral pulses, skin turgor, capillary refill, and oral mucosa. Weigh daily.

Indicators of fluid balance. Reflects level of hydration and effectiveness of fluid replacement therapy.

Collaborative

Administer IV fluids as indicated.

Assists in maintaining hydration/adequate circulating volume and urinary flow.

Monitor electrolytes, ABGs, calcium.

Impaired renal function in patient with intestinal conduit increases risk of severe electrolyte and/or acid/base problems, e.g., hyperchloremic acidosis. Elevated calcium levels increase risk of crystal/stone formation, affecting both urinary flow and tissue integrity.

Prepare for diagnostic testing, procedures as indicated.

Retrograde ileogram may be done to evaluate patency of conduit; nephrostomy tube or stents may be inserted to maintain urine flow until edema/obstruction is resolved.

NURSING DIAGNOSIS: Sexual dysfunction, risk for

Risk factors may include
Altered body structure/function; radical resection/treatment procedures
Vulnerability/psychologic concern about response of SO
Disruption of sexual response pattern, e.g., erection difficulty

Possibly evidenced by
[Not applicable; presence of signs and symptoms establishes an *actual* diagnosis]

DESIRED OUTCOMES/EVALUATION CRITERIA—PATIENT WILL:
Verbalize understanding of relationship of physical condition to sexual problems.
Identify satisfying/acceptable sexual practices and explore alternate methods.
Resume sexual relationship as appropriate.

Independent

Ascertain the patient's/SO's sexual relationship prior to the disease and/or surgery. Identify future expectations and desires.

Mutilation and loss of privacy/control of a bodily function can affect patient's view of personal sexuality. When coupled with the fear of rejection by SO, the desired level of intimacy can be greatly impaired. Sexual needs are very basic, and the patient will be rehabilitated more successfully when a satisfying sexual relationship is continued/developed.

Review with the patient/SO anatomy and physiology of sexual functioning in relation to own situation.

Understanding normal physiology helps patient/SO understand the mechanisms of nerve damage and need for exploring alternative methods of satisfaction.

Reinforce information given by the physician. Encourage questions. Provide additional information as needed.

Reiteration of previously given information assists the patient/SO to hear and process the knowledge again, moving toward acceptance of individual limitations/restrictions and prognosis (e.g., that it may take up to 2 years to regain potency after a radical procedure or that a penile prosthesis may be necessary).

Discuss resumption of sexual activity approximately 6 weeks after discharge, beginning slowly and progressing (e.g., cuddling/caressing until both partners are comfortable with body image/function changes). Include alternate methods of stimulation as appropriate.

Knowing what to expect in progress of recovery helps patient avoid performance anxiety/reduce risk of "failure." If the couple is willing to try new ideas, this can assist with adjustment and may help to achieve sexual fulfillment.

Encourage dialogue between patient/SO. Suggest wearing pouch cover, T-shirt, or shortie nightgown.

Disguising urostomy appliance may aid in reducing feelings of self-consciousness, embarrassment during sexual activity.

Stress awareness of factors that might be distracting (e.g., unpleasant odors and pouch leakage).

Promotes resolution of solvable problems.

Encourage use of a sense of humor.

Laughter can help individuals to deal more effectively with difficult situation and promote a positive sexual experience.

Problem-solve alternative positions for coitus.

Minimizing awkwardness of appliance and physical discomfort can enhance satisfaction.

Discuss/role-play possible interactions or approaches when dealing with new sexual partners.

Rehearsal helps to deal with actual situations when they arise, preventing self-consciousness about "different" body image.

Provide birth control information as appropriate and stress that impotence does not mean the patient is necessarily sterile.

Confusion about impotency and sterility can lead to an unwanted pregnancy.

Collaborative

Arrange meeting with an ostomy visitor if appropriate.

Sharing of how these problems have been resolved by others can be helpful and reduce sense of isolation.

Refer to counseling/sex therapy as indicated.

If problems persist longer than several months after surgery, a trained therapist may be required to facilitate communication between patient and SO.

NURSING DIAGNOSIS: Knowledge deficit [learning need] regarding condition, prognosis, treatment, self care and discharge needs

May be related to
Lack of exposure/recall; information misinterpretation
Unfamiliarity with information resources

Possibly evidenced by
Questions; statement of misconception/misinformation
Inaccurate follow-through of instruction/performance of urostomy care
Inappropriate or exaggerated behaviors (e.g., hostile, agitated, apathetic, withdrawn)

DESIRED OUTCOMES/EVALUATION CRITERIA—PATIENT WILL:
Verbalize understanding of condition/disease process and treatment and prognosis.
Correctly perform necessary procedures, explain reasons for the action.
Initiate necessary lifestyle changes.

ACTIONS/INTERVENTIONS	RATIONALE
Independent	
Evaluate patient's emotional and physical capabilities.	These factors affect patient's ability to master tasks and willingness to assume responsibility for ostomy care.
Review anatomy, physiology, and implications of surgical intervention. Discuss future expectations.	Provides knowledge base on which patient can make informed choices and an opportunity to clarify misconceptions regarding individual situation.
Include written/picture resources.	Provides references after discharge to support patient efforts for independence in self-care.
Instruct patient/SO in stomal care as appropriate. Allot time for return demonstrations and provide positive feedback for efforts.	Promotes positive management and reduces risk of improper ostomy care.
Ensure that stoma and appliance are odorless, nonleaking.	When patient feels confident about urostomy, energy/attention can be focused on other tasks.
Demonstrate padding to absorb urethral drainage; ask patient to report changes in amount, odor, character.	Small amount of leakage may continue for several weeks after prostate surgery with bladder left in place (temporary diversion procedure).
Recommend routine clipping/trimming of hair around stoma to edges of pouch adhesive.	Hair can be pulled out when the pouch is changed causing irritation of hair follicles and increasing risk of local infection.
Encourage patients with Kock pouch to lengthen voiding interval by 1 hour each week unless discomfort noted.	Increases capacity of reservoir to achieve a more normal voiding pattern. Presence of discomfort suggests reservoir is full, necessitating prompt emptying.
Instruct patient in a progressive exercise program to include Kegel's exercises and stop/start of urinary stream.	Improves tone of pelvic muscles and the external sphincter to enhance continence when patient voids through urethra.
Encourage optimal nutrition.	Promotes wound healing, increases utilization of energy to facilitate tissue repair. Anorexia may be present for several months postoperatively requiring conscious effort to meet nutritional needs.

ACTIONS/INTERVENTIONS	RATIONALE

Independent

Discuss use of acid-ash diet (e.g., cranberries, prunes, plums, cereals, rice, peanuts, noodles, cheese, poultry, fish); avoidance of salt substitutes, sodium bicarbonate, and antacids; and cautious use of products containing calcium.

May be useful in acidifying urine to decrease risk of infection and crystal/stone formation. Products containing bicarbonate/calcium potentiate risk of crystal/stone formation affecting both urinary flow and tissue integrity. *Note:* Use of sulfa drugs requires alkaline urine for optimal absorption; so acid-ash diet/vitamin C supplements should be withheld.

Discuss importance of maintaining normal weight.

Changes in weight can affect size of stoma/appliance fit. *Note:* Weight loss of 10–20 lb is not uncommon due to intestinal involvement and anorexia.

Stress necessity of increased fluid intake of at least 2–3 L/d; of cranberry juice or ascorbic acid/vitamin C tablets; avoidance of citrus fruits as indicated.

Maintains urinary output and promotes acidic urine to reduce risk of infection and stone formation. *Note:* Oranges/citrus fruits make urine alkaline and are therefore contraindicated. Large doses of vitamin C can inhibit vitamin B_{12} absorption requiring periodic monitoring of vitamin B_{12} levels.

Discuss resumption of presurgery level of activity and possibility of sleep disturbance, anorexia, loss of interest in usual activities.

Patient should be able to manage same degree of activity as previously enjoyed and in some cases increase activity level except for contact sports. "Homecoming depression" may occur, lasting for up to 3 months after surgery, requiring patience/support and ongoing evaluation.

Encourage regular activity/exercise program.

Immobility/inactivity increases urinary stasis and calcium shift out of bones, potentiating risk of stone formation and resultant urinary obstruction, infection.

Identify signs/symptoms requiring medical evaluation, e.g., changes in character, amount and flow of urine, unusual drainage from wound; fatigue/muscle weakness, anorexia, abdominal distention, confusion.

Early detection and prompt intervention of developing problems such as UTI, stricture, intestinal fistula may prevent more serious complications. Urinary electrolytes (especially chloride) are resorbed in the intestinal conduit, which leads to compensatory bicarbonate loss, lowered serum pH (metabolic acidosis), and potassium deficit.

Stress importance of follow-up appointments.

Monitors healing, disease process; provides opportunity for discussion of appliance fitting problems, generalized health, and adaptation to condition. *Note:* Extensive surgery requires prolonged recuperation for regaining strength and endurance.

Identify community resources, e.g., United Ostomy Association, and local ostomy support group, enterostomal therapist, visiting nurse, pharmacy/medical supply house.

Continued support after discharge is essential to facilitate the recovery process and patient's independence in care. Enterostomal nurse can be very helpful in solving appliance problems and identifying alternatives to meet individual patient needs.

POTENTIAL CONSIDERATIONS following acute hospitalization (dependent on patient's age, physical condition/presence of complications, personal resources, and life responsibilities)

In addition to postsurgical concerns:
Urinary Elimination, altered—anatomic diversion.
Self-Esteem, situational low—loss of/altered control of body function.

BENIGN PROSTATIC HYPERPLASIA (BPH)

Progressive enlargement of the prostate gland (commonly seen in men over age 50) causing varying degrees of urethral obstruction and restriction of urinary flow.

CARE SETTING

Community level, with more acute care provided during outpatient procedures.

RELATED CONCERNS

Renal Failure: Acute, p 555
Psychosocial Aspects of Care, p 783
Prostatectomy, p 621

Patient Assessment Data Base

CIRCULATION

May exhibit: Elevated BP (renal effects of advanced enlargement)

ELIMINATION

May report: Decreased force/caliber of urinary stream; dribbling
Hesitancy in initiating voiding
Inability to empty bladder completely; urgency and frequency of urination
Nocturia, dysuria, hematuria
Sitting to void
Recurrent UTIs, history of calculi (urinary stasis)
Chronic constipation (protrusion of prostate into rectum)

May exhibit: Firm mass in lower abdomen (distended bladder), bladder tenderness
Inguinal hernia; hemorrhoids (result of increased abdominal pressure required to empty
    bladder against resistance)

FOOD/FLUID

May report: Anorexia; nausea, vomiting
Recent weight loss

PAIN/DISCOMFORT

May report: Suprapubic, flank, or back pain; sharp, intense (in acute prostatitis)
Low back pain

SAFETY

May report: Fever

SEXUALITY

May report: Concerns about effects of condition/therapy on sexual abilities
Fear of incontinence/dribbling during intimacy
Decrease in force of ejaculatory contractions

May exhibit: Enlarged, tender prostate

TEACHING/LEARNING

May report: Family history of cancer, hypertension, kidney disease
Use of antihypertensive or antidepressant medications, urinary antibiotics or antibacterial agents, OTC cold/allergy medications containing sympathomimetics

Discharge plan considerations: May need assistance with management of therapy, e.g., catheter

Refer to section at end of plan for postdischarge considerations.

DIAGNOSTIC STUDIES

Urinalysis: Color yellow, dark brown, dark or bright red (bloody); appearance may be cloudy; pH 7 or greater (suggests infection); bacteria, WBCs, RBCs may be present microscopically.

Urine culture: May reveal *Staphylococcus aureus, Proteus, Klebsiella, Pseudomonas,* or *Escherichia coli.*

Urine cytology: To rule out bladder cancer.

BUN/Cr: Elevated if renal function is compromised.

Serum acid phosphatase/prostatic specific antigen: Increased because of cellular growth and hormonal influences in cancer of the prostate (may indicate metastasis to the bone).

Prostate-specific antigen (PSA): Glycoprotein contained in the cytoplasm of prostatic epithelial cells, detected in the blood of adult men. Level is greatly increased in prostatic cancer but can also be somewhat elevated in other prostate disorders.

WBC: May be greater than 11,000, indicating infection if patient is not immunosuppressed.

Uroflowmetry: Assesses degree of bladder obstruction.

IVP with postvoiding film: Shows delayed emptying of bladder, varying degrees of urinary tract obstruction, and presence of prostatic enlargement, bladder diverticuli, and abnormal thickening of bladder muscle.

Voiding cystourethrography: May be used instead of IVP to visualize bladder and urethra because it uses local dyes.

Cystometrogram: Measures pressure and volume in the bladder to identify bladder dysfunction unrelated to BPH.

Cystourethroscopy: To view degree of prostatic enlargement and bladder-wall changes (contraindicated in presence of acute UTI due to risk of gram-negative sepsis when ultrasonography or intravenous urography would be indicated).

Cystometry: Evaluates detrusor muscle function and tone.

Transrectal ultrasound: Measures size of prostate and amount of residual urine; locates lesions unrelated to BPH.

NURSING PRIORITIES

1. Relieve acute urinary retention.
2. Promote comfort.
3. Prevent complications.
4. Help patient to deal with psychosocial concerns.
5. Provide information about disease process/prognosis and treatment needs.

DISCHARGE GOALS

1. Voiding pattern normalized.
2. Pain/discomfort relieved.
3. Complications prevented/minimized.
4. Dealing with situation realistically.
5. Disease process/prognosis and therapeutic regimen understood.
6. Plan in place to meet needs after discharge.

NURSING DIAGNOSIS: Urinary Retention [acute/chronic]

May be related to
Mechanical obstruction; enlarged prostate
Decompensation of detrusor musculature
Inability of bladder to contract adequately

ACTIONS/INTERVENTIONS	RATIONALE
Independent	
Encourage patient to void every 2–4 hours and when urge is noted.	May minimize urinary retention/overdistention of the bladder.
Ask patient about stress incontinence.	High urethral pressure inhibits bladder emptying or can inhibit voiding until abdominal pressure increases enough for urine to be involuntarily lost.
Observe urinary stream, noting size and force.	Useful in evaluating degree of obstruction and choice of intervention.
Have patient document time and amount of each voiding. Note diminished urinary output. Measure specific gravity as indicated.	Urinary retention increases pressure within the upper urinary tract, which may compromise renal function. Any deficit in blood flow to the kidney impairs its ability to filter and concentrate substances.
Percuss/palpate suprapubic area.	A distended bladder can be felt in the suprapubic area.
Encourage oral fluids up to 3000 ml daily, within cardiac tolerance, if indicated.	Increased circulating fluid maintains renal perfusion and flushes kidneys and bladder of bacterial growth. *Note:* Initially, fluids may be restricted to prevent additional bladder distention until adequate urinary flow is reestablished.
Monitor vital signs closely. Observe for hypertension, peripheral/dependent edema, changes in mentation. Weigh daily. Maintain accurate I&O.	Loss of kidney function results in decreased fluid elimination and accumulation of toxic wastes; may progress to complete renal shutdown.
Provide/encourage meticulous catheter and perineal care.	Reduces risk of ascending infection.
Recommend sitz bath as indicated.	Promotes muscle relaxation, decreases edema, and may enhance voiding effort.
Collaborative	
Administer medications as indicated:	
Antispasmodics, e.g., oxybutynin chloride (Ditropan);	Relieves bladder spasms related to irritation by the catheter.
Rectal suppositories (B&O);	Suppositories are absorbed easily through mucosa into bladder tissue to produce muscle relaxation/relieve spasms.
Antibiotics and antibacterials;	Given to combat infection. May be used prophylactically.

615

Independent

Phenoxybenzamine (Dibenzyline);	May be given to make urinating easier by relaxing prostatic smooth muscle and decreasing resistance to flow of urine. Used with caution as it does not shrink the gland and has unpleasant side effects such as dizziness and fatigue.
Alpha-adrenergic antagonists, e.g., prazosin (Minipress), terazosin (Hytrin), dorazosin (Cordura);	Studies indicate that these drugs may be as effective as dibenzyline and have fewer side effects.
Androgen inhibitors, e.g., finasteride (Proscar).	Reduces the size of the prostate and decreases symptoms if taken long-term; however, side effects such as decreased libido and ejaculatory dysfunction may affect patient's choice for long-term use.

Catheterize for residual urine and leave indwelling catheter as indicated.

Relieves/prevents urinary retention and rules out presence of ureteral stricture. *Note:* Bladder decompression should be done in increments of 200 ml to prevent hematuria (rupture of blood vessels in the mucosa of the overdistended bladder) and syncope (excessive autonomic stimulation). Coudé catheter may be required as the curved tip eases passage of the tube through the prostatic urethra.

Irrigate catheter as indicated.

Maintains patency/urinary flow.

Monitor laboratory studies, e.g.:

BUN, Cr, electrolytes;

Prostatic enlargement (obstruction) eventually causes dilatation of upper urinary tract (ureters and kidneys), potentially impairing kidney function and leading to uremia.

Urinalysis and culture.

Urinary stasis potentiates bacterial growth, increasing risk of UTI.

Prepare for/assist with urinary drainage, e.g.:

Cystostomy;

May be indicated to drain bladder during acute episode with azotemia or when surgery is contraindicated because of patient's health status.

Prepare for surgical intervention, e.g.:

Balloon urethroplasty/transurethral dilatation of the prostatic urethra;

Inflation of a balloon-tipped catheter within the obstructed area stretches the urethra and displaces prostatic tissue, thus improving urinary flow.

Transurethral incision of the prostate (TUIP);

A procedure of almost equivalent efficacy to TURP for prostates with estimated resected tissue weight of 30 g or less. It may be performed instead of balloon dilatation with better outcomes. Procedure can be done in ambulatory or short-stay settings. *Note:* Open prostate resection procedures (TURP) are typically performed on patients with very large prostates.

Transurethral hyperthermia.

Heating the central portion of the prostate by the insertion of a heating element through the urethra tends to shrink the prostate. Treatments are carried out 1–2 times/wk for several weeks to achieve desired results. *Note:* This procedure is considered investigational and its efficacy has not been well documented.

NURSING DIAGNOSIS: Pain [acute]

May be related to
Mucosal irritation: Bladder distention, renal colic; urinary infection; radiation therapy

Possibly evidenced by
Reports of pain (bladder/rectal spasm)
Narrowed focus; altered muscle tone, grimacing; distraction behaviors, restlessness
Autonomic responses

DESIRED OUTCOMES/EVALUATION CRITERIA—PATIENT WILL:
Report pain relieved/controlled.
Appear relaxed.
Be able to sleep/rest appropriately.

ACTIONS/INTERVENTIONS	RATIONALE
Independent	
Assess pain, noting location, intensity (scale of 0–10), duration.	Provides information to aid in determining choice/effectiveness of interventions.
Tape drainage tube to thigh and catheter to the abdomen (if traction not required).	Prevents pull on the bladder and erosion of the penile–scrotal junction.
Recommend bed rest as indicated.	Bed rest may be needed initially during acute retention phase; however, early ambulation can help restore normal voiding patterns and relieve colicky pain.
Suggest comfort measures, e.g., back rub; helping patient assume position of comfort; use of relaxation/deep-breathing exercises; diversional activities.	Promotes relaxation, refocuses attention, and may enhance coping abilities.
Encourage use of sitz baths, warm soaks to perineum.	Promotes muscle relaxation.
Collaborative	
Insert catheter and attach to straight drainage as indicated.	Draining bladder reduces bladder tension and irritability.
Instruct in prostatic massage.	Aids in evacuation of ducts of gland to relieve congestion/inflammation. Contraindicated if infection is present.
Administer medications as indicated:	
Narcotics, e.g., meperidine (Demerol);	Given to relieve severe pain, provide physical and mental relaxation.
Antibacterials, e.g., methenamine hippurate (Hiprex);	Reduces bacteria present in urinary tract as well as those introduced by drainage system.
Antispasmodics and bladder sedatives, e.g., flavoxate (Urispas); oxybutynin (Ditropan).	Relieves bladder irritability.

NURSING DIAGNOSIS: Fluid Volume deficit, risk for

Risk factors may include
Postobstructive diuresis from rapid drainage of a chronically overdistended bladder
Endocrine, electrolyte imbalances (renal dysfunction)

617

ACTIONS/INTERVENTIONS	RATIONALE
Independent	
Monitor output carefully. Note outputs of 100–200 ml/h.	Rapid diuresis could cause the patient's total fluid volume to become depleted, because insufficient amounts of sodium are resorbed in renal tubules.
Encourage increased oral intake based on individual needs.	Patient may have restricted oral intake in an attempt to control urinary symptoms, reducing homeostatic reserves and increasing risk of dehydration/hypovolemia.
Monitor BP, pulse. Evaluate capillary refill and oral mucous membranes.	Enables early detection of intervention for systemic hypovolemia.
Promote bed rest with head elevated.	Decreases cardiac workload, facilitating circulatory homeostasis.
Collaborative	
Monitor electrolyte levels, especially sodium.	As fluid is pulled from extracellular spaces, sodium may follow the shift, causing hyponatremia.
Administer IV fluids (hypertonic saline) as needed.	Replaces fluid and sodium losses to prevent/correct hypovolemia following outpatient procedures.

NURSING DIAGNOSIS: Fear/Anxiety [specify level]

May be related to
Change in health status: possibility of surgical procedure/malignancy
Embarrassment/loss of dignity associated with genital exposure before, during, and after treatment; concern about sexual ability

Possibly evidenced by
Increased tension, apprehension, worry
Expressed concerns regarding perceived changes
Fear of unspecific consequences

DESIRED OUTCOMES/EVALUATION CRITERIA—PATIENT WILL:
Appear relaxed.
Verbalize accurate knowledge of the situation.
Demonstrate appropriate range of feelings and lessened fear.
Report anxiety is reduced to a manageable level.

ACTIONS/INTERVENTIONS	RATIONALE
Independent	
Be available to the patient. Establish trusting relation3ship with patient/SO.	Demonstrates concern and willingness to help. Helpful in discussing sensitive subjects.
Provide information about specific procedures and tests, and what to expect afterward, e.g., catheter, bloody urine, bladder irritation. Be aware of how much information the patient wants.	Helps patient understand purpose of what is being done, and reduces concerns associated with the unknown, including fear of cancer. However, overload of information is not helpful and may increase anxiety.
Maintain matter-of-fact attitude in doing procedures/dealing with patient. Protect patient's privacy.	Communicates acceptance and eases patient's embarrassment.
Encourage patient/SO to verbalize concerns and feelings.	Defines the problem, providing opportunity to answer questions, clarify misconceptions, and problem-solve solutions.
Reinforce previous information patient has been given.	Allows the patient to deal with reality, and strengthens trust in caregivers and information presented.

NURSING DIAGNOSIS: Knowledge deficit [learning need] regarding condition, prognosis, treatment, self care and discharge needs

May be related to
Lack of exposure/recall, information misinterpretation
Unfamiliarity with information resources
Concern about sensitive area

Possibly evidenced by
Questions, request for information
Verbalization of the problem/nonverbal indicators
Inaccurate follow-through of instructions, development of preventable complications

DESIRED OUTCOMES/EVALUATION CRITERIA—PATIENT WILL:
Verbalize understanding of disease process/prognosis.
Identify relationship of signs/symptoms to the disease process.
Initiate necessary lifestyle/behavior changes.
Participate in treatment regimen.

ACTIONS/INTERVENTIONS	RATIONALE
Independent	
Review disease process, patient expectations.	Provides knowledge base on which patient can make informed therapy choices.
Encourage verbalization of fears/feelings and concerns.	Helping patient work through feelings can be vital to rehabilitation.
Give information that the condition is not sexually transmitted.	May be an unspoken fear.
Recommend avoiding spicy foods, coffee, alcohol, long automobile rides, rapid intake of fluids (particularly alcohol).	May cause prostatic irritation with resulting congestion. Sudden increase in urinary flow can cause bladder distention and loss of bladder tone, resulting in episodes of acute urinary retention.

ACTIONS/INTERVENTIONS	RATIONALE
Independent	
Address sexual concerns, e.g., during acute episodes of prostatitis, intercourse is avoided, but may be helpful in treatment of chronic condition.	Sexual activity can increase pain during acute episodes but may serve as massaging agent in presence of chronic disease.
Provide information about basic sexual anatomy. Encourage questions and promote a dialogue about concerns.	Having information about anatomy involved helps patient understand the implications of proposed treatments, as they might affect sexual performance.
Review signs/symptoms requiring medical evaluation, e.g., cloudy, odorous urine; diminished urinary output, inability to void; presence of fever/chills.	Prompt interventions may prevent more serious complications.
Discuss necessity of notifying other healthcare providers of diagnosis.	Reduces risk of inappropriate therapy; e.g., use of decongestants, anticholinergics, and antidepressants increases urinary retention and may precipitate an acute episode.
Reinforce importance of medical follow-up for at least 6 months–1 year, including rectal examination, urinalysis.	Recurrence of hypertrophy and/or infection (caused by same or different organisms) is not uncommon and will require changes in therapeutic regimen to prevent serious complications.

POTENTIAL CONSIDERATIONS following acute hospitalization (dependent on patient's age, physical condition/presence of complications, personal resources, and life responsibilities)

Urinary Retention [acute/chronic]—urethral obstruction, decompensation of detrusor musculature, loss of bladder tone

Infection, risk for—urinary stasis, invasive procedure (periodic catheterization)

PROSTATECTOMY

Surgical resection of the portion of the prostate gland encroaching on the urethra to improve urinary flow and relieve acute urinary retention. *Note:* Laser prostatectomy is being done in routine practice; however, there is currently insufficient published data relative to the efficacy of the procedure.

Transurethral resection of the prostate (TURP): Obstructive prostatic tissue of the medial lobe surrounding the urethra is removed by means of a cystoscope/resectoscope introduced through the urethra.

Suprapubic/open prostatectomy: Indicated for masses exceeding 60 g (2 oz). Obstructing prostatic tissue is removed through a low midline incision made through the bladder. This approach is preferred if bladder stones are present.

Retropubic prostatectomy: Hypertrophied prostatic tissue mass (located high in the pelvic region) is removed through a low abdominal incision without opening the bladder.

Perineal prostatectomy: Large prostatic masses low in the pelvic area are removed through an incision between the scrotum and the rectum. This radical procedure is done for cancer and may result in impotence.

CARE SETTING

Inpatient acute surgical unit.

RELATED CONCERNS

Surgical Intervention, p 802
Cancer, p 875
Psychosocial Aspects of Care, p 783

PATIENT ASSESSMENT DATA BASE

Refer to CP: Benign Prostatic Hyperplasia (BPH), p 613, for assessment information.

Discharge plan considerations:

DRG projected mean length of inpatient stay: 3.3–7.1 days

Refer to section at end of plan for postdischarge considerations

NURSING PRIORITIES

1. Maintain homeostasis/hemodynamic stability.
2. Promote comfort.
3. Prevent complications.
4. Provide information about surgical procedure/prognosis, treatment, and rehabilitation needs.

DISCHARGE GOALS

1. Urinary flow restored/enhanced.
2. Pain relieved/controlled.
3. Complications prevented/minimized.
4. Procedure/prognosis, therapeutic regimen, and rehabilitation needs understood.
5. Plan in place to meet needs after discharge.

NURSING DIAGNOSIS: Urinary Elimination, altered

May be related to

Mechanical obstruction: Blood clots, edema, trauma, surgical procedure

Pressure and irritation of catheter/balloon

Loss of bladder tone due to preoperative overdistention or continued decompression

ACTIONS/INTERVENTIONS

Independent

Assess urine output and catheter/drainage system, especially during bladder irrigation.

Assist patient to assume normal position to void, e.g., stand, walk to bathroom at frequent intervals after catheter is removed.

Note time, amount of voiding, and size of stream after catheter is removed. Note reports of bladder fullness; inability to void, urgency.

Encourage patient to void when urge is noted but not more than every 2–4 hours per protocol.

Measure residual volumes via suprapubic catheter if present, or with Doppler ultrasound.

Encourage fluid intake to 3000 ml as tolerated. Limit fluids in evening, after catheter removal.

Instruct patient in perineal exercises, e.g., tightening buttocks, stopping and starting urine stream.

Advise patient that "dribbling" is to be expected after catheter is removed and should resolve as recuperation progresses.

Collaborative

Maintain continuous bladder irrigation (CBI), as indicated in early postoperative period.

RATIONALE

Retention can occur because of edema of the surgical area, blood clots, and bladder spasms.

Encourages passage of urine and promotes sense of normality.

The catheter is usually removed 2–5 days after surgery, but voiding may continue to be a problem for some time because of urethral edema and loss of bladder tone.

Voiding with urge prevents urinary retention. Limiting voids to every 4 hours (if tolerated), increases bladder tone, and aids in bladder retraining.

Monitors effectiveness of bladder emptying. Residuals greater than 50 ml suggest need for continuation of catheter until bladder tone improves.

Maintains adequate hydration and renal perfusion for urinary flow. "Scheduling" fluid intake reduces need to void/interrupt sleep during the night.

Helps to regain bladder/sphincter/urinary control, minimizing incontinence.

Information helps patient to deal with the problem. Normal functioning may return in 2–3 weeks but can take up to 8 months following perineal approach.

Flushes bladder of blood clots and debris to maintain patency of the catheter/urinary flow.

DESIRED OUTCOMES/EVALUATION CRITERIA—PATIENT WILL:
Maintain adequate hydration as evidenced by stable vital signs, palpable peripheral pulses, good capillary refill, moist mucous membranes, and appropriate urinary output.
Display no active bleeding.

ACTIONS/INTERVENTIONS	RATIONALE
Independent	
Anchor catheter, avoid excessive manipulation.	Movement/pulling of catheter may cause bleeding or clot formation and plugging of the catheter, with bladder distention.
Monitor I&O.	Indicator of fluid balance and replacement needs. With bladder irrigations, monitoring is essential for estimating blood loss and accurately assessing urine output. *Note:* Following release of urinary tract obstruction, marked diuresis may occur during initial recovery period.
Observe catheter drainage, noting excessive/continued bleeding.	Bleeding is not unusual during first 24 hours for all but the perineal approach. Continued/heavy bleeding or recurrence of active bleeding requires medical evaluation/intervention.
Evaluate color, consistency of urine, e.g.:	
Bright red with bright red clots;	Usually indicates arterial bleeding and requires aggressive therapy.
Dark burgundy with dark clots, increased viscosity;	Suggests venous source (the most common type of bleeding), which usually subsides on its own.
Bleeding with absence of clots.	May indicate blood dyscrasias or systemic clotting problems.
Inspect dressings/wound drains. Weigh dressings if indicated. Note hematoma formation.	Bleeding may be evident or sequestered within tissues of the perineum.
Monitor vital signs, noting increased pulse and respiration, decreased BP, diaphoresis, pallor, delayed capillary refill, and dry mucous membranes.	Dehydration/hypovolemia requires prompt intervention to prevent impending shock. *Note:* Hypertension, bradycardia, nausea/vomiting suggests "TURP syndrome," requiring immediate medical intervention.
Investigate restlessness, confusion, changes in behavior.	May reflect decreased cerebral perfusion (hypovolemia) or indicate cerebral edema from excessive solution absorbed into the venous sinusoids during TUR procedure ("TURP syndrome").
Encourage fluid intake to 3000 ml/d unless contraindicated.	Flushes kidneys/bladder of bacteria and debris but may result in water intoxication/fluid overload if not monitored closely.
Avoid taking rectal temperatures and use of rectal tubes/enemas.	May result in referred irritation to prostatic bed and increased pressure on prostatic capsule with risk of bleeding.

623

ACTIONS/INTERVENTIONS	RATIONALE
Collaborative	
Monitor laboratory studies as indicated, e.g.:	
Hb/Hct, RBCs;	Useful in evaluating blood losses/replacement needs.
Coagulation studies, platelet count.	May indicate developing complications, e.g., depletion of clotting factors, DIC.
Administer IV therapy/blood products as indicated.	May need additional fluids, if oral intake inadequate, or blood products, if losses are excessive.
Maintain traction on indwelling catheter; tape catheter to inner thigh.	Traction on the 30-ml balloon positioned in the prostatic urethral fossa will create pressure on the arterial supply of the prostatic capsule to help prevent/control bleeding.
Release traction within 4–5 hours. Document period of application and release of traction, if used.	Prolonged traction may cause permanent trauma/problems with urinary control.
Administer stool softeners, laxatives as indicated.	Prevention of constipation/straining for stool reduces risk of rectal–perineal bleeding.

NURSING DIAGNOSIS: Infection, risk for

Risk factors may include
Invasive procedures: Instrumentation during surgery, catheter, frequent bladder irrigation
Traumatized tissue, surgical incision (e.g., perineal)

Possibly evidenced by
[Not applicable; presence of signs and symptoms establishes an *actual* diagnosis]

DESIRED OUTCOMES/EVALUATION CRITERIA—PATIENT WILL:
Achieve timely healing.
Experience no signs of infection.

ACTIONS/INTERVENTIONS	RATIONALE
Independent	
Maintain sterile catheter system; provide regular catheter/meatal care with soap and water, applying antibiotic ointment around catheter site.	Prevents introduction of bacteria and resultant infection/sepsis.
Ambulate with drainage bag dependent.	Avoids backward reflux of urine, which may introduce bacteria into the bladder.
Monitor vital signs, noting low-grade fever, chills, rapid pulse and respiration, restlessness, irritability, disorientation.	Patient who has had cystoscopy and/or TUR of the prostate are at increased risk for surgical/septic shock related to manipulation/instrumentation.
Observe drainage from wounds, around suprapubic catheter.	Presence of drains, suprapubic incision increases risk of infection, as indicated by erythema, purulent drainage.

ACTIONS/INTERVENTIONS

Independent

Change dressings frequently (supra/retropubic and perineal incisions), cleaning and drying skin thoroughly each time.

Use ostomy-type skin barriers.

Collaborative

Administer antibiotics as indicated.

RATIONALE

Wet dressings cause skin irritation and provide media for bacterial growth, increasing risk of wound infection.

Provides protection for surrounding skin, preventing excoriation and reducing risk of infection.

May be given prophylactically due to increased risk of infection with prostatectomy.

NURSING DIAGNOSIS: Pain [acute]

May be related to
Irritation of the bladder mucosa; reflex muscle spasm associated with surgical procedure and/or pressure from bladder balloon (traction)

Possibly evidenced by
Reports of painful bladder spasms
Facial grimacing, guarding, restlessness
Autonomic responses

DESIRED OUTCOMES/EVALUATION CRITERIA—PATIENT WILL:
Report pain is relieved/controlled.
Demonstrate use of relaxation skills and diversional activities as indicated for individual situation.
Appear relaxed, sleep/rest appropriately.

ACTIONS/INTERVENTIONS

Independent

Assess pain, noting location, intensity (0–10 scale).

Maintain patency of catheter and drainage system. Keep tubings free of kinks and clots.

Promote intake of up to 3000 ml/d as tolerated.

Give patient accurate information about catheter, drainage, and bladder spasms.

Provide comfort measures (Therapeutic Touch, position changes, back rub) and diversional activities. Encourage use of relaxation techniques, including deep-breathing exercises, visualization, guided imagery.

Provide sitz baths or heat lamp if indicated.

RATIONALE

Sharp, intermittent pain with urge to void/passage of urine around catheter suggests bladder spasms, which tend to be more severe with suprapubic or TUR approaches (usually decrease by the end of 48 hours).

Maintaining a properly functioning catheter and drainage system decreases risk of bladder distention/spasm.

Decreases irritation by maintaining a constant flow of fluid over the bladder mucosa.

Allays anxiety and promotes cooperation with necessary procedures.

Reduces muscle tension, refocuses attention, and may enhance coping abilities.

Promotes tissue perfusion and resolution of edema, and enhances healing (perineal approach).

625

ACTIONS/INTERVENTIONS

Collaborative

Administer antispasmodics, e.g.:

Oxybutynin chloride (Ditropan), B&O suppositories;

Propantheline bromide (Pro-Banthine).

RATIONALE

Relaxes smooth muscle, to provide relief of spasms and associated pain.

Relieves bladder spasms by anticholinergic action. Usually discontinued 24–48 hours before anticipated removal of catheter to promote normal bladder contraction.

NURSING DIAGNOSIS: Sexual dysfunction, risk for

Risk factors may include
Situational crisis (incontinence, leakage of urine after catheter removal, involvement of genital area)
Threat to self-concept/change in health status

Possibly evidenced by
[Not applicable; presence of signs and symptoms establishes an *actual* diagnosis]

DESIRED OUTCOMES/EVALUATION CRITERIA—PATIENT WILL:
Appear relaxed and report anxiety is reduced to a manageable level.
Verbalize understanding of individual situation.
Demonstrate problem-solving skills.

ACTIONS/INTERVENTIONS

Independent

Provide openings for patient/SO to talk about concerns of incontinence and sexual functioning.

Give accurate information about expectation of return of sexual function.

Discuss basic anatomy. Be honest in answers to patient's questions.

Discuss retrograde ejaculation if transurethral/suprapubic approach is used.

RATIONALE

May have anxieties about the effects of surgery and may be hesitant about asking necessary questions. Anxiety may have affected ability to access information given previously.

Physiologic impotence occurs when the perineal nerves are cut during radical procedures; in other approaches, sexual activity can usually be resumed in 6–8 weeks. *Note:* Penile prosthesis may be recommended to facilitate erection and correct impotence following radical perineal procedure.

The nerve plexus that controls erection runs posteriorly to the prostate through the capsule. In procedures that do not involve the prostatic capsule, impotence and sterility usually are not consequences. Surgical procedure may not provide a permanent cure, and hypertrophy may recur.

Seminal fluid goes into the bladder and is excreted with the urine. This does not interfere with sexual functioning but will decrease fertility and cause urine to be cloudy.

ACTIONS/INTERVENTIONS

Independent

Instruct in perineal and interruption/continuation of urinary stream exercises.

Collaborative

Refer to sexual counselor as indicated.

RATIONALE

Kegel exercises promote regaining muscular control of urinary continence and sexual function.

Persistent/unresolved problems may require professional intervention.

NURSING DIAGNOSIS: Knowledge deficit [learning need] regarding condition, prognosis, treatment, self care and discharge needs

May be related to
Lack of exposure/recall; information misinterpretation
Unfamiliarity with information resources

Possibly evidenced by
Questions, request for information, statement of misconception
Verbalization of the problem
Inaccurate follow-through of instruction/development of preventable complications

DESIRED OUTCOMES/EVALUATION CRITERIA—PATIENT WILL:
Verbalize understanding of surgical procedure and treatment.
Correctly perform necessary procedures and explain reasons for actions.
Initiate necessary lifestyle changes.
Participate in treatment regimen.

ACTIONS/INTERVENTIONS

Independent

Review implications of procedure and future expectations.

Stress necessity of good nutrition; encourage inclusion of fruits, increased fiber in diet.

Discuss initial activity restrictions, e.g., avoidance of heavy lifting, strenuous exercise, prolonged sitting/long automobile trips, climbing more than 2 flights of stairs at a time.

Encourage continuation of perineal exercises.

Instruct in urinary catheter care if present. Identify source for supplies/support.

Instruct patient to avoid tub baths after discharge.

Review signs/symptoms requiring medical evaluation, e.g., erythema, purulent drainage from wound sites; changes in character/amount of urine, presence of urgency/frequency; heavy bleeding, fever or chills.

RATIONALE

Provides knowledge base on which patient can make informed choices.

Promotes healing and prevents constipation, reducing risk of postoperative bleeding.

Increased abdominal pressure/straining places stress on the bladder and prostate, potentiating risk of bleeding.

Facilitates urinary control and alleviation of incontinence.

Promotes independence and competent self-care.

Decreases the possibility of infection, introduction of bacteria.

Prompt intervention may prevent serious complications. *Note:* Urine may appear cloudy for several weeks until postoperative healing occurs and may appear cloudy after intercourse because of retrograde ejaculation.

627

POTENTIAL CONSIDERATIONS following acute hospitalization (dependent on patient's age, physical condition/presence of complications, personal resources, and life responsibilities)

In addition to postsurgical concerns:
Urinary Elimination, altered—loss of bladder tone, possible discharge with catheter in place
Sexual dysfunction—leakage of urine; loss of erectile function following radical procedure

Sample CP: TURP, Hospital. ELOS: 3 Days Urology or Surgical Unit

ND and categories of care	Day 1 — Day of Surgery	Day 2 — POD #1	Day 3 — POD #2
Altered urinary elimination R/T mechanical obstruction, loss of bladder tone, therapeutic intervention	Display urine output individually appropriate, few clots & catheter free-flowing	Verbalize understanding of home care needs, signs/symptoms to report to healthcare provider	Void normal amounts w/o retention Demonstrate behaviors to regain bladder/urinary control Plan in place to meet postdischarge needs
Referrals		Home care	
Additional assessments	Characteristics of urinary drainage Urinary output q8h → Presence of spontaneous voiding →		Voiding frequency, character of urine Amt per void →
Patient education	Foley cath function, hygiene	Perineal exercises Home care needs, activity/dietary restrictions, sexual concerns Signs/symptoms to report to healthcare provider	Provide written instructions, schedule for follow up visits
Additional nursing actions	Foley cath to st drain, irrigate/CBI per protocol Bedrest if CBI Bed flat X 8h if epidural anesthesia	DC Stand to void q2-4h Ambulate as tol Encourage fluids to 3 L/d as indicated	→ per self q4h → ad lib →
Pain R/T increased frequency/force of ureteral contractions, tissue trauma, edema	Report pain relieved/controlled →		→ Verbalize understanding of pain management postdischarge
Additional assessments	Pain characteristics/changes, presence of bladder spasms → Response to interventions →	Return of bowel function →	→ →
Medications Allergies: _____	Analgesic of choice IM/po q4h Antispasmotic prn	→ PO analgesic → D/C Stool softener/laxative	→ →
Patient education	Reporting of pain/effects of intervention Relaxation techniques		
Additional nursing actions	Routine comfort measures → Anchor catheter, avoid manipulation Maintain potency of catheter	Sitz bath as indicated →	→
Risk for fluid volume deficit, R/T nausea and vomiting, postobstructive diuresis	Maintain adequate hydration w/VS stable, palpable pulses, good capillary refill, adequate urinary output → Free of active bleeding		→

628

Sample CP: TURP, Hospital. ELOS: 3 Days Urology or Surgical Unit (*Continued*)

ND and categories of care	Day 1 _____ Day of Surgery	Day 2 _____ POD #1	Day 3 _____ POD #2
Diagnostic studies		Hb/Hct, RBC	
Additional assessments	Characteristics of catheter drainage	→ Charactristics of urine	→
	VS per postop protocol	→ q8h	→
	Peripheral pulses, capillary refill, status of skin q8h	→	→ D/C
	I & O q8h	→	→ D/C
	Mental status/restlessness q4h	→ q8h	→ D/C
	Temp q8h	→	→
Medications	IV therapy/blood products as indicated	→ DC	
Patient education	Fluid needs/restrictions		
Additional nursing actions	Maintain catheter traction as indicated, release q4h per protocol	→ D/C	
	Begin po fluids as tol	→ Advance diet/fluids as tol	→

UROLITHIASIS (RENAL CALCULI)

Kidney stones (calculi) are formed of mineral deposits, most commonly Ca oxalate and Ca phosphate; however, uric acid and other crystals are also calculus formers. Although renal calculi can form anywhere in the urinary tract, they are most commonly found in the renal pelvis and calyces. Renal calculi can remain asymptomatic until passed into a ureter and/or urine flow is obstructed, when the potential for renal damage is acute.

CARE SETTING

Acute episodes may require inpatient treatment on a medical or surgical unit.

RELATED CONCERNS

Metabolic Acidosis (Primary Base Bicarbonate Deficit), p 506
Metabolic Alkalosis (Primary Base Bicarbonate Excess), p 510
Fluid and Electrolyte Imbalances, p 899
Psychosocial Aspects of Care, p 783
Renal Failure: Acute, p 555

Patient Assessment Data Base

Dependent on size, location, and etiology of calculi

ACTIVITY/REST

May report: Sedentary occupation or occupation in which patient is exposed to high environmental temperatures
Activity restrictions/immobility due to a preexisting condition (e.g., debilitating disease, spinal cord injury)

CIRCULATION

May exhibit: Elevated BP/pulse (pain, anxiety, kidney failure)
Warm, flushed skin; pallor

ELIMINATION

May report: History of recent/chronic UTI; previous obstruction (calculi)
Decreased urinary output, bladder fullness
Burning, urgency with urination
Diarrhea

May exhibit: Oliguria, hematuria, pyuria
Alterations in voiding pattern

FOOD/FLUID

May report: Nausea/vomiting, abdominal tenderness
Diet high in purines, calcium oxalate, and/or phosphates
Insufficient fluid intake; does not drink fluids well

May exhibit: Abdominal distention; decreased/absent bowel sounds
Vomiting

PAIN/DISCOMFORT

May report: Acute episode of excruciating, colicky pain. Location is dependent on stone location, e.g., in the flank in the region of the costovertebral angle; may radiate to back, abdomen, and down to the groin/genitalia. Constant dull pain suggests calculi located in the renal pelvis or calyces

Pain may be described as acute, severe, not relieved by positioning or any other measures

May exhibit: Guarding; distraction behaviors

Tenderness in renal areas on palpation

SAFETY

May report: Use of alcohol

Fever; chills

TEACHING/LEARNING

May report: Family history of calculi, kidney disease, hypertension, gout, chronic UTI

History of small-bowel disease, previous abdominal surgery, hyperparathyroidism

Use of antibiotics, antihypertensives, sodium bicarbonate, allopurinol, phosphates, thiazides, excessive intake of calcium or vitamin D

Discharge plan considerations: **DRG projected mean length of inpatient stay: 3.2 days**

Refer to section at end of plan for postdischarge considerations

DIAGNOSTIC STUDIES

Urinalysis: Color may be yellow, dark brown, bloody; commonly shows RBCs, WBCs, crystals (cystine, uric acid, calcium oxalate), casts, minerals, bacteria, pus; pH may be acid (promotes cystine and uric acid stones) or alkaline (promotes magnesium, ammonium phosphate, or calcium phosphate stones).

Urine (24 hour): Cr, uric acid, calcium, phosphorus, oxalate, or cystine may be elevated.

Urine culture: May reveal UTI (*Staphylococcus aureus, Proteus, Klebsiella, Pseudomonas*).

Biochemical survey: Elevated levels of magnesium, calcium, uric acid, phosphates, protein, electrolytes.

Serum and urine BUN/Cr: Abnormal (high in serum/low in urine) secondary to high obstructive stone in kidney causing ischemia/necrosis.

Serum chloride and bicarbonate levels: Elevation of chloride and decreased levels of bicarbonate suggest developing renal tubular acidosis.

CBC: WBC may be increased indicating infection/septicemia.

RBC: Usually normal.

Hb/Hct: Abnormal if patient is severely dehydrated or polycythemia is present (encourages precipitation of solids), or anemic (hemorrhage, kidney dysfunction/failure).

Parathyroid hormone: May be increased if kidney failure present. (PTH stimulates reabsorption of calcium from bones increasing circulating serum and urine calcium.)

KUB x-ray: Shows presence of calculi and/or anatomic changes in the area of the kidneys or along the course of the ureter.

IVP: Provides rapid confirmation of urolithiasis as a cause of abdominal or flank pain. Shows abnormalities in anatomic structures (distended ureter) and outline of calculi.

Cystoureteroscopy: Direct visualization of bladder and ureter may reveal stone and/or obstructive effects.

CT scan: Identifies/delineates calculi and other masses; kidney, ureteral, and bladder distention.

Ultrasound of kidney: To determine obstructive changes, location of stone.

NURSING PRIORITIES

1. Alleviate pain.
2. Maintain adequate renal functioning.
3. Prevent complications.
4. Provide information about disease process/prognosis and treatment needs.

DISCHARGE GOALS

1. Pain relieved/controlled.
2. Fluid/electrolyte balance maintained.
3. Complications prevented/minimized.
4. Disease process/prognosis and therapeutic regimen understood.
5. Plan in place to meet needs after discharge.

NURSING DIAGNOSIS: Pain [acute]

May be related to
Increased frequency/force of ureteral contractions
Tissue trauma, edema formation; cellular ischemia

Possibly evidenced by
Reports of colicky pain
Guarding/distraction behaviors, restlessness, moaning, self-focusing, facial mask of pain, muscle tension
Autonomic responses

DESIRED OUTCOMES/EVALUATION CRITERIA—PATIENT WILL:
Report pain is relieved with spasms controlled.
Appear relaxed, able to sleep/rest appropriately.

ACTIONS/INTERVENTIONS	RATIONALE
Independent	
Document location, duration, intensity (0–10 scale), and radiation. Note nonverbal signs, e.g., elevated BP and pulse, restlessness, moaning, thrashing about.	Helps evaluate site of obstruction and progress of calculi movement. Flank pain often radiates to back, groin, genitalia due to proximity of nerve plexus and blood vessels supplying other areas. Sudden, severe pain may precipitate apprehension, restlessness, severe anxiety.
Explain cause of pain and importance of notifying caregivers of changes in pain occurrence/characteristics.	Provides opportunity for timely administration of analgesia (helpful in enhancing the patient's coping ability and may reduce anxiety) and alerts caregivers to possibility of passing of stone/developing complications. Sudden cessation of pain usually indicates stone passage.
Provide comfort measures, e.g., back rub, restful environment.	Promotes relaxation, reduces muscle tension, and enhances coping.
Assist with/encourage use of focused breathing, guided imagery, diversional activities.	Redirects attention and aids in muscle relaxation.
Encourage/assist with frequent ambulation as indicated and increased fluid intake of at least 3–4 L/d within cardiac tolerance.	Vigorous hydration promotes passing of stone, prevents urinary stasis, and aids in prevention of further stone formation.
Note reports of increased/persistent abdominal pain.	Complete obstruction of ureter can cause perforation and extravasation of urine into perirenal space. This represents an acute surgical emergency.

ACTIONS/INTERVENTIONS

Collaborative

Administer medications as indicated:

Narcotics, e.g., meperidine (Demerol), morphine;

Antispasmodics, e.g., flavoxate (Urispas), oxybutynin (Ditropan);

Corticosteroids.

Apply warm compresses to back.

Maintain patency of catheters when used.

RATIONALE

Usually given during acute episode to decrease ureteral colic and promote muscle/mental relaxation.

Decreasing reflex spasm may decrease colic and pain.

May be used to reduce tissue edema to facilitate movement of stone.

Relieves muscle tension and may reduce reflex spasms.

Prevents urinary stasis/retention, reduces risk of increased renal pressure and infection.

NURSING DIAGNOSIS: Urinary Elimination, altered

May be related to
Stimulation of the bladder by calculi, renal or ureteral irritation
Mechanical obstruction, inflammation

Possibly evidenced by
Urgency and frequency; oliguria (retention)
Hematuria

DESIRED OUTCOMES/EVALUATION CRITERIA—PATIENT WILL:
Void in normal amounts and usual pattern.
Experience no signs of obstruction.

ACTIONS/INTERVENTIONS

Independent

Monitor I&O and characteristics of urine.

Determine patient's normal voiding pattern and note variations.

Encourage increased fluid intake.

Strain all urine. Document any stones expelled and send to laboratory for analysis.

Investigate reports of bladder fullness; palpate for suprapubic distention. Note decreased urine output, presence of periorbital/dependent edema.

RATIONALE

Provides information about kidney function and presence of complications, e.g., infection and hemorrhage. Bleeding may indicate increased obstruction or irritation of ureter. *Note:* Hemorrhage due to ureteral ulceration is rare.

Calculi may cause nerve excitability, which causes sensations of urgent need to void. Usually frequency and urgency increase as calculus nears ureterovesical junction.

Increased hydration flushes bacteria, blood, and debris and may facilitate stone passage.

Retrieval of calculi allows for identification of type of stone and influences choice of therapy.

Urinary retention may develop, causing tissue distention (bladder/kidney) and potentiates risk of infection, renal failure.

ACTIONS/INTERVENTIONS	RATIONALE

Independent

Observe for changes in mental status, behavior, or level of consciousness.	Accumulation of uremic wastes and electrolyte imbalances can be toxic to the CNS.

Collaborative

Monitor laboratory studies, e.g., electrolytes, BUN, Cr.	Elevated BUN, Cr, and certain electrolytes indicate kidney dysfunction.
Obtain urine for culture and sensitivities.	Determines presence of UTI, which may be causing/complicating symptoms.
Administer medications as indicated, e.g.:	
Acetazolamide (Diamox), allopurinol (Zyloprim);	Increases urine pH (alkalinity) to reduce formation of acid stones. Antigout agents such as Zyloprim also lower uric acid production and potential of stone formation.
Hydrochlorothiazide (Esidrix, HydroDIURIL), chlorthalidone (Hygroton);	May be used to prevent urinary stasis and decrease calcium stone formation if not due to underlying disease process such as primary hyperthyroidism or vitamin D abnormalities.
Ammonium chloride; potassium or sodium phosphate (Sal-Hepatica);	Reduces phosphate stone formation.
Antibiotics;	Presence of UTI/alkaline urine potentiates stone formation.
Sodium bicarbonate;	Replace losses incurred during bicarbonate wasting and/or alkalinization of urine; may reduce/prevent formation of some calculi.
Ascorbic acid.	Acidifies urine to prevent recurrence of alkaline stone formation.
Maintain patency of indwelling catheters (ureteral, urethral, or nephrostomy) when used.	May be required to facilitate urine flow/prevent retention and corresponding complications. *Note:* Tubes may be occluded by stone fragments.
Irrigate with acid or alkaline solutions as indicated.	Changing urine pH may help dissolve stones and prevent further stone formation.
Prepare patient for/assist with endoscopic procedures, e.g.:	
Basket procedure;	Calculi in the distal and mid ureter may be removed by endoscopic cystoscope with capture of the stone in a basketing catheter.
Ureteral stents;	Catheters are positioned above the stone to promote urethral dilation/stone passage. Continuous or intermittent irrigation can be carried out to flush kidneys/ureters and adjust pH of urine to permit dissolution of stone fragments following lithotripsy.
Percutaneous or open pyelolithotomy, nephrolithotomy, ureterolithotomy.	Surgery may be necessary to remove stone that is too large to pass through ureters.
Percutaneous ultrasonic lithotripsy.	Invasive shock wave treatment for stones in renal pelvis/calyx or upper ureters.

ACTIONS/INTERVENTIONS

Collaborative

Extracorporeal shock-wave lithotripsy (ESWL).

RATIONALE

Noninvasive procedure in which kidney stones are pulverized by shock waves delivered from outside the body.

NURSING DIAGNOSIS: Fluid Volume deficit, risk for

Risk factors may include

Nausea/vomiting (generalized abdominal and pelvic nerve irritation from renal or ureteral colic)

Postobstructive diuresis

Possibly evidenced by

[Not applicable; presence of signs or symptoms establishes an *actual* diagnosis]

DESIRED OUTCOMES/EVALUATION CRITERIA—PATIENT WILL:

Maintain adequate fluid balance as evidenced by vital signs and weight within patient's normal range, palpable peripheral pulses, moist mucous membranes, good skin turgor.

ACTIONS/INTERVENTIONS

Independent

Monitor I&O.

Document incidence and note characteristics and frequency of vomiting and diarrhea, as well as accompanying or precipitating events.

Increase fluid intake to 3–4 L/d within cardiac tolerance.

Monitor vital signs. Evaluate pulses, capillary refill, skin turgor, and mucous membranes.

Weigh daily.

Collaborative

Monitor Hb/Hct, electrolytes.

Administer IV fluids.

RATIONALE

Comparing actual and anticipated output may aid in evaluating presence/degree of renal stasis/impairment. *Note:* Impaired kidney functioning and decreased urinary output can result in higher circulating volumes with signs/symptoms of HF.

Nausea/vomiting and diarrhea are commonly associated with renal colic because celiac ganglion serves both kidneys and stomach. Documentation may help rule out other abdominal occurrences as a cause for pain or pinpoint calculi.

Maintains fluid balance for homeostasis as well as "washing" action that may flush the stone(s) out. Dehydration and electrolyte imbalance may occur secondary to excessive fluid loss (vomiting and diarrhea).

Indicators of hydration/circulating volume and need for intervention. *Note:* Decreased GFR stimulates production of renin, which acts to raise BP in an effort to increase renal blood flow.

Rapid weight gain may be related to water retention.

Assesses hydration and effectiveness of/need for interventions.

Maintains circulating volume (if oral intake is insufficient) promoting renal function.

635

ACTIONS/INTERVENTIONS

Collaborative

Provide appropriate diet, clear liquids, bland foods as tolerated.

Administer medications as indicated: antiemetics, e.g., prochlorperazine (Compazine).

RATIONALE

Easily digested foods decrease GI activity/irritation and help maintain fluid and nutritional balance.

Reduces nausea/vomiting.

NURSING DIAGNOSIS: Knowledge deficit [learning need] regarding condition, prognosis, treatment, self care and discharge needs

May be related to
Lack of exposure/recall; information misinterpretation
Unfamiliarity with information resources

Possibly evidenced by
Questions; request for information; statement of misconception
Inaccurate follow-through of instructions, development of preventable complications

DESIRED OUTCOMES/EVALUATION CRITERIA—PATIENT WILL:
Verbalize understanding of disease process.
Correlate symptoms with causative factors.
Initiate necessary lifestyle changes and participate in treatment regimen.

ACTIONS/INTERVENTIONS

Independent

Review disease process and future expectations.

Stress importance of increased fluid intake, e.g., 3–4 L/d or as much as 6–8 L/d. Encourage patient to notice dry mouth and excessive diuresis/diaphoresis and to increase fluid intake whether or not feeling thirsty.

Review dietary regimen, as individually appropriate:

    Low-purine diet, e.g., limited lean meat, turkey, legumes, whole grains, alcohol;

    Low-calcium diet, e.g., limited milk, cheese, green leafy vegetables, yogurt;

    Low-oxalate diet, e.g., restrict chocolate, caffeine-containing beverages, beets, spinach.

    Shorr regimen: low-calcium/phosphorus diet with aluminum carbonate gel 30–40 ml, 30 minutes pc/hs.

RATIONALE

Provides knowledge base on which patient can make informed choices.

Flushes renal system, decreasing opportunity for urinary stasis and stone formation. Increased fluid losses/dehydration require additional intake beyond usual daily needs.

Diet depends on the type of stone. Understanding reason for restrictions provides opportunity for patient to make informed choices, increases cooperation with regimen, and may prevent recurrence.

Decreases oral intake of uric acid precursors.

Reduces risk of calcium stone formation. *Note:* Recent research suggests that restricting dietary calcium is not helpful in reducing calcium-stone formation, and researchers, while not advocating high calcium diets, are urging that calcium limitation be reexamined.

Reduces calcium oxalate stone formation.

Prevents phosphatic calculi by forming an insoluble precipitate in the GI tract, reducing the load to the kidney nephron. Also effective against other forms of calcium calculi. *Note:* May cause constipation.

ACTIONS/INTERVENTIONS	RATIONALE
Independent	
Discuss medication regimen, avoidance of OTC drugs, and reading of all product/food ingredient labels.	Drugs will be given to acidify or alkalize urine, dependent on underlying cause of stone formation. Ingestion of products containing individually contraindicated ingredients (e.g., calcium, phosphorus) potentiates recurrence of stones.
Encourage regular activity/exercise program.	Inactivity contributes to stone formation through calcium shifts and urinary stasis.
Active-listen concerns about therapeutic regimen/lifestyle changes.	Helps patient work through feelings and gain a sense of control over what is happening.
Identify signs/symptoms requiring medical evaluation, e.g., recurrent pain, hematuria, oliguria.	With increased probability of recurrence of stones, prompt interventions may prevent serious complications.
Demonstrate proper care of incisions/catheters if present.	Promotes competent self-care and independence.

POTENTIAL CONSIDERATIONS following acute hospitalizations (dependent on patient's age, physical condition/presence of complications, personal resources, and life responsibilities)

Urinary Elimination, altered—recurrence of calculi

11

Reproductive

HYSTERECTOMY

Hysterectomy is the surgical removal of the uterus, most commonly performed for malignancies and certain nonmalignant conditions (e.g., endometriosis/tumors), to control life-threatening bleeding/hemorrhage, and in the event of intractable pelvic infection or irreparable rupture of the uterus.

Abdominal hysterectomy types include the following:

Subtotal (partial): Body of the uterus is removed; cervical stump remains.
Total: Removal of the uterus and cervix.
Total with bilateral salpingo-oophorectomy: Removal of uterus, cervix, fallopian tubes, and ovaries is the treatment of choice for invasive cancer, fibroid tumors that are rapidly growing or produce severe abnormal bleeding, and endometriosis invading other pelvic organs.

Vaginal hysterectomy may be done in certain conditions, such as uterine prolapse, cystocele/rectocele, carcinoma in situ, and high-risk obesity. It is contraindicated if the diagnosis is obscure.

CARE SETTING

Inpatient acute surgical unit, or short-stay unit, depending on type of procedure.

RELATED CONCERNS

Surgical Intervention, p 802 (for general considerations and interventions)
Cancer, p 875
Psychosocial Aspects of Care, p 783
Thrombophlebitis: Deep Vein Thrombosis, p 107

Patient Assessment Data Base

Data is dependent on the underlying disease process/need for surgical intervention (e.g., cancer, prolapse, dysfunctional uterine bleeding, severe endometriosis, or pelvic infections unresponsive to medical management) and associated complications (e.g., anemia).

TEACHING/LEARNING

Discharge plan considerations:	**DRG projected mean length of inpatient stay: 3.5–6.8 days** May need temporary help with transportation; homemaker/maintenance tasks

Refer to section at end of plan for postdischarge considerations.

DIAGNOSTIC STUDIES

Pelvic examination: May reveal uterine/other pelvic organ irregularities such as masses, tender nodules, visual changes of cervix, requiring further diagnostic evaluation.

Pap smear: Cellular dysplasia reflects possibility of/presence of cancer.

Ultrasound or CT scan: Aids in identifying size/location of pelvic mass.

Laparoscopy: Done to visualize tumors, bleeding, known or suspected endometriosis. (Rarely, exploratory laparotomy may be done for staging cancer or to assess effects of chemotherapy.)

D&C with biopsy (endometrial/cervical): Permits histopathologic study of cells to determine presence/location of cancer.

Schiller's test (staining of cervix with iodine): Useful in identifying abnormal cells.

CBC: Decreased Hb may reflect chronic anemia, while decreased Hct suggests active blood loss. WBC elevation may indicate inflammation/infectious process.

NURSING PRIORITIES

1. Support adaptation to change.
2. Prevent complications.
3. Provide information about procedure/prognosis and treatment needs.

DISCHARGE GOALS

1. Dealing realistically with situation.
2. Complications prevented/minimized.
3. Procedure/prognosis and therapeutic regimen understood.
4. Plan in place to meet needs after discharge.

NURSING DIAGNOSIS: Self Esteem, situational low

May be related to

Concerns about inability to have children, changes in femininity, effect on sexual relationship

Religious conflicts

Possibly evidenced by

Expressions of specific concerns/vague comments about result of surgery; fear of rejection or reaction of SO

Withdrawal, depression

DESIRED OUTCOMES/EVALUATION CRITERIA—PATIENT WILL:

Verbalize concerns and indicate healthy ways of dealing with them.

Verbalize acceptance of self in situation and adaptation to change in body/self-image.

ACTIONS/INTERVENTIONS	RATIONALE
Independent	
Provide time to listen to concerns and fears of patient and SO. Discuss patient's perceptions of self related to anticipated changes and her specific lifestyle.	Conveys interest and concern; provides opportunity to correct misconceptions, e.g., women may fear loss of femininity and sexuality, weight gain, and menopausal body changes.

639

ACTIONS/INTERVENTIONS

Independent

Assess emotional stress the patient is experiencing. Identify meaning of loss for patient/SO. Encourage patient to vent feelings appropriately.

Provide accurate information, reinforcing information previously given.

Ascertain individual strengths and identify previous positive coping behaviors.

Provide open environment for patient to discuss concerns about sexuality.

Note withdrawn behavior, negative self-talk, use of denial, or overconcern with actual/perceived changes.

Collaborative

Refer to professional counseling as necessary.

RATIONALE

Nurses need to be aware of what this operation means to the patient to avoid inadvertent casualness or oversolicitude. Depending on the reason for the surgery (e.g., cancer or long-term heavy bleeding), the woman can be frightened or relieved. She may fear inability to fulfill her reproductive role and may experience grief over loss.

Provides opportunity for patient to question and assimilate information.

Helpful to build on strengths already available for patient to use in coping with current situation.

Promotes sharing of beliefs/values about sensitive subject and identifies misconceptions/myths that may interfere with adjustment to situation. (Refer to ND: Sexual dysfunction, risk for, p 643.)

Identifies stage of grief/need for interventions.

May need additional help to resolve feelings about loss.

NURSING DIAGNOSIS: Urinary Elimination, altered/Urinary Retention [acute]

May be related to
Mechanical trauma, surgical manipulation, presence of local tissue edema, hematoma
Sensory/motor impairment: Nerve paralysis

Possibly evidenced by
Sensation of bladder fullness, urgency
Small, frequent voiding or absence of urinary output
Overflow incontinence
Bladder distention

DESIRED OUTCOMES/EVALUATION CRITERIA—PATIENT WILL:
Empty bladder regularly and completely.

ACTIONS/INTERVENTIONS

Independent

Note voiding pattern and monitor urinary output.

Palpate bladder. Investigate reports of discomfort, fullness, inability to void.

Provide routine voiding measures, e.g., privacy, normal position, running water in sink, pouring warm water over perineum.

RATIONALE

May indicate urinary retention if voiding frequently in small/insufficient amounts (<100 ml).

Perception of bladder fullness, distention of bladder above symphysis pubis indicates urinary retention.

Promotes relaxation of perineal muscles and may facilitate voiding efforts.

ACTIONS/INTERVENTIONS

Independent

Provide/encourage good perianal cleansing and catheter care (when present).

Assess urine characteristics, noting color, clarity, odor.

Collaborative

Catheterize when indicated/per protocol if patient is unable to void or is uncomfortable.

Decompress bladder slowly.

Maintain patency of indwelling catheter; keep drainage tubing free of kinks.

Check residual urine volume after voiding as indicated.

RATIONALE

Promotes cleanliness, reducing risk of ascending UTI.

Urinary retention, vaginal drainage, and possible presence of intermittent/indwelling catheter increase risk of infection, especially if patient has perineal sutures.

Edema or interference with nerve supply may cause bladder atony/urinary retention requiring decompression of the bladder. *Note:* Indwelling urethral or suprapubic catheter may be inserted intraoperatively if complications are anticipated.

When large amount of urine has accumulated, rapid bladder decompression releases pressure on pelvic arteries, promoting venous pooling.

Promotes free drainage of urine, reducing risk of urinary stasis/retention and infection.

May not be emptying bladder completely; retention of urine increases possibility for infection and is uncomfortable/painful.

NURSING DIAGNOSIS: Constipation/Diarrhea, risk for

Risk factors may include
Physical factors: Abdominal surgery, with manipulation of bowel, weakening of abdominal musculature
Pain/discomfort in abdomen or perineal area
Changes in dietary intake

Possibly evidenced by
[Not applicable; presence of signs and symptoms establishes an *actual* diagnosis]

DESIRED OUTCOMES/EVALUATION CRITERIA—PATIENT WILL:
Display active bowel sounds/peristaltic activity.
Maintain usual pattern of elimination.

ACTIONS/INTERVENTIONS

Independent

Auscultate bowel sounds. Note abdominal distention, presence of nausea/vomiting.

Assist patient with sitting on edge of bed and walking.

Encourage adequate fluid intake, including fruit juices, when oral intake is resumed.

Provide sitz baths.

RATIONALE

Indicators of presence/resolution of ileus, affecting choice of interventions.

Early ambulation helps stimulate intestinal function and return of peristalsis.

Promotes softer stool; may aid in stimulating peristalsis.

Promotes muscle relaxation, minimizes discomfort.

641

ACTIONS/INTERVENTIONS

Collaborative

Restrict oral intake as indicated.

Maintain NG tube, if present.

Provide clear/full liquids and advance to solid foods as tolerated.

Use rectal tube; apply heat to the abdomen, if appropriate.

Administer medications, e.g., stool softeners, mineral oil, laxatives as indicated.

RATIONALE

Prevents nausea/vomiting until peristalsis returns (1–2 days).

May be inserted in surgery to decompress stomach.

When peristalsis begins, food and fluid intake promote resumption of normal bowel elimination.

Promotes the passage of flatus.

Promotes formation/passage of softer stool.

NURSING DIAGNOSIS: Tissue Perfusion, altered (specify), risk for

Risk factors may include
Hypovolemia
Reduction/interruption of blood flow: Pelvic congestion, postoperative tissue inflammation, venous stasis
Intraoperative trauma or pressure on pelvic/calf vessels: lithotomy position during vaginal hysterectomy

Possibly evidenced by
[Not applicable; presence of signs and symptoms establishes an *actual* diagnosis]

DESIRED OUTCOMES/EVALUATION CRITERIA—PATIENT WILL:
Demonstrate adequate perfusion, as evidenced by stable vital signs, palpable pulses, good capillary refill, usual mentation, individually adequate urinary output.
Be free of edema, signs of thrombus formation.

ACTIONS/INTERVENTIONS

Independent

Monitor vital signs; palpate peripheral pulses, and note capillary refill; assess urinary output/characteristics. Evaluate changes in mentation.

Inspect dressings and perineal pads, noting color, amount, and odor of drainage. Weigh pads and compare with dry weight if patient is bleeding heavily.

Turn patient and encourage frequent coughing and deep-breathing exercises.

Avoid high-Fowler's position and pressure under the knees or crossing of legs.

Assist with/instruct in foot and leg exercises and ambulate as soon as able.

Check for Homans' sign. Note erythema, swelling of extremity, or reports of sudden chest pain with dyspnea.

RATIONALE

Indicators of adequacy of systemic perfusion, fluid/blood needs, and developing complications.

Proximity of large blood vessels to operative site and/or potential for alteration of clotting mechanism (e.g., cancer) increase risk of postoperative hemorrhage.

Prevents stasis of secretions and respiratory complications.

Creates vascular stasis by increasing pelvic congestion and pooling of blood in the extremities, potentiating risk of thrombus formation.

Movement enhances circulation and prevents stasis complications.

May be indicative of development of thrombophlebitis/pulmonary embolus.

ACTIONS/INTERVENTIONS

Collaborative

Administer IV fluids, blood products as indicated.

Apply antiembolus stockings.

Assist with/encourage use of incentive spirometer.

RATIONALE

Replacement of blood losses maintains circulating volume and tissue perfusion.

Aids in venous return; reduces stasis and risk of thrombosis.

Promotes lung expansion/minimizes atelectasis.

NURSING DIAGNOSIS: Sexual dysfunction, risk for

Risk factors may include
Altered body structure/function, e.g., shortening of vaginal canal; changes in hormone levels, decreased libido
Possible change in sexual response pattern, e.g., absence of rhythmic uterine contractions during orgasm; vaginal discomfort/pain (dyspareunia)

Possibly evidenced by
[Not applicable; presence of signs and symptoms establishes an *actual* diagnosis]

DESIRED OUTCOMES/EVALUATION CRITERIA—PATIENT WILL:
Verbalize understanding of changes in sexual anatomy/function.
Discuss concerns about body image, sex role, desirability as a sexual partner with SO.
Identify satisfying/acceptable sexual practices and some alternative ways of dealing with sexual expression.

ACTIONS/INTERVENTIONS

Independent

Listen to comments of patient/SO.

Assess patient/SO information regarding sexual anatomy/function and effects of surgical procedure.

Identify cultural/value factors and conflicts present.

Assist patient to be aware of/deal with stage of grieving.

Encourage patient to share thoughts/concerns with partner.

Problem-solve solutions to potential problems, e.g., postponing sexual intercourse when fatigued, substituting alternate means of expression, positions that avoid pressure on abdominal incision, use of vaginal lubricant.

RATIONALE

Sexual concerns are often disguised as humor and/or offhand remarks.

May have misinformation/misconceptions that can affect adjustment. Negative expectations are associated with poor overall outcome. Changes in hormone levels can affect libido and/or decrease suppleness of the vagina. Although a shortened vagina can eventually stretch, initially intercourse may be uncomfortable/painful.

May affect return to satisfying sexual relationship.

Acknowledging normal process of grieving for actual/perceived changes may enhance coping and facilitate resolution.

Open communication can identify areas of agreement/problems and promote discussion and resolution.

Helps patient to return to desired/satisfying sexual activity.

643

ACTIONS/INTERVENTIONS

Independent

Discuss expected physical sensations/discomforts, changes in response as appropriate to the individual.

Collaborative

Refer to counselor/sex therapist as needed.

RATIONALE

Vaginal pain may be marked following vaginal procedure, or sensory loss may occur due to surgical trauma. Although sensory loss is usually temporary, it may take weeks/months to resolve. In addition, changes in vaginal size, altered hormone levels, and loss of sensation of rhythmic contractions of the uterus during orgasm can impair sexual satisfaction. *Note:* Many women experience few negative effects because fear of pregnancy is gone and relief from symptoms often improves enjoyment of intercourse.

May need additional assistance to promote a satisfactory outcome.

NURSING DIAGNOSIS: Knowledge deficit [learning need] regarding condition, prognosis, treatment, self care and discharge needs

May be related to
Lack of exposure/recall
Information misinterpretation
Unfamiliarity with information resources

Possibly evidenced by
Questions/request for information; statement of misconception
Inaccurate follow-through of instructions, development of preventable complications

DESIRED OUTCOMES/EVALUATION CRITERIA—PATIENT WILL:
Verbalize understanding of condition.
Identify relationship of signs/symptoms related to surgical procedure and actions to deal with them.

ACTIONS/INTERVENTIONS

Independent

Review effects of surgical procedure and future expectations; e.g., patient needs to know she will no longer menstruate or bear children, whether surgical menopause will occur, and the possible need for hormonal replacement.

Discuss complexity of problems anticipated during recovery, e.g., emotional lability and expectation of feelings of depression/sadness; excessive fatigue, sleep disturbances, urinary problems.

RATIONALE

Provides knowledge base on which patient can make informed choices.

Physical, emotional, and social factors can have a cumulative effect, which may delay recovery, especially if hysterectomy was performed because of cancer. Providing an opportunity for problem solving may facilitate the process. Patient/SO may benefit from the knowledge that a period of emotional lability is normal and expected during recovery.

ACTIONS/INTERVENTIONS	RATIONALE

Independent

Discuss resumption of activity. Encourage light activities initially, with frequent rest periods and increasing activities/exercise as tolerated. Stress importance of individual response in recuperation.

Patient can expect to feel tired when she goes home and needs to plan a gradual resumption of activities, with return to work an individual matter. Prevents excessive fatigue; conserves energy for healing/tissue regeneration. *Note:* Some studies suggest that recovery from hysterectomy (especially when oophorectomy is done) may take 4 times as long as recovery from other major surgeries (12 months versus 3 months).

Identify individual restrictions, e.g., avoiding heavy lifting and strenuous activities (such as vacuuming, straining at stool); prolonged sitting/driving. Avoid tub baths/douching until physician allows.

Strenuous activity intensifies fatigue and may delay healing. Activities that increase intra-abdominal pressure can strain surgical repairs, and prolonged sitting potentiates risk of thrombus formation. Showers are permitted, but tub baths/douching may cause vaginal irritation or incisional infections and are a safety hazard.

Review recommendations of resumption of sexual intercourse. (Refer to ND: Sexual dysfunction, risk for, p 643.)

When sexual activity is cleared by the physician, it is best to resume activity easily and gently, using alternate coital positions or expressing sexual feelings in other ways.

Identify dietary needs, e.g., high protein, additional iron.

Facilitates healing/tissue regeneration and helps correct anemia when present.

Review replacement hormone therapy. Discuss possibility of "hot flashes" even though ovaries may remain.

Total hysterectomy with bilateral salpingo-oophorectomy (surgically induced menopause) requires replacement hormones. In addition, hormone replacement may be needed after subtotal procedures because a portion of the blood supply to the ovaries is clamped during the procedure, possibly impairing long-term function.

Encourage taking prescribed drug(s) routinely (e.g., with meals).

Taking hormones with meals establishes routine for taking drug and reduces potential for initial nausea.

Discuss potential side effects, e.g., weight gain, increased skin pigmentation or acne, breast tenderness, headaches, photosensitivity.

Development of some side effects is expected but may require problem solving such as change in dosage or use of sunscreen.

Recommend cessation of smoking when receiving estrogen therapy.

Some studies suggest an increased risk of thrombophlebitis, MI, CVA, and pulmonary emboli associated with smoking and concurrent estrogen therapy.

Review incisional care when appropriate.

Facilitates competent self-care, promoting independence.

Stress importance of follow-up care.

Provides opportunity to ask questions and clear up misunderstandings as well as detect developing complications.

Identify signs/symptoms requiring medical evaluation, e.g., fever/chills, change in character of vaginal/wound drainage; bright bleeding.

Early recognition and treatment of developing complications such as infection/hemorrhage may prevent life-threatening situations. *Note:* Hemorrhage may occur as late as 2 weeks postoperatively.

645

POTENTIAL CONSIDERATIONS following acute hospitalization (dependent on patient's age, physical condition/presence of complications, personal resources, and life responsibilities)

In addition to surgical and cancer concerns (if appropriate):

Sexual dysfunction—altered body structure/function; changes in hormone levels, decreased libido; possible change in sexual response pattern; vaginal discomfort/pain (dyspareunia)

Self-Esteem, situational low—concerns about inability to have children, changes in femininity, effect on sexual relationship; religious conflicts

MASTECTOMY

The choice of treatment for breast cancer depends on tumor type, size, and location, as well as clinical characteristics (staging). Therapy may include surgical intervention with/without radiation, chemotherapy, and hormone therapy. The use of bone marrow transplantation is under investigation.

Types of surgery are generally grouped into three categories: radical mastectomy, total mastectomy, and more limited procedures (e.g., segmental, lumpectomy). Total (simple) mastectomy removes all breast tissue, but all or most axillary lymph nodes and chest muscles are left intact. Modified radical mastectomy (now the most common surgical option) removes the entire breast, some or most lymph nodes, and sometimes the pectoralis minor chest muscles. Major chest muscles are left intact. Radical (Halsted's) mastectomy is a procedure that is rarely performed as it requires removal of the entire breast, skin, major and minor pectoral muscles, axillary lymph nodes, and sometimes internal mammary or supraclavicular lymph nodes. Limited procedures (i.e., lumpectomy) may be done on an outpatient basis, as only the tumor and some surrounding tissue are removed. Lumpectomy is reserved for well-defined nonmetastatic tumors of less than 5 cm in size that do not involve the nipple. The procedure may be diagnostic (determines cell type) and/or curative when combined with radiation therapy.

CARE SETTING

Inpatient acute surgical unit.

RELATED CONCERNS

Cancer, p 875 (for additional nursing interventions regarding cancer treatment)
Psychosocial Aspects of Care, p 783
Surgical Intervention, p 802

Patient Assessment Data Base

ACTIVITY/REST

May report: Work, activity involving frequent/repetitive arm movements
Sleep style (e.g., sleeping on stomach)

CIRCULATION

May exhibit: Unilateral engorgement in affected arm (invaded lymph system)

FOOD/FLUID

May report: Loss of appetite, recent weight loss

EGO INTEGRITY

May report: Constant stressors in work/home life
Stress/fear involving diagnosis, prognosis, future expectations

PAIN/DISCOMFORT

May report: Pain in advanced/metastatic disease (localized pain rarely occurs in early malignancy)
Some experience discomfort or "funny feeling" in breast tissue
Heavy, painful breasts premenstrually usually indicate fibrocystic disease

647

SAFETY

May exhibit: Nodular axillary masses

Edema, erythema of involved skin

SEXUALITY

May report: Presence of a breast lump; changes in breast symmetry or size

Changes in breast skin color or temperature; unusual nipple discharge; itching, burning, or retracted nipple

History of early menarche (younger than age 12); late menopause (after age 50); late first pregnancy (after age 35)

Concerns about sexuality/intimacy

May exhibit: Change in breast contour/mass, asymmetry

Dimpling, puckering of skin; changes in skin color/texture, swelling, redness or heat in breast

Retraction of nipple; discharge from nipple (serous, serosanguinous, sanguinous, watery discharge increase likelihood of cancer, especially when accompanied by lump)

TEACHING/LEARNING

May report: Family history of breast cancer (mother, sister, maternal aunt, or grandmother)

Previous unilateral breast cancer, endometrial or ovarian cancer

Discharge plan considerations: **DRG projected mean length of inpatient stay: 4.1 days**

May need assistance with treatments/rehabilitation, decisions, self-care activities, homemaker/maintenance tasks

Refer to section at end of plan for postdischarge considerations.

DIAGNOSTIC STUDIES

Mammography: Visualizes internal structure of the breast; is capable of detecting nonpalpable cancers or tumors that are in early stages of development.

Galactography (ductography): Contrast mammograms obtained by injecting dye into a draining duct.

Ultrasound: May be helpful in distinguishing between solid masses and cysts and in women whose breast tissue is dense; complements findings of mammography.

Xeroradiography: Reveals increased circulation around tumor site.

Thermography: Identifies rapidly growing tumors as ''hot spots'' because of increased blood supply and corresponding higher skin temperature.

Diaphanography (transillumination): Identifies tumor or mass by differentiating the way that tissues transmit and scatter light. Procedure remains experimental and is considered less accurate than mammography.

CT scan and MRI: Scanning techniques that can detect breast disease, especially larger masses; or tumors in small, dense breasts that are difficult to examine by mammography. These techniques are not suitable for routine screening and are not a substitute for mammography.

Breast biopsy (needle or excisional): Provides definitive diagnosis of mass and is useful for histologic classification, staging, and selection of appropriate therapies.

Hormone receptor assays: Reveal whether cells of excised tumor or biopsy specimens contain hormone receptors (estrogen and progesterone). In malignant cells, the estrogen-plus receptor complex stimulates cell growth and division. About ⅔ of all women with breast cancer are estrogen-receptor positive and tend to respond favorably to the addition of hormone therapy, which extends the disease-free period and increases survival time.

Chest x-ray, liver function studies, CBC, and bone scan: Done to assess for presence of metastasis.

NURSING PRIORITIES

1. Assist patient/SO in dealing with stress of situation/prognosis.
2. Prevent complications.

3. Establish individualized rehabilitation program.
4. Provide information about disease process, procedure, prognosis, and treatment needs.

DISCHARGE GOALS

1. Dealing realistically with situation.
2. Complications prevented/minimized.
3. Exercise regimen initiated.
4. Disease process, surgical procedure, prognosis, and therapeutic regimen understood.
5. Plan in place to meet needs after discharge.

PREOPERATIVE

NURSING DIAGNOSIS: Fear/Anxiety [specify level]

May be related to
Threat of death, e.g., extent of disease
Threat to self-concept: Change of body image; scarring, loss of body part, sexual attractiveness
Change in health status

Possibly evidenced by
Increased tension; apprehension; feelings of helplessness/inadequacy
Decreased self-assurance
Self-focus; restlessness; sympathetic stimulation
Expressed concerns regarding actual/anticipated changes in life

DESIRED OUTCOMES/EVALUATION CRITERIA—PATIENT WILL:
Acknowledge and discuss concerns.
Demonstrate appropriate range of feelings.
Report fear and anxiety are reduced to a manageable level.

ACTIONS/INTERVENTIONS	RATIONALE
Independent	
Ascertain what information patient has about diagnosis, expected surgical intervention, and future therapies. Note presence of denial or extreme anxiety.	Provides knowledge base for the nurse to enable reinforcement of needed information and helps to identify patient with high anxiety, low capacity for information processing, and need for special attention. *Note:* Denial may be useful as a coping method for a time, but extreme anxiety needs to be dealt with immediately.
Explain purpose and preparation for diagnostic tests.	Clear understanding of procedures and what is happening increases feelings of control and lessens anxiety.
Provide an atmosphere of concern, openness, and availability as well as privacy for the patient/SO. Suggest that SO be present as much as possible/desired.	Time and privacy are needed to provide support, discuss feelings of anticipated loss and other concerns. Therapeutic communication skills, open questions, listening, and so forth facilitate this process.

649

ACTIONS/INTERVENTIONS	RATIONALE

Independent

Encourage questions and provide time for expression of fears. Tell patient that stress related to breast cancer can persist for many months and to seek help/support.	Provides opportunity to identify and clarify misconceptions and offer emotional support.
Assess degree of support available to the patient. Give information about community resources, such as Reach to Recovery, YWCA Encore program. Encourage/provide for visit with a woman who has recovered from a mastectomy.	Can be a helpful resource when patient is ready. A peer who has experienced the same process serves as a role model and can provide validity to the comments, hope for recovery/normal future.
Discuss/explain role of rehabilitation after surgery.	Rehabilitation is an essential component of therapy intended to meet physical, social, emotional, and vocational needs so that the patient can achieve the best possible level of physical and emotional functioning.

POSTOPERATIVE

NURSING DIAGNOSIS: Skin/Tissue Integrity, impaired

May be related to
Surgical removal of skin/tissue; altered circulation, presence of edema, drainage; changes in skin elasticity, sensation; tissue destruction (radiation)

Possibly evidenced by
Disruption of skin surface, destruction of skin layers/subcutaneous tissues

DESIRED OUTCOMES/EVALUATION CRITERIA—PATIENT WILL:
Achieve timely wound healing, free of purulent drainage or erythema.
Demonstrate behaviors/techniques to promote healing/prevent complications.

ACTIONS/INTERVENTIONS	RATIONALE

Independent

Assess dressings/wound for characteristics of drainage. Monitor amount of edema, redness, and pain in the incision.	Use of dressings depends on the extent of surgery and the type of wound closure. (Pressure dressings are usually applied initially and are reinforced, not changed.) Drainage occurs because of the trauma of the procedure and manipulation of the numerous blood vessels and lymphatics in the area.
Perform routine assessment of involved arm. Elevate hand/arm above heart per protocol as indicated.	Detection of edema allows for prompt intervention. Elevation of affected arm enhances drainage and resolution of edema.
Monitor temperature.	Early recognition of developing infection can enable rapid institution of treatment.
Place in semi-Fowler's position on back or unaffected side with arm elevated and supported by pillows.	Assists with drainage of fluid through use of gravity.
Do not take BP, inject medications, or insert IVs in affected arm.	Increases potential of constriction, infection, and lymphedema on affected side.

650

ACTIONS/INTERVENTIONS

Independent

Inspect donor/graft site (if done) for color, blister formation; note drainage from donor site.

Empty wound drains, periodically noting amount and characteristics of drainage.

Encourage wearing of loose-fitting/nonconstrictive clothing. Tell patient not to wear wristwatch or other jewelry on affected arm.

Collaborative

Administer antibiotics as indicated.

RATIONALE

Color will be affected by availability of circulatory supply. Blister formation provides a site for bacterial growth/infection.

Drainage of accumulated fluids (e.g., lymph, blood) enhances healing and reduces the susceptibility to infection. Suction devices (e.g., Hemovac, Jackson-Pratt) are often inserted during surgery to maintain negative pressure in wound. Tubes are usually removed around the third day or when drainage ceases.

Reduces pressure on compromised tissues, which may improve circulation/healing.

May be given prophylactically or to treat specific infection and enhance healing.

NURSING DIAGNOSIS: Pain [acute]

May be related to
Surgical procedure; tissue trauma, interruption of nerves, dissection of muscles

Possibly evidenced by
Reports of stiffness, numbness in chest area, shoulder/arm pain; alteration of muscle tone
Self-focusing; distraction/guarding behaviors

DESIRED OUTCOMES/EVALUATION CRITERIA—PATIENT WILL:
Express reduction in pain/discomfort.
Appear relaxed, able to sleep/rest appropriately.

ACTIONS/INTERVENTIONS

Independent

Assess reports of pain, noting location, duration, and intensity (0–10 scale). Note verbal and nonverbal clues.

Discuss normality of phantom breast sensations.

Assist patient to find position of comfort.

RATIONALE

Aids in identifying degree of discomfort and need for/effectiveness of analgesia. The amount of tissue, muscle, and lymphatic system removed can affect the amount of pain experienced. Destruction of nerves in axillary region causes numbness in upper arm and scapular region, which may be more intolerable than surgical pain. *Note:* Pain in chest wall can occur from muscle tension, be affected by extremes in heat and cold, and continue for several months.

Provides reassurance that sensations are not imaginary and that relief can be obtained.

Elevation of arm, size of dressings, and presence of drains affects patient's ability to relax and rest/sleep effectively.

ACTIONS/INTERVENTIONS

Independent

Provide basic comfort measures (e.g., repositioning on back or unaffected side, backrub) and diversional activities. Encourage early ambulation and use of relaxation techniques, guided imagery, Therapeutic Touch.

Splint/support chest during coughing and deep-breathing exercises.

Give appropriate pain medication on a regular schedule before pain is severe and before activities are scheduled.

Collaborative

Administer narcotics/analgesics as indicated.

RATIONALE

Promotes relaxation, helps to refocus attention, and may enhance coping abilities.

Facilitates participation in activity without undue discomfort.

Maintains comfort level and permits patient to exercise arm and to ambulate without pain hindering efforts.

Provides relief of discomfort/pain and facilitates rest, participation in postoperative therapy.

NURSING DIAGNOSIS: Self-Esteem, situational low

May be related to:
Biophysical: Disfiguring surgical procedure
Psychosocial: Concern about sexual attractiveness

Possibly evidenced by:
Actual change in structure/body contour
Verbalization of fear of rejection or of reaction by others, change in social involvement
Negative feelings about body, preoccupation with change or loss, not looking at body, nonparticipation in therapy

DESIRED OUTCOMES/EVALUATION CRITERIA—PATIENT WILL:
Demonstrate movement toward acceptance of self in situation.
Recognize and incorporate change into self-concept without negating self-esteem.
Set realistic goals and actively participate in therapy program.

ACTIONS/INTERVENTIONS

Independent

Encourage questions about current situation and future expectations. Provide emotional support when surgical dressings are removed.

Identify role concerns as woman, wife, mother, career woman, and so forth.

Encourage patient to express feelings, e.g., anger, hostility, and grief.

RATIONALE

Loss of the breast causes many reactions, including feeling disfigured, fear of viewing scar, and fear of partner's reaction to change in body.

May reveal how patient's self-view has been altered.

Loss of body part, disfigurement, and perceived loss of sexual desirability engender grieving process that needs to be dealt with so that patient can make plans for the future. *Note:* Grief may resurface when subsequent procedures are done (e.g., fitting for prosthesis, reconstructive procedure).

ACTIONS/INTERVENTIONS	RATIONALE
Independent	
Discuss signs/symptoms of depression with patient/SO.	Common reaction to this type of procedure and needs to be recognized and acknowledged.
Provide positive reinforcement for gains/improvement and participation in self-care/treatment program.	Encourages continuation of healthy behaviors.
Review possibilities for reconstructive surgery and/or prosthetic augmentation.	If feasible, reconstruction provides less disfiguring/"near-normal" cosmetic result. Variations in skin flap may be done for facilitation of future reconstructive process. *Note:* Although reconstruction is usually not done for 3–6 months, prolonged delay may result in increased tension in relationships and impair patient's incorporation of changes into self-concept. In some cases, the reconstructive procedure is performed at the same time as the mastectomy, and the emotional boost may help the patient get through the more complex surgical recovery process and adjunctive therapies.
Ascertain feelings/concerns of partner regarding sexual aspects, and provide information and support.	Negative responses directed at the patient may actually reflect partner's concern about hurting patient, fear of cancer/death, difficulty in dealing with personality/behavior changes in patient, or inability to look at operative area.
Discuss and refer to support groups including "Men in Our Lives" for SO as appropriate.	Provides a place to exchange concerns and feelings with others who have had a similar experience and identifies ways SO can facilitate patient's recovery.
Collaborative	
Provide temporary soft prosthesis, if indicated.	Prosthesis of nylon and Dacron fluff may be worn in bra until incision heals if reconstructive surgery is not performed at the time of mastectomy. This may promote social acceptance and allow patient to feel more comfortable about body image at the time of discharge.

NURSING DIAGNOSIS: Physical Mobility, impaired

May be related to
Neuromuscular impairment; pain/discomfort; edema formation

Possibly evidenced by
Reluctance to attempt movement
Limited ROM; decreased muscle mass/strength

DESIRED OUTCOMES/EVALUATION CRITERIA—PATIENT WILL:
Display willingness to participate in therapy.
Demonstrate techniques that enable resumption of activities.
Increase strength of affected body parts.

ACTIONS/INTERVENTIONS	RATIONALE

Independent

Elevate affected arm as indicated.	Promotes venous return, lessening possibility of lymphedema.
Begin passive ROM (e.g., flexion/extension of elbow, pronation/supination of wrist, clenching/extending fingers) as soon as possible.	Early postoperative exercises are usually started in the first 24 hours to prevent joint stiffness that can further limit movement/mobility.
Have patient move fingers, noting sensations and color of hand on affected side.	Lack of movement may reflect problems with the intercostal brachial nerve, and discoloration can indicate impaired circulation.
Encourage patient to use affected arm for personal hygiene, e.g., feeding, combing hair, washing face.	Increases circulation, helps minimize edema, and maintains strength and function of the arm and hand. These activities use the arm without abduction, which can stress the suture line in the early postoperative period.
Help with self-care activities as necessary.	Conserves patient's energy; prevents undue fatigue.
Assist with ambulation and encourage correct posture.	Patient will feel unbalanced and may need assistance until accustomed to change. Keeping back straight prevents shoulder from moving forward, avoiding permanent limitation in movement and posture.
Advance exercise as indicated, e.g., active-extension of arm and rotation of shoulder while lying in bed, pendulum swings, rope turning, elevating arms to touch fingertips behind head.	Prevents joint stiffness, increases circulation, and maintains muscle tone of the shoulders and arm.
Progress to hand climbing (walking fingers up wall), clasping hands behind head, and full abduction exercises as soon as patient can manage.	Since this group of exercises can cause excessive tension on the incision, they are usually delayed until healing process is well-established.
Evaluate presence/degree of exercise-related pain and changes in joint mobility. Measure upper arm and forearm if edema develops.	Monitors progression/resolution of complications. May need to postpone increasing exercises and wait until further healing occurs.
Discuss types of exercises to be done at home to regain strength and enhance circulation in the affected arm.	Exercise program needs to be continued to regain optimal function of the affected side.
Coordinate exercise program into self-care and homemaker activities, e.g., dressing self, washing, dusting, mopping; as well as swimming.	Patient is usually more willing to participate or finds it easier to maintain an exercise program that fits into lifestyle and accomplishes tasks as well.
Assist patient to identify signs and symptoms of shoulder tension, e.g., inability to maintain posture, burning sensation in postscapular region. Instruct patient to avoid sitting or holding arm in dependent position for extended periods.	Altered weight and support put tension on surrounding structures.

Collaborative

Administer medications as indicated, e.g.:	
Analgesics;	Pain needs to be controlled prior to exercise or patient may not participate optimally and incentive to exercise may be lost.
Diuretics.	May be useful in treating and preventing fluid accumulation/lymphedema.

ACTIONS/INTERVENTIONS

Collaborative

Maintain integrity of elastic bandages or custom-fitted pressure-gradient elastic sleeve.

Refer to physical/occupational therapist.

RATIONALE

Promotes venous return and decreases risk/effects of edema formation.

Provides individual exercise program. Assesses limitations/restrictions regarding employment requirements.

> **NURSING DIAGNOSIS: Knowledge deficit [learning need] regarding condition, prognosis, treatment, self care and discharge needs**
>
> **May be related to**
> Lack of exposure/recall
> Information misinterpretation
>
> **Possibly evidenced by**
> Questions/request for information; statement of misconception
> Inaccurate follow-through of instructions/development of preventable complications
>
> **DESIRED OUTCOMES/EVALUATION CRITERIA—PATIENT WILL:**
> Verbalize understanding of disease process and treatment.
> Perform necessary procedures correctly and explain reasons for actions.
> Initiate necessary lifestyle changes and participate in treatment regimen.

ACTIONS/INTERVENTIONS

Independent

Review disease process, surgical procedure, and future expectations.

Review/have patient demonstrate care of drains/wound sites, etc.

Discuss necessity for well-balanced, nutritious meals and adequate fluid intake.

Suggest alternating schedule of frequent rest and activity periods, especially in situations when sitting/standing is prolonged.

Instruct patient to protect hands and arms when gardening; use thimble when sewing; use potholders when handling hot items; use plastic gloves when doing dishes; and so forth, and not to carry purse or wear jewelry/wristwatch on affected side.

Warn against having blood withdrawn or receiving IV fluids/medications or BP measurements on the affected side.

Recommend wearing of a medical identification device.

RATIONALE

Provides knowledge base on which patient can make informed choices including participation in radiation/chemotherapy programs.

Shorter hospital stays may result in discharge with drains in place, requiring more complex care by patient/caregivers.

Provides optimal nutrition and maintains circulating volume to enhance tissue regeneration/healing process.

Prevents/limits fatigue, promotes healing, and enhances feelings of general well-being. Positions in which arm is dangling/extended intensify stress on affected structures, creating muscle tension/stiffness, and may interfere with healing.

Compromised lymphatic system causes tissues to be more susceptible to infection and/or injury, which may lead to lymphedema.

May restrict the circulation and increase risk of infection when the lymphatic system is compromised.

Prevents unnecessary trauma (e.g., BPs, injections) to affected arm in emergency situations.

Independent

Demonstrate use of intermittent compression as appropriate.	Pneumatic device aid is occasionally used in managing lymphedema by promoting circulation and venous return.
Suggest gentle massage of healed incision with emollients.	Stimulates circulation, promotes elasticity of skin, and reduces discomfort associated with phantom breast sensations.
Recommend use of sexual positions that avoid pressure on chest wall. Encourage alternate forms of sexual expression (cuddling, touching) during initial healing process/while operative area is still tender.	Promotes feelings of femininity and sense of ability to resume sexual activities.
Encourage regular self-examination of remaining breast. Determine recommended schedule for mammography.	Identifies changes in breast tissue indicative of recurrent/new tumor development.
Stress importance of regular medical follow-up.	Other treatment may be required as adjunctive therapy, such as radiation. Recurrence of malignant breast tumors also can be identified and managed by oncologist.
Identify signs/symptoms requiring medical evaluation, e.g., breast or arm red, warm, and swollen; edema, purulent wound drainage, fever/chills.	Lymphangitis can occur as a result of infection, causing lymphedema.

POTENTIAL CONSIDERATIONS following acute hospitalization (dependent on patient's age, physical condition/presence of complications, personal resources, and life responsibilities)

In addition to surgical and cancer concerns:

Skin/Tissue Integrity, impaired—surgical removal of skin/tissue; altered circulation, presence of edema, drainage; changes in skin elasticity, sensation, tissue destruction (radiation)

Self-Esteem, situational low—biophysical; disfiguring surgical procedure; concern about sexual attractiveness

Self Care deficit (specify)—decreased strength/endurance, pain, muscular impairment

Sample CP: Mastectomy (Modified Radical), Hospital. ELOS: 3 Days Surgical Unit

ND and Categories of Care	Day 1 _____ Day of Surgery	Day 2 _____ POD #1	Day 3 _____ POD #2
Impaired skin/tissue integrity R/T therapeutic interventions	Display wound drainage w/in established limits (___ ml) Maintain usual color, sensation, motion in fingers/hand	Participate in self-care activities/beginning exercise program Identify ways to maximize healing/minimize risk of injury to arm	Display early signs of healing w/minimal erythema, absence of purulent drainage, edema resolving Report plan in place to meet postdischarge needs
Referrals		Physical therapist Occupational therapist Home care	
Additional assessments	Dressing/drainage q2hX4 → q4h → Presence/degree of edema q8h → Donor/graft site if used q4h VS q1hX4 → q4h Neurovasc check affected UE q1hX8 I & O q8h JP drainage q8h	q8h → q8h → q8h → q8h → →	→ Wound characteristics → q12h → D/C → D/C → D/C if less than 30 ml/24h
		Measure upper arm/forearm if edema present qd	→

Sample CP: Mastectomy (Modified Radical), Hospital. ELOS: 3 Days Surgical Unit (*Continued*))

ND and Categories of Care	Day 1 _____ Day of Surgery	Day 2 _____ POD #1	Day 3 _____ POD #2
Medications	Diuretic if edema present	→	→
Patient teaching	Protection of affected arm: shaving, use of deodorant/creams, activity limitations, avoidance of heat/cold, proper posture/positioning of arm, sexual positions to prevent pressure on chest wall, wearing loose-fitting clothing	Graduated exercise program incorporating ADLs/home-making activities General health care needs to promote healing, dietary, fluids, rest/pacing self	Wound care Management of JP drain if not removed Signs/symptoms to report to healthcare provider Gentle massage of healed incision Breast self-exam Use of medical alert device Provide written instructions, schedule for follow-up visits/additional treatment modalities
Additional nursing actions	Position per protocol; HOB elevated 30° or more	→ HOB elevated 30°	→
	BRP/chair w/assist	→ Chair, ambulate as tol	→ Up ad lib
	Elevate affected arm	→	→
	Turn C, DB, Incentive spirometry q2h	→ DB, IS q2hWA	→
	Maintain elastic bandages/custom fitted pressure-gradient sleeve if used	→	→
	Reinforce dressing PRN	→	→ D/C dressing/assist w/dressing change
	Encourage progressive exercises	→	→
	Advance diet as tol	→	→
Pain R/T tissue trauma, muscle dissection	Report pain reduced to manageable level	→	Verbalize understanding of therapeutic regimen
	Participate in activities to manage pain	→	→
Additional assessments	Pain characteristics/changes	→	→
	Response to interventions	→	→
Medications Allergies: _____	Analgesic of choice IM/po	→ po analgesic	→
Patient education	Orient to unit/room Reporting of pain/effects of interventions Initial exercises of fingers/wrist of affected arm; ROM exercises of unaffected limbs Relaxation techniques Splinting of chest w/cough, DB exercise	Signs/symptoms of shoulder tension; possibility of phantom breast pain Progression of exercises as tol	Home exercise program Medication: dose, time/frequency, purpose, side effects
Additional nursing actions	Routine comfort measures	→	→
	Passive ROM/exercises per protocol	→ Advance exercises as tol	→
	Assist w/self-care	→	→
Self-esteem, situational low	Verbalize feelings, verbal/nonverbal communication congruent	→	
		Participate in care/planning for future	→
			View incision, verbalize acceptance of self Plan in place to meet postdischarge needs
Referrals		Social Services Reach to Recovery	

ND and Categories of Care	Day 1 _____ Day of Surgery	Day 2 _____ POD #1	Day 3 _____ POD #2
Additional assessments	Response to surgical procedure by patient and SO Availability/effectiveness of support systems	Future expectations, role concerns, usual coping strategies, past coping successes Understanding of diagnosis	
Patient education	Postop routines Extent/outcome of surgical procedure Future treatment needs	Community resources for pt & SO Use of/sources for temporary prosthesis Possibilities for reconstructive surgery/prosthetic augmentation Healthcare needs for general well-being (diet, rest, exercise)	Signs/symptoms to report to healthcare provider (depression) Written information regarding diagnosis/treatment options
Additional nursing actions	Discuss normalcy of feelings Encourage participation in self-care at level of ability	Provide positive reinforcement for participation in self-care/treatment program Role-play ways of handling responses of others	Identify options for managing home/work responsibilities; importance of taking time for self Provide support/answer questions when dressing removed

Orthopedic

FRACTURES

A fracture is a discontinuity or break in a bone. There are more than 150 fracture classifications. Five major ones are as follows:

1. *Incomplete:* Fracture involves only a portion of the cross-section of the bone. One side breaks; the other usually just bends (greenstick).
2. *Complete:* Fracture line involves entire cross-section of the bone, and bone fragments are usually displaced.
3. *Closed:* The fracture does not extend through the skin.
4. *Open:* Bone fragments extend through the muscle and skin, which is potentially infected.
5. *Pathologic:* Fracture occurs in diseased bone (such as cancer, osteoporosis), with no or only minimal trauma.

Stable fractures are usually treated with casting. Unstable fractures that are unlikely to reduce may require surgical fixation.

CARE SETTING:

Most fractures are managed at the community level. Although a number of the interventions listed here are appropriate for this population, the plan of care addresses more complicated injuries encountered on an in-patient acute medical/surgical unit.

RELATED CONCERNS

Craniocerebral Trauma (Acute Rehabilitative Phase), p 224
Pneumonia: Microbial, p 130
Psychosocial Aspects of Care, p 783
Spinal Cord Injury (Acute Rehabilitative Phase), p 278
Surgical Intervention, p 802
Thrombophlebitis: Deep Vein Thrombosis, p 107

Patient Assessment Data Base

Symptoms of fracture depend on the site, severity, type, and amount of damage to other structures.

ACTIVITY/REST

May exhibit: Restricted/loss of function of affected part (may be immediate, owing to the fracture, or develop secondarily, from tissue swelling, pain)

CIRCULATION

May exhibit: Hypertension (occasionally seen as a response to pain/anxiety) or hypotension (blood loss)

Tachycardia (stress response, hypovolemia)

Pulse reduced/absent distal to injury; delayed capillary refill, pallor of affected part

Tissue swelling or hematoma mass at site of injury

NEUROSENSORY

May report: Loss of motion/sensation, muscle spasms

Numbness/tingling (paresthesias)

May exhibit: Local deformities; abnormal angulation, shortening, rotation, crepitation (grating sound), muscle spasms, visible weakness/loss of function

Agitation (may be related to pain/anxiety or other trauma)

PAIN/DISCOMFORT

May report: Sudden severe pain at the time of injury (may be localized to the area of tissue/skeletal damage; can diminish on immobilization); absence of pain suggests nerve damage

Muscle spasms/cramping (after immobilization)

May exhibit: Guarding/distraction behaviors

Self-focus

SAFETY

May exhibit: Skin lacerations, tissue avulsion, bleeding, color changes

Localized swelling (may increase gradually or suddenly)

TEACHING/LEARNING

May report: Circumstances of injury

Discharge plan considerations: **DRG projected mean length of inpatient stay: Femur 7.8 days; hip/pelvis, 6.7 days; all other, 4.4 days if hospitalization required**

May require assistance with transportation, self-care activities, and homemaker/maintenance tasks

Refer to section at end of plan for postdischarge considerations.

DIAGNOSTIC STUDIES

X-ray examinations: Determine location and extent of fractures/trauma.

Bone scans, tomograms, CT/MRI scans: Visualize fractures; may also be used to identify soft-tissue damage, differentiate between stress fractures and bone neoplasms.

Arteriograms: May be done if vascular damage is suspected.

CBC: Hct may be increased (hemoconcentration) or decreased (signifying hemorrhage at the fracture site or at distant organs in multiple trauma). Increased WBC count is a normal stress response after trauma.

Cr: Muscle trauma increases load of Cr for renal clearance.

Coagulation profile: Alterations may occur owing to blood loss, multiple transfusions, or liver injury.

NURSING PRIORITIES

1. Prevent further bone/tissue injury.
2. Alleviate pain.
3. Prevent complications.
4. Provide information about condition/prognosis and treatment needs.

DISCHARGE GOALS

1. Fracture stabilized.
2. Pain controlled.
3. Complications prevented/minimized.
4. Condition, prognosis, and therapeutic regimen understood.
5. Plan in place to meet needs after discharge.

NURSING DIAGNOSIS: Trauma, risk for [additional]

Risk factors may include
Loss of skeletal integrity (fractures)

Possibly evidenced by
[Not applicable; presence of signs and symptoms establishes an *actual* diagnosis]

DESIRED OUTCOMES/EVALUATION CRITERIA—PATIENT WILL:
Maintain stabilization and alignment of fracture(s).
Demonstrate body mechanics that promote stability at fracture site.
Display callus formation/beginning union at fracture site as appropriate.

ACTIONS/INTERVENTIONS	RATIONALE
Independent	
Maintain bed/limb rest as indicated. Provide support of joints above and below fracture site when moving/turning.	Provides stability, reducing possibility of disturbing alignment/muscle spasms, enhancing healing.
Place a bedboard under the mattress or place patient on orthopedic bed.	Soft or sagging mattress may deform a wet (green) plaster cast, crack a dry cast, or interfere with pull of traction.
Casts/Splints	
Support fracture site with pillows/folded blankets. Maintain neutral position of affected part with sandbags, splints, trochanter roll, footboard.	Prevents unnecessary movement and disruption of alignment. Proper placement of pillows also can prevent pressure deformities in the drying cast.
Use sufficient personnel for turning. Avoid using abduction bar for turning patient with spica cast.	Hip/body or multiple casts can be extremely heavy and cumbersome. Failure to properly support limbs in casts may cause the cast to break.
Evaluate splinted extremity for resolution of edema.	Coaptation splint (e.g., Jones-Sugar tong) may be used to provide immobilization of fracture while excessive tissue swelling is present. As edema subsides, readjustment of splint or application of plaster cast may be required for continued alignment of fracture.
Traction	
Maintain position/integrity of traction (e.g., Buck's, Dunlop, Pearson, Russell).	Traction permits pull on the long axis of the fractured bone and overcomes muscle tension/shortening to facilitate alignment and union. Skeletal traction (pins, wires, tongs) permits use of greater weight for traction pull than can be applied to skin tissues.
Ascertain that all clamps are functional. Lubricate pulleys and check ropes for fraying. Secure and wrap knots with adhesive tape.	Assures that traction setup is functioning properly to avoid interruption of fracture approximation.

661

ACTIONS/INTERVENTIONS	RATIONALE
Independent	
Keep ropes unobstructed with weights hanging free; avoid lifting/releasing weights.	Optimal amount of traction weight is maintained. *Note:* Assuring free movement of weights during repositioning of patient avoids sudden excess pull on fracture with associated pain and muscle spasm.
Assist with placement of lifts under bed wheels if indicated.	Helps maintain proper patient position and function of traction by providing counterbalance.
Position the patient so that appropriate pull is maintained on the long axis of the bone.	Promotes bone alignment and reduced complications (e.g., delayed healing/nonunion).
Review restrictions imposed by therapy, e.g., not bending at waist/sitting up with Buck's traction or not turning below the waist with Russell traction.	Maintains integrity of pull of traction.
Assess integrity of external fixation device.	Hoffman traction provides stabilization and rigid support for fractured bone without use of ropes, pulleys, or weights, thus allowing for greater patient mobility/comfort and facilitating wound care. Loose or excessively tightened clamps/nuts can alter the compression of the frame, causing misalignment.
Collaborative	
Review follow-up/serial x-rays.	Provides visual evidence of beginning callus formation/healing process to determine level of activity and need for changes in/additional therapy.
Administer alendronate (Fosamax) as indicated.	Acts as a specific inhibitor of osteoclast-mediated bone resorption, allowing bone formation to progress at a greater ratio, promoting healing of fractures/decreasing rate of bone turnover in presence of osteoporosis.
Initiate/maintain electrical stimulation if used.	May be indicated to promote bone growth in presence of delayed healing/nonunion.

NURSING DIAGNOSIS: Pain [acute]

May be related to
Muscle spasms
Movement of bone fragments, edema, and injury to the soft tissue
Traction/immobility device
Stress, anxiety

Possibly evidenced by
Reports of pain
Distraction; self-focusing/narrowed focus; facial mask of pain
Guarding, protective behavior; alteration in muscle tone; autonomic responses

DESIRED OUTCOMES/EVALUATION CRITERIA—PATIENT WILL:
Verbalize relief of pain.
Display relaxed manner; able to participate in activities, sleep/rest appropriately.
Demonstrate use of relaxation skills and diversional activities as indicated for individual situation.

ACTIONS/INTERVENTIONS	RATIONALE
Independent	
Maintain immobilization of affected part by means of bed rest, cast, splint, traction. (Refer to ND: Trauma, risk for [additional], p 661.)	Relieves pain and prevents bone displacement/extension of tissue injury.
Elevate and support injured extremity.	Promotes venous return, decreases edema, and may reduce pain.
Avoid use of plastic sheets/pillows under limbs in cast.	Can increase discomfort by enhancing heat production in the drying cast.
Elevate bed covers; keep linens off toes.	Maintains body warmth without discomfort due to pressure of bedclothes on affected parts.
Evaluate reports of pain/discomfort, noting location and characteristics, including intensity (0–10 scale). Note nonverbal pain cues (changes in vital signs and emotions/behavior).	Influences choice of/monitors effectiveness of interventions. Level of anxiety may affect perception of/reaction to pain.
Encourage patient to discuss problems related to injury.	Helps to alleviate anxiety. Patient may feel need to relive the accident experience.
Explain procedures before beginning them.	Allows patient to prepare mentally for activity as well as to participate in controlling level of discomfort.
Medicate before care activities.	Promotes muscle relaxation and enhances participation.
Perform and supervise active/passive ROM exercises.	Maintains strength/mobility of unaffected muscles and facilitates resolution of inflammation in injured tissues.
Provide alternate comfort measures, e.g., massage, backrub, position changes.	Improves general circulation; reduces areas of local pressure and muscle fatigue.
Encourage use of stress management techniques, e.g., progressive relaxation, deep-breathing exercises, visualization/guided imagery, provide Therapeutic Touch.	Refocuses attention, promotes sense of control, and may enhance coping abilities in the management of pain, which is likely to persist for an extended period.
Identify diversional activities appropriate for patient age, physical abilities, and personal preferences.	Prevents boredom, reduces tension, and can increase muscle strength; may enhance self-esteem and coping abilities.
Investigate any reports of unusual/sudden pain or deep, progressive and poorly localized pain unrelieved by analgesics.	May signal developing complications; e.g., infection, tissue ischemia, compartmental syndrome. (Refer to ND: Peripheral Neurovascular dysfunction, risk for, following.)
Collaborative	
Apply cold/ice pack first 24–48 hours and as necessary.	Reduces edema/hematoma formation, decreases pain sensation.
Administer medications as indicated: narcotic and non-narcotic analgesics; injectable NSAID, e.g., ketorolac (Toradol); and/or muscle relaxants, e.g., cyclobenzaprine (Flexeril), hydroxyzine (Vistaril). Administer analgesics around the clock for 3–5 days;	Given to reduce pain and/or muscle spasms. Studies of Toradol have proven it to be effective in alleviating bone pain, with longer action and fewer side effects than narcotic agents. *Note:* Vistaril is often used to potentiate effects of narcotics to improve/prolong pain relief.

663

ACTIONS/INTERVENTIONS

Collaborative

Maintain/monitor PCA when used.

RATIONALE

Routinely administered or PCA maintains adequate blood level of analgesia, preventing fluctuations in pain relief with associated muscle tension/spasms.

NURSING DIAGNOSIS: Peripheral Neurovascular dysfunction, risk for

Risk factors may include
Reduction/interruption of blood flow: Direct vascular injury, tissue trauma, excessive edema, thrombus formation
Hypovolemia

Possibly evidenced by
[Not applicable; presence of signs and symptoms establishes an *actual* diagnosis]

DESIRED OUTCOMES/EVALUATION CRITERIA—PATIENT WILL:
Maintain tissue perfusion as evidenced by palpable pulses, skin warm/dry, normal sensation, usual sensorium, stable vital signs, and adequate urinary output for individual situation.

ACTIONS/INTERVENTIONS

Independent

Remove jewelry from affected limb.

Evaluate presence/quality of peripheral pulse distal to injury via palpation/Doppler. Compare with normal limb.

Assess capillary return, skin color, and warmth distal to the fracture.

Perform neurovascular assessments, noting changes in motor/sensory function. Ask patient to localize pain/discomfort.

Test sensation of peroneal nerve by pinch/pinprick in the dorsal web between the first and second toe, and assess ability to dorsiflex toes if indicated.

Assess tissues around cast edges for rough places/pressure points. Investigate reports of "burning sensation" under cast.

RATIONALE

May restrict circulation when edema occurs.

Decreased/absent pulse may reflect vascular injury and necessitates immediate medical evaluation of circulatory status. Be aware that occasionally a pulse may be palpated even though circulation is blocked by a soft clot through which pulsations may be felt. In addition, perfusion through larger arteries may continue after increased compartment pressure has collapsed the arteriole/venule circulation in the muscle.

Return of color should be rapid (3–5 seconds). White, cool skin indicates arterial impairment. Cyanosis suggests venous impairment. *Note:* Peripheral pulses, capillary refill, skin color, and sensation may be normal even in presence of compartmental syndrome, because superficial circulation is usually not compromised.

Impaired feeling, numbness, tingling, increased/diffuse pain occurs when circulation to nerves is inadequate or nerves are damaged.

Length and position of peroneal nerve increases risk of its injury in the presence of leg fracture, edema/compartmental syndrome, or malposition of traction apparatus.

These factors may be the cause of or be indicative of tissue pressure/ischemia, leading to breakdown/necrosis.

ACTIONS/INTERVENTIONS	RATIONALE
Independent	
Monitor position/location of supporting ring of splints or sling.	Traction apparatus can cause pressure on vessels/nerves, particularly in the axilla and groin, resulting in ischemia and possible permanent nerve damage.
Maintain elevation of injured extremity(ies) unless contraindicated by confirmed presence of compartment syndrome.	Promotes venous drainage/decreases edema. *Note:* In presence of increased compartment pressure, elevation of the extremity actually impedes arterial flow, decreasing perfusion.
Assess entire length of injured extremity for swelling/edema formation. Measure injured extremity and compare with uninjured extremity. Note appearance/spread of hematoma.	Increasing circumference of injured extremity may suggest general tissue swelling/edema but may reflect hemorrhage. *Note:* A 1-inch increase in an adult thigh can equal approximately 1 unit of sequestered blood.
Note reports of pain extreme for type of injury or increasing pain on passive movement of extremity, development of paresthesia, muscle tension/tenderness with erythema, and change in pulse quality distal to injury. Do not elevate extremity. Report symptoms to physician at once.	Continued bleeding/edema formation within a muscle enclosed by tight fascia can result in impaired blood flow and ischemic myositis or compartmental syndrome, necessitating emergency interventions to relieve pressure/restore circulation. *Note:* This condition constitutes a medical emergency and requires immediate intervention.
Investigate sudden signs of limb ischemia, e.g., decreased skin temperature, pallor, and increased pain.	Fracture dislocations of joints (especially the knee) may cause damage to adjacent arteries, with resulting loss of distal blood flow.
Encourage patient to routinely exercise digits/joints distal to injury. Ambulate as soon as possible.	Enhances circulation and reduces pooling of blood, especially in the lower extremities.
Investigate tenderness, swelling, pain on dorsiflexion of foot (positive Homans' sign).	There is an increased potential for thrombophlebitis and pulmonary emboli in patients immobile for several days.
Monitor vital signs. Note signs of general pallor/cyanosis, cool skin, changes in mentation.	Inadequate circulating volume will compromise systemic tissue perfusion.
Test stools/gastric aspirant for occult blood. Note continued bleeding at trauma/injection site(s) and oozing from mucous membranes.	Increased incidence of gastric bleeding accompanies fractures/trauma and may be related to stress or occasionally reflects a clotting disorder requiring further evaluation.
Collaborative	
Apply ice bags around fracture site as indicated.	Reduces edema/hematoma formation, which could impair circulation.
Split/bivalve cast as needed.	May be done on an emergency basis to relieve restriction of circulation resulting from edema formation in injured extremity.
Assist with/monitor intracompartmental pressures as appropriate.	Elevation of pressure (usually to 30 mm Hg or more) indicates need for prompt evaluation and intervention.
Review electromyography (EMG)/nerve conduction velocity (NCV) studies.	May be performed to differentiate between true nerve dysfunction/muscle weakness and reduced use secondary to pain.

665

ACTIONS/INTERVENTIONS	RATIONALE

Collaborative

ACTIONS/INTERVENTIONS	RATIONALE
Prepare for surgical intervention (e.g., fibulectomy/fasciotomy) as indicated.	Failure to relieve pressure/correct compartmental syndrome within 4 to 6 hours of onset can result in severe contractures/loss of function and disfigurement of extremity distal to injury or even necessitate amputation.
Monitor Hb/Hct, coagulation studies, e.g., PT levels.	Assists in calculation of blood loss and needs/effectiveness of replacement therapy.
Administer IV fluids/blood products as needed.	Maintains circulating volume, enhancing tissue perfusion.
Administer sodium warfarin (Coumadin) if indicated.	May be given prophylactically to reduce threat of deep venous thrombus.
Apply antiembolic hose/sequential pressure hose as indicated.	Decreases venous pooling and may enhance venous return, thereby reducing risk of thrombus formation.

NURSING DIAGNOSIS: Gas Exchange, impaired, risk for

Risk factors may include
Altered blood flow; blood/fat emboli
Alveolar/capillary membrane changes: Interstitial, pulmonary edema, congestion

Possibly evidenced by
[Not applicable; presence of signs and symptoms establishes an *actual* diagnosis]

DESIRED OUTCOMES/EVALUATION CRITERIA—PATIENT WILL:
Maintain adequate respiratory function, as evidenced by absence of dyspnea/cyanosis; respiratory rate and ABGs within patient's normal range.

ACTIONS/INTERVENTIONS	RATIONALE

Independent

ACTIONS/INTERVENTIONS	RATIONALE
Monitor respiratory rate and effort. Note stridor, use of accessory muscles, retractions, development of central cyanosis.	Tachypnea, dyspnea, and changes in mentation are early signs of respiratory insufficiency and may be the only indicator of developing pulmonary emboli in the early stage. Remaining signs/symptoms reflect advanced respiratory distress/impending failure.
Auscultate breath sounds, noting development of unequal, hyperresonant sounds; also note presence of crackles/rhonchi/wheezes and inspiratory crowing or croupy sounds.	Changes in/presence of adventitious breath sounds reflects developing respiratory complications, e.g., atelectasis, pneumonia, emboli, ARDS. Inspiratory crowing reflects upper airway edema and is suggestive of fat emboli.
Handle injured tissues/bones gently, especially during first several days.	This may prevent the development of fat emboli (usually seen in first 12–72 hours), which are closely associated with fractures, especially of the long bone and pelvis.
Instruct and assist with deep-breathing and coughing exercises. Reposition frequently.	Promotes alveolar ventilation and perfusion. Repositioning promotes drainage of secretions and decreases congestion in dependent lung areas.

ACTIONS/INTERVENTIONS	RATIONALE
Independent	
Note increasing restlessness, confusion, lethargy, stupor.	Impaired gas exchange/presence of pulmonary emboli can cause deterioration in the patient's level of consciousness as hypoxemia/acidosis develops.
Observe sputum for signs of blood.	Hemoptysis may occur with pulmonary emboli.
Inspect skin for petechiae above nipple line; in axilla, spreading to abdomen/trunk; buccal mucosa, hard palate; conjunctival sacs and retina.	This is the most characteristic sign of fat emboli, which may appear within 2–3 days after injury.
Collaborative	
Assist with incentive spirometry.	Maximizes ventilation/oxygenation and minimizes atelectasis.
Administer supplemental O_2 if indicated.	Increases available O_2 for optimal tissue oxygenation.
Monitor laboratory studies, e.g.:	
Serial ABGs;	Decreased PaO_2 and increased $PaCO_2$ indicate impaired gas exchange/developing failure.
Hb, calcium, ESR, serum lipase, fat screen, platelets.	Anemia, hypocalcemia, elevated ESR and lipase levels, fat globules in blood/urine/sputum, and decreased platelet count (thrombocytopenia) are often associated with fat emboli.
Administer medications as indicated:	
Low-dose heparin;	Blocks the clotting cycle and prevents clot propagation in presence of thrombophlebitis.
Corticosteroids.	Steroids have been used with some success to prevent/treat fat embolus.

NURSING DIAGNOSIS: Physical Mobility, impaired

May be related to
Neuromuscular skeletal impairment; pain/discomfort; restrictive therapies (limb immobilization)
Psychologic immobility

Possibly evidenced by
Inability to move purposefully within the physical environment, imposed restrictions
Reluctance to attempt movement; limited ROM
Decreased muscle strength/control

DESIRED OUTCOMES/EVALUATION CRITERIA—PATIENT WILL:
Regain/maintain mobility at the highest possible level.
Maintain position of function.
Increase strength/function of affected and compensatory body parts.
Demonstrate techniques that enable resumption of activities.

ACTIONS/INTERVENTIONS	RATIONALE
Independent	
Assess degree of immobility produced by injury/treatment and note patient's perception of immobility.	Patient may be restricted by self-view/self-perception out of proportion with actual physical limitations, requiring information/interventions to promote progress toward wellness.
Encourage participation in diversional/recreational activities. Maintain stimulating environment, e.g., radio, TV, newspapers, personal possessions/pictures, clock, calender, visits from family/friends.	Provides opportunity for release of energy, refocuses attention, enhances patient's sense of self-control/self-worth, and aids in reducing social isolation.
Instruct patient in/assist with active/passive ROM exercises of affected and unaffected extremities.	Increases blood flow to muscles and bone to improve muscle tone, maintain joint mobility; prevent contractures/atrophy, and calcium resorption from disuse.
Encourage use of isometric exercises starting with the unaffected limb.	Isometrics contract muscles without bending joints or moving limbs and helps to maintain muscle strength and mass. *Note:* These exercises are contraindicated while acute bleeding/edema is present.
Provide footboard, wrist splints, trochanter/hand rolls as appropriate.	Useful in maintaining functional position of extremities, hands/feet, and preventing complications (e.g., contractures/footdrop).
Place in supine position periodically if possible, when traction is used to stabilize lower limb fractures.	Reduces risk of flexion contracture of hip.
Instruct in/encourage use of trapeze and "post position" for lower limb fractures.	Facilitates movement during hygiene/skin care and linen changes; reduces discomfort of remaining flat in bed. "Post position" involves placing the uninjured foot flat on the bed with the knee bent while grasping the trapeze and lifting the body off the bed.
Assist with/encourage self-care activities (e.g., bathing, shaving).	Improves muscle strength and circulation, enhances patient control in situation, and promotes self-directed wellness.
Provide/assist with mobility by means of wheelchair, walker, crutches, canes as soon as possible. Instruct in safe use of mobility aids.	Early mobility reduces complications of bed rest (e.g., phlebitis), and promotes healing and normalization of organ function. Learning the correct way to use aids is important to maintain optimal mobility and patient safety.
Monitor BP with resumption of activity. Note reports of dizziness.	Postural hypotension is a common problem following prolonged bed rest and may require specific interventions (e.g., tilt table with gradual elevation to upright position).
Reposition periodically and encourage coughing/deep-breathing exercises.	Prevents/reduces incidence of skin and respiratory complications (e.g., decubitus, atelectasis, pneumonia).
Auscultate bowel sounds. Monitor elimination habits and provide for regular bowel routine. Place on bedside commode, if feasible, or use fracture pan. Provide privacy.	Bed rest, use of analgesics, and changes in dietary habits can slow peristalsis and produce constipation. Nursing measures that facilitate elimination may prevent/limit complications. Fracture pan limits flexion of hips and lessens pressure on lumbar region/lower extremity cast.

ACTIONS/INTERVENTIONS	RATIONALE

Independent

Encourage increased fluid intake to 2000–3000 ml/d, including acid/ash juices.

Keeps the body well hydrated, decreasing risk of urinary infection, stone formation, and constipation.

Provide diet high in proteins, carbohydrates, vitamins, and minerals, limiting protein content until after first BM.

In the presence of musculoskeletal injuries, nutrients required for healing are rapidly depleted, often resulting in a weight loss of as much as 20–30 lb during skeletal traction. This can have a profound effect on muscle mass, tone, and strength. *Note:* Protein foods increase contents in small bowel, resulting in gas formation and constipation. Therefore, GI function should be fully restored before protein foods are increased.

Increase the amount of roughage/fiber in the diet. Limit gas-forming foods.

Adding bulk to stool helps prevent constipation. Gas-forming foods may cause abdominal distention, especially in presence of decreased intestinal motility.

Collaborative

Consult with physical/occupational therapist and/or rehabilitation specialist.

Useful in creating individualized activity/exercise program. Patient may require long-term assistance with movement, strengthening, and weight-bearing activities, as well as use of adjuncts, e.g., walkers, crutches, canes; elevated toilet seats; pickup sticks/reachers, special eating utensils.

Initiate bowel program (stool softeners, enemas, laxatives) as indicated.

Done to promote regular bowel evacuation.

Refer to psychiatric nurse, clinical specialist/therapist as indicated.

Patient/SO may require more intensive treatment to deal with reality of current condition/prognosis, prolonged immobility, perceived loss of control.

NURSING DIAGNOSIS: Skin/Tissue Integrity, impaired: actual/risk for

May be related to
Puncture injury; compound fracture; surgical repair; insertion of traction pins, wires, screws
Altered sensation, circulation; accumulation of excretions/secretions
Physical immobilization

Possibly evidenced by (actual)
Reports of itching, pain, numbness, pressure of affected/surrounding area
Disruption of skin surface; invasion of body structures; destruction of skin layers/tissues

DESIRED OUTCOMES/EVALUATION CRITERIA—PATIENT WILL:
Verbalize relief of discomfort.
Demonstrate behaviors/techniques to prevent skin breakdown/facilitate healing as indicated.
Achieve timely wound/lesion healing if present.

ACTIONS/INTERVENTIONS	RATIONALE

Independent

Examine the skin for open wounds, foreign bodies, rashes, bleeding, discoloration, duskiness, blanching.

Provides information regarding skin circulation and problems that may be caused by application and/or restriction of cast/splint or traction apparatus; or edema formation that may require further medical intervention.

Massage skin and bony prominences. Keep the bed dry and free of wrinkles. Place water pads/other padding under elbows/heels as indicated.

Reduces pressure on susceptible areas and risk of abrasions/skin breakdown.

Reposition frequently. Encourage use of trapeze if possible.

Lessens constant pressure on same areas and minimizes risk of skin breakdown. Use of trapeze may reduce risk of abrasions to elbows/heels.

Assess position of splint ring of traction device.

Improper positioning may cause skin injury/breakdown.

Plaster cast application and skin care:

Cleanse skin with soap and water. Rub gently with alcohol and/or dust with small amount of a borate or stearate of zinc powder;

Provides a dry, clean area for cast application. *Note:* Excess powder may cake when it comes in contact with water/perspiration.

Cut a length of stockinette to cover the area and extend several inches beyond the cast;

Useful for padding bony prominences, finishing cast edges, and protecting the skin.

Use palm of hand to apply, hold, or move cast and support on pillows after application;

Prevents indentations/flattening over bony prominences and weight-bearing areas (e.g., back of heels), which would cause abrasions/tissue trauma. An improperly shaped or dried cast is irritating to the underlying skin and may lead to circulatory impairment.

Trim excess plaster from edges of cast as soon as casting is completed;

Uneven plaster is irritating to the skin and may result in abrasions.

Promote cast drying by removing bed linen, exposing to circulating air;

Prevents skin breakdown caused by prolonged moisture trapped under cast.

Observe for potential pressure areas, especially at the edges of and under the splint/cast;

Pressure can cause ulcerations, necrosis, and/or nerve palsies. These problems may be painless when nerve damage is present.

Pad (petal) the edges of the cast with waterproof tape;

Provides an effective barrier to cast flaking and moisture. Helps prevent breakdown of cast material at edges and reduces skin irritation/excoriation.

Cleanse excess plaster from skin while still wet, if possible;

Dry plaster may flake into completed cast and cause skin damage.

Protect cast and skin in perineal area. Provide frequent pericare;

Prevents tissue breakdown and infection by fecal contamination.

Instruct patient/SO to avoid inserting objects inside casts;

"Scratching an itch" may cause tissue injury.

Massage the skin around the cast edges with alcohol;

Has a drying effect, which toughens the skin. Creams and lotions are not recommended because excessive oils can seal cast perimeter, not allowing the cast to "breathe." Powders are not recommended because of potential for excessive accumulation inside the cast.

ACTIONS/INTERVENTIONS	RATIONALE
Independent	
Turn frequently to include the uninvolved side, back, and prone positions (as tolerated) with patient's feet over the end of the mattress.	Minimizes pressure on feet and around cast edges.
Skin traction application and skin care:	
Cleanse the skin with warm, soapy water;	Reduces level of contaminants on skin.
Apply tincture of benzoin;	"Toughens" the skin for application of skin traction.
Apply commercial skin traction tapes (or make some with strips of moleskin/adhesive tape) lengthwise on opposite sides of the affected limb;	Traction tapes encircling a limb may compromise circulation.
Extend the tapes beyond the length of the limb;	Traction is inserted in line with the free ends of the tape.
Mark the line where the tapes extend beyond the extremity;	Allows for quick assessment of slippage.
Place protective padding under the leg and over bony prominences;	Minimizes pressure on these areas.
Wrap the limb circumference, including tapes and padding, with elastic bandages, being careful to wrap snugly but not too tightly;	Provides for appropriate traction pull without compromising circulation.
Palpate taped tissues daily and document any tenderness or pain;	If area under tapes is tender, suspect skin irritation, and prepare to remove the bandage system.
Remove skin traction every 24 hours, per protocol; inspect and give skin care.	Maintains skin integrity.
Skeletal traction/fixation application and skin care:	
Bend wire ends or cover ends of wires/pins with rubber or cork protectors or needle caps;	Prevents injury to other body parts.
Pad slings/frame with sheepskin, foam.	Prevents excessive pressure on skin and promotes moisture evaporation that reduces risk of excoriation.
Collaborative	
Provide foam mattress, sheepskins, flotation pads, or air mattress as indicated.	Because of immobilization of body parts, bony prominences other than those affected by the casting may suffer from decreased circulation.
Monovalve, bivalve, or cut a window in the cast, per protocol.	Allows the release of pressure and provides access for wound/skin care.

NURSING DIAGNOSIS: Infection, risk for

Risk factors may include
Inadequate primary defenses: Broken skin, traumatized tissues; environmental exposure
Invasive procedures, skeletal traction

Possibly evidenced by
[Not applicable; presence of signs and symptoms establishes an *actual* diagnosis]

DESIRED OUTCOMES/EVALUATION CRITERIA—PATIENT WILL:
Achieve timely wound healing, free of purulent drainage or erythema, and be afebrile.

ACTIONS/INTERVENTIONS	RATIONALE

Independent

Inspect the skin for preexisting irritation or breaks in continuity.

Pins or wires should not be inserted through skin infections, rashes, or abrasions (may lead to bone infection).

Assess pin sites/skin areas noting reports of increased pain/burning sensation or presence of edema, erythema, foul odor, or drainage.

May indicate onset of local infection/tissue necrosis, which can lead to osteomyelitis.

Provide sterile pin/wound care according to protocol, and exercise meticulous hand-washing.

May prevent cross-contamination and possibility of infection.

Instruct patient not to touch the insertion sites.

Minimizes opportunity for contamination.

Line perineal cast edges with plastic wrap.

Damp, soiled casts can promote growth of bacteria.

Observe wounds for formation of bullae, crepitation, bronze discoloration of skin, frothy/fruity-smelling drainage.

Signs suggestive of gas gangrene infection.

Assess muscle tone, DTRs, and ability to speak.

Muscle rigidity, tonic spasms of jaw muscles, and dysphagia reflect development of tetanus.

Monitor vital signs. Note presence of chills, fever, malaise, changes in mentation.

Hypotension, confusion may be seen with gas gangrene; tachycardia and chills/fever reflect developing sepsis.

Investigate abrupt onset of pain/limitation of movement with localized edema/erythema in injured extremity.

May indicate development of osteomyelitis.

Institute prescribed isolation procedures.

Presence of purulent drainage will require wound/linen precautions to prevent cross-contamination.

Collaborative

Monitor laboratory/diagnostic studies, e.g.:

    CBC;

Anemia may be noted with osteomyelitis; leukocytosis is usually present with infective processes.

    ESR;

Elevated in osteomyelitis.

    Cultures and sensitivity of wound/serum/bone;

Identifies infective organism.

    Radioisotope scans.

Hot spots signify increased areas of vascularity, indicative of osteomyelitis.

Administer medications as indicated, e.g.;

    IV/topical antibiotics;

Wide-spectrum antibiotics may be used prophylactically or may be geared toward a specific microorganism.

    Tetanus toxoid.

Given prophylactically because the possibility of tetanus exists with any open wound. *Note:* Risk increases when injury/wound(s) occur in ''field conditions'' (outdoor/rural areas, work environment).

Provide wound/bone irrigations and apply warm/moist soaks as indicated.

Local débridement/cleansing of wounds reduces microorganisms and incidence of systemic infection. Continuous antimicrobial drip into bone may be necessary to treat osteomyelitis, especially if blood supply to bone is compromised.

ACTIONS/INTERVENTIONS

Collaborative

Assist with procedures, e.g., incision/drainage, placement of drains, hyperbaric O_2 therapy.

Prepare for surgery, as indicated.

RATIONALE

Numerous procedures may be carried out in treatment of local infections, osteomyelitis, gas gangrene.

Sequestrectomy (removal of necrotic bone) is necessary to facilitate healing and prevent extension of infectious process.

NURSING DIAGNOSIS: Knowledge deficit [learning need] regarding condition, prognosis, treatment, self care and discharge needs

May be related to
Lack of exposure/recall
Information misinterpretation/unfamiliarity with information resources

Possibly evidenced by
Questions/request for information, statement of misconception
Inaccurate follow-through of instructions/development of preventable complications

DESIRED OUTCOMES/EVALUATION CRITERIA—PATIENT WILL:
Verbalize understanding of condition, prognosis, and treatment
Correctly perform necessary procedures and explain reasons for actions

---

ACTIONS/INTERVENTIONS

Independent

Review pathology, prognosis, and future expectations.

Discuss dietary needs.

Discuss individual drug regimen as appropriate.

Reinforce methods of mobility and ambulation as instructed by physical therapist when indicated.

Suggest use of a backpack.

List activities the patient can perform independently and those that require assistance.

RATIONALE

Provides knowledge base on which patient can make informed choices. *Note:* Internal fixation devices can ultimately compromise the bone's strength and intramedullary nails/rods or plates may be removed at a future date.

A low-fat diet with adequate quality protein and rich in calcium promotes healing and general well-being.

Proper use of pain medication and antiplatelet agents can reduce risk of complications. Long-term use of Fosamax may reduce risk of stress fractures. *Note:* Fosamax should be taken on an empty stomach with plain water, since absorption of drug may be altered by food and some medications (e.g., antacids, calcium supplements).

Most fractures require casts, splints, or braces during the healing process. Further damage and delay in healing could occur secondary to improper use of ambulatory devices.

Provides place to carry necessary articles and leave hands free to manipulate crutches; may prevent undue muscle fatigue when one arm is casted.

Organizes activities around need and who is available to provide help.

ACTIONS/INTERVENTIONS	RATIONALE

Independent

Identify available community services, e.g., rehabilitation teams, home nursing/homemaker services.	Provides assistance to facilitate self-care and support independence. Promotes optimal self-care and recovery.
Encourage patient to continue active exercises for the joints above and below the fracture.	Prevents joint stiffness, contractures, and muscle wasting, promoting earlier return to ADLs.
Discuss importance of clinical and therapy follow-up appointments.	Fracture healing may take as long as a year for completion, and patient cooperation with the medical regimen is helpful for proper union of bone to take place. PT/OT may be indicated for exercises to maintain/strengthen muscles and improve function. Additional modalities such as low-intensity ultrasound may be used to stimulate healing of lower-forearm or lower-leg fractures.
Review proper pin/wound care.	Reduces risk of bone/tissue trauma and infection, which can progress to osteomyelitis.
Recommend cleaning external fixator regularly.	Keeping device free of dust/contaminants reduces risk of infection.
Identify signs and symptoms requiring medical evaluation, e.g., severe pain, fever/chills, foul odors; changes in sensation, swelling, burning, numbness, tingling, skin discoloration, paralysis, white/cool toes or fingertips; warm spots, soft areas, cracks in cast.	Prompt intervention may reduce severity of complications such as infection/impaired circulation. *Note:* Some darkening of the skin (vascular congestion) may occur normally when walking on the casted extremity or using casted arm; however, this should resolve with rest and elevation.
Discuss care of "green" or wet cast.	Promotes proper curing to prevent cast deformities and associated misalignment/skin irritation. *Note:* Placing a "cooling" cast directly on rubber or plastic pillows traps heat and increases drying time.
Suggest the use of a blow-dryer to dry small areas of dampened casts.	Cautious use can hasten drying.
Demonstrate use of plastic bags to cover plaster cast during wet weather or while bathing. Clean soiled cast with a slightly dampened cloth and some scouring powder.	Protects from moisture, which softens the plaster and weakens the cast. *Note:* Fiberglass casts are being used more frequently because they are not affected by moisture. In addition, their light weight may enhance patient participation in desired activities.
Stress importance of not adjusting clamps/nuts of external fixator.	Tampering may alter compression and misalign fracture.
Recommend use of adaptive clothing.	Facilitates dressing/grooming activities.
Suggest ways to cover toes, if appropriate, e.g., stockinette or soft socks.	Helps to maintain warmth/protect from injury.
Discuss post–cast removal instructions:	
Instruct the patient to continue exercises as permitted;	Reduces stiffness and improves strength and function of affected extremity.
Inform the patient that the skin under the cast is commonly mottled and covered with scales or crusts of dead skin;	It will be several weeks before normal appearance returns.

674

ACTIONS/INTERVENTIONS

Independent

Wash the skin gently with soap, povidone-iodine (Betadine), or pHisoDerm, and water. Lubricate with a protective emollient;

Inform the patient that muscles may appear flabby and atrophied (less muscle mass). Recommend supporting the joint above and below the affected part and the use of mobility aids, e.g., elastic bandages, splints, braces, crutches, walkers, or canes;

Elevate the extremity as needed.

RATIONALE

New skin is extremely tender because it has been protected beneath a cast.

Muscle strength will be reduced and new or different aches and pains may occur for awhile secondary to loss of support.

Swelling and edema tend to occur after cast removal.

POTENTIAL CONSIDERATIONS following acute hospitalization (dependent on patient's age, physical condition/presence of complications, personal resources, and life responsibilities)

In addition to surgical considerations:

Trauma, risk for—loss of skeletal integrity, weakness, balancing difficulties, reduced muscle coordination, lack of safety precautions, history of previous trauma

Physical Mobility, impaired—neuromuscular skeletal impairment; pain/discomfort, restrictive therapies (limb immobilization); psychologic immobility

Self Care deficit—musculoskeletal impairment, decreased strength/endurance, pain

Infection, risk for—inadequate primary defenses: broken skin, traumatized tissues; environmental exposure; invasive procedures, skeletal traction

AMPUTATION

In general, amputations are caused by accidents, disease, and congenital disorders. For the purpose of this plan of care, amputation refers to the surgical/traumatic removal of a limb. Lower-extremity amputations are performed much more frequently than upper-extremity amputations. Five levels are currently used in lower-extremity amputation: foot and ankle, below knee (BKA), knee disarticulation and above, knee-hip disarticulation; and hemipelvectomy and translumbar amputation. There are two types of amputations: (1) open (provisional), which requires strict aseptic techniques and later revisions and (2) closed, or "flap."

CARE SETTING

Inpatient acute surgical unit and subacute or rehabilitation unit.

RELATED CONCERNS

Surgical Intervention, p 802
Psychosocial Aspects of Care, p 783
Diabetes Mellitus/Diabetic Ketoacidosis, p 422
Cancer, p 875

Patient Assessment Data Base

Data is dependent on underlying reason for surgical procedure, e.g., severe trauma, peripheral vascular/arterial occlusive disease, diabetic neuropathy, osteomyelitis, cancer.

ACTIVITY/REST

May report: Actual/anticipated limitations imposed by condition/amputation

CIRCULATION

May exhibit: Presence of edema; diminished pulses in affected limb/digits

EGO INTEGRITY

May report: Concern about negative effects/anticipated changes in lifestyle, financial situation, reaction of others
Feelings of helplessness, powerlessness

May exhibit: Anxiety, apprehension, irritability, anger, fearfulness, withdrawal, grief, false cheerfulness

SEXUALITY

May report: Concerns about intimate relationships

SOCIAL INTERACTION

May report: Problems related to illness/condition
Concern about role function, reaction of others

TEACHING/LEARNING

Discharge plan considerations: **DRG projected mean length of inpatient stay: 9.7 days (upper extremity), 15 days (lower extremity)**

May require assistance with wound care/supplies, adaptation to prosthesis/ambulatory devices, transportation, homemaker/maintenance tasks, possibly self-care activities and vocational retraining

Refer to section at end of plan for postdischarge considerations.

DIAGNOSTIC STUDIES

Studies are dependent on underlying condition necessitating amputation and are used to determine the appropriate level for amputation.

X-rays: Identify skeletal abnormalities.
CT scan: Identifies neoplastic lesions, osteomyelitis, hematoma formation.
Angiography and blood flow studies: Evaluate alteration in circulation/tissue perfusion and help predict potential for tissue healing after amputation.
Doppler ultrasound, laser Doppler flowmetry: Performed to assess and measure blood flow.
Transcutaneous O$_2$ pressure: Maps out areas of greater and lesser perfusion in the involved extremity.
Thermography: Measures temperature differences in the ischemic limb at two sites, from cutaneous tissue to center of bone. The lower the difference between the two readings, the greater the chance for healing.
Plethysmography: Segmental systolic BP measurements to the lower extremity evaluates arterial blood flow.
Sedimentation rate (ESR): Elevation indicates inflammatory response.
Wound cultures: Identify presence of infection and causative organism.
WBC/differential: Elevation and ''shift to left'' suggest infectious process.
Biopsy: Confirms diagnosis of benign/malignant mass.

NURSING PRIORITIES

1. Support psychologic and physiologic adjustment.
2. Alleviate pain.
3. Prevent complications.
4. Promote mobility/functional abilities.
5. Provide information about surgical procedure/prognosis and treatment needs.

DISCHARGE GOALS

1. Dealing with current situation realistically.
2. Pain relieved/controlled.
3. Complications prevented/minimized.
4. Mobility/function regained or compensated for.
5. Surgical procedure, prognosis, and therapeutic regimen understood.
6. Plan in place to meet needs after discharge.

NURSING DIAGNOSIS: Self Esteem, situational low

May be related to
Loss of body part/change in functional abilities

Possibly evidenced by
Anticipated changes in lifestyle; fear of rejection/reaction by others
Negative feelings about body, focus on past strength, function, or appearance
Feelings of helplessness, powerlessness
Preoccupation with missing body part, not looking at or touching stump
Perceived change in usual patterns of responsibility/physical capacity to resume role

ACTIONS/INTERVENTIONS	RATIONALE
Independent	
Assess/consider the patient's preparation for and view of amputation.	The patient who views amputation as lifesaving or reconstructive will accept the new self more quickly. The patient with traumatic amputation or who considers amputation to be the result of failure in treatment is at greater risk for self-concept disturbances.
Encourage expression of fears, negative feelings, and grief over loss of body part.	Venting emotions helps patient begin to deal with the fact and reality of life without a limb.
Reinforce preoperative information including type/location of amputation, type of prosthetic fitting if appropriate (immediate, delayed), expected post-operative course, including pain control and rehabilitation.	Provides opportunity for patient to question and assimilate information and begin to deal with changes in body image and function, which can facilitate postoperative recovery.
Assess degree of support available to the patient.	Sufficient support by SO and friends can facilitate rehabilitation process.
Discuss patient's perceptions of self related to change and how patient sees self in usual lifestyle/role functioning.	Aids in defining concerns in relation to previous lifestyle and facilitates problem solving. For example, may fear loss of independence, ability to work, and so forth.
Ascertain individual strengths and identify previous positive coping behaviors.	Helpful to build on strengths that are already available for patient to use in coping with current situation.
Encourage participation in ADLs. Provide opportunities to view/care for stump, using the moment to point out positive signs of healing.	Promotes independence and enhances feelings of self-worth. Although integrating of stump into body image can take months or even years, looking at the stump and hearing positive comments (made in a normal, matter-of-fact manner) can help patient with this acceptance.
Encourage/provide for visit by another amputee, especially one who is successfully rehabilitating.	A peer who has been through a similar experience serves as a role model and can provide validity to comments as well as hope for recovery and a normal future.
Provide open environment for patient to discuss concerns about sexuality.	Promotes sharing of beliefs/values about sensitive subject and identifies misconceptions/myths that may interfere with adjustment to situation.
Note withdrawn behavior, negative self-talk, use of denial, or overconcern with actual/perceived changes.	Identifies stage of grief/need for interventions.
Collaborative	
Discuss availability of various resources, e.g., psychiatric/sexual counseling, occupational therapist.	May need assistance for these concerns to facilitate optimal adaptation and rehabilitation.

NURSING DIAGNOSIS: Pain [acute]

May be related to
Physical injury/tissue and nerve trauma
Psychologic impact of loss of body part

Possibly evidenced by
Reports of pain
Narrowed self-focus
Autonomic responses, guarding/protective behavior

DESIRED OUTCOMES/EVALUATION CRITERIA—PATIENT WILL:
Report pain is relieved/controlled.
Appear relaxed and able to rest/sleep appropriately.
Verbalize understanding of phantom pain and methods to provide relief.

ACTIONS/INTERVENTIONS	RATIONALE
Independent	
Document location and intensity of pain (0–10 scale). Investigate changes in pain characteristics, e.g., numbness, tingling.	Aids in evaluating need for and effectiveness of interventions. Changes may indicate developing complications, e.g., necrosis/infection.
Elevate affected part by raising foot of bed slightly or use of pillow/sling for upper-limb amputation.	Lessens edema formation by enhancing venous return; reduces muscle fatigue and skin/tissue pressure. *Note:* After initial 24 hours and in absence of edema, stump may be extended and kept flat.
Acknowledge reality of phantom limb sensations, that they are usually self-limiting, and that various modalities will be tried for pain relief.	Knowing about these sensations allows the patient to understand this is a normal phenomenon that may develop immediately or several weeks postoperatively. Although the sensations usually resolve on their own, some individuals continue to experience the discomfort for several months/years. *Note:* Phantom pain is not well relieved by traditional pain medications. TENS has proven to offer the most effective short-term relief, in addition to managing stump and prosthesis problems.
Provide/promote general comfort measures (e.g., frequent turning, backrub) and diversional activities. Encourage use of stress management techniques (e.g., deep-breathing exercises, visualization, guided imagery) and Therapeutic Touch.	Refocuses attention, promotes relaxation, may enhance coping abilities and may decrease occurrence of phantom-limb pain.
Provide gentle massage to stump as tolerated once dressings are discontinued.	Enhances circulation; reduces muscle tension.
Investigate reports of progressive/poorly localized pain unrelieved by analgesics.	May indicate developing compartmental syndrome, especially following traumatic injury. (Refer to CP: Fractures; ND: Peripheral Neurovascular dysfunction, risk for, p 664.)
Collaborative	
Administer medications, as indicated, e.g.: analgesics, muscle relaxants. Instruct in/monitor use of PCA.	Reduces pain/muscle spasms. PCA provides for timely drug administration, preventing fluctuations in pain with associated muscle tension/spasms.

ACTIONS/INTERVENTIONS	RATIONALE
Collaborative	
Maintain TENS device if used.	Provides continuous low-level nerve stimulation, blocking transmission of pain sensation. *Note:* There is some evidence that abnormal nerve stimuli and feedback mechanisms are present, possibly because of actual interrupted nerve pathways and partly because of abnormal activity of the remaining nerve fibers. Electrical stimulation offers a short-term rerouting or stimulation of different nerve pathways, thus reducing the activity of the usual pain patterns.
Provide topical heat as indicated.	May be used to promote muscle relaxation, enhance circulation, and facilitate resolution of edema.

NURSING DIAGNOSIS: Tissue Perfusion, altered: peripheral, risk for

Risk factors may include:
Reduced arterial/venous blood flow; tissue edema, hematoma formation
Hypovolemia

Possibly evidenced by:
[Not applicable; presence of signs and symptoms establishes an *actual* diagnosis]

DESIRED OUTCOMES/EVALUATION CRITERIA—PATIENT WILL:
Maintain adequate tissue perfusion as evidenced by palpable peripheral pulses, warm/ dry skin, and timely wound healing.

ACTIONS/INTERVENTIONS	RATIONALE
Independent	
Monitor vital signs. Palpate peripheral pulses, noting strength and equality.	General indicators of circulatory status and adequacy of perfusion.
Perform periodic neurovascular assessments, e.g., sensation, movement, pulse, skin color, and temperature.	Postoperative tissue edema, hematoma formation, or restrictive dressings may impair circulation to stump, resulting in tissue necrosis.
Inspect dressings/drainage device, noting amount and characteristics of drainage.	Continued blood loss may indicate need for additional fluid replacement and evaluation for coagulation defect or surgical intervention to ligate bleeder.
Apply direct pressure to bleeding site if hemorrhage occurs. Contact physician immediately.	Direct pressure to bleeding site may be followed by application of a bulk dressing secured with an elastic wrap once bleeding is controlled.
Investigate reports of persistent/unusual pain in operative site.	Hematoma can form in muscle pocket under flap, compromising circulation and intensifying pain.
Evaluate nonoperated lower limb for inflammation, positive Homans' sign.	Increased incidence of thrombus formation in patients with preexisting peripheral vascular disease/diabetic changes.
Encourage/assist with early ambulation.	Enhances circulation, helps prevent stasis and associated complications. Promotes sense of general well-being.

ACTIONS/INTERVENTIONS	RATIONALE
Collaborative	
Administer IV fluids/blood products as indicated.	Maintains circulating volume to maximize tissue perfusion.
Apply antiembolic/sequential hose to nonoperated leg.	May enhance venous return, reducing venous pooling and risk of thrombophlebitis.
Administer low-dose anticoagulant as indicated.	May be useful in preventing thrombus formation without increasing risk of postoperative bleeding/hematoma formation.
Monitor laboratory studies, e.g.:	
Hb/Hct;	Indicators of hypovolemia/dehydration that can impair tissue perfusion.
PT/aPTT.	Evaluates need for/effectiveness of anticoagulant therapy and identifies developing complication, e.g., posttraumatic DIC.

NURSING DIAGNOSIS: Infection, risk for

Risk factors may include
Inadequate primary defenses (broken skin, traumatized tissue)
Invasive procedures; environmental exposure
Chronic disease, altered nutritional status

Possibly evidenced by
[Not applicable; presence of signs and symptoms establishes an *actual* diagnosis]

DESIRED OUTCOMES/EVALUATION CRITERIA—PATIENT WILL:
Achieve timely wound healing; be free of purulent drainage or erythema; and be afebrile.

ACTIONS/INTERVENTIONS	RATIONALE
Independent	
Maintain aseptic technique when changing dressings/caring for wound.	Minimizes opportunity for introduction of bacteria.
Inspect dressings and wound; note characteristics of drainage.	Early detection of developing infection provides opportunity for timely intervention and prevention of more serious complications (e.g., osteomyelitis).
Maintain patency and routinely empty drainage device.	Hemovac, Jackson-Pratt drains facilitate removal of drainage, promoting wound healing and reducing risk of infection.
Cover dressing with plastic when using the bedpan or if incontinent.	Prevents contamination in lower-limb amputation.
Expose stump to air; wash with mild soap and water after dressings are discontinued.	Maintains cleanliness, minimizes skin contaminants, and promotes healing of tender/fragile skin.
Monitor vital signs.	Temperature elevation/tachycardia may reflect developing sepsis.

681

ACTIONS/INTERVENTIONS

Collaborative

Obtain wound/drainage cultures as appropriate.

Administer antibiotics as indicated.

RATIONALE

Identifies presence of infection/specific organisms and appropriate therapy.

Wide-spectrum antibiotics may be used prophylactically, or antibiotic therapy may be geared toward specific organisms.

NURSING DIAGNOSIS: Physical Mobility, impaired

May be related to
Loss of a limb (particularly a lower extremity); pain/discomfort; perceptual impairment (altered sense of balance)

Possibly evidenced by
Reluctance to attempt movement
Impaired coordination; decreased muscle strength, control, and mass

DESIRED OUTCOMES/EVALUATION CRITERIA—PATIENT WILL:
Verbalize understanding of individual situation, treatment regimen, and safety measures.
Display willingness to participate in activities.
Maintain position of function as evidenced by absence of contractures.
Demonstrate techniques/behaviors that enable resumption of activities.

ACTIONS/INTERVENTIONS

Independent

Provide regular stump care, e.g., inspect area, cleanse and dry thoroughly, and rewrap stump with elastic bandage or air splint, or apply a stump shrinker (heavy stockinette sock), for "delayed" prosthesis. Measure circumference periodically.

Rewrap stump immediately with an elastic bandage, elevate if "immediate/early" cast is accidentally dislodged. Prepare for reapplication of cast.

Assist with specified ROM exercises for the affected as well as unaffected limbs beginning early in postoperative stage.

Encourage active/isometric exercises for upper torso and arms.

Provide trochanter rolls as indicated.

Instruct patient to lie in prone position as tolerated at least twice a day with pillow under abdomen and lower-extremity stump.

RATIONALE

Provides opportunity to evaluate healing and note complications (unless covered by immediate prosthesis). Wrapping stump controls edema and helps form stump into conical shape to facilitate fitting of prosthesis. *Note:* Air splint may be preferred, because it permits visual inspection of the wound. Measurement is done to estimate shrinkage to ensure proper fit of sock and prosthesis.

Edema will occur rapidly, and rehabilitation can be delayed.

Prevents contracture deformities, which can develop rapidly and could delay prosthesis usage.

Increases muscle strength to facilitate transfers/ambulation.

Prevents external rotation of lower-limb stump.

Strengthens extensor muscles and prevents flexion contracture of the hip, which can begin to develop within 24 hours of sustained malpositioning.

682

ACTIONS/INTERVENTIONS	RATIONALE
Independent	
Caution against keeping pillow under lower-extremity stump or allowing BKA limb to hang dependently over side of bed or chair.	Use of pillows can cause permanent flexion contracture of hip, and a dependent position of stump impairs venous return and may increase edema formation.
Demonstrate/assist with transfer techniques and use of mobility aids, e.g., trapeze, crutches, or walker.	Facilitates self-care and patient's independence. Proper transfer techniques prevent shearing abrasions/dermal injury related to "scooting."
Assist with ambulation.	Reduces potential for injury. Ambulation after lower-limb amputation is dependent on timing of prosthesis placement. For example: (1) *Immediate postoperative fitting:* A rigid plaster-of-paris dressing is applied to the stump and a pylon and artificial foot are attached. Weight bearing begins within 24–48 hours. (2) *Early postoperative fitting:* Weight bearing does not occur until 10–30 days postoperatively. (3) *Delayed fitting:* More common in areas that do not have facilities available for immediate/early application of prosthesis or when the condition of the stump and/or the patient precludes these choices. *Note:* Amputation of an upper extremity can affect the patient's sense of balance, necessitating monitoring/assistance with ambulation.
Help patient continue preoperative muscle exercises as able/when allowed out of bed; e.g., patient should (while holding on to chair for balance) perform abdominal-tightening exercises and knee bends; hop on foot; stand on toes.	Contributes to gaining improved sense of balance and strengthens compensatory body parts.
Instruct patient in stump-conditioning exercises, e.g., pushing the stump against a pillow initially, then progressing to harder surface.	Hardens the stump by toughening the skin and altering feedback of resected nerves to facilitate use of prosthesis.
Collaborative	
Refer to rehabilitation team, e.g., physical and occupational therapy.	Provides for creation of exercise/activity program to meet individual needs and strengths, and identifies mobility functional aids to promote independence. Early use of a temporary prosthesis promotes activity and enhances general well-being/positive outlook. *Note:* Vocational counseling/retraining also may be indicated.
Provide foam/flotation mattress.	Reduces pressure on skin/tissues that can impair circulation, potentiating risk of tissue ischemia/breakdown.

NURSING DIAGNOSIS: Knowledge deficit [learning need] regarding condition, prognosis, treatment, self care and discharge needs

May be related to
Lack of exposure/recall
Information misinterpretation

Possibly evidenced by
Questions/request for information, verbalization of the problem
Inaccurate follow-through of instructions/development of preventable complications

ACTIONS/INTERVENTIONS	RATIONALE
Independent	
Review disease process/surgical procedure and future expectations.	Provides knowledge base on which patient can make informed choices.
Instruct in dressing/wound care, inspection of stump using mirror to visualize all areas, skin massage, and appropriate wrapping of the stump.	Promotes competent self-care; facilitates healing and fitting of prosthesis and reduces potential for complications.
Discuss general stump care, e.g.:	
Massaging the stump after dressings are discontinued and suture line is healed;	Massage softens scar and prevents adherence to the bone, decreases tenderness, and stimulates circulation.
Avoiding use of lotions/powders;	Although a small amount of lotion may be indicated if skin is dry, emollients/creams soften skin and may cause maceration when a prosthesis is worn. Powder may cake, potentiating skin irritation.
Wearing only properly fitted, clean, wrinkle-free limb sock;	Stump may continue to shrink for up to 2 years, and an improperly fitting sock or one that is mended or dirty can cause skin irritation/breakdown.
Using clean cotton T-shirt under harness for upper-limb prosthesis.	Absorbs perspiration; prevents skin irritation from harness.
Demonstrate care of prosthetic device. Stress importance of routine maintenance/periodic refitting.	Ensures proper fit, reduces risk of complications, and prolongs life of prosthesis.
Encourage continuation of postoperative exercise program.	Enhances circulation/healing and function of affected part, facilitating adaptation to prosthetic device.
Identify techniques to manage phantom pain, e.g., good stump care, properly fitted prosthesis, gentle massage/pressure to stump. Stress control, relaxation training, and various medications that may be used.	Reduces muscle tension and enhances control of situation and coping abilities.
Stress importance of well-balanced diet and adequate fluid intake.	Provides needed nutrients for tissue regeneration/healing, aids in maintaining circulating volume and normal organ function, and aids in maintenance of proper weight (weight changes affect fit of prosthesis).
Recommend cessation of smoking.	Smoking potentiates peripheral vasoconstriction, impairing circulation as well as tissue oxygenation.
Identify signs/symptoms requiring medical evaluation, e.g., edema, erythema, increased/odorous drainage from incision; changes in sensation, movement, skin color; persistent phantom pain.	Prompt intervention may prevent serious complication and/or loss of function. *Note:* Chronic phantom-limb pain may indicate neuroma, requiring surgical resection.

ACTIONS/INTERVENTIONS	RATIONALE
Independent	
Identify community support and rehabilitation, e.g., certified prosthetist-orthotist, amputee groups, home care service, homemaker services as needed.	Facilitates transfer to home, supports independence, and enhances coping.

POTENTIAL CONSIDERATIONS following acute hospitalization (dependent on patient's age, physical condition/presence of complications, personal resources, and life responsibilities)

In addition to considerations in Surgical Intervention plan of care:

Trauma, risk for—balancing difficulties/altered gait, muscle weakness, reduced muscle coordination, lack of safety precautions, hazards associated with use of assistive devices

Self-Esteem, situational low—loss of body part, change in functional abilities

Self Care deficit/Home Maintenance Management, impaired (dependent on location of amputation)—musculoskeletal impairment, decreased strength/endurance, pain, depression

TOTAL JOINT REPLACEMENT

Joint replacement is indicated for irreversibly damaged joints and unremitting pain (e.g., degenerative and rheumatoid arthritis [RA]); selected fractures (e.g., femoral neck), joint instability, and congenital hip disease. The surgery can be performed on any joint except the spine. Hip and knee replacements are the most common procedures. The prosthesis may be metallic or polyethylene (or a combination) and implanted with an acrylic cement, or it may be a porous, coated implant that encourages bony ingrowth.

CARE SETTING

Inpatient acute surgical unit and subacute or rehabilitation unit.

RELATED CONCERNS

Surgical Intervention, p 802
Rheumatoid Arthritis, p 764
Cancer, p 875
Psychosocial Aspects of Care, p 783

Patient Assessment Data Base

ACTIVITY/REST

May report: Difficulty with ambulation; stiffness in joints (worse in the morning or after period of inactivity)
History of occupation/participation in sports activities that wears on particular joint
Inability to participate in occupational/recreational activities at desired level
Interruption of sleep, delayed falling asleep/awakened by pain; does not feel well rested.

May exhibit: Decreased ROM of affected joints; decreased muscle strength/tone

HYGIENE

May report: Difficulty performing ADLs
Use of special equipment/devices
Need for assistance

NEUROSENSORY

May exhibit: Impaired ROM of affected joints

PAIN/DISCOMFORT

May report: Pain (dull, aching, persistent) in affected joint(s), worsened by movement

SAFETY

May report: Traumatic injury/fractures affecting the joint
Bone tumor, congenital deformities
History of inflammatory, debilitating arthritis (RA or osteoarthritis); aseptic necrosis of the joint head

May exhibit: Joint/tissue swelling, decreased ROM, changes in gait

TEACHING/LEARNING

May report: Current medication use, e.g., anti-inflammatory, analgesics/narcotics, steroids

Discharge plan considerations: **DRG projected mean length of inpatient stay: 7.6 days**
May need assistance with transportation, self-care activities, homemaker/maintenance tasks, possible placement in extended-care facility for continued rehabilitation/assistance

Refer to section at end of plan for postdischarge considerations.

DIAGNOSTIC STUDIES

X-rays and scans of bones/joints: Determine extent of degeneration and rule out malignancy.

NURSING PRIORITIES

1. Prevent complications.
2. Promote optimal mobility.
3. Alleviate pain.
4. Provide information about diagnosis, prognosis, and treatment needs.

DISCHARGE GOALS

1. Complications prevented/minimized.
2. Mobility increased.
3. Pain relieved/controlled.
4. Diagnosis, prognosis, and therapeutic regimen understood.
5. Plan in place to meet needs after discharge.

NURSING DIAGNOSIS: Infection, risk for

Risk factors may include
Inadequate primary defenses (broken skin, exposure of joint)
Inadequate secondary defenses/immunosuppression (long-term corticosteroid use, cancer)
Invasive procedures; surgical manipulation; implantation of foreign body
Decreased mobility

Possibly evidenced by
[Not applicable; presence of signs and symptoms establishes an *actual* diagnosis]

DESIRED OUTCOMES/EVALUATION CRITERIA—PATIENT WILL:
Achieve timely wound healing, be free of purulent drainage or erythema, and be afebrile.

ACTIONS/INTERVENTIONS	RATIONALE
Independent	
Promote good hand-washing by staff and patient.	Reduces risk of cross-contamination.
Use strict aseptic or clean techniques as indicated to reinforce/change dressings and when handling drains. Instruct patient not to touch/scratch incision.	Prevents contamination and risk of wound infection, which could require removal of prosthesis.

ACTIONS/INTERVENTIONS	RATIONALE

Independent

Maintain patency of drainage devices (e.g., Hemovac/Jackson-Pratt). Note characteristics of wound drainage.	Reduces risk of infection by preventing accumulation of blood and secretions in the joint space (medium for bacterial growth). Purulent, nonserous, odorous drainage is indicative of infection, and continuous drainage from incision may reflect developing skin tract, which can potentiate infectious process.
Assess skin/incision color, temperature and integrity; note presence of erythema/inflammation, loss of wound approximation.	Provides information about status of healing process and alerts staff to early signs of infection.
Investigate reports of increased wound pain, changes in characteristics of pain.	Deep, dull, aching pain in operative area may indicate infection in joint. *Note:* Infection is devastating because joint cannot be saved once infection sets in and prosthetic loss will occur.
Monitor temperature. Note presence of chills.	Although temperature elevations are common in early postoperative phase, elevations occurring 5 or more days postoperatively and/or presence of chills usually indicates developing infection requiring intervention to prevent more serious complications, e.g., sepsis, osteomyelitis, tissue necrosis, and prosthetic failure.
Encourage fluid intake, high-protein diet with roughage.	Maintains fluid and nutritional balance to support tissue perfusion and provide nutrients necessary for cellular regeneration and tissue healing.

Collaborative

Maintain reverse/protective isolation, if appropriate.	May be done initially to reduce contact with sources of possible infection, especially in elderly, immunosuppressed, or diabetic patient.
Administer antibiotics as indicated.	May be used prophylactically to prevent infection.
Culture drainage routinely/as needed.	Verifies presence of infection; identifies causative organism. Anaerobic or aerobic bacteria may be present, affecting choice of antibiotic and therapy.

NURSING DIAGNOSIS: Physical Mobility, impaired

May be related to
Pain and discomfort, musculoskeletal impairment
Surgery/restrictive therapies

Possibly evidenced by
Reluctance to attempt movement, difficulty purposefully moving within the physical environment
Reports of pain/discomfort on movement
Limited ROM; decreased muscle strength/control

DESIRED OUTCOMES/EVALUATION CRITERIA—PATIENT WILL:
Maintain position of function, as evidenced by absence of contracture.
Display increased strength and function of affected joint and limb.
Verbalize understanding of individual treatment regimen and participate in rehabilitation program.

ACTIONS/INTERVENTIONS	RATIONALE
Independent	
Maintain initial bed rest with affected joint in prescribed position and body in alignment.	Provides time for stabilization of prosthesis and recovery from effects of anesthesia, reducing risk of injury. Length of bed rest depends on joint replaced (e.g., usually 24–72 hours for hip).
Limit use of semi-high-Fowler's position, if indicated.	Prolonged hip flexion may strain/dislocate new prosthesis.
Elevate extremity by raising foot of bed slightly, not knee gatch. Limit movement as indicated, e.g., keep operative leg slightly abducted after total hip or knee replacement to prevent crossing of legs/inward rotation of joint.	Enhances venous return to prevent excessive edema formation; may prevent dislocation of prosthesis. Use of knee gatch or pillow under knee can compromise circulation.
Medicate prior to procedures/activities.	Muscle relaxants, narcotics/analgesics decrease pain, reduce muscle tension/spasm, and facilitate participation in therapy.
Turn on unoperated side using adequate number of personnel and maintaining operated extremity in neutral alignment. Support position with pillows/wedges.	Prevents dislocation of hip prosthesis and prolonged skin/tissue pressure, reducing risk of tissue ischemia/breakdown.
Demonstrate/assist with transfer techniques and use of mobility aids, e.g., trapeze, walker.	Facilitates self-care and patient's independence. Proper transfer techniques prevent shearing abrasions of skin and falls.
Inspect skin; observe for reddened areas. Keep linens dry and wrinkle-free. Massage skin/bony prominences routinely. Protect operative heel, elevating whole length of leg with pillow and placing heel on water glove if burning sensation reported.	Prevents skin irritation/breakdown.
Perform/assist with ROM to unaffected joints.	Patient with degenerative joint disease can quickly lose joint function during periods of restricted activity.
Promote participation in rehabilitative exercise program, e.g.:	
Total hip: Quadriceps and gluteal muscle setting, hip-hiking, isometrics, leg lifts, dorsiflexion, plantar flexion of the foot. *Total knee:* Quadriceps setting, gluteal contraction, flexion/extension exercises, isometrics.	Strengthens muscle groups, increasing muscle tone and mass; stimulates circulation; prevents decubitus. Active use of the joint may be painful but will not injure the joint. In fact, continuous passive motion (CPM) exercise is usually mechanically performed on the knee joint within the first 48–72 hours.
Other joints: Exercises are individually designed, e.g., toes and knee movements (for ankle-joint replacement); arm and unaffected fingers (for finger-joint replacement).	Meets individual needs of the joint that is replaced.
Observe appropriate limitations based on specific joint; e.g., avoid marked flexion/rotation of hip and flexion or hyperextension of leg; adhere to weight-bearing restrictions; wear knee immobilizer as indicated.	Joint stress is to be avoided at all times during stabilization period to prevent dislocation of new prosthesis.
Investigate sudden increase in pain and shortening of limb, as well as changes in skin color, temperature, and sensation.	Indicative of slippage of prosthesis, requiring medical evaluation/intervention.

689

ACTIONS/INTERVENTIONS	RATIONALE
Independent	
Encourage participation in ADLs.	Enhances self-esteem; promotes sense of control and independence.
Provide positive reinforcement for efforts.	Promotes a positive attitude and encourages involvement in therapy.
Collaborative	
Consult with physical/occupational therapists and rehabilitation specialist.	Useful in creating individualized activity/exercise program. Patient may require ongoing assistance with movement, strengthening, and weight-bearing activities as well as use of adjuncts, e.g., walkers, crutches, canes, elevated toilet seat, pickup sticks, and so on.
Provide foam/flotation mattress.	Reduces skin/tissue pressure; limits feelings of fatigue and general discomfort.

NURSING DIAGNOSIS: Tissue Perfusion, altered: peripheral, risk for

Risk factors may include
Reduced arterial/venous blood flow: Trauma to blood vessels; tissue edema, improper location/dislocation of prosthesis; hypovolemia

Possibly evidenced by
[Not applicable; presence of signs and symptoms establishes an *actual* diagnosis]

DESIRED OUTCOMES/EVALUATION CRITERIA—PATIENT WILL:
Demonstrate adequate tissue perfusion as evidenced by palpable pulses, skin warm/dry, stable vital signs.

ACTIONS/INTERVENTIONS	RATIONALE
Independent	
Palpate pulses. Evaluate capillary refill as well as skin color and temperature. Compare with nonoperated limb.	Diminished/absent pulses, delayed capillary refill time, pallor, blanching, cyanosis, and coldness of skin reflect diminished circulation/perfusion. Comparison with unoperated limb provides clues as to whether neurovascular problem is localized or generalized.
Assess motion and sensation of operated extremity.	Increasing pain, numbness/tingling, inability to perform expected movements (e.g., flex foot) suggest nerve injury, compromised circulation, or dislocation of prosthesis, requiring immediate intervention.
Test sensation of peroneal nerve by pinch/pinprick in the dorsal web between first and second toe and assess ability to dorsiflex toes after hip/knee replacement.	Position and length of peroneal nerve increases risk of direct injury or compression by tissue edema/hematoma.

ACTIONS/INTERVENTIONS	RATIONALE

Independent

Monitor vital signs.

Tachycardia and decreasing BP may reflect response to hypovolemia/blood loss or suggest anaphylaxis related to absorption of methyl methacrylate into systemic circulation. *Note:* This occurs less often because of the advent of prosthetics with a porous layer that fosters ingrowth of bone instead of total reliance on adhesives to internally fix the device.

Monitor amount and characteristics of drainage on dressings/from suction device. Note swelling in operative area.

May indicate excessive bleeding/hematoma formation, which can potentiate neurovascular compromise.

Ensure that stabilizing devices (e.g., abduction pillow, trochanter rolls, sling on splint device, traction apparatus) are in correct position and are not exerting undue pressure on skin and underlying tissue. Avoid use of pillow or knee gatch under knees.

Reduces risk of pressure on underlying nerves or compromised circulation to extremities.

Evaluate for calf tenderness, positive Homans' sign, and inflammation.

Early identification of thrombus development and intervention may prevent embolus formation.

Observe for signs of continued bleeding, oozing from puncture sites/mucous membranes, or ecchymosis following minimal trauma.

Depression of clotting mechanisms/sensitivity to anticoagulants may result in bleeding episodes that can affect RBC level and circulating volume.

Observe for restlessness, confusion, sudden chest pain, dyspnea, tachycardia, fever, development of petechiae.

Fat emboli can occur (usually in first 72 hours postoperatively) because of traumatic manipulation of bone marrow during implantation of hip prosthesis.

Collaborative

Administer IV fluids, blood/plasma expanders as needed.

Restores circulating volume to maintain perfusion. *Note:* Drainage collected from operative site during first 6–10 hours following procedure may be reinfused per protocol, reducing need for transfusion from unknown donor.

Monitor laboratory studies, e.g.:

Hct;

Usually done 24–48 hours postoperatively for evaluation of blood loss, which can be quite large because of high vascularity of surgical site.

Coagulation studies.

Evaluates presence/degree of alteration in clotting mechanisms and effects of anticoagulant/antiplatelet agents when used.

Administer medications as indicated, e.g.: sodium warfarin (Coumadin), heparin, aspirin, low-molecular-weight heparin, e.g., enoxaparin (Lovenox).

Anticoagulants/antiplatelet agents may be used to reduce risk of thrombophlebitis and fat emboli.

Apply cold/heat as indicated.

Ice packs are used initially to limit edema/hematoma formation. Heat may then be used to enhance circulation, facilitating resolution of tissue edema.

Apply elastic leg wraps or antiembolic stockings.

Promotes venous return and prevents venous stasis, reducing risk of thrombus formation.

Prepare for surgical procedure as indicated.

Evacuation of hematoma or relocation of prosthesis may be required to correct compromised circulation.

691

ACTIONS/INTERVENTIONS	RATIONALE
Independent	
Assess reports of pain, noting intensity (scale of 0–10), duration, and location.	Provides information on which to base and monitor effectiveness of interventions.
Maintain proper position of operated extremity.	Reduces muscle spasm and undue tension on new prosthesis and surrounding tissues.
Provide comfort measures (e.g., use of lumbar roll, frequent repositioning, backrub) and diversional activities. Encourage stress management techniques (e.g., progressive relaxation, guided imagery, visualization) and use of Therapeutic Touch.	Reduces muscle tension, refocuses attention, promotes sense of control, and may enhance coping abilities in the management of discomfort/pain, which can persist for an extended period.
Medicate on a regular schedule and prior to activities/procedures.	Reduces muscle tension; improves comfort, and facilitates participation.
Investigate reports of sudden, severe joint pain with muscle spasms and changes in joint mobility; sudden, severe chest pain with dyspnea and restlessness.	Early recognition of developing problems, such as dislocation of prosthesis or pulmonary emboli (blood/fat), provides opportunity for prompt intervention and prevention of more serious complications.
Collaborative	
Administer narcotics, analgesics, and muscle relaxants as needed. Instruct in/monitor use of PCA.	Relieves surgical pain and reduces muscle tension/spasm, which contributes to overall discomfort. Narcotic infusion may be given during first 24–48 hours, with oral analgesics added to pain management program as patient progresses. *Note:* Use of Toradol or other NSAIDs is contraindicated when patient is receiving Lovenox therapy.
Apply ice packs as indicated.	Promotes vasoconstriction to reduce bleeding/tissue edema in surgical area and lessens perception of discomfort.
Maintain TENS unit if used.	Provides constant low-level electrical stimulation to nerves blocking transmission of sensations of pain.

ACTIONS/INTERVENTIONS

Initiate/maintain extremity mobilization: e.g., ambulation, physical therapy, exerciser devices, CPM device.

RATIONALE

Increases circulation to affected muscles. Minimizes joint stiffness; relieves muscle spasms related to disuse.

NURSING DIAGNOSIS: Knowledge deficit [learning need] regarding condition, prognosis, treatment, self care and discharge needs

May be related to
Lack of exposure/recall
Information misinterpretation

Possibly evidenced by
Questions/request for information, statement of misconception
Inaccurate follow-through of instructions/development of preventable complications

DESIRED OUTCOMES/EVALUATION CRITERIA—PATIENT WILL:
Verbalize understanding of surgical procedure and prognosis.
Correctly perform necessary procedures and explain reasons for the actions.

ACTIONS/INTERVENTIONS

Independent

Review disease process, surgical procedure, and future expectations.

Encourage alternating rest periods with activity.

Stress importance of continuing prescribed exercise/rehabilitation program within patient's tolerance: crutch/cane walking, weight-bearing exercises, stationary bicycling, or swimming.

Review/instruct in home use of continuous motion exercise program.

Review long-term activity limitations, dependent on joint replaced, e.g., for hip/knee—sitting for long periods or in low chair/toilet seat, jogging, jumping, excessive bending, lifting, twisting or crossing legs.

Discuss need for safe environment in home (e.g., removing scatter rugs and unnecessary furniture) and use of assistive devices (e.g., handrails in tub/toilet, raised toilet seat, cane for long walks).

Review incisional/wound care.

Stress importance of continuing to wear antiembolic stockings.

RATIONALE

Provides knowledge base on which patient can make informed choices.

Conserves energy for healing and prevents undue fatigue, which can increase risk of injury/fall.

Increases muscle strength and joint mobility. Some patients may be involved in formal rehabilitation programs or be followed in extended-care facilities by physical therapists. Muscle aching indicates too much weight bearing or activity, signaling a need to cut back.

Ongoing CPM therapy may be necessary with earlier discharge from hospital care.

Prevents undue stress on implant.

Reduces risk of falls and excessive stress on joints.

Promotes independence in self-care, reducing risk of complications.

Prevents venous pooling; enhances venous return to reduce risk of thrombophlebitis.

693

ACTIONS/INTERVENTIONS	RATIONALE
Independent	
Identify signs/symptoms requiring medical evaluation, e.g., fever/chills, incisional inflammation, unusual wound drainage, pain in calf or upper thigh, or development of "strep" throat/dental infections.	Bacterial infections require prompt treatment to prevent progression to osteomyelitis in the operative area and prosthesis failure, which could occur at any time, even years later.
Review drug regimen, e.g., anticoagulants or antibiotics for invasive procedures (e.g., tooth extraction).	Prophylactic therapy may be necessary for a prolonged period after discharge to limit risk of thromboemboli/infection. Procedures known to cause bacteremia can result in osteomyelitis and prosthesis failure.
Identify bleeding precautions, (e.g., use of soft toothbrush, electric razor, avoidance of trauma/forceful blowing of nose), and necessity of routine laboratory follow-up.	Reduces risk of therapy-induced bleeding/hemorrhage.
Encourage intake of balanced diet including roughage and adequate fluids.	Enhances healing and feeling of general well-being. Promotes bowel and bladder function during period of altered activity.

POTENTIAL CONSIDERATIONS following acute hospitalization (dependent on patient's age, physical condition/presence of complications, personal resources, and life responsibilities)

In addition to considerations in Surgical Intervention plan of care:
Trauma, risk for—balancing difficulties/altered gait, weakness, lack of safety precautions, hazards associated with use of assistive devices
Self Care deficit/Home Maintenance Management, impaired—musculoskeletal impairment, decreased strength/endurance, pain in operative site or other joints

Sample CP: Total Hip Replacement, Hospital. ELOS: 6 Days Orthopedic or Surgical Unit

ND and Categories of Care	Day 1 Day of Surgery	Day 2 POD 1	Day 3 POD 2	Day 4 POD 3	Day 5 POD 4	Day 6 POD 5
Risk for infection R/T broken skin, exposure of joint, long-term steroid use, decreased mobility	Goals: Participate in activities to reduce risk of postop infection	→ Free of purulent drainage; Be afebrile	→	→	→	→ Display early signs of wound healing, free of erythema or drainage
		→			→ Verbalize understanding of healthcare needs to enhance healing, promote wellness	→ Plan in place to meet postdischarge needs, self-care
Diagnostics	Hb/Hct; Pulse oximetry	→ ; → D/C	CBC; Electrolytes			
Additional assessments	VS/Temp-per postop protocol	q4h	q8h	→ BID unless elevated	→ D/C	
	Breath sounds q8h	→	→	→ BID	→ D/C	
	Amt/characteristics of Hemovac drainage q8h	→	→ D/C			
			Characteristics of wound/drainage qd & prn	→	→	→
Medications Allergies:	IV antibiotics	→	→ D/C			
	IV fluids/blood products	→	→ NS lock or D/C	→ D/C lock		
	Tylenol-Temp ≥101°F	→	→	→	→	→
Patient education	Disease process/surgical procedure; Hand-washing technique, avoid touching of dressing/wound	→	→	→ Wound care; Balancing rest/activity		→ Provide written instructions for home care
	Respiratory exercises, incentive spirometry	→	Dietary needs; Signs/symptoms to report to healthcare provider	→	→	→
Additional nursing actions	Aseptic/clean technique	→	→ D/C		→	→
	Protective isolation as indicated	→	→ D/C			
	Reinforce dressing	→	→ Change dressing qd & prn	→ D/C if incision dry	→ Clean incision BID	→
	Encourage po fluids as tol	→	→			
	T, C, DB q2h	→	→ Per self	→	→	→
	Incentive spirometry q2h	→ q2hWA	→ q4hWA	→	→	→
	Supplemental O₂ as indicated	→ D/C	→ High calorie/protein diet	→	→	→

Sample CP: Total Hip Replacement, Hospital. ELOS: 6 Days Orthopedic or Surgical Unit (*Continued*)

ND and Categories of Care	Day 1 Day of Surgery	Day 2 POD 1	Day 3 POD 2	Day 4 POD 3	Day 5 POD 4	Day 6 POD 5
Impaired physical mobility R/T musculoskeletal impairment/discomfort, therapeutic restrictions	Maintain proper alignment & position of function → Participate in rehab/exercise program →			→	→	Independent in ambulation Free of DT/thromboembolitic complications
				Independent in transfers	Display increased strength/function of op limb Establish regular bladder/bowel elimination	
Referrals		PT-assistive devices if not done preop	PT-exercises/ambulation	OT/Rehab specialist SS if placement indi	Home care	
Diagnostic studies		aPTT →	PT/aPTT →	PT →	→	→
Additional assessments	Neurovas-status/ alignment of op leg per postop protocol					
	Skin (especially heels) q8h or per protocol	→ q4h	→ q8h	→ bid	→	→
	Voiding/urinary output q8h	→	→	→ qd	→	→
	Bowel sounds q8h	→	→ bid	→ D/C → qd	→ D/C	
Medications Allergies:	Heparin/Lovenox per protocol q8h	→	→ D/C	→	→	→
		Coumadin qd Stool softener qHS	Laxative if no BM	Suppository/Fleets if no BM	→	→
Patient education	Hip precautions Use of trapeze Initial exercises-ankle pumps, quad/gluteal sets	Transfer techniques	Use of mobility aids Signs/symptoms to report to healthcare provider	Ambulation/wt-bearing exercises Activity level/ restrictions post-discharge Sexual concerns	Home exercise program Coumadin dose, time, purpose, side effects, precautions, monitoring	Provide written instructions
Additional nursing actions	Bedrest/HOB elevated 30°	→ Chair/commode elevate op leg	→ Chair X3	→ Ambulate X3 with assist	→	→
	Legs abducted Turn per protocol q2h ROM to non op side q2h	→ → →	→ Per self	→ prn	→	→
	Initial exercises q1hWA	→	→ Knee exercise X5 q1hWA	→ Leg strengthening	→	→

Sample CP: Total Hip Replacement, Hospital. ELOS: 6 Days Orthopedic or Surgical Unit (*Continued*)

ND and Categories of Care	Day 1 Day of Surgery	Day 2 POD 1	Day 3 POD 2	Day 4 POD 3	Day 5 POD 4	Day 6 POD 5
	Thigh-high TEDS	→	→	→	→	→ Send home
	SCDs	Remove q8h	→	→	D/C if PT 1.3 or above	
	Total care	While in bed	Self care	→	→	→
	Fracture pan	Assist w/care	→	→	Shower as indi	→
	St catch if no void q8h PRN X2	Elevated toilet seat	→	→	→	→
	Insert Foley on #3 if no void	→	D/C Foley-male	D/C Foley female	→	→ Send home
	Foam/special mattress	→	→	→	→	→ Send home
Pain R/T therapeutic interventions, pre-existing chronic joint disease	Verbalize pain within manageable level	→	→	→	→	→
		Participate in actions to decrease pain	→	→	→	→
						Verbalize understanding of medications/ modalities for pain management; Demonstrates proper use adjunct comfort measures (e.g., TENS unit)
Additional assessments	Pain characteristics/ changes	→	→	→	→	→
	Response to interventions					
Medications Allergies: _____	PCA-narcotic of choice	→	IM/PO	→	D/C, IM/po cont	→
	Antiemetic prn	D/C	→	→	→	→
	Muscle relaxant	→	→	→	→	→
			Acetamin PRN for breakthrough pain	→	→	→
Patient education	Orient to unit/room					
	Proper use of PCA					
	Reporting of pain/ effects of interventions					
		Relaxation techniques, guided imagery, breathing exercises				
					Medications: dose, time, route, purpose, side effects TENS unit (if indi)	
						Written instructions for home care needs, equipment resources
Additional nursing actions	Maintain position/ alignment of leg per protocol	→	→	→	→	→
	Ice pack to op site	prn	D/C			
	Routine comfort measures prn	→	→	→	→	→

CHAPTER 13

Integumentary

BURNS: THERMAL/CHEMICAL/ELECTRICAL (ACUTE AND CONVALESCENT PHASES)

Thermal burns: Injuring agent can be flame, hot liquid, or contact with hot object. Flame burns are associated with smoke/inhalation injury.

Chemical burns: Occur from type/content of injuring agent, as well as concentration and temperature of agent.

Electrical burns: Occur from type/voltage of current that generates heat in proportion to resistance offered and travels the pathway of least resistance (i.e., nerves offer the least resistance and bones the greatest resistance). Underlying injury will be more severe than visible injury.

Superficial partial-thickness burns (first degree): Involve only the epidermis. Wounds appear bright pink to red with minimal edema and no blisters. The skin is often warm/dry.

Moderate partial-thickness burns (second degree): Involve the epidermis and dermis. Wounds appear red to pink with moderate edema and moist, weeping blisters.

Deep partial-thickness burns (second degree): Involve the deep dermis. Wounds appear pink to pale ivory with moderate edema and blisters. These wounds are dryer than the moderate partial-thickness burns.

Full-thickness burns (third degree): Involve all layers of skin, subcutaneous fat, and may involve the muscle, nerves, and blood supply. Wound appearance varies from white to cherry red to brown or black, with blistering uncommon. These wounds have a dry, leathery texture.

Full-thickness burns (fourth degree): Involve all skin layers plus muscle, organ tissue, and bone. Charring occurs.

CARE SETTING

The following adult patients are admitted for acute care and during the rehabilitation phase may be cared for in a subacute or rehabilitation unit: those with partial-thickness burns greater than 15% TBSA or high-risk age (over 65 years of age); or full-thickness burn more than 2% of TBSA; burns of face, both hands, perineum or both feet; or inhalation and all electrical burns.

RELATED CONCERNS

Patient Assessment Data Base

Data is dependent on type, severity, and body surface area involved.

ACTIVITY/REST

May exhibit:	Decreased strength, endurance
	Limited ROM of involved areas
	Impaired muscle mass, altered tone

CIRCULATION

May exhibit (with burn injury involving more than 20% TBSA):	Hypotension (shock)
	Peripheral pulses diminished distal to extremity injury; generalized peripheral vasoconstriction with loss of pulses, mottling of skin, and coolness (electrical shock)
	Tachycardia (shock/anxiety/pain)
	Dysrhythmias (electrical shock)
	Tissue edema formation (all burns)

EGO INTEGRITY

May report:	Concerns about family, job, finances, disfigurement
May exhibit:	Anxiety, crying, dependency, denial, withdrawal, hostility

ELIMINATION

May exhibit:	Urinary output decreased/absent during emergent phase. Color may be pink (hemochromogens from damaged RBCs) or reddish black if myoglobin present, indicating deep-muscle damage
	Diuresis (after capillary leak sealed and fluids mobilized back into circulation)
	Bowel sounds decreased/absent, especially in cutaneous burns of greater than 20%, as stress reduces gastric motility/peristalsis

FOOD/FLUID

May exhibit:	Generalized tissue edema (swelling is rapid and may be extreme in early hours after injury)
	Anorexia, nausea/vomiting

NEUROSENSORY

May report:	Mixed areas of numbness, tingling
	Decreased visual acuity (electrical shock)
May exhibit:	Changes in orientation, affect, behavior
	Decreased DTRs in injured extremities
	Seizure activity (electrical shock)
	Corneal lacerations, retinal damage (electrical shock)
	Rupture of tympanic membrane (electrical shock)
	Paralysis (electrical injury to nerve pathways)

PAIN/DISCOMFORT

May report:	Pain varies, e.g., first-degree burns are extremely sensitive to touch, pressure, air movement, and temperature changes; second-degree moderate-thickness burns are very painful, while pain response in second-degree deep-thickness burns is dependent on intactness of nerve endings; third-degree burns are painless.

699

RESPIRATION

May report: Confinement in a closed space, prolonged exposure (possibility of inhalation injury)

May exhibit: Hoarseness, wheezy cough, carbonaceous particles in sputum, drooling/inability to swallow oral secretions, and cyanosis (indicative of inhalation injury)

Thoracic excursion may be limited in presence of circumferential chest burns

Upper airway stridor/wheezes (obstruction due to laryngospasm, laryngeal edema)

Breath sounds: Crackles (pulmonary edema), stridor (laryngeal edema), profuse airway secretions (rhonchi)

SAFETY

May exhibit: **Skin:**

General: Exact depth of tissue destruction may not be evident for 3–5 days due to the process of microvascular thrombosis in some wounds. Unburned skin areas may be cool/clammy, pale, with slow capillary refill in the presence of decreased cardiac output due to fluid loss/shock state.

Flame injury: There may be areas of mixed depth of injury due to varied intensity of heat produced by burning clothing. Singed nasal hairs; dry, red mucosa of nose and mouth; blisters on posterior pharynx; circumoral and/or circumnasal edema.

Chemical injury: Appearance of wound varies according to causative agent. Skin may be yellowish brown with soft leatherlike texture; blisters, ulcers, necrosis, or thick eschar. Injuries are generally deeper than they appear cutaneously, and tissue destruction can continue for up to 72 hours after injury.

Electrical injury: The external cutaneous injury is usually much less than the underlying necrosis. Appearance of wounds varies and may include entry/exit (explosive) wounds of current, arc burns from current moving in close proximity to body, and thermal burns due to ignition of clothing.

Other: Presence of fractures/dislocations (concurrent falls, motor vehicle accident; tetanic muscle contractions due to electrical shock)

TEACHING/LEARNING

Discharge plan considerations: **DRG projected mean length of inpatient stay: 18.4–31.4 days (inclusive)**

May require assistance with treatments, wound care/supplies, self-care activities, homemaker/maintenance tasks, transportation, finances, vocational counseling

Changes in physical layout of home or living facility other than home during prolonged rehabilitation

Refer to section at end of plan for postdischarge considerations.

DIAGNOSTIC STUDIES

CBC: Initial increased Hct suggests hemoconcentration due to fluid shift/loss. Later decreased Hct and RBCs may occur due to heat damage to vascular endothelium. Leukocytosis (decreased WBCs) can occur due to loss of cells at wound site and inflammatory response to injury.

ABGs: Baseline especially important with suspicion of inhalation injury. Reduced PaO_2/increased $PaCO_2$ may be seen with carbon monoxide retention. Acidosis may occur due to reduced renal function and loss of compensatory respiratory mechanisms.

COHb (carboxyhemoglobin): Elevation of greater than 15% indicates carbon monoxide poisoning/inhalation injury.

Serum electrolytes: Potassium may be initially elevated due to injured tissues/RBC destruction and decreased renal function; hypokalemia can occur when diuresis starts; magnesium may be decreased. Sodium may initially be decreased with body water losses; hypernatremia can occur later as renal conservation occurs.

Alkaline phosphatase: Elevated due to interstitial fluid shifts/impairment of sodium pump.

Serum glucose: Elevation reflects stress response.

Serum albumin: Albumin/globulin ratio may be reversed due to loss of protein in edema fluid.

BUN/Cr: Elevation reflects decreased renal perfusion/function; however, Cr can elevate because of tissue injury.

Urine: Presence of albumin, Hb, and myoglobin indicates deep-tissue damage and protein loss (especially seen with serious electrical burns). Reddish-black color of urine is due to presence of myoglobin.

Random urine sodium: Greater than 20 mEq/L indicates excessive fluid resuscitation; less than 10 mEq/L suggests inadequate fluid resuscitation.

Wound cultures: May be obtained for baseline data and repeated periodically.

Chest x-ray: May appear normal in early postburn period even with inhalation injury; however, a true inhalation injury will present as infiltrates, often progressing to whiteout on x-ray (ARDS).

Fiberoptic bronchoscopy: Useful in diagnosing extent of inhalation injury; findings can include edema, hemorrhage, and/or ulceration of upper respiratory tract.

Flow volume loop: Provides noninvasive assessment of effects/extent of inhalation injury.

Lung scan: May be done to determine extent of inhalation injury.

ECG: Signs of myocardial ischemia/dysrhythmias may occur with electrical burns.

Photographs of burns: Provides documentation for later burn-wound healing.

NURSING PRIORITIES

1. Maintain patent airway/respiratory function.
2. Restore hemodynamic stability/circulating volume.
3. Alleviate pain.
4. Prevent complications.
5. Provide emotional support for patient/SO.
6. Provide information about condition, prognosis, and treatment.

DISCHARGE GOALS

1. Homeostasis achieved.
2. Pain controlled/reduced.
3. Complications prevented/minimized.
4. Dealing with current situation realistically.
5. Condition/prognosis and therapeutic regimen understood.
6. Plan in place to meet needs after discharge.

NURSING DIAGNOSIS: Airway Clearance, ineffective, risk for

Risk factors may include

Tracheobronchial obstruction: Mucosal edema and loss of ciliary action (smoke inhalation); circumferential full-thickness burns of the neck, thorax, and chest, with compression of the airway or limited chest excursion

Trauma: Direct upper-airway injury by flame, steam, hot air, and chemicals/gases

Fluid shifts, pulmonary edema, decreased lung compliance

Possibly evidenced by

[Not applicable; presence of signs and symptoms establishes an *actual* diagnosis]

DESIRED OUTCOMES/EVALUATION CRITERIA—PATIENT WILL:

Demonstrate clear breath sounds, respiratory rate within normal range, free of dyspnea/cyanosis.

ACTIONS/INTERVENTIONS	RATIONALE

Independent

Obtain history of injury. Note presence of preexisting respiratory conditions, history of smoking.	Causative agent, duration of exposure, occurrence in closed or open space indicates probability of inhalation injury. Type of material burned (wood, plastic, wool, and so forth) suggests type of toxic gas exposure. Preexisting conditions increase the risk of respiratory complications.
Assess gag/swallow reflexes; note drooling, inability to swallow, hoarseness, wheezy cough.	Suggestive of inhalation injury.
Monitor respiratory rate, rhythm, depth; note presence of pallor/cyanosis and carbonaceous or pink-tinged sputum.	Tachypnea, use of accessory muscles, presence of cyanosis, and changes in sputum suggest developing respiratory distress/pulmonary edema, and need for medical intervention.
Auscultate lungs, noting stridor, wheezing/crackles, diminished breath sounds, brassy cough.	Airway obstruction/respiratory distress can occur very quickly or may be delayed, e.g., up to 48 hours after burn.
Note presence of pallor or cherry-red color of uninjured skin.	Suggests presence of hypoxemia or carbon monoxide.
Elevate head of bed. Avoid use of pillow under head, as indicated.	Promotes optimal lung expansion/respiratory function. When head/neck burns are present, a pillow can inhibit respiration, cause necrosis of burned ear cartilage, and promote neck contractures.
Encourage coughing/deep-breathing exercises and frequent position changes.	Promotes lung expansion, mobilization and drainage of secretions.
Suction (if necessary) with extreme care, maintaining sterile technique.	Helps to maintain clear airway, but should be done cautiously because of mucosal edema and inflammation. Sterile technique reduces risk of infection.
Promote voice rest but assess ability to speak and/or swallow oral secretions periodically.	Increasing hoarseness/decreased ability to swallow suggests increasing tracheal edema and may indicate need for prompt intubation.
Investigate changes in behavior/mentation, e.g., restlessness, agitation, confusion.	Although often related to pain, changes in consciousness may reflect developing/worsening hypoxia.
Monitor 24-hour fluid balance, noting variations/changes.	Fluid shifts or excess fluid replacement increases risk of pulmonary edema. *Note:* Inhalation injury increases fluid demands as much as 35% or more because of obligatory edema.

Collaborative

Administer humidified O_2 via appropriate mode, e.g., face mask.	O_2 corrects hypoxemia/acidosis. Humidity decreases drying of respiratory tract and reduces viscosity of sputum.
Monitor/graph serial ABGs or pulse oximetry.	Baseline is essential for further assessment of respiratory status and as a guide to treatment. PaO_2 less than 50, $PaCO_2$ greater than 50, and decreasing pH reflect smoke inhalation and developing pneumonia/ARDS.
Review serial x-rays.	Changes reflecting atelectasis/pulmonary edema may not occur for 2–3 days after burn.

ACTIONS/INTERVENTIONS

Independent

Provide/assist with chest physiotherapy and incentive spirometry.

Prepare for/assist with intubation or tracheostomy as indicated.

RATIONALE

Chest physiotherapy drains dependent areas of the lung, while incentive spirometry may be done to improve lung expansion, thereby promoting respiratory function and reducing atelectasis.

Intubation/mechanical support is required when airway edema or circumferential burn injury interferes with respiratory function/oxygenation.

NURSING DIAGNOSIS: Fluid Volume deficit, risk for

Risk factors may include
Loss of fluid through abnormal routes, e.g., burn wounds
Increased need: Hypermetabolic state, insufficient intake
Hemorrhagic losses

Possibly evidenced by
[Not applicable; presence of signs and symptoms establishes an *actual* diagnosis]

DESIRED OUTCOMES/EVALUATION CRITERIA—PATIENT WILL:
Demonstrate improved fluid balance as evidenced by individually adequate urinary output with normal specific gravity, stable vital signs, moist mucous membranes.

ACTIONS/INTERVENTIONS

Independent

Monitor vital signs, CVP. Note capillary refill and strength of peripheral pulses.

Monitor urinary output and specific gravity. Observe urine color and hematest as indicated.

Estimate wound drainage and insensible losses.

Maintain cumulative record of amount and type of fluid intake.

RATIONALE

Serves as a guide to fluid replacement needs and assesses cardiovascular response. *Note:* Invasive monitoring is indicated for patients with major burns, smoke inhalation, or preexisting cardiac disease, although there is an associated increased risk of infection, necessitating careful monitoring and care of insertion site.

Generally, fluid replacement should be titrated to ensure average urinary output of 30–50 ml/h (in the adult). Urine can appear red to black with massive muscle destruction, due to presence of blood and release of myoglobin. If gross myoglobinuria is present, minimum urinary output should be 75–100 ml/h to prevent tubular damage/necrosis.

Increased capillary permeability, protein shifts, inflammatory process, and evaporative losses greatly affect circulating volume and urinary output, especially during initial 24–72 hours after burn.

Massive/rapid replacement with different types of fluids and fluctuations in rate of administration requires close tabulation to prevent constituent imbalances or fluid overload.

ACTIONS/INTERVENTIONS	RATIONALE

Independent

Weigh daily.

Fluid replacement formulas partly depend on admission weight and subsequent changes. A 15%–20% weight gain in the first 72 hours during fluid replacement can be anticipated, with return to preburn weight approximately 10 days after burn.

Measure circumference of burned extremities daily as indicated.

May be helpful in estimating extent of edema/fluid shifts affecting circulating volume and urinary output.

Investigate changes in mentation.

Deterioration in the level of consciousness may indicate inadequate circulating volume/reduced cerebral perfusion.

Observe for gastric distention, hematemesis, tarry stools. Hematest NG drainage and stools periodically.

Stress (Curling's) ulcer occurs in up to half of all severely burned patients (can occur as early as first week). Burn patients with greater than 20% TBSA are at risk for mucosal bleeding in the GI tract during the acute phase because of decreased splanchnic blood flow and reflex paralytic ileus.

Collaborative

Insert/maintain indwelling urinary catheter.

Allows for close observation of renal function and prevents stasis or reflux of urine. Retention of urine with its byproducts of tissue-cell destruction can lead to renal dysfunction and infection.

Insert/maintain large-bore IV catheter(s).

Accommodates rapid infusion of fluids.

Administer calculated IV replacement of fluids, electrolytes, plasma, albumin.

Fluid resuscitation replaces lost fluids/electrolytes and helps to prevent complications, e.g., shock, ATN. Replacement formulas vary (e.g., Brooke, Evans, Parkland) but are based on extent of injury, amount of urinary output and weight. *Note:* Once initial fluid resuscitation has been accomplished, a steady rate of fluid administration is preferred to "boluses," which may increase interstitial fluid shifts and cardiopulmonary congestion.

Monitor laboratory studies (e.g., Hb/Hct, electrolytes, random urine sodium).

Identifies blood loss/RBC destruction, and fluid and electrolyte replacement needs. Urine sodium less than 10 mEq/L suggests inadequate fluid resuscitation. *Note:* During first 24 hours postburn, hemoconcentration is common due to fluid shifts into the interstitial space.

Administer medications as indicated:

  Diuretics, e.g., mannitol (Osmitrol);

May be indicated to enhance urinary output and clear tubules of debris/prevent necrosis, if acute renal failure is present.

  Potassium;

Although hyperkalemia often occurs during first 24–48 hours (tissue destruction), subsequent replacement may be necessary because of large urinary losses.

  Antacids, e.g., calcium carbonate (Titrilac), magaldrate (Riopan); histamine inhibitors, e.g., cimetidine (Tagamet)/ranitidine (Zantac).

Antacids may reduce gastric acidity, while histamine inhibitors decrease production of hydrochloric acid to reduce risk of gastric irritation/bleeding.

ACTIONS/INTERVENTIONS

Collaborative

Add electrolytes to water used for wound débridement.

RATIONALE

Washing solution that approximates tissue fluids may minimize osmotic fluid shifts.

NURSING DIAGNOSIS: Infection, risk for

Risk factors may include
Inadequate primary defenses: Destruction of skin barrier, traumatized tissues
Inadequate secondary defenses: Decreased Hb, suppressed inflammatory response
Environmental exposure, invasive procedures

Possibly evidenced by
[Not applicable; presence of signs and symptoms establishes an *actual* diagnosis]

DESIRED OUTCOMES/EVALUATION CRITERIA—PATIENT WILL:
Achieve timely wound healing free of purulent exudate and be afebrile.

ACTIONS/INTERVENTIONS

Independent

Implement appropriate isolation techniques as indicated.

Stress necessity of good hand-washing technique for all individuals coming in contact with patient.

Use gowns, gloves, masks, and strict aseptic technique during direct wound care and provide sterile or freshly laundered bed linens/gowns.

Monitor/limit visitors, if necessary. If isolation is used, explain procedure to visitors. Supervise visitor adherence to protocol as indicated.

Shave/clip all hair from around burned areas to include a 1-in border (excluding eyebrows). Shave facial hair (men) and shampoo head daily.

Examine unburned areas (such as groin, neck creases, mucous membranes) and vaginal discharge routinely.

Provide special care for eyes, e.g., use eye covers and tear formulas as appropriate.

Prevent skin-to-skin surface contact (e.g., wrap each burned finger/toe separately; do not allow burned ear to touch scalp).

RATIONALE

Dependent on type/extent of wounds and the choice of wound treatment (e.g., open versus closed), isolation may range from simple wound/skin to complete or reverse to reduce risk of cross-contamination and exposure to multiple bacterial flora.

Prevents cross-contamination; reduces risk of acquired infection.

Prevents exposure to infectious organisms.

Prevents cross-contamination from visitors. Concern for risk of infection should be balanced against patient's need for family support and socialization.

Hair is a good medium for bacterial growth; however, eyebrows act as a protective barrier for the eyes. Regular shampooing decreases bacterial fallout into burned areas.

Opportunistic infections (e.g., yeast) frequently occur due to depression of the immune system and/or proliferation of normal body flora during systemic antibiotic therapy.

Eyes may be swollen shut and/or become infected by drainage from surrounding burns. If lids are burned, eye covers may be needed to prevent corneal damage.

Prevents adherence to surface it may be touching and encourages proper healing. *Note:* Ear cartilage has limited circulation and is prone to pressure necrosis.

705

ACTIONS/INTERVENTIONS	RATIONALE

Independent

Examine wounds daily, note/document changes in appearance, odor, or quantity of drainage.

Identifies presence of healing (granulation tissue) and provides for early detection of burn-wound infection. Infection in a partial-thickness burn may cause conversion of burn to full-thickness injury.

Monitor vital signs for fever, increased respiratory rate/depth in association with changes in sensorium, presence of diarrhea, decreased platelet count, and hyperglycemia with glycosuria.

Indicators of sepsis (often occurs with full-thickness burn) requiring prompt evaluation and intervention. *Note:* Changes in sensorium, bowel habits, and respiratory rate usually precede fever and alteration of laboratory studies.

Collaborative

Place IV/invasive lines in nonburned area.

Decreased risk of infection at insertion site with possibility of progression to septicemia.

Remove dressings and cleanse burned areas in a hydrotherapy/whirlpool tub or in a shower stall with handheld shower head. Maintain temperature of water at 100°F (37.8°C). Wash areas with a mild cleansing agent or surgical soap.

Water softens and aids in removal of dressings and eschar (slough layer of dead skin or tissue). Sources vary as to whether bath or shower is best. Bath has advantage of water providing support for exercising extremities but may promote cross-contamination of wounds. Showering enhances wound inspection and prevents contamination from floating debris.

Débride necrotic/loose tissue (including ruptured blisters) with scissors and forceps. Do not disturb intact blisters if they are smaller than 2–3 cm, do not interfere with joint function, and do not appear infected.

Promotes healing. Prevents autocontamination. Small, intact blisters help to protect skin and increase rate of reepithelialization unless the burn injury is the result of chemicals (in which case fluid contained in blisters may continue to cause tissue destruction).

Obtain routine cultures and sensitivities of wounds/ drainage.

Allows early recognition and specific treatment of wound infection.

Assist with excisional biopsies when infection is suspected.

Bacteria can colonize the wound surface without invading the underlying tissue; therefore, biopsies may be obtained for diagnosing infection.

Photograph wound initially and at periodic intervals.

Provides baseline and documentation of healing process.

Administer topical agents as indicated, e.g.:

The following agents help to control bacterial growth and prevent drying of wound, which can cause further tissue destruction.

Silver sulfadiazine (Silvadene);

Wide-spectrum antimicrobial that is relatively painless but has less eschar penetration than Sulfamylon and may cause rash or depression of WBCs.

Mafenide acetate (Sulfamylon);

Antibiotic of choice with confirmed invasive burn-wound infection. Useful against gram-negative/gram-positive organisms. Causes burning/pain on application and for 30 minutes thereafter. Can cause rash, metabolic acidosis, and decreased $PaCO_2$.

Silver nitrate;

Effective against *Staphylococcus aureus*, *Escherichia coli*, and *Pseudomonas aeruginosa*, but has poor eschar penetration, is painful, and may cause electrolyte imbalance. Dressings must be constantly saturated. Product stains skin/surfaces black.

ACTIONS/INTERVENTIONS

Collaborative

Povidone-iodine (Betadine);

Hydrogels, e.g., Transorb.

Administer medications as appropriate, e.g.;

Subeschar clysis/systemic antibiotics;

Tetanus toxoid or clostridial antitoxin as appropriate.

RATIONALE

Broad-spectrum antimicrobial but is painful on application, may cause metabolic acidosis/increased iodine absorption, and damage fragile tissues.

Useful for partial- and full-thickness burns: fills dead spaces, rehydrates dry wound beds, and promotes autolytic débridement. May be used when infection is present.

Systemic antibiotics are given to control general infections identified by culture/sensitivity. Subeschar clysis has been found effective against pathogens in granulated tissues at the line of demarcation between viable/nonviable tissue, reducing risk of sepsis.

Tissue destruction/altered defense mechanisms increases risk of developing tetanus or gas gangrene, especially in deep burns such as those caused by electricity.

NURSING DIAGNOSIS: Pain [acute]

May be related to
Destruction of skin/tissues; edema formation
Manipulation of injured tissues, e.g., wound débridement

Possibly evidenced by
Reports of pain
Narrowed focus, facial mask of pain
Alteration in muscle tone; autonomic responses
Distraction guarding behaviors; anxiety/fear

DESIRED OUTCOMES/EVALUATION CRITERIA—PATIENT WILL:
Report pain reduced/controlled.
Display relaxed facial expressions/body posture.
Participate in activities and sleep/rest appropriately.

ACTIONS/INTERVENTIONS

Independent

Cover wounds as soon as possible unless open-air exposure burn care method required.

Elevate burned extremities periodically.

Provide bed cradle as indicated.

RATIONALE

Temperature changes and air movement can cause great pain to exposed nerve endings.

Elevation may be required initially to reduce edema formation; thereafter, changes in position and elevation reduce discomfort as well as risk of joint contractures.

Elevation of linens off wounds may help to reduce pain.

ACTIONS/INTERVENTIONS	RATIONALE

Independent

Wrap digits/extremities in position of function (avoiding flexed position of affected joints) using splints and footboards as necessary.	Position of function reduces deformities/contractures and promotes comfort. Although flexed position of injured joints may feel more comfortable, it can lead to flexion contractures.
Change position frequently and assist with active and passive ROM as indicated.	Movement and exercise reduce joint stiffness and muscle fatigue, but type of exercise is dependent on location and extent of injury.
Maintain comfortable environmental temperature, provide heat lamps, heat-retaining body coverings.	Temperature regulation may be lost with major burns. External heat sources may be necessary to prevent chilling.
Assess reports of pain, noting location/character and intensity (0–10 scale).	Pain is nearly always present to some degree because of varying severity of tissue involvement/destruction but is usually most severe during dressing changes and débridement. Changes in location, character, intensity of pain may indicate developing complications (e.g., limb ischemia) or herald improvement/return of nerve function/sensation.
Provide medication and/or place in hydrotherapy (as appropriate) before performing dressing changes and débridement.	Reduces severe physical and emotional distress associated with dressing changes and débridement.
Encourage expression of feelings about pain.	Verbalization allows outlet for emotions and may enhance coping mechanisms.
Involve patient in determining schedule for activities, treatments, drug administration.	Enhances patient's sense of control and strengthens coping mechanisms.
Explain procedures/provide frequent information as appropriate, especially during wound débridement.	Empathic support can help to alleviate pain/promote relaxation. Knowing what to expect provides opportunity for patient to prepare self and enhances sense of control.
Provide basic comfort measures, e.g., massage of uninjured areas, frequent position changes.	Promotes relaxation; reduces muscle tension and general fatigue.
Encourage use of stress management techniques, e.g., progressive relaxation, deep breathing, guided imagery, and visualization.	Refocuses attention, promotes relaxation, and enhances sense of control, which may reduce pharmacologic dependency.
Provide diversional activities appropriate for age/condition.	Helps to lessen concentration on pain experience and refocus attention.
Promote uninterrupted sleep periods.	Sleep deprivation can increase perception of pain/reduce coping abilities.

Collaborative

Administer analgesics (narcotic and non-narcotic) as indicated.	IV method is often used initially to maximize drug effect. Concerns of patient addiction or doubts regarding degree of pain experienced are not valid during emergent/acute phase of care, but narcotics should be decreased as soon as feasible and alternate methods for pain relief initiated.

ACTIONS/INTERVENTIONS

Collaborative

Provide/instruct in use of PCA.

RATIONALE

PCA provides for timely drug administration, preventing fluctuations in intensity of pain, often at lower total dosage than would be given by conventional methods.

NURSING DIAGNOSIS: Tissue Perfusion, altered/Peripheral Neurovascular dysfunction, risk for

Risk factors may include

Reduction/interruption of arterial/venous blood flow, e.g., circumferential burns of extremities with resultant edema

Hypovolemia

Possibly evidenced by

[Not applicable; presence of signs and symptoms establishes an *actual* diagnosis]

DESIRED OUTCOMES/EVALUATION CRITERIA—PATIENT WILL:

Maintain palpable peripheral pulses of equal quality/strength; good capillary refill and skin color normal in uninjured areas.

ACTIONS/INTERVENTIONS

Independent

Assess color, sensation, movement, peripheral pulses (via Doppler), and capillary refill on extremities with circumferential burns. Compare with findings of unaffected limb.

Elevate affected extremities, as appropriate. Remove jewelry/arm band. Avoid taping around a burned extremity/digit.

Obtain BP in unburned extremity. Remove BP cuff after each reading.

Investigate reports of deep/throbbing ache, numbness.

Encourage active ROM exercises of unaffected body parts.

Investigate irregular pulses.

RATIONALE

Edema formation can readily compress blood vessels, thereby impeding circulation and increasing venous stasis/edema. Comparisons with unaffected limbs aid in differentiating localized versus systemic problems (e.g., hypovolemia/decreased cardiac output).

Promotes systemic circulation/venous return and may reduce edema or other deleterious effects of constriction of edematous tissues. Prolonged elevation can impair arterial perfusion if BP falls or tissue pressures rise excessively.

If BP readings must be obtained on an injured extremity, leaving the cuff in place may increase edema formation/reduce perfusion, and convert partial-thickness burn to a more serious injury.

Indicators of decreased perfusion and/or increased pressure within enclosed space, such as may occur with a circumferential burn of an extremity (compartment syndrome).

Promotes local and systemic circulation.

Cardiac dysrhythmias can occur as a result of electrolyte shifts, electrical injury, or release of myocardial depressant factor, compromising cardiac output/tissue perfusion.

ACTIONS/INTERVENTIONS

Collaborative

Maintain fluid replacement per protocol. (Refer to ND: Fluid Volume deficit, risk for, p 703.)

Monitor electrolytes, especially sodium, potassium, and calcium. Administer replacement therapy as indicated.

Avoid use of IM/SC injections.

Measure intracompartmental pressures as indicated. (Refer to CP: Fractures; ND: Peripheral Neurovascular dysfunction, risk for p 664.)

Assist with/prepare for escharotomy/fasciotomy, as indicated.

RATIONALE

Maximizes circulating volume and tissue perfusion.

Losses/shifts of these electrolytes affect cellular membrane potential/excitability, thereby altering myocardial conductivity, potentiating risk of dysrhythmias, and reducing cardiac output and tissue perfusion.

Altered tissue perfusion and edema formation impair drug absorption. Injections into potential donor sites may render them unusable due to hematoma formation.

Ischemic myositis may develop due to decreased perfusion.

Enhances circulation by relieving constriction caused by rigid, nonviable tissue (eschar) or edema formation.

NURSING DIAGNOSIS: Nutrition: altered, less than body requirements

May be related to
Hypermetabolic state (can be as much as 50%–60% greater than normal proportional to the severity of injury)
Protein catabolism
Anorexia, restricted oral intake

Possibly evidenced by
Decrease in total body weight, loss of muscle mass/subcutaneous fat, and development of negative nitrogen balance

DESIRED OUTCOMES/EVALUATION CRITERIA—PATIENT WILL:
Demonstrate nutritional intake adequate to meet metabolic needs as evidenced by stable weight/muscle-mass measurements, positive nitrogen balance, and tissue regeneration.

ACTIONS/INTERVENTIONS

Independent

Auscultate bowel sounds, noting hypoactive/absent sounds.

Maintain strict calorie count. Weigh daily. Reassess percent of open body surface area/wounds weekly.

Monitor muscle mass/subcutaneous fat as indicated.

RATIONALE

Ileus is often associated with postburn period but usually subsides within 36–48 hours, at which time oral feedings can be initiated.

Appropriate guides to proper caloric intake. As burn wound heals, percentage of burned areas is reevaluated to calculate prescribed dietary formulas, and appropriate adjustments are made.

May be useful in estimating body reserves/losses and effectiveness of therapy.

ACTIONS/INTERVENTIONS	RATIONALE
Independent	
Provide small, frequent meals and snacks.	Helps to prevent gastric distention/discomfort and may enhance intake.
Encourage patient to view diet as a treatment and to make food/beverage choices high in calories/protein.	Calories and proteins are needed to maintain weight, meet metabolic needs, and promote wound healing.
Ascertain food likes/dislikes. Encourage SO to bring food from home, as appropriate.	Provides patient/SO sense of control; enhances participation in care and may improve intake.
Encourage patient to sit up for meals and visit with others.	Sitting helps to prevent aspiration and aids in proper digestion of food. Socialization promotes relaxation and may enhance intake.
Provide oral hygiene before meals.	Clean mouth/clear palate enhances taste and helps promote a good appetite.
Perform fingerstick glucose, urine testing as indicated.	Monitors for development of hyperglycemia related to hormonal changes/demands or use of hyperalimentation to meet caloric needs.
Collaborative	
Refer to dietitian/nutritional support team.	Useful in establishing individual nutritional needs (based on weight and body surface area of injury) and identifying appropriate routes.
Provide diet high in calories/protein with vitamin supplements.	Calories (3000–5000/d), proteins, and vitamins are needed to meet increased metabolic needs, maintain weight, and encourage tissue regeneration. *Note:* Oral route is preferable once GI function returns.
Insert/maintain small feeding tube for enteral feedings and supplements if needed.	Provides continuous/supplemental feedings when patient is unable to consume total daily calorie requirements orally. *Note:* Continuous tube feeding during the night increases calorie intake without decreasing appetite and oral intake during the day.
Administer parenteral nutritional solutions containing vitamins and minerals as indicated.	TPN will maintain nutritional intake/meet metabolic needs in presence of severe complications or sustained esophageal/gastric injuries that do not permit enteral feedings.
Monitor laboratory studies, e.g., serum albumin/prealbumin, Cr, transferrin; urine urea nitrogen.	Indicators of nutritional needs and adequacy of diet/therapy.
Administer insulin as indicated.	Elevated serum glucose levels may develop due to stress response to injury, high caloric intake, pancreatic fatigue.

NURSING DIAGNOSIS: Physical Mobility, impaired

May be related to
Neuromuscular impairment, pain/discomfort, decreased strength and endurance
Restrictive therapies, limb immobilization; contractures

Possibly evidenced by
Reluctance to move/inability to purposefully move
Limited ROM, decreased muscle strength control and/or mass

ACTIONS/INTERVENTIONS	RATIONALE
Independent	
Maintain proper body alignment with supports or splints, especially for burns over joints.	Promotes functional positioning of extremities and prevents contractures, which are more likely over joints.
Note circulation, motion, and sensation of digits frequently.	Edema may compromise circulation to extremities potentiating tissue necrosis/development of contractures.
Initiate the rehabilitative phase on admission.	It is easier to enlist participation when the patient is aware of the possibilities that exist for recovery.
Perform ROM exercises consistently, initially passive, then active.	Prevents progressively tightening scar tissue and contractures; enhances maintenance of muscle/joint functioning and reduces loss of calcium from the bone.
Medicate for pain before activity/exercises.	Reduces muscle/tissue stiffness and tension, enabling patient to be more active and facilitating participation.
Schedule treatments and care activities to provide periods of uninterrupted rest.	Increases patient's strength and tolerance for activity.
Instruct and assist with mobility aids, e.g., cane, walker, crutches as appropriate.	Promotes safe ambulation.
Encourage family/SO support and assistance with ROM exercises.	Enables family/SO to be active in patient care and provides more constant/consistent therapy.
Incorporate ADLs with physical therapy, hydrotherapy, and nursing care.	Combining activities produces improved results by enhancing effects of each.
Encourage patient participation in all activities as individually able.	Promotes independence, enhances self-esteem, and facilitates recovery process.
Collaborative	
Provide foam, water/air mattress or kinetic therapy bed as indicated.	Prevents prolonged pressure on tissues, reducing potential for tissue ischemia/necrosis and decubitus formation.
Excise and cover burn wounds quickly.	Early excision is known to reduce scarring as well as risk of infection, thereby facilitating healing.
Maintain pressure garment when used.	Hypertrophic scarring can develop around grafted areas or at the site of deep partial-thickness wounds. Pressure dressings minimize scar tissue by keeping it flat, soft, and pliable.

ACTIONS/INTERVENTIONS

Collaborative

Consult with rehabilitation, physical, and occupational therapists.

RATIONALE

Normally members of the burn team, these specialists provide integrated activity/exercise program and specific assistive devices based on individual needs. Consultation facilitates intensive long-term management of potential deficits.

NURSING DIAGNOSIS: Skin Integrity, impaired [grafts]

May be related to
Disruption of skin surface with destruction of skin layers (partial-/full-thickness burn) requiring grafting

Possibly evidenced by
Absence of viable tissue

DESIRED OUTCOMES/EVALUATION CRITERIA—PATIENT WILL:
Demonstrate tissue regeneration.
Achieve timely healing of burned areas.

ACTIONS/INTERVENTIONS

Independent

Preoperative

Assess/document size, color, depth of wound, noting necrotic tissue and condition of surrounding skin.

Provide appropriate burn care and infection control measures. (Refer to ND: Infection, risk for, p 705.)

Postoperative

Maintain wound covering as indicated, e.g.:

Biosynthetic dressing (Biobrane);

Synthetic dressings, e.g., DuoDerm;

Op-Site, ACU-Derm.

Elevate grafted area if possible/appropriate. Maintain desired position and immobility of area when indicated.

RATIONALE

Provides baseline information about need for skin grafting and possible clues about circulation in area to support graft.

Prepares tissues for grafting and reduces risk of infection/graft failure.

Nylon fabric/silicon membrane containing collagenous porcine peptides that adheres to wound surface until removed or sloughed off by spontaneous skin reepithelialization. Useful for eschar-free partial-thickness burns awaiting autografts because it can remain in place 2–3 weeks or longer and is permeable to topical antimicrobial agents.

Hydroactive dressing that adheres to the skin to cover small partial-thickness burns and interacts with wound exudate to form a soft gel that facilitates débridement.

Thin, transparent, elastic, waterproof, occlusive dressing (permeable to moisture and air) that is used to cover clean partial-thickness wounds and clean donor sites.

Reduces swelling/limits risk of graft separation. Movement of tissue under graft can dislodge it, interfering with optimal healing.

ACTIONS/INTERVENTIONS	RATIONALE
Independent	
Maintain dressings over newly grafted area and/or donor site as indicated, e.g., mesh, petroleum, nonadhesive.	Areas may be covered by translucent, nonreactive surface material (between graft and outer dressing) to eliminate shearing of new epithelium/protect healing tissue.
Keep skin free from pressure.	Promotes circulation and prevents ischemia/necrosis and graft failure.
Evaluate color of grafted and donor sites; note presence/absence of healing.	Evaluates effectiveness of circulation and identifies developing complications.
Wash sites with mild soap, rinse, and lubricate with cream (e.g., Nivea) several times daily, after dressings are removed and healing is accomplished.	Newly grafted skin and healed donor sites require special care to maintain flexibility.
Aspirate blebs under sheet grafts with sterile needle or roll with sterile swab.	Fluid-filled blebs prevent graft adherence to underlying tissue, increasing risk of graft failure.
Collaborative	
Prepare for/assist with surgical procedure or biologic dressings, e.g.:	
Homograft (allograft);	Skin grafts obtained from living persons or cadavers are used as a temporary covering for extensive burns until person's own skin is ready for grafting (test graft), to cover excised wounds immediately after escharotomy, or to protect granulation tissue.
Heterograft (xenograft, porcine);	Skin grafts may be carried out with animal skin for the same purposes as homografts or to cover meshed autografts.
Autograft.	Skin graft obtained from uninjured part of patient's own skin; may be full-thickness or partial-thickness.

NURSING DIAGNOSIS: Fear/Anxiety

May be related to
Situational crises: Hospitalization/isolation procedures, interpersonal transmission and contagion, memory of the trauma experience, threat of death and/or disfigurement

Possibly evidenced by
Expressed concern regarding changes in life, fear of unspecific consequences
Apprehension; increased tension
Feelings of helplessness, uncertainty, decreased self-assurance
Sympathetic stimulation, extraneous movements, restlessness, insomnia

DESIRED OUTCOMES/EVALUATION CRITERIA—PATIENT WILL:
Verbalize awareness of feelings and healthy ways to deal with them.
Report anxiety/fear reduced to manageable level.
Demonstrate problem-solving skills, effective use of resources.

ACTIONS/INTERVENTIONS	RATIONALE
Independent	
Provide frequent explanations and information about care procedures.	Knowing what to expect usually reduces fear and anxiety, clarifies misconceptions, and promotes cooperation.
Demonstrate willingness to listen and talk to patient when free of painful procedures.	Helps patient/SO to know that support is available and that caregiver is interested in the person, not just care of the burn.
Involve patient/SO in decision-making process whenever possible.	Promotes sense of control and cooperation, decreasing feelings of helplessness/hopelessness.
Assess mental status, including mood/affect, comprehension of events, and content of thoughts, e.g., illusions or manifestations of terror/panic.	Initially, the patient may use denial and repression to reduce and filter information that might be overwhelming. Some patients display calm manner and alert mental status, representing a dissociation from reality, which is also a protective mechanism.
Investigate changes in mentation and presence of hypervigilance/hypovigilance, hallucinations, sleep disturbances (e.g., nightmares), agitation/apathy, disorientation, labile affect, all of which may vary from moment to moment.	Indicators of extreme anxiety/delirium state in which the patient is literally fighting for life. Although cause can be psychologically based, pathologic life-threatening causes (e.g., shock, sepsis, hypoxia) must be ruled out.
Provide constant and consistent orientation.	Helps the patient stay in touch with surroundings and reality.
Encourage the patient to talk about the burn circumstances when ready.	Patient may need to tell the story of what happened over and over to make some sense out of a terrifying situation.
Explain to patient what happened. Provide opportunity for questions and give open/honest answers.	Compassionate statements reflecting the reality of the situation can help the patient/SO acknowledge that reality and begin to deal with what has happened.
Identify previous methods of coping/handling of stressful situations.	Past successful behavior can be used to assist in dealing with the present situation.
Assist the family to express their feelings of grief and guilt.	The family may initially be most concerned about the patient's dying and/or feel guilty, believing that in some way they could have prevented the incident.
Be nonjudgmental in dealing with the patient and family.	Family relationships are disrupted; financial, lifestyle/role changes make this a difficult time for those involved with the patient, and they may react in many different ways.
Encourage family/SO to visit and discuss family happenings. Remind patient of past and future events.	Maintains contact with a familiar reality, creating a sense of attachment and continuity of life.
Collaborative	
Involve entire burn team in care from admission to discharge, including social worker and psychiatric resources.	Provides a wider support system and promotes continuity of care and coordination of activities.
Administer mild sedation as indicated, lorazepam (Ativan) or alprazolam (Xanax).	Antianxiety medications may be necessary for a brief period until patient is more physically stable and internal locus of control is regained.

715

ACTIONS/INTERVENTIONS	RATIONALE
Independent	
Assess meaning of loss/change to patient/SO.	Traumatic episode results in sudden, unanticipated changes, creating feelings of grief over actual/perceived losses. This necessitates support to work through to optimal resolution.
Acknowledge and accept expression of feelings of frustration, dependency, anger, grief, and hostility. Note withdrawn behavior and use of denial.	Acceptance of these feelings as a normal response to what has occurred facilitates resolution. It is not helpful or possible to push patient before ready to deal with situation. Denial may be prolonged and be an adaptive mechanism because patient is not ready to cope with personal problems.
Set limits on maladaptive behavior (e.g., manipulative/aggressive). Maintain nonjudgmental attitude while giving care and help patient to identify positive behaviors that will aid in recovery.	Patient and SO tend to deal with this crisis in the same way in which they have dealt with problems in the past. Staff may find it difficult and frustrating to handle behavior that is disrupting/not helpful to recuperation but should realize that the behavior is usually directed toward the situation and not the caregiver.
Be realistic and positive during treatments, in health teaching, and in setting goals within limitations.	Enhances trust and rapport between patient and nurse.
Provide hope within parameters of individual situation; do not give false reassurance.	Promotes positive attitude and provides opportunity to set goals and plan for future based on reality.
Give positive reinforcement of progress and encourage endeavors toward attainment of rehabilitation goals.	Words of encouragement can support development of positive coping behaviors.
Show slides or pictures of burn care/other patient outcomes, being selective in what is shown as appropriate to the individual situation. Encourage discussion of feelings about what patient has seen.	Allows patient/SO to be realistic in expectations. Also assists in demonstration of importance of/necessity for certain devices and procedures.
Encourage family interaction with each other and with rehabilitation team.	Maintains/opens lines of communication and provides ongoing support for patient and family.

ACTIONS/INTERVENTIONS

Independent

Provide support group for SO. Give information about how SO can be helpful to the patient.

Collaborative

Refer to physical/occupational therapy, vocational counselor, and psychiatric counseling, e.g., clinical specialist psychiatric nurse, social services, psychologist as needed.

RATIONALE

Promotes ventilation of feelings and allows for more helpful responses to the patient.

Helpful in identifying ways/devices to regain and maintain independence. Patient may need further assistance to resolve persistent emotional problems (e.g., post-trauma response).

NURSING DIAGNOSIS: Knowledge deficit [learning need] regarding condition, prognosis, treatment, self care, and discharge needs

May be related to
Lack of exposure/recall
Information misinterpretation
Unfamiliarity with resources

Possibly evidenced by
Questions/request for information, statement of misconception
Inaccurate follow-through of instructions/development of preventable complications

DESIRED OUTCOMES/EVALUATION CRITERIA—PATIENT WILL:
Verbalize understanding of condition, prognosis, and treatment.
Correctly perform necessary procedures and explain reasons for actions.
Initiate necessary lifestyle changes and participate in treatment regimen.

ACTIONS/INTERVENTIONS

Independent

Review condition, prognosis, and future expectations.

Discuss patient's expectations of returning home, to work, and to normal activities.

Review proper burn, skin-graft, and wound-care techniques. Identify appropriate sources for outpatient care and supplies.

Discuss skin care, e.g., use of moisturizers and sunscreens.

Explain scarring process and necessity for/proper use of pressure garments when used.

RATIONALE

Provides knowledge base on which patient can make informed choices.

Patient frequently has a difficult adjustment to discharge. Problems often occur (e.g., sleep disturbances, nightmares, reliving the accident, difficulty with resumption of intimacy/sexual activity, emotional lability) that interfere with successful adjustment to resuming normal life.

Promotes competent self-care after discharge and enhances independence.

Itching, blistering, and sensitivity of healing wounds/graft sites can be expected for an extended time.

Promotes optimal regrowth of skin, minimizing development of hypertrophic scarring and contractures and facilitating healing process. *Note:* Consistent use of the pressure garment over a long period can reduce the need for reconstructive surgery to release contractures and remove scars.

717

ACTIONS/INTERVENTIONS	RATIONALE
Independent	
Encourage continuation of prescribed exercise program and scheduled rest periods.	Maintains mobility, reduces complications, and prevents fatigue, facilitating recovery process.
Identify specific limitations of activity as individually appropriate.	Imposed restrictions are dependent on severity/location of injury and stage of healing.
Stress importance of sustained intake of high-protein/high-calorie diet.	Optimal nutrition enhances tissue regeneration and general feeling of well-being.
Review medications, including purpose, dosage, route, and expected/reportable side effects.	Reiteration allows opportunity for patient to ask questions and be sure understanding is accurate.
Advise patient/SO of potential for exhaustion, boredom, emotional lability, adjustment problems. Provide information about possibility of discussion/interaction with appropriate professional counselors.	Provides perspective to some of the problems patient/SO may encounter and aids awareness that help/assistance is available when necessary.
Identify signs/symptoms requiring medical evaluation, e.g., inflammation, increased or changes in wound drainage, fever/chills; changes in pain characteristics or loss of mobility/function.	Early detection of developing complications (e.g., infection, delayed healing) may prevent progression to more serious/life-threatening situations.
Stress necessity/importance of follow-up care/rehabilitation.	Long-term support with continual reevaluation and changes in therapy is required to achieve optimal recovery.
Provide phone number for contact person.	Provides easy access to treatment team to reinforce teaching, clarify misconceptions, and reduce potential for complications.
Identify community resources, e.g., crisis centers, recovery groups, mental health, Red Cross, visiting nurse, Ambli-Cab, homemaker service.	Facilitates transition to home, provides assistance with meeting individual needs, and supports independence.

POTENTIAL CONSIDERATIONS following acute hospitalization (dependent on patient's age, physical condition/presence of complications, personal resources, and life responsibilities)

Coping, Individual, ineffective—situational crisis; vulnerability

Disuse Syndrome, risk for—severe pain, prescribed immobilization/restrictive therapies

Self-Esteem, situational low—change in health status/independent functioning, perceived loss of control in some aspect of life

Therapeutic Regimen: Individual, ineffective management—complexity of medical regimen, added demands made on individual/family, adequate social supports

Post-trauma Response—catastrophic accident/injury to self and possibly others

Systemic Infections and Immunologic Disorders

SEPSIS/SEPTICEMIA

Sepsis is a syndrome characterized by clinical signs and symptoms of severe infection, which may progress to septicemia and septic shock. Septicemia implies the presence of a systemic infection of the blood caused by rapidly multiplying microorganisms or their toxins, which can result in profound physiologic changes. The pathogens can be bacteria, fungi, viruses, or rickettsiae. The most common causes of septicemia are gram-negative bacteria. If the defense system of the body is not effective in controlling the invading microorganisms, septic shock may result, characterized by altered hemodynamics, impaired cellular function, and multiple system failure.

Patients at risk for bacteremia and septic shock include elderly, very young, and immunosuppressed patients with chronic diseases (e.g., diabetes); postoperative patients, and those with invasive lines and catheters. Signs and symptoms may be vague, and sepsis can develop subtly until sudden, overwhelming septic shock is present, affecting multiple organ systems.

CARE SETTING

Although severely ill patients may require admission to an ICU, this plan addresses care on an inpatient acute medical/surgical unit.

RELATED CONCERNS

Metabolic Acidosis (Primary Base Bicarbonate Deficit), p 506
Fluid and Electrolyte Imbalance, p 899
AIDS, p 739
Peritonitis, p 366
Pneumonia, Microbial, p 130
Psychosocial Aspects of Care, p 783
Pulmonary Tuberculosis (TB), p 190
Renal Failure: Acute, p 555
Total Nutritional Support: Parenteral/Enteral Feeding, p 491

Patient Assessment Data Base

Data is dependent on the type, location, duration of the infective process and organ involvement.

719

ACTIVITY/REST

May report: Fatigue, malaise

May exhibit: Mental status changes, e.g., withdrawn, lethargic
Respiration/heart rate increased with activity

CIRCULATION

May exhibit: BP normal/slightly low-normal range (as long as cardiac output remains elevated)
Peripheral pulses bounding, rapid (hyperdynamic phase); weak/thready/easily obliterated, extreme tachycardia (shock)
Heart sounds: Dysrhythmias and development of S_3 suggest myocardial dysfunction, effects of acidosis/electrolyte imbalance
Skin warm, dry, flushed (vasodilation), pale, cold, clammy, mottled (vasoconstriction)

ELIMINATION

May report: Diarrhea

May exhibit: Changes in character/amount of urine output

FOOD/FLUID

May report: Anorexia; nausea/vomiting

May exhibit: Weight loss, decreased subcutaneous fat/muscle mass (malnutrition)
Urinary output decreased, concentrated; progressing to oliguria, anuria

NEUROSENSORY

May report: Headache; dizziness, fainting

May exhibit: Restlessness, apprehension, confusion, disorientation, delirium/coma

PAIN/DISCOMFORT

May report: Abdominal tenderness, localized pain/discomfort
Generalized urticaria/pruritus

RESPIRATION

May report: Shortness of breath

May exhibit: Tachypnea with decreased respiratory depth, dyspnea
Basilar crackles, rhonchi, wheezes (developing pulmonary complications/onset of cardiac decompensation)

SAFETY

May report: History of recent/current infection, viral illness; cancer therapies, use of corticosteroids/other immunosuppressant medications

May exhibit: Temperature: Usually elevated (101°F or greater) but may be normal in elderly or compromised patient; occasionally subnormal (under 98.6°F)
Shaking chills
Poor/delayed wound healing, purulent drainage, localized erythema
Macular erythematous rash

SEXUALITY

May report: Perineal pruritus
Recent childbirth/abortion

May exhibit: Maceration of vulva, purulent vaginal drainage

TEACHING/LEARNING

May report: Chronic/debilitating health problems, e.g., liver, renal, cardiac disease; cancer, DM, alcoholism
History of splenectomy
Recent surgery/invasive procedures, traumatic wounds
Antibiotic use (recent or long-term)

Discharge plan   **DRG projected mean length of inpatient stay: 7.5 days**
considerations: May require assistance with wound care/supplies, treatments, self-care, and homemaker tasks

Refer to section at end of plan for postdischarge considerations.

DIAGNOSTIC STUDIES

Cultures (wound, sputum, urine, blood): May identify organism(s) causing the sepsis. Sensitivity determines most effective drug choices. Catheter/intravascular line tips may need to be removed and cultured if the portal of entry is unknown.

CBC: Hct may be elevated in hypovolemic states due to hemoconcentration. Leukopenia (decreased WBCs) occurs early, followed by a rebound leukocytosis (15,000–30,000) with increased bands (shift to the left) indicating rapid production of immature WBCs. Neutrophils (also called granulocytes, polys, or PMNs) may be elevated or depressed. Counts below 500/ml indicate immune system exhaustion.

Serum electrolytes: Various imbalances may occur due to acidosis, fluid shifts, and altered renal function.

Clotting studies:

    Platelets: Decreased levels (thrombocytopenia) can occur due to platelet aggregation.

    PT/aPTT: May be prolonged, indicating coagulopathy associated with liver ischemia, circulating toxins, shock state.

Serum lactate: Elevated in metabolic acidosis, liver dysfunction, shock.

Serum glucose: Hyperglycemia occurs, reflecting gluconeogenesis and glycogenolysis in the liver in response to cellular starvation/alteration in metabolism.

BUN/Cr: Increased levels are associated with dehydration, renal impairment/failure, and liver dysfunction/failure.

ABGs: Respiratory alkalosis and hypoxemia may occur early. In later stages, hypoxemia, respiratory acidosis, and metabolic acidosis occur due to failure of compensatory mechanisms.

Urinalysis: Presence of WBCs/bacteria suggests infection. Protein and RBCs are often present.

X-rays: Abdominal and lower chest films indicating free air in the abdomen may suggest infection due to perforated abdominal/pelvic organ.

ECG: May show ST-segment and T-wave changes and dysrhythmia resembling myocardial infarction.

NURSING PRIORITIES

1. Eliminate infection.
2. Support tissue perfusion/circulatory volume.
3. Prevent complications.
4. Provide information about disease process, prognosis, and treatment needs.

DISCHARGE GOALS

1. Infection eliminated/controlled.
2. Homeostasis maintained.
3. Complications prevented/minimized.
4. Disease process, prognosis, and therapeutic regimen understood.
5. Plan in place to meet needs after discharge.

NURSING DIAGNOSIS: Infection, risk for [progression of sepsis to septic shock, development of opportunistic infections]

Risk factors may include
Compromised immune system
Failure to recognize/treat infection and/or exercise proper preventive measures
Invasive procedures, environmental exposure (nosocomial)

Possibly evidenced by
[Not applicable; presence of signs and symptoms establishes an *actual* diagnosis]

DESIRED OUTCOMES/EVALUATION CRITERIA—PATIENT WILL:
Achieve timely healing, be free of purulent secretions/drainage or erythema, and be afebrile.

ACTIONS/INTERVENTIONS	RATIONALE
Independent	
Provide isolation/monitor visitors as indicated.	Body substance isolation should be employed for all infectious patients. Wound/linen isolation and handwashing may be all that is required for draining wounds. Patients with diseases transmitted through air may also need respiratory precautions. Reverse isolation/restriction of visitors may be needed to protect the immunosuppressed patient.
Wash hands before/after each care activity, even if sterile gloves are used.	Reduces risk of cross-contamination.
Encourage/provide frequent position changes, deep-breathing/coughing exercises.	Good pulmonary toilet may reduce respiratory compromise/prevent pneumonia.
Encourage patient to cover mouth and nose with tissue during coughs/sneezes.	Prevents spread of infection via airborne droplets.
Limit use of invasive devices/procedures when possible.	Reduces number of sites for entry of opportunistic organisms.
Inspect wounds/site of invasive devices daily, paying particular attention to parenteral nutrition lines. Note signs of local inflammation/infection, changes in character of wound drainage, sputum, or urine.	May provide clue to portal of entry, type of primary infecting organism(s), as well as early identification of secondary infections. *Note:* High nutrient content of TPN provides excellent medium for bacterial growth.
Maintain sterile technique when changing dressings, suctioning, providing site care, e.g., invasive line, urinary catheter.	Prevents introduction of bacteria, reducing risk of nosocomial infection.

ACTIONS/INTERVENTIONS

Independent

Wear gloves/gowns when caring for open wounds/anticipating direct contact with secretions or excretions.

Dispose of soiled dressings/materials in double bag.

Monitor temperature trends.

Observe for shaking chills and profuse diaphoresis.

Monitor for signs of deterioration of condition/failure to improve with therapy.

Inspect oral cavity for white plaques (thrush). Investigate reports of vaginal/perineal itching or burning.

Collaborative

Obtain specimens of urine, blood, sputum, wound, invasive lines/tubes as indicated for Gram's stain, culture, and sensitivity.

Monitor laboratory studies, e.g., WBC with neutrophil and band counts.

Administer medications as indicated:

Anti-infective agents: broad-spectrum antibiotics, e.g., methicillin (Staphcillin); gram-negative, e.g., ticarcillin disodium (Ticar); gram-positive, e.g., nafcillin (Nafcil), vancomycin (Vancocin); aminoglycosides, e.g., tobramycin (Nebcin), gentamicin (Garamycin); cephalosporins, e.g., cefotaxime (Claforan);

Immune globulins as appropriate.

Assist with/prepare for incision and drainage of wound, irrigation, application of warm/moist soaks as indicated.

RATIONALE

Prevents spread of infection/cross-contamination.

Reduces contamination/soilage of area; limits spread of airborne organisms.

Fever (101°F–105°F/38.5°C–40°C) is the result of endotoxin effect on the hypothalamus and pyrogen-released endorphins. Hypothermia (less than 96°F/36°C) is a grave sign reflecting advancing shock state, decreased tissue perfusion, and/or failure of the body's ability to mount a febrile response.

Chills often precede temperature spikes in presence of generalized infection.

May reflect inappropriate/inadequate antibiotic therapy or overgrowth of resistant or opportunistic organisms.

Depression of immune system and use of antibiotics increases risk of secondary infections, particularly yeast.

Identification of portal of entry and organism causing the septicemia is crucial to effective treatment.

The normal ratio of neutrophils to total WBCs is at least 50%; however, when WBC count is markedly decreased, calculating the absolute neutrophil count is more pertinent to evaluating immune status. Likewise, an initial elevation of band cells reflects the body's attempt to mount a response to the infection, while a decline indicates decompensation.

Specific antibiotics are determined by culture results, but therapy is usually initiated prior to obtaining results, using broad-spectrum antibiotics and/or based on most likely infecting organisms. Concomitant use of antimicrobials is often beneficial, but dosage must be balanced against renal function/clearance.

May boost/provide temporary immunity to general infection or specific illness, e.g., varicella zoster, rabies.

Facilitates removal of purulent material/necrotic tissue and promotes healing.

ACTIONS/INTERVENTIONS	RATIONALE
Independent	
Monitor patient temperature (degree and pattern); note shaking chills/profuse diaphoresis.	Temperature of 102°F–106°F (38.9°C–41.1°C) suggests acute infectious disease process. Fever pattern may aid in diagnosis; e.g., sustained or continuous fever curves lasting more than 24 hours suggest pneumococcal pneumonia, scarlet or typhoid fever; remittent fever (varying only a few degrees in either direction) reflects pulmonary infections; intermittent curves or fever that returns to normal once in 24-hour period suggests septic episode, septic endocarditis, or TB. Chills often precede temperature spikes. *Note:* Use of antipyretics alters fever patterns and may be restricted until diagnosis is made or if fever remains greater than 102°F (38.9°C).
Monitor environmental temperature; limit/add bed linens as indicated.	Room temperature/number of blankets should be altered to maintain near-normal body temperature.
Provide tepid sponge baths; avoid use of alcohol.	May help reduce fever. *Note:* Use of ice water/alcohol may cause chills, actually elevating temperature. In addition, alcohol is very drying to skin.
Collaborative	
Administer antipyretics, e.g., ASA (aspirin), acetaminophen (Tylenol).	Used to reduce fever by its central action on the hypothalamus; however, fever may be beneficial in limiting growth of organisms and enhancing autodestruction of infected cells.
Provide cooling blanket.	Used to reduce fever, usually greater than 104°F–105°F (39.5°C–40°C), when brain damage/seizures can occur.

NURSING DIAGNOSIS: Tissue Perfusion, altered, risk for

Risk factors may include
Relative/actual hypovolemia
Reduction of arterial/venous blood flow: Selective vasoconstriction, vascular occlusion (intimal damage/microemboli)

Possibly evidenced by
[Not applicable; presence of signs and symptoms establishes an *actual* diagnosis]

DESIRED OUTCOMES/EVALUATION CRITERIA—PATIENT WILL:
Display adequate perfusion as evidenced by stable vital signs, palpable peripheral pulses, skin warm and dry, usual level of mentation, individually appropriate urinary output and active bowel sounds.

ACTIONS/INTERVENTIONS	RATIONALE
Independent	
Maintain bed rest; assist with care activities.	Decreases myocardial workload and O_2 consumption, maximizing effectiveness of tissue perfusion.
Monitor trends in BP, noting progressive hypotension and changes in pulse pressure.	Hypotension develops as microorganisms invade the bloodstream, stimulating release or activation of chemical and hormonal substances, which initially results in peripheral vasodilation, decreased systemic vascular resistance, and relative hypovolemia. As shock progresses, cardiac output becomes severely depressed because of major alterations in contractility and preload/afterload, producing profound hypotension.
Monitor heart rate, rhythm. Note dysrhythmias.	Tachycardia occurs due to sympathetic nervous system stimulation secondary to stress response, and to compensate for the relative hypovolemia and hypotension. Cardiac dysrhythmias can occur as a result of hypoxia, acid-base/electrolyte imbalance, and/or low-flow perfusion state.
Note quality/strength of peripheral pulses.	Initially the pulse is strong/bounding due to increased cardiac output. Pulse may become weak/thready because of sustained hypotension, decreased cardiac output, and peripheral vasoconstriction if the shock state progresses.
Assess respiratory rate, depth, and quality. Note onset of severe dyspnea.	Increased respirations occur in response to direct effects of endotoxins on the respiratory center in the brain, as well as developing hypoxia, stress, and fever. Respiration can become shallow as respiratory insufficiency develops, creating risk of acute respiratory failure. (Refer to ND: Gas Exchange, impaired, risk for, p 728.)
Investigate changes in sensorium, e.g., mental cloudiness, agitation, restlessness, personality changes, delirium, stupor, coma.	Changes reflect alterations in cerebral perfusion, hypoxemia, and/or acidosis.

ACTIONS/INTERVENTIONS	RATIONALE
Independent	
Assess skin for changes in color, temperature, moisture.	Compensatory mechanism of vasodilatation results in warm, dry, pink skin, which is characteristic of hyperperfusion in hyperdynamic phase of early septic shock. If shock state progresses, compensatory vasoconstriction occurs, shunting blood to vital organs, reducing peripheral blood flow, and creating cool, clammy, pale/dusky skin.
Record hourly urinary output and specific gravity.	Decreasing urinary output with increased specific gravity indicates diminished renal perfusion related to fluid shifts and selective vasoconstriction. There may be transient polyuria during hyperdynamic phase (while cardiac output is elevated), but this may progress to oliguria.
Auscultate bowel sounds.	Reduced blood flow to the mesentery (splanchnic vasoconstriction) decreases peristalsis and may lead to paralytic ileus.
Monitor gastric pH as indicated. Hematest gastric secretions/stools for occult blood.	Stress of illness and use of steroids increase risk of gastric mucosal erosion/bleeding.
Evaluate lower extremities for local tissue swelling, erythema, positive Homans' sign.	Venous stasis and infectious process may result in the development of thrombosis.
Monitor for signs of bleeding, e.g., oozing from puncture sites/suture lines, petechiae, ecchymoses, hematuria, epistaxis, hemoptysis, hematemesis.	Coagulopathy/DIC may occur related to accelerated clotting in the microcirculation (activation of chemical mediators, vascular insufficiency, and cell destruction), creating a life-threatening hemorrhagic situation/multiple emboli.
Note drug effects, and monitor for signs of toxicity.	Massive doses of antibiotics are often ordered. These have potentially toxic effects when hepatic/renal perfusion is compromised.
Collaborative	
Administer parenteral fluids. (Refer to ND: Fluid Volume deficit, risk for, following.)	To maintain tissue perfusion, large amounts of fluid may be required to support circulating volume.
Administer drugs as indicated:	
Corticosteroids;	Although steroid therapy remains controversial, steroids may be given for the potential advantages of decreased capillary permeability, increased renal perfusion, and inhibition of microemboli formation.
NaHCO$_3$;	Impaired tissue perfusion and production of lactate result in metabolic acidosis, requiring base replacement therapy.
Antacids: e.g., aluminum hydroxide (Amphojel).	Decreases potential for gastric bleeding related to stress response/altered perfusion.
Monitor laboratory studies, e.g., ABGs, lactate levels.	Development of respiratory/metabolic acidosis reflects loss of compensatory mechanisms, e.g., decreased renal perfusion/hydrogen excretion; and accumulation of lactic acid due to circulatory shunting and stagnation.

ACTIONS/INTERVENTIONS

Collaborative

Administer supplemental O_2.

Maintain body temperature, using adjunctive aids as necessary. (Refer to ND: Hyperthermia, p 724.)

Prepare for/transfer to critical care setting as indicated.

RATIONALE

Maximizes O_2 available for cellular uptake.

Temperature elevations increase metabolic/O_2 demands beyond cellular resources, hastening tissue ischemia/cellular destruction.

Progressive deterioration will require more aggressive therapy (e.g., hemodynamic monitoring and vasoactive drugs).

NURSING DIAGNOSIS: Fluid Volume deficit, risk for

Risk factors may include
Marked increase in vascular compartment/massive vasodilatation
Capillary permeability/fluid leaks into the interstitial space (third spacing)

Possibly evidenced by
[Not applicable; presence of signs and symptoms establishes an *actual* diagnosis]

DESIRED OUTCOMES/EVALUATION CRITERIA—PATIENT WILL:
Maintain adequate circulatory volume as evidenced by vital signs within patient's normal range, palpable peripheral pulses of good quality, and individually appropriate urinary output.

ACTIONS/INTERVENTIONS

Independent

Measure/record urinary output and specific gravity. Note cumulative I&O imbalances (including insensible losses), and correlate with daily weight. Encourage oral fluids to tolerance.

Monitor BP and heart rate. Measure CVP if used.

Palpate peripheral pulses.

Assess for dry mucous membranes, poor skin turgor, and thirst.

Observe for dependent/peripheral edema in sacrum, scrotum, back, legs.

Collaborative

Administer IV fluids, e.g., crystalloids (D5W, NS) and colloids (albumin, fresh frozen plasma) as indicated.

RATIONALE

Decreasing urinary output with a high specific gravity suggests hypovolemia. Continued positive fluid balance with corresponding weight gain may indicate third spacing and tissue edema, suggesting need to alter fluid therapy/replacement components.

Reduction in the circulating fluid volume reduces BP/CVP, initiating compensatory mechanisms of tachycardia to improve cardiac output and increase systemic BP.

Weak, easily obliterated pulses suggest hypovolemia.

Hypovolemia/third spacing of fluid gives rise to signs of dehydration.

Fluid losses from the vascular compartment into the interstitial space create tissue edema.

Large volumes of fluid may be required to overcome relative hypovolemia (peripheral vasodilation); replace losses from increased capillary permeability (e.g., sequestration of fluid in the peritoneal cavity) and increased insensible sources (e.g., fever/diaphoresis).

727

ACTIONS/INTERVENTIONS	RATIONALE

Collaborative

Monitor laboratory values, e.g.:

Hct/RBC count;	Evaluates changes in hydration/blood viscosity.
BUN/Cr.	Moderate elevations of BUN reflect dehydration, high values of BUN/Cr may indicate renal dysfunction/failure.
Monitor cardiac output.	CO (and other functional parameters, such as cardiac index, preload/afterload, contractility, and cardiac work) can be measured noninvasively using thoracic electrical bioimpedance (TEB) technique. Useful in determining therapeutic needs/effectiveness.

NURSING DIAGNOSIS: Gas Exchange, impaired, risk for

Risk factors may include

Altered O_2 supply: Effects of endotoxins on the respiratory center in the medulla (resulting in hyperventilation/respiratory alkalosis); hypoventilation

Altered blood flow (changes in vascular resistance), alveolar–capillary membrane changes (increased capillary permeability leading to pulmonary congestion)

Interference with O_2 delivery/utilization in the tissues (endotoxin-induced damage to the cells/capillaries)

Possibly evidenced by

[Not applicable; presence of signs and symptoms establishes an *actual* diagnosis]

DESIRED OUTCOMES/EVALUATION CRITERIA—PATIENT WILL:

Display ABGs and respiratory rate within patient's normal range, with breath sounds clear and chest x-ray clear/improving.

Experience no dyspnea/cyanosis.

ACTIONS/INTERVENTIONS	RATIONALE

Independent

Maintain patent airway. Place patient in position of comfort with head of bed elevated.	Enhances lung expansion, respiratory effort.
Monitor respiratory rate and depth. Note use of accessory muscles/work of breathing.	Rapid/shallow respirations occur because of hypoxemia, stress, and circulating endotoxins. Hypoventilation and dyspnea reflect ineffective compensatory mechanisms and are an indication that ventilatory support is needed.
Auscultate breath sounds. Note crackles, wheezes, areas of decreased/absent ventilation.	Respiratory distress and the presence of adventitious sounds are indicators of pulmonary congestion/interstitial edema, atelectasis. *Note:* Respiratory complications, including pneumonia and ARDS, are a prime cause of death.

ACTIONS/INTERVENTIONS	RATIONALE
Independent	
Note presence of circumoral cyanosis.	Reflects inadequate systemic oxygenation/hypoxemia.
Investigate alterations in sensorium: agitation, confusion, personality changes, delirium, stupor, coma.	Cerebral function is very sensitive to decreases in oxygenation (e.g., hypoxemia/reduced perfusion).
Note cough and purulent sputum production.	Pneumonia is a common nosocomial infection that can occur by aspiration of oropharyngeal organisms or spread from other sites.
Reposition frequently. Encourage coughing and deep-breathing exercises. Suction with lavage, as indicated.	Good pulmonary toilet is necessary for reducing ventilation/perfusion imbalance and for mobilizing and facilitating removal of secretions to maximize gas exchange.
Collaborative	
Monitor ABGs/pulse oximetry.	Hypoxemia is related to decreased ventilation/pulmonary changes (e.g., interstitial edema, atelectasis, and pulmonary shunting) and increased demands (e.g., fever). Respiratory acidosis (pH below 7.35 and $Paco_2$ greater than 40 mm Hg) occurs because of hypoventilation and ventilation-perfusion imbalance. As septic condition worsens, metabolic acidosis (pH below 7.35 and HCO_3 less than 22–24 mEq/L) arises due to buildup of lactic acid from anaerobic metabolism.
Administer supplemental O_2 via appropriate route, e.g., nasal cannula, mask, high-flow rebreathing mask.	Necessary for correction of hypoxemia with failing respiratory effort/progressing acidosis. *Note:* Intubation/mechanical ventilation may be required if respiratory failure develops.
Review serial chest x-rays.	Changes reflect progression/resolution of pulmonary complications, e.g., infiltrates/edema.

NURSING DIAGNOSIS: Knowledge deficit [learning need] regarding illness, prognosis, treatment, self care and discharge needs

May be related to
Lack of exposure/recall; information misinterpretation
Cognitive limitation

Possibly evidenced by
Questions/request for information, statement of misconception
Inaccurate follow-through of instructions/development of preventable complications

DESIRED OUTCOMES/EVALUATION CRITERIA—PATIENT WILL:
Verbalize understanding of disease process and prognosis.
Correctly perform necessary procedures and explain reasons for the actions.
Initiate necessary lifestyle changes.
Participate in treatment regimen.

ACTIONS/INTERVENTIONS	RATIONALE
Independent	
Review disease process and future expectations.	Provides knowledge base on which patient can make informed choices.
Review individual risk factors and mode of transmission/portal of entry of infections.	Glucocorticoid therapy, kidney/liver dysfunction, neoplastic disease, rheumatic heart disease, valve dysfunction, and DM may predispose to septicemia. Awareness of means of infection transmission provides opportunity to plan for/institute protective measures.
Provide information about drug therapy, interactions, side effects, and importance of adherence to regimen.	Promotes understanding of and enhances cooperation in treatment/prophylaxis and reduces risk of recurrence and complications.
Discuss need for good nutritional intake/balanced diet.	Necessary for optimal healing and general well-being.
Encourage adequate rest periods with scheduled activities.	Prevents fatigue, conserves energy, and promotes healing.
Review necessity of personal hygiene and environmental cleanliness.	Helps to control environmental exposure by diminishing the number of pathogens present.
Discuss proper use or avoidance of tampons as indicated.	Superabsorbent tampons/infrequent changing potendtiates risk of *Staphylococcus aureus* infection (toxic shock syndrome).
Identify signs/symptoms requiring medical evaluation, e.g., persistent temperature elevation(s), tachycardia, syncope, rashes of unknown origin, unexplained fatigue, anorexia, increased thirst, and changes in bladder function.	Early recognition of developing/recurring infection allows for timely intervention and reduces risk for progression to life-threatening situation.
Stress importance of prophylactic immunization/antibiotic therapy as needed.	Used for prevention of infection.

POTENTIAL CONSIDERATIONS following acute hospitalization (dependent on patient's age, physical condition/presence of complications, personal resources, and life responsibilities)

Infection, risk for, recurrence/opportunistic—stasis of body fluids, decreased hemoglobin, leukopenia, suppressed inflammatory response, use of anti-infective agents, increased environmental exposure, malnutrition

Nutrition: altered, less than body requirements—increased energy needs (hypermetabolic state), anorexia, continuing GI dysfunction, side effects of medication

Self Care deficit/Home Maintenance Management, impaired—decreased strength/endurance, pain/discomfort, inadequate support systems, unfamiliarity with neighborhood resources

THE HIV-POSITIVE PATIENT

The individual identified as HIV-seropositive is one who is asymptomatic and does not meet the Centers for Disease Control (CDC) definition for AIDS. Studies reveal that persons with HIV-positive status may remain asymptomatic for 10 or more years. While imminent death is not a realistic concern, the patient needs to make major behavioral and lifestyle changes to prolong life expectancy and may have significant problems that require information and assistance. The person who is well-supported medically may survive opportunistic infection episodes for a number of years.

CARE SETTING

Community setting, although development of opportunistic infections may require occasional inpatient acute medical care.

RELATED FACTORS

AIDS, p 739
Pneumonia, Microbial, p 130
Psychosocial Aspects of Care, p 783
Sepsis/Septicemia, p 719

Patient Assessment Data Base

Refer to CP: AIDS, p 739, although patient may be asymptomatic.

Refer to section at end of plan for ongoing considerations.

DIAGNOSTIC STUDIES

ELISA: A positive test result may be indicative of exposure to HIV but is not diagnostic. (Sensitivity varies, with the incidence of false-positive results being approximately 25%).
Western blot test: Confirms diagnosis of HIV from tests previously positive by ELISA screening.
CD$_4$ lymphocyte count (previously T$_4$ helper cells): Reduced. Patients with counts below 500 may benefit from anti-retroviral therapy; counts equal to/or below 200 define progression to AIDS.
Screening tests: PPD: Positive result reflects current or prior exposure to tuberculosis.
 Anergy test (Candida/mumps/tetanus toxoid): Done in combination with PPD to clarify false negatives reflecting cutaneous anergy (inability of immune system to respond to specific antigens).
 RPR/VDRL: Determines current/past exposure to syphilis and need for more specific testing.
 PAP smear: May reveal higher incidence of abnormal cells.
 Pelvic/genital exam: Identifies presence of STD lesions, cervical and vaginal abnormalities.
 Chest x-ray: Abnormalities suggest presence of TB in PPD-positive, anergic, and/or symptomatic individuals. Diagnosis is then verified by sputum cultures.

NURSING PRIORITIES

1. Promote acceptance of reality of diagnosis/condition.
2. Support incorporation of behavioral/lifestyle changes to enhance well-being.
3. Provide information about disease process/prognosis and treatment needs.

DISCHARGE GOALS

1. Patient dealing with current situation realistically.
2. Patient participating in therapeutic regimen.
3. Diagnosis, prognosis, and therapeutic regimen understood.
4. Plan in place to meet needs after discharge.

ACTIONS/INTERVENTIONS	RATIONALE
Independent	
Evaluate patient's ability to understand events and realistically appraise situation.	Provides base to develop plan of action.
Encourage expression of feelings, denial, shock, and fears. Listen without judgment, accepting patient's expressions. Avoid dwelling on future possibilities; rather, focus on positive outcomes.	It is important to convey belief in commonality of patient's fears/feelings. Speculating about the future focuses on the negative aspects of what might happen. By focusing on positive outcomes, the patient is encouraged to take charge of those areas where changes can be made.
Challenge morbid thoughts and reframe into positive statements, i.e., "You know why the virus is going to kill me, I deserve to die for what I've done." Response: "The virus may or may not kill you. It's not smart enough to decide when you may die. The virus is 'just there.' It does not have a mind to know what you have or have not done."	Interrupts morbid thoughts and challenges patient's self-depreciating ideas. As with any potentially terminal disease, this population is likely to experience depression and is at increased risk for suicide, necessitating ongoing evaluation.
Determine available resources or programs.	Addictive behaviors, ability of injection drug user to obtain clean "works," sexual myths, and perceptions of the use of condoms may need to be addressed.
Assess social system as well as presence of support, perception of losses, and stressors.	Partners, friends, and families will have individual responses dependent on acceptance of the person's lifestyle, knowledge of HIV transmission, and belief in myths.
Encourage patient to participate in support groups.	Long-term support is critical to dealing with and effectively coping with the reality of ongoing changes.
Discuss meaning of high-risk behavior and barriers to change.	Sexual behavior may be used to express caring as well as to feel connected and less lonely.
Inform patient about interactions among medications, HIV, and emotions.	Fatigue and depression can be side effects of medications as well as of the infection itself. Knowledge that it is usually of short duration can support informed choices/cooperation and promote hope.

732

ACTIONS/INTERVENTIONS

Independent

Encourage continued or renewed use of familiar effective coping strategies.

Explore and practice the potential use of new and different coping strategies.

Help the patient to use humor to combat stigmatization of the disease.

Reinforce structure in daily life. Include exercise as part of routine.

Assist patient to set limits on sexually risky behaviors.

Assist patient to channel anger to healthy activities.

Inform patient about new medical advances/treatments.

Discuss issues of voluntary disclosure, personal responsibility, needs of others; as well as federal, state, and local reporting requirements.

Collaborative

Refer to nurse practitioner/clinical specialist, psychologist, social worker knowledgeable about HIV.

RATIONALE

Patient is supported and given strokes for past effective behavior. Positive reinforcement enhances self-esteem.

Using new strategies can be uncomfortable and practice fosters self-confidence.

Humor defuses the sense of secretiveness people may place on HIV.

Routines help the person to focus. Exercise improves sense of wellness and enhances immune response.

Needs for love, comfort, and companionship that have been met through sexual expression need to be met through other means that carry a reduced risk of HIV transmission.

The increased energy of anger can be used to accomplish other tasks and enhance feelings of self-esteem.

Promotes hope and helps patient to make informed decisions.

Understanding responsibilities and consequences of disclosure is necessary for patient to make informed decisions.

May need additional help to adjust to difficult situation.

NURSING DIAGNOSIS: Fatigue

May be related to
Decreased metabolic energy production, increased energy requirements (hypermetabolic state)
Overwhelming psychologic/emotional demands
Altered body chemistry: Side effects of medications

Possibly evidenced by
Inability to maintain usual routines, decreased performance, impaired ability to concentrate

DESIRED OUTCOMES/EVALUATION CRITERIA—PATIENT WILL:
Report improved sense of energy.
Identify individual areas of control.
Participate in desired activities at level of ability.

ACTIONS/INTERVENTIONS

Independent

Discuss reality of fatigue. Identify limitations imposed by fatigue state.

RATIONALE

Patients often expect too much of themselves, believing that they *should* be able to do more.

ACTIONS/INTERVENTIONS

Independent

Note daily energy patterns—peaks and valleys.

Determine individual priorities and responsibilities. Assist patient to set realistic goals.

Identify available resources and support systems.

Discuss energy conservation techniques, e.g., sitting instead of standing for activities as appropriate.

Review importance of meeting individual nutritional needs.

Encourage adequate rest periods during day and routine schedule for bedtime/arising.

Instruct in stress management techniques, e.g., breathing exercises, visualization, music therapy.

RATIONALE

Helpful in planning activities within tolerance levels.

Patient may need to alter priorities, delegate some responsibilities in order to manage fatigue and optimize performance.

May require outside assistance with homemaking/maintenance activities, child care, etc.

Enables patient to become aware of ways in which energy expenditure can be maximized to complete necessary tasks.

Adequate nutrition is needed for optimizing energy production.

Helps patient to recoup energy to manage desired activities.

Reduction of stress factors in patient's life can minimize energy output.

NURSING DIAGNOSIS: Nutrition: altered, risk for less than body requirements

Risk factors may include
Reported inadequate food intake less than recommended daily allowance
Lack of interest in food, anorexia
Lack of information, misinformation, misconceptions
Reported altered taste sensation, nausea and other side effects of medications
Sore, inflamed buccal cavity (e.g., thrush, CMV lesions)

Possibly evidenced by
[Not applicable; presence of signs and symptoms establishes an *actual* diagnosis]

DESIRED OUTCOMES/EVALUATION CRITERIA—PATIENT WILL:
Maintain adequate muscle mass.
Maintain weight within 2–3 lb of usual premorbid weight.
Demonstrate laboratory values within normal limits.
Report improved energy level.

ACTIONS/INTERVENTIONS

Independent

Determine usual weight before patient was diagnosed with HIV.

Establish current anthropometric measurements. Measure resting energy expenditure (REE) using indirect calorimetry.

RATIONALE

Early wasting is not readily determined by normal-weight-to-height charts; therefore, determining current weight in relation to prediagnosis weight is more useful. Recent unexplained/involuntary weight loss may be a factor in seeking initial medical evaluation.

Helps to monitor wasting and determine nutritional needs as illness progresses. Indirect calorimetry is more accurate for calculating REE than Harris-Benedict equation, which underestimates the energy needs of these patients.

ACTIONS/INTERVENTIONS	RATIONALE

Independent

Determine patient's current dietary pattern/intake and knowledge of nutrition. Use an in-depth dietary assessment tool.

Identification of these factors helps to plan for individual needs. Patients with HIV infection have documented trace mineral (zinc, magnesium, selenium) deficits. Alcohol and drug abuse interfere with adequate intake.

Discuss/document nutritional side effects of medications.

Commonly used medications cause anorexia and n/v; some interfere with bone marrow production of RBCs.

Provide information about nutritionally dense high-calorie, high-protein, high-vitamin, and high-mineral foods. Help patient plan ways to maintain/improve intake. Identify lactose-free supplements as appropriate.

Having this information helps patient to understand importance of well-balanced diet. Some patients may try macrobiotic or other diets, believing the diarrhea is caused by lactose intolerance. Eliminating dairy products can have detrimental effects when these components are not replaced from other sources.

Stress importance of maintaining balanced/adequate nutritional intake.

Patient may get discouraged with changed status and find it difficult to eat. Knowing how important nutritional intake is to remaining healthy can motivate patient to maintain proper diet.

Assist patient to formulate dietary plan, taking into consideration increased metabolic demands/energy needs.

Provides guidance and feedback while promoting sense of control, enhancing self-esteem, and possibly improving intake. HIV infection is continuously stimulating the immune system, increasing metabolic rate and nutritional needs.

Recommend environment conducive to eating, e.g., avoiding cooking odors if bothersome; keeping room well ventilated, removing noxious stimuli. Suggest use of spices, marinating red meat before cooking, and/or substituting other protein sources for red meat. Stress importance of sharing mealtime with others. Identify someone who can join patient for meals.

Improves nutritional intake. Medications and disease can change sense of smell and taste. Patient may develop an aversion to red meat. Socialization can enhance appetite/food intake.

Discuss use of lactobacillus/acidophilus replacement.

Antibiotics taken for prevention of opportunistic infections cause changes in normal bowel flora, contributing to diarrhea.

Collaborative

Consult with dietitian.

Provides assistance in planning nutritionally sound diet and identifying nutritional supplements to meet individual needs. Liquid supplements (e.g., Advera) have been specifically formulated for the GI manifestations common to the HIV-positive population.

Monitor laboratory values, e.g., Hb, RBCs, albumin/prealbumin, potassium, sodium.

In spite of adequate nutritional intake, fluctuations occur and supplemental feedings or vitamins may be needed to prevent further deterioration. Decreased RBCs (anemia) may require additional interventions, such as use of epoetin alfa (Epogen) to stimulate RBC production.

Provide medications as indicated, e.g.,

    Dronabinol (Marinol), megestrol (Megace);

Antiemetics/appetite stimulants can improve intake to prevent and correct dietary deficiencies.

    Anti-infective agents.

Treatment of opportunistic GI tract infections (MAC, CMV) can enhance oral intake and correct malabsorption related to persistent diarrhea.

NURSING DIAGNOSIS: Knowledge deficit [learning need] regarding disease, prognosis, treatment, self care and discharge needs

May be related to
Lack of exposure/recall
Information misinterpretation
Unfamiliarity with information resources
Cognitive limitation

Possibly evidenced by:
Statement of misconception/request for information
Inaccurate follow-through of instructions/development of preventable complications
Inappropriate/exaggerated behaviors (e.g., hostile, agitated, hysterical, apathetic)

DESIRED OUTCOMES/EVALUATION CRITERIA—PATIENT WILL:
Verbalize understanding of condition/disease process and goals of treatment.
Identify relationship of signs/symptoms to the disease process and correlate symptoms with causative factors.
Initiate necessary lifestyle changes.
Participate in treatment regimen.

ACTIONS/INTERVENTIONS	RATIONALE
Independent	
Determine current understanding and perception of diagnosis. Discuss difference between HIV-positivity and AIDS.	Provides opportunity to clarify misconceptions/myths and make informed choices. Allows for development of individualized plan of care.
Assess emotional ability to assimilate information and understand instructions. Respect patient's need to use "denial" coping techniques initially.	Initial shock and anxiety can block intake of information. Self-esteem, lifestyle, guilt, and denial of possibility of exposure/own responsibility in acquiring disease become issues. *Note:* Some initial denial may serve as a protective mechanism promoting more effective self-care.
Identify/problem-solve potential or actual barriers to accessing healthcare services.	Transportation, distance, child care, work schedule, lack of insurance or finances interfere with accessing needed primary care and prophylactic interventions.
Assess potential for inappropriate/high-risk behavior: continued injection drug abuse, unsafe sexual practices.	High denial/anger, drug addiction may result in behaviors that are high risk for spread of the virus. A person's sexual expression and identity are threatened by the discovery of the diagnosis.
Provide information about normal immune system/response and how HIV affects it, transmission of the virus, behaviors and factors believed to increase probability of progression. Encourage questions.	Patient needs to be aware of own personal risk as well as risk to others in order to make immediate and long-range decisions and establish a basis for goal setting. Also, establishes rapport and provides opportunity to identify concerns and assimilate information.
Provide realistic, optimistic information during each contact with patient.	Necessary to provide realistic hope as most patients have been exposed to media information about AIDS or have friends/lovers who have died of the disease.
Plan short sessions for additional information.	Patient will need time and repeated contacts to absorb information.

ACTIONS/INTERVENTIONS	RATIONALE

Independent

Review signs/symptoms that may be a consequence of HIV infection, e.g., mild persistent fever, anorexia, weight loss, fatigue, night sweats, diarrhea, dry cough, rashes, headaches, and sleep disturbances.

Patient may experience an acute illness 2–6 weeks after becoming infected; however, it is common for infection to be subclinical, with the individual simply feeling unwell.

Discuss signs/symptoms that require medical evaluation, e.g., persistent increasing cough or swollen lymph glands, profound fatigue unrelieved by rest, weight loss of 10 lb in less than 2 months, severe/persistent diarrhea, fever, blurred vision, skin discoloration or rash that persists or spreads, open sores anywhere.

Early recognition of progression of disease/development of opportunistic infections provides for timely intervention and may prevent more serious situations.

Stress necessity of practicing safe sex at all times; also stress need to avoid use of illicit injected drugs or, if unwilling to abstain, to avoid sharing needles and to clean "works" with bleach solution, rinsing carefully with water.

Limits spread of virus. Reduces exposure to other infective agents/additional stress to the immune system.

Discuss active changes in sexual behaviors that the patient can make that may satisfy sexual needs and are designed to prevent transmission.

Promotes a sense of responsibility and control and may reduce sexual tensions.

Provide information about necessary lifestyle changes and health maintenance factors:

Evidence suggests that specific dietary and lifestyle factors may slow the progression of HIV infection along the continuum to AIDS.

Avoid crowds and people with infections;

Early detection and treatment of infection are crucial to delay of further impairment of the immune system and development of opportunistic diseases.

Exercise to limit of ability, alternate rest periods with activity, and get adequate sleep;

Avoids undue fatigue; maintains strength and release of endorphins for sense of well-being. Exercise has also been shown to stimulate the immune system.

Eat regularly, even if appetite is reduced. Try small, frequent meals and snacks;

Physical and psychologic stressors increase metabolic needs; in addition, side effects of medication, presence of n/v, and anorexia often limit oral intake. The result is nutritional deficits that can further impair the immune system.

Practice daily oral hygiene, use a soft toothbrush; examine mouth regularly for sores, white film, or changes in color; have regular dental checkups every 6 months;

Poor oral hygiene/dental care can affect oral intake adversely and increase the risk of opportunistic/systemic infections.

Examine skin for rashes, bruises, breaks in skin integrity;

May indicate developing complications/increase risk of infection.

Stress necessity of follow-up care and evaluations including routine CD_4 counts.

Even though patient may be asymptomatic, periodic evaluation may prevent development of complications/progression of the disease and assist with treatment decisions.

Discuss need for regular gynecologic examinations and/or pregnancy considerations.

HIV-positive women experience a high prevalence of Pap smear, vaginal, and cervical abnormalities. Pregnancy counseling should include review of possible effects of childbirth on maternal health as well as risk of perinatal transmission.

737

ACTIONS/INTERVENTIONS	RATIONALE

Independent

Discuss management strategies for persistent signs and symptoms.	Patient involvement in care increases cooperation and satisfaction with care.
Review drug therapies, side effects, and adverse reactions as appropriate:	
Antiretrovirals, e.g., zidovudine (ZVD/formerly AZT, Retrovir), dideoxyinosine (DDI, Videx), zalcitabine (ddC, Hivid), stavudine (d$_4$T, Zerit), lamivudine (3TC, Epivir), saquinavir (Invirase);	These drugs interfere with the HIV replication process, and early treatment may be considered when CD$_4$ count is near 500, even if individual is asymptomatic. Side effects such as symptoms of peripheral neuropathy or pancreatitis necessitate prompt evaluation and possible discontinuation/change in therapy.
Anti-infectives, e.g., trimethoprim-sulfamethoxazole (TMP/SMX, Bactrim, Septra), foscarnet (Foscavir), rifabutin (Mycobutin).	Focus on prevention of commonly occurring infections, such as PCP, CMV, MAC may prolong general wellness. Primary prophylactic therapy aims to prevent or delay onset of symptoms of reactivated or newly acquired infection. The goal of secondary prophylaxis is to prevent or delay recurrent episodes of particular infection. Prophylaxis continues indefinitely as long as the drug is tolerated.
Provide written information—a few pieces at each visit.	Patient may feel overwhelmed, and written materials allow for later review and reinforcement when patient has had an opportunity to calm down.
Encourage contact with SO, family, and friends. Include in discussions/conferences as appropriate.	Many fear telling SO, family, and friends for fear of rejection; others withdraw as a result of tumultuous feelings. Contact promotes sense of support, concern, involvement, and understanding. Supporting loved ones as they learn of the diagnosis can be beneficial for the long-term support of the patient.
Identify additional resources, e.g.:	
Support groups, peer counselors, and mental health professionals;	Patient will experience a variety of emotional and psychologic responses to the diagnosis and may need additional assistance to promote optimal adjustment.
Case managers.	In early stages of HIV infection, focus may be on social services (e.g., help with housing, employment, finances). Later, as disease progresses, the emphasis switches to medical and related community services).
Provide information about clinical trials available as individually appropriate.	Scientific research requires HIV-positive test subjects. Participation may provide individual with a sense of contributing to body of knowledge/search for cure, in addition to no-cost monitoring and medications for those with limited financial resources.

POTENTIAL ONGOING CONSIDERATIONS (dependent on patient's age, physical condition/presence of complications, personal resources, and life responsibilities)

Fatigue—decreased metabolic energy production, increased energy requirements (hypermetabolic state)

Nutrition: altered, less than body requirements—increased metabolic demands/energy requirements, side effects of medication, anorexia, fatigue

Decisional Conflict—unclear personal values/beliefs, perceived threat to value system, multiple or divergent sources of information, support system deficit, interference with decision making

Infection, risk for—depression of immune system, chronic disease, malnutrition, use of antimicrobial agents

AIDS

As defined by the Centers for Disease Control (CDC) (January 1994) "persons with CD_4 cell count of under 200 (with or without symptoms of opportunistic infection) who are HIV-positive are diagnosed as having AIDS." Research in 1995 showed that the HIV virus replicates rapidly on a daily basis. The half-life of the virus is 2 days, with almost complete turnover in 14 days. Therefore, the immune response is massive throughout the course of HIV disease and pathogenesis is due to destruction of CD_4 cells, not a lack of production of new lymphocytes. Controlling the growth of the virus is the current focus of treatment.

Persons with the acquired immunodeficiency syndrome (AIDS) have generally been found to fall into six categories: homosexual or bisexual men, injection drug users, recipients of infected blood or blood products, heterosexual partners of a person with HIV infection, and children born to an infected mother. The rate of infection is currently most rapidly expanding in minority women.

CARE SETTING

Although many of the interventions listed here are appropriate at the community level, the focus of this plan of care is the acutely ill individual requiring care on an inpatient medical or subacute unit.

RELATED FACTORS

Fluid and Electrolyte Imbalances, p 899
Long-Term Care, p 824
Psychosocial Aspects of Care, p 783
Sepsis/Septicemia, p 719
Total Nutritional Support: Parenteral/Enteral Feeding, p 491
Upper Gastrointestinal/Esophageal Bleeding, p 315
Ventilatory Assistance (Mechanical), p 176

Patient Assessment Data Base

Data is dependent on the organs/body tissues involved and the specific opportunistic infection or cancer.

ACTIVITY/REST

May report: Easily tired, reduced tolerance for usual activities, progressing to profound fatigue and malaise
Altered sleep patterns

May exhibit: Muscle weakness, wasting of muscle mass
Physiologic response to activity, e.g., changes in BP, heart rate, respiration

CIRCULATION

May report: Slow healing (if anemic); bleeding longer with injury (less common)

May exhibit: Tachycardia, postural BP changes
Decreased peripheral pulse volume
Pallor or cyanosis; delayed capillary refill

EGO INTEGRITY

May report: Stress factors related to lifestyle changes, losses, e.g., family support, relationships, finances, and spiritual concerns
Concern about appearance: alopecia, disfiguring lesions, weight loss
Denial of diagnosis, feelings of powerlessness, hopelessness, helplessness, worthlessness, guilt, loss of control, depression

May exhibit: Denial, anxiety, depression, fear, withdrawal
Angry behaviors, dejected body posture, crying, poor eye contact
Failure to keep appointments or multiple appointments for similar symptoms

ELIMINATION

May report: Intermittent, persistent, frequent diarrhea with or without abdominal cramping
Flank pain, burning on urination

May exhibit: Loose-formed to watery stools with or without mucus or blood
Frequent, copious diarrhea
Abdominal tenderness
Rectal, perianal lesions or abscesses
Changes in urinary output, color, character

FOOD/FLUID

May report: Anorexia, changes in taste of foods/food intolerance, nausea/vomiting
Rapid/progressive weight loss
Dysphagia, retrosternal pain with swallowing
Food intolerance: Diarrhea after diary products

May exhibit: Hyperactive bowel sounds
Abdominal distention (hepatosplenomegaly)
Weight loss; thin frame; decreased subcutaneous fat/muscle mass
Poor skin turgor
Lesions of the oral cavity, white patches, discoloration
Poor dental/gum health, loss of teeth
Edema (generalized, dependent)

HYGIENE

May report: Unable to complete ADLs

May exhibit: Disheveled appearance
Deficits in many or all personal care, self-care activities

NEUROSENSORY

May report: Fainting spells/dizziness; headache
Changes in mental status, loss of mental acuity/ability to solve problems, forgetfulness,
poor concentration
Impaired sensation or sense of position and vibration
Muscle weakness, tremors, changes in visual acuity
Numbness, tingling in extremities (feet seem to display earliest changes)
Changes in visual acuity; light flashes/floaters

May exhibit: Mental status changes ranging from confusion to dementia, forgetfulness, poor concen-
tration, decreased alertness, apathy, psychomotor retardation/slowed responses
Paranoid ideation, free-floating anxiety, unrealistic expectations
Abnormal reflexes, decreased muscle strength, ataxic gait
Fine/gross motor tremors, focal motor deficits; hemiparesis, seizures
Retinal hemorrhages and exudates (CMV retinitis)

PAIN/DISCOMFORT

May report: Generalized/localized pain; aching, burning in feet
Headache (CNS involvement)
Pleuritic chest pain

May exhibit: Swelling of joints, painful nodules, tenderness
Decreased ROM, gait changes/limp
Muscle guarding

RESPIRATION

May report: Frequent, persistent URIs
Progressive shortness of breath
Cough (ranging from mild to severe); nonproductive/productive of sputum (earliest sign of PCP may be a spasmodic cough on deep breathing)
Congestion or tightness in chest
History of exposure to/prior episode of active TB

May exhibit: Tachypnea, respiratory distress
Changes in breath sounds/adventitious breath sounds
Sputum: yellow (in sputum-producing pneumonia)

SAFETY

May report: Exposure to infectious diseases e.g., TB, STDs
History of other immune deficiency diseases, e.g., cancer
History of frequent or multiple blood transfusions (e.g., hemophilia, major vascular surgery, traumatic incident)
History of falls, burns, episodes of fainting, slow-healing wounds
Suicidal/homicidal ideation with or without a plan

May exhibit: Recurrent fevers; low grade, intermittent temperature elevations/spikes; night sweats
Changes in skin integrity: Cuts, ulcerations, rashes, e.g., eczema, exanthems, psoriasis; discolorations; changes in size/color of moles; unexplained, easy bruising; multiple injection scars (may be infected)
Rectal, perianal lesions or abscesses
Nodules, enlarged lymph nodes in two or more areas of the body (e.g., neck, armpits, groin)
Decline in general strength, muscle tone, changes in gait
Positive cultures/TB test; decreased CD_4 count

SEXUALITY

May report: History of high-risk behavior, e.g., having sex with a partner who is HIV-positive, multiple sexual partners, unprotected sexual activity, and anal sex
Loss of libido, being too sick for sex
Inconsistent use of condoms
Use of birth control pills (enhanced susceptibility to virus in women who are exposed due to increased vaginal dryness/friability)

May exhibit: Pregnancy or risk for pregnancy (sexually active)
Genitalia: Skin manifestations (e.g., herpes, warts); discharge
Cervical dysplasia; abnormal PAP smear

SOCIAL INTERACTION

May report: Problems related to diagnosis, e.g., loss of family/SO, friends, support; fear of telling others; fear of rejection/loss of income

Isolation, loneliness, close friends or sexual partners who have died of or are sick with AIDS

Questioning of ability to remain independent, unable to plan

May exhibit: Changes in family/SO interaction pattern

Disorganized activities, difficulty with goal setting

TEACHING/LEARNING

May report: Failure to comply with treatment, continued high-risk behavior (e.g., unchanged sexual behavior or injection drug use)

Injection drug use/abuse, current smoking, alcohol abuse

Evidence of failure to improve from last hospitalization

Discharge plan   **DRG projected mean length of stay: 10.2 days**
considerations: May require assistance with finances, medications and treatments, skin/wound care, equipment/supplies; transportation, food shopping and preparation; self-care, technical nursing procedures, homemaker/maintenance tasks, child care; changes in living facilities

Refer to section at end of plan for postdischarge considerations.

DIAGNOSTIC STUDIES

CBC: Anemia and idiopathic thrombocytopenia (maybe profound). WBC: Leukopenia may be present; differential shift to the left suggests infectious process (PCP); shift to the right may be noted. With certain infections, low T-cell count, or with T-cell tumor, no shift may occur.

PPD with anergy panel: Determines exposure and/or active disease (anergy panel identifies false-negative result due to deficient immune response). Of AIDS patients, 100% of those exposed to active *Mycobacterium* TB will develop the disease.

Serologic: *Serum antibody test:* HIV screen by ELISA. A positive test result may be indicative of exposure to HIV but is not diagnostic, as false positives may occur.

Western blot test: Confirms diagnosis of HIV.

T-lymphocyte cells: Total count reduced.

CD$_4$ lymphocyte count (immune system indicator that mediates several immune system processes and signals B cells to produce antibodies to foreign germs): Numbers less than 200 indicate severe immune deficiency response and diagnosis of AIDs.

T8 (cytopathic suppressor cells): Reversed ratio (2:1 or greater) of suppressor cells to helper cells (T8 to T4) indicates immune suppression.

P24 (envelope protein of HIV): Increased quantitative values of this protein indicative of progression of infection with highest levels during aggressive HIV replication. (May not be detectable during very early stages of HIV infection.)

Ig levels: Usually elevated, especially IgG and IgA, with normal to near-normal IgM (indicator of the ability of the body to mount a response to infectious process but is used infrequently because other factors can alter it, e.g., environmental pollutants).

Polymerase chain reaction (PCR) test: Detects HIV DNA; most helpful in testing newborns of HIV-infected mothers. Infants carry maternal HIV antibodies, therefore test positively on ELISA and Western blot, even though infant is not necessarily infected.

STD testing: Hepatitis B envelope and core antibodies, syphilis, and other common STDs may be positive.

Cultures: Histologic, cytologic studies of urine, blood, stool, spinal fluid, lesions, sputum, and secretions may be done to identify the opportunistic infection. Some of the most commonly identified are the following:

Protozoal and helminthic infections: PCP, cryptosporidiosis, toxoplasmosis.

Fungal infections: Candida albicans (candidiasis), *Cryptococcus neoformans* (cryptococcosis); *Histoplasma capsulatum* (histoplasmosis).

Bacterial infections: Mycobacterium avium-intercellulare, miliary mycobacterial TB, *Shigella* (shigellosis), *Salmonella* (salmonellosis).

Viral infections: CMV, MAI, herpes simplex, herpes zoster, etc.

Neurologic studies, e.g., EEG, MRI, CT scans of the brain; EMG/nerve conduction studies: Indicated for changes in mentation, fever of undetermined origin, and/or changes in sensory/motor function.

Chest x-ray: May initially be normal or may reveal progressive interstitial infiltrates from advanced PCP (most common opportunistic disease) or other pulmonary complications/disease processes such as TB.

Pulmonary function tests: Useful in early detection of interstitial pneumonias.

Gallium scan: Diffuse pulmonary uptake occurs in PCP and other forms of pneumonia.

Biopsies: May be done for differential diagnosis of KS or other neoplastic lesions.

Bronchoscopy/tracheobronchial washings: May be done with biopsy when PCP or lung malignancies are suspected (diagnostic confirming test for PCP).

Barium swallow, endoscopy, colonoscopy: May be done to identify opportunistic infection (e.g., *Candida,* CMV) or to stage KS in the GI system.

NURSING PRIORITIES

1. Prevent/minimize infections.
2. Maintain homeostasis.
3. Promote comfort.
4. Support psychosocial adjustment.
5. Provide information about disease process/prognosis and treatment needs.

DISCHARGE GOALS

1. Infection prevented/resolved.
2. Complications prevented/minimized.
3. Pain/discomfort alleviated.
4. Patient is dealing with current situation realistically.
5. Diagnosis, prognosis, and therapeutic regimen understood.
6. Plan in place to meet needs after discharge.

NURSING DIAGNOSIS: Infection, risk for [progression to sepsis/onset of new opportunistic infection]

Risk factors may include

Inadequate primary defenses: Broken skin, traumatized tissue, stasis of body fluids

Depression of the immune system; use of antimicrobial agents

Environmental exposure, invasive techniques

Chronic disease; malnutrition

Possibly evidenced by

[Not applicable; presence of signs and symptoms establishes an *actual* diagnosis]

DESIRED OUTCOMES/EVALUATION CRITERIA—PATIENT WILL:

Identify/participate in behaviors to reduce risk of infection.

Achieve timely healing of wounds/lesions.

Be afebrile and free of purulent drainage/secretions and other signs of infectious conditions.

ACTIONS/INTERVENTIONS	RATIONALE

Independent

Wash hands before and after all care contacts. Instruct patient/SO to wash hands as indicated.

Reduces risk of cross-contamination.

Provide a clean, well-ventilated environment. Screen visitors/staff for signs of infection and maintain isolation precautions as indicated.

Reduces number of pathogens presented to the immune system and reduces possibility of patient contracting a nosocomial infection.

Discuss extent and rationale for isolation precautions and maintenance of personal hygiene.

Promotes cooperation with regimen and may lessen feelings of isolation.

Monitor vital signs, including temperature.

Provides information for baseline data; frequent temperature elevations/onset of new fever indicates that the body is responding to a new infectious process or that medications are not effectively controlling noncurable infections.

Assess respiratory rate/depth; note dry spasmodic cough on deep inspiration, changes in characteristics of sputum, and presence of wheezes/rhonchi. Initiate respiratory isolation when etiology of productive cough is unknown.

Respiratory congestion/distress may indicate developing PCP, the most common opportunistic disease; however, TB is on the rise and other fungal, viral, and bacterial infections may occur that compromise the respiratory system. *Note:* CMV and PCP can reside together in the lungs and, if treatment is not effective for PCP, the addition of CMV therapy may be effective.

Investigate reports of headache, stiff neck, altered vision. Note changes in mentation and behavior. Monitor for nuchal rigidity/seizure activity.

Neurologic abnormalities are common and may be related to the HIV or secondary infections. Symptoms may vary from subtle changes in mood/sensorium (personality changes or depression) to hallucinations, memory loss, severe dementias, seizures, and loss of vision. CNS infections (encephalitis is the most common) may be caused by protozoal and helminthic organisms or fungus.

Examine skin/oral mucous membranes for white patches or lesions. (Refer to ND: Skin Integrity, impaired, actual and/or risk for, p 752–753, and ND: Oral Mucous Membrane, altered, p 754.)

Oral candidiasis, KS, herpes, CMV, and cryptococcosis are common opportunistic diseases affecting the cutaneous membranes.

Clean nails daily. File, rather than cut, and avoid trimming cuticles.

Reduces risk of transmission of pathogens through breaks in skin. *Note:* Fungal infections along the nail plate are common.

Monitor reports of heartburn, dysphagia, retrosternal pain on swallowing, increased abdominal cramping, profuse diarrhea.

Esophagitis may occur secondary to oral candidiasis, CMV, or herpes. Cryptosporidiosis is a parasitic infection responsible for watery diarrhea (often greater than 15 L/d).

Inspect wounds/site of invasive devices, noting signs of local inflammation/infection.

Early identification/treatment of secondary infection may prevent sepsis.

Wear gloves and gowns during direct contact with secretions/excretions or any time there is a break in skin of caregiver's hands. Wear mask and protective eyewear to protect nose, mouth, and eyes from secretions during procedures (e.g., suctioning) or when splattering of blood may occur.

Use of masks, gowns, and gloves is required by OSHA (1992) for direct contact with body fluids, e.g., sputum, blood/blood products, semen, vaginal secretions.

744

ACTIONS/INTERVENTIONS	RATIONALE

Independent

Dispose of needles/sharps in rigid, puncture-resistant containers.

Prevents accidental inoculation of caregivers. Use of needle cutters and recapping is not to be practiced. *Note:* Accidental needle sticks should be reported immediately, with follow-up evaluations done per protocol.

Label blood bags, body fluid containers, soiled dressings/linens, and package appropriately for disposal per isolation protocol.

Prevents cross-contamination and alerts appropriate personnel/departments to exercise specific hazardous materials procedures.

Clean up spills of body fluids/blood with bleach solution (1:10); add bleach to laundry.

Kills HIV and controls other microorganisms on surfaces.

Collaborative

Monitor laboratory studies, e.g.:

CBC/differential;

Shifts in the differential and changes in WBC count indicate infectious process. Low WBC count or other changes in blood count may be related to treatments/medications.

Culture/sensitivity studies of lesions, blood, urine, and sputum.

May be done to identify cause of fever, diagnose infecting organisms, or determine appropriate course of treatment.

Administer medications as indicated:

Anti-infectives, e.g., trimethoprim (TMP/SMX, Bactrim, Septra), nystatin (Mycostatin), ketoconazole (Nizoral), pentamidine (Pentam, Nebupent), rifabutin (Mycobutin), ganciclovir (Cytovene), foscarnet (Foscavir);

Combats illnesses associated with various opportunistic infections. Cytovene is used to prevent blindness/life-threatening dissemination of CMV. Foscavir can also be used to prevent CMV progression, but should be used with caution as it may cause renal toxicity.

Antiretrovirals, e.g., zidovudine (ZVD/formerly AZT, Retrovir), dideoxyinosine (DDI, Videx), zalcitabine (ddc, Hivid), stavudine (d_4T, Zerit), lamivudine (3TC, Epivir), saquinavir (Invirase).

No cure is currently available, but antiviral agents are aimed at blocking replication of the HIV virus and thereby improving immune function.

NURSING DIAGNOSIS: Fluid Volume deficit, risk for

Risk factors may include
Excessive losses: Copious diarrhea, profuse sweating, vomiting
Hypermetabolic state, fever
Restricted intake: Nausea, anorexia; lethargy

Possibly evidenced by
[Not applicable; presence of signs and symptoms establishes an *actual* diagnosis]

DESIRED OUTCOMES/EVALUATION CRITERIA—PATIENT WILL:
Maintain hydration as evidenced by moist mucous membranes, good skin turgor, stable vital signs, individually adequate urinary output.

ACTIONS/INTERVENTIONS	RATIONALE

Independent

Monitor vital signs, including CVP if available. Note hypotension, including postural changes.	Indicators of circulating fluid volume.
Note temperature elevation and duration of febrile episode. Administer tepid sponge baths as indicated. Keep clothing and linens dry. Maintain comfortable environmental temperature.	Increased metabolic demands and excessive diaphoresis associated with fever result in increased insensible fluid losses.
Assess skin turgor, mucous membranes, and thirst.	Indirect indicators of fluid status.
Measure urinary output and specific gravity. Measure/estimate amount of diarrheal loss. Note insensible losses.	Increased specific gravity/decreasing urinary output reflects altered renal perfusion/circulating volume. *Note:* Monitoring fluid balance is difficult because of excessive GI/insensible losses.
Weigh as indicated.	Although weight loss may reflect muscle wasting, sudden fluctuations reflect state of hydration. Fluid losses associated with diarrhea can quickly create a crisis and become life-threatening.
Monitor oral intake and encourage fluids of at least 2500 ml/d.	Maintains fluid balance, reduces thirst, and keeps mucous membranes moist.
Make fluids easily accessible to patient; use fluids that are tolerable to the patient and that replace needed electrolytes, e.g., Gatorade, broth.	Enhances intake. Certain fluids may be too painful to consume (e.g., acidic juices) because of mouth lesions.
Eliminate foods potentiating diarrhea, e.g., spicy/high-fat foods, nuts, cabbage, milk products. Adjust rate/concentration of tube feedings if indicated.	May help reduce diarrhea.

Collaborative

Administer fluids/electrolytes via feeding tube/IV.	May be necessary to support/augment circulating volume, especially if oral intake is inadequate, nausea/vomiting persists.
Monitor laboratory studies as indicated, e.g.:	
Hct;	Useful in estimating fluid needs.
Serum/urine electrolytes;	Alerts to possible electrolyte disturbances and determines replacement needs.
BUN/Cr.	Evaluates renal perfusion/function.
Administer medications as indicated:	
Antiemetics, e.g., prochlorperazine maleate (Compazine), trimethobenzamide (Tigan), metoclopramide (Reglan);	Reduces incidence of vomiting to reduce further loss of fluids/electrolytes.
Antidiarrheals, e.g., diphenoxylate (Lomotil), loperamide (Imodium), paregoric, or antispasmodics, e.g., mepenzolate bromide (Cantil);	Decreases the amount and fluidity of stool; may reduce intestinal spasm and peristalsis. *Note:* Antibiotics may also be used to treat diarrhea if caused by infection.
Antipyretics, e.g., acetaminophen (Tylenol).	Helps to reduce fever and hypermetabolic response, decreasing insensible losses.
Maintain hypothermia blanket if used.	May be necessary when other measures fail to reduce excessive fever.

NURSING DIAGNOSIS: Breathing Pattern, ineffective/Gas Exchange, impaired, risk for

Risk factors may include

Muscular impairment (wasting of respiratory musculature), decreased energy/fatigue, decreased lung expansion

Retained secretions (tracheobronchial obstruction), infectious/inflammatory process; pain

Ventilation perfusion imbalance (PCP/other pneumonias, anemia)

Possibly evidenced by

[Not applicable; presence of signs and symptoms establishes an *actual* diagnosis]

DESIRED OUTCOMES/EVALUATION CRITERIA—PATIENT WILL:

Maintain effective respiratory pattern.

Experience no dyspnea/cyanosis, with breath sounds and chest x-ray clear/improving and ABGs within patient's normal range.

ACTIONS/INTERVENTIONS

Independent

Auscultate breath sounds, noting areas of decreased/absent ventilation and presence of adventitious sounds, e.g., crackles, wheezes, rhonchi.

Note rate/depth of respiration, cyanosis, use of accessory muscles, increased work of breathing and presence of dyspnea, anxiety.

Elevate head of bed. Have patient turn, cough, deep-breathe, as indicated.

Suction airway as indicated, using sterile technique and observing safety precautions, e.g., mask, protective eyewear.

Assess changes in level of consciousness.

Investigate reports of chest pain.

Allow adequate rest periods between care activities. Maintain a quiet environment.

Collaborative

Monitor/graph serial ABGs or pulse oximetry.

Review serial chest x-rays.

RATIONALE

Suggests developing pulmonary complications/infection, e.g., atelectasis/pneumonia. *Note:* PCP is often advanced before changes in breath sounds occur.

Tachypnea, cyanosis, restlessness, and increased work of breathing reflect respiratory distress and need for increased surveillance/medical intervention.

Promotes optimal pulmonary function and reduces incidence of aspiration or infection due to atelectasis.

Assists in clearing the ventilatory passages, thereby facilitating gas exchange and preventing respiratory complications.

Hypoxemia can result in changes ranging from anxiety and confusion to unresponsiveness.

Pleuritic chest pain may reflect nonspecific pneumonitis or pleural effusions associated with malignancies.

Reduces O_2 consumption.

Indicators of respiratory status, treatment needs/effectiveness.

Presence of diffuse infiltrates may suggest pneumonia, while areas of congestion/consolidation may reflect other pulmonary complications, e.g., atelectasis or KS lesions.

ACTIONS/INTERVENTIONS	RATIONALE

Collaborative

Assist with/instruct in use of incentive spirometer. Provide chest physiotherapy, e.g., percussion, vibration, and postural drainage.	Encourages proper breathing technique and improves lung expansion. Loosens secretions, dislodges mucus plugs to promote airway clearance. *Note:* In the event of multiple skin lesions, chest physiotherapy may be discontinued.
Provide humidified supplemental O_2 via appropriate means, e.g., cannula, mask, intubation/mechanical ventilation.	Maintains effective ventilation/oxygenation to prevent/correct respiratory crisis.
Administer medications as indicated:	Choice of therapy is dependent on individual situation/infecting organism(s).
Antimicrobials, e.g.: trimethoprim (Bactrim, Septra), pentamidine isethionate (Pentam);	While Bactrim (TMP/SMX) is the drug of choice for PCP, Pentam can be used in combination or alone when treatment with Bactrim is unsuccessful or contraindicated. *Note:* Bactrim is also used prophylactically.
Foscarnet (Foscavir), ganciclovir (Cytovene);	Effective for treatment of pulmonary CMV infections. *Note:* CMV often coexists with PCP.
Rifabutin (Mycobutin), clarithromycin (Biaxin);	For treatment of mycobacterium avium complex (MAC), a common bacterial infection that frequently disseminates to other organ systems.
Bronchodilators, expectorants, cough depressants.	May be needed to improve/maintain airway patency or help clear secretions.
Prepare/assist with procedures as indicated, e.g., bronchoscopy.	May be required to clear mucus plugs, obtain specimens for diagnosis (biopsies/lavage).

NURSING DIAGNOSIS: Injury, risk for (hemorrhage)

Risk factors may include
Abnormal blood profile: Decreased vitamin K absorption, alteration in hepatic function, presence of autoimmune antiplatelet antibodies, malignancies (KS); and/or circulating endotoxins (sepsis)

Possibly evidenced by
[Not applicable; presence of signs and symptoms establishes an *actual* diagnosis]

DESIRED OUTCOMES/EVALUATION CRITERIA—PATIENT WILL:
Display homeostasis as evidenced by absence of mucosal bleeding and be free of ecchymosis.

ACTIONS/INTERVENTIONS	RATIONALE

Independent

Hematest body fluids, e.g., urine, stool, vomitus, for occult blood.	Prompt detection of bleeding/initiation of therapy may prevent critical hemorrhage.

ACTIONS/INTERVENTIONS	RATIONALE
Independent	
Observe for/report epistaxis, hemoptysis, hematuria, nonmenstrual vaginal bleeding, or oozing from lesions/body orifices/IV insertion sites.	Spontaneous bleeding may indicate development of DIC or immune thrombocytopenia.
Monitor for changes in vital signs and skin color, e.g., BP, pulse, respirations, skin pallor/discoloration.	Presence of bleeding/hemorrhage may lead to circulatory failure/shock.
Monitor for change in level of consciousness and visual disturbances.	Change may reflect cerebral bleeding.
Avoid injections, rectal temperatures/suppositories, rectal tubes.	Protects patient from procedure-related causes of bleeding; e.g., insertion of thermometers, rectal tubes can damage or tear rectal mucosa.
Maintain a safe environment; e.g., keep all necessary objects and call bell within patient's reach and keep bed in low position.	Reduces accidental injury, which could result in bleeding.
Maintain bed/chair rest when platelets are below 10,000 or as individually appropriate. Assess medication regimen.	Reduces possibility of injury, although activity needs to be maintained. May need to discontinue or reduce drug, e.g., AZT. *Note:* Patient can have a surprisingly low platelet count without bleeding.
Collaborative	
Review laboratory studies, e.g., PT, aPTT, clotting time, platelets, Hb/Hct.	Detects alterations in clotting capability; identifies therapy needs. *Note:* Many individuals (up to 80%) display platelet counts below 50,000, and may be asymptomatic, necessitating regular monitoring.
Administer blood products as indicated.	Transfusions may be required in the event of persistent/massive spontaneous bleeding.
Avoid use of aspirin products/NSAIDs especially in presence of gastric lesions.	Reduces platelet aggregation, impairing/prolonging the coagulation process, and may cause further gastric irritation, increasing risk of bleeding.

NURSING DIAGNOSIS: Nutrition: altered, less than body requirements

May be related to

Inability or altered ability to ingest, digest and/or metabolize nutrients: nausea/vomiting, hyperactive gag reflex, intestinal disturbances, GI tract infections, fatigue

Increased metabolic rate/nutritional needs (fever/infection)

Possibly evidenced by

Weight loss, decreased subcutaneous fat/muscle mass (wasting)

Lack of interest in food, aversion to eating, altered taste sensation

Abdominal cramping, hyperactive bowel sounds, diarrhea

Sore, inflamed buccal cavity

Abnormal laboratory results: Vitamin/mineral and protein deficiencies, electrolyte imbalances

DESIRED OUTCOMES/EVALUATION CRITERIA—PATIENT WILL:

Maintain weight or display weight gain toward desired goal.

Demonstrate positive nitrogen balance, be free of signs of malnutrition, and display improved energy level.

ACTIONS/INTERVENTIONS	RATIONALE
Independent	
Assess ability to chew, taste, and swallow.	Lesions of the mouth, throat, and esophagus (often caused by candidiasis, herpes simplex, hairy leukoplakia, KS, and other cancers) may cause dysphagia, limiting patient's ability to ingest food and reducing desire to eat.
Auscultate bowel sounds.	Hypermotility of intestinal tract is common and is associated with vomiting and diarrhea, which may affect choice of diet/route. *Note:* Lactose intolerance and malabsorption (e.g., with CMV, MAC, cryptosporidiosis) contribute to diarrhea and may necessitate change in diet/supplemental formula (e.g., Advera, Resource).
Weigh as indicated. Evaluate weight in terms of premorbid weight. Compare serial weights and anthropometric measurements.	Indicator of nutritional needs/adequacy of intake. *Note:* Because of immune suppression, some blood tests normally used for testing nutritional status are not useful.
Plan diet with patient/SO; suggest "foods from home" if appropriate. Provide small, frequent meals/snacks of nutritionally dense foods and nonacidic foods and beverages, with choice of foods palatable to patient. Encourage high-calorie/nutritious foods, some of which may be considered appetite stimulants. Note time of day when appetite is best, and try to serve larger meal at that time.	Including patient in planning gives sense of control of environment and may enhance intake. Fulfilling cravings for noninstitutional food may also improve intake. *Note:* In this population, foods with a higher fat content may be recommended as tolerated to enhance taste and oral intake.
Note drug side effects.	Prophylactic and therapeutic medications can have side effects affecting nutrition, e.g., ZVD (altered taste, nausea/vomiting), Bactrim (anorexia, glucose intolerance, glossitis), Pentam (altered taste and smell, nausea/vomiting, glucose intolerance).
Limit food(s) that induce nausea/vomiting or are poorly tolerated by the patient because of mouth sores/dysphagia. Avoid serving very hot liquids/foods. Serve foods that are easy to swallow, e.g., eggs, ice cream, cooked vegetables.	Pain in the mouth or fear of irritating oral lesions may cause the patient to be reluctant to eat. These measures may be helpful in increasing food intake.
Schedule medications between meals (if tolerated) and limit fluid intake with meals, unless fluid has nutritional value.	Gastric fullness diminishes appetite and food intake.
Encourage as much physical activity as possible.	May improve appetite and general feelings of well-being.
Provide frequent mouth care, observing secretion precautions. Avoid alcohol-containing mouthwashes.	Reduces discomfort associated with nausea/vomiting, oral lesions, mucosal dryness, and halitosis. Clean mouth may enhance appetite.
Provide rest period before meals. Avoid stressful procedures close to mealtime.	Minimizes fatigue; increases energy available for work of eating.
Remove existing noxious environmental stimuli or conditions that aggravate gag reflex.	Reduces stimulus of the vomiting center in the medulla.
Encourage patient to sit up for meals.	Facilitates swallowing and reduces risk of aspiration.

ACTIONS/INTERVENTIONS	RATIONALE
Independent	
Record ongoing caloric intake.	Identifies need for supplements or alternate feeding methods.
Collaborative	
Review laboratory studies, e.g., BUN, glucose, liver function studies, electrolytes, protein, and albumin.	Indicates nutritional status and organ function, and identifies replacement needs. *Note:* Nutritional tests can be altered because of disease processes as well as response to some medications/therapies.
Maintain NPO status when appropriate.	May be needed to reduce vomiting.
Insert/maintain NG tube as indicated.	May be needed to reduce n/v or to administer tube feedings. *Note:* Esophageal irritation from existing infection (*Candida*, herpes, or KS) may provide site for secondary infections/trauma; therefore, tube should be used with caution.
Consult with dietitian/nutritional support team.	Provides for diet based on individual needs/appropriate route.
Administer enteral/parenteral feedings as indicated.	Occasionally TPN may be required if oral/enteral feedings are not tolerated. TPN is reserved for those whose gut cannot absorb even an elemental formula (such as Vivonex) or those with severe refractory diarrhea. Otherwise enteral feedings are preferred, as they cost less and carry less risk than TPN.
Administer medications as indicated:	
Antiemetics, e.g., dronabinol (Marinol), megestrol (Megace);	Reduces incidence of vomiting; promotes gastric function.
Sucralfate (Carafate) suspension;	Given with meals to relieve mouth pain, enhance intake.
Vitamin supplements;	Corrects vitamin deficiencies resulting from decreased food intake and/or disorders of digestion and absorption in the GI system. *Note:* Avoid megadoses; suggested supplemental level is 2 times the RDA.
Appetite stimulants, e.g., oxandrolone (Oxandrin);	Currently being studied in clinical trials to boost appetite as well as improve muscle mass and strength.
Antidiarrheals, e.g., octreotide (Sandostatin);	Effective treatment for secretory diarrhea (secretion of water and electrolytes by intestinal epithelium).
Antibiotic therapy, e.g., ketoconazole (Nizoral), fluconazole (Diflucan).	May be given to treat/prevent infections involving the GI tract.

NURSING DIAGNOSIS: Pain [acute]/chronic

May be related to

Tissue inflammation/destruction: Infections, internal/external cutaneous lesions, rectal excoriation, malignancies, necrosis

Peripheral neuropathies, myalgias, and arthralgias

Abdominal cramping

ACTIONS/INTERVENTIONS	RATIONALE
Independent	
Assess pain reports, noting location, intensity (0–10 scale), frequency, and time of onset. Note nonverbal cues, e.g., restlessness, tachycardia, grimacing.	Indicates need for/effectiveness of interventions and may signal development/resolution of complications. *Note:* Chronic pain does not produce autonomic changes.
Encourage verbalization of feelings.	Can reduce anxiety and fear and thereby reduce perception of intensity of pain.
Provide diversional activities, e.g., reading, visiting, television.	Refocuses attention; may enhance coping abilities.
Perform palliative measures, e.g., repositioning, massage, ROM of affected joints.	Promotes relaxation/decreases muscle tension.
Apply warm/moist packs to pentamidine injection/IV sites for 20 minutes after administration.	These injections are known to cause pain and sterile abscesses.
Instruct patient in/encourage use of visualization, guided imagery, progressive relaxation, deep-breathing techniques.	Promotes relaxation and feeling of well-being. May decrease the need for narcotic analgesics (CNS depressants) where there is already a neuro/motor degenerative process involved. May not be successful in presence of dementia, even when dementia is minor.
Provide oral care. (Refer to ND: Oral Mucous Membrane, altered, p 754.)	Oral ulcerations/lesions may cause severe discomfort.
Collaborative	
Administer analgesics/antipyretics, narcotic analgesics. Use PCA or provide around-the-clock analgesia with rescue doses prn.	Provides relief of pain/discomfort; reduces fever. Patient-controlled or around-the-clock medication keeps the blood level of analgesia stable, preventing cyclic undermedication or overmedication. *Note:* Drugs such as Ativan may be used to potentiate effects of analgesics.

May be related to (actual)

Immunologic deficit: AIDS-related dermatitis; viral, bacterial, and fungal infections (e.g., herpes, *Pseudomonas, Candida*); opportunistic disease processes (e.g., KS)

Possibly evidenced by

Skin lesions; ulcerations; decubitus ulcer formation

DESIRED OUTCOMES/EVALUATION CRITERIA—PATIENT WILL:

Demonstrate behaviors/techniques to prevent skin breakdown/promote healing.
Display improvement in wound/lesion healing.

ACTIONS/INTERVENTIONS	RATIONALE
Independent	
Assess skin daily. Note color, turgor, circulation, and sensation. Describe lesions and observe changes.	Establishes baseline with which changes in status can be compared and appropriate interventions instituted.
Maintain/instruct in good skin hygiene, e.g., wash thoroughly, pat dry carefully, and massage with lotion or appropriate cream.	Maintaining clean, dry skin provides a barrier to infection. Patting skin dry instead of rubbing reduces risk of dermal trauma to dry/fragile skin. Massaging increases circulation to the skin and promotes comfort. *Note:* Isolation precautions are required, especially when extensive mucocutaneous lesions are present.
Reposition frequently. Use turn sheet as needed. Encourage periodic weight shifts. Protect bony prominences with pillows, heel/elbow pads, sheepskin.	Reduces stress on pressure points, improves blood flow to tissues, and promotes healing.
Maintain clean, dry, wrinkle-free linen.	Skin friction caused by wet or wrinkled sheets leads to irritation and potentiates infection.
Encourage ambulation/out of bed as tolerated.	Decreases pressure on skin from prolonged bed rest.
Cleanse perianal area by removing stool with water and mineral oil or commercial product. Avoid use of toilet paper if vesicles are present. Apply protective creams, e.g., zinc oxide, A and D ointment.	Prevents maceration caused by diarrhea and keeps perianal lesions dry. *Note:* Use of toilet paper may abrade lesions.
File nails regularly.	Long/rough nails increase risk of dermal damage.
Cover open pressure ulcers with sterile dressings or protective barrier, e.g., Tegaderm, DuoDerm, as indicated.	May reduce bacterial contamination, promote healing.
Collaborative	
Provide foam/flotation mattress or bed.	Reduces pressure on skin, tissue, and lesions, decreasing tissue ischemia.
Obtain cultures of open skin lesions.	Identifies pathogens and appropriate treatment choices.

753

ACTIONS/INTERVENTIONS	RATIONALE

Independent

Apply/administer topical/systemic drugs as indicated.	Used in treatment of skin lesions. Use of agents such as Prederm spray can stimulate circulation, enhancing healing process. *Note:* When multidose ointments are used, care must be taken to avoid cross-contamination.
Cover ulcerated KS lesions with wet-to-wet dressings or antibiotic ointment and nonstick dressing (e.g., Telfa) as indicated.	Protects ulcerated areas from contamination and promotes healing.

NURSING DIAGNOSIS: Oral Mucous Membrane, altered

May be related to
Immunologic deficit and presence of lesion-causing pathogens, e.g., *Candida*, herpes, KS
Dehydration, malnutrition
Ineffective oral hygiene
Side effects of drugs, chemotherapy

Possibly evidenced by
Open, ulcerated lesions, vesicles
Oral pain/discomfort
Stomatitis; leukoplakia, gingivitis, carious teeth

DESIRED OUTCOMES/EVALUATION CRITERIA—PATIENT WILL:
Display intact mucous membranes, which are pink, moist, and free of inflammation/ulcerations.
Demonstrate techniques to restore/maintain integrity of oral mucosa.

ACTIONS/INTERVENTIONS	RATIONALE

Independent

Assess mucous membranes/document all oral lesions. Note reports of pain, swelling, difficulty with chewing/swallowing.	Edema, open lesions, and crusting on oral mucous membranes and throat may cause pain and difficulty with chewing/swallowing.
Provide oral care daily and after food intake, using soft toothbrush, nonabrasive toothpaste, nonalcohol mouthwash, floss, and lip moisturizer.	Alleviates discomfort, promotes feeling of well-being, and prevents acid formation associated with retained food particles.
Rinse oral mucosal lesions with saline/dilute hydrogen peroxide or baking soda solutions.	Reduces spread of lesions and encrustations from candidiasis and promotes comfort.
Suggest use of sugarless gum/candy or commercial salivary substitute.	Stimulates flow of saliva to neutralize acids and protect mucous membranes.
Plan diet to avoid salty, spicy, abrasive, and acidic foods or beverages. Check for temperature tolerance of foods. Offer cool/cold smooth foods.	Abrasive foods may open healing lesions. Open lesions are painful and aggravated by salt, spice, acidic foods/beverages. Extreme cold or heat can cause pain to sensitive mucous membranes.
Encourage oral intake of at least 2500 ml/d.	Maintains hydration; prevents drying of oral cavity.
Encourage patient to refrain from smoking.	Smoke is drying and irritating to mucous membranes.

ACTIONS/INTERVENTIONS

Collaborative

Obtain culture specimens of lesions.

Administer medications, as indicated, e.g., nystatin (Mycostatin), ketoconazole (Nizoral).

Refer for dental consultation, if appropriate.

RATIONALE

Reveals causative agents and identifies appropriate therapies.

Specific drug choice is dependent on particular infecting organism(s), e.g., *Candida*.

May require additional therapy to prevent dental losses.

NURSING DIAGNOSIS: Fatigue

May be related to
Decreased metabolic energy production, increased energy requirements (hypermetabolic state)
Overwhelming psychologic/emotional demands
Altered body chemistry: Side effects of medication, chemotherapy

Possibly evidenced by
Unremitting/overwhelming lack of energy, inability to maintain usual routines, decreased performance, impaired ability to concentrate, lethargy/listlessness
Disinterest in surroundings

DESIRED OUTCOMES/EVALUATION CRITERIA—PATIENT WILL:
Report improved sense of energy.
Perform ADLs, with assistance as necessary.
Participate in desired activities at level of ability.

ACTIONS/INTERVENTIONS

Independent

Assess sleep patterns and note changes in thought processes/behaviors.

Plan care to allow for rest periods. Schedule activities for periods when patient has most energy. Involve patient/SO in schedule planning.

Establish realistic activity goals with patient.

Assist with self-care needs; keep bed in low position and travelways clear of furniture; assist with ambulation.

Encourage patient to do whatever possible, e.g., self-care, sit in chair, walk, go out to lunch. Increase activity level as indicated.

Monitor physiologic response to activity, e.g., changes in BP, respiratory rate, or heart rate.

RATIONALE

Multiple factors can aggravate fatigue, including sleep deprivation, CNS disease, emotional distress, and side effects of drugs/chemotherapies.

Frequent rest periods are needed to restore/conserve energy. Planning will allow patient to be active during times when energy level is higher, which may restore a feeling of well-being and a sense of control.

Provides for a sense of control and feelings of accomplishment. Prevents discouragement from fatigue of overactivity.

Weakness may make ADLs almost impossible for the patient to complete. Protects patient from injury during activities.

May conserve strength, increase stamina, and enable patient to become more active without undue fatigue and discouragement.

Tolerance varies greatly depending on the stage of the disease process, nutrition state, fluid balance, and number/type of opportunistic diseases that the patient has been subject to.

ACTIONS/INTERVENTIONS	RATIONALE

Independent

Encourage nutritional intake. (Refer to ND: Nutrition: altered, less than body requirements, p 749.)	Adequate intake/utilization of nutrients is necessary to meet increased energy needs for activity. *Note:* Continuous stimulation of the immune system by HIV infection contributes to a hypermetabolic state.

Collaborative

Provide supplemental O$_2$ as indicated.	Presence of anemia/hypoxemia reduces O$_2$ available for cellular uptake and contributes to fatigue.
Refer to physical/occupational therapy.	Programmed daily exercises and activities help patient to maintain/increase strength and muscle tone, enhance sense of well-being.

NURSING DIAGNOSIS: Thought Processes, altered

May be related to

Hypoxemia, CNS infection by HIV, brain malignancies, and/or disseminated systemic opportunistic infection, CVA/hemorrhage; vasculitis

Alteration of drug metabolism/excretion, accumulation of toxic elements; renal failure, severe electrolyte imbalance, hepatic insufficiency

Possibly evidenced by

Altered attention span; distractibility

Memory deficit

Disorientation; cognitive dissonance; delusional thinking

Sleep disturbances

Impaired ability to make decisions/problem-solve; inability to follow complex commands/mental tasks, loss of impulse control

DESIRED OUTCOMES/EVALUATION CRITERIA—PATIENT WILL:

Maintain usual reality orientation and optimal cognitive functioning.

ACTIONS/INTERVENTIONS	RATIONALE

Independent

Assess mental and neurologic status using appropriate tools.	Establishes functional level at time of admission and provides baseline for future comparison.
Consider effects of emotional distress, e.g., anxiety, grief, anger.	May contribute to reduced alertness, confusion, withdrawal, hypoactivity and require further evaluation and intervention.
Monitor medication regimen and usage.	Actions and interactions of various medications, prolonged drug half-life/altered excretion results in cumulative effects, potentiating risk of toxic reactions. Some drugs may have adverse side effects; e.g., haloperidol (Haldol) can seriously impair motor function in patients with AIDS dementia complex.

ACTIONS/INTERVENTIONS

Independent

Investigate changes in personality, response to stimuli, orientation/level of consciousness; or development of headache, nuchal rigidity, vomiting, fever, seizure activity.

Maintain a pleasant environment with appropriate auditory, visual, and cognitive stimuli.

Provide cues for reorientation, e.g., radio, television, calendars, clocks, room with an outside view. Use patient's name; identify yourself. Maintain consistent personnel and structured schedules as appropriate.

Discuss use of datebooks, lists, other devices to keep track of activities.

Encourage family/SO to socialize and provide reorientation with current news, family events.

Encourage patient to do as much as possible, e.g., dress and groom daily, see friends, and so forth.

Provide support for SO. Encourage discussion of concerns and fears.

Reduce provocative/noxious stimuli. Maintain bed rest in quiet, darkened room if indicated.

Decrease noise, especially at night.

Set limits on maladaptive/abusive behavior; avoid open-ended choices.

Maintain safe environment: e.g., excess furniture out of the way, call bell within patient's reach, bed in low position/rails up; restriction of smoking (unless monitored by caregiver/SO), seizure precautions, soft restraints if indicated.

Provide information about care on an ongoing basis. Answer questions simply and honestly. Repeat explanations as needed.

Discuss causes/future expectations and treatment if dementia is diagnosed. Use concrete terms.

Collaborative

Assist with diagnostic studies, e.g., MRI, CT scan, spinal tap; and monitor laboratory studies as indicated, e.g., BUN/Cr, electrolytes, ABGs.

RATIONALE

Changes may occur for numerous reasons, including development/exacerbation of opportunistic diseases/CNS infection. *Note:* Early detection and treatment of CNS infection may return the patient to near-former cognitive ability.

Providing normal environmental stimuli can help in maintaining some sense of reality orientation.

Frequent reorientation to place and time may be necessary, especially during fever/acute CNS involvement. Sense of continuity may reduce associated anxiety.

These techniques help patient to manage problems of forgetfulness.

Familiar contacts are often helpful in maintaining reality orientation, especially if patient is hallucinating.

Can help to maintain mental abilities for longer period.

Bizarre behavior/deterioration of abilities may be very frightening for SO and makes management of care/dealing with situation difficult. SO may feel a loss of control as stress, anxiety, burnout, and anticipatory grieving impair usual coping abilities.

If the patient is prone to agitation, violent behavior, or seizures, reducing external stimuli may be helpful.

Promotes sleep, reducing cognitive symptoms and effects of sleep deprivation.

Provides sense of security/stability in an otherwise confusing situation.

Decreases the possibility of patient injury.

Can reduce anxiety and fear of unknown; can enhance patient's understanding and involvement/cooperation in treatment when possible.

Obtaining information that ZVD has been shown to improve cognition can provide hope and control for losses.

Choice of tests/studies is dependent on clinical manifestations and index of suspicion, as changes in mental status may reflect a wide variety of causative factors, e.g., CMV meningitis/encephalitis, drug toxicity, electrolyte imbalances, and altered organ function.

ACTIONS/INTERVENTIONS

Collaborative

Administer medications as indicated:

    Amphotericin B (Fungizone);

    ZVD (Retrovir) and other antiretrovirals alone or in combination;

    Antipsychotics, e.g., haloperidol (Haldol), and/or antianxiety agents, e.g., lorazepam (Ativan).

Provide controlled environment/behavioral management.

Refer to counseling as indicated.

RATIONALE

Antifungal useful in treatment of cryptococcosis meningitis.

Shown to improve neurologic and mental functioning for undetermined period of time.

Cautious use may help with problems of sleeplessness, emotional lability, hallucinations, suspiciousness, and agitation.

Team approach may be required to protect patient when mental impairment (e.g., delusions) threatens patient safety.

May help patient gain control in presence of thought disturbances or psychotic symptomatology.

NURSING DIAGNOSIS: Anxiety [specify level]/Fear

May be related to
Threat to self-concept, threat of death, change in health/socioeconomic status, role functioning
Interpersonal transmission and contagion
Separation from support system
Fear of transmission of the disease to family/loved ones

Possibly evidenced by
Increased tension, apprehension, feelings of helplessness/hopelessness
Expressed concern regarding changes in life
Fear of unspecific consequences
Somatic complaints, insomnia; sympathetic stimulation, restlessness

DESIRED OUTCOMES/EVALUATION CRITERIA—PATIENT WILL:
Verbalize awareness of feelings and healthy ways to deal with them.
Display appropriate range of feelings and lessened fear/anxiety.
Demonstrate problem-solving skills.
Use resources effectively.

ACTIONS/INTERVENTIONS

Independent

Assure patient of confidentiality within limits of situation.

Maintain frequent contact with patient. Talk with and touch the patient. Limit use of isolation clothing and masks.

Provide accurate, consistent information regarding prognosis. Avoid arguing about patient's perceptions of the situation.

RATIONALE

Provides reassurance and opportunity for patient to problem-solve solutions to anticipated situations.

Provides assurance that the patient is not alone or rejected; conveys respect for and acceptance of the person, fostering trust.

Can reduce anxiety and enable patient to make decisions/choices based on realities.

ACTIONS/INTERVENTIONS	RATIONALE
Independent	
Be alert to signs of denial/depression (e.g., withdrawal; angry, inappropriate remarks). Determine presence of suicidal ideation and assess potential on a scale of 1–10.	Patient may use defense mechanism of denial and continue to hope that diagnosis is inaccurate. Feelings of guilt and spiritual distress may cause the patient to become withdrawn and believe that suicide is a viable alternative.
Provide open environment in which patient feels safe to discuss feelings or to refrain from talking.	Helps patient to feel accepted in present condition without feeling judged and promotes sense of dignity and control.
Permit expressions of anger, fear, despair without confrontation. Give information that feelings are normal and are to be appropriately expressed.	Acceptance of feelings allows patient to begin to deal with situation.
Recognize and support the stage patient/family is at in the grieving process. (Refer to CP: Cancer, ND: Grieving, anticipatory, p 879.)	Choice of interventions is dictated by stage of grief, coping behaviors, e.g., anger/withdrawal, denial.
Explain procedures, providing opportunity for questions and honest answers. Stay with patient during anxiety-producing procedures and consultations.	Accurate information allows the patient to deal more effectively with the reality of the situation, thereby reducing anxiety and fear of the unknown.
Identify and encourage patient interaction with support systems. Encourage verbalization/interaction with family/SO.	Reduces feeling of isolation. If family support systems are not available, outside sources may be needed immediately, e.g., local AIDS task force.
Provide reliable and consistent information and support for SO.	Allows for better interpersonal interaction and reduction of anxiety and fear.
Include SO as indicated when major decisions are to be made.	Ensures a support system for the patient, and allows the SO the chance to participate in patient's life. *Note:* If patient, family, and SO are in conflict, separate care consultations and visiting times may be needed.
Discuss Advance Directives, end-of-life desires/needs.	May assist patient/SO to plan realistically for terminal stages and death.
Collaborative	
Refer to psychiatric counseling (e.g., clinical nurse specialist, psychiatrist, social worker).	May require further assistance in dealing with diagnosis/prognosis, especially when suicidal thoughts are present.
Provide contact with other resources as indicated, e.g.:	
Spiritual advisor;	Provides opportunity for addressing spiritual concerns.
Hospice staff.	May help relieve anxiety regarding end-of-life care and support for SO.

NURSING DIAGNOSIS: Social Isolation

May be related to
Altered state of wellness, changes in physical appearance, alterations in mental status
Perceptions of unacceptable social or sexual behavior/values
Inadequate personal resources/support systems
Physical isolation

ACTIONS/INTERVENTIONS	RATIONALE
Independent	
Ascertain patient's perception of situation.	Isolation may be partly self-imposed as patient fears rejection/reaction of others.
Spend time talking with patient during and between care activities. Be supportive, allowing for verbalization. Treat with dignity and regard for patient's feelings.	Patient may experience physical isolation due to current medical status and some degree of social isolation secondary to diagnosis of AIDS.
Limit/avoid use of mask, gown, and gloves when possible, e.g., when talking to patient.	Reduces patient's sense of physical isolation and provides positive social contact, which may enhance self-esteem.
Identify support systems available to patient, including presence of/relationship with immediate and extended family.	When patient has assistance from SO, feelings of loneliness and rejection will be diminished. *Note:* Patient may not receive usual/needed support for coping with life-threatening illness and associated grief because of fear and lack of understanding (AIDS hysteria).
Explain isolation precautions/procedures to patient and SO.	Gloves, gowns, mask are not routinely required with a diagnosis of AIDS except when contact with secretions/excretions is expected. Misuse of these barriers enhances feelings of emotional as well as physical isolation. When precautions are necessary, explanations help patient understand reasons for procedures and provide feeling of inclusion in what is happening.
Encourage open visitation (as able), telephone contacts, and social activities within tolerated level.	Participation with others can foster a feeling of belonging.
Encourage active role of contact with SO.	Helps to reestablish a feeling of participation in a social relationship. May lessen likelihood of suicide attempts.
Develop a plan of action with patient: Look at available resources; support healthy risk-taking behaviors. Help patient problem-solve solutions to short-term/imposed isolation.	Having a plan promotes a sense of control over own life and gives patient something to look forward to/actions to accomplish.
Be alert to verbal/nonverbal cues, e.g., withdrawal, statements of despair, sense of aloneness. Ask the patient if thoughts of suicide are being entertained.	Indicators of despair and suicidal ideation are often present; when these cues are acknowledged by the caregiver, the patient is usually willing to talk about thoughts of suicide and sense of isolation and hopelessness.

ACTIONS/INTERVENTIONS

Collaborative

Refer to resources, e.g., social services, counselors, and AIDS organizations/projects (local and national).

Provide for placement in sheltered community when necessary.

RATIONALE

Establishes support systems; may reduce feelings of isolation.

May need more specific care when unable to be maintained at home or when SO cannot manage care.

NURSING DIAGNOSIS: Powerlessness

May be related to
Confirmed diagnosis of a potentially terminal disease, incomplete grieving process
Social ramifications of AIDS; alteration in body image/desired lifestyle; advancing CNS involvement

Possibly evidenced by
Feelings of loss of control over own life
Depression over physical deterioration that occurs despite patient compliance with regimen
Anger, apathy, withdrawal, passivity
Dependence on others for care/decision making, resulting in resentment, anger, guilt

DESIRED OUTCOMES/EVALUATION CRITERIA—PATIENT WILL:
Acknowledge feelings and healthy ways to deal with them.
Verbalize some sense of control over present situation.
Make choices related to care and be involved in self-care.

ACTIONS/INTERVENTIONS

Independent

Identify factors that contribute to the patient's feelings of powerlessness, e.g., diagnosis of a terminal illness, lack of support systems, lack of knowledge about present situation.

Assess degree of feelings of helplessness, e.g., verbal/nonverbal expressions indicating lack of control ("It won't make any difference"), flat affect, lack of communication.

Encourage active role in planning activities, establishing realistic/attainable daily goals. Encourage patient control and responsibility as much as possible. Identify things that the patient can and cannot control.

Encourage living will and durable power of attorney documents, with specific and precise instructions regarding acceptable and unacceptable procedures to prolong life.

RATIONALE

Patients with AIDS are usually aware of the current literature and prognosis. Fear of AIDS (by the general population as well as the patient's family/SO) is the most profound cause of the patient's isolation. For some homosexual patients, this may be the first time that the family has been made aware that the patient lives an alternative lifestyle.

Determines the status of the individual patient and allows for appropriate intervention when the patient is immobilized by depressed feelings.

May enhance feelings of control and self-worth and sense of personal responsibility.

Many factors associated with the treatments used in this debilitating and often fatal disease process place the patient at the mercy of medical personnel and other unknown people who may be making decisions for and about the patient without regard for the patient's wishes, increasing loss of independence.

761

ACTIONS/INTERVENTIONS	RATIONALE
Independent	
Review disease process and future expectations.	Provides knowledge base on which patient can make informed choices.
Determine level of independence/dependence and physical condition. Note extent of care and support available from family/SO and need for other caregivers.	Helps to plan amount of care and symptom management required and need for additional resources.
Review modes of transmission of disease.	Corrects myths and misconceptions; promotes safety for patient/others.
Instruct patient and caregivers concerning infection control, e.g.: good hand-washing techniques for everyone (patient, family, caregivers); use of gloves when handling bedpans, dressings/soiled linens; wearing mask if patient has productive cough; placing soiled/wet linens in plastic bag and separating from family laundry, washing with detergent and hot water; cleaning surfaces with bleach/water solution of 1:10, disinfecting toilet bowl/bedpan with full-strength bleach; preparing patient's food in clean area; washing dishes/utensils in hot soapy water (can be washed with the family dishes).	Reduces risk of transmission of diseases; promotes wellness in presence of reduced ability of immune system to control level of flora.
Stress necessity of daily skin care, including inspecting skin folds, pressure points, and perineum, and of providing adequate cleansing and protective measures, e.g., ointments, padding.	Healthy skin provides barrier to infection. Measures to prevent skin disruption and associated complications are critical.

ACTIONS/INTERVENTIONS

Independent

Ascertain that patient/SO can perform necessary oral and dental care. Review procedures as indicated. Encourage regular dental care.

Review dietary needs (high-protein and high-calorie) and ways to improve intake when anorexia, diarrhea, weakness, depression interfere with intake.

Discuss medication regimen, interactions, and side effects.

Provide information about symptom management that complements medical regimen; e.g., with intermittent diarrhea, take Lomotil before going to social event.

Stress importance of adequate rest.

Encourage activity/exercise at level that patient can tolerate.

Stress necessity of continued health care and follow-up.

Recommend cessation of smoking.

Identify signs/symptoms requiring medical evaluation, e.g., persistent fever/night sweats, swollen glands, continued weight loss, diarrhea, skin blotches/lesions, headache, chest pain, dyspnea.

Identify community resources, e.g., hospice/residential care centers, visiting nurse, home care services, Meals-on-Wheels, peer group support.

RATIONALE

The oral mucosa can quickly exhibit severe, progressive complications. Studies indicate that 65% of AIDs patients have some oral symptoms. Therefore, prevention and early intervention are critical.

Promotes adequate nutrition necessary for healing and support of immune system; enhances feeling of well-being.

Enhances cooperation with/increases probability of success with therapeutic regimen.

Provides patient with increased sense of control, reduces risk of embarrassment, and promotes comfort.

Prevents/reduces fatigue; enhances abilities.

Stimulates release of endorphins in the brain, enhancing sense of well-being.

Provides opportunity for altering regimen to meet individual/changing needs.

Smoking increases risk of respiratory infections and can impair immune system (decrease O_2-combining power with RBCs).

Early recognition of developing complications and timely interventions may prevent progression to life-threatening situation.

Facilitates transfer from acute care setting for recovery/independence, or end-of-life care.

POTENTIAL CONSIDERATIONS in addition to the nursing diagnoses listed in the plan of care

Grieving, anticipatory—loss of physiologic/psychologic well-being, social/lifestyle changes, loss of SO/family, probability of death

Protection, altered—abnormal blood profile (anemia, thrombocytopenia, coagulation), inadequate nutrition, drug therapies (e.g., antineoplastic, immune), chronic disease

Caregiver Role Strain—illness severity of care receiver, significant home care needs, caregiver health impairment, marginal family adaptation or dysfunction, presence of situational stressors, lack of respite for caregiver, caregiver's competing role commitments

RHEUMATOID ARTHRITIS

RA is a chronic, systemic inflammatory disease of unknown cause, involving connective tissue and characterized by destruction and proliferation of the synovial membrane, resulting in joint destruction, ankylosis, and deformity. Immunologic mechanisms appear to play an important role in the initiation and perpetuation of the disease in which spontaneous remissions and unpredictable exacerbations occur. RA is a disorder of the immune system and, as such, is a whole-body disease that can extend beyond the joints, affecting other organ systems.

CARE SETTING

Community level unless surgical procedure is required.

RELATED CONCERNS

Psychosocial Aspects of Care, p 783
Total Joint Replacement, p 686

Patient Assessment Data Base

Data is dependent on severity and involvement of other organs (e.g., eyes, heart, lungs, kidneys), stage (i.e., acute exacerbation or remission), and coexistence of other forms of arthritis/autoimmune diseases.

ACTIVITY/REST

May report:
Joint pain with motion or tenderness worsened by stress placed on joint; morning stiffness, usually occurs bilaterally and symmetrically
Functional limitations affecting lifestyle, leisure time, occupation
Fatigue; sleep disturbances

May exhibit:
Malaise
Limited ROM; muscle atrophy; joint and muscle contractures/deformities
Decreased muscle strength, altered gait/posture

CARDIOVASCULAR

May report:
Intermittent pallor, cyanosis, then redness of fingers/toes before color returns to normal (Raynaud's phenomenon)

EGO INTEGRITY

May report:
Acute/chronic stress factors; e.g., financial, employment, disability, relationship factors
Hopelessness and powerlessness (incapacitating situation)
Threat to self-concept, body image, personal identity (e.g., dependence on others)

FOOD/FLUID

May report:
Inability to obtain/consume adequate food/fluids; nausea
Anorexia
Difficulty chewing (TMJ involvement)

May exhibit:
Weight loss
Dryness of oral mucous membranes, decreased oral secretions; dental caries (Sjögren's syndrome)

HYGIENE

May report:
Varying difficulty performing self-care activities; dependence on others

NEUROSENSORY

May report: Numbness/tingling of hands and feet, loss of sensation in fingers

May exhibit: Symmetric joint swelling

PAIN/DISCOMFORT

May report: Acute episodes of pain (may/may not be accompanied by soft-tissue swelling in joints)
Chronic aching pain and stiffness (mornings are most difficult)

May exhibit: Red, swollen, hot joints

SAFETY

May report: Difficulty managing homemaker/maintenance tasks
Persistent low-grade fever
Dryness of eyes and mucous membranes

May exhibit: Shiny, taut skin; subcutaneous nodules; lesions, leg ulcers
Skin/periarticular local warmth, erythema
Decreased muscle strength, altered gait, reduced ROM

SOCIAL INTERACTION

May report: Impaired interactions with family/others; change in roles; isolation

TEACHING/LEARNING

May report: Familial history of RA (in juvenile onset)
Use of health foods, vitamins, untested arthritis "cures"
History of pericarditis, valvular lesions; pulmonary fibrosis, pleuritis

Discharge plan considerations: **DRG projected mean length of inpatient stay: 4.8 days**
May require assistance with transportation, self-care activities, and homemaker/maintenance tasks; changes in physical layout of home

Refer to section at end of plan for after discharge considerations.

DIAGNOSTIC STUDIES

Rheumatoid factor: Positive in 50%–95% of cases.

Latex fixation: Positive in 75% of typical cases.

Agglutination reactions: Positive in more than 50% of typical cases.

Sedimentation rate (ESR): Usually greatly increased (80–100 mm/h). May return to normal as symptoms improve.

Serum complement: C_3 and C_4 increased in acute onset (inflammatory response). Immune disorder/exhaustion results in depressed total complement levels.

CBC: Usually reveals moderate anemia.

WBC: Elevated when inflammatory processes are present.

Ig (IgM and IgG): Elevation strongly suggests autoimmune process as cause for RA.

X-rays of involved joints: Reveals soft-tissue swelling, erosion of joints, and osteoporosis of adjacent bone (early changes) progressing to bone-cyst formation, narrowing of joint space, and subluxation. Concurrent osteoarthritic changes.

Radionuclide scans: Identify inflamed synovium.

Direct arthroscopy: Visualization of area reveals bone irregularities/degeneration of joint.

Synovial/fluid aspirate: May reveal volume greater than normal; opaque, cloudy, yellow appearance (inflammatory response, bleeding, degenerative waste products); elevated WBCs and leukocytes; decreased viscosity and complement (C_3 and C_4).

Synovial membrane biopsy: Reveals inflammatory changes and development of pannus.

NURSING PRIORITIES

1. Alleviate pain.
2. Increase mobility.
3. Promote positive self-concept.
4. Support independence.
5. Provide information about disease process/prognosis and treatment needs.

DISCHARGE GOALS

1. Pain relieved/controlled.
2. Patient is dealing realistically with current situation.
3. Patient is managing ADLs by self/with assistance as appropriate.
4. Disease process/prognosis and therapeutic regimen understood.
5. Plan in place to meet needs after discharge.

NURSING DIAGNOSIS: Pain [acute]/chronic

May be related to

Injuring agents: Distention of tissues by accumulation of fluid/inflammatory process, destruction of joint

Possibly evidenced by

Reports of pain/discomfort, fatigue
Self-narrowed focus
Distraction behaviors/autonomic responses
Guarding/protective behavior

DESIRED OUTCOMES/EVALUATION CRITERIA—PATIENT WILL:

Report pain is relieved/controlled.
Appear relaxed, able to sleep/rest and participate in activities appropriately.
Follow prescribed pharmacologic regimen.
Incorporate relaxation skills and diversional activities into pain control program.

ACTIONS/INTERVENTIONS	RATIONALE
Independent	
Investigate reports of pain, noting location and intensity (scale of 0–10). Note precipitating factors and nonverbal pain cues.	Helpful in determining pain management needs and effectiveness of program.
Recommend/provide firm mattress or bedboard, small pillow. Elevate linens with bed cradle as needed.	Soft/sagging mattress, large pillows prevent maintenance of proper body alignment, placing stress on affected joints. Elevation of bed linens reduces pressure on inflamed/painful joints.
Suggest patient assume position of comfort while in bed or sitting in chair. Promote bed rest as indicated.	In severe disease/acute exacerbation, total bed rest may be necessary (until objective and subjective improvements are noted) to limit pain/injury to joint.
Place/monitor use of pillows, sandbags, trochanter rolls, splints, braces.	Rests painful joints and maintains neutral position. *Note:* Use of splints can decrease pain and may reduce damage to joint; however, prolonged inactivity can result in loss of joint mobility/function.
Encourage frequent changes of position. Assist patient to move in bed, supporting affected joints above and below, avoiding jerky movements.	Prevents general fatigue and joint stiffness. Stabilizes joint, decreasing joint movement/pain.

ACTIONS/INTERVENTIONS	RATIONALE
Independent	
Recommend that patient take warm bath or shower on arising and/or at bedtime. Apply warm, moist compresses to affected joints several times a day. Monitor water temperature of compress, baths, and so on.	Heat promotes muscle relaxation and mobility, decreases pain, and relieves morning stiffness. Sensitivity to heat may be diminished and dermal injury may occur.
Provide gentle massage.	Promotes relaxation/reduces muscle tension.
Encourage use of stress management techniques, e.g., progressive relaxation, Therapeutic Touch, biofeedback, visualization, guided imagery, self-hypnosis, and controlled breathing.	Promotes relaxation, provides sense of control, and may enhance coping abilities.
Involve in diversional activities appropriate for individual situation.	Refocuses attention, provides stimulation, and enhances self-esteem and feelings of general well-being.
Medicate prior to planned activities/exercises as indicated.	Promotes relaxation, reduces muscle tension/spasms, facilitating participation in therapy.
Collaborative	
Administer medications as indicated, e.g.:	
Acetylsalicylates (aspirin);	ASA exerts an anti-inflammatory and mild analgesic effect, decreasing stiffness and increasing mobility. ASA must be taken regularly to sustain a therapeutic blood level. Research indicates that ASA has the lowest ''toxicity index'' of commonly prescribed NSAIDs.
Other NSAIDs, e.g., ibuprofen (Motrin), naproxen (Naprosyn), sulindac (Clinoril), piroxicam (Feldene), fenoprofen (Nalfon),	May be used when patient does not respond to aspirin or to enhance effects of aspirin. *Note:* These drugs are listed in ascending order of relative severity of side effects (''toxicity index'').
D-penicillamine (Cuprimine);	May control systemic effects of RA if other therapies have not been successful. High rate of side effects (e.g., thrombocytopenia, leukopenia, aplastic anemia) necessitates close monitoring. *Note:* Drug should be given between meals because drug absorption is impaired by food as well as antacids and iron products.
Antacids;	Given with NSAID agents to minimize gastric irritation/discomfort.
Codeine-containing medications.	Although narcotics are generally contraindicated because of chronic nature of condition, short-term use of these products may be required during periods of acute exacerbation to control severe pain.
Assist with physical therapies, e.g., paraffin glove, whirlpool baths.	Provides sustained heat to affected joints. *Note:* Heat may be contraindicated in the presence of hot, swollen joints.
Apply ice or cold packs when indicated.	Cold may relieve pain and swelling during acute episodes.
Maintain TENS unit if used.	Constant low-level electrical stimulus blocks transmission of pain sensations.
Prepare for surgical interventions, e.g., synovectomy.	Removal of inflamed synovium can alleviate pain and limit progression of degenerative changes.

> **NURSING DIAGNOSIS: Physical Mobility, impaired**
>
> **May be related to**
> Skeletal deformity
> Pain, discomfort
> Intolerance to activity; decreased muscle strength
>
> **Possibly evidenced by**
> Reluctance to attempt movement/inability to purposefully move within the physical environment
> Limited ROM, impaired coordination, decreased muscle strength/control and mass [late stages]
>
> **DESIRED OUTCOMES/EVALUATION CRITERIA—PATIENT WILL:**
> Maintain position of function with absence/limitation of contractures.
> Maintain or increase strength and function of affected and/or compensatory body part.
> Demonstrate techniques/behaviors that enable resumption/continuation of activities.

ACTIONS/INTERVENTIONS	RATIONALE
Independent	
Evaluate/continuously monitor degree of joint inflammation/pain.	Level of activity/exercise is dependent on progression/resolution of inflammatory process.
Maintain bed/chair rest when indicated. Schedule activities providing frequent rest periods and uninterrupted nighttime sleep.	Systemic rest is mandatory during acute exacerbations and important throughout all phases of disease to prevent fatigue, maintain strength.
Assist with active/passive ROM as well as resistive exercises and isometrics when able.	Maintains/improves joint function, muscle strength, and general stamina. *Note:* Inadequate exercise leads to joint stiffening, whereas excessive activity can damage joints.
Reposition frequently with adequate personnel. Demonstrate/assist with transfer techniques and use of mobility aids, e.g., trapeze.	Relieves pressure on tissues and promotes circulation. Facilitates self-care and patient's independence. Proper transfer techniques prevent shearing abrasions of skin.
Position with pillows, sandbags, trochanter rolls, splints, braces.	Promotes joint stability (reducing risk of injury) and maintains proper joint position and body alignment, minimizing contractures.
Suggest using small/thin pillow under neck.	Prevents flexion of neck.
Encourage patient to maintain upright and erect posture when sitting, standing, walking.	Maximizes joint function, maintains mobility.
Discuss/provide safety needs, e.g., raised chairs/toilet seat, use of handrails in tub/shower and toilet, proper use of mobility aids/wheelchair safety.	Avoids accidental injuries/falls.

ACTIONS/INTERVENTIONS	RATIONALE
Collaborative	
Consult with physical/occupational therapists and vocational specialist.	Useful in formulating exercise/activity program based on individual needs and in identifying mobility devices/adjuncts.
Provide foam/alternating pressure mattress.	Decreases pressure on fragile tissues to reduce risks of immobility/development of decubitus.
Administer medications as indicated:	
Disease-modifying antirheumatic drugs (DMARDs), e.g., gold, sodium thiomaleate (Myochrysine) or auranofin (Ridaura), methotrexate (Amethopterin, Folex);	These drugs appear to alter the natural history of RA by slowing the progression of bony erosion and cartilage loss. *Note:* Chrysotherapy (gold salts) may produce dramatic/sustained remission but may result in rebound inflammation if discontinued, or serious side effects, e.g., nitritoid crisis with dizziness, blurred vision, flushing, progressing to anaphylactic shock.
Antimalarial agents, e.g., hydroxychloroquine (Plaquenil);	Used for patients with moderately severe RA to provide some disease-modifying and anti-inflammatory effects.
Glucocorticoid steroids.	May be necessary to suppress acute systemic inflammation.
Prepare for surgical interventions, e.g.:	
Arthroplasty for synovectomy and débridement, tendon transfers, osteotomy, or joint replacement;	Can maintain/improve joint function, prevent progressive deformity. Replacement may be needed to restore optimal functioning and mobility. *Note:* Early synovectomy may help prevent recurrent inflammation.
Tunnel release procedures, tendon repair, ganglionectomy;	Corrects associated connective tissue/neuromuscular defects; enhances function and mobility.

NURSING DIAGNOSIS: Body Image disturbance/Role Performance, altered

May be related to
Changes in ability to perform usual tasks
Increased energy expenditure; impaired mobility

Possibly evidenced by
Change in structure/function of affected parts
Negative self-talk; focus on past strength/function, appearance
Change in lifestyle/physical ability to resume roles, loss of employment, dependence on SO for assistance
Change in social involvement; sense of isolation
Feelings of helplessness, hopelessness

DESIRED OUTCOMES/EVALUATION CRITERIA—PATIENT WILL:
Verbalize increased confidence in ability to deal with illness, changes in lifestyle, and possible limitations.
Formulate realistic goals/plans for future.

ACTIONS/INTERVENTIONS	RATIONALE

Independent

Encourage verbalization about concerns of disease process, future expectations.

Provides opportunity to identify fears/misconceptions and deal with them directly.

Discuss meaning of loss/change to patient/SO. Ascertain how patient views self in usual lifestyle functioning, including sexual aspects.

Identifying how illness affects perception of self and interactions with others will determine need for further intervention/counseling.

Discuss patient's perception of how SO perceives limitations.

Verbal/nonverbal cues from SO may have a major impact on how patient views self.

Acknowledge and accept feelings of grief, hostility, dependency.

Constant pain is wearing, and feelings of anger and hostility are common. Acceptance provides feedback that feelings are normal.

Note withdrawn behavior, use of denial, or over-concern with body/changes.

May suggest emotional exhaustion or maladaptive coping methods, requiring more in-depth intervention/psychologic support.

Set limits on maladaptive behavior. Assist patient to identify positive behaviors that will aid in coping.

Helps patient to maintain self-control, which enhances self-esteem.

Involve patient in planning care and scheduling activities.

Enhances feelings of competency/self-worth, encourages independence, and encourages participation in therapy.

Assist with grooming needs as necessary.

Maintaining appearance enhances self-image.

Give positive reinforcement for accomplishments.

Allows patient to feel good about self. Reinforces positive behavior. Enhances self-confidence.

Collaborative

Refer to psychiatric counseling, e.g., clinical specialist psychiatric nurse, psychiatrist/psychologist, social worker.

Patient/SO may require ongoing support to deal with long-term/debilitating process.

Administer medications as indicated, e.g., antianxiety and mood-elevating drugs.

May be needed in presence of severe depression until patient develops more effective coping skills.

NURSING DIAGNOSIS: Self Care deficit: (specify)

May be related to
Musculoskeletal impairment; decreased strength/endurance, pain on movement
Depression

Possibly evidenced by
Inability to manage ADLs (feeding, bathing, dressing, and toileting)

DESIRED OUTCOMES/EVALUATION CRITERIA—PATIENT WILL:
Perform self-care activities at a level consistent with individual capabilities.
Demonstrate techniques/lifestyle changes to meet self-care needs.
Identify personal/community resources that can provide needed assistance.

ACTIONS/INTERVENTIONS	RATIONALE

Independent

Determine usual level of functioning (0–4) prior to onset/exacerbation of illness and potential changes now anticipated.

May be able to continue usual activities with necessary adaptations to current limitations.

Maintain mobility, pain control, and exercise program.

Supports physical/emotional independence.

Assess barriers to participation in self-care. Identify/plan for environmental modifications.

Prepares for increased independence, which enhances self-esteem.

Allow patient sufficient time to complete tasks to fullest extent of ability. Capitalize on individual strengths.

May need more time to complete tasks by self but provides an opportunity for greater sense of self-confidence and self-worth.

Collaborative

Consult with rehabilitation specialists, e.g., occupational therapist.

Helpful in determining assistive devices to meet individual needs, e.g., button hook, long-handled shoe horn, reacher, handheld shower head.

Arrange home-health evaluation prior to discharge with follow-up afterward.

Identifies problems that may be encountered because of current level of disability. Provides for more successful team efforts with others who are involved in care, e.g., occupational therapy team.

Arrange for consult with other agencies, e.g., Meals-on-Wheels, home care service, nutritionist.

May need additional kinds of assistance to continue in home setting.

NURSING DIAGNOSIS: Home Maintenance Management, impaired, risk for

Risk factors may include
Long-term degenerative disease process
Inadequate support systems

Possibly evidenced by
[Not applicable; presence of signs and symptoms establishes an *actual* diagnosis]

DESIRED OUTCOMES/EVALUATION CRITERIA—PATIENT WILL:
Maintain safe, growth-promoting environment.
Demonstrate appropriate, effective use of resources.

ACTIONS/INTERVENTIONS	RATIONALE

Independent

Assess level of physical functioning.

Identifies degree of assistance/support required.

Evaluate environment to assess ability to care for self.

Determines feasibility of remaining in/changing home layout to meet individual needs.

Determine financial resources to meet needs of individual situation. Identify support systems available to patient, e.g., extended family, friends/neighbors.

Availability of personal resources/community supports will affect ability to problem-solve/choice of solutions.

Develop plan for maintaining a clean, healthful environment, e.g., sharing of household repair/tasks between family members or by contract services.

Ensures that needs will be met on an ongoing basis.

ACTIONS/INTERVENTIONS

Independent

Identify sources for necessary equipment, e.g., lifts, elevated toilet seat, wheelchair.

Collaborative

Coordinate home evaluation by occupational therapist.

Identify/meet with community resources, e.g., visiting nurse, homemaker service, social services, senior citizens' groups.

RATIONALE

Provides opportunity to acquire equipment before discharge.

Useful for identifying adaptive equipment, ways to modify tasks to maintain independence.

Can facilitate transfer to/support continuation in home setting.

NURSING DIAGNOSIS: Knowledge deficit [learning need] regarding disease, prognosis, treatment, self care and discharge needs

May be related to
Lack of exposure/recall
Information misinterpretation

Possibly evidenced by
Questions/request for information, statement of misconception
Inaccurate follow-through of instructions/development of preventable complications

DESIRED OUTCOMES/EVALUATION CRITERIA—PATIENT WILL:
Verbalize understanding of condition/prognosis, treatment.
Develop a plan for self-care, including lifestyle modifications consistent with mobility and/or activity restrictions.

ACTIONS/INTERVENTIONS

Independent

Review disease process, prognosis, and future expectations.

Discuss patient's role in management of disease process through diet, medication, and balanced program of exercise and rest.

Assist in planning a realistic and integrated schedule of activity, rest, personal care, drug administration, physical therapy, and stress management.

Stress importance of continued pharmacotherapeutic management.

Recommend use of enteric-coated/buffered aspirin or nonacetylated salicylates, e.g., choline salicylate (Arthropan) or choline magnesium trisalicylate (Trilisate).

Suggest ingestion of medications with meals, milk products, or antacids and at bedtime.

RATIONALE

Provides knowledge base on which patient can make informed choices.

Goal of disease control is to suppress inflammation in joints/other tissues to maintain joint function and prevent deformities.

Provides structure and defuses anxiety when managing a complex chronic disease process.

Benefits of drug therapy are dependent on correct dosage; e.g., aspirin must be taken regularly to sustain therapeutic blood levels of 18–25 mg/dL.

Coated/buffered preparations ingested with food minimize gastric irritation, reducing risk of bleeding/hemorrhage. *Note:* Nonacetylated products have a longer half-life, requiring less frequent administration in addition to producing less gastric irritation.

Limits gastric irritation. Reduction of pain at HS enhances sleep and increased blood level decreases early-morning stiffness.

ACTIONS/INTERVENTIONS	RATIONALE

Independent

Identify adverse drug effects, e.g., tinnitus, gastric intolerance, GI bleeding, purpuric rash.	Prolonged, maximal doses of aspirin may result in overdose. Tinnitus usually indicates high therapeutic blood levels. If tinnitus occurs, the dosage is usually decreased by 1 tablet every 2–3 days until it stops.
Stress importance of reading product labels and refraining from OTC drug usage without prior medical approval.	Many products (e.g., cold remedies, antidiarrheals) contain hidden salicylates that increase risk of drug overdose/harmful side effects.
Review importance of balanced diet with foods high in vitamins, protein, and iron.	Promotes general well-being and tissue repair/regeneration.
Encourage obese patient to lose weight and supply with weight reduction information as appropriate.	Weight loss will reduce stress on joints, especially hips, knees, ankles, feet.
Provide information about/resources for assistive devices, e.g., wheeled dolly/wagon for moving items, pickup sticks, lightweight dishes and pans, raised toilet seats, safety handlebars.	Reduces force exerted on joints and enables individual to participate more comfortably in needed/desired activities.
Discuss energy-saving techniques, e.g., sitting instead of standing to prepare meals and shower.	Prevents fatigue; facilitates self-care and independence.
Encourage maintenance of correct body position and posture both at rest and during activity, e.g., keeping joints extended, not flexed, wearing splints for prescribed periods, avoiding remaining in a single position for extended periods, positioning hands near center of body during use, and sliding rather than lifting objects when possible.	Good body mechanics must become a part of the patient's lifestyle to lessen joint stress and pain.
Review necessity of frequent inspection of skin and meticulous skin care under splints, casts, supporting devices. Demonstrate proper padding.	Reduces risk of skin irritation/breakdown.
Discuss necessity of medical follow-up/laboratory studies, e.g., ESR, salicylate levels, PT.	Drug therapy requires frequent assessment/refinement to assure optimal effect and to prevent overdose/dangerous side effects, e.g., aspirin prolongs PT, increasing risk of bleeding. Chrysotherapy depresses platelets, potentiating risk of thrombocytopenia.
Provide for sexual counseling as necessary.	Information about different positions and techniques and/or other options for sexual fulfillment may enhance personal relationships and feelings of self-worth/self-esteem.
Identify community resources, e.g., Arthritis Foundation.	Assistance/support from others promotes maximal recovery.

POTENTIAL CONSIDERATIONS following acute hospitalization (dependent on patient's age, physical condition/presence of complications, personal resources, and life responsibilities)

Fatigue—increased energy requirements to perform ADLs, states of discomfort

Pain, chronic—accumulation of fluid/inflammation, destruction of joint

Physical Mobility, impaired—skeletal deformity, pain/discomfort, decreased muscle strength, intolerance to activity

Self Care deficit/Home Maintenance Management, impaired—musculoskeletal impairment, decreased strength/endurance, pain on movement, inadequate support systems, insufficient finances, unfamiliarity with neighborhood resources

TRANSPLANTATION (POSTOPERATIVE AND LIFELONG)

With current advances in technology and knowledge of immune responses at the molecular level, organ and tissue transplantation is becoming more commonplace. The most frequently transplanted organs are the kidney, liver, and heart. The major problem to be overcome is the immunologic response of the patient to donor tissues. The ability of the immune system to distinguish between self and nonself is crucial to its proper functioning; therefore, in the process of transplantation, the donor/nonself can be rejected. The three forms of rejection are (1) hyperactive or hyperacute (within 48 hours); (2) acute (usually within 3–6 months); and (3) chronic (can occur months or years after transplant). General postoperative care is similar to that for any other major abdominal or cardiothoracic surgery; however, special considerations necessitate meticulous measures to prevent infection and identify early signs of rejection.

CARE SETTING

Post-ICU; plan of care addresses early recovery and long-term postdischarge community/clinic follow-up phases.

RELATED CONCERNS

Refer to (1) specific surgical plans of care for general considerations (e.g., Cardiac Surgery), and (2) organ-specific plans (e.g., Heart Failure, Renal Failure, Cirrhosis, Hepatitis), relative to issues of target organ problems following transplantation.

Surgical Intervention, p 802
Sepsis/Septicemia, p 719
Peritonitis, p 366
Thrombophlebitis: Deep Vein Thrombosis, p 107
Psychosocial Aspects of Care, p 783

Patient Assessment Data Base

Refer to specific plans of care for data reflecting specific organ failure necessitating transplantation.

EGO INTEGRITY

May report: Feelings of anxiety, fearfulness
Multiple stressors: Impact of condition on personal relationships, ability to perform expected/needed roles, loss of control, required lifestyle changes; financial concerns, cost of procedure/future treatment needs; uncertainty of outcomes/personal mortality, spiritual conflicts; waiting period for suitable donation
Concerns about changes in appearance (e.g., bloating, jaundice, major scars), aesthetic side effects of immunosuppressant medications (e.g., steroids)
Spiritual questioning (e.g., "Why me?" "Why should I benefit from someone else's death?")

SEXUALITY

May report: Loss of libido
Concerns regarding resumption of sexual activity

SOCIAL INTERACTIONS

May report: Reactions of family members

Conflicts regarding family member(s) ability/willingness to participate, e.g., financial, organ/bone marrow donation, postprocedure support

Concern about benefiting from other person's death

Concern for family member who must take on new responsibilities as roles shift

TEACHING/LEARNING

May report: Lack of improvement/deterioration in condition

Beliefs about transplantation

History of alcohol/drug abuse, disease resulting in organ failure

Discharge plan Considerations **DRG projected mean length of inpatient stay: Dependent on organ transplanted, e.g., kidney, 6 days, liver, 8 days**

May need assistance with activities of daily living; shopping, transportation, ambulation; managing medication regimen

Refer to section at end of plan for postdischarge considerations.

DIAGNOSTIC STUDIES (dependent on specific organ involvement)

General preoperative screening studies include:

Chest x-ray: Provides information about status of lungs and heart.

CT/MRI scan: Reveals status of body systems and organs, including size, shape, and general function of major blood vessels; organ size for best match with donor organ; and potential sources of postoperative complications. Rules out presence of cancer, which would contraindicate transplantation.

Total-body bone scan: Evaluates status of skeletal system to determine presence/absence of bone cancer.

Specific blood and tissue typing: As may be required for donor-recipient matching.

Dental evaluation: To rule out oral infection or abscessed teeth.

Ear, nose, and throat evaluation: To rule out sinus infection.

Renal function studies (e.g., IV pyelogram, creatinine clearance): Determines functional status of kidneys.

Pulmonary function studies: Determines lung function and/or limitations that may complicate recovery.

CBC: Identifies anemia, which can reduce oxygen-carrying capacity, and other blood factors that may affect recovery.

Biochemical studies: Various tests done as indicated in addition to electrolytes, immune status.

Screening tests: To detect presence/type of hepatitis; HIV, viral titer (e.g., CMV, herpes).

ECG: Screens cardiac status, e.g., electrical conduction/dysrhythmias, signs of infarcts/hypertrophy.

NURSING PRIORITIES

1. Prevent infection.
2. Maximize organ function.
3. Promote independent functioning.
4. Support family involvement and coping.

DISCHARGE GOALS

1. Free of signs of infection.
2. Signs of rejection absent/minimized.
3. New organ function good or improving.
4. Usual activities resumed.
5. Plan in place to meet individual needs following discharge.

ACTIONS/INTERVENTIONS	RATIONALE
Independent	
Screen visitors/staff for signs of infection; make sure nurse caring for patient with new transplant is not caring for another patient with infection. Maintain protective isolation as indicated.	Reduces possibility of patient's contracting a nosocomial infection. *Note:* Total isolation is usually restricted to patients with lung transplants or individuals with neutropenia.
Demonstrate and emphasize importance of proper hand-washing techniques by patient and caregivers.	First-line defense against infection/cross-contamination.
Inspect all incisions/puncture sites. Evaluate healing progress.	Promotes early identification of onset of infection and prompt intervention.
Provide meticulous care of invasive lines, incisions, wounds.	Minimizes potential for bacteria in order to reduce exposure/risk of infection. *Note:* Invasive lines are removed as early as possible following transplant.
Encourage deep breathing, coughing.	Mobilizes respiratory secretions and reduces risk of respiratory problems.
Provide/assist with frequent oral hygiene.	Meticulous attention to oral mucosa is necessary because immunosuppression/antibiotic therapies increase risk of opportunistic oral/mucosal infections.
Obtain sterile specimens of wound drainage as appropriate.	Identifying organism allows for appropriate treatment.

Possibly evidenced by
Increased tension, apprehension, uncertainty
Expressed concerns
Somatic complaints
Sympathetic stimulation

DESIRED OUTCOMES/EVALUATION CRITERIA—PATIENT WILL:
Appear relaxed and report anxiety is reduced to a manageable level.
Verbalize awareness of feelings.
Identify healthy ways to deal with anxiety.
Use resources/support systems effectively.

ACTIONS/INTERVENTIONS	RATIONALE
Independent	
Discuss patient's posttransplant expectations, including physical appearance and lifestyle changes.	Depending on past experience and exposure to others with transplants, patient may have unrealistic ideas as well as real concerns about what may happen (e.g., organ rejection, effects of medications, including steroid use, limitations associated with immunosuppression). Even with effective preoperative teaching, patient will continue to have new concerns or suppressed thoughts and beliefs, which can surface during recovery.
Encourage patient to discuss feelings and concerns about situation and to express fears.	Helps to identify issues and can lead to problem solving.
Discuss beliefs/concerns that are commonly held regarding source of organ.	Cultural/spiritual beliefs may lead patient to question whether organ from someone of another race or particular group may change own sense of self-identity.
Identify/encourage use of previously successful coping behaviors.	Under stress, patient may not remember what has worked in the past; discussion can refresh memories of successful behaviors and promote repetition.
Help patient to focus on one "problem" at a time.	Dealing with one issue at a time seems to make it more manageable. Provides sense of success and opportunity to build on each success.
Discuss possibility and normalcy of mood swings.	Feelings of euphoria and depression are not uncommon, especially with use of steroids, and are usually short-lived.
Encourage open communication between SO/family and patient within safe environment.	Free expression of feelings/beliefs can lead to clarification and problem solving of different views. When concerns or beliefs are hidden from one another, additional stress/adverse effects may result.

777

ACTIONS/INTERVENTIONS

Independent

Provide opportunity for patient and SO/family to meet with other(s) who have experienced a similar and successful transplant.

Identify possible actions to limit physical effects or manifestations of long-term steroid/cyclosporine use.

Collaborative

Refer to spiritual advisor as indicated.

Refer to social worker, other professionals as indicated.

RATIONALE

Sharing experiences and hearing about successes and universal problems experienced by another can lessen patient/SO anxieties, promote hope, and provide a role model.

Learning about clothing styles, makeup techniques, use of bleach or mild depilatory to reduce facial hair can enhance patient's appearance and reduce anxiety about social rejection.

Facing one's mortality may provoke feelings of anxiety and questioning about one's spiritual beliefs and practices.

Provides assistance with readjustment to life following major life event.

NURSING DIAGNOSIS: Coping, Individual/Family, ineffective, risk for

Risk factors may include
Situational crises
Family disorganization and role changes
Prolonged disease exhausting supportive capacity of SO/family

Possibly evidenced by
[Not applicable; presence of signs and symptoms establishes an *actual* diagnosis]

DESIRED OUTCOMES/EVALUATION CRITERIA—PATIENT/FAMILY WILL:
Assess current situation accurately.
Verbalize awareness of own coping abilities.
Meet psychologic needs as evidenced by appropriate expression of feelings, identifying options and resources.

ACTIONS/INTERVENTIONS

Independent

Encourage and support patient in evaluating lifestyle. Discuss previous occupation and leisure activities and implications for the future.

Assess patient's/family's current functional status and note how transplant is affecting ability to cope.

Determine additional outside stressors (e.g., family, social, work environment, or nursing/health care management).

Provide ongoing information about expected progression of recuperation and potential course of recovery.

RATIONALE

Helps patient to evaluate and choose activities that are important and begin to adjust to new lifestyle of wellness.

Provides a starting point to identify needs and plan care.

Illness and treatment demands may affect all areas of life and problems need to be addressed and resolved to enable patient and SO to manage current situation optimally.

Knowing what to expect helps individuals cope more effectively, encourages planning for future needs/lifestyle changes.

ACTIONS/INTERVENTIONS	RATIONALE

Independent

Discuss normalcy of/monitor progression through stages of acceptance of transplanted organ:

    Foreign body stage—organ feels strange, separate from own body;

    Partial internalization stage—protective of organ, restricts movement/activity, excessive concern regarding organ function/fragility;

    Complete internalization—acceptance of organ into self-concept, discusses organ only in response to direct questioning.

Sense that organ is "outside" body can be very frightening, while fixation on organ can be irritating to others. Understanding normalcy of feelings is reassuring. *Note:* Movement through stages is variable and regression is common, especially during early posttransplant period.

Have individual list previous methods of dealing with life problems and outcomes of actions.

Promotes problem solving in current situation, allows individual to build on past successes.

Active-listen and identify individual's perceptions of what is happening, how transplant has affected view of self/family member.

Helps those involved to recognize own feelings and concerns regarding use of an organ from someone who died.

Encourage discussion between patient/family regarding future expectations.

Period of dependence during illness, concerns over possible organ rejection/life-threatening complications may lead to conflicts regarding patient's return to an independent role.

Collaborative

Refer to spiritual resource and/or psychiatric clinical nurse specialist/psychiatrist, social worker, as indicated.

May be helpful in resolving lingering/difficult concerns.

NURSING DIAGNOSIS: Knowledge deficit [learning need] regarding prognosis, therapeutic regimen, self care and discharge needs

May be related to
Lack of exposure/recall
Information misinterpretation
Unfamiliarity with information resources
Cognitive limitation

Possibly evidenced by
Request for information
Statement of misconception
Development of preventable complication

DESIRED OUTCOMES/EVALUATION CRITERIA—PATIENT WILL:
Participate in the learning process.
Assume responsibility for own learning and begin to look for information and ask questions.
Initiate necessary lifestyle changes and participate in treatment regimen.

In addition to routine postoperative instructions, refer to CP: Surgical Intervention, p 802.

779

ACTIONS/INTERVENTIONS	RATIONALE

Independent

Review general signs/symptoms of rejection and infection (e.g., general malaise/fatigue, dyspnea, sudden weight gain, fever/chills, sore throat, delayed healing of wound, nausea/vomiting, syncope). Review indicators specific to transplanted organ (e.g., liver rejection: pain in liver or back, lighter-colored stools, jaundice, dark-colored urine).

Prompt recognition and timely intervention may limit severity of complication. Acute rejection usually develops within days of transplant or may be delayed for number of months. If detected early, rejection process can be minimized or reversed with changes in drug regimen. *Note:* Chronic rejection developing after months/years is generally irreversible.

Stress necessity of adherence to medical regimen and appropriate follow-up, including routine examinations (e.g., dental, gynecologic) and specialty examinations (e.g., ophthalmology, gastroenterology).

Adherence to regimen is imperative to reduce risk of organ rejection/other complications. Routine monitoring/care by primary care providers is necessary to maximize general well-being and to monitor effects of long-term medication regimen on other organ systems and general well-being. Specialty monitoring (such as gastroenterology for liver transplant) aids in monitoring new organ function and effect on other systems. Additionally, steroids may cause changes in visual acuity or development of cataracts/glaucoma. *Note:* Immunosuppression increases risk of cancer, especially lymphomas and skin lesions.

Discuss need to seek medical attention earlier than was probably done in the past.

Generally a "wait and see" attitude can be detrimental, as a delay in treatment could result in organ damage/rejection.

Recommend that results of laboratory tests/diagnostic studies done locally be faxed to transplant center.

Long-term care is very complex and requires coordination and cooperation between all healthcare providers.

Provide information via multiple media, including written format, dependent on level of comprehension. Include various members of the transplant team as appropriate.

Enhances learning experience and provides references for postdischarge review/verification of recall. Use of team members, e.g., dietitian, physical/occupational therapists, provides for individualization of teaching plan to meet individual needs.

Discuss "Dos and Don'ts" of specific medications, anticipated and adverse effects, interaction with other drugs, appropriate use of OTC products; adjustment of prescribed medication dosage (e.g., prednisone) during periods of stress, or as gradual decrease in immunosuppression occurs over months/years as appropriate.

Multiple medications (often a triple therapy of cyclosporine, prednisone, and azathioprine) are typically required on an ongoing/lifelong basis to prevent organ rejection. Additional drugs may be needed to manage adverse side effects of immunosuppressant therapy, (e.g., infection, osteoporosis, peptic ulcers, hypertension).

Include SO/family members, caregivers in education sessions and discharge planning as appropriate.

Promotes understanding and cooperation among those providing support for/involved in care of the patient.

Recommend wearing an identification tag (bracelet, necklace, etc.).

In emergencies, provides immediate information to care providers relative to surgical/transplant history and medication regimen.

Identify community resources, including transplant club/support groups.

Provides opportunity for patient and SO(s) to share experiences with others who are going through the same process. Providing anticipatory guidance may enhance problem solving.

ACTIONS/INTERVENTIONS	RATIONALE
Independent	
Discuss self-monitoring routine and record keeping, e.g., chart temperature per protocol (e.g., before breakfast/dinner and when not feeling well); weigh daily before breakfast (in like clothing, same scale); blood pressure/pulse, changes in medication dosage, changes in health status/functional ability, etc.	Helps care providers to identify individual needs/development of complications.
Recommend frequent oral/dental care and periodic visual inspection of oral mucosa and gums.	Immunosuppression increases susceptibility to common opportunistic infections affecting the mouth, (e.g., *Candida,* herpes simplex); and ongoing drug regimen (such as cyclosporine) can cause hypertrophy of gums.
Review dietary needs. Determine optimal weight, discuss expected changes associated with medication regimen.	Requirements of normal healing, as well as effects of current stress, medications, and preoperative debilitation can exacerbate nutritional deficiencies/imbalances and cause excessive weight loss; however, undesired weight gain can also occur as food tastes better, dietary restrictions are deleted, and prednisone stimulates appetite.
Identify risk factors/additional safety concerns relative to infections, e.g., avoid changing cat litter box or use of live virus vaccines; use gloves when gardening, and take proper care of wounds/tissue trauma.	Awareness of possible risks (including unusual sources) enable patient/family to plan for avoidance. Cat litter can transmit infectious agents such as *Listeria.* Steroid-induced skin fragility increases risk of injury from minor trauma as a result of immunosuppression.
Discuss necessity of handling skin carefully, use of sunscreen with SPF of 15 or greater.	Steroid therapy results in skin fragility and sun sensitivity. Broken/damaged skin provides an entry for bacteria.
Discuss common postoperative care needs, e.g., avoidance of *heavy* lifting/physical labor or exercise (including contact sports), and activities that stretch or put pressure on incision; when/how to resume driving and sexual activity; dietary and fluid needs/restrictions.	Reduces likelihood of complication, aids patient/SO in determining appropriateness of activities, and enhances patient's sense of control and personal responsibility for altering activity level. *Note:* General advice for early phase: "If it hurts, don't do it."
Encourage continuation of pre-illness daily routines and activities as appropriate.	Enhances general well-being. Promotes focus on returning to "normal life," reducing sense that *everything* is different now.
Discuss participation in planned exercise program and inform about Transplant Olympics as appropriate/desired.	Restores strength, promotes sense of well-being and self-esteem, reduces risk of osteoporosis, inappropriate weight gain, and decreased hypertension.
Identify employment concerns/risks specific to particular transplanted organ, job responsibilities, and workplace environment.	Provides opportunity to problem-solve, plan for modifications, or seek alternative vocational options.
Discuss travel needs, e.g., notify team contact person in advance regarding plans; hand carry medications when traveling by airplane; locate transplant center nearest to travel destination before leaving home.	Frees patient to be involved in travel if desired. May need special instructions/precautions, depending on travel destination.
Stress importance of notifying future care providers of medication regimen.	Status of immune system functioning may require prophylactic therapy for procedures (such as antibiotics with dental care).

781

POTENTIAL CONSIDERATIONS following acute hospitalization (depending on patient's age, physical condition/presence of complications, personal resources, and life responsibilities)

Therapeutic Regimen: Individual, ineffective management—postdischarge concern, complexity of therapeutic regimen, side effects of medications, economic difficulties

Infection, risk for—immunosuppression, antibiotic therapy

Protection, altered—drug therapies (corticosteroid, immune)

Knowledge deficit [learning need]—participation in support groups; ongoing care in collaboration with transplant team; gradual decrease of immunosuppression over months and years

PSYCHOSOCIAL ASPECTS OF CARE

The emotional response of the patient during illness is of extreme importance. The mind-body-spirit connection is well established; for example, when a physiologic response occurs, there is a corresponding psychologic response. Also, there are physiologic conditions that have a psychologic component, for example, the emotional instability of steroid therapy or Cushing's syndrome or the irritability of hypoglycemia. Rapid growth of the field of psychoneuroimmunology is regularly providing new information about these issues.

With expanding technology in health care, ethical issues are more hotly debated. Although the stress of illness is well recognized, the effect on the individual is unpredictable. Values of caregivers and patients/SOs, sensitivity to different cultures, language barriers (including difficulties that people have in talking about their bodies) affect the care a patient expects and receives. It is not necessarily the event that creates problems, but rather the patient's perception of and response to the event, which may result in unmet psychologic needs that drain energy resources needed for healing.

CARE SETTING

Any setting in which nursing contact occurs/care is provided.

RELATED CONCERNS

This is an aspect of all care and plans of care.

Assessment Factors to be Considered

INDIVIDUAL

Age and sex

Religious affiliation: Church attendance, importance of religion in patient's life, belief in life after death

Level of knowledge/education; how the individual accesses information, e.g., auditory, visual, kinesthetic

Patient's dominant language? Is he or she literate?

Patterns of communication with SOs, with healthcare givers? Style of speech?

Perception of body and its functions. When well? In illness? In this illness?

How does patient define and perceive illness?

How is patient experiencing illness versus what illness actually is?

Emotional response to current treatment/hospitalization?
Past experience with illness, hospitalization, and healthcare systems?
Emotional reactions in feeling (sensory) terms: e.g., States, "I feel scared."
Behavior when anxious, afraid, impatient, or angry

SIGNIFICANT OTHERS

Marital status; who are SOs, nuclear family, extended family? Recurring or patterned relationships?
Family development cycle: Just married, children (young, adolescent, leaving/returning home), retired?
What are the interaction processes within the family?
Patient's role in family tasks and functions
How are SOs affected by the illness and prognosis?
Lifestyle differences that need to be considered: Dietary, Spiritual, Sexual preference, other community (e.g., religious order, commune, retirement center)?

SOCIOECONOMIC

Employment; finances
Environmental factors: Home, work, and recreation
Out of usual environment (on vacation, visiting)
Social class; value system
Social acceptability of disease/condition (e.g., STDs, HIV, obesity, substance abuse)

CULTURAL

Ethnic background
Beliefs regarding caring and curing
Health-seeking behaviors; illness referral system
Values related to health and treatment
Cultural factors related to illness in general and to pain response

DISEASE (ILLNESS)

Kind/cause of illness; how has it been treated? How/should it be treated? Anticipated response to treatment? What is the threat to self/others?
Is this an acute or a chronic illness? Is it inherited?
If terminal illness, what do the patient and SO know and anticipate?
Is the condition "appropriate" to the afflicted individual, e.g., multiple sclerosis, DM, cancer?
Illness related to personality factors, such as type A (may be myth or valid)?

NURSE-RELATED

Basic knowledge of human responses and how the current situation is related to response of the individual
Basic knowledge of biologic, psychologic, social, and cultural issues
Knowledge and use of therapeutic communication skills
Knowledge of own value and belief systems, including prejudices, biases

Willingness to look at own behavior in relation to interaction with others and make changes as necessary

Respect of patient's privacy; confidentiality

NURSING PRIORITIES

1. Reduce anxiety/fear.
2. Support grieving process.
3. Facilitate integration of self-concept and body-image changes.
4. Encourage effective coping skills of patient/SO.
5. Promote safe environment/patient well-being.

DISCHARGE GOALS

1. Reports anxiety/fear manageable.
2. Progressing through stages of grieving.
3. Patient/family dealing realistically with current situation.
4. Safe environment maintained.
5. Plan in place to meet needs after discharge.

NURSING DIAGNOSIS: Anxiety [specify level]/Fear

May be related to

Unconscious conflict about essential values

Situational and/or maturational crises; interpersonal transmission and contagion

Threat to self-concept; threat of death; change in health status; unmet needs

Separation from support system; knowledge deficit

Sensory impairment; environmental stimuli

Possibly evidenced by

Reports of increased tension; feelings of helplessness

Inadequacy; apprehension, uncertainty, being scared, overexcitedness

Expressed concern regarding changes in life events; dread of an identifiable problem recognized by the patient; fear of unspecific consequences

Focus on self; fight/flight behavior

Facial tension; sympathetic stimulation; extraneous movements

DESIRED OUTCOMES/EVALUATION CRITERIA—PATIENT WILL:

Acknowledge and discuss fears.

Appear relaxed and report anxiety is reduced to a manageable level.

Verbalize awareness of feelings of anxiety and healthy ways to deal with them.

Demonstrate problem solving and use resources effectively.

ACTIONS/INTERVENTIONS	RATIONALE
Independent	
Note palpitations, elevated pulse/respiratory rate.	Changes in vital signs may suggest the degree of anxiety being experienced by the patient or reflect the impact of physiologic factors, e.g., endocrine imbalances.

785

ACTIONS/INTERVENTIONS	RATIONALE
Independent	
Acknowledge fear/anxieties. Validate observations with patient, e.g., "You seem to be afraid?"	Feelings are real, and it is helpful to bring them out in the open so they can be discussed and dealt with.
Assess degree/reality of threat to patient and level of anxiety (e.g., mild, moderate, severe) by observing behavior such as clenched hands, wide eyes, startle response, furrowed brow, clinging to family/staff, or physical/verbal lashing out.	Individual responses can vary according to culturally learned patterns. Distorted perceptions of the situation may magnify feelings.
Note narrowed focus of attention (e.g., patient concentrates on one thing at a time).	Narrowed focus usually reflects extreme fear/panic.
Observe speech content and patterns: rapidity/slowed, pressured, words used, repetition, laughter.	Provides clues about such factors as the level of anxiety, ability to comprehend, brain damage, or possible language differences.
Assess severity of pain when present. Delay gathering of information if pain is severe.	Severe pain and anxiety leave little energy for thinking and other activities.
Identify patient's/SO's perception(s) of the situation.	Regardless of the reality of the situation, perception affects how each individual deals with the illness/stress.
Acknowledge reality of the situation as the patient sees it, without challenging the belief.	Patient may need to deny reality until ready to deal with it. It is not helpful to force the patient to face facts.
Evaluate coping/defense mechanisms being used to deal with the perceived or real threat.	May be dealing well with the situation at the moment; e.g., denial and regression may be helpful coping mechanisms for a time. However, use of such mechanisms diverts energy the patient needs for healing, and problems need to be dealt with at some point in time.
Review coping mechanisms used in the past, e.g., problem-solving skills, recognizing/asking for help.	Provides opportunity to build on resources the patient/SO may have used successfully.
Assist patient to use anxiety for coping with the situation when possible.	Moderate anxiety heightens awareness and can help the patient to focus on dealing with problems.
Maintain frequent contact with the patient/SO. Be available for listening and talking as needed.	Establishes rapport, promotes expression of feelings, and helps patient and SO look at realities of the illness/treatment without confronting issues they are not ready to deal with.
Acknowledge feelings as expressed (e.g., use of Active-listen, reflection). If actions are unacceptable, take necessary steps to control/deal with behavior. (Refer to ND: Violence, risk for, directed at self/others, p 798.)	Often acknowledging feelings will enable patient to deal more appropriately with situation. May need chemical/physical control for brief periods.
Identify ways in which patient can get help when needed.	Provides assurance that staff/resources are available for assistance/support.

ACTIONS/INTERVENTIONS	RATIONALE
Independent	
Stay with or arrange to have someone stay with patient as indicated.	Continuous support may help patient regain internal locus of control and reduce anxiety/fear to a manageable level.
Provide accurate information as appropriate and when requested by the patient/SO. Answer questions freely and honestly and in language that is understandable by all. Repeat information as necessary; correct misconceptions.	Complex and/or anxiety-provoking information can be given in manageable amounts over an extended period. As opportunities arise and facts are given, individuals will accept what they are ready for. *Note:* Words/phrases may have different meanings for each individual; therefore, clarification is necessary to ensure understanding.
Avoid empty reassurances, with statements of "everything will be all right." Instead, provide specific information: e.g., "Your heart rate is regular, your pain is being easily controlled, and that is what we want," or "Your CD$_4$ count has been stable for the last 3 visits."	It is not possible for the nurse to know how the specific situation will be resolved, and false reassurances may be interpreted as lack of understanding or honesty, further isolating the patient. Sharing observations used in assessing condition/prognosis provides opportunity for patient/SO to feel reassured.
Note expressions of concern/anger about treatment or staff.	Anxiety about self and outcome may be masked by comments or angry outbursts directed at therapy/caregivers.
Ask the patient/SO to identify what he or she can/cannot do about what is happening.	Assists in identifying areas in which control can be exercised as well as those in which control is not possible.
Provide as much order and predictability as possible in scheduling care/activities, visitors.	Helps patient anticipate and prepare for difficult treatments/movements as well as look forward to pleasant occurrences.
Instruct in ways to use positive self-talk, e.g., "I can manage this pain for now," or "My cancer is shrinking."	Internal dialogue is often negative. When this is shared out loud, the patient becomes aware and can be directed in the use of positive self-talk, which can help reduce anxiety.
Encourage patient to develop exercise/activity program.	Helpful in reducing level of anxiety; has been shown to raise endorphin levels to enhance sense of well-being.
Encourage/instruct in mental imagery/relaxation methods; e.g., imaging a pleasant place, use of music/tapes, slow breathing, and meditation.	Promotes release of endorphins and aids in developing internal locus of control, reducing anxiety. May enhance coping skills, allowing body to go about its work of healing.
Provide touch, Therapeutic Touch, massage, and other adjunctive therapies as indicated.	Aids in meeting basic human need, decreasing sense of isolation, and assisting the patient to feel less anxious. *Note:* Therapeutic Touch is a method of using the hands to correct energy field disturbances by redirecting human energies to help or to heal.

787

ACTIONS/INTERVENTIONS

Collaborative

Administer medications as needed: e.g., diazepam (Valium), clorazepate (Tranxene), chlordiazepoxide (Librium), alprazolam (Xanax), buspirone (BuSpar), oxazepam (Serax), lorazepam (Ativan), doxepin (Sinequan), fluoxetine (Prozac), sertraline (Zoloft).

RATIONALE

Antianxiety agents may be useful for brief periods to assist the patient/SO to reduce anxiety to manageable levels, providing opportunity for initiation of patient's own coping skills.

NURSING DIAGNOSIS: Grieving [specify]

May be related to
Actual or perceived loss; chronic and/or fatal illness
Thwarted grieving response to a loss; lack of resolution of previous grieving response/
    absence of anticipatory grieving

Possibly evidenced by
Verbal expression of distress/unresolved issues, difficulty in expressing loss
Denial of loss
Altered eating habits, sleep/dream patterns, activity levels, libido
Crying; labile affect; feelings of sorrow, guilt, anger
Alterations in concentration and/or pursuit of tasks, developmental regression

DESIRED OUTCOMES/EVALUATION CRITERIA—PATIENT WILL:
Identify and express feelings freely/effectively.
Verbalize a sense of progress toward resolution of the grief and hope for the future.
Function at an adequate level, participate in work and ADLs.

ACTIONS/INTERVENTIONS

Independent

Provide open environment in which the patient feels free to realistically discuss feelings and concerns.

Determine patient perception and meaning of loss (current and past). Note cultural factors/expectations.

Identify stage of grieving and effect on function:

Denial: Be aware of avoidance behaviors; anger, withdrawal, and so forth. Allow patient to talk about what he or she chooses, and do not try to force patient to "face the facts";

RATIONALE

Therapeutic communication skills such as Active-listening, silence, being available, and acceptance can allow the patient the opportunity to talk freely and deal with the perceived/actual loss.

May affect patient's responses and need to be acknowledged in planning care.

Awareness allows for appropriate choice of interventions, as individuals handle grief in many different ways.

Denying the reality of diagnosis and/or prognosis is an important phase in which the patient protects self from the pain and reality of the threat of loss. Each person does this in an individual manner based on previous experiences with loss and cultural/religious factors.

ACTIONS/INTERVENTIONS	RATIONALE

Independent

Anger: Note behaviors of withdrawal, lack of cooperation, and direct expression of anger. Be alert to body language and check meaning with the patient, noting congruency with verbalizations. Encourage/allow verbalization of anger with acknowledgment of feelings and setting of limits regarding destructive behavior;

Denial gives way to feelings of anger, rage, guilt, and resentment. Patient may find it difficult to express anger directly and may feel guilty about normal feelings of anger. Although staff may have difficulty dealing with angry behaviors, acceptance allows patient to work through the anger and move on to more effective coping behaviors.

Bargaining: Be aware of statements such as "... if I do this, that will fix my problem." Allow verbalization without confrontation about realities;

Bargaining with care providers or God often occurs and may be helpful in beginning resolution and acceptance. Patient may be working through feelings of guilt about things done or undone.

Depression: Give patient permission to be where he or she is. Provide hope within parameters of individual situation without giving false reassurance. Provide comfort and availability as well as caring for physical needs;

When patient can no longer deny the reality of the loss, feelings of helplessness and hopelessness replace feelings of anger. The patient needs information that this is a normal progression of feelings.

Acceptance: Respect the patient's needs and wishes for quiet, privacy, and/or talking.

Having worked through the denial, anger, and depression, patient often prefers to be alone and does not want to talk much. Patient may still cling to hope, which can be sustaining through whatever is happening at this point.

Active-listen patient's concerns and be available for help as necessary.

The process of grieving does not proceed in an orderly fashion, but fluctuates with various aspects of all stages present at one time or another. If process is dysfunctional or prolonged, more aggressive interventions may be required to facilitate the process.

Determine quality of interactions with others, including family members.

Although periods of withdrawal/loneliness usually accompany grieving, evidence of persistent isolation may indicate deepening depression, necessitating further evaluation/intervention. *Note:* Family/SO may not be dysfunctional but may be intolerant of patient's behaviors.

Identify and problem-solve solutions to existing physical responses, e.g., eating, sleeping, activity levels, and sexual desire.

May need additional assistance to deal with the physical aspects of grieving.

Assess needs of SO and assist as indicated.

Identification of problems indicating dysfunctional grieving allows for individual interventions.

Include family/SO as appropriate when determining future needs.

Depending on patient desires/legal requirements, choices regarding future plans (e.g., living situation, continuation of care, end-of-life decisions, funeral arrangements) can provide guidance and peace of mind.

Discuss healthy ways of dealing with difficult situation.

Provides opportunity to look toward the future and plan family/SO needs (e.g., for life after loss).

789

ACTIONS/INTERVENTIONS	RATIONALE
Collaborative	
Refer to other resources, e.g., support groups, counseling, spiritual/pastoral care, psychotherapy as indicated.	May need additional help to resolve grief, make plans, and look toward the future.

NURSING DIAGNOSIS: Self Esteem, situational low

May be related to

Biophysical, psychosocial, cognitive, perceptual, cultural, and/or spiritual crisis, e.g., changes in health status/body image, role performance, personal identity; loss of control of some aspect of life

Maturational transitions

Perceived/anticipated failure at life event(s)

Possibly evidenced by

Negating self-appraisal in response to life events

Verbalization of negative feelings about the self (helplessness, uselessness); focus on past abilities, strengths, function or appearance; preoccupation with change/loss

Evaluates self as unable to handle situations/events

Fear of rejection/reaction by others

Difficulty making decisions

DESIRED OUTCOMES/EVALUATION CRITERIA—PATIENT WILL:

Verbalize realistic view and acceptance of self in situation.

Identify existing strengths and view self as capable person.

Recognize and incorporate change into self-concept in accurate manner without negating self-esteem.

Demonstrate adaptation to changes/events that have occurred as evidenced by setting of realistic goals and active participation in work/play/personal relationships.

ACTIONS/INTERVENTIONS	RATIONALE
Independent	
Ask what the patient would like to be called.	Shows courtesy/respect and acknowledges person.
Identify SO from whom the patient derives comfort and who should be notified in case of emergency.	Allows provisions to be made for specific person(s) to visit or remain close and provide needed support for patient. *Note:* May or may not be legal next of kin.
Identify basic sense of self-esteem, image patient has of existential, physical, psychologic self. Identify locus of control.	Helpful for determining needs and treatment plan. May provide insight into whether this is a single episode or recurrent/chronic situation.
Determine patient perception of threat to self.	Patient's perception is more important than what is really happening and needs to be dealt with before reality can be addressed.
Active-listen patient concerns and fears.	Conveys sense of caring and can more effectively identify the needs and problems as well as patient's coping strategies and how effective they are. Provides opportunity to duplicate and begin a problem-solving process.

ACTIONS/INTERVENTIONS	RATIONALE

Independent

Encourage verbalization of feelings, accepting what is said.

Helps patient/SO begin to adapt to change and reduces anxiety about altered function/lifestyle.

Discuss stages of grief and the importance of grief work. (Refer to ND: Grieving [specify], p 788.)

Grieving is a necessary step for integration of change/loss into self-concept.

Provide nonthreatening environment.

Promotes feelings of safety, encouraging verbalization.

Observe nonverbal communication, e.g., body posture and movements, eye contact, gestures, use of touch.

Nonverbal language is a large portion of communication and therefore is extremely important. How the person uses touch provides information about how it is accepted and how comfortable the individual is with being touched.

Reflect back to the patient what has been said, for clarification and verification.

Information must be validated by the patient, as assumptions may be inaccurate.

Observe and describe behavior in objective terms.

All behavior has meaning, some of which is obvious and some of which needs to be identified. This is a process of educated guesswork and needs to be validated by the patient.

Identify age and developmental level.

Age is an indicator of the stage of life patient is experiencing, e.g., adolescence, middle age. However, developmental level may be more important than chronologic age in anticipating and identifying some of patient's needs. Some degree of regression occurs during illness, dependent on many factors such as the normal coping skills of the individual and the severity of the illness.

Discuss patient's view of body image and how illness/condition might affect it.

The patient's perception of a change in body image may occur suddenly or over time (e.g., actual loss of a body part through injury/surgery or a perceived loss; heart attack) or be a continuous subtle process (e.g., chronic illness, eating disorders, or aging). Awareness can alert the nurse to the need for appropriate interventions tailored to the individual need.

Encourage discussion of physical changes in a simple, direct, and factual manner. Give realistic feedback and discuss future options, e.g., rehabilitation services.

Provides opportunity to begin incorporating actual changes in an accepting and hopeful atmosphere.

Acknowledge efforts at problem solving, resolution of current situation, and future planning.

Provides encouragement and reinforces continuation of desired behaviors.

Recognize patient's pace for adaptation to demands of current situation.

Failure to acknowledge patient's need to take time and/or pressuring patient to ''get on with it'' conveys a lack of acceptance of the person as an individual and may result in feelings of lowered self-esteem.

Introduce tasks at patient's level of functioning, progressing to more complex activities as tolerated.

Provides for success experiences, reaffirming capabilities and enhancing self-esteem.

Ascertain how the patient sees own role within the family system, e.g., breadwinner, homemaker, husband/wife.

Illness may create a temporary or permanent problem in role expectations. Sexual role and how the patient views self in relation to the current illness also play important parts in recovery.

791

ACTIONS/INTERVENTIONS	RATIONALE
Independent	
Assist patient/SO with clarifying expected roles and those that may need to be relinquished or altered.	Provides opportunity to identify misconceptions and begin to look at options; promotes reality orientation.
Determine patient awareness of own responsibility for dealing with situation, personal growth, and so forth.	Conveys confidence in patient's ability to cope. When patient acknowledges own part in planning and carrying out treatment plan, he or she has more investment in following through on decisions that have been made.
Assess impact of illness/surgery on sexuality.	Sexuality encompasses the whole person in the total environment. Many times problems of illness are superimposed on already existing problems of sexuality and can affect patient's sense of self-worth. Some problems are more obvious than others, such as illness involving the reproductive parts of the body. Others are less obvious, such as sexual values, role in family, e.g., mother, wage earner, single parent, and so on.
Be alert to comments and innuendos, which may mean the patient has a concern in the area of sexuality.	People are often reluctant and/or embarrassed to ask direct questions about sexual/sexuality concerns.
Be aware of caregiver's feelings about dealing with the subject of sexuality.	Nurses/caregivers are often as reluctant and embarrassed in dealing with sexuality issues as most patients.
Provide information and referral to hospital and community resources.	Enables patient/SO to be in contact with interested groups with access to assistive and supportive devices, services and counseling.
Collaborative	
Support participation in group/community activities, e.g., assertiveness classes, volunteer work, support groups.	Promotes skills of coping and sense of self-worth.
Refer to psychiatric support/therapy group, social services, as indicated.	May be needed to assist patient/SO to achieve optimal recovery.
Refer to appropriate resources for sex therapy as need indicates.	May be someone with comfort level and knowledge who is available, or may be necessary to refer to professional resources for additional help and support.

NURSING DIAGNOSIS: Coping, Individual, ineffective/Decisional Conflict

May be related to

Situational crises/personal vulnerability; multiple life changes/maturational crises, age/developmental stage

Inadequate coping methods, support systems

No vacations/inadequate relaxation

Impairment of nervous system; memory loss; impaired adaptive behaviors and problem-solving skills

Severe pain/overwhelming threat to self

Unclear personal values/beliefs; perceived threat to value system; lack of experience/interference with decision making; lack of information

ACTIONS/INTERVENTIONS	RATIONALE
Independent	
Review pathophysiology affecting the patient and extent of feelings of hopelessness/helplessness/loss of control over life, level of anxiety; perception of situation.	Indicators of degree of disequilibrium and need for intervention to prevent or resolve the crisis. *Note:* Impairment of normal functioning for more than 2 weeks, especially in presence of chronic condition, may reflect depression, requiring further evaluation. Studies suggest that up to 85% of all physically ill people are depressed to some degree.
Establish therapeutic nurse-patient relationship.	Patient may feel freer in the context of this relationship to verbalize feelings of helplessness/powerlessness and to discuss changes that may be necessary in the patient's life.
Note expressions of indecision, dependence on others, and inability to manage own ADLs.	May indicate need to lean on others for a time. Early recognition and intervention can help patient regain equilibrium.
Assess presence of positive coping skills/inner strengths, e.g., use of relaxation techniques, willingness to express feelings, use of support systems.	When the individual has coping skills that have been successful in the past, they may be used in the current situation to relieve tension and preserve the individual's sense of control. However, limitations of condition may impact choices available to patient; e.g., playing musical instrument to relieve stress may not be possible for individual with tremors or hemiparesis.
Encourage patient to talk about what is happening at this time and what has occurred to precipitate feelings of helplessness and anxiety.	Provides clues to assist patient to develop coping skills and regain equilibrium.
Evaluate ability to understand events. Correct misperceptions, provide factual information.	Assists in identification and correction of perception of reality and enables problem solving to begin.

793

ACTIONS/INTERVENTIONS	RATIONALE

Independent

Provide quiet, nonstimulating environment. Determine what patient needs, and provide if possible. Give simple, factual information about what patient can expect and repeat as necessary.	Decreases anxiety and provides control for the patient during crisis situation.
Allow patient to be dependent in the beginning, with gradual resumption of independence in ADLs, self-care, and other activities. Make opportunities for patient to make simple decisions about care/other activities when possible, accepting choice not to do so.	Promotes feelings of security (patient will know nurse will provide safety). As control is regained, patient has the opportunity to develop adaptive coping/problem-solving skills.
Accept verbal expressions of anger, setting limits on maladaptive behavior.	Verbalizing angry feelings is an important process for resolution of grief and loss. However, preventing destructive actions (such as striking out at others) preserves patient's self-esteem.
Discuss feelings of self-blame/projection of blame on others.	While these mechanisms may be protective at the moment of crisis, they are counterproductive and intensify feelings of helplessness and hopelessness.
Note expressions of inability to find meaning in life/reason for living, feelings of futility or alienation from God.	Crisis situation may evoke questioning of spiritual beliefs, affecting ability to cope with current situation and plan for the future.
Promote safe and hopeful environment, as needed. Identify positive aspects of this experience and assist patient to view it as a learning opportunity.	May be helpful while patient regains inner control.
Problem-solve solutions for current situation. Provide information/support and reinforce reality as patient begins to ask questions; look at what is happening.	Helping patient/SO to brainstorm possible solutions (giving consideration to the pros and cons of each) promotes feelings of self-control/esteem.
Provide for gradual implementation and continuation of necessary behavior/lifestyle changes. Reinforce positive adaptation/new coping behaviors.	Reduces anxiety of sudden change and allows for developing new and creative solutions.

Collaborative

Refer to other resources as necessary (e.g., clergy, psychiatric clinical nurse specialist/psychiatrist, family/marital therapist, addiction support groups).	Additional assistance may be needed to help patient resolve problems/make decisions.

NURSING DIAGNOSIS: Family Coping: ineffective, compromised or disabling/Caregiver Role Strain, risk for

May be related to

Inadequate or incorrect information or understanding by a primary person; unrealistic expectations

Temporary preoccupation by significant person who is trying to manage emotional conflicts and personal suffering and is unable to perceive or to act effectively with regard to patient's needs; does not have enough resources to provide the care needed

Temporary family disorganization and role changes; feel that caregiving interferes with other important roles in their lives

Patient providing little support in turn for the primary person

Prolonged disease/disability progression that exhausts the supportive capacity of significant persons

Significant person with chronically unexpressed feelings of guilt, anxiety, hostility, despair

Highly ambivalent family relationships; feel stress or nervousness in their relationship with the care receiver

Possibly evidenced by

Patient expressing/confirming a concern or complaint about SO's response to patient's health problem, despair about family reactions/lack of involvement; history of poor relationship between caregiver and care receiver

Neglectful relationships with other family members

SO describing preoccupation about personal reactions; displaying intolerance, abandonment, rejection; caregiver not developmentally ready for caregiver role

SO attempting assistive/supportive behaviors with less than satisfactory results; withdrawing or entering into limited or temporary personal communication with patient; displaying protective behavior disproportionate (too little or too much) to patient's abilities or need for autonomy

DESIRED OUTCOMES/EVALUATION CRITERIA—FAMILY/CAREGIVER WILL:

Identify resources within themselves to deal with situation.

Provide opportunity for patient to deal with situation in own way.

Express more realistic understanding and expectations of the patient; visit regularly and participate positively in care of patient, within limits of abilities.

ACTIONS/INTERVENTIONS	RATIONALE
Independent	
Assess level of anxiety present in family/SO.	Anxiety level needs to be dealt with before problem solving can begin. Individuals may be so preoccupied with own reactions to situation that they are unable to respond to another's needs.
Establish rapport and acknowledge difficulty of the situation for the family.	May assist SO to accept what is happening and be willing to share problems with staff.
Assess pre-illness/current behaviors that are interfering with the care/recovery of the patient.	Information about family problems (e.g., divorce/separation, alcoholism, drug abuse, abusive situation) will be helpful in developing an appropriate plan of care.
Discuss underlying reasons for patient behaviors with family.	When family members know why patient is behaving in different ways, it helps them to understand and accept/deal with unusual behaviors.
Assist family/patient to understand "who owns the problem" and who is responsible for resolution. Avoid placing blame or guilt.	When these boundaries are defined, each individual can begin to take care of own self and stop taking care of others in inappropriate ways.
Determine current knowledge/perception of the situation.	Provides information on which to begin planning care and make informed decisions. Lack of information or unrealistic perceptions can interfere with caregiver's/care receiver's response to illness situation.
Assess current actions of SO and how they are received by patient.	SO may be trying to be helpful but is not perceived as helpful by the patient. SO may be withdrawn or may be too protective.
Involve SO in information giving, problem solving, and care of patient as feasible. Identify other ways of demonstrating support while maintaining patient's independence.	Information can reduce feelings of helplessness and uselessness. Involvement in care enhances feelings of control and self-worth.

795

ACTIONS/INTERVENTIONS	RATIONALE
Independent	
Reframe negative expressions into positives whenever possible.	Promotes more hopeful attitude and helps family/patient look toward the future.
Collaborative	
Refer to appropriate resources for assistance as indicated (e.g., counseling, psychotherapy, financial, spiritual).	May need additional assistance in resolving family issues.

NURSING DIAGNOSIS: Family Coping: potential for growth

May be related to

Basic needs sufficiently gratified and adaptive tasks effectively addressed to enable goals of self-actualization to surface

Willingness to deal with one's own needs and to begin to problem-solve with the patient

Possibly evidenced by

Family member attempting to describe growth impact of crisis on his/her own values, priorities, goals, or relationships

Family member moving in direction of health-promoting and enriching lifestyle and generally choosing experiences that optimize wellness

DESIRED OUTCOMES/EVALUATION CRITERIA—FAMILY WILL:

Express willingness to look at own role in family's growth.

Undertake tasks leading to change.

Verbalize feelings of self-confidence and satisfaction with progress being made.

ACTIONS/INTERVENTIONS	RATIONALE
Independent	
Provide opportunities for family to talk with patient and/or staff.	Reduces anxiety and allows expression of what has been learned and how they are managing, as well as opportunity to make plans for the future and share support.
Listen to family's expressions of hope, planning, effect on relationships/life, change of values.	Provides clues to avenues to explore for assistance with growth.
Provide opportunities for and instruction in how SOs can care for patient. Discuss ways in which they can support patient in meeting own needs.	Enhances feelings of control and involvement in situation in which SOs cannot do many things. Also provides opportunity to learn how to be most helpful when patient is discharged.
Provide a role model with which family may identify.	Having a positive example can help with adoption of new behaviors to promote growth.
Discuss importance of open communication. Role play effective communication skills of Active-listening, "I-messages," and problem solving.	Helps individuals to express needs and wants in ways that will develop family cohesiveness. Promotes solutions in which everyone wins.
Encourage family to learn new and effective ways of dealing with feelings.	Effective recognition and expression of feelings clarify situation for involved individuals.
Encourage seeking help appropriately. Give information about persons and agencies available to them.	Permission to seek help as needed allows them to choose to take advantage of what is available.

ACTIONS/INTERVENTIONS

Collaborative

Refer to specific support group(s) as indicated.

RATIONALE

Provides opportunities for sharing experiences; provides mutual support and practical problem solving; and can aid in decreasing alienation and helplessness.

NURSING DIAGNOSIS: Therapeutic Regimen: Individual, risk for ineffective management

Risk factors may include
Complexity of therapeutic regimen
Decisional conflict: Patient value system, health beliefs, spiritual values, cultural influences
Perceived barriers; economic difficulties; side effects of therapy

Possibly evidenced by
[Not applicable; presence of signs and symptoms establishes an *actual* diagnosis]

DESIRED OUTCOMES/EVALUATION CRITERIA—PATIENT WILL:
Participate in the development of goals and treatment plan.
Verbalize accurate knowledge of disease and understanding of treatment regimen.
Demonstrate behaviors/changes in lifestyle necessary to maintain therapeutic regimen.
Identify/use available resources.

ACTIONS/INTERVENTIONS

Independent

Review patient's/SO's knowledge and understanding of the need for treatment/medication as well as consequences of actions and choices. Note ability to comprehend information, including literacy, level of education, primary language.

Be aware of developmental and chronological age.

Determine cultural, spiritual, and health beliefs.

Note length of illness/prognosis.

Assess availability/use of support systems. Identify additional resources as appropriate.

Review treatment plan with patient/SO.

RATIONALE

Provides opportunities to clarify viewpoints/misconceptions. Verifies that patient/SO has accurate/factual information with which to make informed choices.

Impacts ability to understand own needs/incorporate into treatment regimen.

Provides insight into thoughts/factors related to individual situation. Beliefs will affect patient's perception of situation and participation in treatment regimen. Treatment may be incongruent with patient's social/cultural lifestyle and perceived role/responsibilities.

Patients tend to become passive and dependent in long-term, debilitating illness.

Access to/proper use of helpful resources can assist patient in meeting treatment goals and provide purpose for living. Presence of caring, empathic family/SO(s) can help patient in process of recovery.

Provides opportunities to exchange accurate information and to clarify viewpoints/misconceptions.

797

ACTIONS/INTERVENTIONS	RATIONALE

Independent

Establish graduated goals or modified regimen as necessary; work out alternate solutions.	Promotes patient involvement/independence; provides opportunity for compromise, and may enhance cooperation with regimen. When patient participates in setting goals, there is a sense of investment that encourages cooperation and willingness to follow through with the program.
Contract with the patient for participation in care.	Patient who agrees to own responsibility is more apt to cooperate.
Determine potential problems that may/do interfere with treatment. Assess level of anxiety, locus of control, sense of powerlessness, and so forth.	Many factors may be involved in behavior that is disruptive to the treatment regimen (e.g., fear, denial, pain, anxiety, hypoxemia, chemical imbalance).
Accept the patient's choice/point of view, even it if appears to be self-destructive, e.g., decision to continue smoking.	Patient has the right to make own decisions, and acceptance may give a sense of control, which can help the patient look more clearly at consequences. Confrontation is not beneficial and may actually be detrimental to future cooperation and goal achievement.
Develop a system for self-monitoring. Share data pertinent to patient's condition, e.g., laboratory results, BP readings.	Provides a sense of control, enables patient to follow own progress and make informed choices.
Have same personnel care for patient as much as possible.	Enables relationship to develop in which the patient can begin to trust/participate in care.
Be aware of own/caregiver's response to patient's treatment choices (e.g., refusal of blood or chemotherapy, living will).	Negative feelings regarding these choices may create power struggles and be expressed in judgmental behaviors that block or interfere with patient's wishes, comfort, and/or care.
Listen to/Active-listen patient's reports and comments.	Conveys message of concern, belief in individual's capabilities to resolve situation in positive manner.

NURSING DIAGNOSIS: Violence, risk for, directed at self/others

Risk factors may include
Attempt to deal with the threat to self-concept that illness can represent
Antisocial character; catatonic/manic excitement; panic states; rage reactions
Suicidal ideation/behavior, depression
Hormonal imbalance; temporal lobe epilepsy; toxic reactions to medication
Negative role modeling; developmental crisis

[Possible indicators]
Suspicion of others, paranoid ideation, delusions, hallucinations
Expressed intent or desire to harm self/others (directly or indirectly); hostile verbalizations; plan and possession of/access to destructive means
Body language: Rigid posture, clenched fists, facial expressions
Increased motor activity, excitement, irritability, agitation
Overt and aggressive acts; self-destructive behavior
Substance abuse/withdrawal

DESIRED OUTCOMES/EVALUATION CRITERIA—PATIENT WILL:
Acknowledge realities of the situation.
Verbalize understanding of reason(s) for behavior/precipitating factors.
Express increased self-concept
Demonstrate self-control, as evidenced by relaxed posture, nonviolent behavior.

ACTIONS/INTERVENTIONS	RATIONALE
Independent	
Observe for early signs of distress.	Irritability, pacing, shouting/cursing, lack of cooperation and demanding behavior may all be signs of increasing anxiety.
Maintain straightforward communication and assist patient to learn assertive rather than manipulative, nonassertive/aggressive behavior.	Avoids reinforcing manipulative behavior and enhances positive interactions with others, accomplishing the goal of getting needs met in acceptable ways.
Help patient identify more adequate solutions/behaviors (e.g., motor activities/exercise). Provide directions for actions patient can take.	Promotes release of energies in acceptable ways.
Give as much autonomy as is possible in the situation.	Enhances feelings of power and control in a situation in which many things are not within individual's control.
Provide protection within the environment, e.g., constant observation, removal of objects that might be used to harm self/others.	May need more structure to maintain control until own internal locus of control is regained.
Give permission to express angry feelings in acceptable ways. Make time to listen to verbalization of these feelings.	Encouraging acceptable expression can be helpful in defusing feelings of helplessness and anger, as well as decreasing guilt.
Accept patient's anger without reacting on an emotional basis.	Responding with anger is not helpful in resolving the situation and may result in escalating patient's behavior.
Remain calm and state limits on behavior in a firm manner. Be truthful and nonjudgmental.	Understanding that helplessness and fear underlie this behavior can be helpful.
Assume that the patient has control and is responsible for own behavior.	Often enables the individual to exercise control. *Note:* When violent behavior is the result of drugs, patient may not be able to respond appropriately.
Identify conditions that may interfere with ability to control own behavior.	Acute or chronic brain syndrome, drug-induced or postsurgical confusion may precipitate violent behavior that is difficult to control.
Tell patient to "stop."	May be sufficient to help patient control own actions if exhibiting hostile actions. *Note:* Patient is often afraid of own actions and wants staff to set limits.
Use an organized team approach when necessary to subdue patient with force. Tell patient clearly and concisely what is happening.	Knowing and practicing these actions before they are needed helps to prevent untoward problems. Keeping patient informed can help patient to regain internal control.
Hold patient; place in restraints or seclusion if necessary. Do so in a calm, positive, nonstimulating/nonpunitive manner.	As a last resort, physical restraint may be necessary while the patient regains control. *Note:* These measures are meant to protect the patient, not punish the behavior.
Apply and adjust restraint devices properly.	It is important to maintain body alignment and patient comfort.
Document precise reason for restraints, actions taken. Check restraints frequently per facility protocol, each time documenting the condition and how long the restraints are used.	Restraints are to be used for very specific reasons, which need to be clearly documented to avoid overuse or misuse.

Independent

Monitor for suicidal/homicidal intent, e.g., morbid or anxious feelings while with the patient; warning from the patient, "It doesn't matter, I'd be better off dead"; mood swings, putting affairs in order, previous suicide attempt.

Indicators of need for further assessment, evaluation, and intervention/psychiatric care.

Assess suicidal intent (1–10 scale) by asking directly if patient is thinking of killing self, has plan, means, and so on.

Provides guidelines for necessity/urgency of interventions. Direct questioning is most helpful when done in a caring, concerned manner.

Acknowledge reality of suicide/homicide as an option. Discuss consequences of actions if patient were to follow through on intent. Ask how it will help patient to resolve problems.

Patient is often focused on suicide (or homicide) as the "only" option and this response provides an opening to look at and discuss other options. (*Note:* Be aware of own responsibility under Tarasoff rule when patient is expressing homicidal ideation).

Collaborative

Refer to psychiatric resource(s), e.g., clinical specialist psychiatric nurse, psychiatrist, psychologist, social worker.

More in-depth assistance may be needed to deal with patient and defuse situation.

Administer medications, e.g., antianxiety/antipsychotic agents, sedatives, narcotics.

May be indicated to quiet/control behavior. *Note:* May need to be withheld if they are suspected to be the cause of/contribute to the behavior.

NURSING DIAGNOSIS: Post-trauma Response

May be related to
Disasters (e.g., floods, earthquakes, tornadoes, airplane crashes); wars, epidemics, rape, incest, assault, torture, catastrophic illness or accident, being held hostage

Possibly evidenced by
Reexperiencing traumatic event (may be identified in cognitive, affective, and/or sensory-motor activities, e.g., flashbacks, intrusive thoughts, repetitive dreams or nightmares, excessive verbalization of the traumatic event, verbalization of survival guilt or guilt about behavior required for survival)
Altered lifestyle (self-destructiveness); loss of interest in usual activities; loss of feeling of intimacy/sexuality; development of phobia; poor impulse control/irritability and explosiveness
Disturbance of mood, e.g., depression, anxiety, embarrassment, fear, self-blame, low self-esteem
Cognitive disruption: Confusion, loss of memory/concentration, indecisiveness

DESIRED OUTCOMES/EVALUATION CRITERIA—PATIENT WILL:
Verbalize reduced anxiety/fear.
Demonstrate ability to deal with emotional reactions in an individually appropriate manner.
Express own feelings/reactions; avoid projection.
Demonstrate appropriate changes in lifestyle/getting support from SO as needed.
Participate in plans for follow-up care/counseling.

ACTIONS/INTERVENTIONS	RATIONALE
Independent	
Determine when traumatic event(s) occurred: present or past.	Manifestations of acute and chronic posttrauma responses may require different interventions. *Note:* Event may encompass many forms of trauma, including the diagnosis of life-threatening illness.
Assess physical trauma if present, as well as individual reaction to occurrence, e.g., physical symptoms such as numbness, headache, tightness in chest, and psychologic responses of anger, shock, acute anxiety, confusion, denial.	Provides information on which to develop plan of care, make informed choices.
Evaluate behavior (e.g., calm or agitated, excited/hysterical; inappropriate laughter, crying), expressions of disbelief and/or self-blame.	Indicators of extent of individual response to traumatic incident and degree of disorganization.
Note ethnic background/cultural and religious perceptions and beliefs about the event.	May influence patient's response to what has happened, e.g., may believe it is retribution from God.
Assess signs/stage of grieving.	Patient may be suffering from sense of loss of self and/or others.
Tell patient that painful emotional reactions are normal. Phrase this information in neutral terms: "You may or may not experience. . . ."	Understanding that experiencing these uncomfortable feelings is not unusual after traumatic event may reduce patient's anxiety/fear of "going crazy" and enhance coping.
Discuss things patient can do to feel better, e.g., physical exercise alternated with relaxation; keeping busy with normal activities; talking to others; acknowledging that it is all right to feel upset; writing about the experience in a journal; being kind to yourself.	Enhances sense of control and helps patient achieve resolution of uncomfortable feelings. Often when the patient begins these activities within the first 24 hours of the event, further therapy may not be required.
Assist with learning stress management techniques.	Promotes sense of control and ability to handle existing problems.
Identify supportive persons for patient.	Having positive support systems can help patient reach optimal recovery.
Note signs of severe/prolonged depression; frequency of flashbacks/nightmares; presence of chronic pain, somatic complaints.	If patient did not deal with trauma when it occurred, behavioral manifestations may reveal extent of problem in the present.
Help patient to identify factors that may have created a vulnerable situation/increased likelihood for event.	Even though individual may not be responsible for what has happened, he/she may have created an atmosphere in which negative things occurred. Changes in behaviors/lifestyle may decrease potential for recurrence.
Collaborative	
Refer to support groups, counselors/therapists for further therapy, e.g., psychotherapy (in conjunction with medications); implosive therapy, flooding, hypnosis, eye movement desensitization and reprocessing (EMDR), Rolfing, memory work, or cognitive restructuring as indicated.	When posttrauma response has become chronic, patient may need more in-depth assistance from sensitive, trained individuals who are skilled in dealing with these problems.

POTENTIAL CONSIDERATIONS
Refer to primary diagnosis for postdischarge concerns.

801

SURGICAL INTERVENTION

Surgery may be needed to diagnose or cure a specific disease process, correct a structural deformity, restore a functional process, or reduce level of dysfunction/pain. Although surgery is generally elective or preplanned, potentially life-threatening conditions can arise, requiring emergency intervention. Absence or limitation of preoperative preparation and teaching increases the need for postoperative support in addition to managing underlying medical conditions.

CARE SETTING

May be inpatient on a surgical unit or outpatient/short-stay in an ambulatory surgical setting.

RELATED CONCERNS

Alcoholism [Acute]: Intoxication/Overdose, p 847
Cancer, p 875
Diabetes Mellitus/Diabetic Ketoacidosis, p 422
Fluid and Electrolyte Imbalances, p 899
Hemothorax/Pneumothorax, p 154
Metabolic Acidosis (Primary Base Carbon Deficit), p 506
Metabolic Alkalosis (Primary Base Carbon Excess), p 510
Peritonitis, p 366
Pneumonia, Microbial, p 130
Psychosocial Aspects of Care, p 783
Respiratory Acidosis (Primary Carbonic Acid Excess), p 200
Respiratory Alkalosis (Primary Carbonic Acid Deficit), p 204
Sepsis/Septicemia, p 719
Thrombophlebitis: Deep Vein Thrombosis, p 107
Total Nutritional Support: Parenteral/Enteral Feeding, p 491

Also refer to plan of care for specific surgical procedure performed.

Patient Assessment Data Base

Data is dependent on the duration/severity of underlying problem and involvement of other body systems. Refer to specific plans of care for data and diagnostic studies relevant to the procedure and additional nursing diagnoses.

CIRCULATION

May report:	History of cardiac problems, HF, pulmonary edema, peripheral vascular disease, or vascular stasis (increases risk of thrombus formation)

EGO INTEGRITY

May report:	Feelings of anxiety, fear, anger, apathy Multiple stress factors, e.g., financial, relationship, lifestyle
May exhibit:	Restlessness, increased tension/irritability Sympathetic stimulation

ELIMINATION

May report:	History of kidney/bladder conditions; use of diuretics/laxatives

FOOD/FLUID

May report: Pancreatic insufficiency/DM (predisposing to hypoglycemia/ketoacidosis)
Use of diuretics

May exhibit: Malnutrition (including obesity)
Dry mucous membranes (limited intake/NPO period preoperatively)

RESPIRATION

May report: Infections, chronic conditions/cough, smoking

SAFETY

May report: Allergies or sensitivities to medications, food, tape, latex, and solution(s)
Immune deficiencies (increases risk of systemic infections and delayed healing)
Presence of cancer/recent cancer therapy
Family history of malignant hyperthermia/reaction to anesthesia, autoimmune diseases
History of hepatic disease (affects drug detoxification and may alter coagulation)
History of blood transfusion(s)/transfusion reaction

May exhibit: Presence of existing infectious process; fever

TEACHING/LEARNING

May report: Use of medications such as anticoagulants, steroids, antibiotics, antihypertensives, cardiotonic glycosides, antidysrhythmics, bronchodilators, diuretics, decongestants, analgesics, anti-inflammatories, anticonvulsants, or antipsychotics/antianxiety agents, as well as OTC or street drugs or drugs of abuse
Use of alcohol (risk of liver damage affecting coagulation and choice of anesthesia, as well as potential for postoperative withdrawal)

Discharge plan considerations: **DRG projected mean length of stay: 2.6 days for inpatient procedures, 2–36 hours for outpatient**
May require assistance with transportation, dressing(s)/supplies, self-care, and homemaker/maintenance tasks.
Possible placement in rehabilitation/long-term facility

Refer to section at end of plan for postdischarge considerations.

DIAGNOSTIC STUDIES

General preoperative requirements may include: Urinalysis, CBC, PT, aPTT, chest x-ray. Other studies are dependent on type of operative procedure, current medications, systemic processes, age, and weight, e.g., BUN, Cr, glucose, ABGs, electrolytes; liver function, thyroid, and nutritional studies. Deviations from normal should be corrected if possible prior to safe administration of anesthetic agents.

Urinalysis: Presence of WBCs or bacteria indicates infection.

Pregnancy test: Positive results affect timing of procedure and choice of pharmacologic agents.

CBC: WBC elevation is indicative of inflammatory process (may be diagnostic, e.g., appendicitis); decreased WBC count suggests viral processes (requiring evaluation because immune system may be dysfunctional). Low Hb suggests anemia/blood loss (impairs tissue oxygenation and reduces the Hb available to bind with inhalation anesthetics); may suggest need for cross-match/blood transfusion. Hct elevation may indicate dehydration; decreased Hct suggests fluid overload.

Electrolytes: Imbalances impair organ function, e.g., decreased potassium affects cardiac muscle contractility, leading to decreased cardiac output.

ABGs: Evaluates current respiratory status.

Coagulation times: May be prolonged, interfering with intraoperative/postoperative hemostasis.

Chest x-ray: Should be free of infiltrates, pneumonia; used for identification of masses and COPD.

ECG: Abnormal findings require attention prior to administering anesthetics.

NURSING PRIORITIES

1. Reduce anxiety and emotional trauma.
2. Provide for physical safety.
3. Prevent complications.
4. Alleviate pain.
5. Facilitate recovery process.
6. Provide information about disease process/surgical procedure, prognosis, and treatment needs.

DISCHARGE GOALS

1. Patient is dealing realistically with current situation.
2. Injury prevented.
3. Complications prevented/minimized.
4. Pain relieved/controlled.
5. Wound healing/organ function progressing toward normal.
6. Disease process/surgical procedure, prognosis, and therapeutic regimen understood.
7. Plan in place to meet needs after discharge.

PREOPERATIVE

NURSING DIAGNOSIS: Knowledge deficit [learning need] regarding condition, prognosis, treatment, self care and discharge needs

May be related to
Lack of exposure/recall, information misinterpretation
Unfamiliarity with information resources

Possibly evidenced by
Statement of the problem/concerns, misconceptions
Request for information
Inappropriate, exaggerated behaviors (e.g., agitated, apathetic, hostile)
Inaccurate follow-through of instructions/development of preventable complications

DESIRED OUTCOMES/EVALUATION CRITERIA—PATIENT WILL:
Verbalize understanding of disease process/perioperative process and postoperative expectations.
Correctly perform necessary procedures and explain reasons for the actions.
Initiate necessary lifestyle changes and participate in treatment regimen.

ACTIONS/INTERVENTIONS	RATIONALE
Independent	
Assess patient's level of understanding.	Facilitates planning of preoperative teaching program.
Review specific pathology and anticipated surgical procedure. Verify that appropriate consent has been signed.	Provides knowledge base on which patient can make informed therapy choices and consent for procedure, and presents opportunity to clarify misconceptions.
Use resource teaching materials, audiovisuals as available.	Specifically designed materials can facilitate the patient's learning.

ACTIONS/INTERVENTIONS   **RATIONALE**

Independent

Implement individualized preoperative teaching program:

Preoperative/postoperative procedures and expectations, urinary and bowel changes, dietary considerations, activity levels/transfers, respiratory/cardiovascular exercises; anticipated IV lines and tubes (e.g., NG tubes, drains, and catheters);

Enhances patient's understanding/control and can relieve stress related to the unknown/unexpected.

Preoperative instructions, e.g., NPO time, shower/skin preparation, which routine medications to take/hold;

Helps reduce the possibility of postoperative complications and promotes a rapid return to normal body function. *Note:* Frequently, liquids are allowed up to 2 hours before scheduled procedure.

Intraoperative patient safety, e.g., not crossing legs during procedures performed under local/light anesthesia;

Reduces risk of complications/untoward outcomes, such as injury to the peroneal and tibial nerves with postoperative pain in the calves and feet.

Expected/transient reactions (e.g., low backache, localized numbness and reddening or skin indentations);

Minor effects of immobilization/positioning should resolve in 24 hours. If they persist, medical evaluation is required.

Inform patient/SO about itinerary, physician/SO communications.

Logistical information about OR schedule and places (e.g., recovery room, postoperative room assignment) as well as where and when the surgeon will communicate with SO relieves stress and miscommunications, preventing confusion and doubt over patient's well-being.

Discuss/develop individual postoperative pain management plan. Identify misconceptions patient may have and provide appropriate information.

Increases likelihood of successful pain management. Some patients may expect to be pain-free or fear becoming addicted to narcotic agents.

Provide opportunity to practice coughing, deep-breathing, and muscular exercises.

Enhances learning and continuation of activity postoperatively.

NURSING DIAGNOSIS: Fear/Anxiety (specify level)

May be related to
Situational crisis; unfamiliarity with environment
Threat of death; change in health status
Separation from usual support systems

Possibly evidenced by
Increased tension, apprehension, decreased self-assurance
Expressed concern regarding changes, fear of consequences
Facial tension, restlessness, focus on self
Sympathetic stimulation

DESIRED OUTCOMES/EVALUATION CRITERIA—PATIENT WILL:
Acknowledge feelings and identify healthy ways to deal with them.
Appear relaxed, able to rest/sleep appropriately.
Report decreased fear and anxiety reduced to a manageable level.

ACTIONS/INTERVENTIONS	RATIONALE

Independent

Provide preoperative education, including visit with OR personnel before surgery when possible. Discuss anticipated things that may frighten/concern patient, e.g., masks, lights, IVs, BP cuff, electrodes, bovie pad, feel of oxygen cannula/mask on nose or face, autoclave and suction noises, child crying.	Can provide reassurance and alleviate patient's anxiety, as well as provide information for formulating intraoperative care. Acknowledges that foreign environment may be frightening, alleviates associated fears.
Inform patient/SO of nurse's intraoperative advocate role.	Develops trust/rapport, decreasing fear of loss of control in a foreign environment.
Identify fear levels that may necessitate postponement of surgical procedure.	Overwhelming or persistent fears result in excessive stress reaction, potentiating risk of adverse reaction to procedure/anesthetic agents.
Validate source of fear. Provide accurate, factual information. Active-listen concerns.	Identification of specific fear helps patient to deal realistically with it, e.g., misidentification/wrong operation, dismemberment, disfigurement, loss of dignity/control, or being awake/aware with local anesthesia. Patient may have misinterpreted preoperative information or have misinformation regarding surgery/disease process. Fears regarding previous experiences of self/family/acquaintances may be unresolved.
Note expressions of distress/feelings of helplessness, preoccupation with anticipated change/loss, choked feelings.	Patient may already be grieving for the loss represented by the anticipated surgical procedure/diagnosis/prognosis of illness.
Tell patient anticipating local/spinal anesthesia that drowsiness/sleep occurs, that more sedation may be requested and will be given if needed, and that surgical drapes will block view of the operative field.	Reduces concerns that patient may "see" the procedure.
Introduce staff at time of transfer to operating suite.	Establishes rapport and psychologic comfort.
Compare surgery schedule, chart, patient identification band, and signed operative consent.	Provides for positive identification, reducing fear that wrong procedure may be done.
Prevent unnecessary body exposure during transfer and in OR suite.	Patients are concerned about loss of dignity and inability to exercise control.
Give simple, concise directions/explanations to sedated patient. Review environmental concerns as needed.	Impairment of thought processes makes it difficult for patient to understand lengthy instructions.
Control external stimuli.	Extraneous noises and commotion may accelerate anxiety.

Collaborative

Refer to pastoral spiritual care, psychiatric nurse clinical specialist, psychiatric counseling if indicated.	Professional counseling may be required for patient to resolve excessive fear.

ACTIONS/INTERVENTIONS

Collaborative

Discuss postponement/cancellation of surgery with physician, anesthesiologist, patient, and family as appropriate.

Administer medications as indicated, e.g.:

Sedatives, hypnotics;

IV antianxiety agents.

RATIONALE

May be necessary if overwhelming fears are not reduced/resolved.

Used to promote sleep the evening before surgery; may enhance coping abilities.

May be provided in the outpatient admitting/preoperative holding area to reduce nervousness and provide comfort. *Note:* Respiratory depression/bradycardia may occur, necessitating prompt intervention.

INTRAOPERATIVE

NURSING DIAGNOSIS: Perioperative Positioning Injury, risk for

Risk factors may include
Disorientation; sensory/perceptual disturbances due to anesthesia
Immobilization; musculoskeletal impairments
Obesity/emaciation
Edema

Possibly evidenced by
[Not applicable; presence of signs and symptoms establishes an *actual* diagnosis]

DESIRED OUTCOMES/EVALUATION CRITERIA—PATIENT WILL:
Be free of injury related to perioperative disorientation.
Be free of untoward skin/tissue injury or changes lasting beyond 24–48 hours following procedure.
Report resolution of localized numbness, tingling, or changes in sensation related to positioning within 24–48 hours as appropriate.

ACTIONS/INTERVENTIONS

Interventions

Note anticipated length of procedure and customary position. Be aware of potential complications.

RATIONALE

Supine position may cause low back pain and skin pressure at heels/elbows/sacrum; lateral chest position can cause shoulder and neck pain, plus eye and ear injury on the patient's downside.

ACTIONS/INTERVENTIONS

Independent

Review patient's history, noting age, weight/height, nutritional status, physical limitation/preexisting conditions that may affect choice of position and skin/tissue integrity during surgery.

Stabilize both patient cart and OR table when transferring patient to and from OR table, using adequate numbers of personnel for transfer and support of extremities.

Anticipate movement of extraneous lines and tubes during the transfer and secure or guide them into position.

Secure patient on OR table with safety belt over thighs as appropriate, explaining necessity for restraint.

Protect body from contact with metal parts of the operating table.

Prepare equipment and padding for required position, according to operative procedure and patient's specific needs. Pay special attention to pressure points of bony prominences (e.g., arms, ankles) and neurovascular pressure points (e.g., breasts, knees).

Position extremities so they may be periodically checked for safety, circulation, nerve pressure, and alignment. Periodically check peripheral pulses, skin color/temperature.

Place legs in stirrups simultaneously (when lithotomy position used), adjusting stirrup height to patient's legs, maintaining symmetrical position. Pad popliteal space and heels/feet as indicated.

Provide foot board/elevate drapes off toes. Avoid/monitor placement of equipment, instrumentation on trunk/extremities during procedure.

Reposition slowly at transfer from table and in bed (especially halothane-anesthetized patient).

Determine specific postoperative positioning guidelines, e.g., elevation of head of bed following spinal anesthesia, turn to unoperated side following pneumonectomy.

RATIONALE

Many conditions (such as lack of subcutaneous padding in elderly person, arthritis, thoracic outlet/cubital tunnel syndrome, diabetes, obesity, presence of abdominal stoma, peripheral vascular disease, level of hydration, temperature of extremities) can make individual prone to injury.

Unstabilized cart/table can separate, causing patient to fall. Both side rails must be in the down position for caregiver(s) to assist patient transfer and prevent loss of balance.

Prevents undue tension and dislocation of IV lines, NG tubes, catheters, and chest tubes; maintains gravity drainage when appropriate.

OR tables and arm boards are narrow, and patient or extremity may fall off, causing injury, especially during fasciculation. Sedated or emerging patient may become resistive or combative, furthering potential for injury.

Reduces risk of burns.

Depending on individual patient's size, weight, and preexisting conditions, extra padding materials may be required to protect bony prominences, prevent circulatory compromise/nerve pressure, or allow for optimum chest expansion for ventilation.

Prevents accidental trauma, e.g., hands, fingers, and toes could inadvertently be scraped, pinched, or amputated by moving table attachments; positional pressure of brachial plexus, peroneal, and ulnar nerves can cause serious problems with extremities; prolonged plantar flexion may result in footdrop.

Prevents muscle strain; reduces risk of hip dislocation in elderly patients. Padding helps prevent peroneal and tibial nerve damage. *Note:* Prolonged positioning in stirrups may lead to compartment syndrome in calf muscles.

Continuous pressure may cause neural, circulatory, and skin integrity disruption.

Myocardial depressant effect of various agents increases risk of hypotension and/or bradycardia.

Reduces risk of postoperative complications, e.g., headache associated with migration of spinal anesthesia, or loss of maximal respiratory effort.

ACTIONS/INTERVENTIONS

Collaborative

Recommend position changes to anesthesiologist and/or surgeon as appropriate.

RATIONALE

Close attention to proper positioning can prevent muscle strain, nerve damage, circulatory compromise, and undue pressure on skin/bony prominences. Although the anesthesiologist is responsible for positioning, the nurse may be able to see/have more time to note patient needs, and provide assistance.

NURSING DIAGNOSIS: Injury, risk for

Risk factors may include
Interactive conditions between individual and environment
External environment, e.g., physical design, structure of environment, exposure to equipment, instrumentation, positioning, use of pharmaceutical agents
Internal environment, e.g., tissue hypoxia, abnormal blood profile/altered clotting factors, broken skin

Possibly evidenced by
[Not applicable; presence of signs and symptoms establishes an *actual* diagnosis]

DESIRED OUTCOMES/EVALUATION CRITERIA—CAREGIVER WILL:
Identify individual risk factors.
Modify environment as indicated to enhance safety and use resources appropriately.

ACTIONS/INTERVENTIONS

Independent

Remove partial plates or bridges preoperatively per protocol. Inform anesthesiologist of loose teeth.

Remove artificial devices preoperatively or after induction, dependent on sensory/perceptual alterations and mobility impairment.

Remove jewelry preoperatively.

Verify patient identity and scheduled operative procedure by comparing patient chart, arm band, and surgical schedule. Verbally ascertain correct name, procedure, operative site, and physician.

Give simple and concise directions to the sedated patient.

Prevent pooling of prep solutions under and around patient.

RATIONALE

Foreign bodies may be aspirated during endotracheal intubation/extubation.

Contact lenses may cause corneal abrasions while under anesthesia; eyeglasses and hearing aids are obstructive and may break; however, patients may feel more in control of environment if hearing and visual aids are left on as long as possible. Artificial limbs may be damaged and skin integrity impaired if left on.

Metals conduct electrical current and provide an electrocautery hazard. In addition, loss or damage to patient's personal property can easily occur in the foreign environment.

Assures correct patient, procedure, and appropriate extremity/side.

Impairment of thought process makes it difficult for patient to understand lengthy directions.

Antiseptic solutions may chemically burn skin as well as conduct electricity.

ACTIONS/INTERVENTIONS	RATIONALE
Independent	
Assist with induction as needed; e.g., stand by to apply cricoid pressure during intubation or stabilize position during lumbar puncture for spinal block.	Facilitates safe administration of anesthesia.
Ascertain electrical safety of equipment used in surgical procedure, e.g., intact cords, grounds, medical engineering verification labels.	Malfunction of equipment can occur during the operative procedure, causing not only delays and unnecessary anesthesia but also injury or death, e.g., short circuits, faulty grounds, laser malfunction, or laser misalignment. Periodic electrical safety checks are imperative for all OR equipment.
Place dispersive electrode (electrocautery pad) over greatest available muscle mass, ensuring its contact.	Provides a ground for maximum conductivity to prevent electrical burns.
Verify credentials of laser operators for specific wavelength laser required for particular procedure.	Due to the potential hazards of laser, physician and equipment operators must be certified in the use and safety requirements of specific wavelength laser and procedure, i.e., open, endoscopic, abdominal, laryngeal, intrauterine.
Confirm presence of fire extinguishers and wet fire smothering materials when lasers are used intraoperatively.	Laser beam may inadvertently contact and ignite combustibles outside of surgical field, i.e., drapes, sponges.
Apply patient eye protection before laser activation.	Eye protection for specific laser wavelength must be used to prevent injury.
Protect surrounding skin and anatomy appropriately, i.e., wet towels, sponges, dams, cottonoids.	Prevents inadvertent skin integrity disruption, hair ignition, and adjacent anatomy injury in area of laser beam use.
Monitor I&O during procedure.	Potential for fluid volume deficit exists, affecting safety of anesthesia, organ function, and patient well-being.
Confirm and document correct sponge, instrument, needle, and blade counts.	Foreign bodies remaining in body cavities at closure not only cause inflammation, infection, perforation, and abscess formation, but also may result in disastrous complications, leading to death.
Handle, label, and document specimens appropriately, ensuring proper medium and transport for tests required.	Proper identification of specimens to patient is imperative. Frozen sections, preserved or fresh examination, and cultures all have different requirements. OR nurse advocate must be knowledgeable of specific hospital laboratory requirements for validity of examination.
Collaborative	
Administer antacids preoperatively as indicated.	Neutralizes gastric acidity and may reduce severity of pneumonia should aspiration occur, especially in obese/pregnant patients in whom there is an 85% risk of mortality with aspiration.
Collect blood intraoperatively as appropriate.	Blood lost intraoperatively may be collected, filtered, and infused either intraoperatively or postoperatively.
Limit/avoid use of epinephrine to Fluothane-anesthetized patient.	Fluothane sensitizes the myocardium to catecholamines and may produce dysrhythmias.

> **NURSING DIAGNOSIS: Infection, risk for**
>
> **Risk factors may include**
> Broken skin, traumatized tissues, stasis of body fluids
> Presence of pathogens/contaminants, environmental exposure, invasive procedures
>
> **Possibly evidenced by**
> [Not applicable; presence of signs and symptoms establishes an *actual* diagnosis]
>
> **DESIRED OUTCOMES/EVALUATION CRITERIA—CAREGIVER WILL:**
> Identify individual risk factors and interventions to reduce potential for infection.
> Maintain safe aseptic environment.

ACTIONS/INTERVENTIONS	RATIONALE
Independent	
Adhere to facility infection control, sterilization, and aseptic policies/procedures.	Established mechanisms designed to prevent infection.
Verify sterility of all manufacturers' items.	Prepackaged items may appear to be sterile; however, each item must be scrutinized for manufacturer's statement of sterility, breaks in packaging, environmental effect on package, and delivery techniques. Package sterilization and expiration dates, lot/serial numbers must be documented on implant items for further follow-up if necessary.
Review laboratory studies for possibility of systemic infections.	Increased WBC may indicate ongoing infection, which the operative procedure will alleviate (e.g., appendicitis, abscess, inflammation from trauma); or presence of systemic/organ infection, which may contraindicate surgical procedure and/or anesthesia (e.g., pneumonia, kidney infection).
Verify that preoperative skin, vaginal, and bowel cleansing procedures have been done as needed.	Cleansing reduces bacterial counts on the skin, vaginal mucosa, and alimentary tract.
Prepare operative site according to specific procedures.	Minimizes bacterial counts at operative site.
Examine skin for breaks or irritation, signs of infection.	Disruptions of skin integrity at or near the operative site are sources of contamination to the wound. Careful shaving/clipping is imperative to prevent abrasions and nicks in the skin.
Maintain dependent gravity drainage of indwelling catheters, tubes, and/or positive pressure of parenteral or irrigation lines.	Prevents stasis and reflux of body fluids.
Identify breaks in aseptic technique and resolve immediately on occurrence.	Contamination by environmental/personnel contact renders the sterile field unsterile, thereby increasing the risk of infection.

ACTIONS/INTERVENTIONS

Independent

Contain contaminated fluids/materials in specific site in operating room suite, and dispose of according to hospital protocol.

Apply sterile dressing.

Collaborative

Provide copious wound irrigation, e.g., saline, water, antibiotic, or antiseptic.

Obtain specimens for cultures/Gram's stain.

Administer antibiotics as indicated.

RATIONALE

Containment of blood and body fluids, tissue and materials in contact with an infected wound/patient will prevent spread of infection to environment/other patients or personnel.

Prevents environmental contamination of fresh wound.

May be used intraoperatively to reduce bacterial counts at the site and cleanse the wound of debris, e.g., bone, ischemic tissue, bowel contaminants, toxins.

Immediate identification of type of infective organism by Gram's stain allows prompt treatment, while more specific identification by cultures can be obtained in hours/days.

May be given prophylactically for suspected infection or contamination.

NURSING DIAGNOSIS: Body Temperature, altered, risk for

Risk factors may include
Exposure to cool environment
Use of medications, anesthetic agents
Extremes of age, weight
Dehydration

Possibly evidenced by
[Not applicable; presence of signs and symptoms establishes an *actual* diagnosis]

DESIRED OUTCOMES/EVALUATION CRITERIA—PATIENT WILL:
Maintain body temperature within normal range.

ACTIONS/INTERVENTIONS

Independent

Note preoperative temperature.

RATIONALE

Used as baseline for monitoring intraoperative temperature. Preoperative temperature elevations are indicative of disease process, e.g., appendicitis, abscess, or systemic disease requiring treatment preoperatively and possibly postoperatively. *Note:* Effects of aging on hypothalamus may decrease fever response to infection.

ACTIONS/INTERVENTIONS	RATIONALE
Independent	
Assess environmental temperature and modify as needed, e.g., providing warming and cooling blankets, increasing room temperature.	May assist in maintaining/stabilizing patient's temperature.
Cover skin areas outside of operative field.	Heat losses will occur as skin (e.g., legs, arms, head) is exposed to cool environment.
Provide cooling measures for patient with preoperative temperature elevations.	Cool irrigations and exposure of skin surfaces to air may be required to decrease temperature.
Note rapid temperature elevation/persistent high fever and treat promptly per protocol.	Malignant hyperthermia must be recognized and treated promptly to avoid serious complications.
Increase ambient room temperature (e.g., to 78°F or 80°F) at conclusion of procedure.	Helps limit patient heat loss when drapes are removed and patient is prepared for transfer.
Apply warming blankets at emergence from anesthesia.	Inhalation anesthetics depress the hypothalamus, resulting in poor body temperature regulation.
Collaborative	
Monitor temperature throughout intraoperative phase.	Continuous warm/cool humidified inhalation anesthetics are used to maintain humidity and temperature balance within the tracheobronchial tree. Temperature elevation intraoperatively may indicate adverse response to anesthesia. *Note:* Use of atropine or scopolamine may further increase temperature.
Place warming/cooling blanket under patient. Provide iced saline as indicated.	Maintains steady body temperature in cool environment of OR suite and/or fever. *Note:* Lavage of body cavity with iced saline may help reduce hyperthermic responses.
Obtain dantrolene (Dantrium) for IV administration.	Immediate action to control temperature is necessary to prevent death from malignant hyperthermia.

POSTOPERATIVE

NURSING DIAGNOSIS: Breathing Pattern, ineffective

May be related to
Neuromuscular, perceptual/cognitive impairment
Decreased lung expansion, energy
Tracheobronchial obstruction

Possibly evidenced by
Changes in respiratory rate and depth
Reduced vital capacity, apnea, cyanosis, noisy respirations

DESIRED OUTCOMES/EVALUATION CRITERIA—PATIENT WILL:
Establish a normal/effective respiratory pattern free of cyanosis or other signs of hypoxia.

ACTIONS/INTERVENTIONS	RATIONALE

Independent

Maintain patent airway by head tilt, jaw hyperextension, oral pharyngeal airway.

Prevents airway obstruction.

Auscultate breath sounds. Listen for gurgling, wheezing, crowing, and/or silence after extubation.

Lack of breath sounds is indicative of obstruction by mucus or tongue and may be corrected by positioning and/or suctioning. Diminished breath sounds suggest atelectasis. Wheezing indicates bronchospasm, whereas crowing or silence reflects partial-to-total laryngospasm.

Observe respiratory rate and depth, chest expansion, use of accessory muscles, retraction or flaring of nostrils, skin color; note airflow.

Ascertains effectiveness of respirations immediately so corrective measures can be initiated.

Monitor vital signs continuously.

Increased respirations, tachycardia, and/or bradycardia suggests hypoxia.

Position patient appropriately, dependent on respiratory effort and type of surgery.

Head elevation and left lateral Sims' position prevent aspiration of vomitus; proper positioning enhances ventilation to lower lobes and relieves pressure on diaphragm.

Observe for return of muscle function, especially respiratory.

After administration of intraoperative muscle relaxants, return of muscle function occurs first to the diaphragm, intercostals, and larynx; followed by large muscle groups, neck, shoulders, and abdominal muscles; then by midsize muscles, tongue, pharynx, extensors, and flexors; and finally by eyes, mouth, face, and fingers.

Initiate *stir-up regimen* as soon as patient is reactive and continue into the postoperative period.

Active deep ventilation inflates alveoli, breaks up secretions, increases O_2 transfer, and removes anesthetic gases; coughing enhances removal of secretions from the pulmonary system. *Note:* Respiratory muscles weaken and atrophy with age, hampering patient's ability to cough or deep-breathe effectively.

Observe for excessive somnolence.

Narcotic-induced respiratory depression or presence of muscle relaxants in the system may be cyclical in recurrence, creating sine-wave pattern of depression and reemergence. In addition, Pentothal is absorbed in the fatty tissues, and, as circulation improves, it may be redistributed throughout the bloodstream.

Elevate head of bed as appropriate.

Promotes maximal expansion of lungs.

Suction as necessary.

Airway obstruction can occur because of blood or mucus in throat or trachea.

Collaborative

Administer supplemental O_2 as indicated.

Maximizes O_2 for uptake to bind with Hb in place of anesthetic gases to enhance removal of inhalation agents.

ACTIONS/INTERVENTIONS

Collaborative

Administer IV medications, e.g., naloxone (Narcan) or doxapram (Dopram).

Provide/maintain ventilator assistance.

Assist with use of respiratory aids, e.g., incentive spirometer, blow bottles.

RATIONALE

Narcan reverses narcotic-induced CNS depression and Dopram stimulates respiratory muscles. The effects of both drugs are cyclic in nature and respiratory depression may return.

Dependent on cause of respiratory depression or type of surgery (e.g., pulmonary, extensive abdominal, cardiac), endotracheal tube may be left in place and mechanical ventilation maintained for a time.

Maximal respiratory efforts reduce potential for atelectasis and infection.

NURSING DIAGNOSIS: Sensory-perceptual alterations: (specify)/ Thought Processes, altered

May be related to
Chemical alteration: Use of pharmaceutical agents, hypoxia
Therapeutically restricted environments; excessive sensory stimuli
Physiologic stress

Possibly evidenced by
Disorientation to person, place, time; change in usual response to stimuli; impaired ability to concentrate, reason, make decisions
Motor incoordination

DESIRED OUTCOMES/EVALUATION CRITERIA—PATIENT WILL:
Regain usual level of consciousness/mentation.
Recognize limitations and seek assistance as necessary.

ACTIONS/INTERVENTIONS

Independent

Reorient patient continuously when emerging from anesthesia; confirm that surgery is completed.

Speak in normal, clear voice without shouting, being aware of what you are saying. Minimize discussion of negatives (e.g., patient/personnel problems) within patient's hearing. Explain procedures, even if patient does not seem aware.

Evaluate sensation/movement of extremities and trunk as appropriate.

Use bedrail padding, restraints as necessary.

RATIONALE

As patient regains consciousness, support and assurance will help to alleviate anxiety.

Cannot tell when patient is aware, but sense of hearing returns first; so it is important not to say things that may be misinterpreted. Providing information helps patient to preserve dignity and to prepare for activity.

Return of function following local or spinal nerve blocks is dependent on type/amount of agent used and duration of procedure.

Provides for patient safety during emergence stage. Prevents injury to head and extremities if patient becomes combative while disoriented.

ACTIONS/INTERVENTIONS	RATIONALE
Independent	
Secure parenteral lines, endotracheal tube, catheters, if present, and check for patency.	Disoriented patient may pull on lines and drainage systems, disconnecting or kinking them.
Maintain quiet, calm environment.	External stimuli, such as noise, lights, touch may cause psychic aberrations when dissociative anesthetics (e.g., ketamine) have been administered.
Investigate changes in sensorium.	Confusion, especially in elderly patients, may reflect drug interactions, hypoxia, anxiety, pain, electrolyte imbalances, or fear.
Observe for hallucinations, delusions, depression, or an excited state.	May develop following trauma and indicate delirium, or may reflect "sundowner's syndrome" in elderly patient. In patient who has used alcohol to excess, may suggest impending delirium tremens.
Reassess return of sensory abilities and thought processes thoroughly prior to discharge, as indicated.	Ambulatory surgical patient must be able to care for self with the help of SO (if available) to prevent personal injury after discharge.
Collaborative	
Maintain extended stay in postoperative recovery area prior to discharge as appropriate.	Disorientation may persist, and SO may not be able to protect the patient at home.

NURSING DIAGNOSIS: Fluid Volume deficit, risk for

Risk factors may include
Restriction of oral intake (disease process/medical procedure/presence of nausea)
Loss of fluid through abnormal routes, e.g., indwelling tubes, drains; normal routes, e.g., vomiting
Loss of vascular integrity, changes in clotting ability
Extremes of age and weight

Possibly evidenced by
[Not applicable; presence of signs and symptoms establishes an *actual* diagnosis]

DESIRED OUTCOMES/EVALUATION CRITERIA—PATIENT WILL:
Demonstrate adequate fluid balance, as evidenced by stable vital signs, palpable pulses of good quality, normal skin turgor, moist mucous membranes, and individually appropriate urinary output.

ACTIONS/INTERVENTIONS	RATIONALE
Independent	
Measure and record I&O (including GI losses). Calculate urine specific gravity as appropriate. Review intraoperative record.	Accurate documentation helps identify fluid losses/replacement needs and influences choice of interventions. *Note:* Ability to concentrate urine declines with age, increasing renal losses despite general fluid deficit.

ACTIONS/INTERVENTIONS	RATIONALE

Independent

Assess urinary output specifically for type of operative procedure done.

May be decreased or absent after procedures on the genitourinary system and/or adjacent structures (e.g., ureteroplasty, ureterolithotomy, abdominal or vaginal hysterectomy), indicating malfunction or obstruction of the urinary system.

Provide voiding assistance measures as needed, e.g., privacy, sitting position, running water in sink, pouring warm water over perineum.

Promotes relaxation of perineal muscles and may facilitate voiding efforts.

Monitor vital signs. Calculate pulse pressure.

Hypotension, tachycardia, increased respirations may indicate fluid deficit, e.g., dehydration/hypovolemia. Although a drop in blood pressure is generally a late sign of fluid deficit (hemorrhagic loss), widening of the pulse pressure may occur early, followed by narrowing as bleeding continues and systolic BP begins to fall.

Note presence of nausea/vomiting, patient history of motion sickness.

Women, obese patients, and those prone to motion sickness have a higher risk of postoperative nausea/vomiting. In addition, the longer the duration of anesthesia, the greater the risk for nausea. *Note:* Nausea occurring during first 12 to 24 hours postoperatively is frequently related to anesthesia (including regional anesthesia). Nausea persisting more than 3 days postoperatively may be related to the choice of narcotic for pain control or other drug therapy.

Inspect dressings, drainage devices at regular intervals. Assess wound for swelling.

Excessive bleeding can lead to hypovolemia/circulatory collapse. Local swelling may indicate hematoma formation/hemorrhage. *Note:* Bleeding into a cavity (e.g., retroperitoneal) may be hidden and only diagnosed via vital sign depression, patient reports of pressure sensation in affected area.

Monitor skin temperature, palpate peripheral pulses.

Cool/clammy skin, weak pulses indicate decreased peripheral circulation and need for additional fluid replacement.

Collaborative

Administer parenteral fluids, blood products (including autologous collection), and/or plasma expanders as indicated. Increase IV rate if needed.

Replaces documented fluid loss. Timely replacement of circulating volume decreases potential for complications of deficit, e.g., electrolyte imbalance, dehydration, cardiovascular collapse. *Note:* Increased volume may be required initially to support circulating volume/prevent hypotension because of decreased vasomotor tone following Fluothane administration.

Insert urinary catheter with or without urimeter as necessary.

Provides mechanism for accurate monitoring of urinary output.

Resume oral intake gradually as indicated.

Oral intake is dependent on return of GI function.

817

ACTIONS/INTERVENTIONS

Independent

Administer antiemetics as appropriate.

Monitor laboratory studies, e.g., Hb/Hct, electrolytes. Compare preoperative and postoperative blood studies.

RATIONALE

Relieves nausea/vomiting, which may impair intake and add to fluid losses. *Note:* Naloxone (Narcan) may relieve nausea related to use of regional anesthesia agents, e.g., Duramorph, Sublimaze.

Indicators of hydration/circulating volume. Preoperative anemia and/or low Hct combined with unreplaced fluid losses intraoperatively will further potentiate deficit.

NURSING DIAGNOSIS: Pain [acute]

May be related to
Disruption of skin, tissue, and muscle integrity; musculoskeletal/bone trauma
Presence of tubes and drains

Possibly evidenced by
Reports of pain
Alteration in muscle tone; facial mask of pain
Distraction/guarding/protective behaviors
Self-focusing; narrowed focus
Autonomic responses

DESIRED OUTCOMES/EVALUATION CRITERIA—PATIENT WILL:
Report pain relieved/controlled.
Appear relaxed, able to rest/sleep and participate in activities appropriately.

ACTIONS/INTERVENTIONS

Independent

Note patient's age, weight, coexisting medical/psychologic conditions, idiosyncratic sensitivity to analgesics, and intraoperative course (e.g., size/location of incision, drain placement, anesthetic agents) used.

Review intraoperative/recovery room record for type of anesthesia and medications previously administered.

Evaluate pain regularly (e.g., every 2 hours × 12) noting characteristics, location, and intensity (0–10 scale). Emphasize patient's responsibility for reporting pain/relief of pain.

RATIONALE

Approach to postoperative pain management is based on multiple variable factors.

Presence of narcotics and droperidol in system will potentiate narcotic analgesia, whereas patients anesthetized with Fluothane and Ethrane have no residual analgesic effects. In addition, intraoperative local/regional blocks have varying duration, e.g., 1–2 hours for regionals or up to 2–6 hours for locals.

Provides information about need for/effectiveness of interventions. *Note:* Because of side effects of medication, it may not be possible to eliminate pain; however, medication should reduce pain to a tolerable level. A frontal and/or occipital headache may develop 24–72 hours following spinal anesthesia, necessitating recumbent position, increased fluid intake, and notification of the anesthesiologist.

ACTIONS/INTERVENTIONS

Independent

Note presence of anxiety/fear, and relate with nature of and preparation for procedure.

Assess vital signs, noting tachycardia, hypertension, and increased respiration, even if patient denies pain.

Assess causes of possible discomfort other than operative procedure.

Provide information about transitory nature of discomfort, as appropriate.

Reposition as indicated, e.g., semi-Fowler's; lateral Sims'.

Provide additional comfort measures, e.g., backrub, heat/cold applications.

Encourage use of relaxation techniques, e.g., deep-breathing exercises, guided imagery, visualization, music.

Provide regular oral care, occasional ice chips/sips of fluids as tolerated.

Document effects of analgesia.

Collaborative

Administer medications as indicated:

Analgesics IV (after reviewing anesthesia record for contraindications and/or presence of agents that may potentiate analgesia); provide around-the-clock analgesia with intermittent rescue doses;

RATIONALE

Concern about the unknown (e.g., outcome of a biopsy) and/or inadequate preparation (e.g., emergency appendectomy) can heighten patient's perception of pain.

May indicate acute pain and discomfort. *Note:* Some patients may have a slightly lowered BP, which returns to normal range after pain relief is achieved.

Discomfort can be caused/aggravated by presence of nonpatent indwelling catheters, NG tube, parenteral lines (bladder pain, gastric fluid and gas accumulation, and infiltration of IV fluids/medications).

Understanding the cause of the discomfort (e.g., sore muscles from administration of succinylcholine may persist up to 48 hours postoperatively; sinus headache associated with nitrous oxide and sore throat due to intubation are transitory) provides emotional reassurance. *Note:* Paresthesia of body parts suggests nerve injury. Symptoms may last hours or months and require additional evaluation.

May relieve pain and enhance circulation. Semi-Fowler's position will relieve abdominal muscle tension and arthritic back muscle tension, whereas lateral Sims' will relieve dorsal pressures.

Improves circulation, reduces muscle tension and anxiety associated with pain. Enhances sense of well-being.

Relieves muscle and emotional tension; enhances sense of control and may improve coping abilities.

Reduces discomfort associated with dry mucous membranes due to anesthetic agents, oral restrictions.

Respirations may decrease on administration of narcotic, and synergistic effects with anesthetic agents may occur. *Note:* Migration of epidural analgesia toward head (cephalad diffusion) may cause respiratory depression or excessive sedation.

Analgesics given IV reach the pain centers immediately, providing more effective relief with small doses of medication. IM administration takes longer, and its effectiveness is dependent on absorption rates and circulation. *Note:* Narcotic dosage should be reduced by ¼ to ⅓ after use of Innovar or Inapsine to prevent profound tranquilization during first 10 hours postoperatively. Current research supports need to administer analgesics around the clock instead of prn in order to *prevent* rather than merely treat pain.

ACTIONS/INTERVENTIONS	RATIONALE

Collaborative

Patient-controlled analgesia;	Use of PCA necessitates detailed patient instruction. PCA must be monitored closely but is considered very effective in managing acute postoperative pain with smaller amounts of narcotic and increased patient satisfaction.
Local anesthetics, e.g., epidural block/infusion;	Analgesics may be injected into the operative site, or nerves to the site may be kept blocked in the immediate postoperative phase to prevent severe pain. *Note:* Continuous epidural infusions may be used for 1–5 days following procedures that are known to cause severe pain (e.g., certain types of thoracic or abdominal surgery).
NSAIDs, e.g., aspirin, diflunisal (Dolobid), naproxen (Anaprox).	Useful for mild to moderate pain or as adjuncts to opioid therapy when pain is moderate to severe. Allows for a lower dosage of narcotics, reducing potential for side effects.
Monitor use/effectiveness of transcutaneous electrical nerve stimulation.	TENS may be useful in reducing pain and amount of medication required postoperatively.

NURSING DIAGNOSIS: Skin/Tissue Integrity, impaired

May be related to
Mechanical interruption of skin/tissues
Altered circulation, effects of medication; accumulation of drainage; altered metabolic state

Possibly evidenced by
Disruption of skin surface/layers and tissues

DESIRED OUTCOMES/EVALUATION CRITERIA—PATIENT WILL:
Demonstrate behaviors/techniques to promote healing and to prevent complications.
Achieve timely wound healing.

ACTIONS/INTERVENTIONS	RATIONALE

Independent

Reinforce initial dressing/change as indicated. Use strict aseptic techniques.	Protects wound form mechanical injury and contamination. Prevents accumulation of fluids that may cause excoriation.
Gently remove tape (in direction of hair growth) and dressings when changing.	Reduces risk of skin trauma and disruption of wound.
Apply skin sealants/barriers before tape if needed. Use paper/silk (hypoallergenic) tape or Montgomery straps/elastic netting for dressings requiring frequent changing.	Reduces potential for skin trauma/abrasions and provides additional protection for delicate skin/tissues.
Check tension of dressings. Apply tape at center of incision to outer margin of dressing. Avoid wrapping tape around extremity.	Can impair/occlude circulation to wound as well as distal portion of extremity.

ACTIONS/INTERVENTIONS	RATIONALE

Independent

Inspect wound regularly, noting characteristics and integrity.

Early recognition of delayed healing/developing complications may prevent a more serious situation. Wounds may heal more slowly in elderly patients, as reduced cardiac output decreases capillary blood flow.

Assess amount and characteristics of drainage.

Decreasing drainage suggests evolution of healing process, while continued drainage or presence of bloody/odoriferous exudate suggests complications (e.g., fistula formation, hemorrhage, infection).

Maintain patency of drainage tubes; apply collection bag over drains/incisions in presence of copious or caustic drainage.

Facilitates approximation of wound edges; reduces risk of infection and chemical injury to skin/tissues.

Elevate operative area as appropriate.

Promotes venous return and limits edema formation. *Note:* Elevation in presence of venous insufficiency may be detrimental.

Splint abdominal and chest incisions/area with pillow or pad during coughing/movement.

Equalizes pressure on the wound, minimizing risk of dehiscence/rupture.

Caution patient not to touch wound.

Prevents contamination of wound.

Leave wound open to air as soon as possible, or cover with small gauze/Telfa pad as needed.

Aids in drying wound and facilitates healing processes. Light covering may be necessary to prevent irritation if sutures/wound edges rub against linens.

Cleanse skin surface with diluted hydrogen peroxide, or running water and mild soap after incision is sealed.

Reduces skin contaminants; aids in removal of exudate.

Collaborative

Apply ice if appropriate.

Reduces edema formation that may cause undue pressure on incision during initial postoperative period.

Use abdominal binder if indicated.

Provides additional support for high-risk incisions (e.g., obese patient).

Irrigate wound; assist with débridement as needed.

Removes infectious exudate/necrotic tissue to promote healing.

Monitor/maintain specialty dressings, e.g., vacuum dressing.

Vacuum dressing may be used to hasten healing in large, draining wound/fistula, to increase patient comfort, and to reduce frequency of dressing changes. Also allows drainage to be measured more accurately and analyzed for pH and electrolyte content.

NURSING DIAGNOSIS: Tissue Perfusion, altered, risk for

Risk factors may include
Interruption of flow: Arterial, venous
Hypovolemia

Possibly evidenced by
[Not applicable; presence of signs and symptoms establishes an *actual* diagnosis]

DESIRED OUTCOMES/EVALUATION CRITERIA—PATIENT WILL:
Demonstrate adequate perfusion evidenced by stable vital signs, peripheral pulses present and strong; skin warm/dry; usual mentation and individually appropriate urinary output.

ACTIONS/INTERVENTIONS	RATIONALE

Independent

Change position slowly in bed and at transfer (especially Fluothane-anesthetized patient).	Vasoconstrictor mechanisms are depressed and quick movement may lead to hypotension.
Assist with ROM exercises, including active ankle/leg exercises.	Stimulates peripheral circulation, aids in preventing venous stasis to reduce risk of thrombus formation.
Encourage/assist with early ambulation.	Enhances circulation and return of normal organ function.
Avoid use of knee gatch/pillow under knees. Caution patient against crossing legs or sitting with legs dependent for prolonged period.	Prevents stasis of venous circulation and reduces risk of thrombophlebitis.
Assess lower extremities for erythema, positive Homans' sign.	Circulation may be restricted by some positions used during surgery, while anesthetics and decreased activity alter vasomotor tone, potentiating vascular pooling and increasing risks of thrombus formation.
Monitor vital signs; palpate peripheral pulses; note skin temperature/color and capillary refill. Evaluate urinary output/time of voiding. Document dysrhythmias.	Indicators of adequacy of circulating volume and tissue perfusion/organ function. Effects of medications/electrolyte imbalances may create dysrhythmias, impairing cardiac output and tissue perfusion.
Investigate changes in mentation/failure to achieve usual mental state.	May reflect a number of problems such as inadequate clearance of anesthetic agent, oversedation (pain medication), hypoventilation, hypovolemia, or intraoperative complications (emboli).

Collaborative

Administer IV fluids/blood products as needed.	Maintains circulating volume; supports perfusion.
Apply antiembolic hose as indicated.	Promotes venous return and prevents venous stasis of legs to reduce risk of thrombosis.

NURSING DIAGNOSIS: Knowledge deficit [learning need] regarding condition/situation, prognosis, treatment, self care and discharge needs

May be related to
Lack of exposure/lack of recall, information misinterpretation
Unfamiliarity with information resources
Cognitive limitation

Possibly evidenced by
Questions/request for information
Statement of misconception
Inaccurate follow-through of instructions/development of preventable complications

DESIRED OUTCOMES/EVALUATION CRITERIA—PATIENT WILL:
Verbalize understanding of condition, effects of procedure and treatment.
Correctly perform necessary procedures and explain reasons for actions.
Initiate necessary lifestyle changes and participate in treatment regimen.

ACTIONS/INTERVENTIONS	RATIONALE
Independent	
Review specific surgery performed/procedure done and future expectations.	Provides knowledge base on which patient can make informed choices.
Review and have patient/SO demonstrate dressing/wound/tube care when indicated. Identify source for supplies.	Promotes competent self-care and enhances independence.
Review avoidance of environmental risk factors, e.g., exposure to crowds/persons with infections.	Reduces potential for acquired infections.
Discuss drug therapy, including use of prescribed and OTC analgesics.	Enhances cooperation with regimen; reduces risk of adverse reactions/untoward effects.
Identify specific activity limitations.	Prevents undue strain on operative site.
Recommend planned/progressive exercise.	Promotes return of normal function and enhances feelings of general well-being.
Schedule adequate rest periods.	Prevents fatigue and conserves energy for healing.
Review importance of nutritious diet and adequate fluid intake.	Provides elements necessary for tissue regeneration/healing and support of tissue perfusion and organ function.
Encourage cessation of smoking.	Smoking increases risk of pulmonary infections, causes vasoconstriction, and reduces oxygen-binding capacity of blood, affecting cellular perfusion and potentially impairing healing.
Identify signs/symptoms requiring medical evaluation, e.g., nausea/vomiting; difficulty voiding; fever, continued/odoriferous wound drainage; incisional swelling, erythema or separation of edges; unresolved or changes in characteristics of pain.	Early recognition and treatment of developing complications (e.g., ileus, urinary retention, infection, delayed healing) may prevent progression to more serious or life-threatening situation.
Stress necessity of follow-up visits with providers, including therapists, laboratory.	Monitors progress of healing and evaluates effectiveness of regimen.
Include SO in teaching program/discharge planning. Provide written instructions/teaching materials. Instruct in use of and arrange for special equipment.	Provides additional resource for reference after discharge.
Identify available resources, e.g., homecare services, visiting nurse, Meals-on-Wheels, outpatient therapy, contact phone number for questions.	Enhances support for patient during recovery period and provides additional evaluation of ongoing needs/new concerns.

POTENTIAL CONSIDERATIONS following surgical procedure (dependent on patient's age, physical condition/presence of complications, personal resources, and life responsibilities)

Fatigue—increased energy requirements to perform activities of daily living, states of discomfort

Infection, risk for—broken skin, traumatized tissues, stasis of body fluids; presence of pathogens/contaminants, environmental exposure, invasive procedures

Self Care deficit/Home Maintenance Management, impaired—decreased strength/endurance, pain/discomfort, unfamiliarity with neighborhood resources, inadequate support systems

Refer also to appropriate plans of care regarding underlying condition/specific surgical procedure for additional considerations

LONG-TERM CARE

Patients in the acute care setting may be discharged to an extended care facility. Patients requiring relatively short-term rehabilitation as well as those needing long-term care/permanent nursing care are included in this group. Coordination and knowledge are essential in providing continuity and quality care. The level of care and needs of the patient (e.g., physical, occupational, rehabilitation therapy; IV and respiratory support) are frequently the deciding factors in the choice of placement. Although elderly people are the primary population in extended care facilities, increasing numbers of younger individuals are requiring care for debilitating conditions that they can no longer manage in the home setting.

RELATED CONCERNS

AIDS, p 739
Cancer, p 875
Cerebrovascular Accident/Stroke, p 242
Craniocerebral Trauma (Acute Rehabilitative Phase), p 230
Fractures, p 659
Multiple Sclerosis, p 298
Psychosocial Aspects of Care, p 783
Spinal Cord Injury (Acute Rehabilitative Phase), p 278
Surgical Intervention, p 802
Ventilatory Assistance (Mechanical), p 176

Patient Assessment Data Base

Data is dependent on underlying physical/psychosocial conditions necessitating continuation of structured care.

TEACHING/LEARNING

Discharge plan considerations: **Projected mean length of stay: Dependent on underlying disease/condition and individual care needs. Therefore, this may be temporary or permanent placement.**
May require assistance with treatments, self-care activities, homemaker/maintenance tasks or alternate living arrangements (e.g., group home)

Refer to section at end of plan for postdischarge considerations.

DIAGNOSTIC STUDIES (dependent on age, general health, and medical condition)

ECG: Provides baseline data; detects abnormalities.
Chest x-ray: Reveals size of heart, lung abnormalities/disease conditions, changes of the large blood vessels and bony structure of the chest.
Visual acuity testing: Identifies cataracts/other vision problems.
Tonometer test: Measures intraocular pressure.
CBC: Reveals problems such as infection, anemia, other abnormalities.
Chemistry profile: Evaluates general organ function/imbalances.
Pulse oximetry: Determines oxygenation, respiratory function.
Communicable disease screens: To rule out TB, HIV, RPR, hepatitis.
Drug screen: As indicated by usage to identify therapeutic or toxic levels.
Urinalysis: Provides information about kidney function; determines presence of UTI or diabetes mellitus.

NURSING PRIORITIES

1. Promote physiologic and psychologic well-being.
2. Provide for security and safety.
3. Prevent complications of disease and/or aging process.
4. Promote effective coping skills and independence.
5. Encourage continuation of healthy habits, participation in plan of care to meet individual needs and wishes.

DISCHARGE GOALS

1. Patient dealing realistically with current situation.
2. Homeostasis maintained.
3. Injury prevented.
4. Complications prevented/minimized.
5. Patient meeting ADLs by self/with assistance as necessary.
6. Plan in place to meet needs after discharge as appropriate.

NURSING DIAGNOSIS: Anxiety [specify level]/Fear

May be related to

Change in health status, role functioning, interaction patterns, socioeconomic status, environment

Unmet needs; recent life changes, loss of friends/SO

Possibly evidenced by

Apprehension, restlessness, repetitive questioning; pacing, purposeless activity; insomnia

Various behaviors (appears overexcited, withdrawn, worried, fearful); presence of facial tension, trembling, hand tremors

Expressed concern regarding changes in life events

Focus on self; lack of interest in activity

DESIRED OUTCOMES/EVALUATION CRITERIA—PATIENT WILL:

Verbalize understanding of reasons for change, as able.

Demonstrate appropriate range of feelings and lessened fear.

Participate in routine and special/social events as capable.

Verbalize acceptance of situation.

ACTIONS/INTERVENTIONS	RATIONALE
Independent	
Provide patient/SO with copy of "A Patient's Bill of Rights" and review it with them. Discuss facility's rules, e.g., visiting, off-grounds visits.	Provides information that can foster confidence that individual rights do continue in this setting and the patient is still "his or her own person" and has some control over what happens.
Ascertain if patient has completed Advance Directives. Provide information as appropriate.	Assures patient/family wishes will be known to provide direction to caregivers.

ACTIONS/INTERVENTIONS	RATIONALE
Independent	
Determine patient/SO attitude toward admission to facility and expectations for the future.	If this is expected to be a temporary placement, patient/SO concerns will be different than if placement is permanent. When patient is giving up own home and way of life, feelings of helplessness, loss, and grief are to be expected.
Help family/SO to be honest with patient regarding admission. Be clear about actions/events.	Family may have difficulty dealing with decision/reality of permanent placement and may avoid discussing situation with patient. Honesty decreases "surprises," assists in maintaining trust, and may enhance coping.
Identify support person(s) important to patient and include in care activities, mealtime, and so on, as appropriate.	During adjustment period/times of stress, patient may benefit from presence of trusted individual who can provide reassurance and reduce sense of isolation.
Assess level of anxiety and discuss reasons when possible.	Identifying specific problems will enable individual to deal more realistically with them.
Develop nurse-patient relationship.	Trusting relationships among patient/SO/staff promotes optimal care and support.
Make time to listen to patient about concerns, and encourage free expression of feelings, e.g., anger, hostility, fear, and loneliness.	Being available in this way allows patient to feel accepted, begin to acknowledge and deal with feelings related to circumstances of admission.
Acknowledge reality of situation and feelings of patient. Accept expressions of anger while limiting aggressive, acting-out behavior.	Permission to express feelings allows for beginning resolution. Acceptance promotes sense of self-worth. *Note:* Psychosocial and/or physiologic disturbances can occur as a result of transfer from one environment to another (i.e., relocation stress syndrome).
Identify strengths and successful coping behaviors and incorporate into problem solving.	Building on past successes increases likelihood of positive outcome in present situation. Enhances sense of control and management of current deficits.
Orient to physical aspects of facility, schedules, and activities. Introduce to roommate(s) and staff. Give explanation of roles.	Getting acquainted is an important part of admission. Knowledge of where things are and who patient can expect assistance from can be helpful in reducing anxiety.
Determine patient's usual schedule and incorporate into hospital routine as much as possible.	Consistency provides reassurance and may lessen confusion and enhance cooperation.
Provide above information in written or taped form as well.	Overload of information is difficult to remember. Patient can refer to written or taped material as needed to refresh memory/learn new information.
Give careful thought to room placement. Provide help and encouragement in placing patient's own belongings around room. Do not transfer from one room to another without patient approval/documentable need.	Location, roommate compatibility, and place for personal belongings are important considerations for helping the patient feel "at home." Changes are often met with resistance and can result in emotional upset and decline in physical condition. *Note:* Persons with severe behavioral problems/cognitive dysfunctions may require a private room.

ACTIONS/INTERVENTIONS

Independent

Note behavior, presence of suspiciousness/paranoia, irritability, defensiveness. Compare with SO's description of customary responses.

Collaborative

Refer to social service or other appropriate agency for assistance. Have case manager social worker discuss ramifications of Medicare/Medicaid if patient is eligible for these resources.

RATIONALE

Increased stress, physical discomfort, and fatigue may temporarily exacerbate mental deterioration (cognitive inaccessibility) and further impair communication (social inaccessibility). This represents a catastrophic episode that can escalate into a panic state and violence.

Often patient is not aware of the resources available, and providing current information about individual coverage/limitations and other possible sources of support will assist with adjustment to new situation.

NURSING DIAGNOSIS: Grieving, anticipatory

May be related to
Perceived, actual or potential loss of physiopsychosocial well-being, personal possessions, or SO; cultural beliefs about aging/debilitation

Possibly evidenced by
Denial of feelings, depression, sorrow, guilt
Alterations in activity level, sleep patterns, eating habits, libido

DESIRED OUTCOMES/EVALUATION CRITERIA—PATIENT WILL:
Identify and express feelings appropriately; progress through the grieving process.
Enjoy the present and plan for the future, one day at a time.

ACTIONS/INTERVENTIONS

Independent

Assess emotional state.

Make time to listen to the patient. Encourage free expression of hopeless feelings and desire to die.

Assess suicidal potential.

Involve SO in discussions and activities to the level of their willingness.

RATIONALE

Anxiety and depression are common reactions to changes/losses associated with long-term illness or debilitating condition. In addition, changes in neurotransmitter levels (e.g., increased MAO and serotonin levels with decreased norepinephrine) may potentiate depression in elderly patients.

It is more helpful to allow these feelings to be expressed and dealt with than to deny them.

May be related to physical disease, social isolation, and grief. *Note:* Studies indicate women are three times as likely to attempt suicide; however, men are three times as likely to succeed.

When SOs are involved, there is more potential for successful problem solving. *Note:* SO may not be available or may not choose to be involved.

ACTIONS/INTERVENTIONS

Independent

Provide liberal touching/hugs as individually accepted.

Identify spiritual concerns. Discuss available resources and encourage participation in religious activities as appropriate.

Assist with/plan for specifics as necessary, e.g., advance directives (to determine code status/Living Will wishes), making of will, funeral arrangements.

Collaborative

Refer to other resources as indicated, e.g., clinical specialist nurse, case manager/social worker, spiritual advisor.

RATIONALE

Conveys sense of concern/closeness to reduce feelings of isolation and enhance sense of self-worth. *Note:* Touch may be viewed as a threat by some patients and escalate feelings of anger.

Search for meaning is common to those facing changes in life. Participation in religious/spiritual activities can provide sense of direction and peace of mind.

Having these issues resolved can help patient/SO deal with the grieving process and may provide peace of mind.

May need further assistance to resolve some problems.

NURSING DIAGNOSIS: Thought Processes, altered

May be related to
Physiologic changes of aging, loss of cells/brain atrophy, decreased blood supply, altered sensory input
Pain; effects of medications
Psychologic conflicts: Disrupted life pattern

Possibly evidenced by
Slower reaction times, gradual memory loss, altered attention span; disorientation; inability to follow
Altered sleep patterns
Personality changes

DESIRED OUTCOMES/EVALUATION CRITERIA—PATIENT WILL:
Maintain usual reality orientation.
Recognize changes in thinking and behavior.
Identify interventions to deal effectively with situation/deficits.

ACTIONS/INTERVENTIONS

Independent

Allow adequate time for patient to respond to questions/comments and to make decisions.

Discuss happenings of the past. Place familiar objects in room. Encourage the display of photographs/photo albums, frequent visits from SO/friends.

RATIONALE

Reaction time may be slowed with aging (changes in metabolism/cerebral blood flow) or with brain injuries and some neuromuscular conditions.

Events of the past may be more readily recalled by the elderly patient, because long-term memory usually remains intact. Reminiscence/life review and companionship are beneficial to patients.

ACTIONS/INTERVENTIONS	RATIONALE
Independent	
Note patient's problem of short-term memory loss, and provide with aids (e.g., calendars, clocks, room signs, pictures) to assist in continual reorientation.	Short-term memory loss presents a challenge for nursing care, especially if the patient cannot remember such things as how to use the call bell or how to get to the bathroom. This problem is not in patient's control but may be less frustrating if simple reminders are used. It may be helpful for older person (and family) to know that short-term memory loss is common and is not necessarily a sign of "senility."
Evaluate individual stress level and deal with it appropriately.	Stress level may be greatly increased because of recent losses, e.g., poor health, death of spouse/companion, loss of home. In addition, some conflicts that occur with age come from previously unresolved problems that may need to be dealt with now.
Assess physical status/psychiatric symptoms. Institute interventions appropriate to findings.	Not all mental changes are the result of aging, and it is important to rule out physical causes before accepting these as unchangeable. May be metabolic, toxic, drug-induced (e.g., antiparkinson agents, tricyclic antidepressants), or the result of infectious, cardiac, or respiratory disorders.
Reorient to person/place and time as appropriate.	Helps patient maintain focus.
Have patient repeat verbal/written instructions.	Verifies hearing/ability to read and comprehend.
Note cyclic changes in mentation/behavior, e.g., evening confusion, picking at bedclothes, banging on side rails, pacing, shouting, wandering aimlessly.	"Sundowner syndrome" may occur in response to visual/hearing deficits enhanced by declining light, fatigue, inflexible institution schedules, peak/trough drug levels, dehydration, and electrolyte imbalances.
Involve in regular exercise and activity programs.	Promotes release of endorphins enhancing sense of well-being, and can improve thinking abilities. *Note:* Studies suggest withdrawn and inactive patients are at greater risk of evening confusion.
Schedule at least one rest period per day.	Prevents fatigue; enhances general well-being.
Provide brighter lighting in room/area by midafternoon (e.g., 3 PM) or earlier on cloudy/winter days.	Maximizes visual perception; may limit evening confusion.
Turn off lights at bedtime. Provide night lights where appropriate.	Reinforces "sleep time" while meeting safety needs.
Support patient's involvement in own care. Provide opportunity for choices on a daily basis.	Choice is a necessary component in everyday life. Cognitively impaired patients may respond with aggressive behavior as they lose control in their lives.
Collaborative	
Review results of laboratory/diagnostic tests, e.g., electrolytes, thyroid studies, RPR, full drug screen, CT scan.	Aids in establishing cause of changes in mentation and determining treatment options. *Note:* The latter four tests can identify the causes of dementia in 90% of the cases.

829

ACTIONS/INTERVENTIONS	RATIONALE
Independent	
Introduce staff and provide SO with information about facility and care. Be available for questions. Provide tour of facility.	Helpful to establish beginning relationships. Offers opportunities for enhancing feelings of involvement.
Determine involvement and availability of family/SO.	Clarifies expectations and abilities, identifies needs.
Encourage SO participation in care at level of desire and capability, and within limits of safety. Include in social events/celebrations.	Helps family to feel at ease and allows them to feel supportive and a part of the patient's life.
Accept choices of SO regarding level of involvement in care.	Families may choose to ignore patient or may project feelings of guilt regarding placing patient in LTC by criticizing staff. *Note:* Feelings of dissatisfaction with the staff may be transferred back to the patient.
Evaluate SO's/caregiver's level of stress/coping abilities, especially prior to planning for discharge.	Caring for/about patients with chronic/debilitating conditions places a heavy strain on SO. Although support groups may be very helpful, learning stress management techniques may be more effective in strengthening individual coping as the focus is on the SO rather than the SO-patient relationship.
Identify availability and use of community support systems.	Helps determine areas of need and provides information regarding additional resources to enhance coping.

ACTIONS/INTERVENTIONS

Independent

Be aware of staff's own feelings of anger and frustration about patient's/SO's choices and goals that differ from those of staff, and deal with appropriately.

Collaborative

Inform SO of services available to them (meal tickets, family cooking time, group care conference, visiting nurse, caseworker, social services).

RATIONALE

Group care conferences or individual counseling may be helpful in problem solving.

Promotes feeling of involvement; eases transition in adjustment to patient's admission.

NURSING DIAGNOSIS: Poisoning, risk for [drug toxicity]

Risk factors may include
Reduced metabolism; impaired circulation; precarious physiologic balance, presence of multiple diseases/organ involvement
Use of multiple prescribed/OTC drugs

Possibly evidenced by
[Not applicable; presence of signs and symptoms establishes an *actual* diagnosis]

DESIRED OUTCOMES/EVALUATION CRITERIA—PATIENT WILL:
Maintain prescribed drug regimen free of untoward side effects.

ACTIONS/INTERVENTIONS

Independent

Determine allergies and other drug history.

Review resources (e.g., drug manuals, pharmacist) for information about toxic symptoms and side effects. List drug actions and interactions and idiosyncracies, e.g., medications that are given with or without foods, as well as those that should not be crushed.

Discuss self-administration of/access to OTC products.

Identify swallowing problems or reluctance to take tablets or capsules.

Give pills in a spoonful of soft foods, e.g., applesauce, ice cream; or use liquid form of medication if available.

RATIONALE

Avoids repetition/creation of problems.

Provides information about drugs being taken and identifies possible interactions. Toxicity can be increased in the debilitated and older patient with symptoms not as apparent.

Limits interference with prescribed regimen/desired drug action and organ function. May prevent inadvertent overdosing/toxic reactions. *Note:* Appropriate use of OTC products kept at bedside or via free access at nurses' station fosters independence as well as enhances sense of control and self-esteem.

May not be able to or want to take medication.

Ensures proper dosage if patient is unable to/does not like to swallow pills.

ACTIONS/INTERVENTIONS	RATIONALE
Independent	
Open capsules or crush tablets only when appropriate.	Should not be done unless absolutely necessary as this may alter absorption of medications, e.g., enteric-coated tablets may be absorbed in stomach when crushed, instead of the intestines.
Make sure medication has been swallowed.	Ensures effective therapeutic use of medication and prevents pill hoarding.
Observe for changes in condition/behavior.	Behavior may be only indication of drug toxicity, and early identification of problems provides for appropriate intervention. *Note:* Elderly individuals have increased sensitivity to anticholinergic effects of medications; therefore, use of anticholinergics, antiparkinson agents, benzodiazepines, CNS depressants, and tricyclic antidepressants may cause delirium/confusion.
Use discretion in the administration of sedatives.	A quiet place where the patient can pace, or seclusion, may be more helpful. If patient is destructive or excessively disruptive, pharmacologic or mechanical control measures may be required. Convenience of the staff is never a reason for sedating patient; however, patient safety and rights of other patients need to be taken into consideration.
Collaborative	
Review drug regimen routinely with physician and pharmacist.	Provides opportunity to alter therapy (e.g., reduce dosage, discontinue medications) as patient's needs and organ functions change.
Obtain serum drug levels as indicated.	Determines therapeutic/toxicity levels.

NURSING DIAGNOSIS: Communication, impaired verbal

May be related to

Degenerative changes (e.g., reduced cerebral circulation, hearing loss); progressive neurologic disease (e.g., Parkinson's disease, Alzheimer's disease)

Laryngectomy/tracheostomy; stroke, traumatic brain injury

Possibly evidenced by

Impaired articulation; difficulty with phonation; inability to modulate speech, find words, name, or identify objects

Diminished hearing ability

Aphasia, dysarthria

DESIRED OUTCOMES/EVALUATION CRITERIA—PATIENT WILL:

Establish method of communication by which needs can be expressed.

Demonstrate congruent verbal and nonverbal communication.

ACTIONS/INTERVENTIONS	RATIONALE
Independent	
Assess reason for lack of communication, including CNS and neuromuscular functioning, gag/swallow reflexes, hearing, teeth/mouth problems.	Identification of the problem is essential to appropriate intervention. Sometimes patients do not want to talk, may think they talk when they do not, may expect others to know what they want, may not be able to comprehend or be understood.
Check for excess cerumen.	Hardened earwax may decrease hearing acuity and causes tinnitus.
Ascertain if patient has/uses hearing aid.	Patient may have, but not use, hearing aid (e.g., may not fit well, may need batteries).
Be aware that behavioral problems may indicate hearing loss.	Anger, explosive temper outbursts, frustration, embarrassment, depression, withdrawal, and paranoia may be attempts to deal with communication problems.
Determine whether patient is bilingual or whether English is primary language.	With declining cerebral function/diminished thought processes, increased level of stress, patient may mix languages/revert to original language.
Investigate how SO communicates with the patient.	Provides opportunity to develop/continue effective communication patterns, which have already been established.
Assess patient knowledge base and level of comprehension. Treat the patient as an adult, avoiding pity and impatience.	Knowing how much to expect of the patient can help to avoid frustration and unreasonable demands for performance. However, having an expectation that the patient will understand may help to raise level of performance.
Establish therapeutic nurse-patient relationship through Active-listening, being available for problem solving.	Aids in dealing with communication problems.
Make patient aware of presence when entering the room by turning a light off and on/touching patient or mattress as appropriate.	Getting attention is the first step in communication.
Make eye contact, place self at or below patient's level, and speak face to face.	Conveys interest and promotes contact.
Speak slowly and distinctly, using simple sentences, yes-or-no questions. Avoid speaking loudly or shouting. Supplement with written communication when possible/needed. Allow sufficient time for reply; remain relaxed with patient.	Assists in comprehension and overall communication. Patient may respond poorly to high-pitched sounds; shouting also obscures consonants and amplifies vowels.
Use other creative measures to assist in communication, e.g., picture chart/alphabet board, sign language, lip reading when appropriate.	Many options are available, depending on individual situation. *Note:* Sign language also may be used effectively with other than hearing-impaired individuals.

ACTIONS/INTERVENTIONS	RATIONALE
Collaborative	
Refer to speech therapists, ear, nose, and throat physician, or for audiometry as needed.	Determines extent of hearing loss and whether a hearing aid is appropriate. May be helpful to patient and staff in improving communication. *Note:* Some sources believe 90% of the patients in LTC facilities have some degree of hearing loss (presbycusis), as this is a common age change. Hearing aids are most effective with conductive losses and may help with sensorineural losses.

NURSING DIAGNOSIS: Sleep Pattern disturbance

May be related to
Internal factors: Illness, psychologic stress, inactivity
External factors: Environmental changes, facility routines

Possibly evidenced by
Reports of difficulty in falling asleep/not feeling well-rested
Interrupted sleep, awakening earlier than desired
Change in behavior/performance, increasing irritability, listlessness

DESIRED OUTCOMES/EVALUATION CRITERIA—PATIENT WILL:
Report improvement in sleep/rest pattern.
Verbalize increased sense of well-being and feeling rested.

ACTIONS/INTERVENTIONS	RATIONALE
Independent	
Ascertain usual sleep habits and changes that are occurring.	Determines need for action and helps identify appropriate interventions.
Provide comfortable bedding and some of own possessions, e.g., pillow, afghan.	Increases comfort for sleep as well as physiologic/psychologic support.
Establish new sleep routine incorporating old pattern and new environment.	When new routine contains as many aspects of old habits as possible, stress and related anxiety may be reduced.
Match with roommate who has similar sleep patterns and nocturnal needs.	Decreases likelihood that "night owl" roommate may delay patient's falling asleep or create interruptions that cause awakening.
Encourage some light physical activity during the day. Make sure patient stops activity several hours before bedtime as individually appropriate.	Daytime activity can help patient expend energy and be ready for nighttime sleep; however, continuation of activity close to bedtime may act as a stimulant, delaying sleep.
Promote bedtime comfort regimens, e.g., warm bath and massage, a glass of warm milk, wine, or brandy at bedtime.	Promotes a relaxing, soothing effect. *Note:* Milk has soporific qualities, enhancing synthesis of serotonin, a neurotransmitter that helps patient fall asleep faster and sleep longer.

ACTIONS/INTERVENTIONS	RATIONALE
Independent	
Instruct in relaxation measures.	Helps to induce sleep.
Reduce noise and light.	Provides atmosphere conducive to sleep.
Encourage position of comfort, assist in turning.	Repositioning alters areas of pressure and promotes rest.
Use side rails as indicated; lower bed when possible.	May have fear of falling because of change in size and height of bed. Side rails provide safety and may be used to assist with turning. *Note:* Some people do better with no side rails and tend to fall when climbing over side rails.
Avoid interruptions when possible (e.g., awakening for medications or therapies).	Uninterrupted sleep is more restful, and patient may be unable to return to sleep when wakened.
Collaborative	
Administer sedatives, hypnotics, as indicated.	May be given to help patient sleep/rest during transition period from home to new setting. *Note:* Avoid habitual use, because these drugs decrease REM sleep time.

NURSING DIAGNOSIS: Nutrition: altered, less/more than body requirements

May be related to
Impaired dentition; dulling of senses of smell and taste
Cognitive limitations, depression
Inability to feed self effectively
Sedentary activity level

Possibly evidenced by
Reported/observed dysfunctional eating patterns
Weight under/over ideal for height and frame
Poor muscle tone, pale conjunctiva/mucous membranes
Signs/symptoms of vitamin/protein deficits, electrolyte imbalances

DESIRED OUTCOMES/EVALUATION CRITERIA—PATIENT WILL:
Maintain normal weight or progress toward weight goal with normalization of laboratory values and be free of signs of malnutrition/obesity.
Demonstrate eating patterns/behaviors to maintain appropriate weight.

ACTIONS/INTERVENTIONS	RATIONALE
Independent	
Assess causes of weight loss/gain, e.g., dysphagia due to neurogenic/psychogenic disturbances, tumors, muscular dysfunction, or dysfunctional eating patterns related to depression.	Aids in creating plan of care/choice of interventions.

ACTIONS/INTERVENTIONS	RATIONALE
Independent	
Check state of patient's dental health periodically, including fit and condition of dentures, if present.	Oral infections/dental problems, shrinking gums, and loose-fitting dentures decrease patient's ability to chew.
Weigh on admission and on a regular basis.	Monitors nutritional state and effectiveness of interventions.
Monitor total caloric intake as indicated.	If dietary plan is ineffective in meeting individual goals, calorie count/food diary may help identify problem areas.
Observe condition of skin; note muscle wasting, brittle nails; dry, lifeless hair, and signs of poor healing.	Reflects lack of adequate nutrition.
Evaluate activity pattern.	Extremes of exercise (e.g., sedentary life, continuous pacing) affect caloric needs.
Incorporate favorite foods and maintain as near-normal food consistency as possible, e.g., soft or finely ground food with gravy or liquid added. Avoid baby food whenever possible.	Aids in maintaining intake, especially when mouth and dental problems exist. Baby food is often unpalatable and can decrease appetite and lower self-esteem.
Encourage the use of spices (other than sodium) to patient's personal taste.	Reduction in number and acuity of taste buds results in food tasting bland and decreases enjoyment of food and desire to eat.
Provide small, frequent feedings as indicated.	Decreased gastric motility causes patient to feel full and reduces intake.
Serve hot foods hot and cold foods cold.	Foods served at the proper temperature are more palatable, and enjoyment may increase appetite.
Promote a pleasant environment for eating, with company if possible.	Eating is in part a social event, and appetite can improve with increased socialization.
Have snack foods (e.g., cheese, crackers, soup, fruit) available on a 24-hour basis.	Helps meet individual needs and enhances intake.
Plan for social events; provide for snacks, even when working to reduce total calories.	Eating is part of socialization, and being able to respond to body's needs enhances sense of control and willingness to participate in dietary program.
Encourage exercise and activity program within individual ability.	Promotes sense of well-being and may improve appetite.
Collaborative	
Consult with dietitian.	Aids in establishing specific nutritional program to meet individual patient needs.
Provide balanced diet with individually appropriate protein, complex carbohydrates, and calories. Include supplements between meals as indicated. Administer vitamin/mineral supplements as appropriate.	Adjustments may be needed to deal with the body's decreased ability to process protein, as well as decreased metabolic rate and levels of activity. *Note:* Elderly individuals have delayed insulin release by the pancreas and reduced peripheral sensitivity to insulin, decreasing their glucose tolerance.
Refer for dental care routinely and as needed.	Maintenance of oral/dental health and good dentition can enhance intake.

NURSING DIAGNOSIS: Self Care deficit: (specify)

May be related to

Depression, discouragement, loss of mobility, general debilitation; perceptual/cognitive impairment

Possibly evidenced by

Inability to manage ADLs; unkempt appearance

DESIRED OUTCOMES/EVALUATION CRITERIA—PATIENT WILL:

Perform self-care activities within level of own ability.

Demonstrate techniques/lifestyle changes to meet own needs.

Use resources effectively.

ACTIONS/INTERVENTIONS	RATIONALE
Independent	
Determine current capabilities (0–4 scale) and barriers to participation in care.	Identifies need for/level of interventions required.
Involve patient in formulation of plan of care at level of ability.	Enhances sense of control and aids in cooperation and development of independence.
Encourage self-care. Work with present abilities; do not pressure patient beyond capabilities. Provide adequate time for patient to complete tasks. Have expectation of improvement and assist as needed.	Doing for oneself enhances feeling of self-worth. Failure can produce discouragement and depression.
Provide and promote privacy, including during bathing/showering.	Modesty may lead to reluctance to participate in care or perform activities in the presence of others.
Use specialized equipment as needed, e.g., tub transfer seat, grab bars, raised toilet seat.	Enhances ability to move/perform activities safely.
Give tub bath, using a 2-person or mechanical lift if necessary. Use shower chair and spray attachment, as appropriate. Avoid chilling.	Provides safety for those who cannot get into the tub alone. Shower may be more feasible for some patients, though it may be less beneficial/desirable to the patient. Elderly/debilitated patients are more prone to chilling.
Shampoo/style hair as needed. Provide/assist with manicure.	Aids in maintaining appearance. Shampooing may be required more/less frequently than bathing schedule.
Encourage use of barber/beauty salon if patient is able.	Enhances self-image and self-esteem, preserving dignity of the patient.
Acquire clothing with modified fasteners as indicated.	Use of Velcro instead of buttons/shoe laces can facilitate process of dressing/undressing.
Encourage/assist with routine mouth/teeth care daily.	Reduces risk of gum disease/tooth loss; promotes proper fitting of dentures.
Collaborative	
Consult with physical/occupational therapists and rehabilitation specialist.	Useful in establishing exercise/activity program and in identifying assistive devices to meet individual needs/facilitate independence.

837

> ### NURSING DIAGNOSIS: Skin Integrity, impaired, risk for
>
> **Risk factors may include**
>
> General debilitation; reduced mobility; changes in skin and muscle mass associated
> with aging, sensory/motor deficits
> Altered circulation; edema; poor nutrition
> Excretions/secretions (bladder and bowel incontinence)
> Problems with self-care
>
> **Possibly evidenced by**
>
> [Not applicable; presence of signs and symptoms establishes an *actual* diagnosis]
>
> ### DESIRED OUTCOMES/EVALUATION CRITERIA—PATIENT WILL:
>
> Maintain intact skin.
> Identify individual risk factors.
> Demonstrate behaviors/techniques to prevent skin breakdown/facilitate healing.

ACTIONS/INTERVENTIONS	RATIONALE
Independent	
Anticipate and use preventive measures in patients who are at risk for skin breakdown, such as anyone who is thin, obese, aging, or debilitated.	Decubitus ulcers are difficult to heal, and prevention is the best treatment.
Assess nutritional status and initiate corrective measures as indicated. Provide balanced diet, e.g., adequate protein, vitamins, and minerals.	A positive nitrogen balance and improved nutritional state can help prevent skin breakdown and promote ulcer healing. *Note:* May need additional calories and protein if draining ulcer present.
Maintain strict skin hygiene, using mild, nondetergent soap (if any), drying gently and thoroughly, and lubricating with lotion or emollient.	A daily bath is usually not necessary in elderly patients because there is atrophy of sebaceous and sweat glands, and bathing may create dry-skin problems. However, as epidermis thins with age, cleansing and use of lubricants is needed to keep skin soft/pliable and protect susceptible skin from breakdown.
Change position frequently in bed and chair. Recommend 10 minutes of exercise each hour and/or perform passive ROM.	Improves circulation, muscle tone, and joint motion and promotes patient participation.
Use a rotation schedule in turning patient. Use draw/turn sheet. Pay close attention to patient's comfort level.	Allows for longer periods free of pressure; prevents shearing or tearing motions that can damage fragile tissues. *Note:* Use of prone position is dependent on patient tolerance and should be maintained for only a short time.
Massage bony prominences gently with lotion or cream.	Enhances circulation to tissues, increases vascular tone, and reduces tissue edema. *Note:* Contraindicated if area is pink/red, as cellular damage may occur. Gentle massage *around* area may stimulate circulation to impaired tissues.

ACTIONS/INTERVENTIONS	RATIONALE
Independent	
Keep sheets and bedclothes clean, dry, and free from wrinkles, crumbs, and other irritating material.	Avoids friction/abrasions of skin.
Use elbow/heel protectors, foam/water or gel pads, sheepskin for positioning in bed and when up in chair.	Reduces risk of tissue abrasions and decreases pressure that can impair cellular blood flow. Promotes circulation of air along skin surface to dissipate heat/moisture.
Provide for safety during ambulation.	Loss of muscle control and debilitation may result in impaired coordination.
Limit exposure to temperature extremes/use of heating pad or ice pack.	Decreased sensitivity to pain/heat/cold increases risk of tissue trauma.
Examine feet and nails routinely and provide foot and nail care as indicated:	Foot problems are common among patients who are bedfast/debilitated.
Keep nails cut short and smooth;	Jagged, rough nails can cause tissue damage/infection.
Use lotion, softening cream on feet;	Prevents drying/cracking of skin; promotes maintenance of healthy skin.
Check for fissures between toes. Swab with hydrogen peroxide or dust with antiseptic powder and place a wisp of cotton between the toes;	Prevents spread of infection and/or tissue injury.
Rub feet with witch hazel or a mentholated preparation and have patient wear lightweight cotton stockings.	Even though rash may not be present, burning and itching may be a problem. *Note:* Witch hazel may be contraindicated if skin is dry.
Inspect skin surface/folds (especially when incontinence pad/pants are used) and bony prominences routinely. Increase preventive measures when reddened areas are noticed.	Skin breakdown can occur quickly with potential for infection and necrosis, possibly involving muscle and bone. There is increased risk of redness/irritation around legs due to elastic bands in adult diapers/incontinence pads.
Continue regimen for redness and irritation when break in skin occurs.	Aggressive measures are important because decubitus ulcers can develop in a matter of a few hours.
Observe for decubitus ulcer development, and treat immediately according to protocol.	Timely intervention may prevent extensive damage.
Collaborative	
Provide waterbed, alternating pressure/egg-crate or gel mattress, and pad for chair.	Provides protection and improves circulation by decreasing amount of pressure on tissues.
Monitor Hb/Hct and blood glucose levels.	Anemia, dehydration, and elevated glucose levels are factors in skin breakdown and can impair healing.
Refer to podiatrist as indicated.	May need professional care for such problems as ingrown toenails, corns, bony changes, skin/tissue ulceration.
Provide whirlpool treatments as appropriate.	Increases circulation and has a débriding action.
Assist with topical applications; skin barrier dressings (Duoderm, Op-Site); collagenase therapy; absorbable gelatin sponges (Gelfoam); aerosol sprays.	Although there are differing opinions about the efficacy of these agents, individual or combination use may enhance healing.

839

ACTIONS/INTERVENTIONS

Collaborative

Administer nutritional supplements and vitamins as indicated.

Prepare for/assist with skin grafting. (Refer to CP: Burns: Thermal/Chemical/Electrical (Acute and Convalescent Phases), ND: Skin Integrity, impaired, p 698.)

RATIONALE

Aids in healing/cellular regeneration.

May be needed to close large ulcers.

NURSING DIAGNOSIS: Urinary Elimination, altered, risk for

Risk factors may include
Changes in fluid/nutritional pattern
Neuromuscular changes
Perceptual/cognitive impairment

Possibly evidenced by
[Not applicable; presence of signs and symptoms establishes an *actual* diagnosis]

DESIRED OUTCOMES/EVALUATION CRITERIA—PATIENT WILL:
Maintain/regain effective pattern of elimination.
Initiate necessary lifestyle changes.
Participate in treatment regimen to correct/control situation, e.g., bladder training program or use of indwelling catheter.

ACTIONS/INTERVENTIONS

Independent

Monitor voiding pattern. Identify possible reasons for changes, e.g., disorientation, neuromuscular impairment, psychotropic medications.

Palpate bladder. Observe for "overflow" voiding; determine frequency and timing of dribbling/voiding.

Promote fluid intake of 2000–3000 ml/d within cardiac tolerance; include fruit juices, especially cranberry juice. Schedule fluid intake times appropriately.

Institute bladder program (including scheduled voiding times, Kegel exercise) involving patient and staff in a positive manner.

Assist patient to sit upright on bedpan/commode.

Provide/encourage perineal care daily and prn.

Use adult incontinence pads/pants during day if needed. Keep patient clean and dry. Provide frequent skin care.

RATIONALE

This information is essential to plan for care and influences choice of individual interventions.

Bladder distention indicates urinary retention, which may cause incontinence and infection.

Maintains adequate hydration and promotes kidney function. Acid-ash juices act as an internal pH acidifier, retarding bacterial growth. *Note:* Patient may decrease fluid intake in an attempt to control incontinence and become dehydrated. Instead, fluids may be scheduled to decrease frequency of incontinence (e.g., limit fluids after 6 PM to reduce need to void during the night).

Regular toileting times may help to control incontinence. Program is more apt to be successful when positive attitudes and cooperation are present.

Provides functional position for voiding.

Reduces risk of contamination/ascending infection.

When training is unsuccessful, this is the preferred method of management. *Note:* Using incontinence pads during night exposes skin to air, reducing risk of irritation.

840

ACTIONS/INTERVENTIONS

Independent

Avoid verbal or nonverbal signs of rejection, disgust, or disapproval over failures.

Provide regular catheter care and maintain patency if indwelling catheter is present.

Collaborative

Administer medications as indicated, e.g.:

Oxybutynin chloride (Ditropan);

Vitamin C, methenamine hippurate (Hiprex), methenamine mandelate (Mandelamine).

Maintain indwelling catheter/provide intermittent catheterization.

Irrigate catheter with acetic acid, if indicated.

RATIONALE

Expressions of disapproval lower self-esteem and are not helpful to a successful program.

Prevents infection and/or minimizes reflux.

Promotes bladder sphincter control.

Bladder pH acidifiers retard bacterial growth.

May be used if continence cannot be maintained to prevent skin breakdown and resultant problems.

May be done to maintain acid pH and retard bacterial growth.

NURSING DIAGNOSIS: Constipation/Diarrhea, risk for

Risk factors may include

Changes in/inadequate nutritional or fluid intake; poor muscle tone; change in level of activity

Medication side effects

Perceptual/cognitive impairment, depression

Lack of privacy

Possibly evidenced by

[Not applicable; presence of signs and symptoms establishes an *actual* diagnosis]

DESIRED OUTCOMES/EVALUATION CRITERIA—PATIENT WILL:

Establish/maintain normal patterns of bowel functioning.

Demonstrate changes in lifestyle as necessitated by risk or contributing factors.

Participate in bowel program, as indicated.

ACTIONS/INTERVENTIONS

Independent

Ascertain usual bowel pattern and aids used (e.g., previous long-term laxative use). Compare with current routine.

Assess reasons for problems; rule out medical causes, e.g., bowel obstruction, cancer, hemorrhoids, drugs, impaction.

Determine presence of food/drug sensitivities.

Institute individualized program of exercise, rest, diet, and bowel retraining.

RATIONALE

Determines extent of problem and indicates need for/type of interventions appropriate. Many patients may already be laxative-dependent, and it is important to reestablish as near-normal functioning as possible.

Identification/treatment of underlying medical condition is necessary to achieve optimal bowel function.

May contribute to diarrhea.

Depends on the needs of the patient. Loss of muscular tone reduces peristalsis or may impair control of rectal sphincter.

841

ACTIONS/INTERVENTIONS	RATIONALE

Independent

Provide diet high in bulk in the form of whole-grain cereals, breads, fresh fruits (especially prunes, plums).	Improves stool consistency, promotes evacuation.
Decrease or eliminate foods such as dairy products.	These foods are known to be constipating.
Encourage increased fluid intake.	Promotes normal stool consistency.
Use adult incontinence pads/pants, if needed. Keep patient clean and dry. Provide frequent perineal care. Apply skin protective ointment to anal area.	Prevents skin breakdown.
Keep air freshener in room/at bedside or in bathroom.	Limits noxious odors and may help reduce patient embarrassment/concern.
Give emotional support to patient. Avoid "blaming" (talk/actions) if incontinence occurs.	Decreases feelings of frustration and embarrassment.

Collaborative

Administer medications as indicated:

Bulk-providers/stool softeners, e.g., Metamucil;	Promotes regularity by increasing bulk and/or improving stool consistency.
Camphorated tincture of opium (Paregoric), diphenoxylate with atropine (Lomotil).	May be needed on a short-term basis when diarrhea persists.

NURSING DIAGNOSIS: Physical Mobility, impaired

May be related to
Decreased strength and endurance, neuromuscular impairment
Pain/discomfort
Perceptual/cognitive impairment

Possibly evidenced by
Impaired coordination, limited ROM; decreased muscle mass, strength, control
Reluctance to attempt movement; inability to purposefully move

DESIRED OUTCOMES/EVALUATION CRITERIA—PATIENT WILL:
Verbalize willingness to and participate in desired activities.
Demonstrate techniques/behaviors that enable continuation or resumption of activities.
Maintain/increase strength and function of affected body parts.

ACTIONS/INTERVENTIONS	RATIONALE

Independent

Determine functional ability (0–4 scale) and reasons for impairment.	Identifies need for/degree of intervention required.
Note emotional/behavioral responses to altered ability.	Physical changes and loss of independence often create feelings of anger, frustration, and depression that may be manifested as reluctance to engage in activity.
Plan activities/visits with adequate rest periods as necessary.	Prevents fatigue; conserves energy for continued participation.

ACTIONS/INTERVENTIONS	RATIONALE

Independent

Encourage participation in self-care, occupational/recreational activities.

Promotes independence and self-esteem; may enhance willingness to participate.

Assist with transfers and ambulation if indicated; show patient/SO ways to move safely.

Prevents accidental falls/injury.

Obtain supportive shoes and well-fitting, nonskid slippers.

Assists patient to walk with a firm step/maintain sense of balance and prevents slipping.

Remove extraneous furniture from pathways.

Prevents patient from bumping into furniture and reduces risk of falling/injuring self.

Encourage use of hand rails in hallway, stairwells, and bathrooms.

Promotes independence in mobility; reduces risk of falls.

Review safe use of mobility aids/adjunctive devices, e.g., walker, braces, prosthetics.

Facilitates activity, reduces risk of injury.

Provide chairs with firm, high seats and lifting chairs when indicated.

Facilitates rising from seated position.

Provide for environmental changes to meet visual deficiencies.

Prevents accidents and sensory deprivation. If patient is blind, will need assistance and ongoing orientation to surroundings.

Speak to patient when entering the room, and let patient know when leaving.

Special actions help patient who cannot see to know when someone is there.

Encourage the patient with glasses/contacts to wear them. Be sure glasses are kept clean.

Optimal visual acuity facilitates participation in activities and reduces risk of falls/injury.

Determine reason if glasses are not being worn.

Patient may not be wearing glasses because they need adjustment or change in correction.

Collaborative

Consult with physical/occupational therapists, rehabilitation specialist.

Useful in creating individual exercise/activity program and identifying adjunctive aids.

Arrange for regular eye examinations.

Identifies development/progression of vision problem (e.g., myopia, hyperopia, presbyopia, astigmatism, cataract and glaucoma, tunnel vision, blindness) and specific options for care.

NURSING DIAGNOSIS: Diversional Activity deficit

May be related to
Environmental lack of diversional activity; long-term care requirements
Physical limitations; psychologic condition, e.g., depression

Possibly evidenced by
Statements of boredom, depression, lack of energy
Disinterest, lethargy, withdrawn behavior, hostility

DESIRED OUTCOMES/EVALUATION CRITERIA—PATIENT WILL:
Recognize own response and initiate appropriate coping actions.
Engage in satisfying activities within personal limitations.

843

ACTIONS/INTERVENTIONS	RATIONALE

Independent

Determine avocation/hobbies patient previously pursued. Incorporate activities, if appropriate, into present program.

Encourages involvement and helps to stimulate patient mentally/physically to improve overall condition and sense of well-being.

Encourage participation in mix of activities/stimuli, e.g., music, news program, educational presentations, crafts as appropriate.

Offering different activities helps patient to try out new ideas and develop new interests. Activities need to be personally meaningful for the patient to derive the most enjoyment from them (e.g., talking or Braille books for the blind, closed-captioned TV broadcasts for the deaf/hearing impaired).

Provide change of scenery when possible; alter personal environment; encourage trips to shop/participate in local/family events.

Stimulates energy and provides new outlook for patient.

Collaborative

Refer to occupational therapist, activity director.

Can introduce and design new programs to provide positive stimuli for the patient.

NURSING DIAGNOSIS: Sexuality Patterns, altered, risk for

Risk factors may include
Biopsychosocial alteration of sexuality
Interference in psychologic/physical well-being; self-image
Lack of privacy/SO

Possibly evidenced by
[Not applicable; presence of signs and symptoms establishes an *actual* diagnosis]

DESIRED OUTCOMES/EVALUATION CRITERIA—PATIENT WILL:
Verbalize knowledge and understanding of sexual limitations, difficulties, or changes that have occurred.
Demonstrate improved communication and relationship skills.
Identify appropriate options to meet needs.

ACTIONS/INTERVENTIONS	RATIONALE

Independent

Note patient/SO cues regarding sexuality.

May be concerned that condition/environmental restrictions may interfere with sexual function or ability, but be afraid to ask directly.

Determine cultural and religious/value factors and conflicts that may be present.

Affects patient's perception of existing problems and response of others (e.g., family, staff, other residents). Provides starting point for discussion and problem solving.

Assess developmental and lifestyle issues.

Factors such as menopause and aging, adolescence and young adulthood need to be taken into consideration with regard to sexual concerns about illness and long-term care.

ACTIONS/INTERVENTIONS

Independent

Provide atmosphere in which discussion of sexuality is encouraged/permitted.

Provide privacy for patient/SO.

Collaborative

Refer to sex counselor/therapist, family therapy when needed.

RATIONALE

When concerns are identified and discussed, problem solving can occur.

Demonstrates acceptance of need for intimacy and provides opportunity to continue previous patterns of interaction as much as possible.

May require additional assistance for resolution of problems.

NURSING DIAGNOSIS: Health Maintenance, altered

May be related to
Lack of, or significant alteration in, communication skills
Complete or partial lack of gross and/or fine motor skills
Perceptual/cognitive impairment, lack of ability to make deliberate/thoughtful judgments
Lack of material resources

Possibly evidenced by
Demonstrated lack of knowledge regarding basic health practices
Reported/observed inability to take responsibility for meeting basic health needs; impairment of personal support system
Demonstrated lack of behaviors adaptive to internal or external environmental changes

DESIRED OUTCOMES/EVALUATION CRITERIA—PATIENT WILL:
Verbalize understanding of factors contributing to current situation.
Adopt lifestyle changes supporting individual healthcare goals.
Assume responsibility for own healthcare needs when possible.

ACTIONS/INTERVENTIONS

Independent

Assess level of adaptive behavior; knowledge and skills about health maintenance, environment, and safety.

Provide information about individual healthcare needs.

Note patient's previous use of professional services, and continue as appropriate. Include in choice of new healthcare providers as able.

Maintain adequate hydration and balanced diet with sufficient protein intake.

RATIONALE

Identifies areas of concern/need and aids in choice of interventions.

Provides knowledge base and encourages participation in decision making.

Preserves continuity and promotes independence in meeting own healthcare needs.

Promotes general well-being and aids in disease prevention.

ACTIONS/INTERVENTIONS	RATIONALE

Independent

Schedule adequate rest with progressive activity program.	Prevents fatigue and enhances general well-being.
Promote good hand-washing and personal hygiene. Use aseptic techniques as necessary.	Prevents contamination/cross-contamination, reducing risk of illness/infection.
Protect from exposure to infections; avoid extremes of temperature. Recommend the wearing of masks/other interventions as indicated.	With age, immune protective responses slow down and physiologic reactions to temperature extremes may be impaired. As organ function decreases and natural antibodies decline, patients are at increased risk for infection. Staff and/or visitors with colds or other infections may expose patient to these illnesses.
Encourage cessation of smoking.	Smokers are prone to bronchitis and ineffective clearing of secretions.
Encourage reporting of signs/symptoms as they occur.	Provides opportunity for early recognition of developing complications and timely intervention to prevent serious illness.
Observe for/monitor changes in vital signs, e.g., temperature elevation.	Early identification of onset of illness allows for timely intervention and may prevent serious complications. *Note:* Elderly persons often display subnormal temperatures, so presence of a low-grade fever may be of serious concern.

Collaborative

Administer medications as indicated:	
Immunizations, e.g., *Haemophilus influenzae,* flu, pneumonia;	Reduces risk of acquiring contagious/potentially life-threatening diseases.
Antibiotics.	May be used prophylactically (rare) and to treat infections.
Schedule preventive/routine healthcare appointments based on individual needs, e.g., with cardiologist, podiatrist, ophthalmologist, dentist.	Promotes optimal recovery/maintenance of health.

POTENTIAL CONSIDERATIONS following discharge from care facility

Refer to plan of care for diagnosis that required admission.

ALCOHOLISM [ACUTE]: INTOXICATION/OVERDOSE

Alcohol is a CNS depressant drug that is used socially in our society for many reasons, e.g., to enhance the flavor of food, encourage relaxation and conviviality, for feelings of celebration, and as a sacred ritual in some religious ceremonies. Therapeutically, it is the major ingredient in many OTC/prescription medications. It can be harmless, enjoyable, and sometimes beneficial when used responsibly and in moderation. Like other mind-altering drugs, however, it has the potential for abuse, is the most widely abused drug in the United States (research suggests 5%–10% of adult population), and is potentially fatal.

CARE SETTING

May be inpatient on a behavioral unit or outpatient in community programs.

Although patients are not generally admitted to the acute care setting with this diagnosis, withdrawal from alcohol may occur secondarily during hospitalization for other illnesses/conditions, or a short stay may be required during acute phase due to severity of general condition.

RELATED CONCERNS

Cirrhosis of the Liver, p 466
Upper Gastrointestinal/Esophageal Bleeding, p 315
Heart Failure: Chronic, p 45
Psychosocial Aspects of Care, p 783
Substance Dependence/Abuse Rehabilitation, p 862

Patient Assessment Data Base

Data is dependent on the duration/extent of use of alcohol, concurrent use of other drugs, and degree of organ involvement.

ACTIVITY/REST

May report: Difficulty sleeping, not feeling well rested

CIRCULATION

May exhibit: Generalized tissue edema (due to protein deficiencies)
Peripheral pulses weak, irregular, or rapid
Hypertension common in early withdrawal stage but may become labile/progress to hypotension
Tachycardia common during acute withdrawal; numerous dysrhythmias may be identified.

EGO INTEGRITY

May report: Feelings of guilt/shame; defensiveness about drinking
Denial, rationalization
Multiple stressors/losses (relationships, employment, finances)

ELIMINATION

May report: Diarrhea

May exhibit: Bowel sounds varied (may reflect gastric complications, e.g., hemorrhage)

FOOD/FLUID

May report: Nausea/vomiting; food intolerance

May exhibit: Gastric distention; ascites, liver enlargement (seen in cirrhosis)

Muscle wasting, dry/dull hair, swollen salivary glands, inflamed buccal cavity, capillary fragility (malnutrition)

Bowel sounds varied (reflecting malnutrition, electrolyte imbalances, general bowel dysfunction)

NEUROSENSORY

May report: "Internal shakes"

Headache, dizziness, blurred vision; "blackouts"

May exhibit: Psychopathology, e.g., paranoid schizophrenia, major depression (may indicate dual diagnosis)

Level of consciousness/orientation: Confusion, stupor, hyperactivity, distorted thought processes, slurred/incoherent speech

Memory loss/confabulation

Affect/mood/behavior: May be fearful, anxious, easily startled, inappropriate, silly, euphoric, irritable, physically/verbally abusive, depressed, and/or paranoid

Hallucinations: Visual, tactile, olfactory, and auditory, e.g., patient may be picking items out of air or responding verbally to unseen person/voices

Nystagmus (associated with cranial nerve palsy)

Pupil constriction (may indicate CNS depression)

Arcus senilis (ringlike opacity of the cornea): Although normal in aging populations, suggests alcohol-related changes in younger patients

Fine motor tremors of face, tongue, and hands; seizures (commonly grand mal)

Gait unsteady (ataxia), may be due to thiamine deficiency or cerebellar degeneration (Wernicke's encephalopathy)

PAIN/DISCOMFORT

May report: Constant upper abdominal pain and tenderness radiating to the back (pancreatic inflammation)

RESPIRATION

May report: History of smoking, recurrent/chronic respiratory problems

May exhibit: Tachypnea (hyperactive state of alcohol withdrawal)

Cheyne-Stokes respirations or respiratory depression

Breath sounds: Diminished/adventitious sounds (suggests pulmonary complications, e.g., respiratory depression, pneumonia)

SAFETY

May report: History of recurrent trauma such as falls, fractures, lacerations, burns, blackouts, or automobile accidents

May exhibit: Skin: Flushed face/palms of hands; scars, ecchymotic areas; cigarette burns on fingers, spider nevus (impaired portal circulation), fissures at corners of mouth (vitamin deficiency)

Fractures: Healed or new (signs of recent/recurrent trauma)

Temperature elevation (dehydration and sympathetic stimulation); flushing/diaphoresis (suggests presence of infection)

Suicidal ideation/suicide attempts (some research suggests alcoholic suicide attempts are 30% higher than national average for general population)

SOCIAL INTERACTION

May report: Frequent sick days off from work/school; fighting with others, arrests (disorderly conduct, motor vehicle violations/DUIs)

Denial that alcohol intake has any significant effect on present condition

Dysfunctional family system of origin (generational involvement); problems in current relationships

Mood changes affecting interactions with others

TEACHING/LEARNING

May report: History of alcohol and/or other drug use/abuse

Family history of alcoholism

Ignorance and/or denial of addiction to alcohol, or inability to cut down or stop drinking despite repeated efforts

Large amount of alcohol consumed in last 24–48 hours, previous periods of abstinence/withdrawal

Previous hospitalizations for alcoholism/alcohol-related diseases, e.g., cirrhosis, esophageal varices

Discharge plan considerations: **DRG projected mean length of inpatient stay: 4.5 days**

May require assistance to maintain abstinence and begin to participate in rehabilitation program

Refer to section at end of plan for postdischarge considerations.

DIAGNOSTIC STUDIES

Blood alcohol/drug levels: Alcohol level may/may not be severely elevated, depending on amount consumed and time between consumption and testing. In addition to alcohol, numerous controlled substances may be identified in a poly-drug screen, e.g., amphetamine, cocaine, morphine, Percodan, Quaalude.

CBC: Decreased Hb/Hct may reflect such problems as iron-deficiency anemia or acute/chronic GI bleeding. WBC count may be increased with infection or decreased if immunosuppressed.

Glucose: Hyperglycemia/hypoglycemia may be present, related to pancreatitis, malnutrition, or depletion of liver glycogen stores.

Electrolytes: Hypokalemia and hypomagnesemia are common.

Liver function tests: CPK, LDH, AST, ALT, and amylase may be elevated, reflecting liver or pancreatic damage.

Nutritional tests: Albumin is low and total protein may be decreased. Vitamin deficiencies are usually present, reflecting malnutrition/malabsorption.

Other screening studies (e.g., hepatitis, HIV, TB): Dependent on general condition, individual risk factors, and care setting.

Urinalysis: Infection may be identified; ketones may be present, related to breakdown of fatty acids in malnutrition (pseudodiabetic condition).

Chest x-ray: May reveal right lower lobe pneumonia (malnutrition, depressed immune system, aspiration) or chronic lung disorders associated with tobacco use.

ECG: Dysrhythmias, cardiomyopathies, and/or ischemia may be present owing to direct effect of alcohol on the cardiac muscle and/or conduction system, as well as effects of electrolyte imbalance.

Addiction Severity Index (ASI): An assessment tool that produces a "problem severity profile" of the patient, including chemical, medical, psychologic, legal, family/social, and employment/support aspects, indicating areas of treatment needs.

NURSING PRIORITIES

1. Maintain physiologic stability during acute withdrawal phase.
2. Promote patient safety.
3. Provide appropriate referral and follow-up.
4. Encourage/support SO involvement in "Intervention" (confrontation) process.
5. Provide information about condition/prognosis and treatment needs.

DISCHARGE GOALS

1. Homeostasis achieved.
2. Complications prevented/resolved.
3. Sobriety being maintained on a day-to-day basis.
4. Ongoing participation in rehabilitation program/attending group therapy, e.g., Alcoholics Anonymous.
5. Condition, prognosis, and therapeutic regimen understood.
6. Plan in place to meet needs after discharge.

This plan of care is to be used in conjunction with CP: Substance Dependence/Abuse Rehabilitation.

NURSING DIAGNOSIS: Breathing Pattern, ineffective, risk for

Risk factors may include
Direct effect of alcohol toxicity on respiratory center and/or sedative drugs given to decrease alcohol withdrawal symptoms
Tracheobronchial obstruction
Presence of chronic respiratory problems, inflammatory process
Decreased energy/fatigue

Possibly evidenced by
[Not applicable; presence of signs and symptoms establishes an *actual* diagnosis]

DESIRED OUTCOMES/EVALUATION CRITERIA—PATIENT WILL:
Maintain effective breathing pattern with respiratory rate within normal range, lungs clear; free of cyanosis and other signs/symptoms of hypoxia.

ACTIONS/INTERVENTIONS	RATIONALE
Independent	
Monitor respiratory rate/depth and pattern as indicated. Note periods of apnea, Cheyne-Stokes respirations.	Frequent assessment is important because toxicity levels may change rapidly. Hyperventilation is common during acute withdrawal phase. Kussmaul's respirations are sometimes present due to acidotic state associated with vomiting and malnutrition. However, marked respiratory depression can occur due to CNS depressant effects of alcohol. This may be compounded by drugs used to control alcohol withdrawal symptoms.
Elevate head of bed.	Decreases possibility of aspiration; lowers diaphragm to enhance lung inflation.
Encourage cough/deep-breathing exercises and frequent position changes.	Facilitates lung expansion and mobilization of secretions to reduce risk of atelectasis/pneumonia.
Auscultate breath sounds. Note presence of adventitious sounds, e.g., rhonchi, wheezes.	Patient is at risk for atelectasis related to hypoventilation and pneumonia. Right lower lobe pneumonia is common in alcohol-debilitated patients and is often due to chronic aspiration. Chronic lung diseases are also common, e.g., emphysema, bronchitis.
Have suction equipment, airway adjuncts available.	Sedative effects of alcohol/drugs potentiates risk of aspiration, relaxation of oropharyngeal muscles, and respiratory depression, requiring intervention to prevent respiratory arrest.

ACTIONS/INTERVENTIONS	RATIONALE
Collaborative	
Administer supplemental O$_2$ if necessary.	Hypoxia may occur with CNS/respiratory depression.
Review serial chest x-rays, ABGs/pulse oximetry as indicated.	Monitors presence of secondary complications such as atelectasis/pneumonia; evaluates effectiveness of respiratory effort.

NURSING DIAGNOSIS: Cardiac Output, decreased, risk for

Risk factors may include
Direct effect of alcohol on the heart muscle
Altered systemic vascular resistance
Electrical alterations in rate; rhythm; conduction

Possibly evidenced by
[Not applicable; presence of signs and symptoms establishes an *actual* diagnosis]

DESIRED OUTCOMES/EVALUATION CRITERIA—PATIENT WILL:
Display vital signs within patient's normal range; absence of/reduced frequency of dysrhythmias.
Demonstrate an increase in activity tolerance.
Verbalize understanding of the effect of alcohol on the heart.

ACTIONS/INTERVENTIONS	RATIONALE
Independent	
Monitor vital signs frequently during acute withdrawal.	Hypertension frequently occurs in acute withdrawal phase. Extreme hyperexcitability, accompanied by catecholamine release and increased peripheral vascular resistance, raises BP (and heart rate), but BP may become labile/progress to hypotension. *Note:* May have underlying cardiovascular disease, which is compounded by alcohol withdrawal.
Monitor cardiac rate/rhythm. Document irregularities/dysrhythmias.	Long-term alcohol abuse may result in cardiomyopathy/HF. Tachycardia is common due to sympathetic response to increased circulating catecholamines. Irregularities/dysrhythmias may develop with electrolyte shifts/imbalance. All of these may have an adverse effect on cardiac function/output.
Monitor body temperature.	Elevation may occur due to sympathetic stimulation, dehydration, and/or infections, causing vasodilation and compromising venous return/cardiac output.
Monitor I&O. Note 24-hour fluid balance.	Preexisting dehydration, vomiting, fever, and diaphoresis may result in decreased circulating volume that can compromise cardiovascular function. *Note:* Hydration is difficult to assess in the alcoholic patient because the usual indicators are not reliable, and overhydration is a risk in the presence of compromised cardiac function.

851

ACTIONS/INTERVENTIONS	RATIONALE

Independent

Be prepared for/assist in cardiopulmonary resuscitation.

Causes of death during acute withdrawal stages include cardiac dysrhythmias, respiratory depression/arrest, oversedation, excessive psychomotor activity, severe dehydration or overhydration, and massive infections. Mortality for unrecognized/untreated DTs may be as high as 25%.

Collaborative

Monitor laboratory studies, e.g., serum electrolyte levels.

Electrolyte imbalance, e.g., potassium/magnesium, potentiate risk of cardiac dysrhythmias and CNS excitability.

Administer medications as indicated, e.g.:

Clonidine (Catapres), atenolol (Tenormin);

Although the use of benzodiazepines is often sufficient to control hypertension during initial withdrawal from alcohol, some patients may require more specific therapy.

Potassium.

Corrects deficits that can result in life-threatening dysrhythmias.

NURSING DIAGNOSIS: Injury, risk for [specify]

Risk factors may include
Cessation of alcohol intake with varied autonomic nervous system responses to the system's suddenly altered state
Involuntary clonic/tonic muscle activity (seizures)
Equilibrium/balancing difficulties, reduced muscle and hand/eye coordination

Possibly evidenced by
[Not applicable; presence of signs and symptoms establishes an *actual* diagnosis.]

DESIRED OUTCOMES/EVALUATION CRITERIA—PATIENT WILL:
Demonstrate absence of untoward effects of withdrawal.
Experience no physical injury.

ACTIONS/INTERVENTIONS	RATIONALE

Independent

Identify stage of alcohol withdrawal symptoms; i.e., stage I is associated with signs/symptoms of hyperactivity (e.g., tremors, sleeplessness, nausea/vomiting, diaphoresis, tachycardia, hypertension). Stage II is manifested by increased hyperactivity plus hallucinations and/or seizure activity. Stage III symptoms include DTs and extreme autonomic hyperactivity with profound confusion, anxiety, insomnia, fever.

Prompt recognition and intervention may halt progression of symptoms and enhance recovery/improve prognosis. In addition, recurrence/progression of symptoms indicates need for changes in drug therapy/more intense treatment to prevent death.

ACTIONS/INTERVENTIONS	RATIONALE

Independent

Monitor/document seizure activity. Maintain patent airway. Provide environmental safety, e.g., padded side rails, bed in low position.

Grand mal seizures are most common and may be related to decreased magnesium levels, hypoglycemia, elevated blood alcohol, or preexisting seizure disorder. *Note:* In absence of history of or other pathology causing seizures, they usually stop spontaneously, requiring only symptomatic treatment.

Check deep-tendon reflexes. Assess gait, if possible.

Reflexes may be depressed, absent, or hyperactive. Peripheral neuropathies are common, especially in malnourished patient. Ataxia (gait disturbance) is associated with Wernicke's syndrome (thiamine deficiency) and cerebellar degeneration.

Assist with ambulation and self-care activities as needed.

Prevents falls with resultant injury.

Provide for environmental safety when indicated. (Refer to ND: Sensory-perceptual alterations, following.)

May be required when equilibrium, hand/eye coordination problems exist.

Collaborative

Administer IV/PO fluids with caution, as indicated.

Cautious replacement corrects dehydration and promotes renal clearance of toxins while reducing risk of overhydration.

Administer medications as indicated:

    Benzodiazepines, e.g., chlordiazepoxide (Librium), diazepam (Valium), clonazepam (Klonopin);

Commonly used to control neuronal hyperactivity that occurs as alcohol is detoxified. IV/PO administration is preferred route, as IM absorption is unpredictable. Muscle-relaxant qualities are particularly helpful to patient in controlling "the shakes," trembling, and ataxic quality of movements. Patient may initially require large doses to achieve desired effect, and then drugs may be tapered and discontinued, usually within 96 hours. *Note:* These agents must be used cautiously in patients with hepatic disease as they are metabolized by the liver.

    Oxazepam (Serax);

Although less dramatic for control of withdrawal symptoms, may be drug of choice in patient with liver disease because of its shorter half-life.

    Phenobarbital;

Useful in suppressing withdrawal symptoms as well as an effective anticonvulsant. Use must be monitored so that exacerbation of respiratory depression is prevented.

    Magnesium sulfate.

May reduce tremors and seizure activity by decreasing neuromuscular excitability.

853

ACTIONS/INTERVENTIONS	RATIONALE
Independent	
Assess level of consciousness; ability to speak, response to stimuli/commands.	Speech may be garbled, confused, or slurred. Response to commands may reveal inability to concentrate, impaired judgment, or muscle coordination deficits.
Observe behavioral responses, e.g., hyperactivity, disorientation, confusion, sleeplessness, irritability.	Hyperactivity related to CNS disturbances may escalate rapidly. Sleeplessness is common due to loss of sedative effect gained from alcohol usually consumed prior to bedtime. Sleep deprivation may aggravate disorientation/confusion. Progression of symptoms may indicate impending hallucinations (stage II) or DTs (stage III).
Note onset of hallucinations. Document as auditory, visual, and/or tactile.	Auditory hallucinations are reported to be more frightening/threatening to patient. Visual hallucinations occur more at night and often include insects, animals, or faces of friends/enemies. Patients are frequently observed "picking the air." Yelling may occur if patient is calling for help from perceived threat (usually seen in stage III).
Provide quiet environment. Speak in calm, quiet voice. Regulate lighting as indicated. Turn off radio/TV during sleep.	Reduces external stimuli during hyperactive stage. Patient may become more delirious when surroundings cannot be seen, but some respond better to quiet, darkened room.

ACTIONS/INTERVENTIONS	RATIONALE

Independent

Provide care by same personnel whenever possible.

Promotes recognition of caregivers and a sense of consistency, which may reduce fear.

Encourage SO to stay with patient whenever possible.

May have a calming effect, and may provide a reorienting influence.

Reorient frequently to person, place, time, and surrounding environment as indicated.

May reduce confusion, prevent/limit misinterpretation of external stimuli.

Avoid bedside discussion about patient or topics unrelated to the patient that do not include the patient.

Patient may hear and misinterpret conversation, which can aggravate hallucinations.

Provide environmental safety, e.g., place bed in low position, leave doors in full open or closed position, observe frequently, place call light/bell within reach, remove articles that can harm patient.

Patient may have distorted sense of reality, be fearful, or be suicidal, requiring protection from self.

Collaborative

Provide seclusion, restraints as necessary.

Patients with excessive psychomotor activity, severe hallucinations, violent behavior, and/or suicidal gestures may respond better to seclusion. Restraints are usually ineffective and add to patient's agitation, but occasionally may be required to prevent self-harm.

Monitor laboratory studies, e.g., electrolytes, magnesium levels, liver function studies, ammonia, BUN, glucose, ABGs.

Changes in organ function may precipitate or potentiate sensory-perceptual deficits. Electrolyte imbalance is common. Liver function is often impaired in the chronic alcoholic. Ammonia intoxication can occur if the liver is unable to convert ammonia to urea. Keto-acidosis is sometimes present without glycosuria; however, hyperglycemia or hypoglycemia may occur, suggesting pancreatitis or impaired gluconeogenesis in the liver. Hypoxemia and hypercarbia are common manifestations in chronic alcoholics who are also heavy smokers.

Administer medications as indicated: e.g.:

Minor antianxiety agents as indicated. (Refer to ND: Anxiety [severe/panic]/Fear, p 857);

Reduces hyperactivity, promoting relaxation/sleep. Drugs that have little effect on dreaming may be desired to allow dream recovery (REM rebound) to occur, which has previously been suppressed by alcohol use.

Thiamine, C and B complex, multivitamins, Stress-tabs.

Vitamin deficiency (especially thiamine) is associated with ataxia, loss of eye movement and pupillary response, palpitations, postural hypotension, and exertional dyspnea.

NURSING DIAGNOSIS: Nutrition: altered, less than body requirements

May be related to
Poor dietary intake (replaced by alcohol consumption)
Effects of alcohol on organs involved in digestion, e.g., stomach, pancreas, liver; interference with absorption and metabolism of nutrients and amino acids; and increased loss of vitamins in the urine

ACTIONS/INTERVENTIONS	RATIONALE
Independent	
Evaluate presence/quality of bowel sounds. Note abdominal distention, tenderness.	Irritation of gastric mucosa is common and may result in epigastric pain, nausea, and hyperactive bowel sounds. More serious effects on GI system may occur secondary to cirrhosis and hepatitis.
Note presence of nausea/vomiting, diarrhea.	Nausea/vomiting are often among first signs of alcohol withdrawal and may interfere with achieving adequate nutritional intake.
Assess ability to feed self.	Tremors, altered mentation, or hallucinations may interfere with ingestion of nutrients and indicate need for assistance.
Provide frequent, small, easily digested meals/snacks and advance as tolerated.	May limit gastric distress; may enhance intake and tolerance of nutrients. As appetite and ability to tolerate food increase, diet should be adjusted to provide the necessary calories and nutrition for cellular repair and restoration of energy.
Collaborative	
Review laboratory studies, e.g., AST, ALT, LDH, serum albumin/prealbumin, transferrin.	Assesses liver function, adequacy of nutritional intake; influences choice of diet and need for/effectiveness of supplemental therapy.
Refer to dietitian/nutritional support team.	Useful in establishing individual nutritional program.
Provide diet high in protein with at least half of calories obtained from carbohydrates.	Stabilizes blood sugar, thereby reducing risk of hypoglycemia while providing for energy needs and cellular regeneration.

ACTIONS/INTERVENTIONS	RATIONALE
Collaborative	
Administer medications as indicated, e.g.:	
Antacids, antiemetics, antidiarrheals;	Reduces gastric irritation and limits effects of sympathetic stimulation.
Vitamins, thiamine.	Replace losses. *Note:* All patients should receive thiamine because vitamin deficiencies (either clinical or subclinical) exist in most, if not all, patients with chronic alcoholism.
Institute/maintain NPO status as indicated.	Provides GI rest to reduce harmful effects of gastric/pancreatic stimulation in presence of GI bleeding or excessive vomiting.

NURSING DIAGNOSIS: Anxiety [severe/panic]/Fear

May be related to
Cessation of alcohol intake/physiologic withdrawal
Situational crisis (hospitalization)
Threat to self-concept, perceived threat of death

Possibly evidenced by
Feelings of inadequacy, shame, self-disgust, and remorse
Increased helplessness/hopelessness with loss of control of own life
Increased tension, apprehension
Fear of unspecified consequences; identifies object of fear

DESIRED OUTCOMES/EVALUATION CRITERIA—PATIENT WILL:
Verbalize reduction of fear and anxiety to an acceptable and manageable level.
Express sense of regaining some control of situation/life.
Demonstrate problem-solving skills and use resources effectively.

ACTIONS/INTERVENTIONS	RATIONALE
Independent	
Identify cause of anxiety, involving patient in the process. Explain that alcohol withdrawal increases anxiety and uneasiness. Reassess level of anxiety on an ongoing basis.	Person in acute phase of withdrawal may be unable to identify and/or accept what is happening. Anxiety may be physiologically or environmentally caused. Continued alcohol toxicity will be manifested by increased anxiety and agitation as effects of medication wear off.
Develop a trusting relationship through frequent contact. Project an accepting attitude about alcoholism.	Provides patient with a sense of humanness, helping to decrease paranoia and distrust. Patient will be able to detect biased or condescending attitude of caregivers.

857

ACTIONS/INTERVENTIONS	RATIONALE

Independent

Inform patient about what you plan to do and why. Include patient in planning process and provide choices when possible.

Enhances sense of trust, explanation, and may increase cooperation/reduce anxiety. Provides sense of control over self in circumstance where loss of control is a significant factor. *Note:* Feelings of self-worth are intensified when one is treated as a worthwhile person.

Reorient frequently. (Refer to ND: Sensory-perceptual alterations (specify), p 854.)

Patient may experience periods of confusion, resulting in increased anxiety.

Collaborative

Administer medications as indicated, e.g.:

Benzodiazepines, e.g., chlordiazepoxide (Librium), diazepam (Valium);

Antianxiety agents are given during acute withdrawal to help patient relax, be less hyperactive, and feel more in control.

Barbiturates; e.g., phenobarbital, or possibly secobarbital (Seconal), pentobarbital (Nembutal).

These drugs suppress alcohol withdrawal but need to be used with caution as they are respiratory depressants and REM sleep cycle inhibitors.

Arrange "Intervention" (confrontation) in controlled setting to assist patient to accept that substance use is creating a problem.

Process of intervention, wherein SOs, supported by staff, provide information about how patient's drinking and behavior have affected each one of them, helps patient acknowledge that drinking is a problem and has resulted in current situational crisis.

Provide consultation for referral to detoxification/crisis center for ongoing treatment program as soon as medically stable (e.g., oriented to reality).

Patient is more likely to contract for treatment while still "hurting" and experiencing fear and anxiety from last drinking episode. Motivation decreases as well-being increases and person again feels able to control the problem. Direct contact with available treatment resources provides realistic picture of help. Decreases time for patient to "think about it"/change mind or restructure and strengthen denial systems.

POTENTIAL CONSIDERATIONS following acute care (dependent on patient's age, physical condition/presence of complications, personal resources, and life responsibilities)

Refer to: Substance Abuse/Rehabilitation plan of care, p 862, and plans of care for any specific underlying medical condition(s).

Sample CP: Alcohol Withdrawal Program. ELOS: 7 Days Behavioral Unit

ND and Categories of Care	Time Dimension	Goals/Actions	Time Dimension	Goals/Actions	Time Dimension	Goals/Actions
Risk for injury (varied autonomic and sensory responses)	Day 1	Verbalize understanding of unit policies, procedures, and safety concerns relative to individual needs	Day 3	Vital signs stable I&O balanced	Day 7	Be free of injury resulting from ETOH withdrawal
			Day 4	Display marked decrease in objective symptoms		Display no objective symptoms of withdrawal
		Cooperate with therapeutic regimen				
Referrals	Day 1	RN-NP or MD If indicated: Internist Cardiologist Neurologist				
Diagnostic studies	Day 1	BA level Drug screen (urine & blood) If indicated: CXR Pulse oximetry ECG	Day 2	SMA 20 Serum Mg, amylase RPR UA	Day 4	Repeat of selected studies as indicated
Additional assessments	Day 1	VS, temp, respiratory status/breath sounds q4h	Day 2–3	VS q8h if stable	Day 4–7	VS qd
	Day 1–4	I&O q8h Motor activity, body language, verbalizations, need for/type of restraint				
	Ongoing Stage I	Withdrawal symptoms: Tremors, N/V, hypertension, tachycardia, diaphoresis, sleeplessness				
	Stage II	Increased hyperactivity, hallucinations, seizure activity				
	Stage III	Extreme autonomic hyperactivity, profound confusion, anxiety, fever				
Medications Allergies: _____	Day 1	Librium 200 mg po	Day 3	Librium 120 mg po	Day 5	Librium 40 mg po
	Day 1–4	Thiamine 100 mg IM	Day 4	Librium 80 mg po		
	Day 2	Librium 160 mg po				
Patient education	Day 1	Orient to room/unit, schedule, procedures	Day 5	Need for ongoing therapy Goals/availability of AA program	Day 7	Schedule of follow-up visits if indicated
Additional nursing actions	Day 1	Bed rest 12h if in withdrawal Position change, HOB elevated; C, DB exercises if on bed rest	Day 3–7	Activity as tol		
	Day 1–2	Assist with ambulation, self-care as needed Encourage fluids if free of N/V				

ND and Categories of Care	Time Dimension	Goals/Actions	Time Dimension	Goals/Actions	Time Dimension	Goals/Actions
	Ongoing	Provide environmental safety measures, seizure precautions as indicated Reorient as needed				
Ineffective individual coping R/T personal vulnerability, situational crisis, inadequate coping methods	Day 1–7	Participate in development/evaluation of treatment plan	Day 3	Verbalize understanding of relationship of ETOH abuse to current situation	Day 7	Plan in place to meet needs post-discharge
	Day 2–7	Interact in group sessions	Day 6	Identify/make contact with potential resources, support groups		
Referrals	Day 1	Psychiatrist	Day 5	Community classes: Assertiveness training		
	Day 2–7	Group sessions		Stress management		
Additional assessments	Day 1	Understanding of current situation Drinking pattern, previous withdrawal, other drug use, attitudes toward substance use History of violence	Day 2–3	Previous coping strategies/consequences Perception of drug use on life, employment, legal issues		
	Day 1–2	Relationships with others: personal, work/school Readiness for group activities	Day 3–7	Congruency of actions based on insight		
Medications			Day 5–7	Naltrexone 50 mg/d if indicated		
Patient education	Day 1	Physical effects of ETOH abuse	Day 3–7	Human behavior and interactions with others/transactional analysis (TA)	Day 7	Medication dose, frequency, side effects
	Day 1–2	Types/use of relaxation techniques				Written instructions for therapeutic program
	Day 2	Consequences of ETOH abuse	Day 5–6	Community resources for self/family		
Additional nursing actions	Day 1–7	Support pt's taking responsibility for own recovery Provide consistent approach/expectations for behavior Set limits/confront inappropriate behaviors	Day 2–5	Identify goals for change Discuss alternative solutions Provide positive feedback for efforts		
			Day 2–7	Support during confrontation by peer group Encourage verbalization of feelings, personal reflection		

ND and Categories of Care	Time Dimension	Goals/Actions	Time Dimension	Goals/Actions	Time Dimension	Goals/Actions
Altered nutrition: less than body requirements R/T poor intake, effects of ETOH on digestive system, and hypermetabolic response to withdrawal	Day 2–7	Select foods appropriately to meet individual dietary needs	Day 4	Verbalize understandings of effects of ETOH abuse and reduced dietary intake on nutritional status	Day 7	Display stable weight or initial weight gain as appropriate, and laboratory results WNL
Referrals	Day 1 & prn	Dietitian				
Diagnostic studies	Day 1	CBC, liver function studies Serum albumin, transferrin	Day 2–7	Fingerstick glucose prn		
Additional assessments	Day 1	Weight, skin turgor, condition of mucous membranes, muscle tone			Day 7	Weight
	Day 1–2	Bowel sounds, characteristics of stools				
	Day 1–7	Appetite, dietary intake				
Medications	Day 1–7	Antacid ac & HS Imodium 2 mg prn	Day 2–7	Multivitamin tab/qd		
Patient education	Day 1–2	Individual nutritional needs	Day 4	Principles of nutrition, foods for maintenance of wellness		
Additional nursing actions	Day 1	Liquid/bland diet as tol	Day 2–7	Advance diet as tolerated		
	Day 1–7	Encourage small, frequent, nutritious meals/snacks Encourage good oral hygiene pc & HS				

SUBSTANCE DEPENDENCE/ABUSE REHABILITATION

Many drugs and volatile substances are subject to abuse (as noted in previous plans of care). This disorder is a continuum of phases incorporating a cluster of cognitive, behavioral, and physiologic symptoms that include loss of control over use of the substance and a continued use of the substance despite adverse consequences. A number of factors have been implicated in the predisposition to abuse a substance, e.g., biologic, biochemical, psychologic (including developmental), personality, sociocultural and conditioning, and cultural and ethnic influences. However, no single theory adequately explains the etiology of this problem.

CARE SETTING

Inpatient stay on behavioral unit or outpatient care in a day program or community agency.

RELATED CONCERNS

Alcoholism [Acute]: Intoxication/Overdose, p 847
Psychosocial Aspects of Care, p 783

Patient Assessment Data Base

Refer to appropriate acute plan of care regarding involved substance(s).

TEACHING/LEARNING

Discharge plan considerations:	**DRG projected mean length of inpatient stay: 13.5 days** May need assistance with long-range plan for recovery
	Refer to section at end of plan for postdischarge considerations.

DIAGNOSTIC STUDIES

Drug screen: Identifies drug(s) being used.
Addiction Severity Index (ASI) assessment tool: Produces a "problem severity profile" of the patient, including chemical, medical, psychologic, legal, family/social and employment/support aspects, indicating areas of treatment needs.
Other screening studies (e.g., hepatitis, HIV, TB): Dependent on general condition, individual risk factors, and care setting.

NURSING PRIORITIES

1. Provide support for decision to stop substance use.
2. Strengthen individual coping skills.
3. Facilitate learning of new ways to reduce anxiety.
4. Promote family involvement in rehabilitation program.
5. Facilitate family growth/development.
6. Provide information about condition, prognosis, and treatment needs.

DISCHARGE GOALS

1. Responsibility for own life and behavior assumed.
2. Plan to maintain substance-free life formulated.
3. Family relationships/enabling issues being addressed.
4. Treatment program successfully begun.
5. Condition, prognosis, and therapeutic regimen understood.
6. Plan in place to meet needs after discharge.

NURSING DIAGNOSIS: Denial/Coping, Individual, ineffective

May be related to
Personal vulnerability; difficulty handling new situations
Previous ineffective/inadequate coping skills with substitution of drug(s)
Learned response patterns; cultural factors, personal/family value systems
Anxiety/fear

Possibly evidenced by
Denial; lack of acceptance that drug use is causing the present situation
Use of manipulation to avoid responsibility for self
Altered social patterns/participation
Impaired adaptive behavior and problem-solving skills
Decreased ability to handle stress of illness/hospitalization
Financial affairs in disarray; employment difficulties, e.g., losing time on job/not maintaining steady employment, poor work performance, on-the-job injuries

DESIRED OUTCOMES/EVALUATION CRITERIA—PATIENT WILL:
Verbalize awareness of relationship of substance abuse to current situation.
Identify ineffective coping behaviors/consequences.
Use effective coping skills/problem solving.
Initiate necessary lifestyle changes.
Attend support group (e.g., Cocaine/Narcotics/Alcoholics Anonymous) regularly.

ACTIONS/INTERVENTIONS	RATIONALE
Independent	
Ascertain by what name patient would like to be addressed.	Shows courtesy and respect. Gives sense of orientation and control.
Determine understanding of current situation and previous/other methods of coping with life's problems.	Provides information about degree of denial; identifies coping skills that may be used in present situation. *Note:* Denial is one of the strongest and most resistant symptoms of substance abuse.
Confront and examine denial/rationalization in peer group. Use confrontation with caring.	Because denial is the major defense mechanism in addictive disease, confrontation by peers can help the patient accept the reality of adverse consequences of behaviors and that drug use is a major problem. Caring attitude preserves self-concept and helps decrease defensive response.
Remain nonjudgmental. Be alert to changes in behavior, e.g., restlessness, increased tension.	Confrontation can lead to increased agitation, which may compromise safety of patient/staff.
Provide positive feedback for expressing awareness of denial in self/others.	Positive feedback is necessary to enhance self-esteem and to reinforce insight into behavior.
Maintain firm expectation that patient attend recovery support/therapy groups regularly.	Attendance is related to admitting need for help, to working with denial, and for maintenance of a long-term drug-free existence.

863

ACTIONS/INTERVENTIONS	RATIONALE

Independent

Structure diversional activity that relates to recovery (e.g., social activity within support group), wherein issues of being chemically free are examined.

Discovery of alternative methods of coping with drug hunger can remind patient that addiction is a lifelong process and opportunity for changing patterns is available.

Use peer support to examine ways of coping with drug hunger.

Self-help groups are valuable for learning and promoting abstinence in each member, using understanding and support as well as peer pressure.

Provide information about addictive use versus experimental, occasional use; biochemical/genetic disorder theory (genetic predisposition); use activated by environment; pharmacology of stimulant; compulsive desire as a lifelong occurrence.

Progression of use continuum in the addict is from experimental/recreational to addictive use. Comprehending this process is important in combating denial. Education may relieve patient of guilt and blame, may help awareness of recurring addictive characteristics.

Encourage and support patient's taking responsibility for own recovery (e.g., development of alternative behaviors to drug urge/use). Assist patient to learn own responsibility for recovering.

Denial can be replaced with responsible action when patient accepts the reality of own responsibility.

Set limits and confront efforts to get caregiver to grant special privileges, making excuses for not following through on behaviors agreed on and attempting to continue drug use.

Patient has learned manipulative behavior throughout life and needs to learn a new way of getting needs met. Following through on consequences of failure to maintain limits can help the patient to change ineffective behaviors.

Assist patient to learn/encourage use of relaxation skills, guided imagery, visualizations.

Helps patient to relax, develop new ways to deal with stress, problem-solve.

Be aware of staff attitudes, feelings, and enabling behaviors.

Lack of understanding, judgemental/enabling behaviors can result in inaccurate data collection and non-therapeutic approaches.

Collaborative

Administer medications as indicated, e.g.:

Disulfiram (Antabuse);

This drug can be helpful in maintaining abstinence from alcohol while other therapy is undertaken. By inhibiting alcohol oxidation, the drug leads to an accumulation of acetaldehyde with a highly unpleasant reaction if alcohol is consumed.

Methadone (Dolophine);

This drug is thought to blunt the craving for/diminish the effects of opioids and is used to assist in withdrawal and long-term maintenance programs. It can allow the individual to maintain daily activities and ultimately withdraw from drug use.

Naltrexone (Trexan).

Used to suppress craving for opioids and may help prevent relapse in the patient abusing alcohol. Current research suggests that naltrexone suppresses urge to continue drinking by interfering with alcohol-induced release of endorphins.

Encourage involvement with self-help associations, e.g., Alcoholics/Narcotics Anonymous.

Puts patient in direct contact with support system necessary for managing sobriety/drug-free life.

864

> **NURSING DIAGNOSIS: Powerlessness**
>
> **May be related to**
> Substance addiction with/without periods of abstinence
> Episodic compulsive indulgence; attempts at recovery
> Lifestyle of helplessness
>
> **Possibly evidenced by**
> Ineffective recovery attempts; statements of inability to stop behavior/requests for help
> Continuous/constant thinking about drug and/or obtaining drug
> Alteration in personal, occupational, and social life
>
> **DESIRED OUTCOMES/EVALUATION CRITERIA—PATIENT WILL:**
> Admit inability to control drug habit, surrender to powerlessness over addiction.
> Verbalize acceptance of need for treatment and awareness that willpower alone cannot control abstinence.
> Engage in peer support.
> Demonstrate active participation in program.
> Regain and maintain healthy state with a drug-free lifestyle.

ACTIONS/INTERVENTIONS	RATIONALE
Independent	
Use crisis intervention techniques:	Patient is more amenable to acceptance of need for treatment at this time.
Assist patient to recognize problem exists;	While patient is hurting, it is easier to admit substance use has created negative consequences.
Identify goals for change;	Helpful in planning direction for care, promoting belief that change can occur.
Discuss alternative solutions;	Brainstorming helps creatively identify possibilities and provides sense of control.
Assist in selecting most appropriate alternative;	As possibilities are discussed, the most useful solution becomes clear.
Support decision and implementation of selected alternative(s).	Helps the patient to persevere in process of change.
Discuss need for help in a caring, nonjudgmental way.	A caring confrontive manner is more therapeutic because the patient may respond defensively to a moralistic attitude, blocking recovery.
Discuss ways in which drug has interfered with life occupation, personal/interpersonal relationships.	Awareness of how the drug has controlled life is important in combating denial/sense of powerlessness.
Explore support in peer group. Encourage sharing about drug hunger, situations that increase the desire to indulge, ways that substance has influenced life.	May need assistance in expressing self, speaking about powerlessness, admitting need for help in order to face up to problem and begin resolution.
Assist patient to learn ways to enhance health and structure healthy diversion from drug use, e.g., a balanced diet, adequate rest, acupuncture, biofeedback, deep meditative techniques, exercise (e.g., walking, slow/long distance running).	Learning to empower self in constructive areas can strengthen ability to continue recovery. These activities help restore natural biochemical balance, aid detoxification, and manage stress, anxiety, use of free time. These diversions can increase self-confidence, thereby improving self-esteem. *Note:* Release of endorphins from lengthy exercise can create a feeling of well-being.

865

ACTIONS/INTERVENTIONS	RATIONALE
Independent	
Involve patient in development of treatment plan using problem-solving process in which patient agrees to desired outcomes.	The patient is committed to the outcomes when the decision-making process involves solutions that are promulgated by the individual.
Provide information regarding understanding of human behavior and interactions with others, e.g., transactional analysis.	Understanding these concepts can help the patient to begin to deal with past problems/losses and prevent repeating ineffective coping behaviors and self-fulfilling prophecies.
Assist patient in self-examination of spirituality, faith.	Although not necessary to recovery, surrendering to and faith in a power greater than oneself has been found to be effective for many individuals in substance recovery; may decrease sense of powerlessness.
Assist patient to learn assertive communication.	Effective in assisting in ability to refuse use, to stop relationships with users and dealers, to build healthy relationships, regain control of own life.
Provide treatment information on an ongoing basis.	Helps patient know what to expect. Creates opportunity for patient to be a part of what is happening and make informed choices about participation/outcomes.
Collaborative	
Refer to/assist with making contact with programs for ongoing treatment needs, e.g., partial hospitalization drug treatment programs, Narcotics/Alcoholics Anonymous, peer support group.	Continuing treatment is essential to positive outcome. Follow-through may be easier once initial contact has been made.

NURSING DIAGNOSIS: Nutrition: altered, less than body requirements

May be related to
Insufficient dietary intake to meet metabolic needs for psychologic, physiologic, or economic reasons

Possibly evidenced by
Weight loss; weight below norm for height/body build; decreased subcutaneous fat/muscle mass
Reported altered taste sensation; lack of interest in food
Poor muscle tone
Sore, inflamed buccal cavity
Laboratory evidence of protein/vitamin deficiencies

DESIRED OUTCOMES/EVALUATION CRITERIA—PATIENT WILL:

Demonstrate progressive weight gain toward goal with normalization of laboratory values and absence of signs of malnutrition.
Verbalize understanding of effects of substance abuse, reduced dietary intake on nutritional status.
Demonstrate behaviors, lifestyle changes to regain and maintain appropriate weight.

ACTIONS/INTERVENTIONS	RATIONALE
Independent	
Assess height/weight, age, body build, strength, activity/rest level. Note condition of oral cavity.	Provides information about individual on which to base caloric needs/dietary plan. Type of diet/foods may be affected by condition of mucous membranes and teeth.
Take anthropometric measurements, e.g., triceps skinfold.	Calculates subcutaneous fat and muscle mass to aid in determining dietary needs.
Note total daily calorie intake; maintain a diary of intake, times, and patterns of eating.	Information about patient's dietary pattern will help identify nutritional needs/deficiencies.
Evaluate energy expenditure (e.g., pacing or sedentary), and establish an individualized exercise program.	Activity level affects nutritional needs. Exercise enhances muscle tone, may stimulate appetite.
Provide opportunity to choose foods/snacks to meet dietary plan.	Enhances participation/sense of control and may promote resolution of nutritional deficiencies.
Recommend monitoring weight weekly.	Provides information regarding effectiveness of dietary plan.
Collaborative	
Consult with dietitian.	Useful in establishing individual dietary needs/plan. Provides additional resource for learning.
Review laboratory studies as indicated, e.g., glucose, serum albumin/prealbumin, electrolytes.	Identifies anemias, electrolyte imbalances, other abnormalities that may be present, requiring specific therapy.
Refer for dental consultation as necessary.	Teeth are essential to good nutritional intake and dental hygiene/care is often a neglected area in this population.

NURSING DIAGNOSIS: Self Esteem, chronic low

May be related to

Social stigma attached to substance abuse, expectation that one control behavior

Negative role models; abuse/neglect, dysfunctional family system

Life choices perpetuating failure; situational crisis with loss of control over life events

Biochemical body change (e.g., withdrawal from alcohol/other drugs)

Possibly evidenced by

Not taking responsibility for self/self-care; lack of follow-through; self-destructive behavior

Change in usual role patterns or responsibility (family, job, legal)

Confusion about self, purpose or direction in life

Denial that substance use is a problem, projection of blame/responsibility for problems

DESIRED OUTCOMES/EVALUATION CRITERIA—PATIENT WILL:

Identify feelings and underlying dynamics for negative perception of self.

Verbalize acceptance of self as is and an increased sense of self-esteem.

Set goals and participate in realistic planning for lifestyle changes necessary to live without drugs.

ACTIONS/INTERVENTIONS	RATIONALE

Independent

Provide opportunity for and encourage verbalization/ discussion of individual situation.	Patient often has difficulty expressing self, even more difficulty accepting the degree of importance substance has assumed in life and its relationship to present situation.
Assess mental status. Note presence of other psychiatric disorders (dual diagnosis).	Many patients use substances in an attempt to obtain relief from depression or anxiety, which may predate use and/or be the result of substance use. Approximately 60% of substance-dependent patients have underlying psychologic problems, and treatment for both is imperative.
Spend time with patient. Discuss patient's behavior/ use of substance in a nonjudgmental way.	Presence of the nurse conveys acceptance of the individual as a worthwhile person. Discussion provides opportunity for insight into the problems abuse has created for the patient.
Provide reinforcement for positive actions and encourage patient to accept this input.	Failure and lack of self-esteem have been problems for this patient, who needs to learn to accept self as an individual with positive attributes.
Observe family interactions, SO dynamics/support.	Substance abuse is a family disease, and how the members act and react to the patient's behavior affects the course of the disease and how patient sees self. Many unconsciously become "enablers," helping the individual to cover up the consequences of the abuse. (Refer to ND: Family Process, altered: alcoholism [substance abuse], p 869.)
Encourage expression of feelings of guilt, shame, and anger.	The patient often has lost respect for self and believes that the situation is hopeless. Expression of these feelings helps the patient to begin to accept responsibility for self and take steps to make changes.
Help the patient to acknowledge that substance use is the problem and that problems can be dealt with without the use of drugs. Confront the use of defenses, e.g., denial, projection, rationalization.	When drugs can no longer be blamed for the problems that exist, the patient can begin to deal with the problems and live without substance use. Confrontation helps the patient accept the reality of the problems as they exist.
Ask the patient to list and review past accomplishments and positive happenings.	There are things in everyone's life that have been successful. Often when self-esteem is low, it is difficult to remember these successes or to view them as successes.
Use techniques of role rehearsal.	Assists patient to practice the development of skills to cope with new role as a person who no longer uses or needs drugs to handle life's problems.

Collaborative

Involve in group therapy.	Group sharing helps encourage verbalization, as other members of group are in various stages of abstinence from drugs and can address the patient's concerns/ denial. The patient can gain new skills, hope, and a sense of family/community from group participation.

ACTIONS/INTERVENTIONS

Collaborative

Refer to other resources, such as Narcotics/Alcoholics Anonymous.

Formulate plan to treat other mental illness problems.

Administer antipsychotic medications as necessary.

RATIONALE

One of the oldest and most popular forms of group treatment, which uses a basic strategy known as the Twelve Steps. The patient admits powerlessness over drug, and, although not necessary, may seek help from a "higher power." Members help one another, and meetings are available at many different times and places in most communities. The philosophy of "one day at a time" helps attain the goal of abstinence.

Patients who seek relief for other mental health problems through drugs will continue to do so once discharged. Both the substance use and the mental health problems need to be treated together to maximize abstinence potential.

Prolonged/profound psychosis following LSD or PCP use can be treated with these drugs, as it is probably the result of an underlying functional psychosis that has now emerged. *Note:* Avoid the use of phenothiazines, as they may decrease seizure threshold and cause hypotension in the presence of LSD/PCP.

NURSING DIAGNOSIS: Family Process, altered: alcoholism [substance abuse]

May be related to
Substance abuse
Family history of substance abuse, resistance to treatment
Addictive personality
Inadequate coping skills, lack of problem-solving skills

Possibly evidenced by
Anxiety; anger/suppressed rage; shame/embarrassment
Emotional isolation/loneliness; vulnerability; repressed emotions
Disturbed family dynamics; closed communication systems, ineffective spousal communication/marital problems
Altered role function/disruption of family roles
Manipulation; dependency; criticizing; rationalization/denial of problems
Enabling to maintain drinking (substance abuse); refusal to get help/inability to accept and receive help appropriately

DESIRED OUTCOMES/EVALUATION CRITERIA—FAMILY WILL:
Verbalize understanding of dynamics of enabling behaviors.
Participate in individual family programs.
Identify ineffective coping behaviors/consequences.
Initiate and plan for necessary lifestyle changes.
Take action to change self-destructive behaviors/alter behaviors that contribute to partner's/SO's addiction.

869

ACTIONS/INTERVENTIONS	RATIONALE

Independent

Review family history; explore roles of family members, circumstances involving drug use, strengths, areas for growth.

Determines areas for focus, potential for change.

Explore how the SO has coped with the patient's habit, e.g., denial, repression, rationalization, hurt, loneliness, projection.

The person who enables also suffers from the same feelings as the patient (e.g., anxiety, self-hatred, helplessness, low self-worth, guilt) and needs help in learning new/effective coping skills.

Determine understanding of current situation and previous methods of coping with life's problems.

Provides information on which to base present plan of care.

Assess current level of functioning of family members.

Affects individual's ability to cope with situation.

Determine extent of enabling behaviors being evidenced by family members; explore with individual and patient.

Enabling is doing for the patient what he or she needs to do for self (rescuing). People want to be helpful and do not want to feel powerless to help their loved one to stop substance use and change the behavior that is so destructive. However, the substance abuser often relies on others to cover up own inability to cope with daily responsibilities.

Provide information about enabling behavior, addictive disease characteristics for both user and nonuser.

Awareness and knowledge of behaviors (e.g., avoiding and shielding, taking over responsibilities, rationalizing, and subserving) provide opportunity for individuals to begin the process of change.

Identify and discuss sabotage behaviors of family members.

Even though family member(s) may verbalize a desire for the individual to become substance-free, the reality of interactive dynamics is that they may unconsciously not want the individual to recover, as this would affect the family member(s)' own role in the relationship. Additionally, they may receive sympathy/attention from others (secondary gain).

Provide factual information to patient and family about the effects of addictive behaviors on the family and what to expect after discharge.

Many patients/SOs are not aware of the nature of addiction. If patient is using legally obtained drugs, he or she may believe this does not constitute abuse.

Encourage family members to be aware of their own feelings, look at the situation with perspective and objectivity. They can ask themselves: "Am I being conned? Am I acting out of fear, shame, guilt, or anger? Do I have a need to control?"

When the enabling family members become aware of their own actions that perpetuate the addict's problems, they need to decide to change themselves. If they change, the patient can then face the consequences of his/her own actions and may choose to get well.

Provide support for enabling partner(s). Encourage group work.

Families/SOs need support as much as the person who is addicted in order to produce change.

Assist the partner to become aware that patient's abstinence and drug use are not the partner's responsibility.

Partners need to learn that user's habit may or may not change despite partner's involvement in treatment.

Help the recovering (former user) partner who is enabling to distinguish between destructive aspects of behavior and genuine motivation to aid the user.

Enabling behavior can be partner's attempts at personal survival.

Note how partner relates to the treatment team/staff.

Determines enabling style. A parallel exists between how partner relates to user and to staff, based on partner's feelings about self and situation.

870

ACTIONS/INTERVENTIONS

Independent

Explore conflicting feelings the enabling partner may have about treatment, e.g., feelings similar to those of abuser (blend of anger, guilt, fear, exhaustion, embarrassment, loneliness, distrust, grief, and possibly relief).

Involve family in discharge referral plans.

Be aware of staff's enabling behaviors and feelings about patient and enabling partners.

Collaborative

Encourage involvement with self-help associations, Alcoholics/Narcotics Anonymous, Al-Anon, Alateen, and professional family therapy.

RATIONALE

Useful in establishing the need for therapy for the partner. This individual's own identity may have been lost, s/he may fear self-disclosure to staff, and may have difficulty giving up the dependent relationship.

Drug abuse is a family illness. Because the family has been so involved in dealing with the substance abuse behavior, they need help adjusting to the new behavior of sobriety/abstinence. Incidence of recovery is almost doubled when the family is treated along with the patient.

Lack of understanding of enabling can result in nontherapeutic approaches to patients and their families.

Puts patient/family in direct contact with support systems necessary for continued sobriety and to assist with problem resolution.

NURSING DIAGNOSIS: Sexual dysfunction

May be related to
Altered body function: Neurologic damage and debilitating effects of drug use (particularly alcohol and opiates)

Possibly evidenced by
Progressive interference with sexual functioning
In men: A significant degree of testicular atrophy is noted (testes are smaller and softer than normal); gynecomastia (breast enlargement); impotence/decreased sperm counts
In women: Loss of body hair, thin soft skin, and spider angioma (elevated estrogen); amenorrhea/increase in miscarriages

DESIRED OUTCOMES/EVALUATION CRITERIA—PATIENT WILL:
Verbally acknowledge effects of drug use on sexual functioning/reproduction.
Identify interventions to correct/overcome individual situation.

ACTIONS/INTERVENTIONS

Independent

Assess patient's current information and have patient describe problem in own words.

Encourage and accept individual expressions of concern.

Provide education opportunity (e.g., pamphlets, consultation from appropriate persons) for patient to learn effects of drug on sexual functioning.

RATIONALE

Determines level of knowledge, what patient perceives own needs are.

Most people find it difficult to talk about this sensitive subject and may not ask directly for information.

Much of denial and hesitancy to seek treatment may be reduced as a result of sufficient and appropriate information.

871

Independent

Provide information about individual's condition.

Sexual functioning may have been affected by drug (alcohol) intake, physiologic and/or psychologic factors (such as stress). Information will assist patient to understand own situation and identify actions to be taken.

Provide information about effects of drugs on the reproductive system/fetus (e.g., increased risk of premature birth, brain damage, and fetal malformation). Assess drinking/drug history of pregnant patient.

Awareness of the negative effects of alcohol/other drugs on reproduction may motivate patient to stop using drug(s). When patient is pregnant, identification of potential problems aids in planning for future fetal needs/concerns.

Discuss prognosis for sexual dysfunction, e.g., impotence/low sexual desire.

In about 50% of cases, impotence is reversed with abstinence from drug(s); in 25% the return to normal functioning is delayed; and approximately 25% remain impotent.

Collaborative

Refer for sexual counseling, if indicated.

Patient may need additional assistance to resolve more severe problems/situations. Patient may have difficulty adjusting if drug has improved sexual experience (e.g., heroin decreases dyspareunia in women/premature ejaculation in men). Further, the patient may have engaged enjoyably in bizarre, erotic sexual behavior under influence of the stimulant drug; patient may have found no substitute for the drug, may have driven a partner away, and may have no motivation to adjust to sexual experience without drugs.

Review results of sonogram if pregnant.

Assesses fetal growth and development to identify possibility of fetal alcohol syndrome and future needs.

NURSING DIAGNOSIS: Knowledge deficit [learning need] regarding condition, prognosis, treatment, self care and discharge needs

May be related to
Lack of information; information misinterpretation
Cognitive limitations/interference with learning (other mental illness problems/organic brain syndrome); lack of recall

Possibly evidenced by
Statements of concern; questions/misconceptions
Inaccurate follow-through of instructions/development of preventable complications
Continued use in spite of complications/bad trips

DESIRED OUTCOMES/EVALUATION CRITERIA—PATIENT WILL:
Verbalize understanding of own condition/disease process, prognosis, and treatment plan.
Identify/initiate necessary lifestyle changes to remain drug-free.
Participate in treatment program.

ACTIONS/INTERVENTIONS	RATIONALE

Independent

Be aware of and deal with anxiety of patient and family members.

Anxiety can interfere with ability to hear and assimilate information.

Provide an active role for the patient/SO in the learning process, e.g., discussions, group participation, role playing.

Learning is enhanced when persons are actively involved.

Provide written and verbal information as indicated. Include list of articles and books related to patient/family needs and encourage reading and discussing what they learn.

Helps patient/SO to make informed choices about future. Bibliotherapy can be a useful addition to other therapeutic approaches.

Assess patient's knowledge of own situation, e.g., disease, complications, and needed changes in lifestyle.

Assists in planning for long-range changes necessary for maintaining sobriety/drug-free status. Patient may have street knowledge of the drug but be ignorant of medical facts.

Time activities to individual needs.

Facilitates learning, as information is more readily assimilated when pacing is considered.

Review condition and prognosis/future expectations.

Provides knowledge base on which patient can make informed choices.

Discuss relationship of drug use to current situation.

Often patient has misperception (denial) of real reason for admission to the medical (psychiatric) setting.

Discuss effects of drug(s) used, e.g., PCP is deposited in body fat and may reactivate (flashbacks) even after long interval of abstinence; alcohol use may result in mental deterioration, liver involvement/damage; cocaine can damage postcapillary vessels, increase platelet aggregation, promoting thromboses and infarction of skin/internal organs, causing localized atrophie blanche or sclerodermatous lesions.

Information will help patient understand possible long-term effects of drug use.

Discuss potential for reemergence of withdrawal symptoms in stimulant abuse as early as 3 months or as late as 9–12 months.

While symptoms of intoxication may have passed, patient may manifest denial, drug hunger, and periods of "flare-up," wherein there is a delayed recurrence of withdrawal symptoms, e.g., anxiety, depression, irritability, sleep disturbance, compulsiveness with food (especially sugars).

Inform patient of effects of Antabuse in combination with alcohol intake and importance of avoiding use of alcohol-containing products, e.g., cough syrups or foods/candy.

Interaction of alcohol and Antabuse results in nausea and hypotension, which may produce fatal shock. Individuals on Antabuse are sensitive to alcohol on a continuum, with some being able to drink on the drug, and others having a reaction with only slight exposure, e.g., alcohol-containing foods or products such as aftershave. Reactions appear to be dose-related as well.

ACTIONS/INTERVENTIONS

Independent

Review specific aftercare needs; e.g., PCP user should drink cranberry juice and continue use of ascorbic acid; alcohol abuser with liver damage should refrain from drugs/anesthetics or use of household cleaning products detoxified in the liver.

Discuss variety of helpful organizations and programs that are available for assistance/referral.

RATIONALE

Promotes individualized care related to specific situation. Cranberry juice and ascorbic acid enhance clearance of PCP from the system. Substances that have the potential for liver damage are more dangerous in the presence of an already damaged liver.

Long-term support is necessary to maintain optimal recovery. Psychosocial needs may require addressing as well as other issues.

POTENTIAL CONSIDERATIONS following acute care (dependent on patient's age, physical condition/presence of complications, personal resources, and life responsibilities)

Therapeutic Regimen: Individual/Families, ineffective management—decisional conflicts, excessive demands made on individual or family, family conflict, perceived seriousness/benefits

Coping, Individual, ineffective—vulnerability, situational crises, multiple life changes, inadequate relaxation, inadequate/loss of support systems

Family Coping: potential for growth—needs sufficiently gratified and adaptive tasks effectively addressed to enable goals of self-actualization to surface

(Physical needs are dependent on substance effect on organ systems—refer to appropriate medical plans of care for additional considerations.)

CANCER

Cancer is a general term used to describe a disturbance of cellular growth and refers to a group of diseases and not a single disease entity. There are currently more than 150 different known types of cancer. Because cancer is a cellular disease, it can arise from any body tissue, with manifestations that are the result of failure to control the proliferation and maturation of cells.

There are four main classifications of cancer according to tissue type: (1) lymphomas (cancers originating in infection-fighting organs); (2) leukemias (cancers originating in blood-forming organs); (3) sarcomas (cancers originating in bones, muscle, or connective tissue); and (4) carcinomas (cancers originating in epithelial cells). Within these broad categories, a cancer is classified by histology, stage, and grade.

Through years of observation and documentation, it has been noted that the metastatic behavior of cancers varies according to the primary site of diagnosis. This behavior pattern is known as the "natural history." An example is the metastic pattern for primary breast cancer: breast-bone-lung-liver-brain. Knowledge of the etiology and natural history of a cancer type is important in planning the patient's care and in evaluation of the patient's progress, prognosis, and physical complaints.

CARE SETTING

Cancer centers may focus on staging and major treatment modalities for complex cancers. Treatment for managing adverse effects such as malnutrition and infection may take place in short-stay, ambulatory, or community settings. More cancer patients are receiving care at home because of personal choice and healthcare costs.

RELATED CONCERNS

Fecal Diversions: Postoperative Care of Ileostomy and Colostomy, p 348
Hysterectomy, p 638
Leukemias, p 540
Lung Cancer: Surgical Intervention (Postoperative Care), p 143
Lymphomas, p 549
Mastectomy, p 647
Prostatectomy, p 621
Psychosocial Aspects of Care, p 783
Radical Neck Surgery: Laryngectomy (Postoperative Care), p 162
Sepsis/Septicemia, p 719
Total Nutritional Support: Parenteral/Enteral Feeding, p 491
Urinary Diversions/Urostomy (Postoperative Care), p 601

Patient Assessment Data Base

Refer to appropriate plans of care for additional assessment information.

ACTIVITY/REST

May report: Weakness and/or fatigue
Changes in rest pattern and usual hours of sleep per night; presence of factors affecting sleep, e.g., pain, anxiety, night sweats
Limitations of participation in hobbies, exercise, usual activities

CIRCULATION

May report: Palpitations, chest pain on exertion

May exhibit: Changes in BP

EGO INTEGRITY

May report: Stress factors (financial, job, role changes) and ways of handling stress (e.g., smoking, drinking, delay in seeking treatment, religious/spiritual belief)

875

Concern about changes in appearance, e.g., alopecia, disfiguring lesions, surgery

Denial of diagnosis, feelings of powerlessness, hopelessness, helplessness, worthlessness, guilt, loss of control, depression

May exhibit: Denial, withdrawal, anger

ELIMINATION

May report: Changes in bowel pattern, e.g., blood in stools, pain with defecation

Changes in urinary elimination, e.g., pain or burning on urination, hematuria, frequent micturition

May exhibit: Changes in bowel sounds, abdominal distention

FOOD/FLUID

May report: Poor dietary habits (e.g., low-fiber, high-fat, additives, preservatives)

Anorexia, nausea/vomiting

Food intolerances

May exhibit: Changes in weight; severe weight loss, cachexia, wasting of muscle mass

Changes in skin moisture/turgor; edema

NEUROSENSORY

May report: Dizziness; syncope

Numbness/tingling of extremities; sensation of coldness

PAIN/DISCOMFORT

May report: No pain, or varying degrees, e.g., mild discomfort to severe pain (associated with disease process)

RESPIRATION

May report: Smoking (tobacco, marijuana), living with someone who smokes

Asbestos dust exposure (e.g., coal, sand)

SAFETY

May report: Exposure to toxic chemicals, carcinogens (occupation/profession or environment)

Excessive/prolonged sun exposure

May exhibit: Fever

Skin rashes, ulcerations

SEXUALITY

May report: Sexual concerns, e.g., impact on relationship, change in level of satisfaction

Nulligravida greater than 30 years of age; multigravida

Multiple sex partners, early sexual activity, genital herpes

SOCIAL INTERACTION

May report: Inadequate/weak support system

Marital history (regarding in-home satisfaction, support, or help)

Concerns about role function/responsibility

TEACHING/LEARNING

May report: Family history of cancer, e.g., mother or aunt with breast cancer

Primary site: Of disease, date discovered/diagnosed

Metastatic disease: Additional sites involved (if none, natural history of primary will provide important information for looking for metastasis)

Treatment history: Previous treatment for cancer—place and treatments given

Discharge plan considerations: **DRG projected mean length of stay:** Dependent on specific system affected and therapeutic needs. Refer to appropriate resources.

May require assistance with finances, medications/treatments, wound care/supplies, transportation, food shopping and preparation, self-care, homemaker/maintenance tasks, provision for child care; changes in living facilities/hospice

Refer to section at end of plan for postdischarge considerations.

DIAGNOSTIC STUDIES

Test selection depends on history, clinical manifestations, and index of suspicion for a particular cancer.

Endoscopy: Used for direct visualization of body organs/cavities to detect abnormalities.

Scans (e.g., MRI, CT, gallium) and ultrasound: May be done for diagnostic purposes, identification of metastasis, and evaluation of response to treatment.

Biopsy (aspiration, excision, needle, punch): Done to differentiate diagnosis and delineate treatment and may be taken from bone marrow, skin, organ, and so forth. *Examples:* Bone marrow is done in myeloproliferative diseases for diagnosis; in solid tumors for staging.

Tumor markers (substances produced and secreted by tumor cells and found in serum, e.g., CEA, prostate-specific antigen, alpha-fetoprotein, HCG, prostatic acid phosphatase, calcitonin, pancreatic oncofetal antigen, CA 15-3, CA 19-9, CA 125, and so on): Can help in diagnosing cancer but are more useful as prognostic indices and/or therapeutic monitors. Estrogen and progesterone receptors are assays done on breast tissue to provide information about whether or not hormonal manipulation would be therapeutic in metastatic disease control. *Note:* Any hormone may be elevated, as many cancers secrete inappropriate hormones (ectopic hormone secretion).

Screening chemistry tests: E.g., electrolytes (sodium, potassium, calcium); renal tests (BUN/Cr); liver tests (bilirubin, AST, alkaline phosphatase, LDH); bone tests (ALP isoenzyme, calcium).

CBC with differential and platelets: May reveal anemia, changes in RBCs and WBCs; reduced or increased platelets.

Chest x-ray: Screens for primary or metastatic disease of lungs.

NURSING PRIORITIES

1. Support adaptation and independence.
2. Promote comfort.
3. Maintain optimal physiologic functioning.
4. Prevent complications.
5. Provide information about disease process/condition, prognosis, and treatment needs.

DISCHARGE GOALS

1. Patient is dealing with current situation realistically.
2. Pain alleviated/controlled.
3. Homeostasis achieved.
4. Complications prevented/minimized.
5. Disease process/condition, prognosis, and therapeutic choices and regimen understood.
6. Plan in place to meet needs after discharge.

NURSING DIAGNOSIS: Fear/Anxiety (specify level)

May be related to

Situational crisis (cancer)

Threat to/change in health/socioeconomic status, role functioning, interaction patterns

Threat of death

Separation from family (hospitalization, treatments), interpersonal transmission/contagion of feelings

ACTIONS/INTERVENTIONS	RATIONALE
Independent	
Review patient's/SO's previous experience with cancer. Determine what the doctor has told patient and what conclusion patient has reached.	Clarifies patient's perceptions; assists in identification of fear(s) and misconceptions based on diagnosis and experience with cancer.
Encourage patient to share thoughts and feelings.	Provides opportunity to examine realistic fears as well as misconceptions about diagnosis.
Provide open environment in which patient feels safe to discuss feelings or to refrain from talking.	Helps patient to feel accepted in present condition without feeling judged and promotes sense of dignity and control.
Maintain frequent contact with patient. Talk with and touch patient as appropriate.	Provides assurance that the patient is not alone or rejected; conveys respect for and acceptance of the person, fostering trust.
Be aware of effects of isolation on patient when required for immunosuppression or radiation implant. Limit use of isolation clothing/masks as possible.	Sensory deprivation may result when sufficient stimulation is not available and may intensify feelings of anxiety/fear and alienation.
Assist patient/SO in recognizing and clarifying fears to begin developing coping strategies for dealing with these fears.	Coping skills are often stressed after diagnosis and during different phases of treatment. Support and counseling are often necessary to enable individual to recognize and deal with fear and to realize that control/coping strategies are available.
Provide accurate, consistent information regarding prognosis. Avoid arguing about patient's perceptions of situation.	Can reduce anxiety and enable patient to make decisions/choices based on realities.
Permit expressions of anger, fear, despair without confrontation. Give information that feelings are normal and are to be appropriately expressed.	Acceptance of feelings allows patient to begin to deal with situation.
Explain the recommended treatment, its purpose, and potential side effects. Help patient prepare for treatments.	The goal of cancer treatment is to destroy malignant cells while minimizing damage to normal ones. Treatment may include surgery (curative, preventive, palliative) as well as chemotherapy, radiation (internal, external), or newer/organ-specific treatments such as whole-body hyperthermia or biotherapy. Bone marrow or peripheral progenitor cell (stem cell) transplant may be recommended for some types of cancer.
Explain procedures, providing opportunity for questions and honest answers. Stay with patient during anxiety-producing procedures and consultations.	Accurate information allows patient to deal more effectively with reality of situation, thereby reducing anxiety and fear of the unknown.

ACTIONS/INTERVENTIONS	RATIONALE
Independent	
Provide primary or consistent caregivers whenever possible.	May help reduce anxiety by fostering therapeutic relationship and facilitating continuity of care.
Promote calm, quiet environment.	Facilitates rest, conserves energy, and may enhance coping abilities.
Identify stage/degree of grief patient and SO are currently experiencing. (Refer to ND: Grieving, anticipatory, following.)	Choice of interventions is dictated by stage of grief, coping behaviors, e.g., anger/withdrawal, denial.
Note ineffective coping, e.g., poor social interactions, helplessness, giving up everyday functions and usual sources of gratification.	Identifies individual problems and provides support for patient/SO in using effective coping skills.
Be alert to signs of denial/depression, e.g., withdrawal, anger, inappropriate remarks. Determine presence of suicidal ideation and assess potential on a scale of 1–10.	Patient may use defense mechanism of denial and express hope that diagnosis is inaccurate. Feelings of guilt, spiritual distress, physical symptoms, or lack of cure may cause the patient to become withdrawn and believe that suicide is a viable alternative.
Encourage and foster patient interaction with support systems.	Reduces feelings of isolation. If family support systems are not available, outside sources may be needed immediately, e.g., local cancer support groups.
Provide reliable and consistent information and support for SO.	Allows for better interpersonal interaction and reduction of anxiety and fear.
Include SO as indicated/patient desires when major decisions are to be made.	Ensures a support system for the patient and allows the SO to be involved appropriately.
Collaborative	
Administer antianxiety medications, e.g., lorazepam (Ativan), alprazolam (Xanax), as indicated.	May be useful for brief periods of time to help patient handle feelings of anxiety related to diagnosis/situation and/or during periods of high stress.
Refer to additional resources for counseling/support as needed.	May be useful from time to time to assist patient/SO to deal with anxiety.

NURSING DIAGNOSIS: Grieving, anticipatory

May be related to

Anticipated loss of physiologic well-being (e.g., loss of body part; change in body function); change in lifestyle

Perceived potential death of patient

Possibly evidenced by

Changes in eating habits, alterations in sleep patterns, activity levels, libido, and communication patterns

Denial of potential loss, choked feelings, anger

DESIRED OUTCOMES/EVALUATION CRITERIA—PATIENT WILL:

Identify and express feelings appropriately.

Continue normal life activities, looking toward/planning for the future, one day at a time.

Verbalize understanding of the dying process and feelings of being supported in grief work.

ACTIONS/INTERVENTIONS	RATIONALE

Independent

Expect initial shock and disbelief following diagnosis of cancer and/or traumatizing procedures (e.g., disfiguring surgery, colostomy, amputation).

Few patients are fully prepared for the reality of the changes that can occur.

Assess patient/SO for stage of grief currently being experienced. Explain process as appropriate.

Knowledge about the grieving process reinforces the normality of feelings/reactions being experienced and can help patient deal more effectively with them.

Provide open, nonjudgmental environment. Use therapeutic communication skills of Active-listening, acknowledgment, and so on.

Promotes and encourages realistic dialogue about feelings and concerns.

Encourage verbalization of thoughts/concerns and accept expressions of sadness, anger, rejection. Acknowledge normality of these feelings.

Patient may feel supported in expression of feelings by the understanding that deep and often conflicting emotions are normal and experienced by others in this difficult situation.

Be aware of mood swings, hostility, and other acting-out behavior. Set limits on inappropriate behavior, redirect negative thinking.

Indicators of ineffective coping and need for additional interventions. Preventing destructive actions enables patient to maintain control and sense of self-esteem.

Be aware of debilitating depression. Ask patient direct questions about state of mind.

Studies show that many cancer patients are at high risk for suicide. They are especially vulnerable when recently diagnosed and/or discharged from hospital.

Visit frequently and provide physical contact as appropriate/desired, or provide frequent phone support as appropriate for setting. Arrange for care provider/support person to stay with patient as needed.

Helps reduce feelings of isolation and abandonment.

Reinforce teaching regarding disease process and treatments and provide information as requested/appropriate about dying. Be honest; do not give false hope while providing emotional support.

Patient/SO can benefit from factual information. Individuals may ask direct questions about death, and honest answers promote trust and provide reassurance that correct information will be given.

Review past life experiences, role changes, and coping skills. Talk about things that interest the patient.

Opportunity to identify skills that may help individuals cope with grief of current situation more effectively.

Identify positive aspects of the situation.

Possibility of remission and slow progression of disease and/or new therapies can offer hope for the future.

Discuss ways patient/SO can plan together for the future. Encourage setting of realistic goals.

Having a part in problem solving/planning can provide a sense of control over anticipated events.

Assist patient/SO to identify strengths in self/situation and support systems.

Recognizing these resources provides opportunity to work through feelings of grief.

Encourage participation in care and treatment decisions.

Allows patient to retain some control over life.

Note evidence of conflict; expressions of anger; and statements of despair, guilt, hopelessness, "nothing to live for."

Interpersonal conflicts/angry behavior may be patient's way of expressing/dealing with feelings of despair/spiritual distress and could be indicative of suicidal ideation.

Assess way that patient/SO understand and respond to death, e.g., cultural expectations, learned behaviors, experience with death (close family members/friends), beliefs about life after death, faith in higher being (God).

These factors affect how each individual deals with the possibility of death and influences how they may respond and interact.

ACTIONS/INTERVENTIONS

Independent

Provide open environment for discussion with patient/SO (when appropriate) about desires/plans pertaining to death; e.g., making will, burial arrangements, tissue donation, death benefits, insurance, time for family gatherings, how to spend remaining time.

Be aware of own feelings about cancer, impending death. Accept whatever methods patient/SO have chosen to help each other through process.

Collaborative

Refer to appropriate counselor as needed (e.g., psychiatric clinical nurse specialist, social worker, psychologist, clergyman).

Refer to community hospice program, if appropriate, or visiting nurse, home health agency as needed.

RATIONALE

If the patient/SO are mutually aware of impending death, they may more easily deal with unfinished business, desired activities.

Caregiver's anxiety and unwillingness to accept reality of possibility of own death may block ability to be helpful to the patient/SO, necessitating enlisting the aid of others to provide needed support.

Can help to alleviate distress or palliate feelings of grief to facilitate coping and foster growth.

Provides support in meeting physical and emotional needs of patient/SO and can supplement the care family and friends are able to give.

NURSING DIAGNOSIS: Self Esteem, situational low

May be related to

Biophysical: Disfiguring surgery, chemotherapy or radiotherapy side effects, e.g., loss of hair, nausea/vomiting, weight loss, anorexia, impotence, sterility, overwhelming fatigue, uncontrolled pain

Psychosocial: Threat of death; feelings of lack of control and doubt regarding acceptance by others; fear and anxiety

Possibly evidenced by

Verbalization of change in lifestyle; fear of rejection/reaction of others; negative feelings about body; feelings of helplessness, hopelessness, powerlessness

Preoccupation with change or loss

Not taking responsibility for self-care, lack of follow-through

Change in self-perception/other's perception of role

DESIRED OUTCOMES/EVALUATION CRITERIA—PATIENT WILL:

Verbalize understanding of body changes, acceptance of self in situation.

Begin to develop coping mechanisms to deal effectively with problems.

Demonstrate adaptation to changes/events that have occurred as evidenced by setting of realistic goals and active participation in work/play/personal relationships as appropriate.

ACTIONS/INTERVENTIONS

Independent

Discuss with patient/SO how the diagnosis and treatment are affecting the patient's personal life/home and work activities.

RATIONALE

Aids in defining concerns to begin problem-solving process.

Independent

Review anticipated side effects associated with a particular treatment, including possible effects on sexual activity and sense of attractiveness/desirability, e.g., alopecia, disfiguring surgery. Tell patient that not all side effects occur, and others may be minimized/controlled.

Anticipatory guidance can help patient/SO begin the process of adaptation to new state and to prepare for some side effects, e.g., buy a wig before radiation, schedule time off from work as indicated. (Refer to ND: Sexuality Patterns, altered, risk for, p 895.)

Encourage discussion of/problem-solve concerns about effects of cancer/treatments on role as homemaker, wage earner, parent, and so forth.

May help reduce problems that interfere with acceptance of treatment or stimulate progression of disease.

Acknowledge difficulties patient may be experiencing. Give information that counseling is often necessary and important in the adaptation process.

Validates reality of patient's feelings and gives permission to take whatever measures are necessary to cope with what is happening.

Evaluate support structures available to and used by patient/SO.

Helps with planning for care while hospitalized as well as after discharge.

Provide emotional support for patient/SO during diagnostic tests and treatment phase.

Although some patients adapt/adjust to cancer effects or side effects of therapy, many need additional support during this period.

Use touch during interactions, if acceptable to patient, and maintain eye contact.

Affirmation of individuality and acceptance is important in reducing patient's feelings of insecurity and self-doubt.

Collaborative

Refer patient/SO to supportive group programs (e.g., CanSurmount, I Can Cope, Reach to Recovery, Encore).

Group support is usually very beneficial for both patient/SO, providing contact with other patients with cancer at various levels of treatment and/or recovery, validating feelings and assisting with problem solving.

Refer for professional counseling as indicated.

May be necessary to regain and maintain a positive psychosocial structure if patient/SO support systems are deteriorating.

NURSING DIAGNOSIS: Pain [acute]/chronic

May be related to
Disease process (compression/destruction of nerve tissue, infiltration of nerves or their vascular supply, obstruction of a nerve pathway, inflammation)
Side effects of various cancer therapy agents

Possibly evidenced by
Reports of pain
Self-focusing/narrowed focus
Alteration in muscle tone; facial mask of pain
Distraction/guarding behaviors
Autonomic responses, restlessness (acute pain)

DESIRED OUTCOMES/EVALUATION CRITERIA—PATIENT WILL:
Report maximal pain relief/control with minimal interference with ADLs.
Follow prescribed pharmacologic regimen.
Demonstrate use of relaxation skills and diversional activities as indicated for individual situation.

ACTIONS/INTERVENTIONS	RATIONALE

Independent

Determine pain history, e.g., location of pain, frequency, duration, and intensity (0–10 scale), and relief measures used. Believe patient's report.

Information provides baseline data to evaluate need for/effectiveness of interventions. Pain of more than 6 months' duration constitutes chronic pain, which may affect therapeutic choices. Recurrent episodes of *acute* pain can occur within chronic pain, requiring increased level of intervention. *Note:* The pain experience is an individualized one composed of both physical and emotional responses.

Evaluate/be aware of painful effects of particular therapies, i.e., surgery, radiation, chemotherapy, biotherapy. Provide information to patient/SO about what to expect.

A wide range of discomforts are common (e.g., incisional pain, burning skin, low back pain, headaches) depending on the procedure/agent being used. Pain is also associated with invasive procedures to diagnose/treat cancer.

Provide basic comfort measures (e.g., repositioning, backrub) and diversional activities (e.g., music, television).

Promotes relaxation and helps refocus attention.

Encourage use of stress management skills (e.g., relaxation techniques, visualization, guided imagery, biofeedback), laughter, music, and Therapeutic Touch.

Enables patient to participate actively in nondrug treatment of pain and enhances sense of control. Pain produces stress and, in conjunction with muscle tension and internal stressors, increases patient's focus on self, which in turn increases the level of pain.

Provide cutaneous stimulation, e.g., heat/cold, massage.

May decrease inflammation, muscle spasms, reducing associated pain. *Note:* Heat may increase bleeding/edema following acute injury, whereas cold may further reduce perfusion to ischemic tissues.

Be aware of barriers to cancer pain management related to patients, as well as the healthcare system.

Patients may be reluctant to report pain for reasons such as fear that disease is worse, worry about unmanageable side effects of pain medications. Healthcare system problems include factors such as inadequate assessment of pain, concern about controlled substances/patient addiction, inadequate reimbursement/cost of treatment modalities.

Evaluate pain relief/control at regular intervals. Adjust medication regimen as necessary.

Goal is maximum pain control with minimum interference with ADLs. *Note:* Opioid tolerance requires ongoing readjustment of dosage and use of combination therapy.

Inform patient/SO of the expected therapeutic effects and discuss management of side effects.

This information helps to establish realistic expectations, confidence in own ability to handle what happens.

Discuss alternative/complementary therapies, e.g., acupuncture/acupressure.

May provide reduction/relief of pain without drug-related side effects.

Collaborative

Develop individualized pain management plan with the patient and physician. Provide written copy of plan to patient, family/SO, and care providers.

An organized plan beginning with the simplest dosage schedules and least invasive modalities improves chance for pain control. Particularly with chronic pain, patient/SO must be active participant in pain management and all care providers need to be consistent.

ACTIONS/INTERVENTIONS	RATIONALE
Collaborative	
Administer analgesics as indicated, e.g.:	A wide range of analgesics and associated agents may be employed around the clock to manage pain. *Note:* Addiction to or dependency on drug is not a concern.
NSAID, acetaminophen (Tylenol);	Useful for mild to moderate pain, can be combined with opioids and other modalities. *Note:* Ketorolac (Torodol) may be given IM briefly (up to 5 days) for acute exacerbations of pain.
Opioids, e.g., codeine, morphine (MS Contin), hydrocodone (Vicodin), hydromorphone (Dilaudid), methadone (Dolophine), fentanyl (Duragesic); oxymorphone (Numorphan);	Effective for localized and generalized moderate to severe pain, with long-acting/controlled-release forms available. Routes of administration include oral, transdermal, nasal, rectal, and infusions (subcutaneous, IV, intraventricular), which may be delivered via PCA. *Note:* IM use is not recommended as absorption is not reliable, in addition to being painful and inconvenient.
Corticosteroids;	May be effective in controlling pain associated with inflammatory process (e.g., bone pain).
Anticonvulsants, e.g., phenytoin (Dilantin), valproic acid (Depakote), clonazepam (Klonopin);	Useful for peripheral pain syndromes associated with neuropathic pain, especially shooting pain.
Antidepressants, e.g., imipramine (Tofranil), doxepin (Sinequan), trazodone (Desyrel);	Effective for neuropathic pain (e.g., tingling, burning pain) as well as pain resulting from surgery, chemotherapy, or nerve infiltration.
Antihistamines, e.g., hydroxyzine (Atarax, Vistaril);	Mild anxiolytic agent with sedative and analgesic property. May produce additive analgesia with therapeutic doses of opioids and may be beneficial in limiting opioid-induced nausea/vomiting.
Provide/instruct in use of patient-controlled analgesics (PCA) as appropriate.	PCA provides for timely drug administration, preventing fluctuations in intensity of pain, often at lower total dosage than would be given by conventional methods.
Instruct in use of TENS unit.	Transcutaneous electrical nerve stimulation blocks nerve transmission of pain stimulus, providing reduction/relief of pain without drug-related side effects. Can be used in combination with other modalities.
Prepare for/assist with procedures, e.g., nerve blocks, cordotomy, commissural myelotomy, radiation therapy.	May be used in severe/intractable pain unresponsive to other measures. *Note:* Radiation is especially useful for bone metastasis and may provide fast onset of pain relief, even with only one treatment.
Refer to structured support group, psychiatric clinical nurse specialist/psychologist, spiritual advisor counseling as indicated.	May be necessary to reduce anxiety and enhance patient's coping skills, decreasing level of pain. *Note:* Hypnosis can heighten awareness and help to focus concentration to decrease perception of pain.

NURSING DIAGNOSIS: Nutrition: altered, less than body requirements

May be related to

Hypermetabolic state associated with cancer

Consequences of chemotherapy, radiation, surgery, e.g., anorexia, gastric irritation, taste distortions, nausea

Emotional distress, fatigue, poorly controlled pain

Possibly evidenced by

Reported inadequate food intake, altered taste sensation, loss of interest in food, perceived/actual inability to ingest food

Body weight 20% or more under ideal for height and frame, decreased subcutaneous fat/muscle mass

Sore, inflamed buccal cavity

Diarrhea and/or constipation, abdominal cramping

DESIRED OUTCOMES/EVALUATION CRITERIA—PATIENT WILL:

Demonstrate stable weight/progressive weight gain toward goal with normalization of laboratory values and free of signs of malnutrition.

Verbalize understanding of individual interferences to adequate intake.

Participate in specific interventions to stimulate appetite/increase dietary intake.

ACTIONS/INTERVENTIONS	RATIONALE
Independent	
Monitor daily food intake; have patient keep food diary as indicated.	Identifies nutritional strengths/deficiencies.
Measure height, weight, and tricep skinfold thickness (or other anthropometric measurements as appropriate). Ascertain amount of recent weight loss. Weigh daily or as indicated.	If these measurements fall below minimum standards, patient's chief source of stored energy (fat tissue) is depleted.
Assess for pallor, delayed wound healing, enlarged parotid glands.	Helps in identification of protein-calorie malnutrition, especially when weight and anthropometric measurements are less than normal.
Encourage patient to eat high-calorie, nutrient-rich diet, with adequate fluid intake. Encourage use of supplements and frequent/smaller meals spaced throughout the day.	Metabolic tissue needs are increased as well as fluids (to eliminate waste products). Supplements can play an important role in maintaining adequate caloric and protein intake.
Adjust diet prior to and immediately after treatment, e.g., clear, cool liquids, light/bland foods, dry crackers, toast, carbonated drinks. Give liquids 1 hour before or 1 hour after meals.	The effectiveness of diet adjustment is very individualized in relief of posttherapy nausea. Patients must experiment to find best solution/combination. Avoiding fluids during meals minimizes becoming "full" too quickly.
Control environmental factors (e.g., strong/noxious odors or noise). Avoid overly sweet, fatty, or spicy foods.	Can trigger nausea/vomiting response.
Create pleasant dining atmosphere; encourage patient to share meals with family/friends.	Makes mealtime more enjoyable, which may enhance intake.
Encourage use of relaxation techniques, visualization, guided imagery, moderate exercise before meals.	May prevent onset or reduce severity of nausea, decrease anorexia, and enable patient to increase oral intake.

ACTIONS/INTERVENTIONS	RATIONALE

Independent

Identify the patient who experiences anticipatory nausea/vomiting and take appropriate measures.

Psychogenic nausea/vomiting occurring before chemotherapy begins generally does not respond to antiemetic drugs. Change of treatment environment or patient routine on treatment day may be effective.

Encourage open communication regarding anorexia problem.

Often a source of emotional distress, especially for SO who wants to feed patient frequently. When patient refuses, SO may feel rejected/frustrated.

Administer antiemetic on a regular schedule before/during and after administration of antineoplastic agent as appropriate.

Nausea/vomiting are frequently the most disabling and psychologically stressful side effects of chemotherapy.

Evaluate effectiveness of antiemetic.

Individuals respond differently to all medications. First-line antiemetics may not work, requiring alteration in or use of combination drug therapy.

Hematest stools, gastric secretions.

Certain therapies (e.g., antimetabolites) inhibit renewal of epithelial cells lining the GI tract, which may cause changes ranging from mild erythema to severe ulceration with bleeding.

Collaborative

Review laboratory studies as indicated, e.g., total lymphocyte count, serum transferrin, and albumin/prealbumin.

Helps identify the degree of biochemical imbalance/malnutrition and influences choice of dietary interventions. *Note:* Anticancer treatments can also alter nutrition studies, so all results must be correlated with the patient's clinical status.

Administer medications as indicated:

$5-HT_3$ receptor antagonists, e.g., ondansetron (Zofran), granisetron (Kytril); phenothiazines, e.g., prochlorperazine (Compazine), thiethylperazine (Torecan); antidopaminergics, e.g., metoclopramide (Reglan); antihistamines, e.g., diphenhydramine (Benadryl);

Most antiemetics act to interfere with stimulation of true vomiting center, and chemoreceptor trigger zone agents also act peripherally to inhibit reverse peristalsis. These medications are often prescribed routinely during chemotherapy to prevent nausea and vomiting.

Corticosteroids, e.g., dexamethasone (Decadron); cannabinoids, e.g., 9-tetrahydrocannabinol; benzodiazepines, e.g., diazepam (Valium);

Combination therapy (e.g., Torecan with Decadron or Valium) is often more effective than single agents.

Vitamins, especially A, D, E, and B_6;

Prevents deficit related to decreased absorption of fat-soluble vitamins. Deficiency of B_6 can contribute to/exacerbate depression, irritability.

Antacids.

Minimizes gastric irritation and reduces risk of mucosal ulceration.

Refer to dietitian/nutritional support team.

Provides for specific dietary plan to meet individual needs and reduce problems associated with protein/calorie malnutrition and micronutrient deficiencies.

Insert/maintain NG or feeding tube for enteric feedings, or central line for TPN if indicated.

In the presence of severe malnutrition (e.g., loss of 25%–30% body weight in 2 months), or if patient has been NPO for 5 days and is unlikely to be able to eat for another week, tube feeding or TPN may be necessary to meet nutritional needs. *Note:* TPN is used with caution as it is associated with a more than 4-fold increase in the risk of significant infection.

NURSING DIAGNOSIS: Fluid Volume deficit, risk for

Risk factors may include
Excessive losses through normal routes (e.g., vomiting, diarrhea) and/or abnormal routes (e.g., indwelling tubes, wounds)
Hypermetabolic state
Impaired intake of fluids

Possibly evidenced by
[Not applicable; presence of signs and symptoms establishes an *actual* diagnosis]

DESIRED OUTCOMES/EVALUATION CRITERIA—PATIENT WILL:
Display adequate fluid balance as evidenced by stable vital signs, moist mucous membranes, good skin turgor, prompt capillary refill, and individually adequate urinary output.

ACTIONS/INTERVENTIONS	RATIONALE
Independent	
Monitor I&O and specific gravity; include all output sources, e.g., emesis, diarrhea, draining wounds. Calculate 24-hour balance.	Continued negative fluid balance, decreasing renal output and concentration of urine suggest developing dehydration and need for increased fluid replacement.
Weigh as indicated.	Sensitive measurement of fluctuations in fluid balance.
Monitor vital signs. Evaluate peripheral pulses, capillary refill.	Reflects adequacy of circulating volume.
Assess skin turgor and moisture of mucous membranes. Note reports of thirst.	Indirect indicators of hydration status/degree of deficit.
Encourage increased fluid intake to 3000 ml/d as individually appropriate/tolerated.	Assists in maintenance of fluid requirements and reduces risk of harmful side effects, e.g., hemorrhagic cystitis in patient receiving cyclophosphamide (Cytoxan).
Observe for bleeding tendencies, e.g., oozing from mucous membranes, puncture sites; presence of ecchymosis or petechiae.	Early identification of problems (which may occur as a result of cancer and/or therapies) allows for prompt intervention.
Minimize venipunctures (e.g., combine IV starts with blood draws). Encourage patient to consider central venous catheter placement.	Reduces potential for hemorrhage and infection associated with repeated venous puncture.
Avoid trauma and apply pressure to puncture sites.	Reduces potential for bleeding/hematoma formation.
Collaborative	
Provide IV fluids as indicated.	Given for general hydration as well as to dilute antineoplastic drugs and reduce adverse side effects, e.g., nausea/vomiting, or nephrotoxicity.
Administer antiemetic therapy. (Refer to ND: Nutrition: altered, less than body requirements, p 885.)	Alleviation of nausea/vomiting decreases gastric losses and allows for increased oral intake.
Monitor laboratory studies, e.g., CBC, electrolytes, serum albumin.	Provides information about level of hydration and corresponding deficits. *Note:* Malnutrition and effects of decreased albumin levels potentiates fluid shifts/edema formation.

ACTIONS/INTERVENTIONS

Collaborative

Administer transfusions as indicated, e.g.:

RBCs;

Platelets.

Avoid use of aspirin, gastric irritants, or platelet inhibitors.

RATIONALE

May be needed to restore blood count and prevent manifestations of anemia often present in cancer patients, e.g., tachycardia, tachypnea, dizziness, and weakness.

Thrombocytopenia (which may occur as a side effect of chemotherapy, radiation, or cancer process) increases the risk of bleeding from mucous membranes and other body sites. Spontaneous bleeding may occur with platelet count of 5000.

Negatively affect clotting mechanism and/or risk of bleeding.

NURSING DIAGNOSIS: Fatigue

May be related to
Decreased metabolic energy production, increased energy requirements (hypermetabolic state)
Overwhelming psychologic/emotional demands
Altered body chemistry: Side effects of medications, chemotherapy

Possibly evidenced by
Unremitting/overwhelming lack of energy, inability to maintain usual routines, decreased performance, impaired ability to concentrate, lethargy/listlessness
Disinterest in surroundings

DESIRED OUTCOMES/EVALUATION CRITERIA:—PATIENT WILL:
Report improved sense of energy.
Perform ADLs and participate in desired activities at level of ability.

ACTIONS/INTERVENTIONS

Independent

Plan care to allow for rest periods. Schedule activities for periods when patient has most energy. Involve patient/SO in schedule planning.

Establish realistic activity goals with patient.

Assist with self-care needs when indicated; keep bed in low position, pathways clear of furniture; assist with ambulation.

Encourage patient to do whatever possible, e.g., self-bath, sitting up in chair, walking. Increase activity level as individual is able.

Monitor physiologic response to activity, e.g., changes in BP or heart/respiratory rate.

RATIONALE

Frequent rest periods are needed to restore/conserve energy. Planning will allow patient to be active during times when energy level is higher, which may restore a feeling of well-being and a sense of control.

Provides for a sense of control and feelings of accomplishment.

Weakness may make ADLs difficult to complete or place the patient at risk for injury during activities.

Enhances strength/stamina and enables patient to become more active without undue fatigue.

Tolerance varies greatly depending on the stage of the disease process, nutrition state, fluid balance, and reaction to therapeutic regimen.

ACTIONS/INTERVENTIONS

Independent

Encourage nutritional intake. (Refer to ND: Nutrition: altered, less than body requirements, p 885.)

Collaborative

Provide supplemental O_2 as indicated.

Refer to physical/occupational therapy.

RATIONALE

Adequate intake/use of nutrients is necessary to meet energy needs for activity.

Presence of anemia/hypoxemia reduces O_2 available for cellular uptake and contributes to fatigue.

Programmed daily exercises and activities help patient to maintain/increase strength and muscle tone, enhance sense of well-being. Use of adaptive devices may help conserve energy.

NURSING DIAGNOSIS: Infection, risk for

Risk factors may include
Inadequate secondary defenses and immunosuppression, e.g., bone marrow suppression (dose-limiting side effect of both chemotherapy and radiation)
Malnutrition, chronic disease process
Invasive procedures

Possibly evidenced by
[Not applicable; presence of signs and symptoms establishes an *actual* diagnosis]

DESIRED OUTCOMES/EVALUATION CRITERIA—PATIENT WILL:
Identify and participate in interventions to prevent/reduce risk of infection.
Remain afebrile and achieve timely healing as appropriate.

ACTIONS/INTERVENTIONS

Independent

Promote good hand-washing procedures by staff and visitors. Screen/limit visitors who may have infections. Place in reverse isolation as indicated.

Emphasize personal hygiene.

Monitor temperature.

Assess all systems (e.g., skin, respiratory, genitourinary) for signs/symptoms of infection on a continual basis.

Reposition frequently; keep linens dry and wrinkle-free.

Promote adequate rest/exercise periods.

RATIONALE

Protects patient from sources of infection, such as visitors and staff who may have URI.

Limits potential sources of infection and/or secondary overgrowth.

Temperature elevation may occur (if not masked by corticosteroids or anti-inflammatory drugs) because of various factors, e.g., chemotherapy side effects, disease process, or infection. Early identification of infectious process enables appropriate therapy to be started promptly.

Early recognition and intervention may prevent progression to more serious situation/sepsis.

Reduces pressure and irritation to tissues and may prevent skin breakdown (potential site for bacterial growth).

Limits fatigue, yet encourages sufficient movement to prevent stasis complications, e.g., pneumonia, decubitus, and thrombus formation.

ACTIONS/INTERVENTIONS

Independent

Stress importance of good oral hygiene.

Avoid/limit invasive procedures. Adhere to aseptic techniques.

Collaborative

Monitor CBC with differential WBC and granulocyte count, and platelets as indicated.

Obtain cultures as indicated.

Administer antibiotics as indicated.

RATIONALE

Development of stomatitis increases risk of infection/secondary overgrowth.

Reduces risk of contamination, limits portal of entry for infectious agents.

Bone marrow activity may be inhibited by effects of chemotherapy, the disease state, or radiation therapy. Monitoring status of myelosuppression is important for preventing further complications (e.g., infection, anemia, or hemorrhage) and scheduling drug delivery. *Note:* The nadir (point of lowest drop in blood count) is usually seen 7–10 days after administration of chemotherapy.

Identifies causative organism(s) and appropriate therapy.

May be used to treat identified infection or given prophylactically in immunocompromised patient.

NURSING DIAGNOSIS: Oral Mucous Membrane, altered, risk for

Risk factors may include
Side effect of some chemotherapeutic agents (e.g., antimetabolites) and radiation
Dehydration, malnutrition, NPO restrictions for more than 24 hours

Possibly evidenced by
[Not applicable; presence of signs and symptoms establishes an *actual* diagnosis]

DESIRED OUTCOMES/EVALUATION CRITERIA—PATIENT WILL:
Display intact mucous membranes, which are pink, moist, and free of inflammation/ulcerations.
Verbalize understanding of causative factors.
Demonstrate techniques to maintain/restore integrity of oral mucosa.

ACTIONS/INTERVENTIONS

Independent

Assess dental health and oral hygiene on admission and periodically.

Assess oral cavity daily, noting changes in mucous membrane integrity (e.g., dry, reddened). Ascertain whether patient notices burning in the mouth, changes in voice quality, ability to swallow, sense of taste, development of thick/viscous saliva.

RATIONALE

Identifies prophylactic treatment needs prior to initiation of chemotherapy or radiation and provides baseline data of current oral hygiene for future comparison.

Inflammation of the oral mucosa (stomatitis) generally occurs 7–14 days after treatment begins, but signs may be seen as early as day 3 or 4, especially if there were any preexisting oral problems. The range of response extends from mild erythema to severe ulceration, which can be very painful, inhibit oral intake, and be potentially life-threatening. Early identification enables prompt treatment.

ACTIONS/INTERVENTIONS	RATIONALE

Independent

Discuss with patient areas needing improvement and demonstrate methods for good oral care.

Good care is critical during treatment to control stomatitis complications.

Initiate oral hygiene program to include:

Avoidance of commercial mouthwashes, lemon/glycerine swabs;

Products containing alcohol or phenol may exacerbate mucous membrane dryness/irritation.

Use of mouthwash made from warm saline, dilute solution of hydrogen peroxide or baking soda and water;

May be soothing to the membranes. Rinsing before meals may improve the patient's sense of taste. Rinsing after meals and at bedtime dilutes oral acids and relieves xerostomia.

Brush with soft toothbrush or toothette;

Prevents trauma to delicate/fragile tissues. *Note:* Toothbrush should be changed at least every 3 months.

Floss gently or use WaterPik cautiously;

Removes food particles that can promote bacterial growth.

Keep lips moist with lip gloss or balm, K-Y Jelly, Chapstick, and so forth;

Promotes comfort and prevents drying/cracking of tissues.

Encourage use of mints/hard candy or artificial saliva (Ora-Lube, Salivart) as indicated.

Stimulates secretions/provides moisture to maintain integrity of mucous membranes, especially in presence of dehydration/reduced saliva production.

Instruct regarding dietary changes: e.g., avoid hot or spicy foods, acidic juices; suggest use of straw; ingesting soft or blenderized foods, Popsicles, and ice cream as tolerated.

Severe stomatitis may interfere with nutritional and fluid intake leading to negative nitrogen balance or dehydration. Dietary modifications may make foods easier to swallow and feel soothing.

Encourage fluid intake as individually tolerated.

Adequate hydration helps keep mucous membranes moist, preventing drying/cracking.

Discuss limitation of smoking and alcohol intake.

May cause further irritation and dryness of mucous membranes. *Note:* May need to compromise if these activities are important to patient's emotional status.

Monitor for and explain to patient signs of oral superinfection (e.g., thrush).

Early recognition provides opportunity for prompt treatment.

Collaborative

Refer to dentist before initiating chemotherapy or head/neck radiation.

Prophylactic examination and repair work prior to therapy reduce risk of infection.

Culture suspicious oral lesions.

Identifies organism(s) responsible for oral infections and suggests appropriate drug therapy.

Administer medications as indicated, e.g.:

Analgesic rinses, topical lidocaine (Xylocaine) jelly;

Aggressive analgesia program may be required to relieve intense pain.

Antimicrobial mouthwash preparation, e.g., nystatin (Mycostatin).

May be needed to treat/prevent secondary oral infections, such as *Candida, Pseudomonas,* herpes simplex.

891

ACTIONS/INTERVENTIONS

Independent

Assess skin frequently for side effects of cancer therapy; note breakdown/delayed wound healing. Stress importance of reporting open areas to caregiver.

Bathe with lukewarm water and mild soap.

Encourage patient to avoid scratching and to pat skin dry instead of rubbing.

Turn/reposition frequently.

Review skin care protocol for patient receiving radiation therapy:

Avoid rubbing or use of soap, lotions, creams, ointments, powders, or deodorants on area; avoid applying heat or attempting to wash off marks/tattoos placed on skin to identify area of irradiation;

Recommend wearing soft, loose clothing next to area; have female patient avoid wearing bra if it creates pressure;

Apply cornstarch to area as needed and Eucerin (or other recommended cream) to area twice daily after radiation is completed;

Encourage liberal use of sunscreen/block.

Review skin care protocol for patient receiving chemotherapy, e.g.:

Use appropriate peripheral or central venous catheter, dilute anticancer drug per protocol and ascertain that IV is infusing well;

RATIONALE

A reddening and/or tanning effect (radiation reaction) may develop within the field of radiation. Dry desquamation (dryness and pruritus), moist desquamation (blistering), ulceration, hair loss, loss of dermis and sweat glands may also be noted. In addition, skin reactions (e.g., allergic rashes, hyperpigmentation, pruritus, and alopecia) may occur with some chemotherapy agents.

Maintains cleanliness without irritating the skin.

Helps prevent skin friction/trauma.

Promotes circulation and prevents undue pressure on skin/tissues.

Designed to minimize trauma to area of radiation therapy.

Can potentiate or otherwise interfere with radiation delivery. May actually increase irritation/reaction.

Skin is very sensitive during and after treatment, and all irritation should be avoided to prevent dermal injury.

Helps to control dampness or pruritus. Maintenance care is required until skin/tissues have regenerated and are back to normal.

Protects skin from ultraviolet rays and reduces risk of recall reactions.

Reduces risk of tissue irritation/extravasation of agent into tissues.

892

ACTIONS/INTERVENTIONS	RATIONALE

Independent

Instruct patient to notify caregiver promptly of discomfort at IV insertion site;

Development of irritation indicates need for alteration of rate/dilution of chemotherapy and/or change of IV site to prevent more serious reaction.

Assess skin/IV site and vein for erythema, edema, tenderness; weltlike patches, itching/burning; or swelling, burning, soreness, blisters progressing to ulceration/tissue necrosis.

Presence of phlebitis, vein flare (localized allergic reaction) or extravasation requires immediate discontinuation of antineoplastic agent and medical intervention.

Wash skin immediately with soap and water if antineoplastic agents are spilled on unprotected skin (patient or caregiver).

Dilutes drug to reduce risk of skin irritation/chemical burn.

Advise patients receiving 5-fluorouracil (5-FU) and methotrexate to avoid sun exposure. Withhold methotrexate if sunburn present.

Sun can cause exacerbation of burn spotting (a side effect of 5-fluorouracil) or can cause a red "flash" area with methotrexate, which can exacerbate drug's effect.

Review expected dermatologic side effects seen with chemotherapy, e.g., rash, hyperpigmentation, and peeling of skin on palms.

Anticipatory guidance helps decrease concern if side effects do occur.

Inform patient that if alopecia occurs, hair could grow back after completion of chemotherapy, but may/may not grow back after radiation therapy.

Anticipatory guidance may help adjustment to/preparation for baldness. Men are often as sensitive to hair loss as women. Radiation's effect on hair follicles may be permanent, depending on rad dosage.

Collaborative

Administer appropriate antidote if extravasation of IV should occur, e.g.:

Reduces local tissue damage.

Topical DMSO;

May be useful for mitomycin, doxorubicin (Adriamycin)/daunorubicin. *Note:* Injection of Benadryl may relieve symptoms of vein flare.

Hyaluronidase (Wydase);

Injected subcutaneously for vincristine infiltration.

NaHCO$_3$;

Injected IV and/or into surrounding tissues for Bisantrene.

Thiosulfate.

Injected subcutaneously for nitrogen mustard.

Apply topical ointment, e.g., silver sulfadiazine (Silvadene) as appropriate.

May be used to prevent infection/facilitate healing if chemical burn (extravasation) occurs.

Apply ice pack/warm compresses per protocol.

Controversial intervention is dependent on type of agent used. Ice restricts blood flow, keeping drug localized, while heat enhances dispersion of neoplastic drug/antidote, minimizing tissue damage.

NURSING DIAGNOSIS: Constipation/Diarrhea, risk for

Risk factors may include
Irritation of the GI mucosa from either chemotherapy or radiation therapy; malabsorption of fat
Hormone-secreting tumor, carcinoma of colon
Poor fluid intake, low-bulk diet, lack of exercise, use of opiates/narcotics

893

ACTIONS/INTERVENTIONS	RATIONALE
Independent	
Ascertain usual elimination habits.	Data required as baseline for future evaluation.
Assess bowel sounds and monitor/record bowel movements including frequency, consistency (particularly during first 3–5 days of *Vinca* alkaloid therapy).	Defines problem, i.e., diarrhea, constipation. *Note:* Constipation is one of the earliest manifestations of neurotoxicity.
Monitor I&O and weight.	Dehydration, weight loss, and electrolyte imbalance are complications of diarrhea. Inadequate fluid intake may potentiate constipation.
Encourage adequate fluid intake (e.g., 2000 ml/24 h), increased fiber in diet; regular exercise.	May reduce potential for constipation by improving stool consistency and stimulating peristalsis; can prevent dehydration (diarrhea).
Provide small, frequent meals of foods low in residue (if not contraindicated), maintaining needed protein and carbohydrates (e.g., eggs, cooked cereal, bland cooked vegetables).	Reduces gastric irritation. Use of low-fiber foods can decrease irritability and provide bowel rest when diarrhea present.
Adjust diet as appropriate: avoid foods high in fat (e.g., butter, fried foods, nuts); foods with high-fiber content; those known to cause diarrhea or gas (e.g., cabbage, baked beans, chili); food/fluids high in caffeine; or extremely hot or cold food/fluids.	GI stimulants that may increase gastric motility/frequency of stools.
Check for impaction if patient has not had BM in 3 days or if abdominal distention, cramping, headache are present.	Further interventions/alternative bowel care may be needed.
Collaborative	
Monitor laboratory studies as indicated, e.g., electrolytes.	Electrolyte imbalances may be the result of/contribute to altered GI function.
Administer IV fluids;	Prevents dehydration, dilutes chemotherapy agents to diminish side effects.
Antidiarrheal agents;	May be indicated to control severe diarrhea.
Stool softeners, laxatives, enemas as indicated.	Prophylactic use may prevent further complications in some patients (e.g., those who will receive *Vinca* alkaloid, have poor bowel pattern prior to treatment, or have decreased motility).

NURSING DIAGNOSIS: Sexuality Patterns, altered, risk for

Risk factors may include

Knowledge/skill deficit about alternative responses to health-related transitions, altered body function/structure, illness, and medical treatment

Overwhelming fatigue

Fear and anxiety

Lack of privacy/SO

Possibly evidenced by

[Not applicable; presence of signs and symptoms establishes an *actual* diagnosis]

DESIRED OUTCOMES/EVALUATION CRITERIA—PATIENT WILL:

Verbalize understanding of effects of cancer and therapeutic regimen on sexuality and measures to correct/deal with problems.

Maintain sexual activity at a desired level as possible.

ACTIONS/INTERVENTIONS	RATIONALE
Independent	
Discuss with patient/SO the nature of sexuality and reactions when it is altered or threatened. Provide information about normality of these problems and that many people find it helpful to seek assistance with adaptation process.	Acknowledges legitimacy of the problem. Sexuality encompasses the way men and women view themselves as individuals and how they relate between and among themselves in every area of life.
Advise patient of side effects of prescribed cancer treatment that are known to affect sexuality.	Anticipatory guidance can help patient and SO begin the process of adaptation to new state.
Provide private time for hospitalized patient. Knock on door and receive permission from patient/SO before entering.	Sexual needs do not end because the patient is hospitalized. Intimacy needs continue and an open and accepting attitude for the expression of those needs is essential.

NURSING DIAGNOSIS: Family Processes, altered, risk for

Risk factors may include

Situational/transitional crises: Long-term illness, change in roles/economic status

Developmental: Anticipated loss of a family member

Possibly evidenced by

[Not applicable; presence of signs and symptoms establishes an *actual* diagnosis]

DESIRED OUTCOMES/EVALUATION CRITERIA—FAMILY WILL:

Express feelings freely.

Demonstrate individual involvement in problem-solving process directed at appropriate solutions for the situation.

Encourage and allow member who is ill to handle situation in own way.

ACTIONS/INTERVENTIONS	RATIONALE

Independent

Note components of family, presence of extended family and others, e.g., friends/neighbors.	Helps patient and caregiver to know who is available to assist with care, provide respite and support.
Identify patterns of communication in family and patterns of interaction between family members.	Provides information about effectiveness of communication and identifies problems that may interfere with family's ability to assist patient and adjust positively to diagnosis/treatment of cancer.
Assess role expectations of family members and encourage discussion about them.	Each person may see the situation in own individual manner, and clear identification and sharing of these expectations promote understanding.
Assess energy direction, e.g., are efforts at resolution/problem solving purposeful or scattered?	Provides clues about interventions that may be appropriate to assist patient and family in directing energies in a more effective manner.
Note cultural/religious beliefs.	Affects patient/SO reaction and adjustment to diagnosis, treatment, and outcome of cancer.
Listen for expressions of helplessness.	Helpless feelings may contribute to difficulty adjusting to diagnosis of cancer and cooperating with treatment regimen.
Deal with family members in a warm, caring, respectful way. Provide information (verbal/written), and reinforce as necessary.	Provides feeling of empathy and promotes individual's sense of worth and competence in ability to handle current situation.
Encourage appropriate expressions of anger without reacting negatively to them.	Feelings of anger are to be expected when individuals are dealing with the difficult/potentially fatal illness of cancer. Appropriate expression enables progress toward resolution of the stages of the grieving process.
Acknowledge difficulties of the situation, e.g., diagnosis and treatment of cancer, possibility of death.	Communicates acceptance of the reality the patient/family are facing.
Identify and encourage use of previous successful coping behaviors.	Most people have developed effective coping skills that can be useful in dealing with current situation.
Stress importance of continuous open dialogue between family members.	Promotes understanding and assists family members to maintain clear communication and resolve problems effectively.

Collaborative

Refer to support groups, clergy, family therapy as indicated.	May need additional assistance to resolve problems of disorganization that may accompany diagnosis of potentially terminal illness (cancer).

NURSING DIAGNOSIS: Knowledge deficit [learning need] regarding illness, prognosis, treatment, self care and discharge needs

May be related to
Lack of exposure/recall; information misinterpretation, myths
Unfamiliarity with information resources
Cognitive limitation

Possibly evidenced by
Questions/request for information, verbalization of problem
Statement of misconception
Inaccurate follow-through of instructions/development of preventable complications

ACTIONS/INTERVENTIONS	RATIONALE
Independent	
Review with patient/SO understanding of specific diagnosis, treatment alternatives, and future expectations.	Validates current level of understanding, identifies learning needs, and provides knowledge base on which patient can make informed decisions.
Determine patient's perception of cancer and cancer treatment(s); ask about patient's own/previous experience or experience with other people who have (or had) cancer.	Aids in identification of ideas, attitudes, fears, misconceptions, and gaps in knowledge about cancer.
Provide clear, accurate information in a factual but sensitive manner. Answer questions specifically, but do not bombard with unessential details.	Helps with adjustment to the diagnosis of cancer by providing needed information along with time to absorb it. *Note:* Rate and method of giving information may need to be altered in order to decrease patient's anxiety and enhance ability to assimilate information.
Provide anticipatory guidance with patient/SO regarding treatment protocol, length of therapy, expected results, possible side effects. Be honest with patient.	Patient has the "right to know" (be informed) and participate in decision tree. Accurate and concise information helps to dispel fears and anxiety, helps clarify the expected routine, and enables patient to maintain some degree of control.
Ask patient for verbal feedback, and correct misconception about individual's type of cancer and treatment.	Misconceptions about cancer may be more disturbing than facts and can interfere with treatments/delay healing.
Outline normally expected limitations (if any) on ADLs (e.g., limit sun exposure, alcohol intake; loss of work time because of in-hospital treatments).	Enables patient/SO to begin to put limitations into perspective and plan/adapt as indicated.
Provide written materials about cancer, treatment, and available support systems.	Anxiety and preoccupation with thoughts about life and death often interfere with patient's ability to assimilate adequate information. Written, take-home materials provide reinforcement and clarification about information as patient needs it.
Review specific medication regimen and use of OTC drugs.	Enhances ability to manage self-care and avoid potential complications, drug reactions/interactions.
Address specific home care needs, e.g., ability to live alone, perform necessary treatments/procedures, and acquire supplies.	Provides information regarding changes that may be needed in current plan of care to meet therapeutic needs.
Do predischarge home evaluation as indicated.	Aids in transition to home setting by providing information about needed changes in physical layout, acquisition of needed supplies.

897

ACTIONS/INTERVENTIONS	RATIONALE

Independent

Refer to community resources as indicated: e.g., social services, home health, Meals-on-Wheels, local American Cancer Society chapter, hospice center/services.	Promotes competent self-care and optimal independence. Maintains patient in desired/home setting.
Review with patient/SO the importance of maintaining optimal nutritional status.	Promotes well-being, facilitates recovery, and is critical in enabling the patient to tolerate treatments.
Encourage diet variations and experimentation in meal planning and food preparation, e.g., cooking with sweet juices, wine; serving foods cold or at room temperature as appropriate (egg salad, ice cream).	Creativity may enhance flavor and intake, especially when protein foods taste bitter.
Recommend cookbooks that are designed for cancer patients.	Helps to provide specific menu/recipe ideas.
Recommend increased fluid intake and fiber in diet as well as routine exercise.	Improves consistency of stool and stimulates peristalsis.
Instruct patient to assess oral mucous membranes routinely, noting erythema, ulceration.	Early recognition of problems promotes early intervention, minimizing complications that may impair oral intake and provide avenue for systemic infection.
Advise patient concerning skin and hair care: e.g., avoid harsh shampoos, hair dyes, permanents, salt water, chlorinated water; avoid exposure to strong wind and extreme heat or cold; avoid sun exposure to target area for 1 year after end of radiation treatments; and regularly apply sunblock (SPF 15 or greater).	Prevents additional hair damage and skin irritation; may prevent recall reactions.
Review signs and symptoms requiring medical evaluation, e.g., infection, delayed healing, drug reactions, increased pain (dependent on individual situation).	Early identification and treatment may limit severity of complications.
Stress importance of continuing medical follow-up.	Provides ongoing monitoring of progression/resolution of disease process and opportunity for timely diagnosis and treatment of complications. *Note:* Some complications can develop long after therapy is completed, e.g., pathologic fractures, radiation cystitis/nephritis.
Encourage periodic review of advance directives. Promote inclusion of family/SO in decision-making process.	Patient/family/SO need to reevaluate choices as condition changes (for better/worse) and treatment options become available or are exhausted.

POTENTIAL CONSIDERATIONS following acute hospitalization (dependent on patient's age, physical condition/presence of complications, personal resources, and life responsibilities)

In addition to Potential Considerations in specific plans of care:
Coping, Individual, impaired—situational crises, vulnerability
Self Care deficit/Home Maintenance Management, impaired—decreased strength and endurance, pain/discomfort, depression, insufficient finances, unfamiliarity with neighborhood resources, inadequate support systems
Caregiver Role Strain, risk for—illness severity of care receiver, significant home care needs, situational stressors, complexity/amount of caregiving tasks
Pain—disease process (compression/destruction of nerve tissue, infiltration of nerves, or their vascular supply, obstruction of a nerve pathway, inflammation)
Therapeutic Regimen: Individual, ineffective management—complexity of therapeutic regimen, economic difficulties, decisional conflict, perceived barriers, powerlessness, social support deficits

FLUID AND ELECTROLYTE IMBALANCES

The body is equipped with homeostatic mechanisms to keep the composition and volume of body fluids within narrow limits of normal. Organs involved in this mechanism include the kidneys, lungs, heart, blood vessels, adrenal glands, parathyroid glands, and pituitary gland. Total body water, essential for metabolism, declines with age. It constitutes about 80% of an infant's body weight, 60% of an adult's, and as little as 40% of an older person's weight. *Note:* Because fluid and electrolyte imbalances usually occur in conjunction with other medical conditions, the following information is offered as a reference. The interventions are presented in a general format for inclusion in the primary plan of care.

RELATED CONCERNS

Plans of care specific to underlying health condition causing imbalance
Metabolic Acidosis (Primary Base Bicarbonate Deficit), p 506
Metabolic Alkalosis (Primary Base Bicarbonate Excess), p 510
Renal Dialysis, p 580
Respiratory Acidosis (Primary Carbonic Acid Excess), p 200
Respiratory Alkalosis (Primary Carbonic Acid Deficit), p 204

NURSING PRIORITIES

1. Restore homeostasis.
2. Prevent/minimize complications.
3. Provide information about condition/prognosis and treatment needs as appropriate.

DISCHARGE GOALS

1. Homcostasis restored.
2. Free of complications.
3. Condition/prognosis and treatment needs understood.
4. Plan in place to meet needs after discharge.

Hypervolemia (Extracellular Fluid Volume Excess)

PREDISPOSING/CONTRIBUTING FACTORS

Excess sodium intake including sodium-containing foods, medications, fluids (po/IV)
Excessive, rapid administration of isotonic parenteral fluids
Increased release of ADH; excessive ACTH production, hyperaldosteronism
Decreased plasma proteins as may occur with chronic liver disease with ascites, major abdominal surgery, mal-nutrition/protein depletion
Chronic kidney disease/ARF
Heart failure

Patient Assessment Data Base

ACTIVITY/REST

May report: Fatigue, generalized weakness

899

CIRCULATION

May exhibit: Hypertension, elevated CVP
Pulse full/bounding; tachycardia usually present; bradycardia (late sign of cardiac decompensation)
Extra heart sounds (S_3)
Edema: Dependent, pitting, facial, periorbital, anasarca
Neck and peripheral vein distention

ELIMINATION

May report: Decreased urinary output, polyuria if renal function is normal

FOOD/FLUID

May report: Anorexia, nausea/vomiting; thirst (may be absent, especially in elderly)

May exhibit: Abdominal girth increased with visible fluid wave on palpation (ascites)
Sudden weight gain, often in excess of 5% of total body weight
Edema: Initially dependent, may progress to general/anasarca

NEUROSENSORY

May exhibit: Changes in level of consciousness, from confusion to coma; aphasia
Seizure activity

PAIN/DISCOMFORT

May report: Headache
Abdominal cramps

RESPIRATION

May report: Shortness of breath

May exhibit: Tachypnea with/without dyspnea, orthopnea; productive cough
Crackles

SAFETY

May exhibit: Fever
Skin changes in color, temperature, turgor, e.g., taut and cool where edematous

TEACHING/LEARNING

Refer to predisposing/contributing factors

Discharge plan considerations: **DRG projected mean length of inpatient stay: 4.1 days (dependent on underlying condition)**

May require assistance with changes in therapeutic regimen, dietary management

Refer to plan of care concerning underlying medical/surgical condition for possible postdischarge considerations.

DIAGNOSTIC STUDIES

CBC: Hb/Hct and RBC usually decreased (hemodilution).
Serum sodium: May be high, low, or normal.
Serum potassium and BUN: Normal or decreased, unless renal damage present.

Total protein: Plasma proteins/albumin may be decreased.
Serum osmolality: Usually unchanged, although hypo-osmolality may occur.
Urine sodium: May be low because of sodium retention.
Urine specific gravity: Decreased.
Chest x-ray: May reveal signs of congestion.

NURSING DIAGNOSIS: Fluid Volume excess

May be related to
Excess fluid/sodium intake
Compromised regulatory mechanism

Possibly evidenced by
Signs/symptoms noted in data base

DESIRED OUTCOMES/EVALUATION CRITERIA—PATIENT WILL:
Demonstrate stabilized fluid volume as evidenced by balanced I&O, vital signs within
    patient's normal range, stable weight, and absence of signs of edema.
Verbalize understanding of individual dietary/fluid restrictions.
Demonstrate behaviors to monitor fluid status and prevent/limit recurrence.

ACTIONS/INTERVENTIONS	RATIONALE
Independent	
Monitor vital signs, also CVP if available.	Tachycardia and hypertension are common manifestations. Tachypnea usually present with/without dyspnea. Elevated CVP may be noted before dyspnea and adventitious breath sounds occur.
Auscultate lungs and heart sounds.	Adventitious sounds (crackles) and extra heart sounds (S_3) are indicative of fluid excess. Pulmonary edema may develop rapidly.
Assess for presence/location of edema formation.	Edema may be generalized or localized in dependent areas. Elderly patients may develop dependent edema with relatively little excess fluid. *Note:* Patients in a supine position can have an increase of 4–8 L of fluid before edema is readily detected.
Note presence of neck and peripheral vein distention, along with pitting edema, dyspnea.	Signs of cardiac decompensation/heart failure.
Maintain accurate I&O. Note decreased urinary output, positive fluid balance on 24-hour calculations.	Decreased renal perfusion, cardiac insufficiency, and fluid shifts may cause decreased urinary output and edema formation.
Weigh as indicated. Be alert for acute or sudden weight gain.	1 L of fluid retention equals a weight gain of 2.2 lb.
Give oral fluids with caution. If fluids are restricted, set up a 24-hour schedule for fluid intake.	Fluid restrictions, as well as extracellular shifts, can cause drying of mucous membranes, and patient may desire more fluids than are prudent.
Monitor infusion rate of parenteral fluids closely; administer via control device/pump as necessary.	Sudden fluid bolus/prolonged excessive administration potentiates volume overload/risk of cardiac decompensation.

ACTIONS/INTERVENTIONS	RATIONALE
Independent	
Encourage coughing/deep-breathing exercises.	Pulmonary fluid shifts potentiate respiratory complications.
Maintain semi-Fowler's position if dyspnea or ascites is present.	Gravity improves lung expansion by lowering diaphragm and shifting fluid to lower abdominal cavity.
Turn, reposition, and provide skin care at regular intervals.	Reduces pressure and friction on edematous tissue, which is more prone to breakdown than normal tissue.
Encourage bed rest. Schedule care to provide frequent rest periods.	Limited cardiac reserves result in fatigue/activity intolerance. In addition, lying down favors diuresis and reduction of edema.
Provide safety precautions as indicated, e.g., use of side rails, bed in low position, frequent observation, soft restraints (if required).	Fluid shifts may cause cerebral edema/changes in mentation, especially in the geriatric population.
Collaborative	
Assist with identification/treatment of underlying cause.	Refer to listing of predisposing/contributing factors to determine treatment needs.
Monitor laboratory studies as indicated, e.g., electrolytes, BUN, ABGs.	Extracellular fluid shifts, sodium/water restriction and renal function all affect serum sodium levels. Potassium deficit may occur with diuretic therapy. BUN may be increased as a result of renal dysfunction/failure. ABGs may reflect metabolic acidosis.
Provide balanced protein, low-sodium diet. Restrict fluids as indicated.	In presence of decreased serum proteins (e.g., malnutrition), increasing level of serum proteins can enhance colloidal osmotic gradients and promote return of fluid to the vascular space. Restriction of sodium/water decreases extracellular fluid retention.
Administer diuretics: i.e., loop diuretic, e.g., furosemide (Lasix); thiazide diuretic, e.g., hydrochlorothiazide (Esidrix); potassium-sparing diuretic, e.g., spironolactone (Aldactone).	To achieve excretion of excess fluid, either a single diuretic (e.g., thiazide) or a combination of agents may be selected (e.g., thiazide and spironolactone). The combination can be particularly helpful when two drugs have different sites of action and allow more effective control of fluid excess.
Replace potassium losses as indicated.	Potassium deficit may occur especially if patient is receiving potassium-wasting diuretic. This can cause lethal cardiac dysrhythmias if untreated.
Prepare for/assist with dialysis or ultrafiltration, if indicated.	May be done to rapidly reduce fluid overload, especially in the presence of severe cardiac/renal failure.

Hypovolemia (Extracellular Fluid Volume Deficit)

PREDISPOSING/CONTRIBUTING FACTORS

Excessive losses: Vomiting, gastric suctioning, diarrhea, polyuria, diaphoresis, wounds or burns, intraoperative fluid loss, hemorrhage
Insufficient/decreased fluid intake, e.g., preoperative/postoperative NPO status
Systemic infections, fever

Intestinal obstruction or fistulas
Pancreatitis, peritonitis, cirrhosis/ascites; adrenal insufficiency
Kidney disease, diabetic ketoacidosis, HHNC, diabetes insipidus

Patient Assessment Data Base

ACTIVITY/REST

May report: Fatigue, generalized weakness

CIRCULATION

May exhibit: Hypotension, including postural changes
Pulse weak/thready; tachycardia
Neck veins flattened; CVP decreased

ELIMINATION

May report: Constipation or occasionally diarrhea, abdominal cramps

May exhibit: Urine volume decreased, dark/concentrated color; oliguria (severe fluid depletion)

FOOD/FLUID

May report: Thirst, anorexia, nausea/vomiting

May exhibit: Weight loss often exceeding 2%–8% of total body weight
Abdominal distention
Mucous membranes dry, furrows on tongue; decreased tearing and salivation
Skin dry with poor turgor; or pale, moist, clammy (shock)

NEUROSENSORY

May report: Tingling of the extremities, vertigo, syncope

May exhibit: Behavior change, apathy, restlessness, confusion

RESPIRATION

May exhibit: Tachypnea, rapid/shallow breathing

SAFETY

May exhibit: Temperature usually subnormal, although fever may occur

TEACHING/LEARNING

Refer to predisposing/contributing factors

Discharge plan considerations: **DRG projected mean length of inpatient stay: 4.1 days (dependent on underlying cause)**
May require assistance with changes in therapeutic regimen, dietary management

Refer to plan of care concerning underlying medical/surgical condition for possible considerations after discharge.

DIAGNOSTIC STUDIES

Serum Sodium: May be normal, high, or low.

Urine Sodium: Usually decreased (less than 10 mEq/L when losses are from external causes; usually greater than 20 mEq/L if the cause is renal or adrenal).

CBC: Hb/Hct and RBC usually increased (hemoconcentration); decrease suggests hemorrhage.

Serum glucose: Normal or elevated.

Serum protein: Increased.

BUN and Cr: Increased, with BUN out of proportion to Cr.

Urine specific gravity: Increased.

NURSING DIAGNOSIS: Fluid Volume deficit

May be related to

Active fluid loss, e.g., hemorrhage, vomiting/gastric intubation, diarrhea, burns, wounds, fistulas

Regulatory failure, e.g., adrenal disease, recovery phase of ARF; DKA, HHNC, diabetes insipidus; systemic infections

Possibly evidenced by

Signs/symptoms noted in patient data base

DESIRED OUTCOMES/EVALUATION CRITERIA—PATIENT WILL:

Maintain fluid volume at a functional level as evidenced by individually adequate urinary output with normal specific gravity, stable vital signs, moist mucous membranes, good skin turgor, and prompt capillary refill.

Verbalize understanding of causative factors and purpose of therapeutic interventions.

Demonstrate behaviors to monitor and correct deficit as appropriate.

ACTIONS/INTERVENTIONS	RATIONALE
Independent	
Monitor vital signs and CVP. Note presence/degree of postural BP changes. Observe for temperature elevations/fever.	Tachycardia is present as well as varying degree of hypotension, depending on degree of fluid deficit. CVP measurements are useful in determining degree of fluid deficit and response to replacement therapy. Fever increases metabolism and exacerbates fluid loss.
Palpate peripheral pulses; note capillary refill, skin color/temperature; assess mentation.	Conditions that contribute to extracellular fluid deficit can result in inadequate organ perfusion to all areas and may cause circulatory collapse/shock.
Monitor urinary output. Measure/estimate fluid losses from all sources, e.g., gastric losses, wound drainage, diaphoresis.	Fluid replacement needs are based on correction of current deficits and ongoing losses. *Note:* A diaphoretic episode requiring a full linen change may represent a fluid loss of as much as 1 L. A decreased urinary output may indicate insufficient renal perfusion/hypovolemia, or polyuria can be present, requiring more aggressive fluid replacement.

ACTIONS/INTERVENTIONS	RATIONALE

Independent

Weigh daily and compare with 24-hour fluid balance. Mark/measure edematous areas, e.g., abdomen, limbs.

Changes in weight may not accurately reflect intravascular volume; e.g., third-space fluid accumulation cannot be used by the body for tissue perfusion.

Evaluate patient's ability to swallow.

Impaired gag/swallow reflexes, anorexia/nausea, oral discomfort, and changes in level of consciousness/cognition are among the factors that affect patient's ability to replace fluids orally.

Ascertain patient's beverage preferences, and set up a 24-hour schedule for fluid intake. Encourage foods with high fluid content.

Relieves thirst and discomfort of dry mucous membranes and augments parenteral replacement.

Turn frequently, massage skin, and protect bony prominences.

Tissues are susceptible to breakdown because of vaesoconstriction and increased cellular fragility.

Provide skin and mouth care. Bathe every other day using mild soap. Apply lotion as indicated.

Skin and mucous membranes are dry, with decreased elasticity, because of vasoconstriction and reduced intracellular water. Daily bathing may increase dryness.

Provide safety precautions as indicated, e.g., use of side rails, bed in low position, frequent observation, soft restraints (if required).

Decreased cerebral perfusion frequently results in changes in mentation/altered thought processes, requiring protective measures to prevent patient injury.

Investigate reports of sudden/sharp chest pain, dyspnea, cyanosis, increased anxiety, restlessness.

Hemoconcentration (sludging) and increased platelet aggregation may result in systemic emboli formation.

Monitor for sudden/marked elevation of BP, restlessness, moist cough, dyspnea, basalar crackles, frothy sputum.

Too rapid a correction of fluid deficit may compromise the cardiopulmonary system, especially if colloids are used in general fluid replacement (increased osmotic pressure potentiates fluid shifts).

Collaborative

Assist with identification/treatment of underlying cause.

Refer to listing of predisposing/contributing factors to determine treatment needs.

Monitor laboratory studies as indicated, e.g., electrolytes, glucose, pH/P_{CO_2}, coagulation studies.

Depending on the avenue of fluid loss, differing electrolyte/metabolic imbalances may be present/require correction; e.g., use of glucose solutions in patients with underlying glucose intolerance may result in serum glucose elevation and increased urinary water losses.

Administer IV solutions as indicated:

Isotonic solutions, e.g., 0.9% NaCl (normal saline), 5% dextrose/water;

Crystalloids provide prompt circulatory improvement, although the benefit may be transient (increased renal clearance).

0.45% NaCl (half-normal saline), lactated Ringer's solution;

As soon as the patient is normotensive, a hypotonic solution (0.45% NaCl) may be used to provide both electrolytes and free water for renal excretion of metabolic wastes. *Note:* Buffered crystalloids (LR) are used with caution as they may potentiate the risk of metabolic acidosis.

905

ACTIONS/INTERVENTIONS

Collaborative

RATIONALE

Colloids, e.g., dextran, Plasmanate/albumin, heta-starch (Hespan);

Corrects plasma protein concentration deficits, thereby increasing intravascular osmotic pressure and facilitating return of fluid into vascular compartment.

Whole blood/packed RBC transfusion, or autologous collection of blood.

Indicated when hypovolemia is related to active blood loss.

Administer sodium bicarbonate, if indicated.

May be given to correct severe acidosis while correcting fluid balance.

Provide tube feedings, including free water as appropriate.

Enteral replacement can provide proteins and other needed elements in addition to meeting general fluid requirements when swallowing is impaired.

Sodium

Sodium is the major cation of extracellular fluid and is primarily responsible for osmotic pressure in that compartment. Sodium enhances neuromuscular conduction/transmission of impulses and is essential for maintaining acid/base balance. Normal serum range is 135–145 mEq/L; intracellular, 10 mEq/L. Chloride is carried by Na and will display the same imbalances. Normal serum chloride range is 95–105 mEq/L.

Hyponatremia (Sodium Deficit)

PREDISPOSING/CONTRIBUTING FACTORS

Primary hyponatremia (loss of sodium): Lack of sufficient dietary sodium, severe malnutrition, infusion of sodium-free solutions; excessive sodium loss through heavy sweating (e.g., heat exhaustion), wounds/trauma (hemorrhage), burns, gastric suctioning, vomiting, diarrhea, small-bowel obstruction, peritonitis, salt-wasting renal dysfunction, adrenal insufficiency (Addison's disease)

Dilutional hyponatremia (water gains): Excessive water intake, electrolyte-free IV infusion, water intoxication (IV therapy, tap-water enemas), gastric irrigations with electrolyte-free solutions, presence of tumors or CNS disorders predisposing to SIADH, HF, renal failure/nephrotic syndrome, hepatic cirrhosis, DM (hyperglycemia), freshwater near-drowning; use of certain drugs, e.g., hypoglycemia medications, barbiturates, antipsychotics, aminophylline, morphine (may stimulate pituitary gland to secrete excessive amounts of ADH), anticonvulsants, some antineoplastic agents, or NSAIDs

Note: A pseudohyponatremia may occur in presence of multiple myeloma, hyperlipidemia, or hypoproteinemia but does not reflect an actual abnormality of water metabolism

Patient Assessment Data Base

(Patient may be asymptomatic until serum sodium level is less than 125 mEq/L, dependent on rapidity of onset.)

General

ACTIVITY/REST

May report: Malaise
Generalized weakness, faintness, muscle cramps

EGO INTEGRITY

May report: Anxiety

May exhibit: Restlessness, apprehension

FOOD/FLUID

May report: Nausea, anorexia, thirst
Low-sodium diet
Diuretic use

NEUROSENSORY

May report: Headache, blurred vision, vertigo

May exhibit: Loss of coordination, stupor, personality changes

TEACHING/LEARNING

Refer to predisposing/contributing factors
Use of oral hypoglycemic agent, potent diuretics, NSAIDs, other drugs that impair renal
water excretion

Discharge plan
considerations: **DRG projected mean length of inpatient stay: 4.1 days (dependent on underlying cause)**
May require assistance with changes in therapeutic regimen, dietary management

Refer to plan of care concerning underlying medical/surgical condition for possible
considerations after discharge.

SODIUM/WATER DEFICIT (Na less than 135 mEq/L; urine specific gravity elevated, serum osmolality normal)

CIRCULATION

May exhibit: Hypotension, tachycardia
Peripheral pulses diminished
Pallid, clammy skin

ELIMINATION

May report: Abdominal cramping, diarrhea

May exhibit: Urinary output decreased

FOOD/FLUID

May report: Anorexia, nausea/vomiting

May exhibit: Poor skin turgor; soft/sunken eyeballs
Mucous membranes dry, decreased saliva/perspiration

907

NEUROSENSORY

May report: Dizziness

May exhibit: Muscle twitching
Lethargy, restlessness, confusion, stupor

RESPIRATION

May exhibit: Tachypnea

SAFETY

May exhibit: Skin flushed, dry, hot
Fever

SODIUM DEFICIT/WATER EXCESS (Na less than 135 mEq/L; urine specific gravity low; serum osmolality decreased)

CIRCULATION

May exhibit: Hypertension
Generalized edema

ELIMINATION

May exhibit: Urinary output increased

NEUROSENSORY

May exhibit: Muscle twitching, restlessness, changes in mentation (more severe when problem is acute/develops rapidly)

PAIN/DISCOMFORT

May report: Headache, abdominal cramps

SEVERE SODIUM DEFICIT (Na less than 120 mEq/L)

CIRCULATION

May exhibit: Hypotension with vasomotor collapse
Rapid thready pulse
Cold/clammy skin, fingerprinting on sternum; cyanosis

NEUROSENSORY

May exhibit: Hyporeflexia
Convulsions/coma

DIAGNOSTIC STUDIES (Dependent on associated fluid level)

Serum sodium: Decreased, less than 135 mEq/L. (However, signs and symptoms may not occur until level is less than 120 mEq/L.)

Urine sodium: Less than 15 mEq/L indicates renal conservation of sodium due to sodium loss from a nonrenal source unless sodium-wasting nephropathy is present. Urine sodium greater than 20 mEq/L indicates SIADH.

Serum potassium: May be decreased as the kidneys attempt to conserve sodium at the expense of potassium.

Serum chloride/bicarbonate: Levels are decreased, depending on which ion is lost with the sodium.

Serum osmolality: Commonly low, but may be normal (pseudohyponatremia) or high (HHNC).

Urine osmolality: Usually less than 100 mOsm/L unless SIADH present, in which case it will exceed serum osmolality.

Urine specific gravity: May be decreased (less than 1.010) or increased (greater than 1.020) if SIADH is present.

Hct: Is dependent on fluid balance, e.g., fluid excess versus dehydration.

ACTIONS/INTERVENTIONS	RATIONALE
Independent	
Identify the patient at risk for hyponatremia and the specific cause, e.g., sodium loss or fluid excess.	Provides clues for early intervention. Hyponatremia is a common imbalance and may range from mild to severe. Severe hyponatremia can cause neurologic damage or death if not treated promptly.
Monitor I&O. Calculate fluid balance. Weigh daily.	Indicators of fluid balance are important, because either fluid excess or deficit may occur with hyponatremia.
Assess level of consciousness/neuromuscular response.	Sodium deficit may result in decreased mentation (to point of coma), as well as generalized muscle weakness/cramps, convulsions.
Maintain quiet environment; provide safety/seizure precautions.	Reduces CNS stimulation and risk of injury from neurologic complications, e.g., seizures.
Note respiratory rate and depth.	Co-occurring hypochloremia may produce slow/shallow respirations as the body compensates for metabolic alkalosis.
Encourage foods and fluids high in sodium, e.g., milk, meat, eggs, carrots, beets, and celery. Use fruit juices and bouillon instead of plain water.	Unless sodium deficit causes serious symptoms requiring immediate IV replacement, the patient may benefit from slower replacement by oral method or removal of previous salt restriction.
Irrigate NG tube (when used) with normal saline instead of water.	Isotonic irrigation will minimize loss of GI electrolytes.
Observe for signs of circulatory overload as indicated.	Administration of sodium-containing IV fluids in presence of heart failure increases risk.
Collaborative	
Assist with identification/treatment of underlying cause.	Refer to listing of predisposing/contributing factors to determine treatment needs.
Monitor serum and urine electrolytes, osmolality.	Evaluates therapy needs/effectiveness.
Provide/restrict fluids dependent on fluid volume status.	In presence of hypovolemia, volume losses are replaced with isotonic saline (e.g., normal saline), or, on occasion, hypertonic solution (3% NaCl) when hyponatremia is life-threatening. In the presence of fluid volume excess, or SIADH, fluid restriction is indicated. *Note:* Too rapid/excessive administration of hypertonic solutions can be lethal.

909

ACTIONS/INTERVENTIONS	RATIONALE
Independent	
Administer medications as indicated, e.g.:	
Furosemide (Lasix);	Effective in reducing fluid excess to correct sodium/water balance.
Sodium chloride;	Used to replace deficits/prevent recurrence in the presence of chronic/ongoing losses.
Potassium chloride;	Corrects potassium deficit, especially when diuretic is used.
Demeclocycline (Declomycin);	Useful in treating chronic SIADH, or when severe water restriction may not be tolerated, e.g., COPD. *Note:* May be contraindicated in patients with liver disease, as nephrotoxicity may occur.
Captopril (Capoten).	May be used in combination with a loop diuretic (e.g., Lasix) to correct fluid volume excess, especially in the presence of heart failure.
Prepare for/assist with dialysis as indicated.	May be done to restore sodium balance without increasing fluid level when hyponatremia is severe or response to diuretic therapy is inadequate.

Hypernatremia (Sodium Excess)

PREDISPOSING/CONTRIBUTING FACTORS

Excessive water losses: Polyuria (as may occur with diabetes insipidus); use of osmotic diuretics (such as mannitol); presence of fever, profuse sweating, vomiting, diarrhea; extracellular fluid volume excesses: e.g., renal disease, heart failure, primary aldosteronism, excessive steroids/Cushing's disease; excessive ingestion or infusion of sodium; salt water near-drowning

Insufficient water intake: Administration of tube feedings/high-protein diets with minimal fluid intake, ulcer diets primarily using half and half/whole milk

Patient Assessment Data Base

SODIUM EXCESS/WATER DEFICIT (Na greater than 145 mEq/L; elevated urine specific gravity)

ACTIVITY/REST

May report:	Weakness
May exhibit:	Muscle rigidity/tremors, generalized weakness

CIRCULATION

May exhibit:	Decreased blood pressure, postural hypotension
	Tachycardia

ELIMINATION

May exhibit:	Decreased urinary output

FOOD/FLUID

May report: Thirst

May exhibit: Mucous membranes dry, sticky; tongue dry, swollen, rough

NEUROSENSORY

May exhibit: Irritability, lethargy/coma (dependent on rapidity of onset rather than actual serum sodium level)
Delusions, hallucinations
Muscle irritability, seizure activity

SAFETY

May exhibit: Hot, dry, flushed skin
Fever

SODIUM/WATER EXCESS (Na greater than 145 mEq/L; urine specific gravity decreased)

CIRCULATION

May exhibit: Elevated BP, hypertension

ELIMINATION

May exhibit: Polyuria

FOOD/FLUID

May report: Thirst

May exhibit: Skin pale, moist, taut with pitting edema
Weight gain

NEUROSENSORY

May exhibit: Confusion, lethargy
Delusions, hallucinations

RESPIRATION

May exhibit: Dyspnea

SODIUM EXCESS/WATER DEFICIT OR EXCESS

TEACHING/LEARNING

Refer to predisposing/contributing factors

Discharge plan considerations: **DRG projected mean length of inpatient stay: 4.1 days (dependent on underlying cause)**
May require assistance with changes in therapeutic regimen, dietary management

Refer to plan of care concerning underlying medical/surgical condition for possible considerations after discharge.

DIAGNOSTIC STUDIES

Serum sodium: Increased, greater than 145 mEq/L. Serum levels greater than 160 mEq/L may be accompanied by severe neurologic signs.

Serum chloride: Increased, greater than 106 mEq/L.

Serum potassium: Decreased.

Serum osmolality: Greater than 295 mOsm/L when dehydrated; lower in presence of extracellular fluid excess, and less than 200 mOsm/L with excessive polyuria.

Hct: May be normal or elevated.

Urine sodium: Less than 50 mEq/L.

Urine chloride: Less than 50 mEq/L.

Urine osmolality: Greater than 800 mOsm/L.

Urine specific gravity: Increased, greater than 1.015, if water deficit present; or less than 1.005 when hypernatremia is due to polyuria.

ACTIONS/INTERVENTIONS	RATIONALE
Independent	
Monitor BP.	Either hypertension or hypotension may be present, depending on the fluid status. Presence of postural hypotension may affect activity tolerance.
Identify patient at risk for hypernatremia and likely cause, e.g., water deficit, sodium excess.	Early identification and intervention prevents serious complications associated with this problem.
Note respiratory rate, depth.	Deep, labored respirations with air hunger suggest metabolic acidosis (hyperchloremia), which can lead to cardiopulmonary arrest if not corrected.
Monitor I&O, urine specific gravity. Weigh daily. Assess presence/location of edema.	These parameters are variable depending on fluid status and are indicators of therapy needs/effectiveness.
Evaluate level of consciousness and muscular strength, tone, movement.	Sodium imbalance may cause changes that vary from confusion and irritability to seizures and coma. In presence of water deficit, rapid rehydration may cause cerebral edema.
Maintain safety/seizure precautions, as indicated, e.g., bed in low position, use of padded side rails.	Sodium excess/cerebral edema increases risk of convulsions.
Assess skin turgor, color, temperature, and mucous membrane moisture.	Water-deficit hyponatremia manifests by signs of dehydration.
Provide/encourage meticulous skin care and frequent repositioning.	Maintains skin integrity.
Provide frequent oral care. Avoid use of mouthwash/rinse that contains alcohol.	Promotes comfort and prevents further drying of mucous membranes.
Offer debilitated patient fluids at regular intervals. Give free water to patient receiving enteral feedings.	May prevent hypernatremia in patient who is unable to perceive or respond to thirst.
Recommend avoidance of foods high in sodium, e.g., canned soups/vegetables, processed foods, snack foods, and condiments.	Reduces risk of sodium-associated complications.
Collaborative	
Assist with identification/treatment of underlying cause.	Refer to listing of predisposing/contributing factors to determine treatment needs.

912

ACTIONS/INTERVENTIONS	RATIONALE
Collaborative	
Monitor serum electrolytes, osmolality, and ABGs as indicated.	Evaluates therapy needs/effectiveness. *Note:* Co-occurring hyperchloremia may cause metabolic acidosis, requiring buffering, e.g., sodium bicarbonate.
Increase PO/IV fluid intake, e.g., 5% dextrose (in H_2O in presence of dehydration); 0.90% NaCl (if extracellular deficit is present).	Replacement of total body water deficit will gradually restore sodium/water balance. *Note:* Rapid reduction of serum sodium level with corresponding decrease in serum osmolality can cause cerebral edema/convulsions.
Restrict sodium intake and administer diuretics as indicated.	Restriction of sodium intake while promoting renal clearance lowers serum sodium levels in the presence of extracellular fluid excess.

Potassium

Potassium is the major cation of the intracellular fluid and is responsible for maintaining intracellular osmotic pressure. Potassium also regulates neuromuscular excitability, aids in maintenance of acid/base balance, synthesis of protein, and metabolism of carbohydrates. Normal serum range is 3.5–5.0 mEq/L (body total of 42 mEq/L).

Hypokalemia (Potassium Deficit)

PREDISPOSING/CONTRIBUTING FACTORS

Renal loss: Use of potassium-wasting diuretics, diuretic phase of ATN, healing phase of burns; diabetic acidosis; Cushing's syndrome; nephritis, hypomagnesemia; use of sodium penicillins, amphotericin B, carbenicillin steroids; licorice abuse
GI loss: Profuse vomiting, excessive diarrhea, laxative abuse, prolonged gastric suction, inflammatory bowel disease, fistulas
Inadequate dietary intake: Anorexia nervosa, starvation, high-sodium diet
Shift into cells: TPN, alkalosis, or excessive secretion or administration of insulin
Other: Liver disease.

Patient Assessment Data Base

ACTIVITY/REST

May report: Generalized weakness, lethargy, fatigue

CIRCULATION

May exhibit: Hypotension
Pulses weak/diminished, irregular
Heart sounds distant
Dysrhythmias: PVCs, ventricular tachycardia/fibrillation

ELIMINATION

May exhibit: Nocturia, polyuria if factors contributing to hypokalemia include HF or DM
Bowel sounds diminished, decreased bowel motility, paralytic ileus
Abdominal distention

913

FOOD/FLUID

May report: Anorexia, nausea/vomiting
Thirst

NEUROSENSORY

May report: Paresthesias

May exhibit: Depressed mental state/confusion, apathy, drowsiness, irritability, coma
Hyporeflexia, tetany, paralysis (flaccid quadriparesis)

PAIN/DISCOMFORT

May report: Muscle pain/cramps

RESPIRATION

May exhibit: Hypoventilation/decreased respiratory depth due to muscle weakness/paralysis of diaphragm; apnea, cyanosis

TEACHING/LEARNING

Refer to predisposing/contributing factors

Discharge plan considerations: **DRG projected mean length of inpatient stay: 4.1 days (dependent on underlying cause)**
May require assistance with changes in therapeutic regimen, dietary management

Refer to plan of care concerning underlying medical/surgical condition for possible considerations after discharge.

DIAGNOSTIC STUDIES

Serum potassium: Decreased, less than 3.5 mEq/L.
Serum chloride: Often decreased, less than 98 mEq/L.
Serum glucose: May be slightly elevated.
Plasma bicarbonate: Increased, greater than 29 mEq/L.
Urine osmolality: Decreased.
ABGs: pH and bicarbonate may be elevated (metabolic alkalosis).
ECG: Low voltage; flat or inverted T wave, appearance of U wave, depressed ST segment, peaked P waves; prolonged Q-T interval, ventricular dysrhythmias.

ACTIONS/INTERVENTIONS	RATIONALE
Independent	
Monitor heart rate/rhythm.	Changes associated with hypokalemia include abnormalities in both conduction and contractility. Tachycardia may develop, and potentially life-threatening atrial and ventricular dysrhythmias, e.g., PVCs, sinus bradycardia, AV blocks, AV dissociation, ventricular tachycardia.
Monitor respiratory rate, depth, effort. Encourage cough/deep-breathing exercises; reposition frequently.	Respiratory muscle weakness may proceed to paralysis and eventual respiratory arrest.

ACTIONS/INTERVENTIONS	RATIONALE

Independent

Assess level of consciousness and neuromuscular function, e.g., strength, sensation, movement.

Apathy, drowsiness, irritability, tetany, paresthesias, and coma may occur.

Auscultate bowel sounds, noting decrease/absence or change.

Paralytic ileus commonly follows gastric losses through vomiting/gastric suction, protracted diarrhea.

Maintain accurate record of urinary, gastric, and wound losses.

Guide for calculating fluid/potassium replacement needs.

Monitor rate of IV potassium administration using microdrop or pump infusion devices. Check for side effects. Provide ice pack as indicated.

Ensures controlled delivery of medication to prevent bolus effect and reduce associated discomfort, e.g., burning sensation at IV site. When solution cannot be administered via central vein and slowing rate is not possible/effective, ice pack to infusion site may help relieve discomfort.

Encourage intake of foods and fluids high in potassium, e.g., bananas, oranges, dried fruits, red meat, turkey, salmon, coffee, colas, tea, leafy vegetables, peas, baked potatoes, tomatoes, winter squash. Discuss use of potassium chloride salt substitutes for patient receiving long-term diuretics.

Potassium may be replaced/level maintained through the diet when the patient is allowed oral food and fluids. Dietary replacement of 40–60 mEq/L/day is typically sufficient if no abnormal losses are occurring.

Review drug regimen for potassium-wasting drugs, e.g., furosemide (Lasix), hydrochlorothiazide (Diamox), IV catecholamines, gentamicin (Garamycin), carbenicillin (Geocillin), amphotericin B (Fungizone).

If alternate agents (e.g., potassium-sparing diuretics such as Aldactone, Dyrenium, Midamor) cannot be administered or when high-dose sodium drugs are administered (e.g., carbenicillin), close monitoring and replacement of potassium are necessary.

Discuss preventable causes of condition, e.g., nutritional choices, proper use of laxatives.

Provides opportunity for patient to prevent recurrence. Also, dietary control is more palatable than oral replacement medications.

Dilute liquid and effervescent K supplements (K-Tab, K-Lyte/Cl) with 4 oz water/juice and give after meals.

May prevent/reduce GI irritation and saline laxative effect.

Watch for signs of digitalis intoxication when used (e.g., reports of nausea/vomiting, blurred vision, increasing atrial dysrhythmias, and heart block).

Low potassium enhances effect of digitalis, slowing cardiac conduction. *Note:* Combined effects of digitalis, diuretics, and hypokalemia may produce lethal dysrhythmias.

Observe for signs of metabolic alkalosis, e.g., hypoventilation, tachycardia, dysrhythmias, tetany, changes in mentation.

Frequently associated with hypokalemia.

Collaborative

Assist with identification/treatment of underlying cause.

Refer to listing of predisposing/contributing factors to determine treatment needs. *Note:* Hypokalemia is life-threatening, early detection is crucial.

Monitor laboratory studies, e.g.:

   Serum potassium;

Levels should be checked frequently during replacement therapy, especially in the presence of insufficient renal function. Sudden excess/elevation may cause cardiac dysrhythmias.

915

ACTIONS/INTERVENTIONS	RATIONALE
Collaborative	
ABGs;	Correction of metabolic alkalosis will raise serum potassium level and reduce replacement needs. Correction of acidosis will drive potassium back into cells, resulting in decreased serum levels and increased replacement needs.
Serum magnesium;	Hypomagnesemia exacerbates potassium loss and sodium retention, altering cell membrane excitability (affects cardiac as well as neuromuscular function).
Serum chloride.	Use of diuretics, e.g., Lasix, HydroDIURIL, may cause chloride as well as potassium depletion.
Administer oral and/or IV potassium.	May be required to correct deficiencies when changes in medication, therapy and/or dietary intake are insufficient. *Note:* Parenteral replacement should not exceed 40 mEq/2 h. Dietary supplementation may also be used to produce a gradual equilibration if patient is able to take oral food and fluids.

Hyperkalemia (Potassium Excess)

PREDISPOSING/CONTRIBUTING FACTORS

Potassium retention: Decreased renal excretion (e.g., renal disease/acute failure, hypoaldosteronism, Addison's disease), hypovolemia, use of potassium-conserving diuretics, especially when associated with potassium supplements, use of NSAIDs

Excessive potassium intake: Salt substitutes, drugs containing potassium (e.g., penicillin), improper use of oral potassium supplements, too rapid IV administration of potassium, massive transfusion of banked blood

Shift or release of potassium out of cells: Severe catabolism, burns, crush injuries, MI, severe hemolysis, rhabdomyolysis, chemotherapy with cytotoxic drugs, respiratory or metabolic acidosis, anoxia, hyperglycemia with insulin deficiency, use of some β-adrenergic blockers, profound digitalis toxicity

Other: Use of certain medications such as captopril, heparin, cyclosporin.

Patient Assessment Data Base

Data is dependent on degree of elevation as well as length of time condition has existed.

ACTIVITY/REST

May report:	Vague muscular weakness
May exhibit:	Restlessness, irritability

CIRCULATION

May exhibit:	Irregular pulse, bradycardia, heart block, asystole

EGO INTEGRITY

May report:	Apprehension

ELIMINATION

May report: Intermittent abdominal cramps, diarrhea

May exhibit: Urine volume decreased
Hyperactive bowel sounds

FOOD/FLUID

May report: Nausea/vomiting

NEUROSENSORY

May report: Paresthesias (often of face, tongue, hands, feet)
Slurred speech

May exhibit: Decreased deep-tendon reflexes; progressive, ascending flaccid paralysis; twitching, seizure activity
Apathy, confusion

PAIN/DISCOMFORT

May report: Muscle cramps/pain

TEACHING/LEARNING

Refer to predisposing/contributing factors

Discharge plan considerations: **DRG projected mean length of inpatient stay: 4.1 days (dependent on underlying cause)**
May require assistance with changes in therapeutic regimen, dietary management

Refer to plan of care concerning underlying medical/surgical condition for possible considerations after discharge.

DIAGNOSTIC STUDIES

Serum potassium: Increased, greater than 5.0 mEq/L.
Renal function studies: May be altered, indicating failure.
Leukocyte or thrombocyte count: Elevation may cause a pseudohyperkalemia, affecting choice of interventions.
ECG changes: T waves tall and peaked/tented, prolonged P-R interval, loss of P waves, widening of QRS complex, shortened Q-T interval, and ST-segment depression; atrial/ventricular dysrhythmias, e.g., bradycardia, atrial arrest, complete heart block, ventricular fibrillation, cardiac arrest.

ACTIONS/INTERVENTIONS	RATIONALE
Independent	
Identify the patient at risk; or the cause of the hyperkalemia, e.g., excessive intake of potassium or decreased excretion.	Influences choice of interventions. Early identification and treatment can prevent complication. *Note:* A major cause of hypokalemia is decreased renal excretion.
Instruct patient in use of potassium-containing salts (salt substitutes), taking potassium supplements safely, and so forth.	The patient is often able to prevent hyperkalemia through management of supplements, diets, and other medications.
Monitor respiratory rate and depth. Elevate head of bed. Encourage cough/deep-breathing exercises.	Patients may hypoventilate and retain CO_2, leading to respiratory acidosis. Muscular weakness can affect respiratory muscles and lead to complications of respiratory infection/failure.

ACTIONS/INTERVENTIONS	RATIONALE
Independent	
Monitor heart rate/rhythm. Be aware that cardiac arrest can occur.	Excess potassium depresses myocardial conduction. Bradycardia can progress to cardiac fibrillation/arrest.
Monitor urinary output.	In kidney failure, potassium is retained because of improper excretion. Potassium should not be given if oliguria or anuria is present.
Assess level of consciousness, neuromuscular function, e.g., movement, strength, sensation.	Patient is usually awake and alert; however, muscular paresthesia, weakness, and flaccid paralysis may occur.
Encourage/assist with ROM exercises as tolerated.	Improves muscular tone and reduces muscle cramps and pain.
Encourage frequent rest periods; assist with care activities, as indicated.	General muscle weakness decreases activity tolerance.
Review drug regimen for medications containing/affecting potassium excretion, e.g., penicillin G, Aldactone, Midamor, Dyazide, Maxzide.	Requires regular monitoring of potassium levels, and may require alternate drug choices or changes in dosage/frequency.
Identify/discontinue dietary sources of potassium, e.g., tomatoes, broccoli, orange juice, bananas, bran, chocolate, coffee, tea, eggs, dairy products, dried fruits.	Facilitates reduction of potassium level and may prevent recurrence of hyperkalemia.
Recommend an increase in carbohydrates/fats and foods low in potassium, e.g., canned fruits, refined cereals, apple/cranberry juice.	Reduces exogenous sources of potassium and prevents catabolic tissue breakdown with release of cellular potassium.
Stress importance of patient's notifying future caregivers when chronic condition potentiates development of hyperkalemia, e.g., oliguric renal failure.	May help prevent recurrence.
Collaborative	
Assist with identification/treatment of underlying cause.	Refer to listing of predisposing/contributing factors to determine treatment needs.
Monitor laboratory results, e.g., serum potassium, ABGs, BUN/Cr, glucose as indicated.	Evaluates therapy needs/effectiveness. *Note:* Hypoventilation may result in respiratory acidosis, thereby increasing serum potassium levels.
Administer medications as indicated:	
Diuretics, e.g., furosemide (Lasix);	Loop or thiazide diuretics promote renal clearance and excretion of potassium.
IV glucose with insulin, sodium bicarbonate;	Short-term emergency measure to move potassium into the cell, thus reducing toxic serum level. *Note:* Use with caution in presence of HF or hypernatremia. Use of glucose is contraindicated in patients who are hyperkalemic.
Calcium gluconate;	Temporary stopgap measure that antagonizes toxic potassium depressant effects on heart and stimulates cardiac contractility. *Note:* Calcium is contraindicated in patients on digitalis because it increases the cardiotonic effects of the drug and may cause dysrhythmias.

ACTIONS/INTERVENTIONS	RATIONALE

Collaborative

Sodium polystyrene sulfonate (Kayexalate, SPS suspension), orally, per NG tube, or rectally.	Resin that removes potassium by exchanging potassium for sodium or calcium in the GI tract. Sorbitol enhances evacuation. *Note:* Use cautiously in patients with HF, edema, and in the elderly because it increases sodium level. In addition, Kayexalate may cause hyperchloremia.
β-Adrenergic agonist, e.g., albuterol (Proventil).	Nebulizer administration has been effective in patients receiving hemodialysis, and may also attenuate the hypoglycemic effect of insulin administration.
Infuse potassium-based medication/solutions slowly.	Prevents administration of concentrated bolus, allows time for kidneys to clear excess free potassium.
Provide fresh blood or washed RBCs (when possible) if transfusions required.	Fresh blood has less potassium than banked blood, because breakdown of older RBCs releases potassium.
Prepare for/assist with dialysis (peritoneal or hemodialysis).	May be required when more conservative methods fail or are contraindicated, e.g., severe HF.

Calcium

Calcium is involved in bone formation/reabsorption, neural transmission/muscle contraction, regulation of enzyme systems, and is a coenzyme in blood coagulation. Normal serum levels are 4.5–5.3 mEq/L, 8.5–10.5 mg/dL (total) or 2.1–2.6 mEg/L (ionized). The ionized calcium is physiologically active and clinically important, especially in critically ill patients. The total serum calcium is directly related to the serum albumin, follows it, and must be considered if only total serum readings are available. Some factors that alter the percentage of ionized calcium are changes in pH (affects how much calcium is bound to protein) or increased serum levels of fatty acids, lactate, and bicarbonate.

Hypocalcemia (Calcium Deficit)

PREDISPOSING/CONTRIBUTING FACTORS

Primary or surgical hypoparathyroidism; transient hypocalcemia following thyroidectomy; hyperphosphatemia, hypomagnesemia

Massive subcutaneous tissue infections, acute pancreatitis, burns, peritonitis, malignancies

Excessive GI losses: Draining fistula, diarrhea, fat malabsorption syndromes, chronic laxative use (particularly phosphate-containing laxatives/enemas)

Extreme stress situations with mobilization and excretion of calcium

Diuretic and terminal phase of renal failure

Inadequate dietary intake, lack of milk/vitamin D, excessive protein diet

Alcoholism: Primary effect of ethanol, plus intestinal malabsorption, hypomagnesemia, hypoalbuminemia, and pancreatitis

Use of anticonvulsants, antibiotics, corticosteroids; loop diuretics, drugs that lower serum magnesium (e.g., cisplatin, gentamycin)

Infusion of citrated blood, calcium-free infusions; rapid infusion of Plasmanate

Malignant neoplasms with bone metastases

Alkalotic states

Decreased ultraviolet exposure

Patient Assessment Data Base

Data are dependent on duration, severity, and rate of onset of hypocalcemia.

CIRCULATION

May exhibit: Hypotension
Pulses weak/decreased, irregular (weak cardiac contraction/premature dysrhythmias)

ELIMINATION

May report: Diarrhea, abdominal pain

May exhibit: Abdominal distention (paralytic ileus)

FOOD/FLUID

May report: Nausea/vomiting

May exhibit: Difficulty swallowing

HYGIENE

May exhibit: Coarse, dry skin; alopecia (chronic)

NEUROSENSORY

May report: Circumoral paresthesia, numbness and tingling of fingers and toes; muscle cramps

May exhibit: Anxiety, confusion, irritability, alteration in mood, impaired memory, depression, hallucinations, psychoses
Muscle spasms (carpopedal and laryngeal), increased deep-tendon reflexes; tetany, tonic/clonic seizure activity, positive Trousseau's and Chvostek's signs

RESPIRATION

May exhibit: Labored shallow breathing; stridor (spasm of laryngeal muscles)

SAFETY

May exhibit: Bleeding with no or minimal trauma

TEACHING/LEARNING

Refer to predisposing/contributing factors

Discharge plan considerations: **DRG projected mean length of inpatient stay: 4.1 days (dependent on underlying cause)**
May require assistance with changes in therapeutic regimen, dietary management

Refer to plan of care concerning underlying medical/surgical condition for possible considerations after discharge

DIAGNOSTIC STUDIES

Serium calcium: Decreased, less than 4.5 mEq/L or 8.5 mg/dl (total), 2.1 mEq/L (ionized)
Urine Sulkowitch test: Shows light or no precipitate.
ECG: Prolonged Q-T interval (characteristic but not necessarily diagnostic). In severe deficiency, T waves may flatten or invert, giving appearance of hypokalemia or myocardial ischemia; ventricular tachycardia may develop.

ACTIONS/INTERVENTIONS	RATIONALE

Independent

Monitor heart rate/rhythm.

Calcium deficit along with associated hypomagnesemia weakens cardiac muscle/contractility.

Assess respiratory rate, rhythm, effort. Have tracheostomy equipment available.

Laryngeal stridor may develop and result in respiratory emergency/arrest.

Observe for neuromuscular irritability, e.g., tetany, seizure activity. Assess for presence of Chvostek's/Trousseau's signs.

Calcium deficit causes repetitive and uncontrolled nerve transmission leading to muscle spasms and hyperirritability.

Provide quiet environment and seizure precautions as appropriate.

Reduces CNS stimulation and protects patient from potential injury.

Encourage relaxation/stress reduction techniques, e.g., deep-breathing exercises, guided imagery, visualization.

Tetany can be potentiated by hyperventilation and stress. *Note:* Direct pressure on the nerves (e.g., tightening BP cuff) may also cause tetany.

Check for bleeding from any source (mucous membranes, puncture sites, wounds/incisions, and so on). Note presence of ecchymosis, petechiae.

Alterations in coagulation can occur as a result of calcium deficiency.

Review patient's drug regimen, e.g., use of insulin, mithramycin, parathyroid injection, digitalis.

Some drugs can lower magnesium levels, affecting calcium level. The effect of digitalis is enhanced by calcium, and, in patients receiving calcium, digitalis intoxication may develop.

Discuss use of laxatives/antacids.

Those containing phosphate may negatively affect calcium metabolism.

Review dietary intake of vitamins and fat.

Insufficient ingestion of vitamin D and fat impairs absorption of calcium.

Identify sources to increase calcium and vitamin D in diet, e.g., dairy products, beans, cauliflower, eggs, oranges, pineapples, sardines, shellfish. Restrict intake of phosphorus, e.g., barley, bran, whole wheat, rye, liver, nuts, chocolate.

Vitamin D aids in absorption of calcium from intestinal tract. Phosphorus competes with calcium for intestinal absorption.

Encourage use of calcium-containing antacids if needed (e.g., Titralac, Dicarbosil, Tums).

Possible sources for oral replacement to help maintain calcium levels, especially in patients at risk for osteoporosis.

Stress importance of meeting calcium needs.

Adverse effects of long-term deficiency include tooth decay, eczema, cataracts, and osteoporosis.

Collaborative

Assist with identification/treatment of underlying cause.

Refer to listing of predisposing/contributing factors to determine treatment needs.

Monitor laboratory studies, e.g.:

Serum calcium and magnesium; serum albumin, ABGs;

Evaluates therapy needs/effectiveness. *Note:* Low serum albumin levels or serum pH affects calcium levels, e.g., a low albumin level causes a deceptively low calcium level; alkalosis causes surplus bicarbonate to bind with free calcium, impairing function; acidosis frees calcium, potentiating hypercalcemia.

PT, platelets.

Calcium is an essential part of the clotting mechanism and deficit may lead to excessive bleeding.

ACTIONS/INTERVENTIONS	RATIONALE
Collaborative	
Administer the following:	
Calcium gluconate/gluceptate/chloride IV;	Provides rapid treatment in acute calcium deficit (especially in presence of tetany/convulsions). *Note:* Calcium chloride is not used as often because it is more irritating to the vein and can cause tissue sloughing if it leaks into tissues.
Oral preparations, e.g., calcium lactate/carbonate;	Oral preparations are useful in correcting subacute deficiencies.
Magnesium sulfate IV/PO if indicated;	Hypomagnesemia is a precipitating factor in calcium deficit.
Vitamin D supplement (e.g., calcitriol).	May be used in combination with calcium therapy to enhance calcium absorption once concomitant phosphate deficiency is corrected.

Hypercalcemia (Calcium Excess)

PREDISPOSING/CONTRIBUTING FACTORS

Hyperparathyroidism, hyperthyroidism, multiple myeloma/other malignancies (e.g., cancer of breast, lung); renal disease, skeletal muscle paralysis, parathyroid tumor, sarcoidosis, adrenal insufficiency, TB

Excessive/prolonged use of vitamins A and D and calcium-containing antacids; prolonged use of thiazide diuretics, theophylline, lithium

Multiple fractures, bone tumors, osteoporosis, osteomalacia, prolonged immobilization causing imbalance between the rate of bone formation and resorption

Milk-alkali syndrome as a side effect of prolonged milk/antacid self-medication for gastric pain/ulcer

Hypophosphatasia, hyperproteinemia

Anticancer drugs, e.g., tamoxifen, androgens/estrogens

Patient Assessment Data Base

ACTIVITY/REST

May report:	General malaise, fatigue/weakness Lethargy
May exhibit:	Incoordination, ataxia

CIRCULATION

May exhibit:	Hypertension Irregular pulse, dysrhythmias, bradycardia

ELIMINATION

May report:	Constipation or diarrhea
May exhibit:	Polyuria, nocturia Kidney stones/calculi

FOOD/FLUID

May report:	Anorexia, nausea/vomiting Thirst Abdominal pain
May exhibit:	Poor skin turgor, dry mucous membranes

NEUROSENSORY

May report:	Headache
May exhibit:	Hypotonicity/muscular relaxation, flaccid paralysis, depressed/absent deep-tendon reflexes Drowsiness, apathy, paranoia, personality changes, decreased attention span, memory loss, depression, inappropriate/bizarre behaviors, psychosis, confusion, stupor/coma (with high calcium levels) Slurred speech

PAIN/DISCOMFORT

May report:	Epigastric, deep flank pain, or bone/joint pain

TEACHING/LEARNING

Refer to predisposing/contributing factors

Discharge plan considerations:	**DRG projected mean length of inpatient stay: 4.1 days (dependent on underlying cause)** May require assistance with changes in therapeutic regimen, dietary management

Refer to plan of care concerning underlying medical/surgical condition for possible considerations after discharge.

DIAGNOSTIC STUDIES

Serum calcium: Increased, greater than 2.6 mEq/L (ionized) or 10.5 mg/dl (total).
BUN: Increased (calculi can damage kidney).
Serum phosphorus: Decreased levels may be noted.
Urine Sulkowitch test: Shows heavy precipitate.
Urine calcium: Increased.
Urine osmolality: Decreased.
Urine specific gravity: Decreased.
X-ray: May reveal evidence of bone cavitation, pathologic fracture, osteoporosis, urinary calculi.
ECG changes: Shortened Q–T interval, inverted T waves. In severe deficit, QRS may widen, P–R interval lengthen, and ventricular prematurities develop.

ACTIONS/INTERVENTIONS	RATIONALE
Independent	
Monitor cardiac rate/rhythm. Be aware that cardiac arrest can occur in hypercalcemic crisis.	Overstimulation of cardiac muscle occurs with resultant dysrhythmias and ineffective cardiac contraction. Sinus bradycardia, sinus dysrhythmias, wandering pacemaker, and AV block may be noted. Hypercalcemia creates a predisposition to cardiac arrest.

ACTIONS/INTERVENTIONS	RATIONALE

Independent

Assess level of consciousness and neuromuscular status, e.g., muscle movement, strength, tone.	Nerve and muscle activity is depressed. Lethargy and fatigue can progress to convulsion/coma.
Monitor I&O; calculate fluid balance.	Efforts to correct original condition may result in secondary imbalances/complications.
Encourage fluid intake of 3–4 L/d, including sodium-containing fluids, (within cardiac tolerance) and use of acid-ash juices, e.g., cranberry and prune if kidney stones present or suspected.	Reduces dehydration, encourages urinary flow and clearance of calcium, reduces risk of stone formation. *Note:* Sodium favors calcium excretion and can be used if not contraindicated by other conditions.
Strain urine if flank pain occurs.	Large amount of calcium present in kidney parenchyma may lead to stone formation.
Auscultate bowel sounds.	Hypotonicity leads to constipation when the smooth muscle tone is inadequate to produce peristalsis.
Maintain bulk in diet.	Constipation may be a problem because of decreased GI tone.
Encourage frequent repositioning and ROM and/or muscle-setting exercises with caution. Promote ambulation if patient is able.	Muscle activity may reduce calcium shifting from the bones that occurs during immobilization. *Note:* Increased risk for pathologic fractures exists due to calcium shifts out of the bones.
Provide safety measures, e.g., gentle handling when moving/transferring patient.	Reduces risk of injury/pathologic fractures.
Review drug regimen, noting use of calcium-elevating drugs, e.g., heparin, tetracyclines, methicillin, phenytoin.	May affect drug choice or require reduction in oral sources of calcium.
Identify/restrict sources of calcium intake, e.g., dairy products, eggs, and spinach; calcium-containing antacids (Titralac, Dicarbosil, Tums).	Foods or drugs containing calcium may need to be limited in chronic conditions causing hypercalcemia.

Collaborative

Assist with identification/treatment of underlying cause.	Refer to listing of predisposing/contributing factors to determine treatment needs.
Monitor laboratory studies, e.g., calcium, magnesium, phosphate.	Monitors therapy needs/effectiveness. *Note:* Phosphate levels may be low when parathyroid hormone inversely promotes calcium uptake and calcium competes with phosphate for absorption/transport with vitamin D.
Administer isotonic saline and sodium sulfate IV/orally.	Emergency measures in severe hypercalcemia used to dilute extracellular calcium concentration and inhibit tubular reabsorption of calcium, thereby increasing urinary excretion.
Administer medications as indicated:	
Diuretics, e.g., furosemide (Lasix);	Diuresis promotes renal excretion of calcium and reduces risks of fluid excess from isotonic saline infusion.

ACTIONS/INTERVENTIONS	RATIONALE
Collaborative	
Sodium bicarbonate;	Induces alkalosis, thereby reducing the ionized calcium fraction.
Phosphate;	Rapid-acting agent that induces calcium excretion and inhibits resorption of bone.
Glucocorticoid therapy;	Inhibits intestinal absorption of calcium and reduces inflammation and associated stress response that mobilizes calcium from the bone.
Mithramycin (Mithracin);	Cytotoxic antibiotic that lowers serum calcium by inhibiting inappropriate bone resorption, typically seen in malignancies or hyperparathyroidism.
Disodium edetate (EDTA);	Chelating action lowers serum calcium level.
Calcitonin;	Promotes movement of serum calcium into bones, temporarily reducing serum calcium levels especially in the presence of increased parathyroid hormone.
Neutra-Phos, Fleet Phospho-Soda.	These drugs bind calcium in the GI tract, promoting excretion.
Prepare for/assist with hemodialysis.	Rapid reduction of serum calcium may be necessary to correct life-threatening situation.

Magnesium

Magnesium influences carbohydrate metabolism, secretion of parathyroid hormone, sodium/potassium transport across the cell membrane, and synthesis of protein and nucleic acid. Magnesium activates ATP and mediates neural transmission within the CNS. Magnesium deficit is often associated with hypokalemia and promotes intracellular potassium loss and sodium accumulation, altering and exacerbating membrane excitability. Normal serum range is 1.5–2.5 mEq/L or 1.8–3.0 mg/dl.

Hypomagnesemia (Magnesium Deficit)

PREDISPOSING/CONTRIBUTING FACTORS

GI losses: Biliary/intestinal fistula; surgery (bowel resection, small-bowel bypass); severe, protracted diarrhea, laxative abuse, impaired GI absorption/malabsorption syndrome, gastric/colon cancer, prolonged gastric suction

Protein/calorie malnutrition. Feeding (enteral or parenteral) without adequate magnesium replacement

Prolonged IV infusion of magnesium-free solutions, multiple transfusions with citrated blood products

Chronic alcoholism, alcohol withdrawal; pancreatitis

Hyperaldosteronism: Primary or secondary (e.g., cirrhosis or heart failure)

Toxemia of pregnancy

Renal losses: Severe renal disease/diuretic phase of ARF; vigorous and/or prolonged diuresis with mercurial thiazides or loop diuretics; SIADH

Drugs that affect magnesium balance: Aminoglycosides (gentamicin, tobramycin), antifungals (amphotericin B); chemotherapy agents (cisplatin); antirejection agents (cyclosporine), and excessive doses of calcium or vitamin D supplements

Diabetic ketoacidosis, malignancies causing hypercalcemic states, severe burns, sepsis, hypothermia; hypoparathyroidism, hypercalcemia, hyperthyroidism

Patient Assessment Data Base

ACTIVITY/REST

May report: Generalized weakness, insomnia
                    Ataxia, vertigo

CIRCULATION

May exhibit: Tachycardia, dysrhythmias
                    Hypotension (vasodilation); occasional hypertension

FOOD/FLUID

May report: Anorexia, nausea/vomiting, diarrhea

NEUROSENSORY

May report: Paresthesia (legs, feet)
                    Vertigo

May exhibit: Nystagmus
                    Musculoskeletal fasciculations/tremors, neuromuscular irritability/spasticity, spontane-
                       ous carpopedal spasms, hyperactive deep-tendon reflexes, clonus
                    Tetany, convulsions; positive Babinski's, Chvostek's, and Trousseau's signs
                    Disorientation, apathy, depression, irritability, agitation, hallucinations/psychoses, coma

TEACHING/LEARNING

Refer to predisposing/contributing factors

Discharge plan   DRG projected mean length of inpatient stay: 4.1 days (dependent on underlying cause)
considerations: May require assistance with changes in therapeutic regimen, dietary management

                     Refer to plan of care concerning underlying medical/surgical condition for possible
                     postdischarge considerations.

DIAGNOSTIC STUDIES

Serum magnesium: Decreased, less than 1.5 mEq/L or 1.8 mg/dl. *Note:* Usually symptoms do not appear until
    level is less than 1 mEq/L.
Calcium: May be decreased, unless there is a hypercalcemic condition causing the magnesium deficit.
Potassium: Decrease associated with severe hypomagnesemia.
ECG: Prolonged P-R and Q-T intervals, widened QRS complex, ST-segment depression, T-wave inversion.

ACTIONS/INTERVENTIONS	RATIONALE
Independent	
Monitor cardiac rate/rhythm, noting tachydysrhythmias and characteristic ECG changes.	Magnesium influences sodium/potassium transport across the cell membrane and affects excitability of cardiac tissue.
Monitor for signs of digitalis intoxication when used (e.g., reports of nausea/vomiting, blurred vision; increasing atrial dysrhythmias and heart block).	Magnesium deficit may precipitate digitalis toxicity.

ACTIONS/INTERVENTIONS	RATIONALE

Independent

Assess level of consciousness and neuromuscular status, e.g., movement, strength, reflexes/tone; note presence of Chvostek's/Trousseau's signs.

Confusion, irritability, and psychosis may occur. However, more common manifestations are muscular, e.g., hyperactive deep-tendon reflexes, muscle tremors, spasticity, generalized tetany.

Monitor status of airway and swallowing.

Laryngeal stridor and dysphagia can occur when depletion is moderate to severe.

Take seizure/safety precautions, e.g., padded side rails, bed in low position, frequent observation as indicated.

Changes in mentation or the development of seizure activity in severe hypomagnesemia increases the risk of patient injury.

Provide quiet environment and subdued lighting.

Reduces extraneous stimuli; promotes rest.

Encourage ROM exercises as tolerated.

Reduces deleterious effects of muscle weakness/spasticity.

Place footboard/cradle on bed.

Elevation of linens may reduce spasms.

Auscultate bowel sounds.

Muscle weakness/spasticity may reduce peristalsis and bowel function.

Encourage intake of dairy products, whole grains, green leafy vegetables, meat, and fish.

Provides oral replacement of mild magnesium deficits; may prevent recurrence.

Instruct patient in proper use of laxatives and diuretics.

Deficit may be the result of abuse of these drugs.

Observe for signs of magnesium toxicity during replacement therapy, e.g., thirst, feeling hot and flushed, diaphoresis, anxiety, drowsiness, hypotension, increased muscular and nervous system irritability, loss of patellar reflex.

Rapid, excessive IV replacement may lead to toxicity and life-threatening complications.

Collaborative

Assist with identification/treatment of underlying cause.

Refer to listing of predisposing/contributing factors. *Note:* Studies have shown that chronic alcoholism with malnutrition is the most common cause of hypomagnesemia in the United States.

Monitor laboratory studies, e.g., serum magnesium, calcium, and potassium levels.

Evaluates therapy needs/effectiveness. *Note:* These electrolytes are interrelated, symptoms may be similar, and deficits of more than one may be present.

Administer medications as indicated:

Magnesium sulfate or magnesium chloride IV:

IV replacement is preferred in severe deficit because absorption of magnesium from intestinal tract varies inversely with calcium absorption. *Note:* Calcium gluconate is the antidote should hypermagnesemia be evidenced by depressed deep-tendon reflexes or respiratory depression and hypotension (late sign).

Magnesium sulfate IM, or magnesium hydroxide PO (Amphojel, milk of magnesia)

May be given for mild deficit or in nonemergent situations. Injections should be deep IM to decrease local tissue reaction.

Magnesium-based antacids, e.g., Mylanta, Maalox, Gelusil, Riopan.

Can supplement dietary replacement. *Note:* Use of these products may cause diarrhea, which can be alleviated by concurrent use of aluminum-containing products, e.g., Amphojel, Basaljel.

Hypermagnesemia (Magnesium Excess)

PREDISPOSING/CONTRIBUTING FACTORS

Reduced renal function (e.g., acute processes or age), chronic renal disease/failure; or dialysis with hard water

Excessive intake/absorption: e.g., too-rapid replacement of magnesium (as in pregnancy-induced hypertension or premature labor, excessive use of magnesium-containing drugs/products, e.g., Maalox, milk of magnesia, Epsom salts

Untreated diabetic ketoacidosis

Hyperparathyroidism, aldosterone deficiency, adrenal insufficiency

Extracellular fluid volume depletion (e.g., after diuretic abuse)

Salt-water near-drowning, hypothermia, shock

Chronic diarrhea; diseases that interfere with gastric absorption

Patient Assessment Data Base

ACTIVITY/REST

May report: Generalized weakness, lethargy

May exhibit: Drowsiness, lethargy, stupor

CIRCULATION

May exhibit: Hypotension (mild to severe)
Pulses weak/irregular, bradycardia, cardiac arrest

FOOD/FLUID

May report: Nausea/vomiting

NEUROSENSORY

May exhibit: Skin flushing, sweating
Depressed deep tendon reflexes progressing to flaccid paralysis
Decreased level of consciousness, lethargy progressing to coma
Slurred speech

RESPIRATION

May exhibit: Hypoventilation progressing to apnea

SAFETY

May exhibit: Skin flushing, sweating

TEACHING/LEARNING

Refer to predisposing/contributing factors

Discharge plan considerations: **DRG projected mean length of inpatient stay: 4.1 days (dependent on underlying cause)**
May require assistance with changes in therapeutic regimen, dietary management

Refer to plan of care concerning underlying medical/surgical condition for possible considerations after discharge.

DIAGNOSTIC STUDIES

Serum magnesium: Symptomatic levels greater than 3 mEq/L (increase to 10–20 mEq/L results in respiratory depression, coma, and cardiac arrest).

ECG: Prolonged P-R and Q-T intervals, wide QRS, elevated T waves, development of heart block, cardiac arrest.

ACTIONS/INTERVENTIONS	RATIONALE
Independent	
Monitor cardiac rate/rhythm.	Bradycardia and heart block may develop, progressing to cardiac arrest as a direct result of hypermagnesemia on cardiac muscle.
Monitor BP.	Hypotension unexplained by other causes is an early sign of toxicity.
Assess level of consciousness and neuromuscular status, e.g., reflexes/tone, movement, strength.	CNS and neuromuscular depression can cause decreasing level of alertness, progressing to coma, and depressed muscular responses, progressing to flaccid paralysis.
Monitor respiratory rate/depth/rhythm. Encourage cough/deep-breathing exercises. Elevate head of bed as indicated.	Neuromuscular transmissions are blocked by magnesium excess, resulting in respiratory muscular weakness and hypoventilation, which may progress to apnea.
Check patellar reflexes.	Absences suggest magnesium levels about 7 mEq/L. If untreated, cardiac/respiratory arrest can occur.
Encourage increased fluid intake if appropriate.	Increased hydration enhances magnesium excretion, but fluid intake must be cautious in event of renal/cardiac failure.
Monitor urinary output and 24-hour fluid balance.	Renal failure is the primary contributing factor in hypermagnesemia; and, if it is present, fluid excess can easily occur.
Promote bed rest, assist with personal care activities as needed.	Flaccid paralysis, lethargy, and decreased mentation reduce activity tolerance/ability.
Recommend avoidance of magnesium-containing antacids, e.g., Maalox, Mylanta, Gelusil, Riopan, in patient with renal disease. Caution patients with renal disease to avoid OTC drug use without first discussing with healthcare provider.	Limits oral intake to help prevent hypermagnesemia.
Collaborative	
Assist with identification/treatment of underlying cause.	Refer to listing of predisposing/contributing factors to determine treatment needs. *Note:* Most frequently occurs in patients with advanced renal failure.
Monitor laboratory studies as indicated: serum magnesium and calcium levels.	Evaluates therapy needs/effectiveness.
Administer IV fluids and thiazide diuretics as indicated.	Promotes renal clearance of magnesium (if renal function is normal).
Administer 10% calcium chloride or gluconate IV.	Antagonizes action/reverses symptoms of magnesium toxicity to improve neuromuscular transmission.
Assist with dialysis as needed.	In the presence of renal disease/failure, dialysis may be needed to lower serum levels.

929

APPENDIX

Key to Abbreviations

A-a DO$_2$ ratio: alveolar to arterial oxygen diffusion gradient
ABG: arterial blood gas
a.c.: before meals
ACE: angiotensin-converting enzyme
ACh RAb: acetylcholine receptor antibody
ACT: activated clotting time
ACTH: adrenocorticotropic hormone
AD: autonomic dysreflexia
ADA: American Diabetes Association
ADH: antidiuretic hormone
ADLs: activities of daily living
ADRDA: Alzheimer's Disease and Related Disorders Association
AED: antiepileptic drug
AF: atrial fibrillation
AI: aortic valve insufficiency
AICD: automatic implantable cardioverter defibrillator
AIDS: acquired immunodeficiency syndrome
ALP: alkaline phosphatase
ALS: amyotrophic lateral sclerosis
ALT: alanine aminotransferase (equivalent SGPT)
ANA: antinuclear antibody
Anti-DNA: deoxyribonuclease
AP: anterior-posterior
aPTT: activated partial thromboplastin time
AR: aortic valve regurgitation
ARDS: adult respiratory distress syndrome
ARF: acute renal failure
AS: aortic valve stenosis
ASA: acetylsalicylic acid
ASI: addiction severity index
ASHD: arteriosclerotic heart disease
ASL: antistreptolysin
ASO: antistreptolysin-O titer

AST: aspartate aminotransferase (equivalent SGOT)
ATN: acute tubular necrosis
AV: aortic valve: atrioventricular; arteriovenous
AVF: augmented unipolar foot lead of electrocardiogram

BAERs: brainstem auditory evoked responses
BBB: bundle branch block
BEAM: brain electrical activity map
BEE: basal energy expenditure
BFP: biologically false positive
bid: twice a day
BKA: below-knee amputation
BM: bowel movement
BMR: basal metabolic rate
B&O: belladonna and opium
BP: blood pressure
BPH: benign prostatic hypertrophy
BPM: beats per minute
BSP: Bromsulphalein
BUN: blood urea nitrogen

C: centigrade
Ca: calcium ion
CABG: coronary artery bypass graft
CAD: coronary artery disease
CAPD: continuous ambulatory peritoneal dialysis
CAVH: continuous arteriovenous hemofiltration
CBC: complete blood count
cc: cubic centimeters
CCPD: continuous cycling peritoneal dialysis
CEA: carcinogenic embryonic antigen
CHI: creatinine height index
CI: cardiac index
Cl$^-$: chloride ion
cm: centimeter
CMV: cytomegalovirus
CNS: central nervous system

CO: cardiac output; carbon monoxide
CO_2: carbon dioxide
CO_3: carbonate
COHb: carboxyhemoglobin
COPD: chronic obstructive pulmonary disease
CPB: cardiopulmonary bypass (machine)
CPK: creatinine phosphokinase
CPK-MB: creatinine phosphokinase isoenzyme
CPP: cerebral perfusion pressure
CPR: cardiopulmonary resuscitation
CPT: chest physiotherapy
Cr: creatinine
CRF: chronic renal failure
CRP: C-reactive protein
C&S: culture and sensitivities
CSF: cerebrospinal fluid
CT: computerized axial tomography
CTZ: chemoreceptor trigger zone
cu: cubic
CVA: cerebrovascular accident; costovertebral angle
CVP: central venous pressure

DAT: dementia of the Alzheimer's type
DI: diabetes insipidus
DIC: disseminated intravascular coagulation
DIPs: distal interphalangcal joints
DKA: diabetic ketoacidosis
dl: deciliter
DM: diabetes mellitus
D&C: dilation and curettage
DOB: date of birth
DOM: dimethoxymethylamphetamine, STP (used as street drug)
DRG: diagnosis-related group
DSA: digital subtraction angiography
DST: dexamethasone suppression test
DT: delirium tremens
DTIC: dicarbazine (synthetic chemotherapeutic agent)
DTRs: deep-tendon reflexes
DUI: driving under the influence
D5W: dextrose 5% water
DVT: deep vein thrombosis
DVWR: (ventilatory weaning response, dysfunctional)

EACA: epsilon-aminocaproic acid
ECF: extracellular fluid
ECG: electrocardiogram
ECT: electroconvulsive therapy
EEG: electroencephalogram
EGD: esophagogastroduodenoscopy
ELISA: enzyme-linked immunosorbent assay
ELOS: estimated length of stay
EMDR: eye movement desensitization and reprocessing
EMG: electromyography
ENG: electronystagmogram

ERCP: endoscopic retrograde cholangiopancreatography
ESR: erythrocyte sedimentation rate
ESWL: extracorporeal shock-wave lithotripsy
ET: endotracheal tube

F: Fahrenheit
FAS: fetal alcohol syndrome
FBS: fasting blood sugar
FEV_1: forced expiratory volume in 1 second
FFP: fresh frozen plasma
FIo_2: fraction of inspired oxygen
FRC: functional reserve capacity
FVC: forced vital capacity

GF: glomerular filtration
GFR: glomerular filtration rate
GH: growth hormone
GI: gastrointestinal
Gly-Hb: glycosylated hemoglobin
g: gram
GU: genitourinary

H: hydrogen
HAA: hepatitis associated antigen
HAV: hepatitis A virus
Hb: hemoglobin
Hb/Hct: hemoglobin and hematocrit
HBIg: hepatitis B immunoglobulin
HBsAg: hepatitis B surface antigen
HBV: hepatitis B virus
HCG: human chorionic gonadotropin
HCl: hydrochloric acid
HCO_3: bicarbonate
Hct: hematocrit
HCV: hepatitis C virus
HDL: high-density lipoproteins
HF: heart failure
Hg: mercury
HHNC: hyperglycemic, hyperosmotic nonketotic coma
HIV: human immunodeficiency virus
HOB: head of bed
HNP: herniated nucleus pulposus (disc)
H_2O: water
HR: heart rate
HS: hour of sleep
HSV: herpes simplex virus

IABP: intraaortic balloon pump
ICF: intracellular fluid
ICP: intracranial pressure
ICU: intensive care unit
ID: iron deficiency (anemia)
I&D: incision and drainage
IDDM: insulin-dependent diabetes mellitus (type I)

I:E: inspiratory/expiratory ratio
Ig: immune globulin
IHSS: idiopathic hypertrophic subaortic stenosis
IICP: increased intracranial pressure
IM: intramuscular
IMV: intermittent mandatory ventilation
INR: international normalized ratio
I&O: intake and output
IOL: intraocular lens
IOP: intraocular pressure
IP: identified patient
IPPB: intermittent positive pressure breathing
IV: intravenous
IVP: intravenous pyelogram

JVD: jugular vein distention

K: potassium
kg: kilogram
KS: Kaposi's sarcoma
KUB: kidneys, ureters, bladder x-ray

L: liter
LAP: leucine aminopeptidase
LDH: lactate dehydrogenase
LDL: low-density lipoprotein
LE cell: neutrophil
LOC: level of consciousness
LP: lumbar puncture
LR: lactated Ringer's solution
LSD: D-lysergic acid (used as street drug)
LTC: long-term care
LUQ: left upper quadrant
LV: left ventricle
LVEDP: left ventricular end-diastolic pressure
LVF: left ventricular failure

MAO: monoamine oxidase inhibitors
MAP: mean arterial pressure
MAT: multiple atrial tachycardia
MCL$_1$: modified chest lead (V$_1$)
MCL$_6$: modified chest lead (V$_6$)
MCT: medium chain triglycerides
MCV: mean corpuscular volume
MDA: methylenedioxymethamphetamine
MDF: myocardial depressant factor
mEq: milliequivalent
Mg: magnesium
mg: milligram
MG: myasthenia gravis
MI: myocardial infarction, mitral valve insufficiency
min: minute
ml: milliliter
mm: millimeter
mOsm: milliosmol
MR: mitral valve regurgitation
MRI: magnetic resonance imaging

MS: mitral valve stenosis; multiple sclerosis
MSG: monosodium glutamate
MSH: melanocyte-stimulating hormone
MTM: modified-Thayer-Martin (culture medium for gonococcus)
MUGA: multigated acquisition (radioactive heart scan)
MV: mitral valve
MVP: mitral valve prolapse

Na: sodium
NaHCO$_3$: sodium bicarbonate
NANDA: North American Nursing Diagnosis Association
NG: nasogastric
NIDDM: non-insulin-dependent diabetes mellitus (type II)
NMR: nuclear magnetic resonance
NPO: nothing by mouth
NS: normal saline
NSAID: nonsteroid anti-inflammatory drug
NSR: normal sinus rhythm
NSU: nonspecific urethritis
NTG: nitroglycerin
n/v: nausea/vomiting

O$_2$: oxygen
OR: operating room
Osm: osmolality
OTC: over-the-counter (drugs)
OT: occupational therapy

PA: posterior-anterior
PAC: premature atrial contraction
PaCO$_2$: arterial carbon dioxide pressure
PAO$_2$: alveolar oxygen pressure
PaO$_2$: arterial oxygen pressure
PAP: pulmonary artery pressure
PAT: paroxysmal atrial tachycardia
PAWP: pulmonary artery wedge pressure
pc/hs: after meals and at bedtime
PCA: patient-controlled analgesia
PCO$_2$: partial pressure of carbon dioxide
PCP: *Pneumocystis carinii* pneumonia; phencyclidine (used as street drug)
PCWP: pulmonary capillary wedge pressure
PE: pulmonary embolus; physical examination
PEEP: positive end-expiratory pressure
PEG: percutaneous esophagogastritis
PET: positron emission tomography
PG: phosphatidylglycerol
pH: degree of acidity or alkalinity
PI: phosphatidylinositol, pulmonary insufficiency
PIPs: proximal interphalangeal joints
PJC: premature junctional contraction
PMI: point of maximal impulse
PMS: premenstrual syndrome

PND: paroxysmal nocturnal dyspnea
po: per os (by mouth)
PO_2: partial pressure of oxygen
PO_4: phosphate
PPD: purified protein derivative
prn: as necessary
PS: pulmonary valve stenosis
PT: prothrombin time; physical therapy
PTCA: percutaneous transluminal coronary angioplasty
PTH: parathyroid hormone
PTHC: percutaneous transhepatic cholangiography
PTT: partial thromboplastin time
PTU: propylthiouracil
PUL: percutaneous ultrasonic lithotripsy
PVC: premature ventricular contractions
PWP: pulmonary wedge pressure

qid: four times a day
QP/QS: shunt measurement pulmonary versus systemic flow
Qs/Qt: quality shunted/quantity total (respiratory shunt measurement)
QRS: electrocardiogram measure of electrical activity of ventricle

R: electrocardiogram wave representing ventricular innervation
RA: rheumatoid arthritis
Rad: right axis deviation; radiation dosage
RAI: radioactive iodine
RAP: right atrial pressure
RBC: red blood cell
RCVA: right cerebral vascular accident
REM: rapid eye movement
RIA: radioimmunoassay
RL: renal electrolytes
ROM: range of motion
RPR: rapid plasma reagin (serologic test)
RSD: reflex sympathetic dystrophy
RUQ: right upper quadrant
RV: right ventricle
RVF: right ventricular failure

S_1, S_2, S_3, S_4: heart sounds
SA: sinoatrial
SB: sinus bradycardia
SC: subcutaneous
SCI: spinal cord injury
sec: second
SGOT: serum glutamic-oxaloacetic transaminase
SGPT: serum glutamic pyruvic transaminase
SIADH: syndrome of inappropriate antidiuretic hormone
SIMV: synchronized intermittent mandatory ventilation
SLE: systemic lupus erythematosus

SMA: serum chemistry profile
SO: significant other(s)
SPF: sun protective factor
SR: sinus rhythm
ST: sinus tachycardia, electrocardiographic wave representing ventricular repolarization
STD: sexually transmitted disease
STP: (serendipity, tranquility, peace) dimethoxymethylamphetamine (used as a street drug)
ST/T: segment/interval measure on ECG
SVO_2: systemic venous oxygen level
SVR: systemic vascular resistance

T_3: triiodothyronine
T_4: thyroxine
TB: tuberculosis
TBSA: total body surface area
TCDB: turn, cough, deep-breathe
TENS: transcutaneous electrical nerve stimulator
THC: tetrahydrocannabinol (used as a street drug)
TI: tricuspid valve insufficiency
TIA: transient ischemic attacks
TIBC: total iron-binding capacity
tid: three times a day
TKO: to keep open
TLC: total lung capacity
TMJ: temporomandibular joint
TPN: total parenteral nutrition
TRF: thyrotropin-releasing factor
TRH: thyrotropin-releasing hormone
TS: tricuspid stenosis
TSH: thyroid-stimulating hormone
TUR: transurethral resection
TVC: true vomiting center
T-tube: T-shaped drainage tube generally for the common bile duct

UA: urinalysis
UC: ulcerative colitis
UO: urinary output
URI: upper respiratory infection
UTI: urinary tract infection

V, V_1, V_5, V_6: electrocardiogram chest leads
$\dot{V}_E$: minute ventilation
VC: vital capacity
VCU: voiding cystourethrogram
V_d/V_t: dead space/tidal volume
VF: ventricular fibrillation
VMA: vanillylmandelic acid
VPD: ventricular premature depolarization
V/Q: ventilation/perfusion
VS: vital signs
V_T: tidal volume
VT: ventricular tachycardia

WBC: white blood cell
WNL: within normal limits

BIBLIOGRAPHY

General References

Electronic Media

Medical Housecall: Interactive Home Medical Guide and Symptom Analysis, Applied Medical Informatics (AMI), 1994.

Books

Belcher, A: Cancer Nursing. Mosby Year Book, CV Mosby, St Louis, 1992.

Benign Prostatic Hyperplasia: Diagnosis and Treatment. Quick Reference Guide for Clinicians. AHCPR, Pub 94-0583, US Department of Health and Human Services, Public Health Service Agency for Health Care Policy and Research, Rockville, MD, February, 1994.

Berkow, R (ed): The Merck Manual, ed 16. Merck & Co., Inc., Rahway, NJ, 1992.

Black, J and Matassarin-Jacobs, E (eds): Luckmann and Sorensen's Medical-Surgical Nursing, A Psychophysiologic Approach, ed 4. WB Saunders, Philadelphia, 1993.

Carnevali, DL and Thomas, MD: Diagnostic Reasoning and Treatment: Decision-Making in Nursing, JB Lippincott, Philadelphia, 1993.

Carpenito, L: Nursing Diagnosis: Application to Clinical Practice, ed 6. JB Lippincott, Philadelphia, 1995.

Cataract in Adults: Management of Functional Impairment. Clinical Practice Guidelines, number 4. AHCPR Pub 93-0542, US Department of Health & Human Services, Public Health Agency for Health Care Policy and Research, February, 1993.

Condon, RE and Nyhus, LM (eds): Manual of Surgical Therapeutics, ed 8. Little, Brown & Co, Boston, 1993.

Cox, H, Hinz, M, Lubno, M, et al: Clinical Applications of Nursing Diagnosis: Adult, Child, Women's, Psychiatric, Gerontic and Home Health Considerations, ed 2. FA Davis, Philadelphia, 1993.

Deglin, JH and Vallerand, AH: Davis's Drug Guide for Nurses, ed 5. FA Davis, Philadelphia, 1997.

DeVita, V, Hellman, S and Rosenberg, S: Cancer: Principles & Practice of Oncology, ed 4. JB Lippincott, Philadelphia, 1993.

Doenges, M and Moorhouse, M: Nurse's Pocket Guide: Nursing Diagnoses with Interventions, ed 5. FA Davis, Philadelphia, 1996.

Doenges, M, Moorhouse, M and Burley, J: Application of Nursing Process and Nursing Diagnosis, ed 2. FA Davis, Philadelphia, 1995.

Doenges, M, Moorhouse, M and Townsend, M: Psychiatric Care Plans: Guidelines for Planning and Documenting Client Care, ed 2. FA Davis, Philadelphia, 1995.

Epilepsy: Questions and answers about seizure disorders. Epilepsy Foundation of America, Landover, MD, 1994.

Ewald, GA and McKenzie, CR (eds): Manual of Medical Therapeutics, ed 28. Little, Brown & Co, Boston, 1995.

Fischbach, F: A Manual of Laboratory and Diagnostic Tests, ed 4. JB Lippincott, Philadelphia, 1992.

Guyton, AC: Textbook of Medical Physiology, ed 8. WB Saunders, Philadelphia, 1991.

Heart Failure: Evaluation and Care of Patients with Left-Ventricular Systolic Dysfunction. AHCPR Pub 94-0612, US Department of Health and Human Services, Public Health Service Agency for Health Care Policy and Research, June, 1994.

High Quality Mammography, Information for Referring Providers. Quick Reference Guide for Clinicians, number 13, AHCPR, Pub 95-633, US Department of Health and Human Services, Public Health Service Agency for Health Care Policy and Research, Rockville, MD, October, 1994.

Ignatavicius, DD and Hausman, KA: Clinical Pathways for Collaborative Practice. WB Saunders, Philadelphia, 1995.

Introducing Imitrex: A Clinical Demonstration of Migraine Relief You Can See in Minutes. Cerenex and Glaxo Pharmaceuticals, IMX177, March, 1993.

Kee, JL: Laboratory & Diagnostic Tests with Nursing Implications, ed 4. Appleton & Lange, Norwalk, Conn, 1995.

Lampe, S: Focus Charting. Creative Nursing Management, Inc., Minneapolis, 1988.

Living With Transplantation, Patient Education Manual. Sandoz Pharmaceuticals Corporation, East Hanover, NJ, 1989.

Management of Cancer Pain: Adult Quick Reference Guide, number 9. AHCPR, Pub 94-0593, US Department of Health and Human Services, Public Health Service Agency for Health Care Policy and Research, Rockville, MD, March, 1994.

Mathewson-Kuhn, M: Pharmacotherapeutics: A Nursing Process Approach, ed 3. FA Davis, Philadelphia, 1994.

McCance, KL and Huether, SE: Pathophysiology: The Biologic Basis for Disease in Adults and Children, ed 2. Mosby, St. Louis, 1994.

McCloskey, JC and Bulechek, GM (ed): Nursing Interventions Classification (NIC). CV Mosby, St. Louis, 1992.

Metheny, NM: Fluid and Electrolyte Balance: Nursing Considerations, ed 2. JB Lippincott, Philadelphia, 1992.

NANDA Nursing Diagnoses: Definitions and Classifications. North American Nursing Diagnosis Association, St. Louis, 1994.

Nicholi, AM, The New Harvard Guide to Psychiatry. Belknap Press of Harvard Univ. Press, Cambridge, 1988.

(No author): Chronic hepatitis B and chronic hepatitis, Non-A, Non-B/C: Two Common Forms, One Effective Therapy. Schering Corp, Kenilworth, NJ, 1992.

(No author): Orthopaedic Nursing Practice Guidelines. NAON, 1992.

Otto, S: Oncology Nursing, ed 2. CV Mosby, St Louis, 1994.

Post-Stroke Rehabilitation: Assessment, Referral, and Patient Management. Clinical Practice Guideline Number 16, AHCPR Pub 95-0663, US Department of Health & Human Services, Public Health Services Agency for Health Care and Research, May, 1995.

Prevention Magazine (eds): Listen to Your Body: How to Read Its Signals for Better Health. Rodale, Emmaus, PA, 1987.

Richard, RL, et al: Burn Care and Rehabilitation: Principles and Practice. FA Davis, Philadelphia, 1994.

Seidel, HM, et al: Mosby's Guide to Physical Examination, ed 2. Mosby-Year Book, St. Louis, 1991.

Shore, LS: Nursing Diagnosis: What It Is and How to Do It: A Programmed Text. Medical College of Virginia Hospitals, Richmond, VA, 1988.

Sickle Cell Disease: Comprehensive Screening and Management in Newborns and Infants. Quick Reference Guide for Clinicians, Number 6, AHCPR Pub 93-0563, US Department of Health and Human Services, Public Health Service Agency for Health Care Policy and Research, April, 1993.

Slye, DA and Theis, LM: An Introduction to Orthopaedic Nursing: An Orientation Module. NAON, 1991.

TB/HIV, the Connection: What Health Care Workers Should Know. US Dept. Health & Human Services, CDC, Atlanta (no date).

Thelan, LA, Davie, J, Urden, L, et al: Critical Care Nursing: Diagnosis & Management, ed 2. CV Mosby, St. Louis, 1994.

Thomas, CL (ed): Taber's Cyclopedic Medical Dictionary, ed 17. FA Davis, Philadelphia, 1993.

Thompson, J, et al: Mosby's Manual of Clinical Nursing, ed 2. CV Mosby, St. Louis, 1989.

Townsend, M: Psychiatric Mental Health Nursing: Concepts of Care, ed 2. FA Davis, Philadelphia, 1993.

Tucker, SM, et al: Patient Care Standards, ed 5. Mosby, St Louis, 1992.

Unstable Angina: Diagnosis and Management. AHCPR Pub 94-0602, US Department of Health and Human Services, Public Health Service Agency for Health Care Policy and Research, Rockville, MD, 1994.

Urinary Incontinence in Adults. Clinical Practice Guideline. AHCPR Pub 92-0038, US Department of Health and Human Services, Public Health Service Agency for Health Care Policy and Research, Rockville, MD, 1992.

Watson, J and Jaffe, M: Nurse's Manual of Laboratory and Diagnostic Tests, ed 2. FA Davis, Philadelphia, 1995.

Wyatt, LK: Living & Loving with Arthritis. Rheumatoid Arthritis Foundation, 2(3), 1981.

Chapter References

Chapter 1

Decker, S: Computer networks advance traditional nursing. Reflections, 21(2):13, Summer, 1995.

Foust, JB: Creating a future for nursing through interactive planning at the bedside. Image: Journal of Nursing Scholarship, 26(2):129, Summer, 1994.

Friese, B, Howard, M and Stanton, J: It's about time: Shortened rehab times offer challenges for case managers. Continuing Care, 14(5):24, May/June, 1995.

Lee, S: Clinical pathways for case management. Continuing Care, 14(6):12, July/August, 1995.

O'Grady, TP: Nursing at millennium. Taped presentation at Chautauqua 95, Colorado Nurses' Association, Vail, CO, 1995.

Chapter 2

Leuner, JD, et al: Mastering the Nursing Process: A Case Study Approach. FA Davis, Philadelphia, 1990.

Nursing's Social Policy Statement. American Nurses' Association, St. Louis, 1995.

Standards of Clinical Nursing Practice. American Nurses' Association, St. Louis, 1991.

Chapter 3

Loomis, ME and Conco, D: Patient's perception of health, chronic illness, and nursing diagnosis. Nursing Diagnosis, 2(4):162, 1991.

Chapter 4

Bolz, MA: Nurses guide to identifying cardiac rhythms. Nursing94, 24(4):54, April, 1994.

Bone, LA: Now! Surgery for heart failure. RN, 58(5):26, May 1995.

Bright, LD: Deep vein thrombosis. AJN, 95(6):48, June, 1995.

Brown, LM and Brown, AS: Transesophageal echocardiography: Implications for the critical care nurse. Crit Care Nurse, 14(3):55, June, 1994.

Collins, MA: When your patient has an implantable cardioverter defibrillator. AJN, 94(3):34, March, 1994.

Cuddy: RP: Hypertension, keeping dangerous blood pressure down. Nursing95, 25(8):35, August, 1995.

Dracup, K, Dunbar, SB and Baker, DW: Rethinking heart failure. AJN, 95(7):22, July, 1995.

Fowler, JP, From chronic to acute: When CHF turns deadly. Nursing95, 25(1):54, January, 1995.

Karnes, N, Adenosine: a quick fix for PSVT. Nursing95, 25(7):55, July, 1995.

Lewandowski, DM: Clinical snapshot: Congestive heart failure. AJN, 95(5):36, May, 1995.

Moser, SA, Crawford, D and Thomas, A: Updated care guidelines for patients with automatic implantable cardioverter defibrillators. Crit Care Nurse, 13(2):62, April, 1993.

Murphy, TG: Digoxin toxicity: Ventricular dysrhythmias to watch for. AJN, 93(12):37, December, 1993.

(No author): A stable approach to unstable angina. RN, 58(7):29, July, 1995.

(No author): Postoperative care: A leg up on preventing thromboembolism. AJN, 95(6):9, June, 1995.

Owen, A: Tracking the rise and fall of cardiac enzymes. Nursing95, 25(5):34, May, 1995.

Raimer, J and Thomas, M: Clot stoppers: Using anticoagulants safely and effectively. Nursing95, 25(3):34, March, 1995.

Stahl, L: How to manage common arrhythmias in medical patients. AJN, 95(3):36, March, 1995.

Strimike, CL: Caring for a patient with an intracoronary stent. AJN, 95(1):40, January, 1995.

Yacone-Morton, LA: Antiarrhythmics. RN, 58(4):26, April, 1995.

Chapter 5

Avalos-Bock, S: Getting a rise out of tuberculosis with the PPD skin test. Nursing94, 24(8):51, August, 1994.

Bolton, PJ and Kline, KA: Understanding modes of mechanical ventilation. AJN, 94(9):36, June, 1994.

Boutotte, J: TB the second time around . . . and how you can help to control it. Nursing93, 23(5):42, May, 1993.

Brenner, ZR and Addona, C: Caring for the pneumonectomy patient: Challenges and changes. Crit Care Nurs, 15(5):65, October, 1995.

Carroll, P: A med/surg nurse's guide to mechanical ventilation. RN, 58(2):26, February, 1995.

Catania, U: Monitoring coumadin therapy. RN, 57(2):29, February, 1994.

Colizza, DF: Action stat! Dislodged chest tube. Nursing95, 25(9):33, September, 1995.

Dabbs, AD, Olslund, L: The new alternative to intubation. AJN, 94(8):42, August, 1994.

Glass, CA and Grap, MJ: Ten tips for safer suctioning. AJN, 95(5):51, May, 1995.

Hamner, J: Challenging diagnosis: Adult respiratory distress syndrome. Crit Care Nurs, 15(5):46, October, 1995.

Keep, NB: Emergency! Identifying pulmonary embolism. AJN, 95(4):52, April, 1995.

Jablonski, RA: If ventilator patients could talk. RN, 58(2):32, February, 1995.

Lavell, DR and Higgins, VR: Lung surgery when less is more. RN, 58(7):40, July, 1995.

Mays, D: Turn ABGs into child play. RN, 58(1):36, January, 1995.

McKinney, B: COPD & depression: Treat them both. RN, 57(4):48, April, 1994.

Mee, CL: Ventilator alarms: How to respond with confidence. Nursing95, 25(7):61, July, 1995.

Mergaert, S: S.T.O.P. and assess chest tubes the easy way. Nursing94, 24(2):52, February, 1994.

(No author): Boosting survival rates in MDR-TB AIDS patients. TB Monitor, p 41, April, 1995.

Repasky, TM: Emergency! Tension pneumothorax. AJN, 94(9):47, September, 1994.

Rutter, KM: Action stat! Tension pneumothorax: How to restore normal breathing. Nursing95, 25(4):33, April, 1995.

Smith, RN, Fallentine, J and Kessel, S: Underwater chest drainage: Bringing the facts to the surface. Nursing95, 25(2):60, February, 1995.

Tasota, FJ and Wesmiller, SW: Assessing ABGs: Maintaining the delicate balance. Nursing94, 24(4):34, May, 1994.

Witta, KM: When gauging respiratory status is critical. RN, 56(11):40, November, 1993.

Chapter 6

Blake, K: The social isolation of young men with quadriplegia. Rehab Nursing, 20(1):17, January/February, 1995.

Bronstein, KS and Chadwick, LR: Ticlopidine Hydrochloride: Its current use in cerebrovascular disease. Rehab Nursing, 19(1):17, January/February, 1994.

Caine, RM: The cutting edge in neuroscience. Crit Care Nurse [Supp], June, 1993.

Cole-Arvin, C, Notich, L and Underhill, A: Identifying & managing dysphagia. Nursing94, 24(1):48, January, 1995.

Del Zoppo, G, et al: Recombinant tissue plasminogen activator in acute thrombotic and embolic stroke. Ann Neurol, 32: 78, 1992.

Donohue, J and Gebbard, P (eds): Special techniques and adaptations. The Kinsey/Indiana University report on sexuality and spinal cord injury. Sexuality and Disability, 13(1):77, Spring, 1995.

Dreyer, EB: Glaucoma: Preserving eyesight with foresight. Harvard Health Letter, 19(12):4, October, 1994.

Dunleavy, KJ: Protecting patients after a right CVA. AJN, 95(6):24F, June, 1995.

Fairly, TM: Caring for chronic pain patients. Continuing Care, 13(4):14, May, 1994.

Fettner, AG: Low back pain: If it ain't broke . . . Harvard Health Letter, 20(7):6, May, 1995.

Gauvitz, DF: How to protect the dysphagic stroke patient. AJN, 95(8):34, August, 1995.

Gless, PA: Applying the Roy adaptation model to the care of clients with quadriplegia. Rehab Nursing, 20(1):11, January/February, 1995.

Huston, CJ: Autonomic dysreflexia. AJN, 95(6):55, June, 1995.

Junker, J: Understanding and assessing cognitive function. Multiple Sclerosis Milestones, 4(9):2, September, 1995, Multiple Sclerosis Society of Colorado Springs.

Laskowski-Jones, L: Acute SCI, how to minimize the damage. AJN, 93(12):23, December, 1993.

Masel, B: Common medical issues in postacute brain injury. The Case Manager, 6(3):55, July/Aug/Sept, 1995.

Meissner, JE: Caring for patients with multiple sclerosis. Nursing94, 25(7):50, August, 1995.

(No author) Many diets touted for MS, but no proven winners. Environmental Nutrition, 17(3):7, March, 1994.

(No author): Opening your eyes to intraocular administration. (Adapted from Giving Drugs by Advanced Techniques [copyright, Springhouse]). Nursing94, 24(6):44, June, 1994.

Pierce, L, et al: Frequently selected nursing diagnoses for the rehabilitation client with stroke. Rehab Nursing, 20(3):138, May/June, 1995.

Sandler, RL: Clinical snapshot: Glaucoma. AJN, 95(3):34, March, 1995.

Seachrist, L: Mimicking the brain: Using computers to investigate neurological disorder. Science News, 148(4):62, July 22, 1995.

Travis, J: MS families: It's genes, not a virus. Science News. 148(12):180, September 16, 1995.

Zasler, N: Neurorehabilitation: Issues in post-concussive disorders. Continuing Care, 14(3):31, April, 1995.

Chapter 7

Angelucci: P: T.I.P.S. for controlling bleeding. Nursing95, 25(7):43, July, 1995.

Barnie, DC and Currier, J: What's that GI tube being used for? RN, 58(8):45, August, 1995.

Chase, SL: OTC Interactions—Antacids. RN, 56(8):46, RN, August, 1993.

Chase, SL: OTC Interactions—GI remedies. RN, 56(10):30, October, 1993.

Doherty, MM and Carver, DK: New relief for esophageal varices. AJN, 93(4):58, April, 1993.

Doughty, DB: What you need to know about inflammatory bowel disease. AJN, 94(7):24, July, 1994.

Flynn, M: Update your nutrition vocabulary with environmental nutrition. Nutrition's A-to-Z Guide to Healthy Eating, 18(1):1, January, 1995.

Jess, LW: Acute abdominal pain: Revealing the source. Nursing93, 23(9):34, September, 1993.

Krasner, D: Six steps to successful stoma care. RN, 56(7):32, July, 1993.

Marchiondo, K: When the Dx is diverticular disease. RN, 57(2):42, February, 1994.

McConnell, EA: Loosening the grip of intestinal obstructions. Nursing94, 24(3):34, March, 1994.

Meissner, JE: Caring for patients with ulcerative colitis. Nursing94, 24(7):54, July, 1994.

(No author): Bug and guts. Men's Confidential: Healthy sex and fitness news for men. Rodale Press, Emmaus, October, 1995.

Ondrusek, RS: Cholecystectomy: An update. RN, 56(1):28, January, 1993.

Paulford-Lecher, N: Teaching your patient stoma care. Nursing93, 23(9):47, September, 1993.

Surratt, S, et al: Troubleshooting a sump tube. AJN, 93(1):42, January, 1993.

Weant, CA: Easing the pain of esophageal surgery. RN, 58(8):26, August, 1995.

Chapter 8

Anderson, S: 7 care tips for managing patients with diabetes. AJN, 94(9):36, September, 1994.

Angelucci, P: T.I.P.S. for controlling bleeding, Nursing95, 25(7):43, July, 1995.

Arbour, R: Action Stat! Acute hypoglycemia: Responding quickly to prevent hypoglycemic seizures, Nursing94, 24(1):33, January, 1994.

Bockus, S: When your patient needs tube feedings: Making the right decision. Nursing93, 23(7):34, July 1993.

Brotman, AW: What works in the treatment of anorexia nervosa?, The Harvard Mental Health Letter, 10(7):8, January, 1994.

Butler, RO: Managing the complications of cirrhosis. AJN, 94(3):46, March, 1994.

Castrone, L: Making friends with food. Rocky Mountain News, Spotlight, p1D, Tuesday, August 15, 1995.

Deakins, DA: Teaching elderly patients about diabetes. AJN, 94(4):38, April, 1994.

Eisenberg, PG: A nurse's guide to tube feeding: Feeding formulas. RN, 57(12):46, December, 1994.

Eisenberg, PG: A nurse's guide to tube feeding: Gastrostomy and jejunostomy tubes. RN, 57(11):54, November, 1994.

Eisenberg, PG: A nurse's guide to tube feeding: Nasoenteral tubes, RN, 57(10):62, October, 1994.

Faller, N and Lawrence, KG: Comparing low-profile gastrostomy tubes. Nursing93, 23(12):46, December, 1993.

Hennessey, B, Fitzgerald, A and Graham, D: Venous air embolism: Keeping your patient out of danger. AJN, 93(11):54, November, 1993.

Hoyson, PM: Diabetes 2000: Oral medications. RN, 58(5):34, May, 1995.

Jackson, MM and Rymer, TE: Viral hepatitis: Anatomy of a diagnosis. AJN, 94(1):43, January, 1994.

Kestel, F: Are you up to date on diabetes medications? AJN, 94(7):48, July, 1994.

Lammon, CA and Hart, G: Action Stat! Recognizing thyroid crisis. Nursing93, 23(4):33, April, 1993.

Machea, MKK: Diabetic hypoglycemia: Keeping the threat at bay. AJN, 93(4):26, April, 1993.

Marx, JF: Viral hepatitis: Unscrambling the alphabet. Nursing93, 23(1):34, January, 1993.

Murray, R: Home before dark: One nurse's personal experience with diabetic neuropathy. AJN, 93(11):36, November, 1993.

(No author): Caring for a Gastrostomy: Guidelines and troubleshooting tips. Nursing94, 24(8):48, August, 1994.

(No author): Childhood sexual abuse and eating disorders, The Harvard Mental Health Letter, 11(10):7, April, 1995.

(No author): Diabetes Update93. Nursing93, 23(8):59, August, 1993.

(No author): Living with diabetes: Diet and exercise. RN, 58(4):23, April, 1995.

(No author): Living with diabetes: Insulin therapy. RN, 58(4):35, June, 1995.

(No author): Living with diabetes: Monitoring. RN, 58(3):43, March, 1995.

(No author): Living with diabetes: Oral medications. RN, 58(5):39, May, 1995.

Noone, J: Acute pancreatitis: An Orem approach to nursing assessment and care. Crit Care Nurse, 15(4):27, August, 1995.

Norton, RA: Diabetes 2000: The right mix of diet and exercise. RN, 58(4):20, April, 1995.

Owen, SV and Fullerton, ML: Would it make a difference? A discussion group in a behaviorally oriented inpatient eating disorder program. Psychosoc Nurs, 33(1):35, November, 1995.

Pergallo, Dittko, V: Diabetes: 2000: Acute complications, RN, 58(8):36, August, 1995.

Reising, DL: Acute hypoglycemia: Keeping the bottom from falling out. Nursing95, 25(2):41, February, 1995.

Ricciardi, E and Brown, D: Managing PEG tubes. AJN, 94(10):29, October, 1994.

Robertson, C and Cerrato, PL: Managing diabetes: A major study injects good news. RN, 56(10):26, October, 1993.

Roesler, TA, et al: Bulimia recovery linked to caring relationships. The Menninger Letter, 2(9):1, September, 1994.

Shapiro, M and Stegall, MD: When insulin isn't enough. RN, 58(7):34–37, July, 1995.

Siconolfi, LA: Clarifying the complexity of liver function tests. Nursing 95, 25(5):39, May, 1995.

Strowig, S: Diabetes 2000 Insulin therapy. RN, 58(6):30, June, 1995.

Tomky, D: Diabetes 2000 Advances in monitoring. RN, 58(3):37, RN, March, 1995.

Viall, C: Taking the mystery out of TPN: Part 1. Nursing95, 25(4):34, April, 1995.

Viall, C: Taking the mystery out of TPN: Part 2. Nursing95, (25)5:56, May, 1995.

Wilson, JP: New diabetes nutrition guidelines: Do you know the score? Nursing95, 25(7):65–66, July, 1995.

Chapter 9

Crouch, MA: Current concepts in autologous bone marrow transplantation. Seminar Oncology Nursing, 10(2):12, February, 1994.

Fackelmann, K: Drug wards off sickle-cell attacks. Science News, 147(5):68, February 4, 1995.

Ferrell, G and Rhiner, M: Managing Cancer Pain: A three step approach, Nursing94, 24(7):56, July, 1994.

Franco, T: Allogenic bone marrow transplantation. Seminar Oncology Nursing, 10(1):3, February, 1994.

Fromm, CG and Metzler, DJ: Preparing your older patient for surgery. RN, 56(1):38, January, 1993.

Geissler, A (In press): Aplastic anemias. In Sommers, MS and Johnson, S. (eds): Davis's Manual of Diseases and Disorders. FA Davis, Philadelphia, (pub Fall, 1996).

Held, J: Cancer Care: Managing fatigue. Nursing94, 24(2):26, February, 1994.

Yeager, K and Miaskowski, C: Advances in understanding the mechanisms & management of acute myelogenous leukemia. Oncology Nursing Forum, 21(3):541, March, 1994.

Ziegler, TR, et al: Nutrition notes: An amino acid helps bone-marrow transplant patients. RN, 56(1):72, January, 1993.

Chapter 10

Byers, JF and Goshorn, J: How to manage diuretic therapy. AJN, 95(2):38, February, 1995.

Dunn, SA: How to care for the dialysis patient. AJN, 93(6):26, June, 1993.

King, BA: Detecting acute renal failure. RN, 57(3):34, March, 1994.

McKinney, BC: Cut your patient's risk of nosocomial UTI. RN, 58(11):20, November, 1995.

Mondoux, L: Patient's won't ask. RN, 57(2):35, February, 1994.

Moore, S, Newton, M, Grant, E, et al: Treating bladder cancer: New methods, new management. AJN, 93(5):32, May, 1993.

Moore, S, Newton, M and Yancey, R: How to irrigate a nephrostomy tube. AJN, 93(7):63, July, 1993.

(No author): Bladder volume: Measuring up: New ultrasound device reduces urinary tract infections. Nursing95, 25(10):61, October, 1995.

(No author): Clinical News: About face on calcium and kidney stones. AJN, 93(5):10, May, 1993.

(No author): Prostate Cancer: The big chill. Harvard Health Letter, 20(11):4, September, 1995.

(No author): Urinary Tract Infections. Harvard Women's Health Watch, 1(7):6, March, 1994.

Resnick, B: Retraining the bladder after catheterization. AJN, 93(11):46, November, 1993.

Ruth-Sahd, LA: Emergency! Renal Calculi. AJN, 95(11):50, November, 1995.

Wood, JM and Bosley, C: Acute postrenal failure: Reversing the problem. Nursing95, 25(3):48, March, 1995.

Chapter 11

Anderson, BL and Elliot, ML: Sexuality for women with cancer: Assessment, theory, and treatment. Sexuality and Disability, 11(1):7, Spring, 1993.

Baron, RH and Walsh, A: 9 facts everyone should know about breast cancer. AJN, 95(7):29, July, 1995.

Dest, VM and Fisher, SM: Breast cancer: Dreaded diagnosis, complicated care. RN, 57(6):48, June, 1994.

Granda, C: Nursing management of patients with lymphedema associated with breast cancer therapy. Cancer Nursing, 17(3):229, March, 1994.

Holm, K, Penckofer, S and Chandler, P: Deciding on hormone replacement therapy. AJN, 95(8):57, August, 1995.

Ivey, CL: When your patient has ovarian cancer. RN, 57(11):26, November, 1995.

Ivey, CL and Gordon, SI: Breast reconstruction: New image, new hope. RN, 57(7):48, July, 1994.

Johnson, JR: Caring for the woman who's had a mastectomy. AJN, 94(5):25, May, 1994.

Moutos, DM and Rock, JA: Six gynecologic uses for GnRH agonists. Medical Aspects of Human Sexuality, 26(2):67, February, 1992.

Sciartelli, CH: Using a clinical pathway approach to document patient teaching for breast cancer surgical procedure. Oncology Nursing Forum, 22(1):131, January, 1995.

Whitman, M, McDaniel, RW: Preventing lymphedema, an unwelcome sequel to breast cancer. Nursing93, 23(12):36, December, 1993.

Chapter 12

Altizer, L: Total hip arthroplasty. Orthopaedic Nursing, 14(4):7, Jul/Aug, 1995.

Bailey, MM and Michalski, J: Close-up on scaphoid fracture. Nursing93, 23(3):49, March, 1993.

Bright, LD and George, S: How to protect your patient from DVT. AJN, 94(12):28, December, 1994.

Clay, KL and Stirn, ML: Documentation of discharge teaching of patients who have had hip surgery. Orthopaedic Nursing, 5(6):22, Nov/Dec, 1986.

Clutter, P, Easter, A, et al: Help! She's been shot! RN, 57(9):45, September, 1994.

Dykes, PC: Minding the five Ps of neurovascular assessment. AJN, 93(6):38, June, 1993.

Grant, E, Newton, M and Moore, S: Keeping patients on the right track. Nursing95, 25(8):57, August, 1995.

Gray, MA: NSAIDs revisited. Orthopaedic Nursing, 14(1):52, Jan/Feb, 1995.

Halverson, PB: Extraarticular manifestations of rheumatoid arthritis. Orthopaedic Nursing, 14(4):47, July/August, 1995.

Johnson, J, et al: Roller traction: Mobilizing patients with acetabular fractures. Orthopaedic Nursing, 14(1):21, Jan/Feb, 1995.

Kendrick, DW: Now I stand up for my patients. RN, 56(4):37, April, 1993.

Monk, HL: Fractures are never simple. RN 56(4):30, April, 1993.

Mornhinweg, GC and Voigneir, RR: Holistic nursing interventions. Orthopaedic Nursing, 14(4):20, Jul/Aug, 1995.

Naden, BA: When bone disappears. RN, 58(10):26, October, 1995.

(No author): Bonewise: Living with osteoporosis. Public Information Pamphlet, National Osteoporosis Foundation, Washington, DC, 1991.

(No author): Stand up to osteoporosis: Your guide to staying healthy and independent through prevention and treatment. National Osteoporosis Foundation, Washington, DC, 1994.

Pellino, TA: How to manage hip fractures. AJN, 94(4):46, April, 1994.

Rankin, JA: Pathophysiology of the rheumatoid joint. Orthopaedic Nursing 14(4):39, July/August, 1995.

Styrcula, L: Orthopaedic essentials: Traction basics series. Orthopaedic Nursing, 13(2):2, March-December, 1994.

Chapter 13

Allwood, JS: The primary care management of burns. Nurse Pract, 20(8):74, August, 1995.

Calistro, AM: Burn care basics and beyond. RN, 56(3):26, March, 1993.

Carliste, D: Face value. Nursing Times, 87(42):26, October, 16–22, 1991.

Carroll, P: Bed selection: Help patients rest easy. RN, 58(5):44, May, 1995.

Erwin-Toth, Panel Hocevar, BJ: Wound Care: Selecting the right dressing. AJN, 95(2):46, February, 1995.

Krasner, D: Wound Care: How to use the red-yellow-black system. AJN, 95(5):44, May, 1995.

Partridge, J: Staring prejudice in the face. Nursing Times, 87(42):28, Oct. 16–22, 1991.

Chapter 14

Anastasi, JK and Thomas, F: Dealing with HIV-related pulmonary infections. Nursing94, 24(11):60, November, 1994.

Anastasi, JK and Sun Lee, V: HIV wasting: How to stop the cycle. AJN, 94(6):18, June, 1994.

Anastasi, JK and Rivera, J: Understanding prophylactic therapy for HIV infections. AJN, 94(2):36, February, 1994.

Baigis-Smith, J, Gordon, D, McGuire, DB, et al: Healthcare needs of HIV-infected persons in hospital, outpatient, home and long-term care settings. JANAC, 6(6):21, Nov-Dec, 1995.

Beyer, L: Preparing for your transplant. LifeTIMES, Issue 3, 1995.

Blanford, NL: Renal transplantation: A case study of the ideal. Crit Care Nurse, 13(1):46, February, 1993.

Brown, KK: Critical interventions in septic shock. AJN, 94(10):20, October, 1994.

Brown, KK: Septic shock: How to stop the deadly cascade. AJN, 94(9):20, September, 1994.

Cerney, MS: Solving the organ donor shortage by meeting the bereaved family's needs. Crit Care Nurse, 13(2):32, February, 1993.

Chabalewski, R and Gaedeke-Norris, MK: The gift of life: Talking to families about organ and tissue donation. AJN, 94(6):28, June, 1994.

Erwin-Toth, P and Hocevar, BJ: Wound Care: Selecting the right dressing. AJN, 95(2):46, February, 1995.

Fackelmann, K: People with HIV get immune-reviving drug. Science News, 147(9):135, March 4, 1995.

Giddens, JF, et al: Risks and rewards of kidney transplant. RN, 56(6):56, June, 1993.

Halverson, PB: Extraarticular manifestations of rheumatoid arthritis. Orthopaedic Nursing, 14(4):47, July/August, 1995.

Horvath, TA, Patsdaughter, CA, Bumbalo, JA, et al: Dementia-related behaviors in Alzheimer's and AIDS. J Psychosoc Nurs, 33(1):35, January, 1995.

Hricik, DE: Advice to transplant recipients: Know your immunosuppressant medications. LifeTIMES, Issue 3, 1995.

Kirton, CA: AIDS: When your patient refuses HIV testing. AJN, 94(11):48, November, 1994.

Krasner, D: Wound care: How to use the red-yellow-black system. AJN, 95(5):44, May, 1995.

Lyons, M: Immunosuppressive therapy after cardiac transplantation: Teaching pediatric patients and their families. Crit Care Nurse, 13(1):39, February, 1993.

(No author): Aids and Mental Health—Part II. The Harvard Mental Health Letter, 10(8):1, February, 1994.

(No author): AIDSFILE: Quick screen for HIV dementia. AJN, 95(7):12, July, 1995.

(No author listed): An HIV battle plan. RN, 58(3):18, March, 1995.

Partridge, J: Staring prejudice in the face. Nursing Times, 87(42):28, Oct. 16–22, 1991.

Pedersen, A, Groves, JL, Coleman, RB, et al: Intramuscular administration of RATG in the heart transplant patient. Crit Care Nurse, 13(1):22, February, 1993.

Porche, DJ: Treatment review: Zerit. JANAC, 6(5):50, Sept–Oct, 1995.

Price, N: The role of the consultation-liaison nurse—caring for patients with AIDS dementia comlex. J of Psychosoc Nurs, 33(12):31, Dec, 1995.

Rankin, JA: Arthophysiology of the Rheumatoid Joint. Orthopaedic Nursing. 14(4):39, Jul/Aug, 1995.

Russell, S: Septic shock: Can you recognize the clues? Nursing94, 24(4):40, April, 1994.

Schred, E: Future care of rheumatoid arthritis. Bulletin of the Rheumatic Diseases, 42(7):1, November, 1993.

Sipos, DA: MP Implants for Rheumatoid Arthritis of the hand. Orthopedic Nursing. 12(5):7, Sept/Oct, 1993.

Smith, SL: The cutting edge in organ transplantation. Crit Care Nurse/supplement, p 10, June, 1993.

Travis, J: Science News of the Week: Body's proteins suppress AIDS virus. Science News, 1148(24):388, December 9, 1995.

Zurlinden, J and Verheggen, R: HIV vaccines: A report from the front. RN, 57(1):36, January, 1994.

Chapter 15

Advice, P.R.N., (no author), Outpatient surgery: Relaxing the hard fast rule. Nursing95, 25(8):9, August, 1995.

Antai-Otong, D: Helping the alcoholic patient recover. AJN, 95(8):22, August, 1995.

Badger, JM: Calming the anxious patient. AJN, 94(5):46, May, 1994.

Belcaster, A: Caring for the alcohol abuser. Nursing94, 24(2):56, February, 1994.

Bove, LA: How fluid and electrolytes shift after surgery. Nursing94, 24(8):34, August, 1994.

Bove, LA: Restoring electrolyte balance: Sodium and chloride. RN, 59(1):25, January, 1996.

Bower, B: Brain data fuel alcoholism gene clash. Science News, 148(2):20, July 8, 1995.

Bryce, J: Action stat! S.I.A.D.H. Recognizing and treating syndrome of inappropriate antidiuretic hormone secretion. Nursing94, 24(4):33, April, 1994.

Burke, MM and Walsh, MB: New opportunities in gerontologic nursing. Nursing93, 23(12):40, December, 1993.

DiStasio, SA: Zofran makes chemo bearable. RN, 56(5):56, May, 1993.

Ferszt, GG: Cancer Care: Performing a crisis assessment. Nursing95, 25(5):88, May, 1995.

Ferrell, B and Rhiner, M: Managing cancer pain. Nursing94, 24(7):57, July, 1994.

Flavell, C: Combating hemorrhagic shock. RN, 57(12):26, December, 1994.

Gore, MJ: Laboratory tests for the elderly patient: How aging changes body chemistry. The Consultant Pharmacist, 9(8):839, August, 1994.

Hall, RWC; Beresford, TP and Kirkland, RG: Aging in America: Dementia, the growing problem. Medical Aspects of Human Sexuality, 24(5):29, May, 1990.

Hambleton, NE: Dealing with complications of epidural analgesia. Nursing94, 24(10):55, October, 1994.

Holbrook-West, E: Did Henry deserve more from us? RN, 56(10):42, October, 1993.

Hser, Y, Anglin, D and Powers, K: Follow-up on addicts. The Harvard Mental Health Letter, 10(8):7, February, 1994.

Irons, RR: Addiction affects all member of family. The Menninger Letter, 2(12):3, December, 1994.

Janowski, MJ: Managing cancer pain. RN, 58(9):30, September, 1995.

Jost, KE. Psychosocial care: Document it. AJN, 95(7):46–49, July, 1995.

Kendler, KS, Neale, MC, Heath, AC, et al: Genetics of female alcoholism. The Harvard Mental Health Letter, 11(5):7, November, 1994.

Marshall, M: Postoperative confusion: Helping your patient emerge from the shadows. Nursing93, 24(4):44, January, 1993.

McCaffrey, M and Ferrell, BR: How to use the new AHCPR cancer pain guidelines. AJN, 94(4):34, April, 1995.

McCarron, EG: Supporting the families of cancer patients. Nursing95, 25(6):48, June, 1995.

McDivitt, MJ: A(TENS)tion! Nursing95, 25(12):46, December, 1995.

McLaughlin-Hagan, M and Baird, SB: Predicting future trends in oncology nursing. Nursing93, 23(5):55, May, 1993.

Messner, RL and Lewis, S: Double trouble: Managing chronic illness and depression. Nursing95, 25(8):46, August, 1995.

Metzler, DJ and Fromm, CG: Laying out a care plan for the elderly postoperative patient Nursing93, 23(4):67, April, 1993.

Myer, C: 'End-of-life' care: Patients' choices, nurses' challenges. AJN, 93(2):40, February, 1993.

(No author): Cancer update94. Nursing94, 24(4):59, April, 1994.

(No author): Geriatric update94. Nursing94, 24(3)59, March, 1994.

(No author): Home health care update95. Nursing95, 25(7):57, July, 1995.

(No author) Treatment of drug abuse and addiction—Part I. The Harvard Mental Health Letter, 12(2):1, August, 1995.

(No author). Treatment of drug abuse and addiction—Part II. The Harvard Mental Health Letter, 12(3):1, September, 1995.

(No author). Treatment of drug abuse and addiction—Part III. The Harvard Mental Health Letter, 12(4):1, October, 1995.

O'Donnell, ME: Assessing fluid and electrolyte balance in elders. AJN, 95(11):40, November, 1995.

Perez, A: Restoring electrolyte balance: Hypokalemia. RN, 58(12):33, December, 1995.

Perez, A: Electrolytes: Restoring the balance: Hyperkalemia. RN, 58(11):32, November, 1995.

Raimer, F: How to identify electrolyte imbalances on your patient's ECG. Nursing94, 24(6):54, June, 1994.

Robins, LN: Lessons from the Vietnam heroin experience. The Harvard Mental Health Letter, 11(6):5, December, 1994.

Russell, S: Hypovolemic shock: Is your patient at risk? Nursing94, 24(4):34, April, 1994.

Schoenbeck, SB: Exploring the mystery of near-death experiences. AJN, 93(5):43, May, 1995.

Schuckit, MA: Are alcoholics insensitive to alcohol? The Harvard Mental Health Letter, 10(12):7, June, 1994.

Valenta, AL: Using the vacuum dressing alternative for difficult wounds. AJN, 94(4):44, April, 1994.

Valente, SM: Recognizing depression in elderly patients. AJN, 94(12):18, December, 1994.

Walsh, J: Postop effects of OR positioning. RN, 56(2):50, February, 1993.

Weber, MS: Clinical snapshot: Chemotherapy-induced nausea and vomiting. AJN 95(4):34, April, 1995.

Willens, JS: Giving Fentanyl for pain outside the OR. AJN, 94(2):24, February, 1994.

Wilson, SA: Can you spot an alcoholic patient. RN, 57(1):46, January, 1994.

Woodin, LM: Cutting postop pain. RN, 56(8):26, August, 1993.

INDEX OF NURSING DIAGNOSES

Cardiac Output, decreased—*Continued*
   sion: severe and, risk for, 35; hyperthyroidism (thyrotoxicosis, Graves' disease) and, risk for, 439; myocardial infarction and, risk for, 78; renal failure:
   acute and, risk for, 560; renal failure: chronic and,
   risk for, 571
Caregiver Role Strain, risk for: multiple sclerosis and,
   306; psychosocial aspects of care and, 794
Communication, impaired verbal: cerebrovascular ac-
   cident/stroke and [and/or written], 249; long-term
   care, and, 832; radical neck surgery: laryngectomy
   (postoperative care) and, 166; thyroidectomy and,
   450; ventilatory assistance (mechanical) and, 181
Confusion, acute, risk for: cirrhosis of the liver and,
   475
Constipation: anemias (iron deficiency, pernicious,
   aplastic, hemolytic) and, 521, cancer and, risk for,
   893; disc surgery and, 272; fecal diversions: postoperative care of ileostomy and colostomy and, risk
   for, 356; hysterectomy and, risk for, 641; long-term
   care and, risk for, 841; renal dialysis and, risk for,
   584; spinal cord injury (acute rehabilitative phase)
   and, 290
Coping, Individual, ineffective: cerebrovascular acci-
   dent/stroke, 254; herniated nucleus pulposus (ruptured intervertebral disc) and, [chronic], 263; hypertension: severe and, 40; inflammatory bowel
   disease: ulcerative colitis, regional enteritis
   (Crohn's disease, ileocolitis) and, 345; multiple sclerosis and, risk for, 309; psychosocial aspects of care
   and, 792; substance dependence/abuse rehabilitation and, 863; transplantation (postoperative and
   lifelong) and, 778
Decisional Conflict (specify): psychosocial aspects of
   care and, 792
Denial, ineffective: substance dependence/abuse rehabilitation and, 863
Diarrhea: anemias (iron deficiency, pernicious, aplastic, hemolytic) and, 521; cancer and, risk for, 893;
   fecal diversions: postoperative care of ileostomy and
   colostomy and, risk for, 356; hysterectomy and, risk
   for, 641; inflammatory bowel disease: ulcerative colitis, regional enteritis (Crohn's disease, ileocolitis)
   and, 337; long-term care and, risk for, 841; obesity:
   surgical interventions (gastric partitioning/gastro-
   plasty, gastric bypass) and, 418
Diversional Activity deficity: long-term care and, 843
Dysreflexia, risk for: spinal cord injury (acute rehabilitative phase) and, 293
Family Coping: ineffective, compromised: long-term
   care and, 830; multiple sclerosis and, 310; psychosocial aspects of care and, risk for, 794
Family Coping: ineffective, disabling: multiple sclerosis and, 310; psychosocial aspects of care and, risk
   for, 794
Family Coping, potential for growth: psychosocial aspects of care and, 796

Family Process, altered: alcoholism [substance abuse],
   substance dependence/abuse rehabilitation and,
   869
Family Processes, altered: cancer and, risk for, 895;
   craniocerebral trauma (acute rehabilitative phase)
   and, 238; eating disorders: anorexia nervosa/bu-
   limia nervosa and, 398
Fatigue: AIDS and, 755; cancer and, 888; diabetes mel-
   litus/diabetic ketoacidosis and, 431; the HIV-positive patient and, 733; hyperthyroidism (thyrotoxicosis, Graves' disease) and, 442; multiple sclerosis
   and, 301; total nutritional support: parenteral/en-
   teral feeding and, 502
Fear: AIDS and, 758; alcoholism [acute]: intoxica-
   tion/overdose and, 857; benign prostatic hyperplasia (BPH) and, 618; burns: thermal/chemical/elec-
   trical (acute and convalescent phases) and, 714;
   cancer and, 877; hepatitis and, 457; long-term care
   and, 825; lung cancer: surgical intervention (postoperative care) and, 150; mastectomy and, 649;
   myocardial infarction and, 77; peritonitis and, 372;
   psychosocial aspects of care and, 785; renal dialysis
   and, 586; surgical intervention and, 805; transplantation (postoperative and lifelong) and, 776; upper
   gastrointestinal/esophageal bleeding and, 323; ventilatory assistance (mechanical) and, 182
Fluid Volume [fluctuation], risk for: total nutritional
   support: parenteral/enteral feeding and, 501
Fluid Volume deficit [active loss]: hypovolemia (extracellular fluid volume deficit) and, 902; peritonitis
   and, 369; upper gastrointestinal/esophageal bleeding and, 318
Fluid Volume deficit [regulatory failure]: diabetes
   mellitus/diabetic ketoacidosis and, 425
Fluid Volume deficit, risk for: acute hemodialysis and,
   598; AIDS and, risk for, 745; appendectomy and,
   363; benign prostate hyperplasia (BPH) and, 617;
   burns: thermal/chemical/electrical (acute and convalescent phases) and, 703; cancer and, 887; cholecystectomy and, 383; cholecystitis with cholelithiasis
   and, 378; eating disorders: anorexia nervosa/bu-
   limia nervosa and, 393; fecal diversions: postoperative care of ileostomy and colostomy and, 353; hepatitis and, 459; inflammatory bowel disease:
   ulcerative colitis, regional enteritis (Crohn's disease, ileocolitis) and, 339; leukemias and, 544; obesity: surgical interventions (gastric partitioning/gas-
   troplasty, gastric bypass) and, 415; pancreatitis and,
   485; pneumonia: microbial and, 138; prostatectomy
   and, 622; renal dialysis: peritoneal and, 592; renal
   failure: acute and, 564; sepsis/septicemia and, 727;
   sickle cell crisis and, 533; surgical intervention and,
   816; urolithiasis (renal calculi) and, 635
Fluid Volume excess: acute hemodialysis and, risk for,
   599; cirrhosis of the liver and, 470; heart failure:
   chronic and, 52; hypervolemia (extracellular fluid
   volume excess) and, 899; myocardial infarction and,

Nutrition: altered, risk for less than body requirements: cholecystitis with cholelithiasis and, 379; craniocerebral trauma (acute rehabilitative phase) and, 237; fecal diversions: postoperative care of ileostomy and colostomy and, 354; the HIV-positive patient and, 734; hyperthyroidism (thyrotoxicosis, Graves' disease) and, 443; obesity: surgical interventions (gastric partitioning/gastroplasty, gastric bypass) and, 416; peritonitis and, 371; pneumonia: microbial and, 137; renal failure: acute and, 562; subtotal gastrectomy/gastric resection and, 328

Nutrition: altered, less than body requirements: AIDS and, 749; alcoholism [acute]: intoxication/overdose and, 855; anemias (iron deficiency, pernicious, aplastic hemolytic) and, 519; burns: thermal/chemical/electrical (acute and convalescent phases) and, 710; cancer and, 885; chronic obstructive pulmonary disease (COPD) and, 125; cirrhosis of the liver and, 468; diabetes mellitus/diabetic ketoacidosis and, 427; eating disorders: anorexia nervosa/bulimia nervosa and, 390; hepatitis and, 458; inflammatory bowel disease: ulcerative colitis, regional enteritis (Crohn's disease, ileocolitis) and, 340; long-term care and, 835; pancreatitis and, 487; pneumonia: microbial and, 137; pulmonary tuberculosis (TB) and, 196; radical neck surgery: laryngectomy (postoperative care) and, 171; renal dialysis and, 581; substance dependence/abuse rehabilitation and, 866; subtotal gastrectomy/gastric resection and, risk for, 328; total nutritional support: parenteral/enteral feeding and, 494; ventilatory assistance (mechanical) and, 184

Nutrition: altered, more than body requirements: eating disorders: obesity and, 405; hypertension: severe and, 39; long-term care and, 835

Oral Mucous Membrane, altered: AIDS and, 754; cancer and, risk for, 890; radical neck surgery; laryngectomy (postoperative care) and, 169; renal failure: chronic and, risk for, 576; ventilatory assistance (mechanical) and, risk for, 184

Pain [acute]: AIDS and, 751; amputation and, 679; angina pectoris and, 63; appendectomy and, 364; benign prostatic hyperplasia (BPH) and, 617; burns: thermal/chemical/electrical (acute and convalescent phases) and, 707; cancer and, 882; cardiac surgery: coronary artery bypass graft; cardiomyoplasty; valve replacement (postoperative care) and, 100; cholecystitis with cholelithiasis and, 376; disc surgery and, 270; fecal diversions; postoperative care of ileostomy and colostomy and, 351; fractures and, 662; herniated nucleus pulposus (ruptured intervertebral disc) and, 260; hypertension: severe and, headache, 38; inflammatory bowel disease: ulcerative colitis, regional enteritis (Crohn's disease, ileocolitis) and, 343; leukemias and, 546; lung cancer: surgical intervention (postoperative care) and,

148; mastectomy and, 651; myocardial infarction and, 74; pancreatitis and, 483; peritonitis and, 370; pneumonia: microbial and, 137; prostatectomy and, 625; radical neck surgery: laryngectomy (postoperative care) and, 170; renal dialysis: peritoneal and, 593; rheumatoid arthritis and, 766; sickle cell crisis and, 534; spinal cord injury (acute rehabilitative phase) and, 286; surgical intervention and, 818; thyroidectomy and, 452; thrombophlebitis: deep vein thrombosis and, 111; total joint replacement and, 692; upper gastrointestinal/esophageal bleeding and, 324; urinary diversions/urostomy (postoperative care) and, 605; urolithiasis (renal calculi) and, 632

Pain, chronic: AIDS and, 751; cancer and, 882; rheumatoid arthritis and, 766; sickle cell crisis and, 534; upper gastrointestinal/esophageal bleeding and, 324

Perioperative Positioning Injury, risk for: surgical intervention and, 807

Peripheral Neurovascular dysfunction, risk for: burns: thermal/chemical/electrical (acute and convalescent phases) and, 709; fractures and, 664

Personal Identity disturbance: seizure disorders/epilepsy and, 220

Physical Mobility, impaired: amputation and, 682; burns: thermal/chemical/electrical (acute and convalescent phases) and, 711; cerebrovascular accident/stroke and, 247; craniocerebral trauma (acute rehabilitative phase) and, 235; disc surgery and, 272; fractures and, 667; herniated nucleus pulposus (ruptured intervertebral disc) and, 262; long-term care and, 842; mastectomy and, 653, renal dialysis, and 582; rheumatoid arthritis and, 768; sickle cell crisis and, 535; spinal cord injury (acute rehabilitative phase) and, 283; total joint replacement and, 688

Post-Trauma Response: psychosocial aspects of care and, 800

Powerlessness: AIDS and, 761; diabetes mellitus/diabetic ketoacidosis and, 432; multiple sclerosis and [specify degree], 307; substance dependence/abuse rehabilitation and, 865

Role Performance, altered: burns: thermal/chemical/electrical (acute and convalescent phases) and, 716; cardiac surgery: coronary artery bypass graft; cardiomyoplasty; valve replacement (postoperative care) and, 101; radical neck surgery: laryngectomy (postoperative care) and, 173; rheumatoid arthritis and, 769

Self Care Deficit: feeding, bathing/hygiene, dressing/grooming, toileting: cerebrovascular accident/stroke and, 253; long-term care and, 837; multiple sclerosis and, 303; renal dialysis and, 583; rheumatoid arthritis and, 770

Self Esteem, chronic low: eating disorders: anorexia nervosa/bulimia nervosa and, 395; eating disorders:

obesity and, 408; substance dependence/abuse rehabilitation and, 867

Self Esteem disturbance: cirrhosis of the liver and, 477; multiple sclerosis and, 305; seizure disorders/ epilepsy and, 220; substance dependence/rehabilitation and, 869

Self Esteem, situational low: amputation and, 652; cancer and, 881; hepatitis and, 461; hysterectomy and, 639; mastectomy and, 652; psychosocial aspects of care and, 790; renal dialysis and, 587; spinal cord injury (acute rehabilitative phase) and, 289

Sensory/Perceptual alterations (specify): visual, auditory, kinesthetic, gustatory, tactile, olfactory: alcoholism [acute]: intoxication/overdose and, 854; cerebrovascular accident/stroke and, 251; craniocerebral trauma (acute rehabilitative phase) and, 231; diabetes mellitus/diabetic ketoacidosis and, risk for, 430; glaucoma and, 210; spinal cord injury (acute rehabilitative phase) and, 285; surgical intervention and, 815

Sexual dysfunction: fecal diversions: postoperative care of ileostomy and colostomy and, risk for, 357; hysterectomy and, risk for, 643; prostatectomy and, 626; substance dependence/abuse rehabilitation and, 871; urinary diversions/urostomy (postoperative care) and, risk for, 609

Sexuality Patterns, altered, risk for: cancer and, 895; long-term care and, 844

Skin Integrity, impaired: AIDS and, 752; burns: thermal/chemical/electrical (acute and convalescent phases) and, 713; cardiac surgery: coronary bypass graft; cardiomyoplasty; valve replacement (postoperative care) and, 104; cholecystectomy and, 384; eating disorders: anorexia nervosa/bulimia nervosa and, 397; fecal diversions: postoperative care of ileostomy and colostomy and, 353; fractures and, 669; mastectomy and, 650; obesity: surgical interventions (gastric partitioning/gastroplasty, gastric bypass) and, 417; radical neck surgery: laryngectomy (postoperative care) and, 167; surgical intervention and, 820

Skin Integrity, impaired, risk for: AIDS and, 752; cancer and, 892; cirrhosis of the liver and, 472; eating disorders: anorexia nervosa/bulimia nervosa and, 397; fractures and, 669; heart failure: chronic and, 55; hepatitis and, 463; long-term care and, 638; obesity: surgical interventions (gastric partitioning/gastroplasty, gastric bypass), 417; renal failure: chronic and, 575; sickle cell crisis and, 536; spinal cord injury (acute rehabilitative phase) and, 294; urinary diversions/urostomy (postoperative care) and, 602

Sleep Pattern disturbance: fecal diversions: postoperative care of ileostomy and colostomy and, 355; long-term care and, 834

Social Interaction, impaired: eating disorders: obesity and, 410

Social Isolation: AIDS and, 759

Spontaneous Ventilation, inability to sustain: ventilatory assistance (mechanical) and, 177

Suffocation, risk for: hemothorax/pneumothorax and, 159; seizure disorders/epilepsy and, 217

Swallowing, impaired, risk for: cerebrovascular accident/stroke and, 255

Therapeutic Regimen: individual, ineffective management, risk for: psychosocial aspects of care and, 797

Thought Processes, altered: AIDS and, 756; craniocerebral trauma (acute rehabilitative phase) and, 233; eating disorders: anorexia nervosa/bulimia nervosa and, 394; hyperthryoidism (thyrotoxicosis, Graves' disease) and, risk for, 445; long-term care and, 828; renal dialysis and, 585; renal failure: chronic and, 574; surgical intervention and, 815

Tissue Integrity, impaired: cancer and, 892; cholecystectomy and, 384; fecal diversions: opostoperative care of ileostomy and colostomy and, 353; fractures and, 669; hepatitis and, risk for, 463; hyperthyroidism (thyrotoxicosis, Graves' disease) and, 446; mastectomy and, 650; radical neck surgery: laryngectomy (postoperative care) and, 167; surgical intervention and, 820

Tissue Perfusion, altered (specify) (cerebral, cardiopulmonary, renal, gastrointestinal, peripheral): amputation and, 680; burns: thermal/chemical/electrical (acute and convalescent phases) and, 709; cerebrovascular accident/stroke and, 245; craniocerebral trauma (acute rehabilitative phase) and, 226; disc surgery and, 267; hysterectomy and, 642; myocardial infarction and, risk for, 80; obesity: surgical interventions (gastric partitioning/gastroplasty, gastric bypass) and, peripheral, risk for, 414; sepsis/septicemia and, 725; sickle cell crisis and, 531; surgical intervention and, 821; thrombophlebitis: deep vein thrombosis and, 107; total joint replacement and, 690; upper gastrointestinal/esophageal bleeding and, risk for, 325

Trauma, risk for: disc surgery and, 268; fractures and, 268; hemothorax/pneumothorax and, 159; renal dialysis: peritoneal and, 593; seizure disorders/epilepsy and, 217; spinal cord injury (acute rehabilitative phase) [additional spinal injury] and, 282

Urinary Elimination, altered: hysterectomy and, 640; long-term care and, 840; multiple sclerosis and, 312; prostatectomy and, 621; spinal cord injury (acute rehabilitative phase) and, 292; urinary diversions/ urostomy (postoperative care) and, 608; urolithiasis (renal calculi) and, 633

Urinary Retention [acute/chronic]: benign prostatic hyperplasia (BPH) and, 614; disc surgery and, 273; hysterectomy and, 640

Ventilatory Weaning Response, dysfunctional (DVWR), risk for: ventilatory assistance (mechanical) and, 186

Violence, risk for, directed at self/others: psychosocial aspects of care and, 798

CLASSIFICATION OF NANDA NURSING DIAGNOSES BY GORDON'S FUNCTIONAL HEALTH PATTERNS*

HEALTH PERCEPTION—HEALTH MANAGEMENT PATTERN
Altered health maintenance
Effective management of individual therapeutic regimen
Ineffective management of individual therapeutic regimen
Ineffective management of therapeutic regimen: community
Ineffective management of family therapeutic regimen
Total health management deficit
Health management deficit (specify)
Noncompliance (specify)
High risk for noncompliance (specify)
Health-seeking behaviors (specify)
Risk for infection
Risk for injury (trauma)
Risk for poisoning
Risk for suffocation
Altered protection

NUTRITIONAL-METABOLIC PATTERN
Adaptive capacity, intracranial: decreased
Altered nutrition: potential for more than body requirements or high risk for obesity
Altered nutrition: more than body requirements or exogenous obesity
Altered nutrition: less than body requirements or nutritional deficit (specify)
Ineffective breastfeeding
Effective breastfeeding
Interrupted breastfeeding
Ineffective infant feeding pattern
Risk for aspiration
Impaired swallowing or uncompensated swallowing impairment
Altered oral mucous membrane
Risk for fluid volume deficit
Fluid volume deficit
Fluid volume excess
Risk for impaired skin integrity or high risk for skin breakdown
Impaired skin integrity
Pressure ulcer (specify stage)
Impaired tissue integrity
Risk for altered body temperature
Ineffective thermoregulation
Hyperthermia
Hypothermia

ELIMINATION PATTERN
Constipation or intermittent constipation pattern
Colonic constipation
Perceived constipation
Diarrhea
Bowel incontinence
Altered urinary elimination pattern
Functional incontinence
Reflex incontinence
Stress incontinence
Urge incontinence
Total incontinence
Urinary retention

ACTIVITY-EXERCISE PATTERN
Risk for activity intolerance
Activity intolerance (specify level)
Fatigue
Impaired physical mobility (specify level)
Risk for disuse syndrome
Risk for joint contractures
Total self-care deficit (specify level)
Self–bathing-hygiene deficit (specify level)
Self–dressing-grooming deficit (specify level)
Self–feeding deficit (specify level)
Self–toileting deficit (specify level)
Altered growth and development: self-care skills (specify)
Diversional activity deficit
Impaired home maintenance management (mild, moderate, severe, potential, chronic)
Infant behavior, disorganized
Risk for disorganized infant behavior
Potential for enhanced organized infant behavior
Dysfunctional ventilatory weaning response (DVWR)
Inability to sustain spontaneous ventilation
Ineffective airway clearance
Ineffective breathing pattern
Impaired gas exchange
Decreased cardiac output
Altered tissue perfusion (specify)
Dysreflexia
Risk for peripheral neurovascular dysfunction
Altered growth and development

SLEEP-REST PATTERN
Sleep-pattern disturbance

COGNITIVE-PERCEPTUAL PATTERN
Pain
Chronic pain
Acute confusion
Chronic confusion
Pain self-management deficit (acute, chronic)
Uncompensated sensory deficit (specify)
Sensory-perceptual alterations: input deficit or sensory deprivation
Sensory-perceptual alterations: input excess or sensory overload
Unilateral neglect
Impaired environmental interpretation syndrome
Impaired thought processes
Knowledge deficit (specify)
Uncompensated short-term memory deficit
Risk for cognitive impairment
Decisional conflict (specify)

SELF-PERCEPTION–SELF-CONCEPT PATTERN
Fear (specify focus)
Anxiety
Mild anxiety
Moderate anxiety
Severe anxiety (panic)
Anticipatory anxiety (mild, moderate, severe)
Fatigue
Reactive depression (situational)
Hopelessness
Powerlessness (severe, low, moderate)
Self-esteem disturbance
Chronic low self-esteem
Situational low self-esteem
Body image disturbance
Risk for self-mutilation
Personal identity confusion

ROLE-RELATIONSHIP PATTERN
Anticipatory grieving
Dysfunctional grieving
Disturbance in role performance
Unresolved independence-dependence conflict
Social isolation or social rejection
Social isolation
Impaired social interaction
Altered growth and development: social skills (specify)
Relocation stress syndrome
Altered family processes
Altered family process: alcoholism
Altered parenting
Risk for altered parent-infant-child attachment
Risk for altered parenting
Parental role conflict
Parent-infant separation
Weak mother-infant or parent-infant attachment
Caregiver role strain
Risk for caregiver role strain
Impaired verbal communication
Altered growth and development: communication skills (specify)
Risk for loneliness
High risk for violence

SEXUALITY-REPRODUCTIVE PATTERN
Sexual dysfunction (specify type)
Altered sexuality patterns
Rape trauma syndrome
Rape trauma syndrome: compound reaction
Rape trauma syndrome: silent reaction

COPING-STRESS TOLERANCE PATTERN
Coping, ineffective (individual)
Avoidance coping
Defensive coping
Ineffective denial or denial
Impaired adjustment
Post-trauma response
Family coping: potential for growth
Ineffective family coping: compromised
Ineffective family coping: disabling
Ineffective community coping
Potential for enhanced community coping
Risk for self-harm
Risk for self-abuse
Risk for self-mutilation
Risk for suicide
Risk for violence

VALUE-BELIEF PATTERN
Spiritual distress (distress of the human spirit)
Potential for enhanced spiritual well-being

---

* Based on Gordon, M: Nursing Diagnosis: Process and Applications. McGraw Hill, New York, 1996, with permission.